# Nutrition
# in Health
# and Disease

# Nutrition in Health and Disease

**17th Edition**

**Linnea Anderson, M.P.H.**
Associate Professor
Medical Dietetics Division
School of Allied Medical Professions
The Ohio State University
Columbus, Ohio

**Marjorie V. Dibble, M.S., R.D.**
Chairperson and Professor
Department of Human Nutrition
College for Human Development
Syracuse University
Syracuse, New York

**Pirkko R. Turkki, Ph.D., R.D.**
Professor
Department of Human Nutrition
College for Human Development
Syracuse University
Syracuse, New York

**Helen S. Mitchell, Ph.D., Sc.D.**
Dean, Emeritus
School of Home Economics
University of Massachusetts
Amherst, Massachusetts

**Henderika J. Rynbergen, M.S.**
Professor of Science, Emeritus
School of Nursing
Cornell University—New York Hospital
New York, New York

with 6 contributors

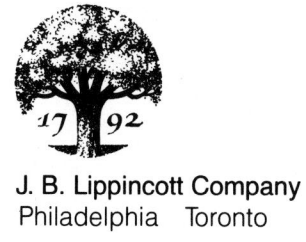

**J. B. Lippincott Company**
Philadelphia   Toronto

# Contents

## Part 3  Diet in Disease

# Contributors

**Linda J. Boyne, M.S., R.D.**
Instructor
Medical Dietetics Division
School of Allied Medical Professions
The Ohio State University
Columbus, Ohio

**Therese A. Dolecek, M.S., R.D.**
Chief Nutritionist
Department of Preventive Medicine
Rush-Presbyterian–St. Luke's Medical Center
Chicago, Illinois

**Clair Agriesti Johnson, Ph.D., R.D.**
Associate Professor
Medical Dietetics Division
School of Allied Medical Professions
The Ohio State University
Columbus, Ohio

**Rosita Schiller, Ph.D., R.D.**
Director and Associate Professor
Medical Dietetics Division
School of Allied Medical Professions
The Ohio State University
Columbus, Ohio

**Lois Schroeder, Ph.D., R.D.**
Assistant Professor
Department of Human Nutrition
College for Human Development
Syracuse University
Syracuse, New York

**Margaret Knight Snowman, Ph.D., R.D.**
Associate Professor
Department of Human Nutrition
College for Human Development
Syracuse University
Syracuse, New York

# Preface

Medicine arose from dietetics: the Pythagoreans (including Hippocrates) used diet to prevent and cure diseases, and drugs only if these failed.

H.M. Sinclair*

The preface of the first edition of *Nutrition in Health and Disease*, written by Lenna F. Cooper, Edith M. Barber, and Helen S. Mitchell and published by J. B. Lippincott Company in 1928, states

> This book presents the newer ideas in both the principles of nutrition and the practice of dietetics, based upon the most recent experimentation and study as well as upon the established knowledge of earlier research findings.

Over 50 years later, the authors and contributors of the 17th edition have worked to achieve the same purpose as the original authors. As in previous editions the text presents a comprehensive overview of the principles of nutrition as they apply to individuals and groups throughout the life span, as well as the dietary needs of individuals with metabolic aberrations due to pathological conditions.

This book is a basic text for college students in normal and clinical nutrition courses who are planning to enter the health professions. It will also serve the members of the health professions—dietitians/nutritionists, nurses and physicians, and their assistants—who share responsibility for the nutritional care and counseling of individuals and their families. The central focus is on the client with emphasis on those knowledges, attitudes, and abilities required of the professional person to be an effective nutrition counselor.

When supplemented with current literature, this book can also serve as a reference for advanced courses in nutrition that focus primarily on vitamins, minerals, and metabolism. The reader is reminded that professional

*In Birch GG et al (eds): Health and Food, p 23. New York, John Wiley & Sons, 1972

practice in the late 20th century is related to basic bio-medical and psychosocial principles and that the nutritional component of practice derives not only from physiology, anatomy, nutritional biochemistry, genetics, and food science, but as well from sociology, psychology, and anthropology. Pertinent principles from these disciplines are repeated only for clarity where these are essential for bridging the gap between theory and practice.

In Part One, Principles of Nutrition, there are major revisions and additions to Chapter 1, Introduction to Nutrition Counseling; Chapter 2, Carbohydrates; Chapter 3, Fats and Other Lipids; Chapter 5, Water and Electrolyte Metabolism; Chapter 6, Mineral Metabolism; Chapter 7, Fat-soluble Vitamins; Chapter 8, Water-soluble Vitamins; Chapter 9, Nutrient Utilization: Digestion, Absorption, and Metabolism; Chapter 10, Energy Metabolism; Chapter 11, Meeting Nutritional Norms; Chapter 14, Regional, Cultural, and Religious Food Patterns; and Chapter 15, Ecology of Food.

In Chapter 1, discussions of HANES and of the National Food Consumption Survey 1977–78 have been added. A section on U.S. dietary guidelines is also presented in the first chapter. Chapter 2 has an expanded section on dietary fiber, with tables on the components of dietary fiber by structure and possible physiologic function, and on dietary fiber in foods. The increased use of fructose as a sweetener is also discussed, and the information on alcohol metabolism has been brought up to date. In Chapter 3, "Essential Fatty Acids—Role of Lipids in Health" includes a discussion on prostaglandins and a figure of the simplified pathways of essential fatty acid metabolism as related to prostaglandin synthesis.

Chapter 5, Water and Mineral Metabolism, 16th edition, has been rewritten and expanded to two chapters: Chapter 5, Water and Electrolyte Metabolism; and Chapter 6, Mineral Metabolism. Chapter 5 includes a discussion of acidosis and alkalosis, and Chapter 6 presents in detail a discussion of the functions and utilization of the trace elements as well as of calcium, phosphorus, and iron. A method for estimating iron availability from different types of meals is also included in Chapter 6. Chapters 7 and 8 have expanded discussions on the functions and utilization of the fat- and water-soluble vitamins. Several new figures have been added to these four chapters which further enhance the usefulness of this book as a basic text in courses that emphasize these topics.

Chapter 8, Energy, 16th edition, has been moved to Chapter 10, thus following instead of preceding Chapter 9, Nutrient Utilization: Digestion, Absorption, and Metabolism. The section on biologic oxidation now is included in Chapter 9, and a discussion on energy balance has been added to Chapter 10.

The 1980 revised Recommended Dietary Allowances are included in Chapter 11. Dietary habits in Arab countries and in South and Southeast Asia and Islamic and Hindu food patterns have been added to Chapter 14. Additions to Chapter 15 include vibrio infections, infant botulism, and *Bacillus cereus* foodborne illness.

In Part Two, Application of Nutrition to Critical Periods Throughout the Life Span, significant changes and additions of new material have been made in Chapter 16, Growth and Development; Chapter 17, Nutrition in Pregnancy and Lactation; Chapter 18, Nutrition During Infancy and Early Childhood—from Birth to 3 Years; Chapter 19, Nutrition for Children and Youth; and Chapter 20, Nutrition for Older Persons.

In Chapter 16, the section on nutrition in brain development and behavior has been revised, and information on neurotransmitters has been added. A discussion on alcohol and caffeine consumption and smoking during pregnancy has been included in Chapter 17. Expanded discussions on iron status during infancy and on breast-feeding, including the use of drugs during lactation, are to be found in Chapter 18. Also in this chapter the section on introduction of semisolid foods has been revised to conform with current practice. Sections on oral contraceptives, alcohol and drugs, and athletics have been added to Chapter 19. Chapter 20 has been extensively revised and includes discussions of the physiology of aging and the programs of preventive care and group care for the older person.

The chapter titles in Part Three, Diet in Disease, continue to reflect disease processes rather than metabolic problems. However, the sequence of the chapters continues to reflect related metabolic problems. Numerous changes and additions have been made in this section. Chapter 22, Nutritional Care and Diet Therapy for the Hospitalized Patient, includes a section on quality assurance and standards of practice. Chapter 23, Assessment of Patient Needs, has a section on the methodology for assessment of nutritional status used to identify the hospitalized patient malnourished at the time of admission or at risk for developing malnutrition. The 1976 revision of the Exchange System used to calculate energy-controlled diets is in Chapter 24, Food Composition—A Basic Tool of Diet Therapy. The original Exchange System Food Lists published in 1950 are reproduced in Part 4, Tabular Material and Bibliography, for the convenience of the counselor who is working with clients who are familiar with these lists and do not wish, or need, to change to the newer lists. A section on parenteral and enteral alimentation has been added to Chapter 27, Nutrition Care—Surgery and Burn Therapy.

In Chapter 30, Atherosclerosis, the Exchange System has been revised to reflect newer information available on the polyunsaturated fatty acid composition of foods. Chapter 32, Renal Disease: Nephrolithiasis, has been extensively revised. The Exchange System reflects the need to calculate phosphorus as well as the protein, sodium, and potassium content of diet plans for patients with chronic renal failure. Chapter 34, Cancer and Special Problems, presents the feeding problems encountered by patients receiving various cancer therapies.

Chapter 35, Nutrition in Diseases of Infancy and Childhood, and Chapter 36, Inborn Errors of Metabolism in Infancy and Childhood, have been extensively revised. Chapter 35 includes a section on the nutritional care of the infant, the newborn intensive care unit, and the role of the nutrition counselor on the child abuse team. In Chapter 36, the nutrient values of foods used to calculate diet plans for infants with phenylketonuria or maple syrup urine disease have been updated.

The tables in Part Four, Tabular Material and Bibliography, have also been revised. The nutrient values in Table 1, Nutritive Values of the Edible Part of Foods, are those in the USDA Home and Garden Bulletin No. 72. Table 2, Cholesterol in Common Foods, has been revised where new figures are available. It is strongly advised that, as the USDA Handbook 8 series becomes available, the values of the amino acid content of foods used to calculate diet plans be derived from these publications, not Table 3, Amino Acid Content of Foods per 100 Grams—Edible Portion. Table 6, Vitamin E Content of

Food; Table 12, Dietary Standard for Canada; and Table 13, Canada's Food Guide, are new additions to this section.

Special attention is drawn to the Bibliography and Glossary. The Bibliography has been included to assist the student who wishes to pursue a subject in more depth than the space in this book allows. However, the student is cautioned that the Bibliography contains citations only through mid-1981. The Glossary has been revised and expanded, although many readers may require a standard medical dictionary for those medical terms found in Part Three.

For the convenience of both students and instructors, a complete list of abbreviations used in this edition is to be found on page 777.

Linnea Anderson
Marjorie V. Dibble
Pirkko R. Turkki
Helen S. Mitchell
Henderika J. Rynbergen

# *Acknowledgments*

The authors and contributors wish to express their sincere appreciation to their colleagues and friends for the generous help given during the preparation of the 17th edition of *Nutrition in Health and Disease* and to various investigators and authors for permission to use material from their research and work. Special commendation goes to the graduate and undergraduate students whose diligent literature searches to document term papers or modes of clinical intervention have been of inestimable value to the authors and contributors. Without their assistance no basic textbook would ever be written.

In this edition the authors and contributors are indebted to many persons: Jean Bowering, Ph.D., R.D., Associate Professor of Human Nutrition, College for Human Development, Syracuse University, for her critical review of the section on iron in Chapter 6, Mineral Metabolism; Anne L. Babic, M.S.W., Lecturer, Community Services, and E. Helen Howard, M.S., R.D., Lecturer, Human Nutrition, College for Human Development, Syracuse University, for their contribution to and critical review of Chapter 20, Nutrition for Older Persons; Marian F. Chase, M.A., L.P.T., Chief, Physical Therapy, and Patricia A. Lubas, M.S., R.D., Nutritionist, Nisonger Center, The Ohio State University, for revising sections of Chapter 25, Handicapping Problems—Self-Feeding, Chewing, Swallowing; and Debra Wright, M.S., R.D., Assistant Director of Dietetics, and Melody Thompson, R.D., Neonatal Nutritionist, Columbus Children's Hospital, for their assistance with the revision of Chapter 35, Nutrition in Diseases of Infancy and Childhood, and Chapter 36, Inborn Errors of Metabolism. James A. Schoenberger, M.D., Professor and Chairman, Department of Preventive Medicine, Rush-Presbyterian–St. Luke's Medical Center, Chicago, assisted Therese Dolecek, R.D., with the revision of Chapter 30, Atherosclerosis, and E.T. Schroeder, M.D., Chief, Nephrology Section, SUNY, Upstate Medical Center at Syracuse, assisted Lois Schroeder, Ph.D., with the revision of Chapter 32, Renal Disease: Nephrolithiasis.

Lastly, the authors and contributors wish to acknowledge the patience and skill of their editor, Bernice Heller, in converting the manuscript into a book.

To these persons, as well as to others who have assisted in the preparation of this textbook, the authors and contributors express gratitude and recognize that factual errors which may appear in the text are solely their own responsibility.

# Principles of Nutrition

# Part 1

# Introduction to Nutrition Counseling

*1*

**CSFP:** Commodity Surplus Food Program
**FNIC:** Food and Nutrition Information
    Center
**HANES:** Health and Nutrition Examination
    Survey
**HNIS:** Human Nutrition Information
    Service
**NFCS:** National Food Consumption
    Survey
**NSLP:** National School Lunch Program
**PIR:** Poverty Income Ratio
**PNS:** Preschool Nutrition Survey
**TSNS:** Ten-state Nutrition Survey
**WIC:** Special Supplementary Program for
    Women, Infants and Children

## Why do we need nutrition counseling?

### Evidence that adequate diets affect health

Early in this century the application of nutrition research demonstrated the importance of adequate nutrient intake to the promotion of normal growth and development in infants and young children and to the protection of all segments of society against deficiency diseases. In 1932 Bowles, an anthropologist, showed that freshmen students entering Harvard College were taller and heavier than their fathers were on admission to the same school in the early 1900s. Better food intake during infancy and childhood was one factor accounting for the difference between these two generations. Control of acute and chronic infectious diseases and better obstetrical care were also important factors.

In another study Ito[1] demonstrated that Japanese women born and reared in California were taller and heavier than relatives born and reared in Hawaii, whereas those born and reared in Japan were smaller and lighter than the other two groups. The differences in these three groups could be accounted for in part by the quantity and quality of the food consumed during infancy and childhood. More recently Mitchell[2] has observed that when the nutritional needs of the adolescent are not met, stature potential is not realized. In Japan during World War II, food shortages resulted in a reduction in height among Japanese youth at all ages, compared to the prewar stature of that age group. With increased prosperity resulting in more and better food after 1950, Japanese youth has grown taller than ever before.

These and similar observations have demonstrated to health workers that an adequate intake of nutrients during infancy and childhood is required if a healthy person is to achieve his growth potential.

In 1915, Goldberger reported on his success in curing and preventing pellagra, a deficiency of the B vitamin niacin, by adding animal and leguminous protein foods to a diet of cereals and vegetables served to an institutionalized population. Prior to World War I, workers in England and the United States showed that the addition of cod-liver oil to an infant's diet protected against rickets. The factor in the cod-liver oil was later proven to be vitamin D.

### The importance of nutrition counseling

Throughout this century and up to the present day, many other studies have continued to demonstrate the importance of an adequate diet to health. Unfortunately, however, even today medical, dietetic, and nursing students can observe the effects of inadequate feeding on the growth and development of infants in the pediatric units of general and teaching hospitals. The infant admitted with the diagnosis of failure to thrive (FTT), who is shown to have no organic disease and who, following treatment in the hospital, gains weight daily in excess of any norm, is seen too frequently in U.S. hospitals. If the knowledge of the relationship of adequate diet to health, discovered in the past, is to benefit today's infants and children and their families, each generation must receive nutrition counseling.

Dietary modification is also an important factor in the prevention and treatment of many diseases. There still exist unsolved nutritional problems such as obesity and atherosclerosis. Diet therapy is important in the treatment of diabetes mellitus and in other metabolic and endocrine disorders. Diseases affecting the gastrointestinal tract and the kidney and certain inborn errors of metabolism require nutritional management as a major part of the treatment.

*The Surgeon General's Report on Health Promotion and Prevention,*[3] published in 1979, states:

> Although evidence keeps mounting that certain food factors and current dietary habits may be linked with health problems as diverse as heart disease, tooth decay, obesity, and some types of cancer, consumers often find it difficult to make informed choices about food.
>
> Most know that good nutrition can make a substantial contribution to health and development of infants and children and that healthy eating patterns should be firmly established in adolescents and young adults. Most also are aware that good nutrition is particularly important for pregnant women and the elderly.
>
> But food choices are influenced by many complex factors, and the consumer is often bombarded with an overload of somewhat confusing—and even conflicting—information from books, newspapers, magazine articles, and advertising.

As a result, the need for scientifically sound and effective nutritional counseling continues to be of prime importance in protecting and promoting good health.

## Nutritional status in the United States
### Nutritional status surveys

A comprehensive nutritional status survey must be so designed that it reflects the relationship between the intake of food, the utilization of the nutrients in the food, and the total health status of the subjects studied. The components of a comprehensive nutritional status survey are: the clinical assessment of the persons being studied, including medical history, physical examination, anthropometric studies, and x-ray measurements; biochemical measurements performed on samples of blood and urine collected under standard conditions; dental examinations; evaluation of dietary intake to obtain information on the level of nutrients, food habits, food preparation practices, and food attitudes; and socioeconomic data including such items as income, availability of food and government food distribution programs, health and education facilities and their use, and the ethnic and cultural characteristics of the subjects. Determining the nutritional status of any population requires an adequate number of cooperative subjects; a representative sample of the population as a whole; a team of knowledgeable investigators; and the appropriate equipment for both the collection and analysis of the data.

The U.S. Public Health Service conducted nutritional status surveys in the late 1940s in various parts of the country. From 1947 to 1958 several studies were sponsored by the Cooperative State Agriculture Experiment Stations and the Agricultural Research Service of the U.S. Department of Agriculture (USDA). These surveys indicated that the population as a whole consumed diets adequate in essential nutrients and was free from symptoms of frank deficiency diseases. There were signs, however, that the nutritional status of pregnant women, infants, preschool children, and adolescent girls merited special concern.

In 1967, a group of concerned citizens raised the question of hunger "in our midst." Congressional hearings pointed to the probability of problems of serious hunger and malnutrition in the United States. In December of 1967, Congress directed the Secretary of Health, Education, and Welfare to make a comprehensive survey of the incidence and location of hunger and malnutrition and related health problems in the United States. The survey undertaken to carry out this mandate is known as the *Ten-State Nutrition Survey, 1968 to 1970.* At approximately the same time the Maternal and Child Health Service in the Health Services and Mental Health Administration, Public Health Service, contracted with a research team for a *Preschool Nutrition Survey* to study a cross-sectional sample of children 1 to 6 years of age in the United States.

#### Ten-state nutrition survey (TSNS), 1968 to 1970[4]

The TSNS was conducted in low income areas in ten states widely distributed throughout the nation and reflects the nutritional problems related to specific ethnic groups and income levels. The Poverty Income Ratio (PIR) was calculated for each family according to certain characteristics of the family (size, farm or nonfarm, sex of the head of the household) compared with family income. A PIR of 1.0 indicated that a family was living at the poverty line. Although all the subjects studied had low incomes, those who lived in Texas, Louisiana, South Carolina, Kentucky, and West Virginia had a median PIR below the overall median for the ten states, whereas those who resided in Massachusetts, New York, Michigan, Washington, and California had a median PIR above the overall median. Therefore, the first five states are referred to as low income states and the other five as high income states in the survey reports.

The outcomes of the TSNS indicate that the growth and development of children 0 to 9 years of age appear to present a relatively important problem for both sexes in all ethnic groups (white, black, Spanish-Americans in Texas), regardless of income ratio. Obesity was an important nutritional problem in women 17 years of age and older in all ethnic groups. The black female population seems to present a greater problem than the white population in this regard. Iron nutriture was a problem in all age and ethnic groups, with the black population in the low income ratio states and the pregnant and lactating women in all states presenting a more important problem than the rest of the survey sample. The Spanish-American population (primarily the Mexican-Americans residing in Texas) presented an important problem in vitamin A nutriture.

### Preschool nutrition survey (PNS), 1968 to 1970[5]

The subjects in this study represented all socioeconomic and ethnic groups in the United States. The outcomes of this survey also indicate that it is the children in the lowest socioeconomic group who are most at risk, demonstrated by their lower dietary intakes, lower biochemical indices, and smaller physical size for age compared with the rest of the subjects. It was concluded that the major nutritional problem is insufficient food for the children in the lowest socioeconomic group. The nutritional quality of the intake might have been adequate if the quantity of food eaten had been sufficient. Approximately one-third of the children in the lowest socioeconomic group consumed diets inadequate in total calories. Their intake of protein was not a problem. The level of ascorbic acid intake was also related to the socioeconomic status of the family. More than half of all children in the survey consumed diets inadequate in iron.

## Nutritional status monitoring

Since 1956, the National Center for Health Statistics in the Department of Health, Education, and Welfare (DHEW) has been responsible for the Health Examination Survey. Nutritional status surveillance has become a component of the Health Examination Survey, and the program is now known as the Health and Nutrition Examination Survey (HANES).[6]

### Plan and operation of Hanes I, 1971 to 1974

The HANES I survey of over 20,000 people was the first nationwide, scientifically designed sample representing the noninstitutionalized civilian population, ages 1 to 74 years. Differential sampling of high-risk groups was designed to permit estimates of the total population and more detailed analysis of specific groups at high risk for malnutrition—the poor, preschool children, women of childbearing age, and the elderly.

Specially constructed Mobile Examination Centers were moved into a central location in each of the 65 primary sampling units. The survey included a medical history; a general medical examination for indicators of nutritional deficiencies; dermatological, ophthalmic, and dental examinations; audiometric tests; anthropometric measurements; x-ray studies of chest, hand-wrist, knee, and hip; a dietary interview consisting of a food frequency questionnaire and a recall of food consumption over a 24-hour period; *Health Care Needs and General Well-being* questionnaires; and numerous laboratory tests on blood and urine. An *Augmentation Survey* of HANES I,[7] which visited another 35 primary sampling units (PSU), was continued from July, 1974, through September, 1975.

The Poverty Income Ratio (PIR) is used to express the income status of each person in the sample. The dietary standards used for evaluation of the HANES I data are designed for the maintenance of good nutrition in healthy persons in the United States.[8]

***Principal findings of HANES I.*** Since the data from HANES I continue to be published periodically, the nutrition counselor should be aware of the sources of these reports. Early release of selected findings are reported in *Advance Data from Vital and Health Statistics of the National Center for Health Statistics*. Detailed reports follow in the *Vital and Health Statistics, Series 11*.

***Height and weight of adults 18 to 74 years of age in the United States.***[9,10] The mean weight of men aged 18 to 74 years was 172 lb, 29 lb more than the mean weight of women, which was 143 lb. Men aged 18 to 24 years weighed 165 lb; those aged 35 to 44 years were 178 lb, an increase of 13 lb. Male mean weight decreased to 175 lb in the age group 45 to 54 years, to 171 lb at 55 to 64 years, and to a low of 161 lb in the age group 65 years and over. Women aged 18 to 24 years weighed 132 lb, but weight increased to a high of 149 lb in the 45 to 64 age group and declined to 146 lb in the oldest age group.

Both men and women in the youngest age group had the highest mean height, 69.7 in and 64.3 in, respectively. Mean height decreased 2.0 to 2.4 in between the youngest and oldest age group, approximately one-half in per decade over the age range of 18 to 74 years.

Men and women were both slightly taller in 1971 to 1974 than in 1960 to 1962. Men were an average of 6 lb heavier and women 3 lb heavier in 1970 to 1974 compared to 1960 to 1962. Approximately 30% of the middle-aged women and 15% of the middle-aged men were obese in the 1971 to 1974 survey.

***Dietary intake of persons 1 to 74 years of age.*** [8,11] The dietary intakes from the 24-hour recall records were analyzed for calories, protein, calcium, iron, vitamin A, thiamin, riboflavin, and ascorbic acid. All groups, regardless of level of income, race, sex, and age, showed adequate or more than adequate mean intakes for thiamin and riboflavin. The mean intakes for vitamins A and C also met the standards for males and females in all age groups, regardless of income level. Women in age groups 25 years and over who were below the poverty level and women over 45 years in both income levels had consistently lower than standard mean intakes for calcium. Mean protein intakes were below standard for men in age groups over 55 years and for women in age groups 15 to 17 years and over 20 years who were in the below poverty income level. Women over 55 years who were in the above poverty level also had mean protein intakes slightly below the standard. The mean dietary intakes of calories and iron were below the standards for most population subgroups. With the exception of the younger child, calorie intake was below the standards for all groups, regardless of sex, race, and income level. Iron intake was generally below the standard for all groups of women and for boys aged 1 to 3 years and 12 to 19 years. The report of HANES I Caloric and Nutrient Values points out that the anthropometric measures belie the extent of low energy intake indicated by the 24-hr dietary recall and reveal that a much smaller extent of iron inadequacy was shown when physiological measures were evaluated. They urge delaying any conclusions on the amount of malnutrition until all measures can be interpreted together.

Differences in food selection, that is, nutrient density rather than the total amount of food consumed, appear to account for higher mean intakes of vitamins A and C among the black population compared to the white groups. Similarly, differences in nutrient intake between men and women pertained to the specific sources of protein, calcium, vitamins A and C, thiamin, and riboflavin rather than to the amount of food consumed. [12]

***Hemoglobin and selected iron-related findings of persons 1 to 74 years.*** [13] Men had hemoglobin levels of 11.9 g per dl at 1 year. The levels increased to 15.8 g per dl at 18 to 19 years and remained relatively constant until the later ages, declining only slightly to 15.3 g per dl at 65 to 74 years. The pattern for mean hemoglobin levels in women was different. At 1 year they had levels of 12.0 g per dl, which gradually increased to a maximum value of 14.1 g per dl at 55 to 64 years when there was a slight drop in the

age group 65 to 74 years. The greatest difference between the mean hemoglobin levels of men and women was at ages 18 to 24 years. The hemoglobin pattern for black and white men and women was similar, although at all ages whites had higher hemoglobin levels than blacks.

The prevalence rate for anemia was 10% to 20% or more of the U.S. population. Meyers and Habicht[14] have suggested that if the criteria for diagnosing anemia in blacks and whites were different, the cases of anemia reported would be fewer.

### Hanes II

Although data from HANES I were still being released, HANES II survey began in 1976. The age range includes from 6 months to 74 years. Many of the same procedures used in HANES I will be followed so that changes in nutritional status over time can be examined. Although nutritional status surveys are useful to the nutrition counselor in that they indicate nutrition problems or the lack of them in general, the data derived from them cannot be used to predict the nutritional status of any individual client or group of clients.

### Nutritional status surveillance

The Center for Disease Control (CDC), Public Health Service, provides a continuous process of nutritional surveillance for 20 states. The states collect the data on height, weight, age, and blood analysis for populations at risk. The data are then sent to CDC, which collects, collates, and analyzes them rapidly. Once the analysis is returned, the state or local health department can then assess the population at greatest need for nutrition services and evaluate the effectiveness of the programs.

## Trends in food consumption

Information about trends in food consumption in the United States are also available to the nutrition counselor. There are two methods of collecting these data: (1) household food consumption surveys, and (2) statistics on the availability of food for civilian consumption. These data give information about what the public eats but none about other aspects of nutritional status. The information has been used to identify areas where improvement in nutrition is needed and to give direction to programs improving the national food supply. For example, the data from one of the household food consumption surveys were responsible for the initiation of bread and flour enrichment (see Chap. 11).

### Household food consumption surveys

A nationwide survey of the food consumption and dietary levels of households and of food and nutrient intake of individuals in the population was made in the United States in 1977-78. Earlier surveys were made in 1936, 1942, 1948, 1955, and 1965–66. In 1977–78 data on household food use and individual intake were collected from at least 15,000 households in the 48 conterminous states and the District of Columbia. Additional surveys were also made during this period as part of the 1977–78 *National Food Consumption Survey* (NFCS). A *bridging survey* of 1200 households using the 1965–66 procedures was conducted to enable comparisons between the results of the 1965–66 and 1977–78 surveys. Data were also collected from 1200 Alaskan, 1200 Hawaiian, and 3000 Puerto Rican households and their members. Household and individual intake data were also gathered from 5000 households with one or more members 65 years or older. Finally, 5000 low-income households, which were either receiving or were eligible to receive food stamps, were surveyed.

Just as previous surveys have shown changes in the pattern of food consumption, it is expected that similar trends will be seen when the data from the 1977–78 survey are completely analyzed. Between 1955 and 1965 there was a shift in food consumption to foods requiring less preparation in the home, for example, more frozen and chilled than fresh citrus juices, more processed potatoes, and more commercial bakery products. A greater use of foods associated with snacking was also observed.[15] It is anticipated that the 1977–78 survey will reflect some of the changes in American life-style as well as technological innovations in the food industry. It can be predicted that fast food restaurants and take-out chains will have an impact on family food consumption patterns as will the sharp increase in the number of women employed outside the home. The popularity of vegetarianism among certain groups may affect consumption patterns. The impact of new or greatly expanded federal nutrition programs such as the WIC program for women, infants, and children, the Nutrition for the Elderly Program, those programs under the Child Nutrition Act, the Food Stamp Program, and Nutritional Labeling may be reflected in the nutritional quality of diets.[16]

Preliminary findings of the 1977–78 NFCS are periodically being released by the United States Department of Agriculture (USDA). To date, they show that about three-fourths of the money spent for food was spent for food consumed at home and that one-fourth was for food bought and eaten away from home; however, 85% of the meals were eaten at home. A meal purchased away from home cost about two and one-half times more than a home-prepared meal. In terms of nutritional quality, the lower income households received the most nutrient return for their food dollar for food consumed at home (Table 1-1). This is of particular importance because they also spent less money for food.[17]

In households where women worked outside the home, only slightly more money was spent for food than in other households, but almost 50% more was spent for food away from home. Moreover, the nutrient return per

dollar's worth of food was slightly lower for each of the 11 nutrients in the households of working women. The nutrition counselor should also note that the man's role in shopping, planning, and preparing food did not differ greatly in the households where the women worked compared to those where she did not. In both types of households he was likely to participate in shopping, but less than 15% of the men helped in planning and preparing food in households where women worked compared to about 7% in other households.[18]

The elderly spent about the same amount of money per person as other households but bought fewer meals outside the home. However, when they ate out, they spent considerably more for the meal than others in the survey. Their nutrient return per dollar's worth of food indicated that they probably bought less milk, as their dollar return was less than that for other households only in protein, calcium, phosphorus, and riboflavin.[18]

Substantially more money was spent in 1977–78 compared to 1965–66 for soft drinks, punches, and desserts. Much larger quantities of alcoholic beverages, probably representing more beer and wine, were reported in 1977–78 than in former surveys.

The fact that the lowest income families spent approximately the same amount for food per member as the three middle-income household groups seems to indicate that the Food Stamp Program is effectively assisting the poor to obtain their food needs. Certain food groups appeared to be more closely related to income than others; for instance, the greater the income a family had, the greater the portion of the food dollar spent for alcoholic beverages and for the milk, cream, and cheese group. Lower income groups used a higher proportion of their food money for eggs and dry legumes. All income groups spent about the same for grain products and fats and oils.[19]

### Table 1-1. Nutrients Per Dollar's Worth of Food Used at Home by Housekeeping Households, Spring 1977

| Nutrient | Unit | Household Income (1976) Before Taxes | |
|---|---|---|---|
| | | *Under $5000* | *$20,000 and Over* |
| Protein | g | 45 | 41 |
| Calcium | mg | 470 | 440 |
| Iron | mg | 9.1 | 7.7 |
| Vitamin A value | IU | 3720 | 2930 |
| Thiamin | mg | 0.89 | 0.72 |
| Riboflavin | mg | 1.2 | 1.0 |
| Ascorbic acid | mg | 61 | 56 |

(From Rizek RL, Peterkin BB: Food Costs of U.S. Households, Spring, 1977. Family Economics Review, Washington, DC, USDA, Agricultural Research Service, Fall 1979)

Table 1-2 compares the nutrient level of foods used in households in 1965–77. The data reflect a slight decrease in the consumption of milk and dairy products, pork, luncheon meats, eggs, dried beans, breads and cereals, potatoes, sugar, syrup, jelly and candy, and fats and oils and an increase in dark green vegetables, fruit, especially citrus and ascorbic acid-fortified fruit drinks, punches and ades, and desserts and soft drinks. In general, these changes are reflected in all income groups.[20]

Because the average values of per capita nutrient consumption patterns for 1977 are similar to the HANES I results, they raise the same questions about calories and iron intake.[21] As Hegsted[22] points out in discussing the implications of the NFCS, certain results are encouraging, whereas others are cause for concern; equally important are the many questions that the survey leaves unanswered, which indicate a number of areas where more research effort is required before any conclusions can be drawn. Recognition of the importance of these results in future planning is acknowledged. At the same time the nutritional counselor must understand the limitations of such a study, especially as it applies to any individual client or to groups of clients.

### Food available for civilian consumption

Table 1-3 shows the trends in the consumption of nutrients in the United States from 1969 to 1979. These trends are derived by the Agricultural Research Service of the USDA from its statistics on the quantities of foods that are available in the retail market each year. It is interesting to note the increase in all nutrients except calcium, vitamin A, and $B_{12}$. The caloric content of the diet increased to the highest level since 1909 because all three energy-yielding nutrients showed gains—protein because of the increased use of poultry and peanuts; fat because of greater consumption of salad and cooking oils, shortening, pork, and poultry; and carbohydrates as a result of much greater use of corn syrup in commercially prepared products and of smaller increases in grain products. Changes in thiamin, niacin, and riboflavin values are accounted for by the increased enrichment of white flour, which became effective in 1975. The increase in ascorbic acid is due to the greater use of frozen and chilled orange juice and other citrus products as well as the vitamin C-fortification of many fruit drinks, punches, and ades. Phosphorus, iron, magnesium, and vitamin $B_6$ levels are higher due to increased consumption of grain products, fruits, poultry, and peanuts. Reduced use of carrots and liver resulted in a slight decrease in vitamin A. The lower level of vitamin $B_{12}$ was due to a decreased availability of meat, especially beef.[23]

### Nutrition Canada

A national survey of the nutritional status of Canadians was completed in 1972.[24] Findings of the survey included a general problem of obesity among the adult population, high prevalence of elevated cholesterol among both men and women, low intakes of protein among preschool children and pregnant women, and a shortage of calcium and vitamin D in the diets of many infants, children, and adolescents. Eskimos and Indians were found to be at higher risk than the general population in ascorbic acid and vitamin A deficiencies. To meet the problems identified in this survey, priorities were recommended in government policies, industry's action, and consumer attitudes. In line with these recommendations, increased emphasis has been given to nutritional education of the public, revision of Canada's Food Guide, and the initiation of mandatory enrichment of certain foods by the government.

### World nutrition problems

Ever since World War II scientists in technically advanced countries have become increasingly aware of world food problems. Surveys have been made in many of the developing countries in an effort to understand their specific problems in food production, distribution, conservation, and the nutrient content of the local food supply. The public press has repeatedly reported that the world food supply is not keeping pace with the population explosion.

In considering world nutrition problems today, one must recognize the many complex factors that affect food

### Table 1-2. Comparison of Nutrient Level in Food Used in Housekeeping Households in the United States, Spring 1965–1977

| | Average Per Person Per Day* | | |
| --- | --- | --- | --- |
| *Nutrient* | *1965* | *1977* | *Percent Change from 1965†* |
| *Food energy (cal)* | 3210 | 2900 | −10 |
| *Protein (g)* | 106 | 102 | −4 |
| *Fat (g)* | 154 | 140 | −9 |
| *Carbohydrate (g)* | 353 | 307 | −13 |
| *Calcium (mg)* | 1110 | 1070 | −4 |
| *Iron (mg)* | 20 | 20 | 2 |
| *Vitamin A (IU)* | 7020‡ | 7520 | 7 |
| *Thiamin (mg)* | 1.6 | 1.9 | 18 |
| *Riboflavin (mg)* | 2.4 | 2.6 | 7 |
| *Preformed niacin (mg)* | 25 | 27 | 8 |
| *Ascorbic acid (mg)* | 100 | 135 | 35 |

*Average is calculated using a population ratio procedure; twenty-one meals from household food supplies in a week is equivalent to one person.

†Calculated prior to rounding.

‡Adjustment made to reflect revised vitamin A value for eggs.

(From Cronin FJ: Nutrient Levels and Food Used by Households, 1977 and 1965. Family Economics Review, Washington, DC, USDA, Agricultural Research Service, Spring, 1980)

production, distribution, and availability. In 1972 adverse weather conditions drastically reduced crops in Africa, India, the Philippines, Australia, and the Soviet Union. This caused a sharp increase in the price of cereal grains, and famines in those countries too poor to buy grain in the world market. In addition, the effects of the "green revolution," which had previously increased grain production in certain Asian nations, were reduced by the recent petroleum shortage; it sharply raised the price of fertilizer, which further reduced grain production in India, Pakistan, and Bangladesh. Although the world's food situation is less serious now than it was in 1972–74, the anticipated food deficit of approximately 100 million tons in developing countries by 1985 makes it more precarious unless their food production rate can be significantly increased.[25]

Some of the problems that must be faced in attempts to relieve the problems of hunger in developing countries are the following: arable land for growing crops is reaching its limits; untapped fresh water supplies for irrigation are shrinking; fertilizers, pesticides, and petroleum are costly and not constantly available; population growth continues to undermine gains in food production; the higher consumption levels of the affluent nations put pressure on the world's food and energy resources; distribution problems within countries with food deficits are such that 20% of the population may control half of the national wealth; lack of technical assistance and training for small farmers is related to widespread unemployment and migration to urban areas.[25] It is generally agreed that the realistic approach is to give the kind of aid that will help the developing countries help themselves. One example of the aid that the United States can give is help in setting up agricultural research and extension services. In the United States, the Agricultural Extension Service worked with rural families during the 1920s and 1930s to increase food production by improving agricultural procedures. The lessons learned in this country from extension methods, an example of nutrition counseling of population groups, could be more efficiently practiced than is presently done among rural and village people in many undeveloped countries. In the meantime, there is a need for a World Food Reserve to help the countries most deficient in food until their agriculture improves as well as a need for emergency assistance at the first signs of impending famine.

There is reason to believe that if an intense international effort were made to improve conventional agriculture, annual food production could be doubled throughout the world, and if at the same time an equal effort were made to achieve zero population growth, the food gap between the have and have-not nations could be reduced. All of humanity would reap the benefits.[26]

Overfishing and pollution are also reducing the supply of fish, which in the past has contributed significantly to meeting the world's food needs. International regulations and conservation techniques must be applied to the sea and inland waterways if these sources are to continue their yields in the future.

Research and development of nonconventional methods of providing additional food sources should also be encouraged. These include aquaculture and organized fishing systems, utilization of solar and geothermal energy, genetic improvement of biological species, creation of new biological species through genetic manipulations, control of pests and pathogens, and utilization of single-cell protein.

To help formulate a world food plan which would deal effectively with the food crisis, a World Food Conference was held in Rome in November, 1974. Action was called for on five fronts—accelerating food production in developing countries, improving distribution and financing, enhancing food quality, increasing the production of present food exporters, and insuring security against food emergencies.

In 1977 the President of the United States recognized the "importance of meeting basic human needs—in particular, the alleviation of world hunger and malnutri-

### Table 1-3. Nutrients Available for Consumption Per Capita Per Day *

| Nutrient (Unit) | 1969 | 1979† | 1979 as a Percentage of 1969 |
|---|---|---|---|
| Food energy (cal) | 3310 | 3500 | 106 |
| Protein (g) | 100 | 104 | 104 |
| Fat (g) | 156 | 168 | 108 |
| Carbohydrate (g) | 381 | 400 | 105 |
| Calcium (g) | 0.95 | 0.95 | 100 |
| Phosphorus (g) | 1.54 | 1.57 | 102 |
| Iron (mg) | 17.6 | 18.5 | 105 |
| Magnesium (mg) | 343 | 352 | 102 |
| Vitamin A value (IU) | 8100 | 8000 | 99 |
| Thiamin (mg) | 1.92 | 2.17 | 113 |
| Riboflavin (mg) | 2.31 | 2.44 | 105 |
| Niacin (mg) | 23.6 | 26.7 | 113 |
| Vitamin $B_6$ (mg) | 1.95 | 2.05 | 105 |
| Vitamin $B_{12}$ (mcg) | 9.7 | 9.3 | 97 |
| Ascorbic Acid (mg) | 108 | 120 | 111 |

*Quantities of nutrients computed by Science and Education Administration, Consumer and Food Economics Institute, on the basis of estimates of per capita food consumption (retail weight), including estimates of produce of home gardens, prepared by the Economics, Statistics, and Cooperatives Service. No deduction made in nutrient estimates for loss or waste of food in the home, use for pet food, or for destruction or loss of nutrients during the preparation of food. Civilian consumption. Data include iron, thiamin, riboflavin, and niacin added to flour and cereal products; other nutrients added primarily as follows: vitamin A value to margarine, milk of all types, flavored milk extenders; vitamin $B_6$ to cereals, meat replacements, infant formulas; vitamin $B_{12}$ to cereals; ascorbic acid to fruit juices and drinks, flavored beverages and dessert powders, flavored milk extenders, and cereals. Nutrient data reflect for the first time poultry values from *Composition of foods—poultry products . . . raw, processed, prepared*, AH-8-5 (1979).

†Preliminary.

(From Marston RM, Peterkin BB: Nutrient Content of the National Food Supply. National Food Review, Washington, DC, USDA, Economics, Statistics, and Cooperatives Service, Winter, 1980)

tion—as a major goal of United States foreign policy."[25] He defined the goals as follows:

- To provide more equitable access to available food and to improve nutritional wellbeing
- To increase the supply of food relative to need
- To offer food assistance to those unable to purchase enough food for adequate nutrition
- To ensure a decision-making process, management, and resources adequate to implement world hunger policies.

## National nutrition policy

In the United States, the National Nutrition Consortium published its proposed Guidelines for a National Nutrition Policy in 1974.[27] Because nutrition counselors can function more effectively if they understand their role in terms of the overall nutrition policy, counselors are urged to review the following guidelines carefully.

The goals of a national nutrition policy should be to

1. Assure an adequate, wholesome food supply at reasonable cost to meet the needs of all segments of the population, this supply being available at a level consistent with the affordable life-style of the area
2. Maintain food resources sufficient to meet emergency needs and to fulfill a responsible role as a nation in meeting world food needs
3. Develop a level of sound public knowledge and responsible understanding of nutrition and foods that will promote maximal nutritional health
4. Maintain a system of quality and safety control that justifies public confidence in its food supply
5. Support research and education in foods and nutrition with adequate resources and reasoned priorities to solve important current problems and to permit exploratory basic research

To attain these goals, it is essential to

1. Maintain surveillance of the nutritional status of the population and determine the nature of nutritional problems observed
2. Develop programs within the health care system that will prevent and rectify nutritional problems
3. Assist the health professions in coordinated efforts to improve the nutritional status of the population throught the life cycle
4. Develop programs for nutrition education for both health professionals and the general public
5. Identify areas in which nutrition knowledge is inadequate and foster research to provide this knowledge
6. Assemble information on the food supply, including food production and distribution, and provide a nutritional input in the regulation of foreign agricultural trade
7. Determine the nutrient composition of foods and promote and monitor food quality and safety
8. Cooperate with other nations and international agencies in developing measures for solving the world food and nutrition problems

Following the introduction of various plans (see Dietary Guidelines for Americans) to implement a national nutrition policy, the National Nutrition Consortium reviewed and updated its statement in 1980.

The Consortium Board reaffirms its recommendations for a sound national nutrition policy put forward in 1974. It endorses the principle of dietary guidelines which emphasize weight control, and stress moderation in the use of alcohol, fat, sugar and salt.

The Consortium Board believes that there is a need for the development of quantitative guidelines for healthful diets dealing with the intake of non-essential nutrients (for example, saturated fat, sugar, fiber and cholesterol) and essential nutrients above the requirement (for example, water, salt, vitamins, trace minerals, and polyunsaturated fats). The Consortium Board is concerned, however, about the strength of the data base which underlies some of the recommendations currently being made to the American people. . . .

The Consortium Board believes that nutritional guidelines cannot be the sole basis of a national nutrition policy. It urges continuing research to define quantitatively the optimum levels of fat, carbohydrate, protein, salt, sugar, and fiber needed to maximize health and improve the quality of life for all segments of our population. Continuing research into the causes and pathogenesis of the major degenerative diseases should go hand in hand with nutritional investigations.

It believes that nutritional guidelines, in line with all public health policies, will be evolutionary with the advent of new scientific information and clinical experience and will require periodic review and updating. Risk–benefit considerations for any recommended change in the American diet or lack of such change, should be a part of all nutrition policy decisions.

Finally the Consortium Board supports strong nutrition education programs which are scientifically based, forthright with response to controversy and well-formulated in order to keep the public informed about the current state of knowlege with respect to diet and the prevention of disease.[28]

## U.S. dietary guidelines

*Dietary Goals for the United States* was issued by the Senate Select Committee on Nutrition and Human Needs in February, 1977.[29] There was an immediate reaction; those who supported the goals felt they were straightforward in dealing with some of the contemporary health problems caused by dietary excesses and were long overdue; others had equally strong opinions that the goals were premature in terms of current scientific knowledge and could cause economic problems in parts of the food industry and agricultural system.[30,31] The American Dietetic Association endorsed the goals with the following recommendations: continuous re-evaluation of their specificity; investigation of the role of diet in preventing disease and restoring health; determination of their impact on institutional and home food services; and adoption of a Nutrition Policy to establish a framework for the implementation of programs to promote the optimal nutritional health of the public.[32] The Dietary Goals were rejected by the American Medical Association, which declared: "There is insufficient evidence at this time for assuming that benefits will be derived from the adoption of such universal goals."[33] In December, 1977, the Senate Select Committee published the following slightly revised *Dietary Goals for the United States:*[34]

1. To avoid overweight, consume only as much energy (calories) as is expended; if overweight, decrease energy intake and increase energy expenditure.
2. Increase consumption of complex carbohydrates and "naturally occurring" sugars from about 28% to 48% of energy intake; and
   Reduce the consumption of refined and processed sugars by about 45% to account for about 10% of total energy intake.
3. Reduce overall fat consumption from approximately 40% to about 30% of energy intake.
4. Reduce saturated fat consumption to account for about 10% of total energy intake; and balance that with polyunsaturated and monounsaturated fats, which should each account for about 10% of energy intake.
5. Reduce cholesterol consumption to about 300 mg per day.
6. Limit sodium intake by reducing salt intake to about 5 g a day.

These changes are to be accomplished by making the following alterations in food selection and preparation:

1. Increase consumption of fruits, vegetables, and whole grains.
2. Decrease consumption of refined and other processed sugars and foods high in such sugars.
3. Decrease consumption of food high in total fat and partially replace saturated fats, whether obtained from animal or vegetable sources, with polyunsaturated fats.
4. Decrease consumption of animal fat, and choose meat, poultry, and fish that will reduce saturated fat intake.
5. Except for young children, substitute lowfat and nonfat milk for whole milk, and lowfat dairy products for highfat dairy products.
6. Decrease consumption of butterfat, eggs, and other high cholesterol sources.

7. Decrease consumption of salt and foods high in salt content.

The controversy over the dietary goals has continued, however. One of the most positive effects that the publication of these goals has had was making the public and the government aware of nutrition and its role in health and disease. Moreover, in recent years several government agencies have published their own goals, guides, or guidelines. In July, 1979, the Surgeon General's Report included the following statement on nutrition:[3]

Good nutrition is an essential component of good health. People should adopt prudent dietary habits, consuming:

- Only sufficient calories to meet body needs (fewer calories if the person is overweight)
- Less saturated fat and cholesterol
- Less salt
- Less sugar
- Relatively more complex carbohydrates, such as whole grains, cereals, fruits and vegetables, and
- Relatively more fish, poultry, legumes (*e.g.*, peas, beans, peanuts), and less red meat

In September, 1979, the USDA published *Food*, which presented a Daily Food Guide of five food groups compared to the previous four food groups:[35]

- Vegetable and Fruit Group—four basic servings daily. Include one good vitamin C source each day. Also frequently include deep yellow or dark green vegetables (for vitamin A) and unpeeled fruits and vegetables and those with edible seeds, such as berries (for fiber).
- Bread and Cereal Group—four basic servings daily. Select only whole grain and enriched or fortified products. (But include some whole grain bread or cereals for sure!) Check labels.
- Milk and Cheese Group—basic servings daily based on servings of fluid milk.
  Children under 9—2 or 3 servings
  Children 9 to 12—3 servings
  Teens—4 servings
  Adults—2 servings
  Pregnant women—3 servings
  Nursing mothers—4 servings
- Meat, Poultry, Fish and Beans Group—two basic servings. Two to 3 oz of lean, cooked meat, poultry or fish without bone or equivalent in eggs, beans, peanut butter, nuts, or seeds equals a serving.
- Fats, Sweets, and Alcohol Group—no serving sizes are defined because a basic number of servings is not suggested.

It is pointed out that the suggested number of servings in the food guide will average about 1200 calories and that you can "personalize the guide by fitting it to your caloric needs."[35] The guide also leaves the choice of making changes in the diet up to the individual.

More recently, *Dietary Guidelines for Americans* was issued jointly by the Department of Health, Education, and Welfare and the Department of Agriculture in February, 1980.[36] The joint guidelines are:

- Eat a variety of food
- Maintain ideal weight
- Avoid too much fat, saturated fat, and cholesterol
- Eat foods with adequate starch and fiber
- Avoid too much sugar
- Avoid too much sodium
- If you drink alcohol, do so in moderation

The latest set of guidelines was released by the Food and Nutrition Board of the National Research Council, National Academy of Sciences, in their publication, *Toward Healthful Diets*.[37] Their recommendations for adults are:

> Select a nutritionally adequate diet from the foods available by consuming each day appropriate servings of dairy products, meats or legumes, vegetables and fruits, and cereals and breads.
>
> Select as wide a variety of foods in each of the major food groups as is practicable in order to ensure a high probability of consuming adequate quantities of all essential nutrients.
>
> Adjust dietary energy intake and energy expenditure so as to maintain appropriate weight for height; if overweight, achieve appropriate weight reduction by decreasing total food and fat intake and by increasing physical activity.
>
> If the requirement for energy is low (*e.g.*, reducing diet), reduce consumption of foods such as alcohol, sugars, fats and oils, which provide calories but few other essential nutrients.
>
> Use salt in moderation; adequate but safe intakes are considered to range between 3 g and 8 g of sodium chloride.

Although the recent introduction of a series of different dietary goals, guides, and guidelines initially may seem confusing to the nutrition counselor, they represent the primary step in establishing a nutrition policy, which first focuses on the health needs of the American population, then adjusts the agricultural system to deliver the appropriate quantity and quality of foods to meet these needs. The USDA, as previously mentioned, has indicated the changes in the per capita consumption pattern that would be necessary to meet the Select Committee's Dietary Goals.[38]

Perhaps it is even more important for the nutrition counselor to make sure that all of the goals, guides, and guidelines recognize some of the obvious excesses in the American diet and call for moderation in food consumption. There is little or no disagreement that total calories should be such as to prevent or reduce the prevalence of obesity. Reduction in the consumption of fat, refined sugar, and alcohol is the obvious way to accomplish this goal. Reasonable agreement is also found for avoiding too much salt. The nutrition counselor should also recognize that the moderation in diet, which is suggested by the

goals, guides, and guidelines, will not be harmful to the health of the consumer and may be beneficial for some in reducing the risk of certain diseases such as hypertension, coronary heart disease, and diabetes. It is equally important for the counselor to understand that as our knowledge of the relationships among diet, health and disease prevention increases there very well may be changes in the guidelines. Further application of the various guidelines, as they relate to food selection and preparation, is discussed in the following chapters.

## Definition of nutrition

Although one may find nutrition defined in a variety of ways, the following definition by the American Medical Association is used because it covers the broad scope of the term as it is referred to in the text.

> Nutrition is the science of food, the nutrients and other substances therein, their action, interaction, and balance in relation to health and disease, and the process by which the organism ingests, digests, absorbs, transports, utilizes, and excretes food substances. In addition, nutrition must be concerned with social, economic, cultural, and psychological implications of food and eating.[39]

## The nutrition counselor
### Role of the nutrition counselor

The nutrition counselor is responsible for guiding the food choices of people, either as individuals or as members of a group, wherever they enter the health-care system. Within our present health care system, nutrition counseling may take place in a community health agency, a perinatal center, a Woman, Infant, and Children Program (WIC), a Headstart Project, a health maintenance organization, a pediatrician's or other physician's or dentist's office, a general hospital or its ambulatory care facilities, an extended care facility, or a rehabilitation institute for the handicapped.

Nutrition counseling focuses on the promotion of normal growth and development in infants, children, and adolescents; on the health maintenance of adults, including the special needs of the pregnant and lactating woman; and on the modifications of food intake in the treatment or rehabilitation of the acutely or chronically ill in any age group. To be effective in guiding individuals and groups, the nutrition counselor must be truly committed not only to the doing aspect of professional practice, but also to the knowing and caring which underlie effective doing.

### Knowing

Basic to effective nutrition counseling—as to any professional practice—is that body of knowledge that is unique to the discipline. In this case, it is a knowledge of the sciences of food and human nutrition as well as the biomedical sciences, coupled with a comprehension of fundamental concepts from the behavioral and social sciences and of the limitations of the individual and his circumstances.

The science of human nutrition provides the counselor with an understanding of the qualitative and quantitative nutrient needs of people at any point in their life spans under a wide variety of conditions. Food science provides an understanding of the qualitative and quantitative components of the nutrient composition of foods and the ways in which societies make food available to their consumers. From the biomedical sciences the nutrition counselor gains knowledge of the utilization of nutrients at the cellular level and the effect of diseases on nutrient utilization. The social and behavioral sciences help the counselor to understand the psychosocial conditions which affect food choices and to perceive ways of influencing these choices.

### Caring

The nutrition counselor enters into a helping relationship with an individual or with a group to assist people to meet their health needs. To establish this relationship, the counselor must accept the client as a human being with rights, values, and a life-style, which may be similar to or different from the counselor's, and with the potential to achieve reasonable progress toward his (the client's) goals. To be effective, the counselor must be sensitive to age, sex, and social class differences and to various life-styles in order to avoid setting up barriers to communication with clients. The counselor must not only accept the client but must perceive the situation as the client sees it and work in partnership with him. In other words, the counselor makes a commitment to assist the client to meet his needs, not to meet the counselor's needs.

### Doing

The counselor applies both knowing and caring abilities in guiding and teaching the client. Recognizing that behavioral changes are made slowly, the counselor plans *with* the client and offers optional solutions to problems in an effort to move the client toward reasonable practices. The client participates by choosing the solution that most nearly meets his need. Evaluation of the client's progress is a very important aspect of the helping process and implies continuity of client–counselor contact. It also implies a team approach, by which various members can share the client's progress and give support to each other's roles. The helping process in nutrition counseling is discussed in more detail in Chapter 13.

## Who is the nutrition counselor?

### The physician

As the individual responsible for health care, the physician identifies and makes recommendations concerning the nutritional component of health counseling.

He may undertake the role of nutrition counselor, or, more frequently, he refers the client to the appropriate team member.

### The dietitian-nutritionist

The dietitian-nutritionist is the primary nutrition counselor on the health care team. The Study Commission on Dietetics has described the dietitian as the "translator of the science of nutrition into the skill of furnishing optimal nourishment to people."[40] Through education and supervised clinical experience, he becomes the member of the team who is the specialist in applied human nutrition. He may share these functions with another member of the health-care team such as the nurse, social worker, dietetic technician, or dietetic assistant. However, the ultimate responsibility for the quality of the nutritional care rendered by any health care team rests with the physician and the dietitian-nutritionist.

### The nurse

The nurse in any health care delivery setting may be of great assistance in helping a client understand and accept his nutritional care plan. The nurse may consult with the dietitian-nutritionist when assisting a client to establish his plan or may be the member of the team who refers the client to the dietitian-nutritionist. The nurse working in the community health agency has many opportunities to carry nutrition services into clients' homes when these services would not otherwise be available. The nurse's function may be largely educational, or it may involve giving bedside care or directing the home health aide.

### The social worker

In many health care settings, the social worker is concerned with the socioeconomic functioning of clients. He is frequently as involved with the socioeconomic and psychological aspects of nutritional care as any other member of the health care team.

### Other members of the team

Health educators and health or nutrition aides supplement and extend the nutrition counseling services to the client, whereas health planners help to identify needs and resources and to structure the environment for the delivery of all health care services, including nutrition.

## How does the nutrition counselor function?

### Establishing and maintaining the relationship

The first task of the nutrition counselor is to establish communication with the client. This is a talking *with* process, not a talking *to* process. Establishment of communication leads to the next task, gathering and assessing information.

## Collecting and assessing information

The nutrition counselor is responsible for collecting accurate data regarding the client's food practices in relation to his needs. In many instances the counselor also needs to collect the same information about the client's family. Because there are many patterns of eating that can provide adequate nutrient intake, dietary practices which do not conform to established food guides should not be judged inappropriate without careful estimation of their actual nutrient value.

Estimating the nutrient value of a client's usual daily intake is a particularly difficult task today when food processing removes, replaces, and adds nutrients to basic foods during processing, as well as fabricates new foods from resources not formerly used. For example, a TV dinner may have more or less calories as the same dinner prepared at home from the same foods, or the same size serving of breaded veal cutlet may contain 200 calories in one restaurant and 300 calories in another.

Not only is the total daily nutrient intake of concern to the counselor but also the distribution of the nutrient intake throughout the day. Recent research indicates that nutrient utilization by the body is more consistent when meals of relatively equal value are consumed throughout the day rather than when one large meal per day is consumed.

An assessment of a client's nutritional needs should also take into consideration information about height and weight and any laboratory data such as hemoglobin, hematocrit, glucose, cholesterol, and triglycerides. Also, it must be recognized that any indication of less than adequate nutritional status may be secondary to an acute or chronic disease, which prevents an appropriate nutrient intake or adversely affects nutrient utilization.

Essential to any nutritional care planning is the knowledge of the client's economic resources, living situation, daily routines, emotional maturity, and ability to learn. All of these factors have an important impact on what and when an individual eats.

The same elements of the assessment process used to identify an individual client's nutritional needs are applicable to identifying those of a group. The counselor's next step is planning with the individual and his family or with the group to meet these needs.

## Planning with the client

In many instances the first step in the planning process is to give priority to the client's needs. Dibble and Lally[41] showed that the problem for one mother was not what to feed her infant so much as it was finding the money to purchase food. Also, the client's involvement in the assessment process can result in his identifying his own needs.

Planning with the client demonstrates to him that the counselor accepts him as an individual with rights and respects his values and life-style. It is during the planning stage that the counselor must be capable of offering the client viable alternatives.

## Implementation—teaching the client

The client who has been involved in assessment and planning is more likely to recognize his need for information to solve his nutritional problem, and the counselor who has involved him in the processes is better able to provide him with specific information. All the information that most clients need to achieve reasonable performance cannot be given in one contact with the nutrition counselor. Continuity of contact is required to give the client the information he needs in the proper sequence at the right time. For example, the mother of a 2-week-old infant, her first child, will want to know today what and how to feed him next week, not what to feed him when he is 1 yr old.

## Evaluation

In the evaluation, the nutrition counselor identifies the client's progress toward achieving his goals. Evaluation also leads to reassessment, replanning, and reteaching as the client's situation changes. At the same time, evaluation of the client's progress can help the counselor to evaluate her own effectiveness.

See Chapter 13 for more detail on these functions.

# Resources for the nutrition counselor

Numerous federal, state, and local government agencies, private agencies, and industrial and educational institutions are engaged in various phases of nutrition research and education. Their publications are generally available, and many of them are valuable aids to professional education, or for use in educational programs with the lay public. A few of the groups from which reliable information can be obtained are listed in the following paragraphs.

## Official agencies

The USDA has many divisions concerned with food and nutrition. The Food and Nutrition Service administers the Child Nutrition Programs, which include the National School Lunch Program (NSLP), School Breakfast, Child Care Food and Summer Food Service Programs, the Nutrition Education and Training Program, the Special Supplemental Food Program for Women, Infants, and Children, the Commodity Supplemental Food Program (CSFP), and the Food Distribution Program. A new Human Nutrition Information Service (HNIS) was established in 1981. HNIS includes the Consumer Nutrition Center which conducts the Nationwide Food Consumption Survey, and the Food and Nutrition Information Center (FNIC) of the National Agricultural Library. USDA publishes the *Family Econom-*

*ics Review*, a quarterly research report, which is most helpful to the nutrition counselor. It also publishes the *Composition of Foods: Raw, Processed, and Prepared*, a handbook on nutritive values of food, which is currently being revised as a series of publications rather than one handbook. The nutrition counselor should have the series when they are available.

The Department of Health and Human Services (HHS) has several units involved in nutrition research or service. The Maternal and Child Health Service is concerned with health services to mothers and children, including the nutritional needs of pregnant women, infants, and children. The Food and Drug Administration (FDA) through its regulations is involved in protecting the safety of our food and drugs. The Public Health Service (PHS) is involved both in nutrition research and service. It carries on and supports research through the National Institutes of Health, and through state and local health agencies is involved in service programs.

The U.S. Government Printing Office prints numerous publications for a variety of U.S. government agencies and makes them available at nominal charge through its Public Documents Department. The monthly publication, *Selected U.S. Government Publications*, which is free of charge and includes an order form, makes it convenient for health workers to acquire a wide variety of materials as they are published.

## Other agencies, professional societies, and institutions

The Food and Nutrition Board of the National Academy of Sciences–National Research Council was established in 1940 to consider questions pertaining to nutrition measures necessary during World War II. The Academy is a quasigovernmental agency. The Food and Nutrition Board has taken the leadership in promoting nutrition research and its application to health. The Recommended Dietary Allowances, the yardstick to good nutrition, was one of their first accomplishments and has been revised at about 5-yr intervals since it was first published in 1941.

The American Institute of Nutrition (AIN) is a professional society for nutrition scientists and publishes the *Journal of Nutrition*. The American Society of Clinical Nutrition, a division of the AIN, publishes the *American Journal of Clinical Nutrition*.

The Nutrition Today Society was initiated in 1974 to disseminate reliable nutrition information to various professional groups interested in nutrition.

For those persons who are interpreters of nutritional sciences and motivators for the development of good nutritional practices, the Society for Nutrition Education publishes the *Journal of Nutrition Education*.

The Nutrition Foundation, Inc., established in 1941 by the food and allied industries, "seeks to make essential contributions to the advancement of nutrition knowledge and its effective application, and thus serve the health and welfare of the public." Since 1942 the Foundation has published *Nutrition Reviews*—abstracts of current scientific literature in nutrition. Throughout the years the Foundation has also published semipopular brochures on nutrition topics of current interest.

The American Dietetic Association (ADA), the professional society for dietitians, was founded in 1917 during World War I by pioneers in the then-emerging profession of dietetics. The Association began publication of the *Journal of the American Dietetic Association* in 1925, and continues to report research and studies in food and nutrition and in the administration of food service. In addition, the Association publishes educational materials, which are as useful to nurses, doctors, teachers, and others in related professions as to dietitians.

*The Community Nutrition Institute Report*, a weekly report of the Community Nutrition Institute (CNI), publishes current news, especially regarding legislation and other government activities pertaining to food and nutrition. The Center for Science in the Public Interest, a consumer advocacy group, is also responsible for a variety of publications for the consumer.

### Unreliable organizations

In recent years several widely advertised organizations, which were deliberately given names similar to those of organizations mentioned above, have issued unreliable publications in the field of nutrition and dietetics. They have even led some professionally trained people to accept fads and false ideas about food requirements, vitamin and mineral supplements, and the "dangers" of commercial fertilizers and food additives. Food fads and unreliable sources are discussed more fully in Chapter 14.

## Study questions and activities

1. What are the components of a nutritional status survey?
2. What evidence do we have that nutrition influences the physical growth of population groups?
3. List the specific population groups which are at greatest risk of nutritional inadequacies in the United States and Canada.
4. Explain the present trend in food consumption in the United States as it affects the nutrients available in the diet.
5. Collect articles from newspapers and magazines on the world food situation during the next month. Post them on the bulletin board.
6. List four different sets of goals, guides, or guidelines recommending modifications in the American diet. Indicate the group responsible for each of the plans. Discuss their similarities and differences.

7. Define nutrition and the role of the nutrition counselor. Explain what is meant by "doing," "knowing," and "caring" as they relate to nutrition counseling.
8. Describe your role as a nutrition counselor. What other professional or paraprofessional workers share your responsibility for providing nutritional care? What do they do?
9. Begin compiling a list of reliable source material for nutrition information. Start with the suggestions in this chapter and add to it during the term.
10. Select a recent pamphlet or popular book concerned with nutrition and evaluate its content and appropriateness for the lay public.

## References

1. Ito PK: Hum Biol 14:279, 1942
2. Mitchell HS: J Am Diet Assoc 44:165, 1966
3. Healthy People—The Surgeon General's Report on Health Promotion and Disease Prevention. DHEW Publ. No. (PHS) 79-55071, 1979
4. Highlights, Ten-State Nutrition Survey. DHEW Publ. No. (HSM) 72-8134, 1972
5. Owen GM et al: Pediatrics (Suppl) 53: Apr, 1974
6. Plan and Operation of the Health and Nutrition Examination Survey, U.S., 1972–73. DHEW Publ. No. (HSM) 73-1310, Vital and Health Statistics Series 1–10 (a&b), 1973
7. Plan and Operation of the HANES I Augmentation Survey of Adults 25–74 Years, U.S., 1974–75. DHEW Publ. No. (PHS) 78-1314, Vital and Health Statistics Series 1, No. 14, 1978
8. Dietary Intake Findings, U.S., 1971–74. DHEW Publ. No. (HRA) 77-1647, Vital and Health Statistics Series 11, No. 202, 1977
9. Height and Weight of Adults 18–74 Years of Age in the United States. Advance Data—Vital and Health Statistics. DHEW (PHS, HRA) Nov 19, 1976
10. Weight and Height of Adults 18–74 Years of Age: U.S., 1971–74. DHEW Publ. No. (PHS) 79-1659, Vital and Health Statistics Series 11, No. 211, 1979
11. Caloric and Selected Nutrient Values for Persons 1–74 Years of Age: U.S., 1971–74. DHEW Publ. No. (PHS) 79-1657, Vital and Health Statistics Series 11, No. 209, 1979
12. Food Consumption Profiles of White and Black Persons Aged 1–74 Years: U.S., 1971–74. DHEW Publ. No. (PHS) 79-1658, Vital and Health Statistics Series 11, No. 210, 1979
13. Hemoglobin and Selected Iron-Related Findings of Persons 1–74 Years of Age: U.S., 1971–74. Advance Data—Vital and Health Statistics, DHEW (PHS) Jan 26, 1979
14. Nutrition Newsletter. Ithaca, NY, Cornell University, Division of Nutritional Sciences, Winter, 1979–80
15. Household Food Consumption Survey Report No. 1. Washington, DC, USDA, 1965–1966
16. Rizek RL: Family Economics Review, Fall, 1978
17. Rizek RL, Peterkin BB: Family Economics Review, Fall, 1979
18. Rizek RL, Peterkin BB: Family Economics Review, Winter, 1980
19. Hama MY: Family Economics Review, Spring, 1980
20. Cronin FJ: Family Economics Review, Spring, 1980
21. Pao EM: Family Economics Review, Spring, 1980
22. Hegsted DM: Family Economics Review, Spring, 1980
23. Marston RM, Peterkin BB: National Food Review, Winter, 1980
24. Nutrition: A National Priority. Report of Nutrition Canada to the Department of National Health and Welfare. Ottawa, Information Canada, 1973
25. Report to the President by the World Hunger Working Group: World Hunger and Malnutrition: Improving the U.S. Response. Washington, DC, The White House. Spring, 1978
26. Hammar JG: Nutr Rev 32:97, 1974
27. National Nutrition Consortium: Nutr Rev 32:153, 1974
28. National Nutrition Consortium: Nutr Rev 38:96, 1980
29. U.S., Senate. Select Committee on Nutrition and Human Needs: Dietary Goals for the United States, 1977
30. Twenty commentaries. Nutr Today 12:11, 1977
31. U.S. dietary goals. J Nutr Educ 9:152, 1977
32. Dietary goals. J Am Diet Assoc, 71:227, 1977
33. American Medical Association statement to Select Committee on Nutrition and Human Needs, Apr 18, 1977. J Am Diet Assoc 71:227, 1977
34. U.S., Senate. Select Committee on Nutrition and Human Needs: Dietary Goals for the United States, 2nd ed. Washington, DC, 1978
35. Food, Home and Garden Bulletin No. 228. Washington, DC, USDA, United States Government Printing Office, 1979
36. Nutrition and Your Health. Washington, DC, USDA-DHEW, 1980
37. Food and Nutrition Board, National Research Council: Toward Healthful Diets. Washington, DC, National Academy of Sciences, 1980
38. LeBovit C, Boehm WT: National Food Review, Fall, 1979
39. Council on Food and Nutrition: JAMA 183:955, 1963
40. Study Commission on Dietetics: The Profession of Dietetics. Chicago, American Dietetic Association, 1972
41. Dibble MV, Lally JR: J Nutr Educ 5:200, 1973

## Supplementary readings

American Dietetic Association Position Paper: Nutrition component of health services delivery systems. J Am Diet Assoc 58:538, 1971

American Dietetic Association Position Paper: Nutrition services in health maintenance organizations. J Am Diet Assoc 60:317, 1972

American Dietetic Association Position Paper: Scope and thrust of nutrition education. J Am Diet Assoc 72:302, 1978

American Dietetic Association Statement: The dietitian in primary health care. J Am Diet Assoc 70:587, 1977

Brewster L, Jacobson MF: The Changing American Diet. Washington, DC, Center for Science in the Public Interest, 1978

Dietary Goals for the United States—American Dietetic Association Reaction Statement. J Am Diet Assoc 74:529, 1979

Dwyer JT: Point of view: Challenges in nutrition education of the public. J Am Diet Assoc 72:53, 1978

Food, Home and Garden Bulletin No. 228. Washington, DC, USDA, United States Government Printing Office, 1979

Glanz K: Strategies for nutritional counseling: Dietitians' attitudes and practices. J Am Diet Assoc 74:431, 1979

Healthy People—The Surgeon General's Report on Health Promotion and Disease Prevention. Washington, DC, DHEW, United States Government Printing Office, 1979

Hegsted DM: Food and nutrition policy: Probability and practicality. J Am Diet Assoc 74:534, 1979

Lee PR: Nutrition policy—From neglect and uncertainty to debate and action. J Am Diet Assoc 72:581, 1978

Mayer J: The dimension of human hunger. Sci Am 235:40, 1976

Mayer J, Dwyer JT: Food and Nutrition Policy in a Changing World. New York, Oxford University Press, 1979

McNutt K: Dietary advice to the public: 1957–1980. Nutr Rev 38:353, 1980

National Nutrition Consortium: Guidelines for a national nutrition policy. Nutr Rev 32:153, 1974

National Nutrition Consortium: Guidelines for a national nutrition policy. Nutr Rev 38:96, 1980

Nationwide Food Consumption Survey Results. Family Economics Review, Washington, DC, USDA, Spring, 1980

Peterkin BB, Shore CJ, Kerr RL: Some diets that meet the Dietary Goals for the United States. J Am Diet Assoc 74:423, 1979

Simopoulos AP: The scientific basis of the "Goals." What can be done now? J Am Diet Assoc 74:539, 1979

Trithart ES, Noel MB: New dimensions: The dietitian in private practice. J Am Diet Assoc 73:60, 1978

Twenty commentaries—The McGovern Dietary Goals. Nutr Today 12:10, 1977

U.S. Dietary Goals: For—Michael Latham, Lani S. Stephenson; Against—Alfred E. Harper. J Nutr Educ 9:152, 1977

World Hunger Working Group: World Hunger and Malnutrition: Improving the U.S. Response. Washington, DC, The White House, United States Government Printing Office, 1978

Zifferblatt SM, Welbur CS: Dietary counseling: Some realistic expectations and guidelines. J Am Diet Assoc 74:539, 1979

*For further references see Bibliography in Part 4.*

# Carbohydrates

## 2

## Man's major source of energy

Carbohydrates, chiefly in the form of cereal grains and root vegetables, are the major sources of energy for most peoples of the world. They provide from 45% to 50% of the calories of the American diet and a far higher percentage for many other peoples. They are the cheapest and the most easily digested form of human and animal energy. The protein-sparing function of carbohydrates, whereby they supply the energy needs and "spare" protein for other purposes, is an important consideration if the supply of protein is limited. "Carbohydrate, the fuel of life" applies to more people than does the more common phrase, "Bread, the staff of life."

The proportion of total calories derived from common carbohydrate foods around the world throws light on the respective standards of living in various countries. Most of the peoples of Asia, the Middle Eastern countries, Africa, and Latin America derive over 80% of their calories from grains and potatoes or other root vegetables.

As economic standards have gone up, especially in the United States, the amount of sugar in the diet has increased whereas the amount of starch from cereal grains has decreased proportionately. Approximately 53% of the carbohydrate in the American diet is consumed as sugar. As shown in Table 2-1, refined cane and beet sugars and other caloric sweeteners supply approximately 18% of the total calories. Corn syrup, especially high-fructose corn syrup (HFCS) used in soft drinks (see p. 32), accounts for the increase in the latter category. As mentioned in Chapter 1, the Dietary Goals suggest that the consumption of refined sugars including caloric sweeteners be reduced to 10% of total calories. This would mean a reduction in the amount of sugar-sweetened soft drinks, cereals, baked products, and candy consumed by the United States public. The typical grains and other carbohydrate foods used in different countries are mentioned as the food sources are discussed. (Energy metabolism is discussed in Chapter 10.)

**HFCS:** High-fructose Corn Syrup

## Photosynthesis

Carbohydrates are the chief form in which plants store potential energy. They are compounds of carbon, hydrogen, and oxygen which, with the aid of the sun, are synthesized from the water in the soil and the carbon dioxide in the air by the chlorophyll in the chloroplasts of green plants (Fig. 2-1). This process, which converts solar energy into chemical energy, is known as photosynthesis. The reaction is so complex that science has yet to fully understand and duplicate the chemical laboratory of the green leaf.

The greatest proportion of the sun's energy that is transformed into potential energy by plants appears as some form of carbohydrate. Monosaccharides, particularly glucose, are synthesized first, then combined to form disaccharides and polysaccharides. The chemical energy formed in this process can be utilized for the biosynthesis of fat, certain amino acids, and other essential substances in the plant.

## Simple sugars

**Monosaccharides** (Fig. 2-2) are the simplest carbohydrate units and are classified according to whether they are aldehyde or ketone derivatives and the number of carbon atoms in the molecule. Hexoses, sugars containing six carbon atoms, are the nutritionally significant sugars found in foods, whereas others, particularly the pentoses, ribose, and deoxyribose, which each contain five carbon atoms, are produced in the metabolism of foodstuffs. The single hexoses—glucose, fructose, and galactose—require no digestion and are readily absorbed from the intestine directly into the bloodstream (see Chap. 9).[4]

*Glucose,* also called dextrose, is a moderately sweet sugar found in fruits and vegetables. Linked with another molecule of a monosaccharide it is a component of all the disaccharides and is the basic structural unit of the polysaccharides starch and cellulose. It is prepared commercially as corn syrup by the acid hydrolysis of starch. Fermentation of glucose by the enzyme zymase in yeast results in the formation of carbon dioxide and ethyl alcohol. Glucose is the form of carbohydrate to which all other carbohydrates are eventually converted for transport in the blood and for utilization by the cells of the body. The following terms are used to describe the blood glucose level in the body: *normoglycemia,* which refers to a blood glucose level within normal range (65–115 mg/dl), *hyperglycemia,* which indicates a blood glucose level above normal range, and *hypoglycemia,* which means a blood glucose level below normal range.

*Fructose,* also called levulose or fruit sugar, is found associated with glucose in many fruits and vegetables, and especially in honey. It is a highly soluble sugar and in water solution appears to be the sweetest of the simple sugars. It is fermented by yeast. It is combined with glucose to form sucrose and is the structural unit in inulin, a polysaccharide found in certain roots (Jerusalem artichoke) and bulbs (onions and garlic). Inulin, however, has limited dietary significance because very little is digested in the gastrointestinal tract.

### Table 2-1. Percentage of Calories Provided by Sugars

| Year | Total Sugars* | Naturally Occurring Sugar | Refined Cane and Beet Sugar | Other Caloric Sweeteners† |
|------|------|------|------|------|
| | | | (Percent) | |
| 1909–1913 | 18.0 | 5.9 | 10.6 | 1.5 |
| 1925–1929 | 22.9 | 6.4 | 14.2 | 2.3 |
| 1967 | 24.1 | 7.4 | 14.1 | 2.6 |
| 1969 | 24.2 | 7.2 | 14.2 | 2.7 |
| 1970 | 24.4 | 7.1 | 14.6 | 2.7 |
| 1971 | 24.3 | 7.0 | 14.5 | 2.8 |
| 1972 | 24.4 | 6.9 | 14.5 | 3.0 |
| 1973 | 24.9 | 7.1 | 14.5 | 3.5 |
| 1974 | 24.3 | 6.9 | 13.9 | 3.6 |
| 1975 | 24.6 | 7.4 | 12.9 | 4.3 |
| 1976 | 24.7 | 7.1 | 13.0 | 4.5 |
| 1977 | 24.7 | 6.9 | 13.1 | 4.8 |
| 1978 | 24.3 | 6.6 | 12.6 | 5.1 |
| 1979‡ | 24.4 | 6.7 | 12.2 | 5.5 |

*Components may not add to total because of rounding.

†Includes syrups, corn sugar (dextrose), honey, molasses, sorghum, and maple products.

‡Preliminary.

(From Marston RM, Peterkin BB: Nurtrient Content of the National Food Supply. National Food Review, Washington, DC, USDA, Economics, Statistics, and Cooperatives Service, Winter, 1980.)

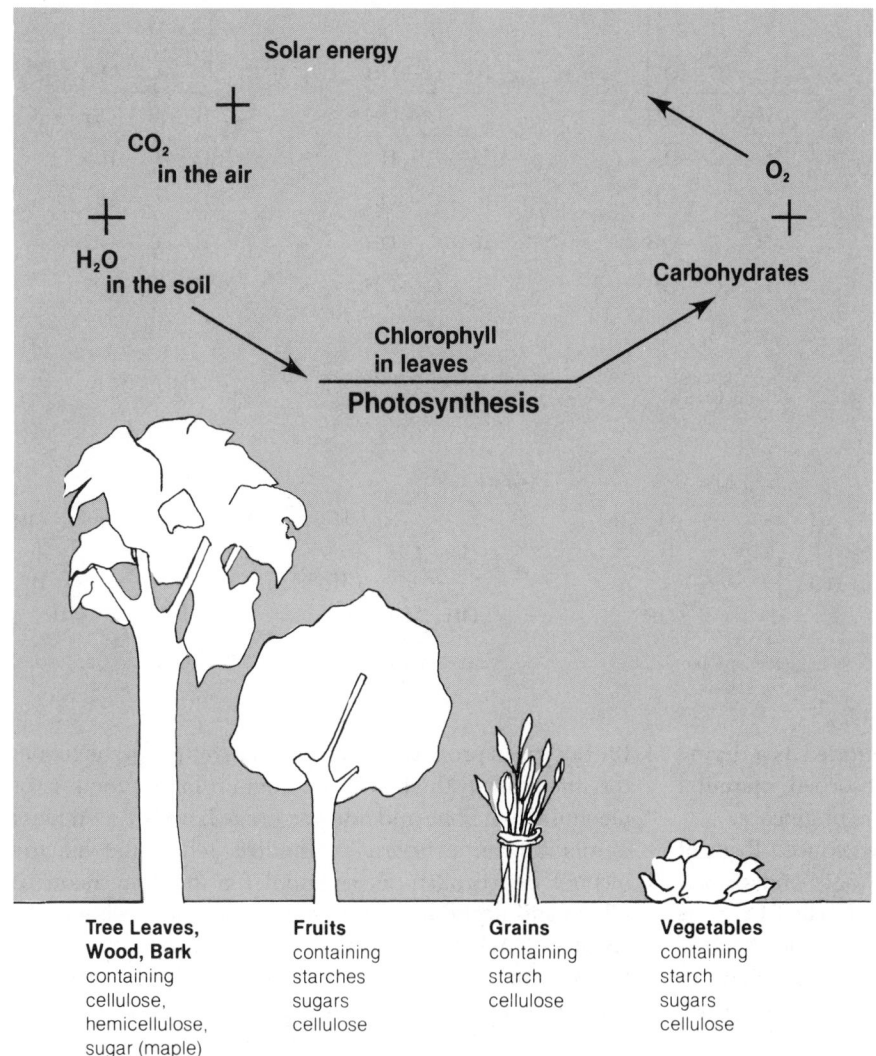

| Tree Leaves, Wood, Bark | Fruits | Grains | Vegetables |
|---|---|---|---|
| containing cellulose, hemicellulose, sugar (maple) | containing starches sugars cellulose | containing starch cellulose | containing starch sugars cellulose |

**Fig. 2–1.** Synthesis of carbohydrates in plants.

Now that a commercially economical method of separating glucose from fructose in digested sucrose has been developed, fructose is now available in liquid, powder, and tablet form. Because of its sweetness, it has been suggested that fructose replace saccharin as a sweetener in diabetic and low-calorie diets. Although fructose does not require insulin to enter the cell, in insulin deficiency, fructose can lead to increased glucose production[1] (see Chap. 9, *Carbohydrate Metabolism*). As the long-term effects on metabolic function of substituting fructose for glucose in the diet are not known, caution is recommended. Moreover, the sweetness of fructose varies to such a degree in different products,[2] depending on the temperature, acidity, flavor, and other characteristics, that the reduction in sugar and, hence, calories may be minimal. Its significance in calorie-restricted diets, therefore, depends on how much of the low-calorie product is consumed and its total calorie content. High-fructose corn syrup (HFCS), which is from 42% to 90% fructose, is also being used in many commercial products.[3]

*Galactose* is seldom found free in nature but is derived chiefly by hydrolysis from the disaccharide lactose found in milk. It is less soluble in water and less sweet than glucose. Some galactosans, also called galactans, occur in food. Since little is known about the digestibility of these galactose-containing polysaccharides, they are frequently excluded in the dietary treatment of galactosemia (see Chap. 36). Galactose is also a constituent of the glycolipids and glycoproteins found in many tissues. In the body, glucose is changed to galactose so that the mammary glands can produce lactose.

***Sugar alcohols*** called *sorbitol, mannitol,* and *xylitol* have a sweetening effect similar to glucose. Sorbitol, which is made commercially from glucose by hydrogenation and also is found in many fruits and vegetables, is very slowly absorbed into the bloodstream and can apparently be metabolized without insulin. It has the same caloric value as glucose, the sugar from which it is derived. Mannitol, obtained commercially by hydrogenation of mannose, occurs naturally in pineapples, olives, as-

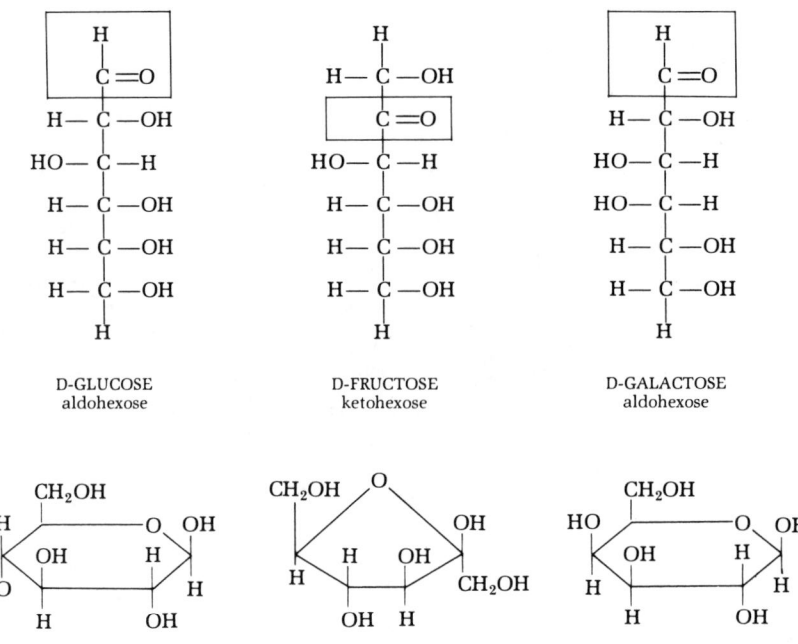

**Fig. 2-2.** Chemical structure of the monosaccharides glucose, fructose, and galactose in the straight chain form (above) and the ring form (below). Each of these sugars is a hexose containing 6 carbon atoms, 12 hydrogen atoms, and 6 oxgyen atoms. Glucose and galactose are aldoses, and fructose is a ketose (boxed-in areas). Glucose and galactose are shown below in the pyranose ring form and fructose in the furanose ring form.

paragus, and carrots, and may also be added as a drying agent to other foods. Since it is poorly absorbed, mannitol supplies about one-half the energy value of glucose.

*Xylitol,* a five-carbon sugar, is the reduced form of xylose. It is equal to sucrose in sweetness and caloric content. Although it is found naturally in such foods as raspberries, strawberries, spinach, and cauliflower, it is commercially produced from birch tree chips. Because metabolism of xylitol is independent of insulin, its possible use in diabetic diets was suggested. Also, its lower cavity-causing potential led to its use in chewing gum. Recently, however, food and gum manufacturers have ceased using xylitol because of reports of its carcinogenic effects. The status of xylitol is currently under review by the Food and Drug Administration.[3]

*Inositol* occurs in many foods, especially in the bran of cereal grains. Inositol, when combined with certain phosphate groups, forms phytic acid, which reduces the absorption of calcium and iron from the intestines. *Dulcitol,* obtained from galactose by hydrogenation, is sometimes added to foods.

***Alcohol*** or ***ethanol*** is produced from the fermentation of glucose by the enzymes in yeast and may, for certain individuals consuming large quantities of alcoholic beverages, represent a significant part of the total energy intake. One g of alcohol yields 7 kilocalories (kcal). One jigger, approximately 1 oz (30 ml), of 100-proof alcohol (50% alcohol) contains about 15 g of alcohol, which contributes 105 kcal (see Table 7, Part 4).

Ethanol requires no digestion and can be absorbed throughout the gastrointestinal tract. Its concentration in the body is in proportion to the water content of the tissue; for this reason, the blood can contain large amounts of alcohol while bone and adipose tissue have little. Alcohol is metabolized primarily in the liver where the enzyme alcohol dehydrogenase, essential for the conversion of ethanol to acetaldehyde, is found. Because alcohol also requires $NAD^+$ (nicotinamide adenine dinucleotide) (see Chap. 9) for this reaction, the rate of alcohol metabolism is increased by the simultaneous metabolism of carbohydrate (*pyruvate*). For the same reason, fasting or starvation decreases the rate of alcohol metabolism.

Another enzyme system for metabolizing ethanol oxidizes ethanol and NADPH (see Chap. 9) so that the first step in oxidation consumes metabolic energy. It depends on two enzymes, cytochrome P-450 and a reductase, and is associated with the endoplasmic reticulum of cells. In chronic alcoholics who consume a pint or more of alcohol a day, this pathway may account for much of the metabolism of ethanol. Tolerance to alcohol may occur from an increase in the enzyme cytochrome P-450 as a result of the frequent consumption of large amounts of alcohol. Moreover, due to the metabolic inefficiency of this system, the alcoholic derives fewer calories per gram of alcohol. Because the same system is also responsible for the metabolism of barbiturates, it is not surprising that there is an interaction beween alcohol and drugs.[4]

The ***disaccharides*** (Fig. 2-3)—sugars containing two hexose units—that are commonly encountered in foods include: sucrose (cane or beet sugar), maltose (malt sugar), and lactose (milk sugar). Disaccharides are hydrolyzed by specific enzymes in the digestive tract into monosaccharides or, commercially, by acid hydrolysis. Each of the three disaccharides has distinct characteristics that are of interest in human nutrition.

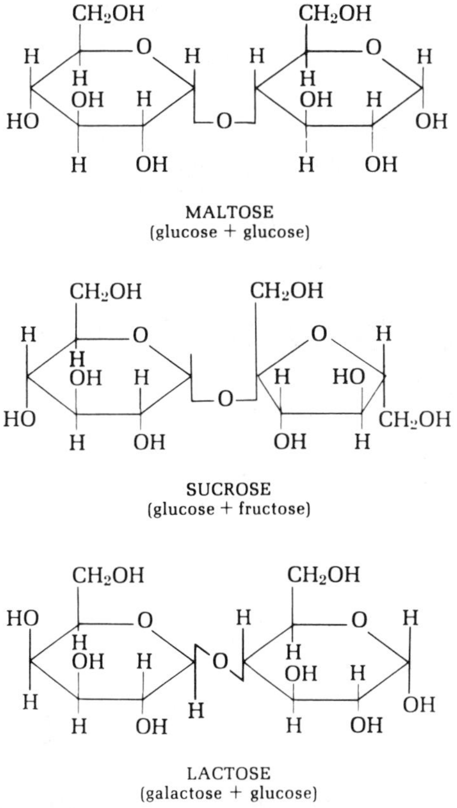

*Sucrose*—ordinary granulated, powdered, or brown sugar and molasses—is one of the sweetest forms of sugar. It is also found free in most fruits and vegetables. It is very soluble and on hydrolysis yields equal amounts of fructose and glucose, or invert sugar, as this mixture is commonly called.

*Maltose,* or malt sugar, does not occur free in nature but is manufactured from starch by enzyme or acid hydrolysis. It is less sweet than sucrose and very soluble in water. Two molecules of glucose are formed by the hydrolysis of maltose. In the body it is an intermediate product in starch digestion.

Maltose, easily used by the body, is sometimes used in combination with dextrin, a polysaccharide, as an ingredient in home-prepared infant formulas, where it is desirable to have a soluble form of carbohydrate which does not readily ferment in the digestive tract.

*Lactose,* or milk sugar, is the only one of the common sugars not found in plants. It is not very soluble and is the least sweet of the sugars, only about one-sixth as sweet as sucrose; this gives milk its blandness. It is formed only in the mammary glands of lactating mothers, animal or human. When lactose is hydrolyzed, a molecule of glucose and a molecule of galactose are formed. In the souring or fermenting of milk to make buttermilk or yogurt, some of the lactose can be converted to lactic acid. For this reason these products generally contain less lactose than milk.

A **trisaccharide** called *raffinose*, containing the three hexoses—glucose, fructose, and galactose—is found along with sucrose in molasses. *Maltotriose,* an intermediate product formed during the digestion of starch, contains three glucose units.

## Complex carbohydrates

For more stable and efficient storage of potential energy, plants and animals pack carbohydrate energy into units much larger than the sugars—dextrin, starch, cellulose, and glycogen. All of these are *polysaccharides*, the molecules of which may contain several hundred times as many glucose units as those of the sugars. Consequently they are much less soluble and more stable but differ markedly among themselves in digestibility and resistance to spoilage. Because there is so much moisture in all growing plants, one essential characteristic of a storage material is insolubility. To be suitable for human food, however, a carbohydrate must be subject to digestion by the enzymes of the digestive tract. Starches and dextrins fall into this category, but celluloses and hemicelluloses, which also occur in food, cannot be digested by humans.

*Dextrins* occur mostly as intermediate products in the partial hydrolysis of starch by enzymatic action or in

**Fig. 2–3.** Disaccharides in their ring forms. Maltose contains two glucose molecules, sucrose one glucose and one fructose molecule, and lactose one glucose and one galactose molecule.

cooking. They are made up of many glucose units joined together with the same linkages as starch. The individual molecules are smaller than those of starch, and they do not have the thickening property of starch. They are water soluble and, depending on their color reaction with iodine, are classified as soluble starch (blue), amylodextrin (purple), erythrodextrin (red), and achrodextrin (colorless). Dextrins are formed when bread or cereals are toasted or flour is browned. They are also used in some infant formula preparations and in products used in soda fountain beverages.

$\alpha$-Limit dextrins are formed in the digestion of the amylopectin form of starch because beta-amylase cannot split the branched chain linkage.

*Starch,* the chief form of carbohydrate in the diet, occurs in two forms (Fig. 2-4): (1) amylose, a straight chain polysaccharide of glucose units linked together the same as maltose (1,4 glucosidic bonds) and (2) amylopectin, a branched structure of glucose units with a linkage different from maltose at the branchings (1,6 glucosidic bonds) but similar throughout the rest of the chain. Starch is found in cereal grains, vegetables, and other plants. The starch of the grain is mostly in the endosperm (Fig. 2-5), encased in a protective covering of cellulose (the bran or

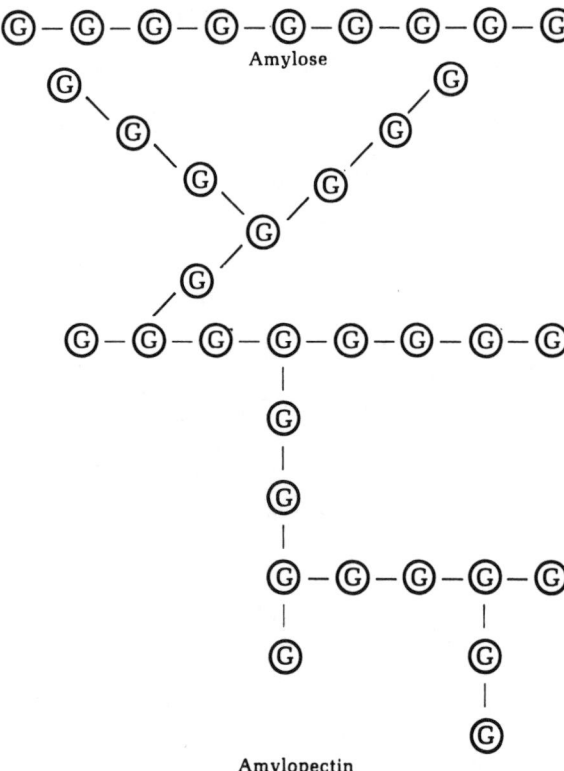

**Fig. 2–4.** Simplified diagrams of amylose and amylopectin, the two forms of starch found in foods. Amylose molecules consist of 250 to 300 units of glucose in a straight chain. Amylopectin, in addition to containing the straight chain units of amylose, also has branched chains and is composed of over 1000 glucose units.

the husk). The starch granule in the endosperm consists of tiny particles of starch usually arranged in concentric layers in a pattern of characteristic shape and appearance. The starch granules in turn may be enclosed in cells of larger size. This storage of starch in plants may be compared to warehouse storing of small packages of prepared cereal in cartons, with the cartons in turn packed in larger containers for ease in handling.

Before starch can be used readily by the body, the outer membrane must be broken, either by grinding or cooking. By the application of heat and moisture the outer cellulose envelope is ruptured, and the moisture permeates the starch granules themselves. Starch granules have an affinity for water, absorbing it like a sponge and increasing greatly in volume. The thickening property of a starch varies according to the source: for example, that of potato starch is greater than those of corn or wheat. After rupture of the cellulose wall by cooking, the starch is in a form that can be acted on more easily by digestive enzymes.

Cooking may carry the breakdown of starch to the dextrin stage if continued long enough. Starch granules break down most rapidly when moisture is present. Long application of dry heat, such as in baking or toasting, will also change starch to soluble dextrins. The palatable fla-

vor of the brown crust of rolls or bread or the brown part of toast or of toasted cereals is due partly to forms of dextrin.

*Modified food starches* are natural starches, which have been chemically or physically modified to provide special properties desirable in food processing. The types of modification include crossbonding with phosphates, derivatization such as esterification, conversion by acid or enzyme activity, and pregelatinization. Depending on their treatment, modified starches may have greater viscosity, more resistance to syneresis (weeping or leaking), improved clarity, or the ability to be dispersed in cold water. They are used in the processing of sauces for canned and frozen foods, frozen fruit pies, infant foods, canned and instant puddings, and gumdrops.

*Cellulose,* found in the framework of plants, is also a polysaccharide of glucose units but with linkages different from those of maltose and starch. It is the chief constituent of wood, stalks and leaves of all plants, and the outer coverings of seeds and cereals. Cellulose forms the more or less porous walls of cells in which water, starch, minerals, and other substances are stored in the plant much as honey is held in the comb.

No cellulose-splitting enzyme is secreted by the mucosa of the human gastrointestinal tract, but bacterial fermentation or disintegration may play a role in dissolving the substances that bind the cellulose fibers or particles together.

The indigestibility of cellulose is its major asset, as the undigested fiber furnishes the bulk necessary for efficient and normal peristaltic action (muscular contraction) of the intestines. Research has demonstrated that the normal colon performs better when a reasonable amount (4 g–7 g) of bulk or residue is present.

*Methylcellulose* and other cellulose derivatives that absorb large quantities of water may be used in manufacturing low calorie foods, such as imitation syrups and salad dressings.

*Glycogen,* or "animal starch," is the form in which the animal stores carbohydrate. It is a polysaccharide similar to amylopectin but with more branched chains and higher molecular weight. When more glucose than can be immediately metabolized enters the bloodstream, the healthy person combines many glucose molecules (up to 30,000) to form glycogen. By the same token, when glucose is needed, glycogen is broken down and glucose becomes quickly available for energy (see Chap. 9). In the living mammal both the liver and muscle store glycogen. Approximately three-quarters of a pound of glycogen can be stored by the adult male, one-quarter pound in the liver and one-half pound in muscles. The liver glycogen is the more quickly available for replenishing blood sugar. The muscle glycogen is used primarily as fuel for the muscles. In muscle meat when purchased little glycogen is present because it disappears during

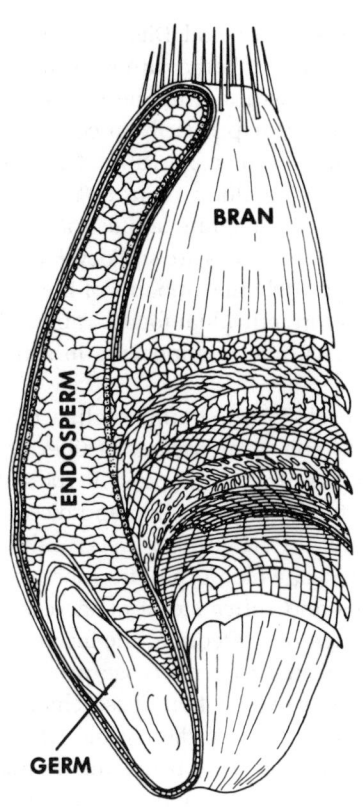

**Endosperm** . . . about 83% of the kernel
Source of white flour. Of the nutrients in the whole kernel the endosperm contains about:

70-75% of the protein
43% of the pantothenic acid
32% of the riboflavin
12% of the niacin
6% of the pyridoxine
3% of the thiamin

} B-complex vitamins

Enriched flour products contain added quantities of riboflavin, niacin and thiamin, plus iron, in amounts equal to or exceeding whole wheat—according to a formula established on the basis of popular need of those nutrients.

**Bran** . . . about 14½% of the kernel
Included in whole wheat flour. Of the nutrients in whole wheat, the bran, in addition to indigestible cellulose material contains about:

86% of the niacin
73% of the pyridoxine
50% of the pantothenic acid
42% of the riboflavin
33% of the thiamin
19% of the protein

**Germ** . . . about 2½% of the kernel
The embryo or sprouting section of the seed, usually separated because it contains fat which limits the keeping quality of flours. Available separately as human food. Of the nutrients in whole wheat, the germ contains about:

64% of the thiamin
26% of the riboflavin
21% of the pyridoxine
8% of the protein
7% of the pantothenic acid
2% of the niacin

**Fig. 2–5.** A cross section of a kernel of wheat and the nutrients in each of the three parts—endosperm, bran, and germ (Kansas Wheat Commission).

rigor mortis. Scallops, oysters, and other shellfish contain significant amounts of glycogen.

*Other polysaccharides,* such as the pectic substances, agar, alginates, carrageenans (Irish moss), and vegetable gums, cannot be digested but are used in various foods because of their colloidal property, that is, the ability to absorb water and form a gel. Commercial pectin, prepared from cull apple peels and cores or the albedo of lemons and available as liquid or powder, is used primarily for making fruit jellies. Agar is used as a thickening agent in candy manufacturing and in processing meats; the alginates and carrageenans are used in the manufacture of ice cream to give body and smooth consistency and as stabilizing agents in other food processing. Carrageenans, which have the unique ability to stabilize milk proteins, are used in evaporated and flavored milks. Vegetable gums, including arabic, tragacanth, guar, and xanthan, are also used in a variety of products as water-binders, thickeners, and stabilizers.

In the process of human metabolism *mucopolysaccharides,* such as hyaluronic acid and chondroitin sulfate, are synthesized and found in the ground substance of connective tissue where they have structural importance.

## Role of carbohydrates in health

### Energy

Carbohydrates are a major source of energy in the human diet; approximately 4 kcal are provided by each gram of carbohydrate. Although fat and protein can replace carbohydrate as a source of energy for most of the cells of the body, some carbohydrate is essential for humans. Brain, nerve, and lung tissue require glucose as their source of energy. If the blood glucose level falls (hypoglycemia) and the brain is deprived of glucose, convulsions may result. It should be pointed out, however, that certain amino acids and part of the fat molecule can also contribute to the total amount of glucose available in the body and in this way provide a source of energy for these tissues. Also, as is discussed in Chapter 9, carbohydrates, especially sugars, are converted to fats (triglycerides) in the liver and become available to cells for energy or storage in adipose tissue. In transamination reactions, intermediary products of carbohydrate metabolism can be converted into amino acids and used for protein synthesis.

Although a diet free of carbohydrate is seldom found,

people who, as participants in experimental studies, have consumed such diets have developed many of the same symptoms as people on a starvation regimen. These symptoms include abnormal fat metabolism, breakdown of body protein, increased sodium excretion, loss of energy, and fatigue. Relatively small amounts (50 g–100 g) of carbohydrate appear to prevent these symptoms.[5]

## Detoxification

Glucuronic acid, an oxidation product of glucose metabolism, is important in the detoxification of a number of intermediary products of normal metabolism and of certain drugs. Morphine, salicylic acid, and the sulfa drugs are but a few of the drugs that are detoxified by combining with and being excreted as glucuronic acid derivatives.

## Dental caries

Carbohydrates, primarily sucrose, are easily fermented and can produce weak inorganic acids capable of dissolving the mineral constituents of the enamel and dentin of the teeth. The combination of sugar and certain bacteria found in plaque, a sticky, colorless film of nonpathogenic oral bacteria that forms on teeth, results in the production of acids, which can attack the tooth and lead to decay. Foods that adhere to the teeth and sticky sweets, such as caramels, pastries, and candied apples, are the most damaging. Soft drinks and sweetened juices, however, can also be harmful to dental health. Frequency of sugar intake may be even more important in caries development than the total amount of sugar consumed. Good oral hygiene, less frequent consumption of sweets, and limiting certain forms of snack foods are practices that will help reduce the incidence of dental caries.[6]

## Fiber in the diet

In recent years the role of fiber in the diet has become a topic of much concern and controversy. Epidemiological evidence has been used to show the differences between the prevalence of many degenerative diseases among population groups, particularly in Africa, who consume a diet high in fiber and similar groups whose dietary intake of fiber is much lower.[7] These diseases include appendicitis, diverticular disease, hiatus hernia, hemorrhoids, cancer of the colon, atherosclerosis, ischemic heart disease, and diabetes. One of the first questions raised by the theory that fiber is related to the etiology of diseases so varied and different as diverticulosis and atherosclerosis was, "What is meant by dietary fiber?" Although there is still lack of general agreement among various research workers in defining terms, there is almost total agreement that the term "crude fiber," which is found in food composition tables, has little meaning in determining the actual amount of dietary fiber present in a food. Dietary fiber has been defined as the plant materials that are resistant to the action of the digestive enzymes of the human small intestine.[8] These materials occur primarily in cell walls and include the components shown in Table 2-2. The values given for "crude fiber" exclude about 80% of the hemicellulose, 50% to 90% of the lignin, and as much as 50% of the cellulose in food. Scientists are still developing methods to determine accurately the amounts of the different components of fiber in individual foods. Table 2-3 shows certain major dietary fiber components in some common foods.

The nutrition counselor also should realize that many functions of the different components of fiber are still under investigation. However, some possible roles of dietary fiber in relation to health protection and disease prevention have been described. High-fiber diets result in increased retention of water, which promotes more frequent bowel movements and softer stools of increased weight. It has also been demonstrated that the increased bulk and decreased fecal viscosity decrease pressure within the bowel. Burkitt suggests that these changes within the bowel from a high-fiber diet would afford protection against such diseases as appendicitis, hiatus hernia, hemorrhoids, varicose veins, and diverticulosis, even if other dietary factors or nondietary factors were the causative agents.[9]

Pectin and guar flour have recently been shown to have a positive effect in controlling blood glucose by regulating insulin release.[10] In another study using apples, apple puree, and apple juice, the responses of insulin and blood glucose to the differences in fiber paralleled the individuals' response to satiety.[11] Dietary fiber appears to slow down the gastric emptying time, increasing the feeling of satiety and reducing both blood insulin and glucose levels.

Although cellulose has been shown to have little effect on reducing serum cholesterol levels,[12] pectin[13] and guar gum[14] have been demonstrated to possess significant cholesterol-lowering properties. The mechanisms for this action are not clearly understood, but this hypocholesterolemic effect may indicate a possible link between atherosclerosis and dietary fiber.

There is still little clinical evidence to relate cancer of the colon to the diet. However, it has been postulated that if a foreign material, such as a virus or a chemical, causes cancer, this substance would remain in the intestinal tract longer and, as a result, be capable of doing more harm in people consuming low-fiber diets. In conflict with this theory is the fact that constipation does not appear to be a predisposing factor in colon cancer.

Other investigators have warned of some of the hazards of excessive dietary fiber. There is evidence of increased mineral losses in the feces when dietary fiber is increased. Volvulus (intestinal obstruction due to a knotting and twisting of the bowel), a rare disease in the United States, is not uncommon among rural African populations consuming high-fiber diets.

There is much interest in fiber, not only by the nutrition counselor but also by research investigators. As more and more laboratory and clinical studies are published, the fiber story will be unravelled. In the meantime, a reasonable increase in dietary fiber such as that suggested by the various goals and guidelines (see Chap. 1) would be appropriate for promoting health in the population of the United States.

## Plant sources of carbohydrates
### Cereal grains

The ancient Romans called Demeter, the Greek goddess of the grains and harvests, Ceres, and from her name the word *cereal* is derived. Because of their wide cultivation, good keeping qualities, bland flavor, and great variety, cereals have continued to be the staple of the human diet from prehistoric times to the present. Most of them belong to the botanic family of grasses, with the exception of buckwheat. Each of the cereals has characteristic properties and uses.

**Table 2-2. Components of Dietary Fiber by Structure and Possible Physiologic Function**

| Fiber Component | Chemical Structure of Main Chain | Possible Physiologic Function |
|---|---|---|
| 1. Cellulose (principal cell wall constituent) | Glucose straight chain polymer | Retains water in feces<br>Increases bulk and weight of feces<br>Promotes colonic peristalsis<br>Decreased fecal transit time<br>Increased number of bowel actions<br>Reduces colonic intraluminal pressure<br>May increase zinc, calcium, magnesium, phosphorus, and iron excretion |
| 2. Noncellulosic polysaccharides Hemicelluloses (found in cell wall) | Xylose branched chain polymers<br>Glucose and mannose branched chain polymers<br>Galactose and mannose branched chain polymers<br>Galactose, glucose, and mannose branched chain polymers | Retains water in feces<br>Increases bulk and weight of feces<br>Reduces elevated colonic intraluminal pressure<br>Increases bile acid excretion |
| Pectin substances (intercellular cement) | Methylated galacturonic acid branched chain polymer | Absorbs water<br>Slows gastric emptying<br>Provides fermentable substrate for colonic bacteria with production of gas and volatile fatty acids<br>Binds bile acids and increases their excretion<br>Lowers plasma cholesterol levels<br>Improves glucose tolerance in diabetics |
| Algal polysaccharides (from algae and seaweeds) | Mannose, xylose, glucuronic acid, and glucose | Slows gastric emptying time<br>Provides fermentable substrate for colonic bacteria with production of gas and volatile fatty acids<br>Binds bile acids |
| Gums (secretions) | Galacturonic acid and mannose<br>Galacturonic acid and rhamnose<br>Arabinose and galacturonic acid | Slows gastric emptying time<br>Provides fermentable substrate for colonic bacteria with production of gas and volatile fatty acids<br>Binds bile acids<br>Lowers plasma cholesterol levels (guar gum)<br>Improves glucose tolerance in diabetics (guar flour) |
| Mucilages (secretions of plant seeds) | Galactose and mannose<br>Galacturonic acid and rhamnose<br>Arabinose and xylose | Slows gastric emptying time<br>Provides fermentable substrate for colonic bacteria with production of gas and volatile fatty acids<br>Binds bile acids |
| 3. Lignin (woody parts of plants) | Phenylpropane branched chain polymer | Acts as antioxidant<br>May bind minerals<br>Increase bile acid excretion<br>Lowers plasma cholesterol levels? |

## Table 2-3.  Dietary Fiber in Foods (g/100 g)

| Food | Total Dietary Fiber | Noncellulosic Polysaccharides | Cellulose | Lignin |
|---|---|---|---|---|
| *Flour* | | | | |
| White | 3.15 | 2.52 | 0.60 | 0.03 |
| Brown | 7.87 | 5.70 | 1.42 | 0.75 |
| Whole-meal | 9.51 | 6.25 | 2.46 | 0.80 |
| Bran | 44.0 | 32.7 | 8.05 | 3.23 |
| *Bread* | | | | |
| White | 2.72 | 2.01 | 0.71 | tr |
| Brown | 5.11 | 3.63 | 1.33 | 0.15 |
| Whole-meal | 8.50 | 5.95 | 1.31 | 1.24 |
| *Cereals* | | | | |
| All-Bran | 26.7 | 17.82 | 6.01 | 2.88 |
| Cornflakes | 11.0 | 7.26 | 2.42 | 1.32 |
| Grapenuts | 7.0 | 5.14 | 1.28 | 0.58 |
| Rice Krispies | 4.47 | 3.47 | 0.78 | 0.22 |
| Puffed Wheat | 15.14 | 10.35 | 2.59 | 2.47 |
| Sugar Puffs | 6.08 | 4.00 | 0.99 | 1.09 |
| Shredded Wheat | 12.26 | 8.79 | 2.63 | 0.84 |
| Special K | 5.45 | 3.68 | 0.72 | 1.05 |
| *Vegetables* | | | | |
| Broccoli tops | 4.10 | 2.92 | 1.15 | 0.03 |
| Brussels sprouts | 2.86 | 1.99 | 0.80 | 0.07 |
| Cabbage | 2.83 | 1.76 | 0.69 | 0.38 |
| Cauliflower | 1.80 | 0.67 | 1.13 | tr |
| Lettuce | 1.53 | 0.47 | 1.06 | tr |
| Onions | 2.10 | 1.55 | 0.55 | tr |
| Carrots | 3.70 | 2.22 | 1.48 | tr |
| Parsnips | 4.90 | 3.77 | 1.13 | tr |
| Rutabagas | 2.40 | 1.61 | 0.79 | tr |
| Turnips | 2.20 | 1.50 | 0.70 | tr |
| Potato | 3.51 | 2.49 | 1.02 | tr |
| Peppers (cooked) | 0.93 | 0.59 | 0.34 | tr |
| Tomato (fresh) | 1.40 | 0.65 | 0.45 | 0.30 |
| Sweet corn (canned) | 5.69 | 4.97 | 0.64 | 0.08 |
| *Legumes* | | | | |
| Beans, baked | 7.27 | 5.67 | 1.41 | 0.19 |
| Beans, green | 3.35 | 1.85 | 1.29 | 0.21 |
| Peas (canned) | 7.85 | 5.20 | 2.30 | 0.35 |
| *Fruits* | | | | |
| Apples (flesh) | 1.42 | 0.94 | 0.48 | 0.01 |
| (skin) | 3.71 | 2.21 | 1.01 | 0.49 |
| Bananas | 1.75 | 1.12 | 0.37 | 0.26 |
| Cherries | 1.24 | 0.92 | 0.25 | 0.07 |
| Grapefruit | 0.44 | 0.34 | 0.04 | 0.06 |
| Peaches | 2.28 | 1.46 | 0.20 | 0.62 |
| Pears (flesh) | 2.44 | 1.32 | 0.67 | 0.45 |
| (skin) | 8.59 | 3.72 | 2.18 | 2.67 |
| Plums | 1.52 | 0.99 | 0.23 | 0.30 |
| Strawberries | 2.12 | 0.98 | 0.33 | 0.81 |
| *Nuts* | | | | |
| Brazils | 7.73 | 3.60 | 2.17 | 1.96 |
| Peanuts | 9.30 | 6.40 | 1.69 | 1.21 |
| Peanut Butter | 7.55 | 5.64 | 1.91 | tr |

(Adapted from Shipley EA: Dietary fiber content of foods. In Spiller GA, Amen RJ (eds): Dietary Fiber Research, pp 203–212. New York, Plenum Press, 1978)

The "green revolution," which combined modern agricultural methods with new high-yielding varieties of cereals, has produced a dramatic increase in cereal grain production throughout certain areas of the world. Asian countries, particularly India, have benefited most. In 1973, 40% of India's grain production came from new varieties and was grown on only 20% of the total grain acreage. The continuation and spread of the "green revolution" offers great hope that more and more of the developing nations can become self-sufficient in their food production. Unfortunately, recent shortages of fertilizers, made from petrochemicals which are at present expensive and in short supply, have counteracted some of the benefits of the "green revolution."

**Rice** is the most widely used cereal in the world. It is the staple food for Asia, the Near East, and some Latin American and African countries. It provides as much as 70% to 80% of the calories for the greater part of the population of these areas and is widely used elsewhere.

About 80% of the billion and a half Asians are involved in the production and distribution of rice. To meet the ever increasing demand for rice, the International Rice Research Institute in the Philippines directs work on improving rice production and was involved in the development of a new strain with improved yield and drastically reduced growing time.

Rice is usually milled as *regular* white rice, the form preferred by most people, although much of the vitamin and mineral content is lost in the milling. When the ancient home milling process, which involves parboiling or steaming before polishing, is used, some of the vitamins and minerals are forced into the center of the kernel and are thus conserved. The *parboiled* or converted rice available in the United States, which is commercially parboiled by special steam processing before milling, retains a somewhat higher vitamin and mineral content than regular white rice. Parboiled rice supplies about twice as much calcium, phosphorus, and potassium per serving as regular. However, enriched regular and enriched parboiled rice contain approximately the same amounts of iron, thiamin, and niacin. These amounts are based on minimum levels of enrichment as specified by U.S. government regulations. Enriched *precooked* (instant) rice, which requires a minimum of preparation time, is also available in the United States and has the same level of enrichment as regular and parboiled rice.

A high-vitamin *premix* is being used in Japan and the Philippines. The premix, which is heavily fortified with certain B vitamins, is applied to the white rice together with a protective coating that is highly resistant to cooking losses.

Unpolished brown rice and wild rice, both of which contain more of the original minerals and vitamins than does white rice, have limited use because of their different flavor, poor keeping quality, and high price. Rice-eating countries do not use rice to make bread but in place of bread. Rice flour is used in making a wide variety of snack foods in some of the Oriental countries and is available in the United States for use in modified diets.

**Wheat** is the next most common cereal used throughout the world and the most widely used in the Americas and Europe. High-yielding varieties of wheat have been developed through research sponsored by the Rockefeller and Ford Foundations at the International Maize and Wheat Improvement Center in Mexico. When the new Mexican wheat was planted in India and Pakistan the annual increase in yield per acre was doubled.

Wheat can be milled for a variety of uses—as breakfast cereals, as flour for bread, cakes, pastries, and crackers, and macaroni products. It lends itself to making bread better than other grains because of its high gluten content, which is necessary for yeast breads that demand kneading. Wheat flour is equally good for baking-powder breads, cakes, and cookies. Certain varieties of wheat are preferred for bread flour, others for cake flour, but for both the flour is manufactured by roller- or impact-milling—complicated processes designed to produce a pure white flour containing none of the bran or the germ. The final product represents 70% or less of the wheat kernel. The outer coatings and the germ, which contain the bulk of the minerals and vitamins, are sold mostly as stock feed. A small amount of pure wheat germ is processed for human consumption. Some bran is also processed for use as high-roughage breakfast cereals.

A small proportion of our wheat crop in the United States is milled as whole-wheat or Graham flour and some as whole-wheat breakfast cereal. Hard winter wheat is milled as semolina for the manufacture of macaroni, spaghetti, vermicelli, and noodles. A wide variety of these products are used in Italy and elsewhere in Europe as well as in the Americas and the Orient.

**Rye** is similar to wheat in many respects; rye flour may be used with wheat or by itself for breadmaking. Rye breads, such as pumpernickel or Swedish rye, are used in northern and central Europe and in Russia more commonly than in the United States.

**Triticale,** a hybrid cereal produced by crossbreeding wheat and rye, has been known since the late 1880s but has not been grown to any extent until recently. Research at the International Maize and Wheat Improvement Center in cooperation with the University of Manitoba has led to the development of high-yielding varieties of triticale which can be milled into flour to make bread, rolls, and pasta products, such as macaroni, noodles, and spaghetti.[15] In the future we may have in the United States a very mild rye-flavored white bread made from triticale.

**Corn** (or maize) is used for human food in many countries of the world; some areas, for example in Central and South America, depend on corn as the staple food. To people in these areas the research currently being done in

Mexico City at the International Maize and Wheat Improvement Center to develop new varieties of corn is especially important. By genetic manipulation a new maize variety with increased amounts of the essential amino acid lysine has been developed, thereby improving the protein quality of the corn (see Chap. 4).[16]

Corn is processed from several different varieties of mature field corn into many forms: cornmeal, white and yellow; hominy grits; samp, or hulled corn; popcorn; cornflakes or similar ready-to-eat cereals; and as a source of cornstarch, corn syrup, and corn oil. Yellow or white cornmeal is cooked as mush or grits and is used in pancakes or in cornmeal breads, corn pone, muffins, johnny-cakes and, in Central and South America, tamales and tortillas. Cornstarch is sold commercially as a thickening agent used in cooking. Waxy cornstarch, which contains only the branched or amylopectin fraction, provides thickening without retrogradation. Because it is relatively stable to freezing and thawing, it can be used as a thickening agent in prepared frozen dishes.

New high-amylose cornstarches are also now available to food processors; because of their unique properties they are being used in a variety of food products. Due to their linear structure they have the ability to form films, which act as oxygen and fat barriers on food and packaging materials, to form quick-setting structurally stable gels, and to bind other materials into stable extruded shapes. The consumer will find increased use of these starches in partially fried foods such as French fried potatoes; textured protein products (see Chap. 4); gelatin molds; gumdrops; textured pastes, such as tomato paste; applesauce; and edible or readily biodegradable food packaging.

Enzymatically produced cornstarch hydrolysates having properties intermediate between cornstarch and corn syrup are also available to the food processor for use in fabricated foods. They are soluble, nonsweet, eaily digestible, and may be used to improve the body and texture of certain food items.

Corn sugar and syrup are made by hydrolyzing the starch in the corn, that is, breaking it down into dextrins, maltose, and glucose. A new HFCS is now being manufactured from corn syrup by enzymatically (glucose isomerase) converting glucose to fructose. The syrup contains 42% to 90% fructose, has a sweet flavor, and is highly fermentable. It is used extensively in soft drinks.

Corn oil is extracted from the corn germ by a carefully controlled commercial process. The special properties of corn oil are discussed in Chapter 3.

***Oats*** are used chiefly in the form of rolled oats or oatmeal in the United States and western Europe. In recent years some ready-to-eat cereals have been processed from oats. Oat products carry more of the original kernel than do most other processed cereals and for this reason lose fewer nutrients between field and table than products of any other cereal.

***Granola-type*** cereals are usually mixtures of whole oats and wheat with brown sugar, raisins, nuts, and other ingredients added.

***Barley*** is used mostly as "pearled" barley, which is the kernel left after the bran and the germ have been removed. Barley flour is made by grinding the "pearls." In the United States pearl barley has limited use in soups. In some other countries, such as Korea and Japan, barley is raised and used as a low-cost substitute for rice.

***Buckwheat*** is not a true cereal botanically, that is, it does not belong to the grasses as do the other cereals, but it serves the same purpose for human food. The bran, or the husk, is removed, and the rest of the kernel is rolled and bolted to produce buckwheat flour. In the United States its most common use is in buckwheat pancakes, waffles, and ready-to-eat cereals; in Japan buckwheat is used in noodles. In Europe buckwheat is used in making heavy breads, puddings, cakes, and beer.

***Millet*** is a staple food for millions of people in India, Russia, China, and Africa but is little known in the United States. It can be raised where land is too poor and the climate too dry to grow wheat, rice, corn, or most other grains. Millet is used is eastern Europe for making flat bread and porridge. Russian "kasha" (cereal), often made from millet, may also be made from wheat or buckwheat.

## Milling of grains

Natural grains carry not only the store of carbohydrates already mentioned but also protein and certain minerals and vitamins essential for good nutrition. They also are an excellent source of dietary fiber. The vitamin B complex factors present in the natural whole grains are usually present in sufficient amounts to help form the enzymes necessary for the metabolism of the carbohydrate in grain. The balance of nature is upset when we find it desirable to modify natural grains by milling them to produce a whiter, more easily digested flour with better keeping qualities. In doing so, some of the minerals and vitamins are lost or discarded in the millings. It is interesting to note that the latter find excellent use as animal feed. Attempts to educate people accustomed to white-flour products to return to whole-grain products have never been successful. Consequently, the enrichment of bread and flour was initiated in the United States during World War II, with other cereal products of various types added to the list later. Thiamin, riboflavin, niacin, and iron are the factors added (see Chap. 11). Bread and flour enrichment is of primary importance because bread and products made from flour constitute some of the main sources of energy in the diet of the United States.

## Fruits

Fruits and vegetables constitute a less concentrated source of carbohydrates than do the cereals because of their high water content. In fruits the carbohydrate is found mostly in the form of the monosaccharides, glucose, and fructose. The disaccharide, sucrose, may be found in a few fresh fruits, and most canned fruits contain added sucrose or glucose unless specifically labeled "canned without added sugar." The soluble sugars along with their acids and traces of volatile oils give fruits their odor and appetite appeal, which is further enhanced by color and texture.

The sugar content of fresh fruits may vary from 6% to 20%, that of cantaloupe and watermelon being the lowest and that of banana one of the highest. Of course, dried fruits, such as prunes, apricots, raisins, dates, and figs, have a much higher sugar content (near 70%) due to their low moisture content. The energy value of fruits—fresh, canned, or frozen—is determined largely by their sugar content.

Although most fruits are considered highly desirable raw, plantains, which are related to but larger than the banana, are not palatable unless cooked. Because of their high starch content these fruits are an important source of carbohydrates in many tropical countries and when boiled, baked, or fried are frequently used in the main course of the meal.

The avocado pear and the olive are different from all other fruits because of their high fat content, which gives them a comparatively high energy value in spite of their low carbohydrate content.

Most fresh fruits also contain some dietary fiber, which together with the fruit acids, seems to stimulate intestinal motility in many people.

## Vegetables

Under the term *vegetables* are grouped foods representing practically every part of the plant—leaves, stems, seeds, seed pods, flowers, fruits, roots, and tubers. They vary as widely in composition as they do in their function in the plant and may contain anywhere from 3% to 35% of carbohydrate in the forms of starch, sugars, cellulose, and non-cellulosic polysaccharides.

Obviously, the energy value of vegetables varies with the percentage of carbohydrate present, but, in general, the high water and fiber content of leaf, flower, and stem vegetables puts them in the low-calorie class. This includes all the green leafy vegetables, plus celery, asparagus, cauliflower, broccoli, and Brussels sprouts. The roots, tubers, and seeds of plants have a higher starch and sugar content and less water; for this reason they provide more calories per unit of weight. In this group are found all kinds of potatoes, beets, carrots, turnips, parsnips, peas, beans, and lentils.

Root vegetables often provide much of the carbohydrate in the diets of certain African, Latin American, and Asian peoples. Because these vegetables are for the most part very poor in protein, their wide use creates certain nutrition problems, particularly in infant feeding, where

### Table 2-4. Carbohydrates in Common Foods

| Starches | Percent |
|---|---|
| Barley, pearled | 79 |
| Breads, all types | 52–58 |
| Cassava, meal and flour | 85 |
| Cornmeal and grits | 74–78 |
| Crackers | 71–74 |
| Macaroni, spaghetti, and noodles | 73–77 |
| Oatmeal or oat cereals | 70 |
| Potatoes, cooked | 19 |
| Rice or rice cereals | 79 |
| Rye flour | 68–78 |
| Wheat flour | 69–79 |
| Wheat cereals | 72–80 |

| Sugars | Percent |
|---|---|
| Cakes * | 56–62 |
| Candies | 56–99 |
| Cookies * | 60–80 |
| Dried fruits | 75–88 |
| Honey | 80 |
| Jams and jellies | 65–71 |
| Syrups | 74 |
| Cane or beet sugar | 100 |

* Also include starch.

they may take the place of more nutritious foods. Cassava, also called manioc or yuca, has a long root (1–3 in thick). It is frequently grated, dried, and powdered as a "meal"— tapioca or arrowroot. Taro, which is also grown in tropical and subtropical countries, can be baked or boiled like a potato. The Hawaiians boil the eddoes (as the roots are called), then peel and grind them with water to make *poi*, the sticky pastelike food so popular in the Islands. Other roots and tubers such as sweet potatoes, yams, turnips, and Jerusalem artichokes may also be used as staple foods at certain times by various peoples. To improve agricultural production of certain tropical crops the International Center of Tropical Agriculture in Colombia and the International Institute of Tropical Agriculture in Nigeria have been established.

## Nuts

Nuts seldom are thought of as a source of carbohydrate because of their high content of fat and protein. However, because of their low moisture content, they contain from 10% to 27% total carbohydrate. They also contain significant amounts of dietary fiber. Peanuts, which are really legumes, are usually classed with the nuts because of their composition and common usage.

Due to their high fat content, nuts digest slowly. Chopping or grinding improves digestibility. In the form of nut butter and combined with other foods, there is usually no difficulty with digestion. Peanut butter may be used in sandwiches or as an ingredient of a recipe.

### Other plant sources of carbohydrates

*Common table sugar*—the refined white granulated or powdered sugar or brown sugar—is processed from either sugar cane or sugar beets.

Sucrose is the chief source of sweetening used in most desserts, ice creams, candies, and soft drinks. The average per capita consumption of sugar in the United States is estimated at approximately 2 lb per week. This means, of course, that some people use much more than this, and others consume far less. Because sugar is 99.9% carbohydrate and furnishes almost 4 calories to the gram, those who use the average amount or more are getting more than 3500 empty calories per week. Sugar is concentrated fuel but furnishes no other nutrients. Furthermore, candies and other sweets are reputed to aggravate dental caries, a major health problem. Sugar consumption in the form of candies, soft drinks, and rich desserts is certainly a contributing factor to the great problem of obesity in the United States (see Chap. 28).

*Molasses* is a by-product of sugar refining and carries more of the mineral content of the original plant than do the refined sugars.

*Maple syrup and sugar* are made by boiling down the sap from sugar maples. This was one of the first kinds of sugar used in America—the Indians, who knew how to obtain and process it, taught their techniques to the early settlers. Despite differences in flavor or color, which are due to traces of other factors, the sugar in all of these products is disaccharide sucrose.

*Corn syrup,* made from field corn by hydrolysis of the starch, is mostly glucose and maltose. A HFCS made by converting 42% to 90% of the glucose to fructose has become widely used in commercial processing, particularly in the beverage industry.

*Honey,* made by bees from flower nectars, contains a mixture of the two monosaccharides, glucose amd fructose. The fructose in honey makes it taste sweeter than other sugars because fructose has a sweeter taste than sucrose, glucose, or maltose.

*Sorghum syrup* is made from the sweet juice of the grain sorghum stem, and its use is confined largely to the southeastern and south central states. Grain sorghums are also used for food in parts of India, China, and Africa.

*Other forms* of plant life not usually classed as vegetables are the seaweeds used for food in many countries, notably Japan. Certain varieties of seaweed are sources of *agar, alginates,* and *carrageenans.*

### Change of form

Interchanges among the different forms of carbohydrate in the plant world are interesting and significant factors in food quality and keeping properties. As growth proceeds, there is constant exchange from one form to another. In fruits such as the banana the carbohydrate is in the form of starch in the maturing fruit, but some of it is changed to sugar as the fruit ripens. In some vegetables sugar synthesized by the leaves is stored as starch, as in potatoes and in mature beans, peas, and corn. Connoisseurs of fresh garden vegetables are aware how quickly the sugar of corn and green peas disappears after harvesting, and how much more delicious they are when used immediately after picking. This change is due to the enzymes that are present in the vegetables, and the change is stopped as soon as the enzymes are destroyed by heating. This is the reason that frozen vegetables that have been blanched promptly after harvesting and before freezing may have better flavor than so-called fresh vegetables that have been shipped long distances and stored before appearing at market.

## Animal sources of carbohydrates

Most animal foods, such as meats, poultry, and fish, contain only traces of carbohydrate in the form of *glycogen,* used for muscle contraction. Eggs also contain mere traces of carbohydrate. Only liver contains an appreciable amount, and this is in the form of glycogen. In all animals the liver serves as a temporary storehouse of quickly available fuel for the body, and it may contain from 2% to 6% of glycogen. Another source of glycogen in foods is scallops, which are the muscles of shellfish and contain about 3% of glycogen.

Fresh milk contains about 5% of carbohydrate in the form of *lactose,* a disaccharide. When consumed in amounts greater than those ordinarily present in milk, some lactose may not be digested. An undigested residue of lactose in the large intestine has a laxative action which may be desirable in certain instances but in excess causes diarrhea. Lactose is an excellent medium for the growth of certain useful acid-tolerant bacteria and has been used therapeutically to increase this type of bacterial flora in the large intestines. Lactose also seems to increase the absorption or utilization of calcium, and often this finding is cited as the reason for the efficient utilization of calcium from milk. Sometimes lactose is given as an accompaniment of calcium salts prescribed for persons who have an allergy to milk and must obtain their calcium in another form.

A summary of the types and amounts of carbohydrates found in various foods was compiled by Hardinge and co-workers.[17]

## Study questions and activities

1. Name the monosaccharides and give some food sources of each. What are their chemical similarities and differences?
2. What are the two forms of starch? How do they differ in structure and in use?
3. Why is it important to include alcohol consumption when food intake is calculated? Explain why a meta-

bolic interreaction between alcohol and barbiturates may occur.

4. Explain the commercial sources for sucrose, fructose, and glucose. List the sugar alcohols that may be used for sweetening.

5. In what way is the sugar of milk unique? How is it classified chemically?

6. Which carbohydrates are most common in fruits? In root vegetables?

7. What type of food provides the most common source of carbohydrate and energy for the world's people? What are some of the regional or national preferences?

8. What is another name for "animal starch"? Where is it found? Of what significance is it in animal nutrition?

9. What is meant by dietary fiber? List the components of dietary fiber. What foods are considered good sources of dietary fiber? Describe three possible physiologic functions of dietary fiber.

10. Collect four boxes of ready-to-eat breakfast cereals. List the first three ingredients shown on the package. From the nutrition information label, list the number of calories per serving (1 oz). Determine the cost per serving by dividing the total cost of the box by the number of servings per box. Which cereal is the "better buy"? Why? From the carbohydrate information label determine the percent of carbohydrate from sucrose and other sugars and from starch and related carbohydrates. Do any of the labels include information regarding dietary fiber?

11. List the carbohydrate-containing foods you consumed in the past 24 hours. For each food indicate whether it contained starch, naturally occurring sugars, added sugars or syrups, and dietary fiber. Do you need to make changes to meet dietary goals or guidelines?

## References

1. Brunzell JD: J Am Diet Assoc 73:499, 1978
2. Hardy SL et al: J Am Diet Assoc 74:41, 1979
3. Lecos C: FDA Consumer, 14:21, Mar, 1980
4. Boeker EA: J Am Diet Assoc 76:550, 1980
5. Council on Foods and Nutrition: JAMA 224:1415, 1973
6. Nizel AE: Today's Health, Oct, 1973
7. Burkitt DP: JAMA 299:1068, 1974
8. Trowell HC et al: Lancet 1:967, 1976
9. Burkitt DP: In Heaton KW (ed): Dietary Fiber: Current Developments of Importance to Health, p 35. Westport, CT, Technomic, 1979
10. Jenkins DJA et al: Ann Intern Med 86:20, 1977
11. Haber GB: Lancet 2:679, 1977
12. Story JA et al: Artery 3:154, 1977
13. Kay RM, Truswell AS: Am J Clin Nutr 30:171, 1977
14. Jenkins DJA et al: Lancet 1:1116, 1975
15. Lorenz K: Food Tech 26:66, 1972
16. Mertz ET: Nutr Rev 32:129, 1974
17. Hardinge MG et al: J Am Diet Assoc 46:197, 1965

## Supplementary readings

Bing FC: Dietary fiber—In historical perspective. J Am Diet Assoc 69:498, 1976

Boeker EA: Metabolism of ethanol. J Am Diet Assoc 76:550, 1980

Brown AT: The role of dietary carbohydrate in plaque formation and oral disease. In Hegsted DM et al (eds): Present Knowledge of Nutrition, 4th ed, pp 488–503. New York, Nutrition Foundation, 1976

Burkitt DP: Relationships between diseases and their etiological significance. Am J Clin Nutr 30:262, 1977

Connor WE, Connor SL: Sucrose and carbohydrate. In Hegsted DM et al (eds): Present Knowledge of Nutrition, 4th ed, pp 33–42. New York, Nutrition Foundation, 1976

Food and fiber. Nutr Rev 35:6, 1977

Halsted CH: Nutritional implications of alcohol. In Hegsted DM et al (eds): Present Knowledge of Nutrition, 4th ed, pp 467–477. New York, Nutrition Foundation, 1976

Hollingsworth DF: Translating nutrition into diet. Food Tech 31:38, 1977

Kelsay JL: A review in effects of fiber intake on man. Am J Clin Nutr 31:142, 1978

Trowell H: Definition of dietary fiber and hypothesis that it is a protective factor in certain diseases. Am J Clin Nutr 29:417, 1976

Wang Y-M, van Eys J: Nutritional significance of fructose and sugar alcohols. Ann Rev Nutr 1:437, 1981

*For further references see Bibliography in Part 4.*

# Fats and Other Lipids

# 3

**EFA:** Essential Fatty Acids
**FFA:** Free Fatty Acids
**HDL:** High-density Lipoprotein
**LDL:** Low-density Lipoprotein
**MCT:** Medium-chain Triglycerides
**PG:** Prostaglandins
**PL:** Phospholipids
**PUFA:** Polyunsaturated Fatty Acids
**TG:** Triglycerides
**VLDL:** Very Low Density Lipoprotein

## Fats in the human diet

Fats are a form of stored energy in animals as important as carbohydrates are in plants. They serve multiple purposes in the diet. In addition to their high energy value, they contain essential fatty acids and act as carriers for the fat-soluble vitamins. That fat makes a meal more satisfying is due partially to its slow gastric emptying time and therefore its satiety value, and partially to the flavor it gives to other foods.

There is no physiological evidence that the human body needs as much fat as Americans consume, and many experts recommend a moderate reduction of fat in the diet. In many countries of the Orient, the Middle East, and Africa the average diet provides less than 20% of the total calories in the form of fat, compared with over twice that amount in the American diet.

Because Americans differ so widely in their patterns of food preparation and in their eating practices in regard to fat, reliable information on the actual individual consumption of this nutrient is difficult for the nutrition counselor to obtain. Some homemakers use considerable amounts of fat for frying and flavoring foods; others use methods of preparation, especially in the cooking of meats and poultry, which markedly reduce the amount of fat in the cooked food. Habits vary in regard to the eating or discarding of fat on meat, the use of table fats on breads and cream on cereals, and the use of salad dressings. When people are made aware of the amount of fat that they are consuming and of its caloric value, they frequently modify their intake without making major adjustments in their eating habits.

## Structure and characteristics of lipids

Fats, oils, and fatlike substances, because of similar solubilities, are classified as lipids (Table 3-1). They are insoluble in water and soluble in one or more of the so-called fat solvents, ether, chloroform, benzene, and acetone. Like carbohydrates, fats are composed of carbon, hydrogen, and oxygen but in proportions that greatly

## Table 3-1. Classification of Lipids

*1. Simple Lipids*
  A.  Triglycerides—esters of fatty acids with glycerol
  B.  Esters of fatty acids with high-molecular-weight alcohols
      Waxes
      Cholesterol esters
      Vitamin A and D esters

*2. Compound Lipids*
  A.  Phospholipids—phosphorus-containing lipids
      Lecithins
      Cephalins
      Sphingomyelins
  B.  Glycolipids—sugar-containing lipids
      Cerebrosides
      Gangliosides
  C.  Sulfolipids—sulfur-containing lipids
  D.  Lipoproteins—protein-containing lipids
  E.  Lipopolysaccarides—polysaccharide-containing lipids.

*3. Derived Lipids*
  A.  Fatty acids
  B.  Alcohols
      Glycerol
      High-molecular-weight alcohols
  C.  Mono- and diglycerides
  D.  Sterols
      Cholesterol
      Ergosterol
      Bile acids
      Steroid hormones
      Vitamin D
  E.  Hydrocarbons
      Squalene
      Carotenoids
      Aliphatic hydrocarbons
  F.  Fat-soluble vitamins
      Vitamin A
      Vitamin E
      Vitamin K

increase their energy value. Fats that are fluid at room temperature are usually called oils, whereas those that are solid are called fats. Both are primarily mixtures of triglycerides.

*Triglycerides (TG)* are esters of glycerol with three fatty acids (Fig. 3-1). A new chemical name, triacylglycerols, is also used to describe a true fat. Triglycerides usually contain a mixture of two or three different fatty acids rather than three identical ones. The large number of fatty acids in natural foods and the mixing of them makes possible a large number of different triglycerides in any individual fat. Milk fat is said to have the possibility of containing almost 125,000 different triglycerides.

There is current interest in the positioning of the fatty acids in the triglyceride molecule because the position, as well as the chain length and degree of saturation of the fatty acids, affects the melting point and, thereby, the digestibility and absorption of the fat. The number 2 position on the triglyceride molecule is the central position and is occupied by different types of fatty acids depending on the origin of the fat. Seed fats, such as cottonseed oil, usually have unsaturated fatty acids (oleic or linoleic acids) in this position.

Hydrolysis of triglycerides by heat or by the fat-splitting enzymes, lipases, yields glycerol, fatty acids, diglycerides, and monoglycerides. If an alkali agent (NaOH) is used, soaps are formed; this process is called *saponification.*

*Glycerol* is an alcohol containing three carbon atoms and three hydroxyl groups. The latter are the reactive groups, which can combine with fatty acids to form mono-, di-, and triglycerides (Fig. 3-1).

*Fatty acids.*   The type and configuration of the fatty acids in fats are responsible for differences in flavor,

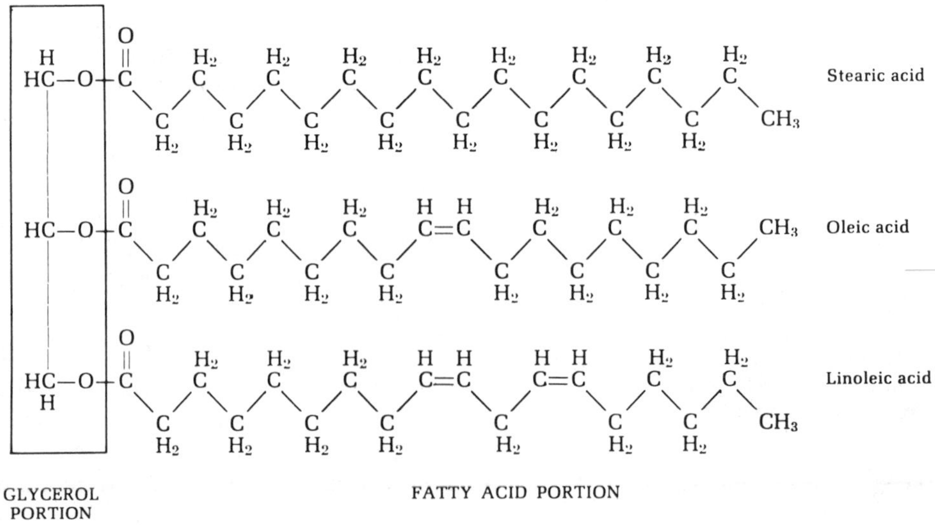

**Fig. 3-1.** The three fatty acids—stearic (saturated), oleic (monounsaturated), and linoleic (polyunsaturated)—combined in ester linkage with glycerol to form a triglyceride or fat.

texture, melting point, absorption, essential fatty acid activity, and other characteristics. Fatty acids vary in length from four to about 24 carbon atoms including, with few exceptions, only the even-numbered members of the series. They are referred to as *short chain* (4 to 6 carbons), *medium chain* (8 to 12 carbons) and *long chain* (more than 12 carbons). Reference may also be made to extra long chain fatty acids, or those over 20 carbons. Natural fats contain 16 and 18 carbon fatty acids in the largest quantities, although short chain fatty acids are found in butterfat and coconut oil. In addition to their presence in relatively small amounts in natural fats, triglycerides containing medium chain fatty acids (MCT) are commercially prepared from such fats as coconut oil. The ease with which fats with medium chain fatty acids are hydrolyzed, absorbed, and transported has made them useful in treating patients with certain types of malabsorption syndromes (see Chaps. 9 and 26).

Fatty acids are also classified as *saturated* or *unsaturated*, depending on the presence or absence of double bonds. A double bond occurs when two adjoining carbons each have one less hydrogen atom than they normally hold. Then a double bond between the two carbons satisfies the carbon valence of 4. Fatty acids, such as oleic, are called *monounsaturated* because they contain one double bond, whereas linoleic, linolenic, and arachidonic acids, which contain two, three, and four double bonds respectively, are called *polyunsaturated* (Fig. 3-1). Table 3-2 shows the nomenclature for some of the common fatty acids. The polyunsaturated fatty acids (PUFA) have been shown in certain instances to lower blood cholesterol level, whereas saturated fatty acids tend to raise the serum cholesterol level. Table 3-3 shows the fatty acid composition of some common animal and vegetable fats. Saturated fatty acids, particularly the long chain fatty acids and their glycerides, have higher melting points and accordingly tend to be solid in form at room temperature. These fats are found in greater amounts in animal sources (Table 3-3). Oils, for the most part, contain large amounts of unsaturated fatty acids, have lower melting points, and are chiefly of vegetable origin. Coconut oil, however, is a notable exception because it is almost 90% saturated; short and medium chain acids account for its being an oil. Animals, including humans, are metabolically able to increase or decrease the chain length of fatty acids by the addition or removal of two carbon fragments and can convert the saturated fatty acid stearic to the monounsaturated fatty acid oleic by removal of two hydrogens. Humans, however, cannot synthesize the polyunsaturated fatty acid, linoleic; for this reason, linoleic is considered to be an essential fatty acid (EFA).

In addition to the length of the fatty acid chain and the degree of saturation, the *configuration*, or isomeric form, of the fatty acid at the double bond and the position of the double bonds are factors that determine the role of fats in nutrition. The fatty acids in most natural fats are in the *cis* form; this means that at the double bond the molecule turns back on itself ⌐___. In processed fats such as margarine much of the fatty acid has been changed into the *trans* form, whereby the chain is stretched out ___⌐. For example, the trans form (isomer) of oleic acid is elaidic acid. This increases the melting point so that a desirable consistency for a table or cooking fat is accomplished with a low degree of saturation. Cis isomers cannot be packed together closely like the trans form or the straight chains of the saturated acids. Trans forms of PUFA do not show essential fatty acid activity nor do they possess the ability to lower plasma cholesterol levels.

Hydrogenation, the addition of hydrogen atoms to unsaturated fats, increases the degree of saturation and changes a liquid oil to a solid fat. These changes in the configuration and degree of saturation of fats have been found not to affect their energy value.

*Mono-* and *diglycerides* are esters of glycerol containing one and two fatty acids, respectively, and are produced from triglycerides in the process of digestion (see Chap. 9). They are also used commercially in prepared baked and processed foods to improve the texture.

*Nonnutritive oils.* A clear distinction should be kept in mind between oils that are true fats and the hydrocarbons derived from petroleum, such as lubricating oil or purified mineral oil. The latter contain carbon and hydrogen but no oxygen. Mineral oil is completely indigestible in the animal body and cannot be classified as a food. Formerly, it was used in place of true fats in certain low calorie diets. This procedure is generally discouraged because mineral oil tends to interfere with the absorption of the fat-soluble vitamins. It is particularly detrimental

### Table 3-2. Nomenclature for Some Common Fatty Acids

| Common Name | Chemical Name | Abbreviation |
|---|---|---|
| Capric | Decanoic | $C_{10:0}$ * |
| Lauric | Dodecanoic | $C_{12:0}$ |
| Myristic | Tetradecanoic | $C_{14:0}$ |
| Palmitic | Hexadecanoic | $C_{16:0}$ |
| Stearic | Octadecanoic | $C_{18:0}$ |
| Oleic | 9-octadecenoic † | $C_{18:1\,\omega9}$ ‡ |
| Linoleic | 9-12-octadecadienoic | $C_{18:2\,\omega6}$ |
| Linolenic | 9,12,15-octadecatrienoic | $C_{18:3\,\omega3}$ |
| Arachidonic | 5,8,11,14-eicosatetraenoic | $C_{20:4\,\omega6}$ |

*First number indicates the number of carbon atoms in the molecule; second number indicates the number of double bonds.

†Number indicates double bond position numbered from the carboxyl end of the molecule.

‡Number indicates the position of the first double bond numbered from the methyl end. Those with their first double bond at $\omega9$ are n-9 acids; those with the first double bond at $\omega6$ are n-6 acids; those with the double bond at $\omega3$ are n-3 acids. Enzymes can only insert double bonds on the carboxylic side of an existing double bond; for this reason, linoleic acid can be desaturated to arachidonic, whereas oleic acid cannot.

### Table 3-3. Fatty Acid Composition of Selected Foods from Animal and Plant Origin

| Food | Total Fat | Fatty Acids | | | | | | | | | | |
| --- | --- | --- | --- | --- | --- | --- | --- | --- | --- | --- | --- | --- |
| | | Saturated | | | | | Unsaturated | | | | | |
| | | | | | | | | | | Monounsaturated | Polyunsaturated | |
| | | Total | 12:0 | 14:0 | 16:0 | 18:0 | Total | 16:1 | 18:1 | 18:2 | 18:3 | Other |
| | | *g/100 g of Food* | | | | | | | | | | |
| **Animal origin** | | | | | | | | | | | | |
| Butter | 80.1 | 49.8 | 2.2 | 8.1 | 21.1 | 9.7 | 26.1 | 1.8 | 20.1 | 1.8 | 1.2 | |
| Cheddar cheese | 32.9 | 20.2 | 0.74 | 3.3 | 8.94 | 3.78 | 10.7 | 1.01 | 8.24 | 0.51 | 0.42 | |
| Cottage cheese | 4.0 | 2.6 | 0.09 | 0.43 | 1.20 | 0.44 | 1.2 | 0.12 | 0.91 | 0.09 | 0.03 | |
| Cream cheese | 33.8 | 21.2 | 0.67 | 3.49 | 9.92 | 3.71 | 10.6 | 0.90 | 8.08 | 0.79 | 0.45 | |
| Light cream | 20.6 | 12.8 | 0.58 | 2.07 | 5.42 | 2.50 | 6.7 | 0.47 | 5.18 | 0.47 | 0.30 | |
| Ice cream | 12.3 | 7.7 | 0.34 | 1.24 | 3.23 | 1.49 | 4.0 | 0.28 | 3.09 | 0.28 | 0.18 | |
| Milk (whole) | 3.5 | 2.2 | 0.10 | 0.35 | 0.92 | 0.42 | 1.1 | 0.08 | 0.88 | 0.08 | 0.05 | |
| Eggs | 11.3 | 3.4 | | 0.03 | 2.51 | 0.87 | 6.0 | 0.38 | 4.16 | 1.26 | 0.03 | 0.14 |
| Beef, arm chuck braised | 19.2 | 8.0 | | 0.7 | 5.0 | 2.1 | 10.1 | 1.1 | 7.7 | 0.5 | 0.2 | 0.5 |
| Beef, sirloin broiled | 42.2 | 17.6 | | 1.6 | 11.2 | 4.4 | 22.4 | 2.5 | 17.3 | 0.9 | 0.6 | 0.8 |
| Lamb, leg (roasted) | 21.2 | 9.57 | 0.02 | 0.73 | 4.72 | 3.39 | 9.7 | 0.40 | 7.92 | 0.79 | 0.34 | 0.29 |
| Chicken, breast (roasted) | 6.38 | 1.86 | | 0.06 | 1.36 | 0.44 | 3.66 | 0.27 | 1.77 | 1.27 | 0.07 | 0.32 |
| Pork, loin (roasted) | 28.1 | 9.84 | | 0.44 | 6.33 | 2.91 | 16.5 | 1.02 | 12.12 | 2.63 | 0.24 | 0.65 |
| Frankfurters | 29.1 | 11.2 | | 0.8 | 6.5 | 3.8 | 15.8 | 1.8 | 12.3 | 0.9 | 0.3 | 0.6 |
| Bacon, cooked | 49.0 | 18.09 | | 0.72 | 11.42 | 5.85 | 28.39 | 1.54 | 21.25 | 4.70 | 0.63 | 0.37 |
| Tuna, albacore | 8.0 | | | 0.22 | 1.6 | 0.32 | | 0.39 | 1.4 | 0.15 | 0.19 | 3.07 |
| Soup (beef noodle, 1:1 dilution) | 1.3 | 0.48 | | 0.02 | 0.26 | 0.16 | 0.71 | 0.04 | 0.45 | 0.17 | 0.02 | 0.06 |
| Soup (cream of chicken, 1:1 dilution) | 3.0 | 0.85 | | 0.06 | 0.53 | 0.17 | 1.94 | 0.12 | 1.20 | 0.57 | 0.03 | 0.05 |
| **Plant origin** | | | | | | | | | | | | |
| Soybean oil | 100.0 | 15.0 | 0.10 | 0.16 | 10.7 | 3.87 | 80.60 | 0.29 | 22.8 | 50.80 | 6.76 | |
| Safflower oil | 100.0 | 9.40 | | 0.11 | 6.38 | 2.45 | 86.2 | 0.57 | 11.9 | 73.30 | 0.46 | |
| Cottonseed oil | 100.0 | 26.10 | 0.38 | 0.79 | 22.00 | 2.24 | 69.6 | 0.78 | 18.1 | 50.3 | 0.40 | |
| Corn oil | 100.0 | 12.70 | | | 10.7 | 1.74 | 83.0 | 0.14 | 24.6 | 57.40 | 0.83 | |
| Peanut oil | 100.0 | 17.40 | | | 9.50 | 2.27 | 77.7 | | 45.6 | 31.00 | | |
| Olive oil | 100.0 | 14.20 | | | 11.50 | 2.32 | 81.4 | 0.97 | 71.5 | 8.23 | 0.72 | |
| Coconut oil | 100.0 | 86.30 | 43.70 | 16.40 | 8.22 | 2.97 | 7.86 | 0.38 | 5.65 | 1.83 | | |
| Peanuts | 49.7 | 9.43 | | | 5.31 | 1.32 | 37.80 | | 22.9 | 14.40 | 0.55 | |

(Adapted from Comprehensive evaluation of fatty acids in foods, I–XIII. J Am Diet Assoc 66:482; 67:35, 111, 351, 1975; 68:224, 335; 69:44, 243, 517, 1976; 70:53; 71:412, 521, 1977; 72:48, 1978)

when used in a food, as in salad dressing, and when taken with meals. Vegetable gums are now frequently used in low-calorie salad dressings to achieve the desired consistency.

*Phospholipids (PL),* structural compounds found in cell membranes, are essential components of certain enzyme systems, are involved in the transport of lipids in the plasma and are a source of energy. Their chemical structure is similar to that of fats except that a phosphoric acid radical and a nitrogen-containing base have replaced one of the fatty acids.

*Lecithins,* phosphatidylcholine, are the most abundant of the phospholipids in both tissues and foods where, because of their emulsifying properties, they serve as solubilizers and stabilizers. Lecithins are made commercially from soybeans and egg yolks and may be added as emulsifiers to margarines, cheese products, and other processed foods. There is no justification for the food faddists' recommendation of dietary supplements of lecithins. They are found in a wide variety of foods from both animal and vegetable sources—liver, egg yolks, and soybeans are especially rich in lecithins. Of even more importance, the cells of the body are capable of synthesizing lecithins as needed.

*Choline,* a part of the lecithin molecule, prevents the accumulation of fat in the liver. Other substances, such as the essential amino acid, methionine, and its derivatives, also have a function in preventing fatty liver. Such substances are called lipotrophic because they have the ability to move or mobilize fat.

Other phospholipids, *cephalin* and *sphingomyelin*, are also present in most tissues, the latter primarily in brain and nerve tissue as a constituent of the myelin sheaths.

*Cholesterol and other sterols.* Cholesterol, an essential constituent of many animal cells, especially the myelin sheath around nerve fibers and in glandular tissues, is found in high concentration in the liver, where it is synthesized and stored. Cholesterol, both free and esterified, is also present in the plasma lipoproteins.

Egg yolks and brains are particularly rich sources of cholesterol in the diet. Other important food sources include butter, cream, cheese, heart, kidneys, liver, sweetbreads, lobster, shrimp, crab, and fish roe. For additional food sources, see Table 2, Part 4.

In normal individuals the body compensates for the level of cholesterol intake in the diet through changes in the synthesis, degradation, and excretion of the compound. Cholesterol synthesis from acetate through mevalonate and squalene occurs mainly in the liver but also in the intestinal tract and may vary from 0.5 g to 2 g per day (see Chap. 9). Conversion in the liver to bile acids, which appears to require adequate tissue levels of ascorbic acid, is the chief method of degradation and excretion, but cholesterol as such may also leave the body through the feces by excretion into the bile. Although as much as 50% of the cholesterol synthesized each day in the body may be secreted with the bile into the intestines, after having been temporarily stored in the gallbladder, much of it may also be reabsorbed in the process of fat absorption.

The maintenance of a normal level of blood cholesterol is of great physiological importance. It is a precursor of vitamin D (see Chap. 7) and closely related to the steroid hormones in the body, the corticoids, androgens, and estrogens. It should not therefore be considered an abnormal substance in the body but one that has vital functions to perform. The Food and Nutrition Board's Report on Dietary Fat and Human Health states:

Evidence to support the concept that increased plasma concentrations of cholesterol are atherogenic is considerable but not conclusive. The type and quantity of dietary fat and the amount of cholesterol eaten influence the cholesterol concentration in the blood. Fats high in saturated fatty acids support a somewhat higher plasma cholesterol concentration than do those rich in polyunsaturated fatty acids. Many, but not all, population studies indicate that diets high in fat, among other nutrients, are correlated with higher concentrations of plasma cholesterol and with increased prevalence of cardiovascular disease. However, proof of a causal relationship is lacking.[1]

Further discussion of the relationship of blood cholesterol levels to atherosclerotic disease is included in Chapter 30.

Plant sterols, phytosterols, are 28 and 29 carbon steroid alcohols and distinct from the 27 carbon cholesterol. Although the nutritional role of the phytosterols is not well understood, they appear to be poorly absorbed themselves and to prevent the absorption of cholesterol. In large amounts they have been shown to reduce plasma cholesterol. The major plant sterols are divided into β-sitosterol, campesterol, and stigmasterol; and the minor plant sterols into $\delta^5$-avenasterol, $\delta^7$-stigmasterol, $\delta^7$-avenasterol, and α-spinasterol. The sterol content of foods of plant origin was published by Weihrauch and Gardner.[2]

Ergosterol, a plant sterol found in yeast and fungi, can be converted by ultraviolet light into vitamin $D_3$, ergocalciferol.

*Lipoproteins.* Since lipids are insoluble in water, they are transported in the blood in the form of lipoproteins, water-soluble fat-protein complexes. Lipoproteins are classified according to their electrophoretic mobility and density as alpha-lipoproteins or high-density lipoproteins (HDL), beta-lipoproteins or low-density lipoproteins (LDL), prebeta-lipoproteins or very low-density lipoproteins (VLDL), and chylomicrons. They all contain protein (apoproteins A, B, and C[3]), triglycerides, phospholipids, and cholesterol but in varying amounts (Table 3-4). Two procedures are used most frequently for the separation and classification of the plasma lipoproteins: ultracentrifugation and electrophoresis. Ultracentrifugation separates them according to their weight or rate of flotation, which is designated as Svedberg flotation units, $S_f$. The lower the density the higher the $S_f$, hence chylomicrons, which consist primarily of triglycerides, have $S_f$ values of 400 or above. In an electrophoretic technique a drop of plasma is placed on a filter paper and put into an electrophoretic cell containing buffer solution with albumin. The electric field causes the lipoproteins to migrate on the paper strip at different rates. Distinct bands

**Table 3-4. The Percent Composition (Dry Weight) of Plasma Lipoproteins**

| Lipoproteins | Protein | Phospholipids | Cholesterol | Triglycerides |
|---|---|---|---|---|
| Chylomicrons $S_f$ 400* and above | 0.5–2.5 | 3–15 | 2–12 | 79–95 |
| Very-low-density (VLDL) $S_f$ 20–400 (prebeta-) | 2–13 | 10–25 | 9–24 | 50–80 |
| Low-density (LDL) $S_f$ 0–20 (beta-) | 20–25 | 22 | 43 | 10 |
| High-density (HDL) (alpha-) | 45–55 | 30 | 18 | 5–8 |

*$S_f$ refers to flotation rate–Svedberg units.

are formed as a result of differences in the migration rates of the various lipoproteins and give rise to the expression, *prebeta-, beta-,* and *alpha-lipoprotein bands.*

Chylomicrons synthesized in the intestinal mucosa consist primarily of triglycerides from dietary fat. They are removed very quickly by lipoprotein lipases, mainly in adipose tissue and muscle. The creamy layer, which the presence of triglycerides produces in plasma, is cleared in the normal person's blood in a few hours after a meal. Small amounts of protein (apoprotein B and C), cholesterol, free and esterified, and a covering layer of phospholipid are also found in chylomicrons.

Prebeta-lipoproteins (VLDL) are the result of endogenous synthesis of triglycerides from carbohydrate and fatty acids in the liver; these, too, are taken up in a few hours by the same lipoprotein lipases that act on the chylomicrons. This is seen by the loss of turbidity in the normal person's blood in the fasting state. VLDL are measured after an overnight fast.

The beta-lipoproteins (LDL) are rich in cholesterol and appear to come from the intravascular degradation of VLDL. LDL change less readily in relationship to food intake and are the lipoproteins most reflective of the blood cholesterol level.

Alpha-lipoprotein (HDL) carries about 20% of the total plasma cholesterol but is not involved in triglyceride transport. It contains a large proportion of protein, mainly apoprotein A with some C. Concentrations of HDL vary much less than those of LDL. Individuals with high HDL levels have been found to have a lower risk of coronary heart disease.[4]

Free fatty acids (FFA) are transported from adipose tissue to the muscle and liver in the blood, where they are bound to plasma albumins. Although the concentration of FFA in the blood at any one time is low, the rate of turnover is rapid, and several thousand calories may be transported each day in this manner.

## Food sources of lipids

### Animal sources (see Fig. 3-2)

The body fat of each form of animal life is typical of the species but varies with function in the body and temperature of the environment. The fat of cold-blooded animals—fish, for example—is a soft fat which remains plastic in the low-temperature environment in which the fish live. The fats of warm-blooded animals have higher melting points but are also plastic at the body temperature of each species. As a rule, the fat of herbivorous animals is harder than the fat of carnivorous animals. When adipose tissue of animals is subjected to heat, the fat liquefies and separates from the connective-tissue cells in which it was stored. Thus pork fat is "tried out" in the manufacture of lard. Sheep have the hardest body fat of any domestic animal; when extracted, it is known as mutton tallow. Poultry fats are intermediate between

meat and fish fats both in hardness and in the content of polyunsaturated fatty acids.

The quantity of fat in meat also varies with different animals. Beef, pork, and lamb are approximately equal in fat content (15%–30%); veal is lower and is comparable to chicken (6%–15%). If all visible fat is trimmed from lean cuts of meat and a cooking method such as broiling or roasting, which increases fat losses, is employed, the amount of fat consumed with meat can be reduced considerably.

The fat of fish is always fluid at cold temperatures and is therefore called an oil. Fish fats can contain a higher proportion of polyunsaturated extra long chain fatty acids than do the meat or poultry fats (see Table 3-3). However, there is a great difference in the fat content of fish, which varies from less than 1% to more than 12%. For this reason, fish are classified as either low in fat or high in fat. The amount in all fish varies somewhat with the season of the year, with the time of spawning, and with changes in feeding conditions. It may be noted that certain fish, which have very little fat in the edible portion, have a comparatively large amount in the liver. Fish-liver oils are extracted and refined for use as rich sources of vitamins A and D.

Milk fat is in an unstable emulsion which breaks (*i.e.,* separates) on standing and allows the cream to rise. Homogenization of milk produces a more stable emulsion with smaller fat globules, and in which the cream does not separate. Butter is the milk fat plus some moisture and milk solids separated by churning; the finished product contains about 80% fat. Butter contains very little polyunsaturated fatty acid, as is noted in Table 3-3. Butter is valued as a good source of vitamin A.

### Plant sources (see Fig. 3-2)

All fats in the plant kingdom are oils at room temperature. Most vegetables and fruits contain less than 1% fat, with the exception of avocados and olives, as can be seen in Figure 3-2. The nuts and the seeds have a higher fat content. Seed oils are mostly extracted or expressed for use as salad and cooking oils. Many of these have a high proportion of linoleic acid, as can be seen in Table 3-3. Olive and peanut oils are exceptions, because both contain more oleic acid than the other salad and cooking oils.

Margarines and cooking fats are usually made from vegetable oils, cottonseed, safflower, soybean, and corn oils by the process of hydrogenation. This chemical process involves the introduction of hydrogen into the fat molecule under carefully controlled conditions to produce a fat with exactly the right melting point and other properties for culinary purposes. Hydrogenation also results in transforming part of the fat to the *trans* form to obtain the desired consistency. Fat treated in this way is homogenized to form a smooth, creamy product, but evidence of its being a mixture is given by the grainy texture of such a fat once it has been melted and allowed to harden again—

## Amounts of Fat in Average Servings

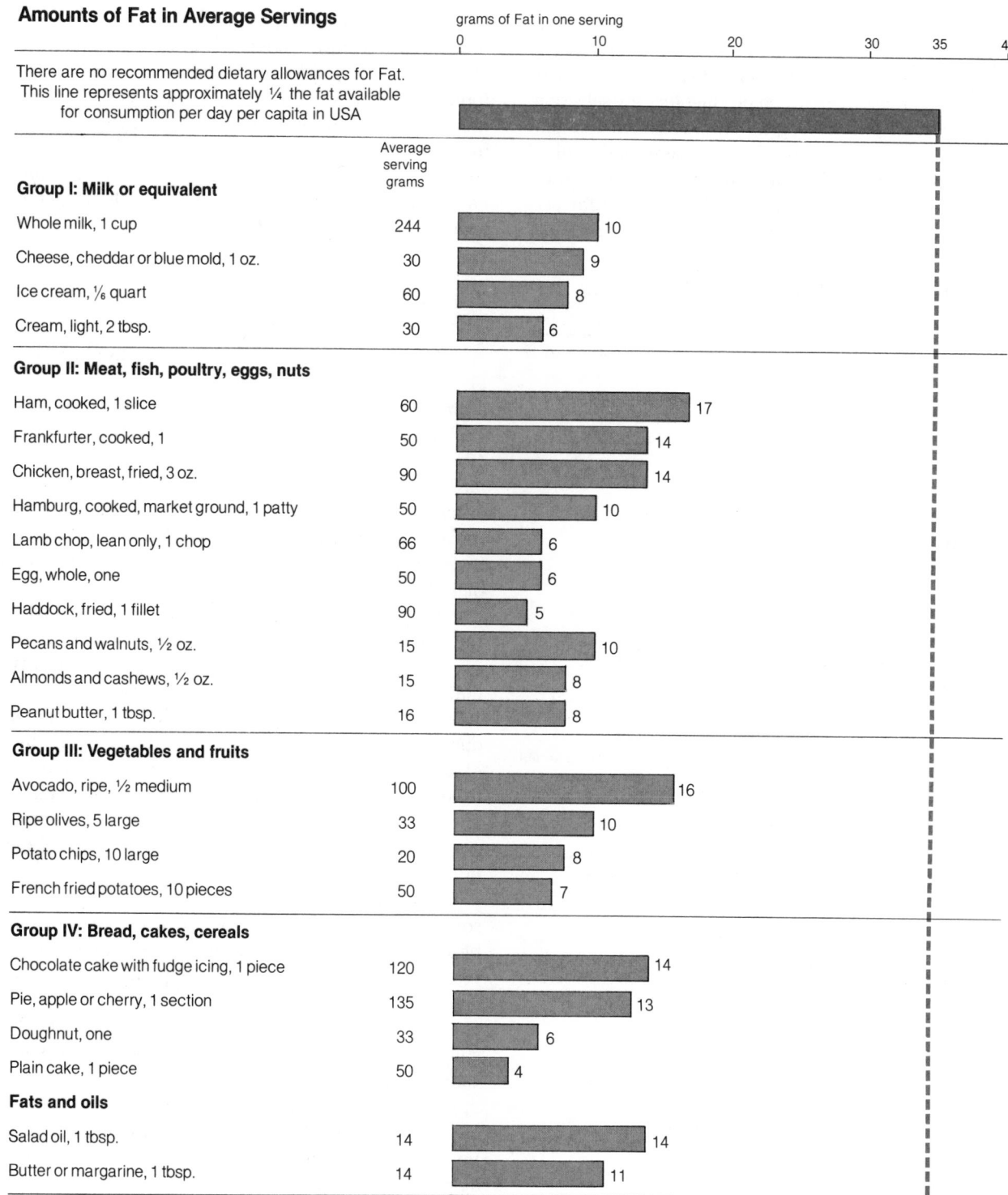

grams of Fat in one serving

There are no recommended dietary allowances for Fat.
This line represents approximately ¼ the fat available
for consumption per day per capita in USA

| | Average serving grams | grams of fat |
|---|---|---|
| **Group I: Milk or equivalent** | | |
| Whole milk, 1 cup | 244 | 10 |
| Cheese, cheddar or blue mold, 1 oz. | 30 | 9 |
| Ice cream, ⅙ quart | 60 | 8 |
| Cream, light, 2 tbsp. | 30 | 6 |
| **Group II: Meat, fish, poultry, eggs, nuts** | | |
| Ham, cooked, 1 slice | 60 | 17 |
| Frankfurter, cooked, 1 | 50 | 14 |
| Chicken, breast, fried, 3 oz. | 90 | 14 |
| Hamburg, cooked, market ground, 1 patty | 50 | 10 |
| Lamb chop, lean only, 1 chop | 66 | 6 |
| Egg, whole, one | 50 | 6 |
| Haddock, fried, 1 fillet | 90 | 5 |
| Pecans and walnuts, ½ oz. | 15 | 10 |
| Almonds and cashews, ½ oz. | 15 | 8 |
| Peanut butter, 1 tbsp. | 16 | 8 |
| **Group III: Vegetables and fruits** | | |
| Avocado, ripe, ½ medium | 100 | 16 |
| Ripe olives, 5 large | 33 | 10 |
| Potato chips, 10 large | 20 | 8 |
| French fried potatoes, 10 pieces | 50 | 7 |
| **Group IV: Bread, cakes, cereals** | | |
| Chocolate cake with fudge icing, 1 piece | 120 | 14 |
| Pie, apple or cherry, 1 section | 135 | 13 |
| Doughnut, one | 33 | 6 |
| Plain cake, 1 piece | 50 | 4 |
| **Fats and oils** | | |
| Salad oil, 1 tbsp. | 14 | 14 |
| Butter or margarine, 1 tbsp. | 14 | 11 |

**Fig. 3-2.**   Fat in average servings of foods classified according to the four food groups.

the high and the low melting point ingredients are no longer evenly mixed.

The public demand for unsaturated fat has prompted margarine manufacturers to reduce the amount of hydrogenation to a minimum in order to retain as much of the polyunsaturated fatty acid as possible.

Margarines are manufactured either by partially hydrogenating the total amount of vegetable oil to the desired consistency or by adding liquid vegetable oil to a more completely hydrogenated solid fat. The latter type contains approximately twice the amount of linoleic acid. Certain of the "soft" margarines marketed in bowl-like containers rather than in sticks contain two to four times the amount of polyunsaturated as saturated fatty acids. The first ingredient named on the label of the margarine package tells consumers which product they are selecting: "liquid corn oil plus hydrogenated corn oil" means that the margarine has been processed by the second method and as a result would have a higher ratio of polyunsaturated to saturated fatty acids (Table 3-5). The fat prepared this way is churned with cultured milk and other ingredients to give the product the flavor of butter. All brands are now fortified with vitamin A to the equivalent of average butter, and some have vitamin D added. Therefore, margarine is the nutritional equivalent of butter and is frequently preferred because of its higher content of unsaturated fatty acids and usually slightly lower cost. All states now permit the sale of margarine to which coloring has been added; Wisconsin in 1967 was the last state to legalize such sales.

### Table 3-5. Selected Fatty Acids in Margarines

| Types of Margarine (First Ingredient Named on Label) | Amount in 100 g | | | |
|---|---|---|---|---|
| | | Total Saturated Fatty Acids (g) | Unsaturated Fatty Acids | |
| | Total Fat (g) | | Oleic (g) | Linoleic (g) |
| Hydrogenated or hardened fat | 81 | 18 | 47 | 14 |
| Liquid oil | 81 | 19 | 31 | 29 |

(Data from Watt BK, Merrill LA: Composition of Foods: Raw, Processed and Prepared. Agriculture Handbook No. 8. Washington, DC, USDA, 1963)

### Table 3-6. Trends in Fat Consumption During Selected Periods—U.S.

| Period | Calories Per Capita Per Day | Fat Per Capita Per Day (g) | Fat Calories (Percent) |
|---|---|---|---|
| 1909–1913 | 3490 | 125 | 32.2 |
| 1935–1939 | 3270 | 133 | 36.6 |
| 1964 | 3170 | 147 | 41.4 |
| 1973 | 3290 | 156 | 42.7 |
| 1979 | 3500 | 168 | 43.2 |

(Data adapted from Friend B: Nutritive Value of Food for Consumption, United States, 1909–64. Washington, DC, USDA, Agricultural Research Service 62-14, 1966; Nutritional Review, National Food Situation, Washington, DC, USDA, Economic Research Service, 1973; and National Food Review, Washington, DC, USDA, Economics, Statistics, and Cooperatives Service, Winter, 1980)

### Table 3-7. Percent of Total Fat Contributed by Each Food Group in 1979—U.S.

| Food Group | Percent |
|---|---|
| Meat, poultry, fish | 35.2 |
| Eggs | 2.7 |
| Dairy products (excluding butter) | 11.8 |
| Fats and oils (including butter) | 42.7 |
| Fruits | 0.4 |
| Vegetables | 0.5 |
| Dried beans, peas, nuts, soya flour | 4.4 |
| Flour and cereal products | 1.3 |
| Sugars and sweeteners | 0.0 |
| Miscellaneous | 1.1 |

(Data adapted from National Food Review, Washington, DC, USDA, Economics, Statistics, and Cooperatives Service, Winter, 1980)

## Trends in fat consumption in the United States

Although there are wide differences among individuals and regions, surveys indicate that today Americans as a group consume more than 43% of their calories as fat (Table 3-6) compared to 32% in 1909 to 1913 and 39% in 1947 to 1949. Visible fats from such sources as butter, lard, margarine, shortening, and salad and cooking oils account for about 43% of the fat intake, whereas the fats of meats, eggs, cheese, nuts, and cereals, often referred to as invisible fats, contribute about 57% of the total fat in the diet (Table 3-7).

In the last 70 years the percentage of fat available to the American consumer from animal sources has decreased from 83% in 1909 to 1913 to 57% in 1978, whereas that from vegetable sources has increased from 17% in 1909 to 1913 to 42% in 1978 (see Table 3-8). This change is due in large measure to the significant increase in the use of salad and cooking oils. From the fats and oils group, ten times more fat was supplied from salad and cooking oils and six times more from margarine in 1978 compared with 1909 to 1913; lard usage decreased eightfold, and butter consumption decreased by more than 80%.[5]

There are other trends in the American food consumption pattern of which the nutrition counselor should be aware today. In 1979 slightly less red meat (beef, pork, veal, lamb, and mutton) but more poultry and fish were consumed compared to 1969. Among the dairy products cheese consumption has increased 63% since 1969; consumption of fluid whole milk has decreased 28%, whereas that of lowfat milks has increased 96%.[5] Fewer eggs also appear in the market basket in this decade than in the last.

These changes have led to differences in the composition of total fat in the diet. Since 1909 to 1913 the percentage of calories from saturated fats has increased approximately 2%, from 13% to 15%; calories from oleic acid (monounsaturated) increased from 13% to 16%, whereas calories from linoleic acid (polyunsaturated) increased almost 5%, from 2% to 7%. The ratio of polyunsaturated to saturated fatty acids (P:S) has increased from 0.33 in 1963 to approximately 0.45 in 1978. The cholesterol content of the American diet, about 500 mg per capita, is about the same as that in 1909 to 1913; however, it was higher in 1947 to 1949 and has gradually decreased to its former level over the last 30 years.

Most of the dietary goals and guidelines suggest a reduction in calories from fat. Because it is primarily the saturated fat that should be reduced, according to present advice, most of the reduction needs to be made in the red meat group, chiefly pork and beef, and in the dairy products, whole milk, cheese, and eggs. A shift in this direction would also result in a P:S ratio closer to 1 and a lower cholesterol intake.

## Role of lipids in health
### Essential fatty acids (EFA)

An essential fatty acid (EFA) is one that is necessary for normal nutrition and that cannot be synthesized by the body from other substances. Linoleic acid, the polyunsaturated fatty acid most abundant in nature, is the main essential fatty acid to be considered. Arachidonic acid, which is effective in curing EFA deficiency symptoms, can be synthesized in the body from linoleic acid (Fig. 3-3). The possible role of linolenic acid, which cannot be synthesized by humans and which does not relieve the dermatitis of essential fatty acid deficiency, remains unclear at present; but if there is a need for linolenic acid, it apparently is met by diets with adequate amounts of linoleic acid.

Essential fatty acids are an integral part of the phospholipids, which make up the structure of all cell membranes. The beta or number 2 position of the phospholipid is normally esterified with one of the highly unsaturated members of the linoleic acid family (Fig. 3-3). In EFA deficiency the essential fatty acid is replaced in the phospholipids by $C_{20:4\omega9}$ from the oleic acid family (Fig. 3-3), and deleterious effects on membrane function and integrity result. This occurrence has led to the diagnostic test for EFA deficiency. The triene (eicosatrienoic acid, $C_{20:3\omega9}$): tetraene (arachidonic acid, $C_{20:4\omega6}$) ratio in EFA deficiency is 0.4 or above, whereas in a normal population the average is approximately 0.1.[6]

Two derivatives of linoleic acid, dihomo-$\gamma$-linolenic and arachidonic acids, are the precursors of the prostaglandins (PG), which regulate production of cyclic AMP and for this reason are considered hormone-like compounds. They are widely distributed in tissues and produce a variety of metabolic effects. Because there is much current investigation in this area, both in the laboratory and in clinical trials, the diagram, Figure 3-3, of some of the metabolic pathways is presented to assist the nutrition counselor in following research reports in the literature.

Activation of phospholipase $A_2$, an enzyme which releases the fatty acid in the beta position of the cell membrane phospholipids, occurs when a tissue is stimulated. Arachidonic acid (dihomo-$\gamma$-linolenic acid has similar pathways) is quickly converted into the endoperoxides, $PGG_2$ and $PGH_2$, by cyclo-oxygenase enzyme in the membrane. The endoperoxide $PGH_2$ can then follow one of three pathways: it can be transformed into prostaglandins $PGE_2$, $F_{2a}$, $D_2$; thromboxanes $TXA_2$ and $TXB_2$ can be formed by the enzyme, thromboxane synthetase; or prostacyclin $PGI_2$ and 6-keto-$PGF_2$ can be formed.[7] The action of these various compounds has been found to affect the formation of blood clots by inducing ($PGG_2$, $PGH_2$, $TXA_2$, $PGE_2$) or inhibiting ($PGE_1$, $PGI_2$, $PGI_3$) platelet aggregation in the blood vessels. It also has been found to cause constriction ($TXA_2$) or dilatation ($PGI_2$) of the blood vessels. In the kidneys $PGE_1$, $PGI_2$, and $PGD_2$ also cause increased water and sodium losses. The contractility of the heart is induced by $PGE_1$, $PGE_2$, $PGF_{1a}$, and $PGF_{2a}$.[6-8] As a result, it has been postulated that the EFAs may play a role in preventing atherosclerosis, hypertension, and ischemic heart disease by promoting synthesis of the prostaglandins. EFA also helps regulate cholesterol metabolism, especially its transport, degradation, and excretion.

Demonstration of an EFA deficiency in animals requires the rigid exclusion of fat from the diet. Therefore, it is not surprising that evidence of EFA deficiencies in adult humans has not been recognized except in hospitalized patients maintained exclusively on intravenous feeding for long periods of time.[9,10] However, Hansen, Wiese, and associates[11,12] have demonstrated a fatty acid deficiency in infants, which proves beyond a doubt that EFAs are required by humans. Dry and scaly skin, similar to the symptoms of EFA deficiency seen in animals, were the most frequent findings among the infants receiving formulas low in linoleic acid. Infants also seemed to grow

**Table 3-8. Fat in the Diet from Animal and Vegetable Sources Per Capita Per Day for Selected Periods—U.S.**

| | *Animal Sources* | | | | | | | *Vegetable Sources* | | | | | |
| *Period* | *Meat, Poultry, Fish* | *Eggs* | *Dairy Products (Excluding Butter)* | *Butter, Lard, Edible Beef Fat* | *Total* | *Percent* | *Other Fats and Oils* | *Dry Beans, Peas, Nuts, Soy Products* | *Flour and Cereal Products* | *Other Foods* | *Total* | *Percent* |
| | *Grams* | | | | | | | | *Grams* | | | |
| *1909–1913* | 46.4 | 4.8 | 18.6 | 33.8 | 103.5 | 83 | 12.3 | 2.4 | 4.8 | 1.8 | 21.3 | 17 |
| *1947–1949* | 46.8 | 6.0 | 24.5 | 27.4 | 104.8 | 75 | 25.1 | 4.7 | 2.6 | 3.3 | 35.8 | 25 |
| *1967* | 52.2 | 5.2 | 20.2 | 19.6 | 97.3 | 65 | 41.6 | 5.5 | 2.1 | 3.3 | 52.5 | 35 |
| *1978* | 53.5 | 4.4 | 19.8 | 13.4 | 91.2 | 57 | 55.5 | 7.2 | 2.1 | 3.2 | 67.9 | 42 |

(Adapted from Marston R, Page L: Nutrient Content of the National Food Supply. National Food Review, Washington, DC, USDA, Economics, Statistics, and Cooperatives Service, Dec, 1978)

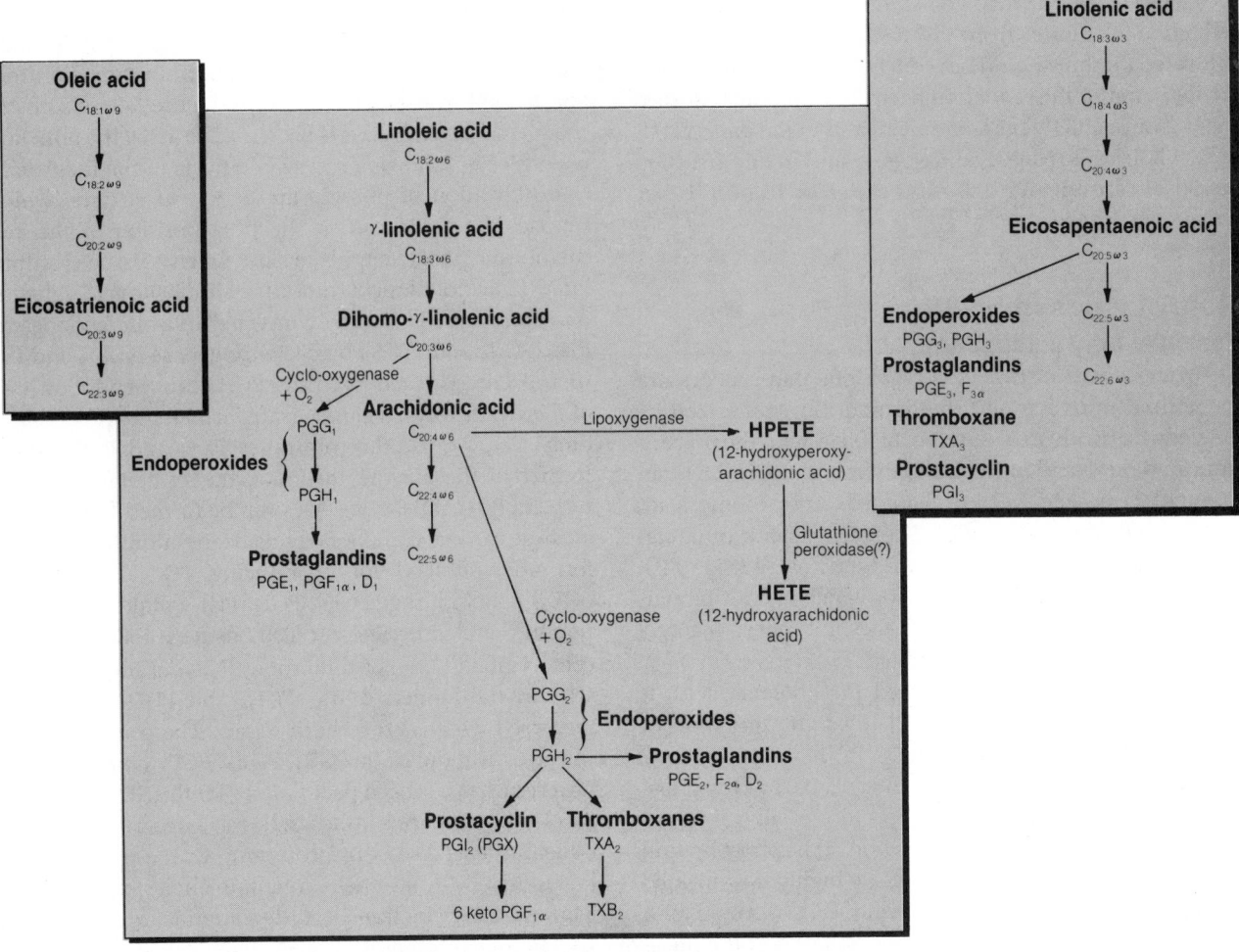

**Fig. 3-3.** Simplified pathways of essential fatty acid metabolism as related to prostaglandin synthesis.

better and required fewer calories for growth when there was an adequate supply of EFA.

Although evaporated milk has proved satisfactory in infant feeding, Wiese and co-workers[13] suggest that the amount of linoleic acid supplied by evaporated milk formulas (1%–2% of total calories) may be considered minimal, whereas breast milk, which is four to five times higher in linoleic acid, contains optimal amounts of EFA. Attention was called by these authors to the infrequent incidence of eczema and other skin manifestations in breast-fed infants when compared with those on cow's milk. Analysis of the linoleic acid content of commercial infant formulas indicates that there is a wide variation in linoleic acid content depending on the source of the fat. Safflower, soy, and corn oils are rich in linoleic acid.[14]

Although the adult human requirement for EFA is not known, the Food and Nutrition Board of the National Research Council suggests that

> For the general population, 3 percent of energy as linoleic acid should be a satisfactory minimum recommended intake for groups with relatively low fat intakes (below 25

percent of calories). For those consuming diets high in fat, as currently are found in most of the United States, there is evidence that a higher intake of linoleic acid may have beneficial health effects for a significant fraction of the population. These health effects relate primarily to coronary heart disease and other conditions related to elevated blood lipids . . . a total fat intake not to exceed 35 percent of dietary energy is recommended for the high risk population. Of this, approximately one fourth to one third, or about 8–10 percent of total calories, should be polyunsaturated (essential) fatty acid.[15]

Similarly, the American Academy of Pediatrics recommended 3% of calories from EFA in infant formulas.[16]

### Fats as a concentrated source of energy

Fats are the most concentrated source of energy for the human body; 1 g of fat yields 9 calories, compared to 4 calories/g from carbohydrate and protein. Thus, relatively small amounts of high-fat foods contribute large amounts of calories to the diet. The percentage of total calories derived from fat in the American diet has increased to 43%; this increase was accompanied by a similar increase in total calories consumed. These trends are of concern to the nutrition counselor because any excess energy consumed is stored as adipose tissue and eventually leads to obesity. To avoid excessive weight gain and its accompanying health risks, it is necessary to balance energy needs with food intake carefully. This implies for most Americans who have sedentary living patterns only moderate consumption of fried foods, pies, pastries, and cakes, butter, margarine, and cream. When weight gain is a problem, it is often indicative that the amount of fat in the diet is higher than desirable. Obesity and its dietary treatment are discussed in Chapter 28.

For people who are underweight, a moderate increase in the amount of fat in the diet would help achieve desirable weight status.

### Lipids and cardiovascular disease

Since there is evidence of increased susceptibility to coronary heart disease among individuals with elevated levels of cholesterol and triglycerides or both, attention is focused on those food constituents that appear to affect these levels—the total fat and sugar intake and the proportion of saturated to polyunsaturated fatty acids and cholesterol. Although there is reasonable agreement among most medical authorities about the treatment of the hyperlipoproteinemias (elevated lipid levels in the blood), discussed in Chapter 30, there is still much controversy among nutrition scientists about the kind and amount of diet modification that should be recommended for the population as a whole. The Committee on Dietary Allowances of the Food and Nutrition Board recommended that fat intake should not be more than 35% of total calories, particularly in diets below 2000 kcal. They also endorsed the additional recommendation of the American Heart Association that less than 10% of total calories should come from saturated fatty acids and up to 10% from polyunsaturated fatty acids; this would probably provide a diet conducive to better health in the population of the United States.[15] Complex carbohydrates rather than simple sugars should replace the fat in the diet, and weight reduction for overweight people would also be desirable. In order to apply these recommendations, the foods selected would need to include more cereal grains, legumes, vegetables, fish, and vegetable oils and less animal fat and sugar. Nutrition counselors should continue to emphasize the need for a diet adequate in all the essential nutrients.

### Study questions and activities

1. What can be said about the human requirement for fat in the diet? How does American consumption compare with that of some other countries?
2. What changes have occurred in the consumption and selection of fats by American consumers? Explain why there may be large differences in the amount of fat consumed by individual families.
3. What is meant by saturated and polyunsaturated fatty acids? Give illustrations of each.
4. Which of the polyunsaturated fatty acids is most widely distributed in foods? What types of foods contribute the most of this factor?
5. From what sources are margarine and some of the cooking fats manufactured and by what process?
6. Is there evidence that the level of fat in the diet of Americans may be a hazard to health? In what way?
7. Name the essential fatty acid. Why is it called essential?
8. Besides its use for energy, what other functions does fat perform in the body?
9. What are phospholipids? Sterols? Where are they found in the body? Which sterols may be converted to vitamin D?
10. What are the normal functions of cholesterol in the body? How is the excess excreted?
11. Name the plasma lipoproteins. What lipids do they contain? Which one contains the most cholesterol; triglycerides from dietary fat; triglycerides from liver synthesis?

### References

1. Dietary Fat and Human Health. National Research Council Publ. No. 1147. Washington, DC, 1966
2. Weihrauch JL, Gardner JM: J Am Diet Assoc 73:39, 1978
3. Jackson RL et al: Physiol Rev 56:259, 1976
4. Castelli WP et al: Circulation 55:767, 1977
5. Marston R, Page L: Nutrient Content of the National Food Supply. National Food Review, Washington, DC, USDA, Dec, 1978
6. Vergroesen MD: Nutr Rev 35:1, 1977
7. Nutr Rev 36:10, 1978
8. Nutr Rev 37:316, 1979
9. Collins FD et al: Nutr Metab 13:150, 1971
10. Paulrud JR et al: Am J Clin Nutr 25:897, 1972
11. Hansen AE, Wiese HF: J Nutr 52:367, 1954
12. Hansen AE et al: Pediatrics 31:171, 1963
13. Wiese HF et al: J Nutr 66:555, 1963
14. Hawley LE et al: J Am Diet Assoc 72:170, 1978
15. Food and Nutrition Board: Recommended Dietary Allowances, 9th rev ed. Washington, DC, NAS-NRC, 1980
16. American Academy of Pediatrics: Commentary on breast feeding and infant formulas, including standards for formulas. Pediatrics 57:278, 1976

### Supplementary readings

Cuthbertson WFJ: Essential fatty acid requirements in infancy. Am J Clin Nutr 29:559, 1976
Feeley RM, Criner PE, Watt BK: Cholesterol content of foods. J Am Diet Assoc 61:134, 1972
Lee JB, Patek RV, Mookerjee BK: Renal prostaglandins and the regulation of blood pressure and sodium and water homeostasis. Am J Med 60:798, 1976

Nazir DJ, Moorecroft BJ, Meshkel MA: Fatty acid composition of margarines. Am J Clin Nutr 29:331, 1976

Subbiah MTR: Dietary plant sterols: Current status in human and animal metabolism. Am J Clin Nutr 26:219, 1973

Vergroesen AJ: Physiological effects of dietary linoleic acid. Nutr Rev 35:1, 1977

Willis AL: Nutritional and Pharmacological Factors in Eicosanoid Biology. Nutr Rev 39:289, 1981

Wilson RB, Hutcheson DR, Wideman L: Dimethylhydrazine-induced colon tumors in rats fed diets containing beef fat or corn oil with or without bran. Am J Clin Nutr 30:176, 1977

Zeisel SH: Dietary choline: biochemistry, physiology, and pharmacology. Ann Rev Nutr 1:95, 1981

*For further references see Bibliography in Part 4.*

# *Proteins*

**4**

**INCAP:** Institute of Nutrition in Central
  America and Panama
**NPU:** Net Protein Utilization
**PER:** Protein Efficiency Ratio
**TPN:** Total Parenteral Nutrition
**BE:** Biologic Value

## Vital importance and world use

All animals, including humans, must have an adequate source of protein in order to grow and maintain themselves.

Proteins have long been recognized as the fundamental structural element of every cell of the body. More recently, specific proteins and protein derivatives have been identified as the functional elements in certain specialized cells, glandular secretions, enzymes, and hormones. In their role as enzymes, proteins control the breakdown of food for energy and the synthesis of new compounds for maintenance and repair of body tissues. When they are supplied in amounts greater than necessary for growth and maintenance, proteins contribute to the energy pool of the body and, similarly, if carbohydrates and fats are not sufficient to meet energy demands, protein will be diverted for this purpose. For this reason, protein well deserves its name, which is of Greek derivation, meaning "of first importance." Because proteins are the principal constituents of the active tissues of the body, and the body is, in turn, dependent upon food protein for these indispensable substances, the quality and the quantity of proteins in the daily diet are of prime importance.

In many parts of the world, the developing countries particularly, food sources of protein, especially proteins of good quality, are extremely scarce. There is some evidence that in countries where the quality and the quantity of protein and other nutrients are inadequate, the stature of whole groups of people may be affected. When height and weight growth curves of groups of preschool children in Mexico, Lebanon (Arab refugees), Hong Kong, and Thailand were compared with those of United States (Iowa) children, growth retardation was evident in the former groups. Children in Ethiopia, Jordan, and Vietnam were also shorter and weighed less than Iowa children between the ages of 1 and 17 years.[1] The increased stature of Japanese youths has paralleled increases in the Japanese diet of both total protein and protein from animal sources[2] (see Chap. 19). Similarly, Japanese who have lived in the United States for a generation or more have shown a marked increase in stature—clear evidence that heredity is not the determining factor.[3] Moreover, Australians and New Zealanders, perhaps the heaviest meat eaters on the globe, have large physiques.

The United States has ample sources of protein available (approximately 100 g per capita per day), and more than two-thirds of it comes from meat, fish, poultry, eggs, and dairy products. Although surveys indicate that most of the North American population consumes an adequate amount, there are still people who, for economic, social, cultural, or other reasons, may not get enough protein.[4]

## Classification and structure of proteins and other nitrogen-containing compounds

### Proteins

Proteins, like fats and carbohydrates, are composed of carbon, hydrogen, and oxygen; in addition, they must contain nitrogen. Most proteins contain about 16% nitrogen; for this reason, nitrogen determination is used to study protein metabolism and protein content of foods. Nitrogen content is multiplied by 6.25 to calculate the protein content. Often sulfur and phosphorus and sometimes other elements such as iron (in hemoglobin) and iodine (in thyroxin) are incorporated into the protein molecule.

Molecular nitrogen is "fixed" or converted into nitrogen compounds by certain bacteria living on the root nodules of plants such as clover or peas. The reaction produces ammonia, which is converted into more complex nitrogen-containing molecules by the plant. Plants that do not themselves have nitrogen-fixing bacteria need to be fertilized with ammonia or nitrates.

Plants can then synthesize proteins from the nitrates and the ammonia in soil and decaying vegetable matter. Water and carbon dioxide from the air provide the necessary carbon, hydrogen, and oxygen. Animals are dependent on plants for this synthesis because animal cells cannot use simpler forms of nitrogen to any great extent, and animal metabolism of protein, in turn, eventually

yields the forms of nitrogen, which only plant life and microorganisms can utilize. This sequence of events is called the *nitrogen cycle.*

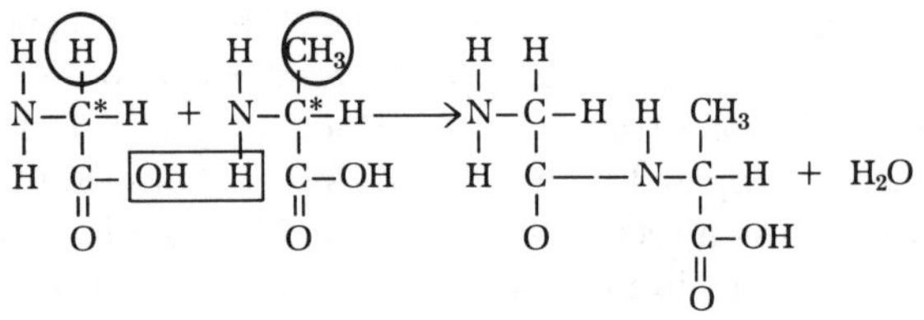

Proteins are made up of some 22 or more nitrogen-containing compounds known as *amino acids.* These amino acids are joined together by chemical linkages called peptide bonds in which the acid group of the first amino acid is attached to the nitrogen group of the next amino acid (Fig. 4-1). Two amino acids so linked are called a dipeptide; three amino acids, tripeptides. Polypeptides are composed of 10 to 100 amino acids. Those polypeptide molecules containing over 100—sometimes several thousand—amino acids are referred to as proteins. The order in which all these amino acids are arranged is determined by the genetic code—the DNA (deoxyribonucleic acid) found in the nucleus of every cell (see Chap. 9).

### Classification

Proteins may be classified according to their chemical structure.

*Simple proteins* yield only amino acids or their derivatives when they are hydrolyzed by acids, alkalies, or enzymes. They are further subdivided according to their solubility and other properties.

*Albumins,* which are soluble in water, and globulins, which are soluble in dilute salt solutions, are globular proteins (see *Structure,* below), and are found in the fluids of animals and plants. They are coagulated by heat and easily digested, as for example, lactalbumin in milk.

*Glutelins* and *prolamins* are the chief plant proteins. Glutelins are soluble in dilute acid and alkali but insoluble in neutral solutions, for example, glutenin in wheat. Prolamins are soluble in alcohols but not in water, for example, gliadin in wheat. Gluten, which is responsible for the structure in breads and other bakery products, is formed from a mixture of glutenin and gliadin in water.

*Albuminoids* or *scleroproteins,* which are insoluble in water and other common solvents, are for the most part indigestible. They are fibrous in structure and include the keratin in hair, collagen in connective tissue, fibrin in blood clot, and myosin in muscle.

*Conjugated proteins* are polypeptides that contain some nonprotein parts called prosthetic groups, for example, nucleoproteins.

*Derived proteins* are substances that result from the breakdown, such as hydrolysis, of simple or conjugated proteins, for example, dipeptides.

### Structure

The first step in determining the structure of a protein is to hydrolyze it and determine the kind and amount of amino acids that it contains. Since some proteins consist of more than one polypeptide chain, it is necessary to find out the number of these chains in each protein mole-

**Fig. 4-1.** Amino acids, glycine and alanine, joined by peptide linkage to form the dipeptide glycylalanine.

*Central carbon atom. The side chain that distinguishes individual amino acids is circled.

cule. The final step is to determine the sequence of amino acids in each polypeptide chain. The *primary structure* refers to the ordinary structural formula, which includes the sequence of amino acids linked by peptide bonds and any other additional prosthetic groups and their linkages.

*Secondary* and *tertiary structures* refer to the shape of the protein molecule. A particular conformation is preferred because it facilitates hydrogen bonding. The most important secondary structure is the alpha-helix, a right- or left-handed spiral made rigid by intramolecular hydrogen bonds between carbonyl oxygen and amide nitrogen. In more complex proteins it is not unusual to find several helixes. The spatial arrangement of these helixes in relationship to one another is called the tertiary structure. Tertiary structures may be stabilized by other types of bonds, especially sulfide bonds. Proteins are classed as fibrous or globular depending on the tertiary spatial arrangement. Fibrous proteins such as those in muscle fiber (myosin), hair (keratin), and connective tissue (collagen and elastin) tend to be formed into relatively long molecules. The globular proteins are spherical and include hemoglobin, myoglobin, albumins, and globulins.

The *quaternary structure* is the aggregation of subunits in the final protein particle, maintained by electrostatic attraction. The oxygen-binding activity of hemoglobin is indicative of the biologic activity of the quaternary structure.

*Denaturation* of proteins is any alteration of the naturally-ordered conformation to a randomly-structured molecule. Denaturation occurs before proteins coagulate and is caused by the application of heat, the addition of acids or alkalies, or mechanical action. The changes that occur in the protein when an egg is cooked or an acid is added to milk are examples of denaturation. Enzymes, for instance, lose their specific properties when they are denatured.

Because protein molecules are so large, with molecular weights ranging from 5000 to several million, they have certain properties in common with colloidal solutions; the fact that protein molecules are too large to pass through cell membranes is important in physiology. For example, plasma proteins, because they cannot penetrate the capillary membranes, remain in the blood vessels and have an important effect on regulating water balance in the body (see Chap. 5).

## Amino acids

All the amino acids are organic acids containing at least one acid group (COOH) and one amino group ($NH_2$) attached to the same central carbon atom. They differ from each other in terms of the side group (R) that is carried on the central carbon atom (Fig. 4-1). Certain amino acids have two acid groups (acidic), others have two amino groups (basic), and still others contain ring structures (aromatic) or sulfur groups in the side chain.

The first amino acid was identified over 145 years ago; the last of the 22 listed in Table 4-1 was isolated and identified in 1935 by W. C. Rose. During the century between these discoveries much of the basic chemistry and physiological significance of proteins came to be understood. When it was realized that the constituent amino acids were important factors in determining the nutritive value of a protein, many investigations were conducted to find out which of them were indispensable and which could be excluded safely from the diet without interfering with normal growth and body function.

## Other nitrogen-containing compounds

*Ammonia* ($NH_3$) is formed as a result of deamination (removal of the amino group) of amino acids in the liver and to some extent in the kidneys. The ammonia formed by deamination is converted to *urea*—$(NH_2)_2CO_2$—in the liver and excreted in the urine. It is the chief end product of protein metabolism and for individuals on a normal or high-protein diet comprises 85% to 92% of the total urinary nitrogen. On a low-protein diet the amount may be decreased to 60%. In acidosis the kidney converts part of the urea back to ammonia and the nitrogenous wastes are excreted as ammonium salts to neutralize the excess acids that are present.

*Creatine* and *creatinine* are also nitrogen-containing compounds found in the urine. Most of the creatine is synthesized in the body but it also may be obtained from creatine in food. It is found chiefly in the muscle, where part of it is converted to creatinine and later excreted in the urine. The amount of creatinine varies in proportion to the amount of muscle in the individual.

*Purines* ($C_5H_4N_4$) are nitrogen-containing ring structures widely distributed in nature, especially in nucleic acids.

### Table 4-1. Classification of Amino Acids with Respect to Their Essentiality

| Essential | | Nonessential | |
|---|---|---|---|
| Histidine * | (His) † | Alanine | (Ala) |
| Isoleucine | (Ile) | Arginine | (Arg) |
| Leucine | (Leu) | Asparagine | (Asn) |
| Lysine | (Lys) | Aspartic acid | (Asp) |
| Methionine | (Met) | Cysteine | (Cys) |
| Phenylalanine | (Phe) | Cystine | (Cys-Cys) |
| Threonine | (Thr) | Glutamic acid | (Glu) |
| Tryptophan | (Trp) | Glutamine | (Gln) |
| Valine | (Val) | Glycine | (Gly) |
| | | Hydroxyproline | (Hyp) |
| | | Proline | (Pro) |
| | | Serine | (Ser) |
| | | Tyrosine | (Tyr) |

*Histidine is required for infants, but its essentiality for adults has not been clearly established.
†Abbreviations are in parentheses.

*Uric acid,* an end product of purine metabolism, is excreted in the urine. It is formed from purines consumed in the diet (exogenous) and from body purines as a result of the breakdown of nucleic acids (endogenous). Abnormal uric acid metabolism is called gout.

## Protein requirements

It is necessary to separate consideration of protein needs into two categories. One is the requirement for the essential amino acids. The other is the requirement for total protein—or total nitrogen, as it is sometimes called—which must be available to the body for the synthesis of the nonessential amino acids and for other nitrogen-containing tissue constituents. For adult humans, approximately 20% of the nitrogen required must be supplied by the essential amino acids.

### Essential amino acids

Amino acids that the body cannot synthesize in adequate amounts are called *essential* or *indispensable* because they must be supplied by the diet in proper proportions and amounts to meet the requirements for maintenance and growth of tissue. Nonessential or dispensable amino acids are those that the body can synthesize in sufficient amounts to meet its needs if the total amount of nitrogen supplied by protein is adequate (Table 4-1). The process by which the body synthesizes nonessential amino acids is called *transamination* and refers to the shifting of the amino group from an amino

acid to a keto acid (Chap. 9). The enzyme required for this reaction contains vitamin $B_6$.

*Nitrogen balance studies* have been used to determine the amounts of essential amino acids required by various groups. An individual is in nitrogen equilibrium or balance when the nitrogen intake from protein or amino acids is approximately equal to the nitrogen lost in the feces and urine. Rose[5] fed young men a well-balanced mixture of all known amino acids in a diet otherwise adequate in vitamins, minerals, and energy from fat and carbohydrate. During succeeding periods he omitted different amino acids, one at a time, and observed the effect on nitrogen balance. If the missing amino acid could be synthesized by the body, nitrogen equilibrium was maintained; if, however, the body could not synthesize the omitted amino acid, negative nitrogen balance followed. This meant that more nitrogen was lost than was consumed because tissues requiring the essential amino acid could not be maintained but were broken down and their nitrogen excreted. Nitrogen equilibrium was again attained when the missing essential amino acid was supplied in amounts adequate to maintain tissues. Positive nitrogen balance, that is, nitrogen intake from protein greater than nitrogen loss in urine and feces, occurs only when new tissues are synthesized, as in growth and pregnancy, or in replacement of tissue loss due to injury or disease.

Nine amino acids are essential for maintenance of nitrogen equilibrium in humans. The estimated essential amino acid requirements for infants, children, and adults are given in Table 4-2. Infants[6] and children[7] have proportionally greater demands for essential amino acids than adults. In addition, infants require histidine as an essential amino acid.

Factors in addition to the age, sex, and physiological condition of an individual influence the requirements for specific amino acids. If total protein intake is low, small surpluses of certain amino acids can increase the need for others. Similarly, amino acid imbalance must be guarded against in the formulation of feedings for total parenteral nutrition (TPN), where increased or decreased amounts of different amino acids are appropriate treatment for specific clinical conditions.

The nonessential amino acids in protein also affect the quality of the protein. For example, the amount required of the sulfur-containing essential amino acid, methionine, may be somewhat reduced if cystine, a sulfur-containing nonessential amino acid, is supplied in the diet. Similarly, the presence in the diet of tyrosine, a nonessential amino acid similar in structure to phenylalanine, may reduce the requirement for phenylalanine. Thus, much definitive work on amino acid requirements has been accomplished, but pieces of the puzzle are still missing.

## Table 4-2. Estimated Amino Acid Requirements of Man

| | REQUIREMENT (mg/kg OF BODY WEIGHT/DAY) | | | Amino Acid Pattern for High-Quality Proteins, |
|---|---|---|---|---|
| AMINO ACID | Infant (3–6 Months) | Child (10–12 Years) | Adult | mg/g of Protein* |
| Histidine | 33 | ? | ? | 17 |
| Isoleucine | 80 | 28 | 12 | 42 |
| Leucine | 128 | 42 | 16 | 70 |
| Lysine | 97 | 44 | 12 | 51 |
| Total S-containing amino acids | 45 | 22 | 10 | 26 |
| Total aromatic amino acids | 132 | 22 | 16 | 73 |
| Threonine | 63 | 28 | 8 | 35 |
| Tryptophan | 19 | 4 | 3 | 11 |
| Valine | 89 | 25 | 14 | 48 |

*2 g/kg of body weight per day of protein of the quality listed in the last column would meet the amino acid needs of the infant.

(From Food and Nutrition Board, National Research Council: Improvement of Protein Nutriture. Washington, DC, National Academy of Sciences, 1973)

## Total protein

Although nitrogen balance studies can also be used to determine the total protein needs, the "factorial method" has been applied more recently to estimate the minimal amount of total protein or total nitrogen required for maintenance of the adult.[8,9] The obligatory losses of nitrogen in human urine and feces,[10,11] as well as the losses of nitrogen in sweat, hair, sloughed skin, and various secretions and excretions of the body,[12] have been determined for young adults consuming a highly digestible protein-free diet. After nitrogen output has fallen to a near plateau level, these losses amount to approximately 70 mg of nitrogen per kg of body weight or 0.45 g per kg of body protein per kg of body weight.[8] Because the body is not 100% efficient in its use of even the highest quality protein (egg protein) and because quality (see below) varies from protein to protein, the actual adult requirement for protein is considerably above the level (see recommended dietary allowances). Adjustments in protein needs also must be made for growth, pregnancy, and lactation.

## Quality of protein

Osborne and Mendel in their pioneer work with rats showed that individual proteins differed in their ability to maintain life and support the growth of their animals (Fig. 4-2). Casein (milk protein), when fed at a level of 18% of the total calories, both maintained life and supported growth; for this reason it was classified as a complete protein. Gliadin (wheat protein), because it maintained life but did not support growth, was called a partially incomplete protein. Incomplete proteins, such as zein (corn protein), were those which could not even maintain life because they were lacking in one or more of the essential amino acids. Because casein was found to be only half as effective in supporting growth when fed at the 9% level as it was at the 18% level, it was recognized that quality and quantity were both important in determining the effectiveness of proteins.

As a result of early research, proteins were classed as complete, partially incomplete, and incomplete. These terms are still used by some authors to describe protein quality. Animal proteins, such as meats, poultry, fish, eggs, milk, and cheese, provide good quality protein in liberal amounts and are termed complete proteins. The exception to this is gelatin, the protein derived from animal connective tissue, which, because of its lack of tryptophan, is classified as an incomplete protein. Proteins from plant sources are usually not of as good quality as those from animal sources because one or more of the following essential amino acids are in short supply: lysine, methionine, threonine, and tryptophan. They are therefore incomplete or partially incomplete. The best quality plant proteins are found in legumes, such as beans, peas, lentils, and peanuts, and in nuts. The proteins in bread,

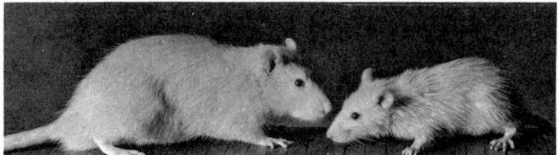

**Fig. 4-2.** Adequate and inadequate protein (18% vs. 4%) in rats of the same litter. This deficiency produces stunted growth but no deformities.

cereals, vegetables other than those mentioned, and fruit are all incomplete. These proteins, nevertheless, are an important part of the food intake because their amino acids contribute to the total nitrogen of the body that must be available for nonessential amino acids and other nitrogen-containing compounds in the tissues.

Protein quality is a measure of the efficiency with which a protein is used for growth or maintenance and depends primarily on the essential amino acid composition of the protein. When the diet is adequate in energy and total nitrogen (protein), protein quality can be calculated by comparing the essential amino acids in an unknown protein with those in a reference protein. The amino acid score (chemical score) can be calculated as follows:

$$\text{amino acid score} = \frac{\text{mg of amino acid in 1 g of test protein}}{\text{mg of amino acid in reference protein}} \times 100$$

The amino acid score for the protein would be the score for the most limiting essential amino acid. If the most limiting essential amino acid is 80% of the reference pattern, then the amino acid score is considered to be 80. The proteins in egg and human milk have been used as the protein reference patterns, but the most recent report of the Joint FAO/WHO Committee also suggests a theoretical protein pattern (Table 4-3).[8]

The FAO/WHO 1973 recommendations for protein requirements make adjustments of the "safe level of protein intake," according to the amino acid score of the protein in the diet. The committee also states that

> Available information on amino acid scores of national diets supports the assumption that the diets of rich countries have a quality relative to that of milk or eggs of about 80%, and those of poor countries about 70%. Situations may exist, particularly with diets in which 70% to 80% of the protein comes from such foods as cassava and maize and virtually none from animal foods, where the relative quality may be as low as 60%.[8]

Biologic value (BV) is another term used to describe protein quality and is defined as the percentage of absorbed nitrogen retained by the body. This is determined by a carefully standardized assay in which the nitrogen intake and losses of rats are measured to determine the efficiency of utilization. Net protein utilization (NPU) is a measure of the efficiency of utilization of the ingested protein. If proteins are completely digested, the BV and NPU are the same; for proteins less well digested, the NPU will be less. Animal proteins in eggs, milk, cheese, meat, poultry, and fish have high biologic values compared with lower values for most of the vegetable proteins. The NPU values vary from the BV in terms of the coefficient of digestibility of the protein food. The amino acid score should correspond with the biologic value for proteins that are completely digested.

Another method of evaluating protein quality is the protein efficiency ratio (PER). The PER is a measure of the weight gain per amount of protein consumed by a growing animal. It is the method used to determine protein quality for food labeling.

Fortunately, most of our foods contain a mixture of proteins, one of which often supplements another. More to the point, however, is the fact that we combine several different foods in a meal in which the proteins tend to supplement one another because of their varying amino acid content. For instance, cereals, which are low in lysine, are usually eaten with milk, which provides a generous amount of this substance. For this reason, cereal and milk or bread and cheese are good combinations. It is obvious that this type of complementary value among foods makes a varied diet more desirable than a restricted one.

The concept of protein supplementation has also been applied in areas where animal proteins are not readily available. Attempts to provide palatable low-cost foods with an adequate amino acid balance from inexpensive indigenous foods have resulted in combinations of various types of vegetable proteins. One such product is "Incaparina," developed by the Institute of Nutrition in Central America and Panama (INCAP). It consists of a mixture of ground maize, sorghum, cottonseed flour, torula yeast, and vitamin A.[13] A number of other countries in Asia, the Near East, and Africa have developed similar products from indigenous foods to meet the protein needs of young infants. Small amounts of animal protein, such as skim milk or fish meal, have also been added to mixtures of vegetable proteins to improve their quality. Another example is seen in the enrichment of cereal grains with one or more of the amino acids, which are the limiting factors, such as the addition of lysine to wheat. These mixtures provide a relatively good source of protein, particularly for the growing child, who suffers the most from poor quality and inadequate protein intake.

The genetic improvement of plant crops both to increase the quality of their protein, such as the hybrid corn with increased lysine, and to increase their yield offers hope for the future.

## Protein allowances

Any quantitative estimate of protein requirement must take into account the quality of the proteins involved. The Food and Nutrition Board[19] recommends a daily intake of 0.8 g protein per kg of body weight for adults consuming the mixed protein diet of the United States. Hence, the recommendation for the 70-kg man is 56 g of protein and for the 55-kg woman, 44 g.

The recommended dietary allowance of protein for infants is based upon the amount of milk protein that is known to produce a satisfactory growth rate. An additional amount of protein to allow for growth has been included in the allowance for children in age groups from 1 to 18 years.

An additional 30 g per day for pregnancy has also been added from the second month to the end of gestation. The allowance for pregnant adolescents is proportionately higher depending on age. Twenty additional g are recommended during lactation to cover the milk produced. As shown in Table 4-4, the Food and Nutrition Board's recommended dietary allowances are similar (except those for the pregnant woman) to the FAO/WHO "safe levels of intake" for people who consume diets with a protein score of 70%.[8] Both groups have emphasized that these recommendations for protein depend on satisfaction of energy needs.

In general, these protein allowances are much lower than the amounts consumed by most Americans, and may not be adequate if energy intakes are low. Calloway[14] also points out that, "the recommended allowances for protein are incompatible with sound nutrition planning." By limiting the quantity of protein-rich foods, adequate amounts of trace minerals and vitamin $B_6$ may not be provided in the diet because only about 8% to 9% of the

**Table 4-3. The FAO/WHO Pattern and the Proteins of Egg, Human Milk, and Cow's Milk (mg/g of Protein)**

| Essential Amino Acids | 1973 FAO/WHO Pattern | Egg | Human Milk | Cow's Milk |
|---|---|---|---|---|
| Histidine | | 22 | 26 | 27 |
| Lysine | 55 | 70 | 66 | 78 |
| Leucine | 70 | 86 | 93 | 95 |
| Isoleucine | 40 | 54 | 46 | 47 |
| Methionine + cystine | 35 | 57 | 42 | 33 |
| Phenylalanine + tyrosine | 60 | 93 | 72 | 102 |
| Threonine | 40 | 47 | 43 | 44 |
| Tryptophan | 10 | 17 | 17 | 14 |
| Valine | 50 | 66 | 55 | 64 |
| Total | 360 | 512 | 460 | 504 |

(Adapted from Report of a Joint FAO/WHO Committee: Energy and Protein Requirements. WHO Tech Rep Ser, no. 522. Geneva, World Health Organization, 1973)

## Table 4-4.  Protein Standards of the Recommended Dietary Allowances and FAO/WHO

| | RECOMMENDED DIETARY ALLOWANCES | | | | FAO/ WHO SAFE LEVEL OF INTAKE | | | |
| --- | --- | --- | --- | --- | --- | --- | --- | --- |
| | | | | Protein (g/day) | | | Protein (g/kg/day) | |
| Age (Years) | Body Weight kg | lbs | Per Person | Per kg | Age (Years) | Body Weight kg | Reference* | Score 70* |
| **Infants** | | | | | | | | |
| 0–0.5 | 6 | 14 | | 2.2 | 0–0.5 | | Breast-feeding recommended | |
| 0.5–1 | 9 | 20 | | 2.0 | 0.5–1 | 7.3 | 1.53 | 2.2 |
| **Children** | | | | | | | | |
| 1–3 | 13 | 28 | 23 | 1.8 | 1–3 | 13.4 | 1.19 | 1.7 |
| 4–6 | 20 | 44 | 30 | 1.5 | 4–6 | 20.2 | 1.01 | 1.4 |
| 7–10 | 30 | 66 | 36 | 1.2 | 7–9 | 28.1 | 0.88 | 1.3 |
| **Males** | | | | | | | | |
| 11–14 | 44 | 97 | 44 | 1.0 | 10–12 | 36.9 | 0.81 | 1.2 |
| 15–18 | 61 | 134 | 54 | 0.9 | 13–15 | 51.3 | 0.72 | 1.0 |
| 19–22 | 67 | 147 | 52 | 0.8 | 16–19 | 62.9 | 0.60 | 0.9 |
| 23–50 | 70 | 154 | 56 | 0.8 | adult | 65.0 | 0.57 | 0.8 |
| 51+ | 70 | 154 | 56 | 0.8 | | | | |
| **Females** | | | | | | | | |
| 11–14 | 44 | 97 | 44 | 1.0 | 10–12 | 38.0 | 0.76 | 1.1 |
| 15–18 | 54 | 119 | 48 | 0.9 | 13–15 | 49.9 | 0.63 | 0.9 |
| 19–22 | 58 | 128 | 46 | 0.8 | 16–19 | 54.4 | 0.55 | 0.8 |
| 23–50 | 58 | 128 | 46 | 0.8 | adult | 55.0 | 0.52 | 0.7 |
| | | | | | | Per person per day | | |
| Pregnant | | | +30 | 1.3 | Pregnant | | + 9 | +13 |
| Lactating | | | +20 | | Lactating | | +17 | +24 |

*Reference protein is milk or egg; score 70 refers to protein utilized 70% as efficiently as the reference protein.
(Adapted from Calloway DH: Recommended dietary allowances for protein and energy, 1973. J Am Diet Assoc 64:157, 1974)

total calories in the diet would then come from protein, as compared with the present 11% to 13%. This may be a particular problem when recommended dietary allowances are used by social welfare agencies to set family food allowances or to plan low-cost institutional menus. The assumption is that those Americans who can afford to will continue to consume amounts of protein in excess of recommended allowances and that this is probably a good practice until more is known about trace nutrients in food and how essential they are to good health. Thus, the calcium allowance set by the Food and Nutrition Board is based on a protein intake greater than the protein allowance for adults (see Chap. 6).

It is highly desirable that at least one-third of the daily protein intake be derived from animal sources, which is usually the case in the average diet in the United States. It is also strongly recommended that some good quality protein be included in every meal because the tissues must have all of the essential amino acids present at one time for tissue synthesis. If they are not there when needed, those that are may be deaminized and oxidized for energy. This rule applies particularly to breakfast and lunch, for these are the meals that most often contain limited amounts of protein. It is also worth noting that, since protein foods with high protein scores are the most expensive class of foods in the diet, there is a tendency

among low-income groups to consume less than recommended amounts of proteins, both quantitatively and qualitatively.

A basic dietary pattern for a day (see Chap. 11) is useful in planning menus. This dietary pattern (Table 4-5)

### Table 4-5.  Protein in Pattern Dietary for 1 Day

| Food Group | Amount g | Household Measure | Energy kcal | Protein g |
| --- | --- | --- | --- | --- |
| *Milk or equivalent* | 488 | 2 cups | 320 | 17 |
| *Meat, fish, poultry, egg* | 120 | 4 oz cooked | 376 | 30 |
| *Vegetables:* | | | | |
| *Potato, cooked* | 100 | 1 medium | 65 | 2 |
| *Green or yellow* | 75 | 1 serving | 27 | 2 |
| *Other* | 75 | 1 serving | 45 | 2 |
| *Fruits:* | | | | |
| *Citrus* | 100 | 1 serving | 43 | 1 |
| *Other* | 100 | 1 serving | 85 | |
| *Bread, white enriched* | 100 | 4 slices | 270 | 9 |
| *Cereal, whole grain or enriched* | 30 | 1 oz dry or | | |
| | 130 | 2/3 cup cooked | 89 | 3 |
| *Butter or margarine* | 14 | 1 tbsp | 100 | — |
| | | Total | 1420 | 66 |

For basis of calculation, see Pattern Dietary in Chapter 11.

of approximately 1400 calories provides a liberal amount of protein, more than two-thirds of which is derived from animal sources. Additional foods chosen to supply the extra calories should also provide more protein.

Protein requirement may be modified by certain pathologic conditions. During convalescence from debilitating diseases or surgery, extra protein is required for nutritional rehabilitation. For this reason, the earlier tendency to reduce protein intake in many diseases, with a few exceptions, has been reversed. The nutrition counselor, however, should recognize that certain diseases (see Chaps. 32, 33, and 36) may require limiting the total amount of protein or the amount of a specific amino acid in a patient's diet.

## Food sources of protein

From the bar chart of average servings (Fig. 4-3), it is evident that the first two food groups supply the most protein per serving and also the best quality proteins. Dry legumes and nuts are included as meat alternates in Group II because they contain the best quality plant proteins.

### Animal sources of protein
#### Group I. Milk and milk products

The foods listed in this group—milk, cheese, and ice cream—all derive their protein from milk. The proteins of milk are casein and lactalbumin; they are both complete, that is, they contain a good balance of amino acids. Milk is the protein food that nature provides for the young of the species, and around the world milk from many different mammals is used for human food. Milk is almost essential for the infant; it is equally good as a source of protein for older children and adolescents during the growing years. Adults also should get some of their protein from milk and milk products. Nonfat dry milk, better known as dried skim milk, is an excellent source of milk protein and calcium at comparatively low cost.

Cheese is the term applied to any product made from the concentrated curd of milk. Cheese is thought to have been the first manufactured food, the process for which was probably discovered accidentally when milk was stored in a bag made from the stomach of a cow, which contains rennin. The action of rennin on milk causes the curds to form and the whey to separate. Although a certain amount of the milk nutrients remain in the whey, the majority remains in the curd, which provides a large amount of the natural food value in milk in concentrated form. The curd in cottage cheese is formed by the development of or addition of lactic acid bacteria to milk.

Both food value and flavor of the many kinds of cheese that are available today depend on the composition and the methods of ripening which are used in production.

#### Group II. Meat, poultry, and fish

Meat, poultry, and fish are forms of animal tissue protein synthesized by each species to meet its specific needs for growth and maintenance. Such proteins are remarkably similar in amino acid content to the amino acid requirements of humans. Meat, poultry, and seafoods vary in protein content in inverse ratio to the moisture content: veal 28 g, beef 25 g, lamb 24 g, poultry 20 g, and fish 15 g to 20 g of protein per 100 g of fresh product.

*Variety meats* is a term applied to the organs and the glands of animals. They include tongue, liver, kidney, sweetbreads (thymus gland of calf or lamb), beef or calf heart, and beef brains. Organ meats tend to be much richer in vitamins and minerals than muscle meats. Popular luncheon meats, such as spiced ham, pressed meat loaves, liverwurst, and various types of cold sausages, such as bologna and frankfurters, are sometimes classed as variety meats. They contain from 11% to 17% protein in a convenient form for quick lunches.

*Poultry* is a general term covering a variety of domestic birds including chickens, turkeys, geese, and ducks. After roasting, the protein content of the lean meat of most poultry is about 30%; after frying or broiling the proportion of the protein content is slightly less than it is after roasting, because less moisture is lost.

*Fish, including shellfish,* compare favorably with meats and poultry as good sources of protein and in many countries are the chief source of animal protein. In the United States an effort is being made to stimulate the use of more varieties of both saltwater and freshwater fish. In other countries such products as fish sausage, fish flour and meal, and other processed fish foods of high protein value are being developed to improve the protein supply. Shellfish are low in fat and somewhat lower in protein ratio than fish because of their higher water content.

#### Egg

Egg protein contains the essential amino acids in proportion so nearly like the theoretical ideal protein that it is often used experimentally as the reference standard in evaluating the protein of other foods (Table 4-2). Eggs contain 13% protein—less than meats, poultry, or fish because of their higher water content. The egg white is one of the best examples of a pure colloidal solution of a protein (ovalbumin), containing 11% protein and 89% water. The protein of the yolk is more concentrated (16%) and much more complex. It contains lipoprotein, phosphoprotein, nucleoprotein, and possibly others, all of which provide nourishment for the embryo chick.

### Plant sources of protein
#### Group III. Vegetables

Vegetables are poor sources of protein; the only group that provides more than 1% or 2% are the legumes. These may run as high as 5% or 6% when they are fresh and still

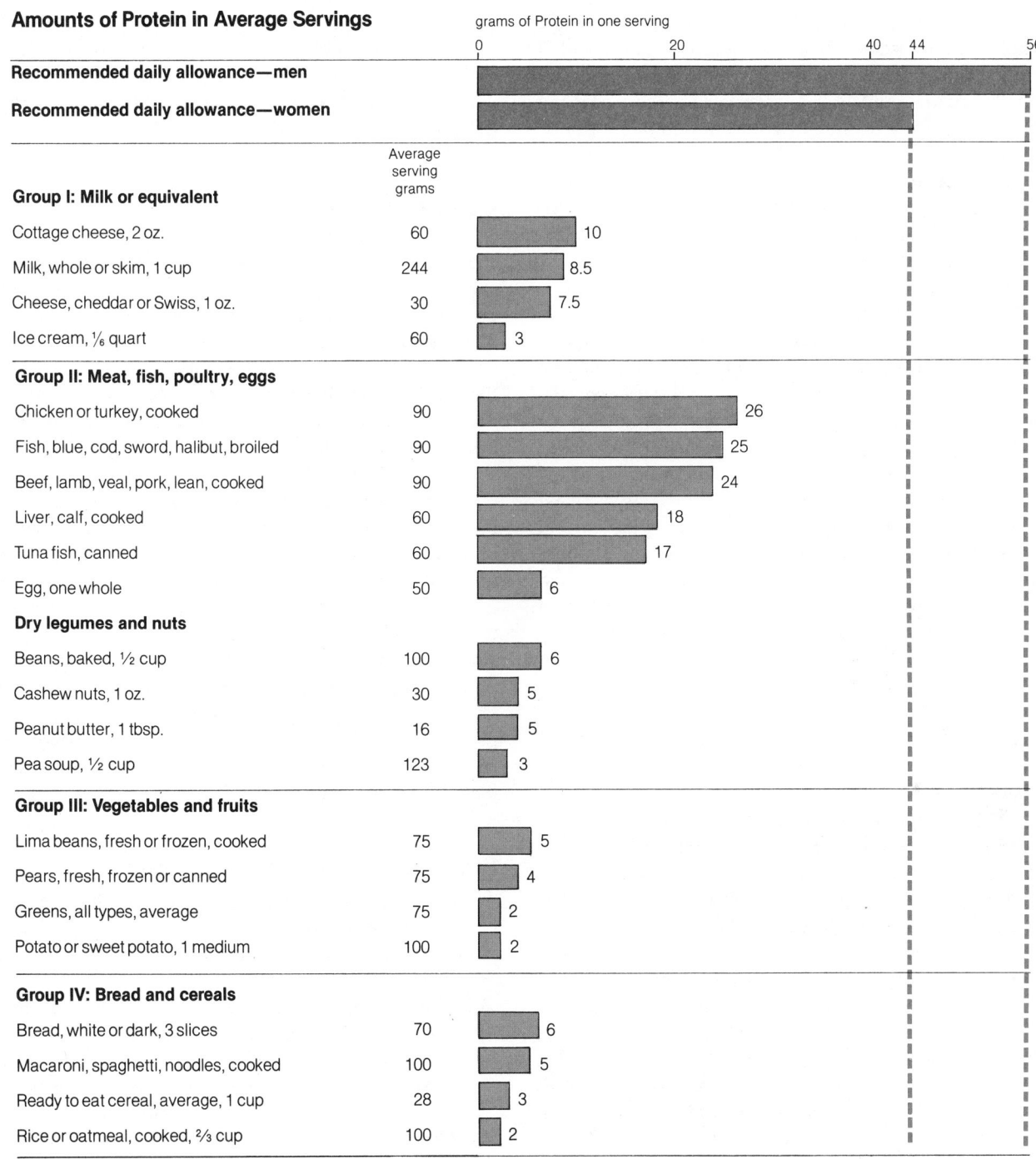

**Amounts of Protein in Average Servings**

grams of Protein in one serving

| | Average serving grams | grams of Protein |
|---|---|---|
| **Recommended daily allowance—men** | | |
| **Recommended daily allowance—women** | | |
| **Group I: Milk or equivalent** | | |
| Cottage cheese, 2 oz. | 60 | 10 |
| Milk, whole or skim, 1 cup | 244 | 8.5 |
| Cheese, cheddar or Swiss, 1 oz. | 30 | 7.5 |
| Ice cream, ⅙ quart | 60 | 3 |
| **Group II: Meat, fish, poultry, eggs** | | |
| Chicken or turkey, cooked | 90 | 26 |
| Fish, blue, cod, sword, halibut, broiled | 90 | 25 |
| Beef, lamb, veal, pork, lean, cooked | 90 | 24 |
| Liver, calf, cooked | 60 | 18 |
| Tuna fish, canned | 60 | 17 |
| Egg, one whole | 50 | 6 |
| **Dry legumes and nuts** | | |
| Beans, baked, ½ cup | 100 | 6 |
| Cashew nuts, 1 oz. | 30 | 5 |
| Peanut butter, 1 tbsp. | 16 | 5 |
| Pea soup, ½ cup | 123 | 3 |
| **Group III: Vegetables and fruits** | | |
| Lima beans, fresh or frozen, cooked | 75 | 5 |
| Pears, fresh, frozen or canned | 75 | 4 |
| Greens, all types, average | 75 | 2 |
| Potato or sweet potato, 1 medium | 100 | 2 |
| **Group IV: Bread and cereals** | | |
| Bread, white or dark, 3 slices | 70 | 6 |
| Macaroni, spaghetti, noodles, cooked | 100 | 5 |
| Ready to eat cereal, average, 1 cup | 28 | 3 |
| Rice or oatmeal, cooked, ⅔ cup | 100 | 2 |

**Fig. 4-3.**  Protein in average servings of foods classified according to the four food groups.

higher in the dried form. For this reason, and because they provide one of the better quality plant proteins, they are listed as meat alternates in the food group chart. Soybeans, which have the highest protein content of the legumes, are now available in the United States in a variety of forms suitable for use in the fabrication of foods. They are also important sources of protein in many countries where animal foods are scarce. Soybean milk, curd, cheese, and flour are a few of the soybean products used by Orientals. In India, pulses (legumes) and beans could be produced and used more extensively than at present with great advantage because of their high nutritive value. They are especially important in a country where animal protein is scarce, or the population is largely vegetarian.

*Peanuts* are really legumes although they are often classed as nuts. Roasted peanuts and peanut butter contain about 26% protein, although roasting reduces the availability or destroys about 10% of three of the essential amino acids present. Peanuts, or groundnuts, as they are called in many countries, are often used without roasting or with much less heating than is common in the United States.

*Nuts* in general are good sources of protein of fairly high quality. Because they are expensive they are seldom eaten in sufficient quantity to make an important contribution to the protein of the diet.

### Group IV. Breads and cereals

Breads and cereals make an important contribution to the protein of the diet, not only because of their liberal consumption but also because many of their uses encourage or increase the consumption of animal proteins, such as milk, eggs, meat, and fish. The protein of uncooked grains ranges from 7% to 14%. The grain proteins are low in one or more essential amino acids; for example, wheat is low in lysine, corn in tryptophan, rice in tryptophan and the sulfur-containing amino acids, cystine and methionine. Plant proteins, however, may supplement each other in such a way that a combination may provide a better balance of amino acids than any one food alone.

A protein-fortified enriched macaroni product (wheat + soy flour) is now allowed to replace up to half the meat alternate requirement when served with meat, poultry, fish, or cheese in the School Lunch Program.

### Textured protein products

Textured protein products are a new type of protein food made from one or more of the following sources: cottonseed, peanuts, sesame seed, soybeans, sunflower seed, and wheat. At the present time, they are derived chiefly from soybeans. These products have similar appearance, taste, and texture to the foods they simulate—ground beef, ham, bacon, chicken, fish, cheese.

The textured protein products, also called *analogs*, are manufactured by making a fiber from one or more of the vegetable sources. The fiber can then be spun into a form that simulates the texture of meat. Flavor additives are used to make them taste like the products they imitate. They may take the form of fiber, shred, chunk, bit, or slice. Some dehydrated forms are also available which may be rehydrated to serve as extenders to mix with ground meat.

The Food and Drug Administration has proposed the establishment of a definition and standard of identity for this new class of foods. Analogs have also been suggested as a food to be considered in nutritional guidelines to be set by the National Research Council. Because they may take the place of meat in the diet, their nutritional value should be comparable. They must supply a specific quantity and quality of protein as well as certain vitamins and minerals.

In 1971 the USDA authorized the use of textured vegetable protein fortified with vitamins and minerals in meals served under the School Lunch Program. The ratio of hydrated vegetable protein to uncooked meat, poultry, or fish in combination must not exceed 30 parts to 70 parts, respectively, on a weight basis. Many supermarkets today sell a blend of ground meat and textured vegetable protein.

### Liquid protein diets

A number of sudden deaths due to cardiac arrhythmias and arrest have been associated with very low-calorie liquid protein diets. These cases have primarily involved obese women who had subsisted on this type of diet without other food for weeks or months. Because autopsy revealed that the coronary arteries were free of disease which could account for sudden death, there was every reason to assume that the liquid protein diets were at least a contributing factor in the deaths.[15]

Liquid protein diets are made from predigested collagen or gelatin obtained from animal hides, tendons, and bones. They contain about 60 calories per ounce serving; 3 oz to 7 oz is usually suggested. Although some may be fortified with a variety of vitamins and minerals, none are nutritionally complete. The theory behind the protein-type low-calorie diet is that a person consuming 500 calories on such a diet loses less lean body mass than a person on another type of diet. Perhaps the extremely obese patient may benefit from such a regimen, but that person should be under close medical supervision and receive appropriate supplements.[15] Chapter 28 discusses diets for weight control.

## Study questions and activities

1. Why is good quality protein important for breakfast as well as for other meals?
2. For what specific purposes are proteins used in the body?
3. What is meant by the terms nitrogen equilibrium, limiting factor, and polypeptide?
4. The structural components of proteins are amino acids. How many of these are known? Do tissues vary in the requirements for specific amino acids?
5. What is meant by "essential amino acids"? How is the amino acid score of a protein calculated?
6. Explain three ways that proteins may be supplemented to improve the quality of the diet. What is meant by net protein utilization? by biologic value?
7. What theory is suggested as to why most Australians and New Zealanders are taller than people of similar racial strains living elsewhere?
8. What are the best food sources of complete proteins? Which food groups furnish the most protein? Compare the quality of protein from plant and animal foods.
9. Explain the factorial method of determining total protein requirements.

10. What are the National Research Council recommendations for protein? Which foods must be included in the daily dietary, and how much of each, in order to ensure good nutrition?
11. The high-protein foods listed in Fig. 4-3 contain appreciable amounts of other food constituents. Look at the Pattern Dietary in Chapter 11 and see what each supplies.
12. What are textured protein products? How are they used to extend animal protein foods?

## References

1. Pre-School Child Malnutrition—Primary Deterrent to Human Progress. NAS-NRC Publ. No. 1282, Washington, DC, 1966
2. Mitchell HS: J Am Diet Assoc 40:521, 1962
3. Gruelich WW: Science 127:515, 1958
4. Chopra JG et al: J Am Diet Assoc 72:253, 1978
5. Rose WC et al: Nutr Abstr Rev 27:631, 1957
6. Holt LE, Snyderman SE: Nutr Abstr Rev 35:1, 1965
7. Nakagawa IT et al: J Nutr 83:115, 1964
8. Joint FAO/WHO Committee: Energy and protein requirements. WHO Tech Rep Ser, No. 522. Geneva, World Health Organization, 1973
9. Food and Nutrition Board: Recommended Dietary Allowances, 9th rev ed. Washington, DC, NAS-NRC, 1980
10. Calloway DH, Margen S: J Nutr 101:205, 1971
11. Scrimshaw NS et al: J Nutr 102:1595, 1972
12. Calloway DH et al: J Nutr 101:775, 1971
13. Scrimshaw NS, Bressani R: Fed Proc 20:80, 1961
14. Calloway DH: J Am Diet Assoc 64:157, 1974
15. FDA Consumer 11:26, Dec, 1977-Jan, 1978

## Supplementary readings

Bessman SP: The justification theory: The essential nature of the nonessential amino acids. Nutr Rev 37:209, 1979

Broquist HP: Amino acid metabolism. Nutr Rev 34:289, 1976

Chopra JG, Forbes AL, Habicht J-P: Protein in the U.S. diet. J Am Diet Assoc 72:253, 1978

Food and Nutrition Board: Improvement of Protein Nutriture. Washington, DC, National Research Council, 1973

Hegsted DM: Balance studies. J Nutr 106:307, 1976

Mitchell HS, Santo S: Nutritional improvement in Japanese orphans. J Am Diet Assoc 72:506, 1978

Munro HN: Major gaps in nutrient allowances. The status of the elderly. J Am Diet Assoc 76:137, 1980

Scrimshaw NS: Through a glass darkly: Discerning the practical implications of human dietary–energy interrelationships. Nutr Rev 35:321, 1977

*For further references see Bibliography in Part 4.*

# Water and Electrolyte Metabolism

**5**

**ECW:** Extracellular Water
**ICW:** Intracellular Water
**ISW:** Interstitial Water
**TBW:** Total Body Water

## Fluids and Electrolytes

### Water and body function

Water is more essential to life than food, for a person may live weeks without food but only days without water. It is an essential component of blood, lymph, the secretions of the body, the interstice (extracellular fluid) and of every cell in the body (intracellular fluid). More than half the adult's weight is water, 60% for men, 54% for women. The difference reflects the fact that women have a higher content of body fat than men. In general, body water decreases, and fat increases with age. In premature infants, 70% to 80% of total body weight is water.

The internal environment of the body is bathed in fluids (which contain certain electrolytes) held in compartments of the body (extracellular and intracellular spaces) divided by semipermeable membranes (Fig. 5-1). The intracellular fluid accounts for 55% to 60% of total body water, and the remainder is distributed between the subcompartments of the extracellular fluid. Plasma and interstitial fluid (including lymph) are the two active compartments of extracellular fluid responsive to changes in the body's water and electrolyte balance, whereas the other subcompartments do not readily exchange with the rest of the body fluids. Transcellular water is composed of small heterogeneous fluids such as glandular secretions, cerebrospinal and peritoneal fluids, and digestive juices.

### Measurement of body water

Total body water content and the size of the various compartments can be estimated by the dilution technique. A known amount of a substance that distributes itself throughout the compartment to be measured is administered and, after an equilibration period, its concentration is determined in a plasma sample. From the extent of its dilution the volume of the compartment can be calculated. Heavy water ($D_2O$), tritiated water ($^3H_2O$), and antipyrine diffuse rapidly throughout the body and are used to estimate total body water (TBW). Substances that do not penetrate cell membranes but pass through

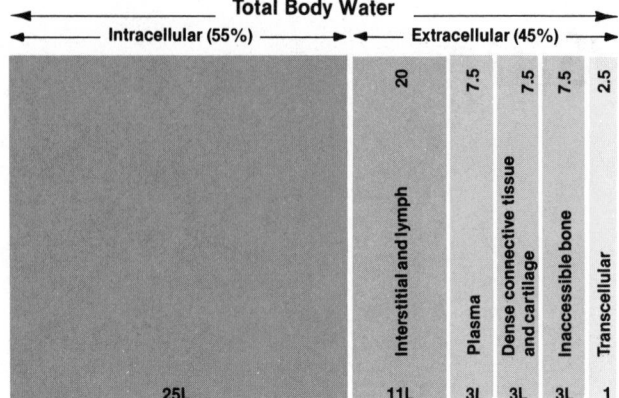

**Fig. 5-1.** Major body fluid compartments and their approximate size in an "average" adult male. (Data from Edelman IS, Leibman J: Am J Med 27:256)

the capillary endothelium are used to determine extracellular water (ECW); mannitol, inulin, thiosulfate, thiocyanide, and $^{24}$Na are examples of such substances. Evans blue dye, $^{131}$I-labelled albumin, and $^{32}$P- or $^{51}$Cr-labelled erythrocytes injected intravenously diffuse within but do not leave the vascular space, and have been used to esti-

mate plasma volume. Intracellular (ICW) and interstitial fluid volumes are obtained by the difference: ICW = TBW − ECW; interstitial water (ISW) = ECW − plasma. The method is simpler in theory than in practice, as the substances used do not behave ideally; they may not remain totally in the compartment measured, or they may not diffuse evenly within the compartment.

### Functions of water

Fluid is necessary for the functioning of every organ in the body. It is a structural component of cells. When cells lose their water they lose their shape. It is the universal medium in which the various chemical changes of the body take place. As a carrier it aids in digestion, absorption, circulation, and excretion; it is essential in the regulation of body temperature; it plays an important part in mechanical functions, such as the lubrication of joints and the movement of the viscera in the abdominal cavity. Waste products from the tissues are transferred to the blood in watery solutions; they are carried by the blood, which is about 80% water; and they are excreted through the kidneys in urine, about 97% water (Fig. 5-2).

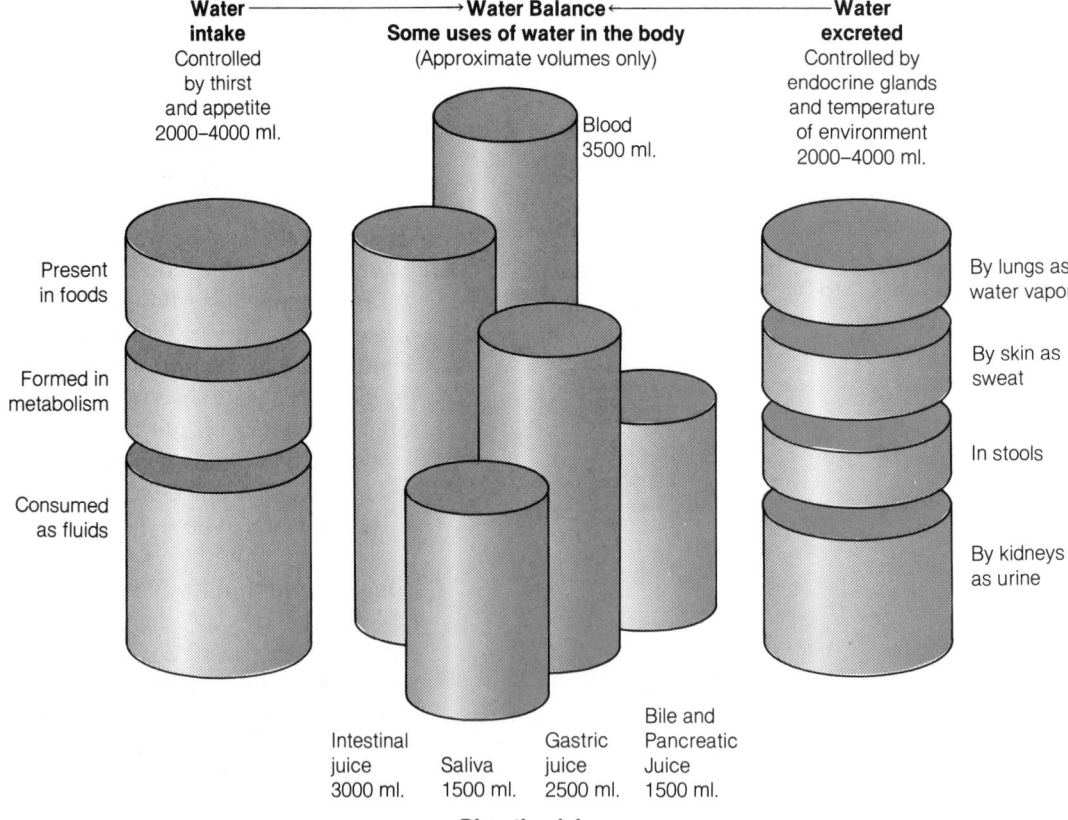

**Fig. 5-2.** Use and balance of body water. Water intake and output can vary greatly between individuals and in an individual from day to day. However, healthy people can maintain water balance over a relatively large range of intakes. The daily use of water by the body exceeds many times the daily intake. Recycling is possible because of the effective intestinal and renal reabsorption of water that flows through the intestine and the kidneys.

The same water is reused many times and for different purposes. Approximately 8 liters of digestive juices are produced and secreted by the glands in 24 hours (see Chap. 9). The water that carries the enzymes into the digestive tract is used during absorption to carry the digested nutrients into the blood and lymph. Over 3 liters of water are always circulating in the bloodstream. Water is the carrier of nutrients throughout the body. It is estimated that some 50 liters of water cross cell membranes in a day. To eliminate wastes from the body, the blood flows repeatedly through the kidneys where it is filtered by the glomeruli, producing a filtrate that is essentially protein-free plasma. Of the approximately 180 liters of filtrate produced in an adult per day, practically all of the water and nonwaste solutes are reabsorbed by the elaborate renal tubular system, except the 1 to 2 liters that are used to remove the waste materials as urine. The volume of urine normally varies with the load of solutes that must be excreted and with the amount of excess water ingested in relation to the water lost through routes other than urine.

## Water intake and output

Normally, the body loses water through four routes—from the skin, as sensible and insensible perspiration; from the lungs, as water vapor in the expired air; from the kidneys, as urine; and from the intestines, in the feces. A minimum of 800 ml of water is lost daily through the skin and lungs, and this amount may increase in hot, dry environments. The kidney eliminates approximately 1000 ml to 1500 ml of water in the urine; fecal losses approximate 200 ml daily but increase greatly when diarrhea occurs. Large water losses also result from excessive perspiration due to fever, vomiting, burns, or hemorrhage (Fig. 5-3).

Fluids are replaced by the ingestion of liquids and foods containing water. Some water is formed within the body as an end product of food metabolism (0.6 g per g glucose; 0.41 g per g protein; 1.07 g per g fat; from mixed diet, approximately 14 ml per 100 calories). Even so, 4 to 6 cups (1–1¹/₂ liters) of water or other liquids should be consumed daily in order to ensure a sufficient amount of water for body functions. Many foods contain a high percentage of water (Fig. 5-4) and may provide as much as 1 liter a day. Once ingested, water is absorbed rapidly from the digestive tract into the blood and lymph, although enough water is retained with food residues in the colon to produce a soft stool.

### Homeostasis—water balance

Water balance is carefully regulated within the body and normally a balance between intake and output is maintained, provided that there is free access to water. The weight of a man may vary by as much as 2 kg in 48 hours due to changes in the amounts of water and salts.

## Water and Electrolytes Loss

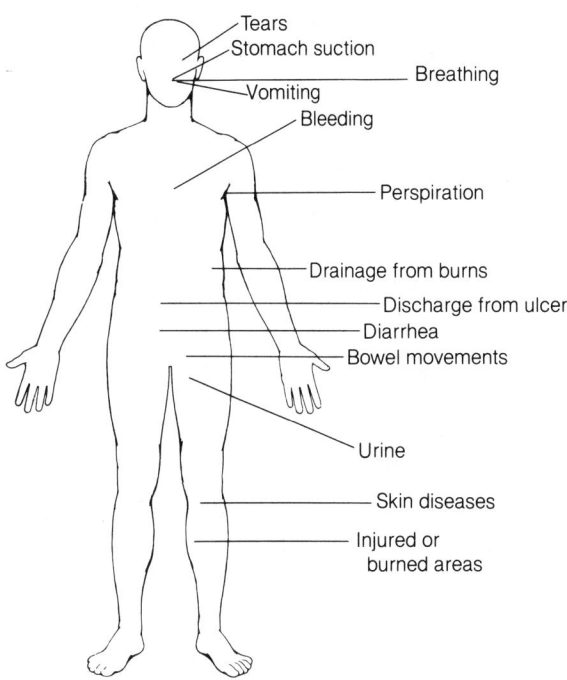

**Fig. 5-3.** Ways in which water and electrolytes may be lost from the body.

When water losses are increased due to excessive sweating or diarrhea, for example, the kidneys conserve water by making less urine. This action of the kidneys is under the control of the pituitary antidiuretic hormone (ADH), which stimulates the renal tubules to increase the reabsorption of water (Fig. 5-5).

Excessive loss of water also results in sensations of extreme thirst. The mechanisms for stimulating thirst are located in the hypothalamus and are activated by an increase in the solute concentration in body fluid. Thirst is a sensation of dryness at the root of the tongue and the back part of the throat and is nature's signal that liquid intake must be increased.

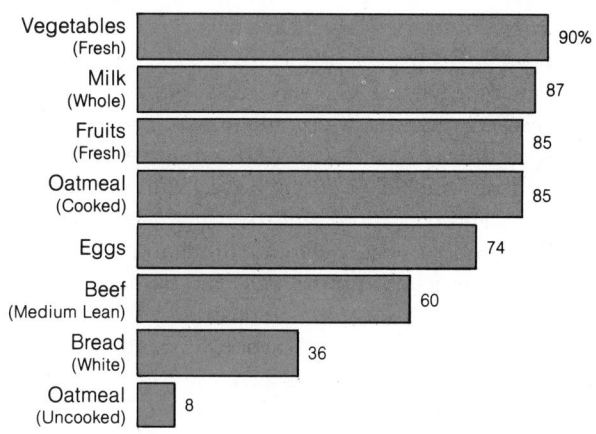

**Fig. 5-4.** Percentage of water in common foods.

**The integrated thirst circuit**

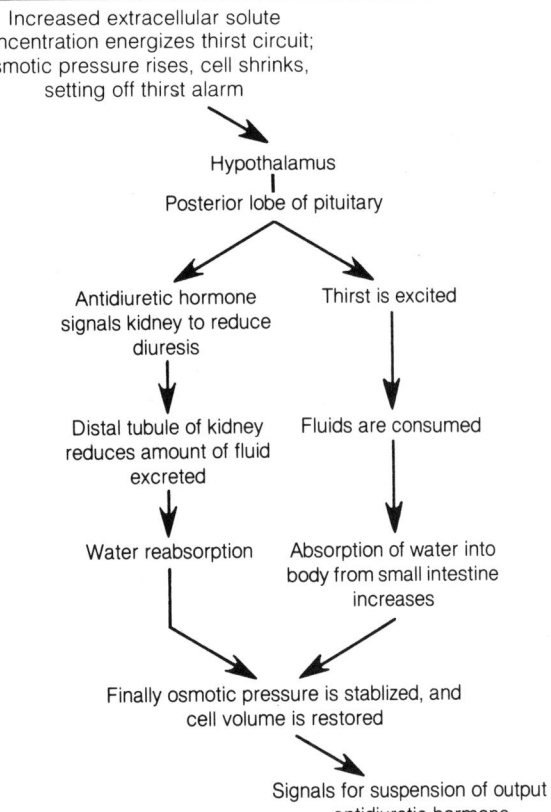

Increased extracellular solute concentration energizes thirst circuit; osmotic pressure rises, cell shrinks, setting off thirst alarm

Hypothalamus

Posterior lobe of pituitary

Antidiuretic hormone signals kidney to reduce diuresis

Thirst is excited

Distal tubule of kidney reduces amount of fluid excreted

Fluids are consumed

Water reabsorption

Absorption of water into body from small intestine increases

Finally osmotic pressure is stablized, and cell volume is restored

Signals for suspension of output of antidiuretic hormone

**Fig. 5-5.** Mechanism for the maintenance of body fluid volume. (Adapted from Robinson JR: Water, the indispensable nutrient. Nutr Today 5:16, 1970. Reproduced with permission of Nutrition Today, P.O. Box 1899, Annapolis, MD 21404, © Spring, 1970)

### Dehydration

Dehydration may be fatal, a fact that further emphasizes the importance of water in the body. The German physiologist Rubner stated that humans can lose all their reserve glycogen, all reserve fat, and about one-half of the body protein without great danger, but that a loss of 10% of the body water is serious and a loss of from 20% to 22% is fatal.

The term, *dehydration*, implies more than a change in water balance—there are always accompanying changes in electrolyte balance. When the water supply is restricted or when losses are excessive, the rate of water loss exceeds the rate of electrolyte loss. The extracellular fluid becomes concentrated, and osmotic pressure draws water from the cells into the extracellular fluid to compensate. This condition is called *intracellular dehydration* and is accompanied by extreme thirst and nausea.

The tremendous nutritional and physiologic importance of water is easy to demonstrate.[1] To evaluate the relative effect of water and carbohydrate supplements on work performance, six dogs were run to exhaustion on a treadmill. When they ran without food or water supplement 17 hours after the last meal, they were able to

expend an average of 1190 calories. With a carbohydrate supplement without water they could expend 1300 calories. When allowed to drink while running, each dog consumed 1.5 liters of water during the run and increased his endurance until he expended 2140 calories. It has also been noted that Sir Edmund Hillary, the first person to climb Mt. Everest, attributed the success of his expedition during the last few days of the ascent to an adequate supply of water, which other expeditions had lacked.

## Electrolyte and fluid balance

Chemical compounds that dissociate in water, breaking up into separate particles called *ions*, are known as *electrolytes*, and the process is referred to as *ionization*. Salts, acids, and bases are electrolytes; compounds, such as glucose and urea, are called *nonelectrolytes* because they are molecules that do not ionize.

Each ion, the dissociated particle of an electrolyte, carries an electric charge, either positive or negative. Positive ions (cations) in the body fluids include sodium ($Na^+$), potassium ($K^+$), calcium ($Ca^{++}$), and magnesium ($Mg^{++}$). The negative ions (anions) include chloride ($Cl^-$), bicarbonate ($HCO_3^-$), phosphate ($HPO_4^=$), sulfate ($SO_4^=$), ions of organic acids, such as lactate, pyruvate and acetoacetate. At the $p$H of the body fluids, some amino acid residues of proteins also carry negative charges; proteins, therefore, contribute significantly to the total anion content of plasma and intracellular fluids, as is shown in Figure 5-6. Electrical balance is always maintained in the fluid compartments of the body. To measure the total combining power of electrolytes in solution, a unit of measure related to the number of electrical charges carried by the ions present in solution must be used. This unit is referred to as milliequivalent (mEq).

One milliequivalent weight of an ion is its atomic weight in milligrams divided by the number of its electrical charges (*e.g.*, Awt. of $Na^+$ is 23, and Awt. of $Mg^{++}$ is 24; 1 mEq of $Na^+$ = 23 mg, and 1 mEq of $Mg^{++}$ = 24 ÷ 2 = 12 mg). The cations and anions in each fluid compartment of the body, as measured in milliequivalents, are equal.

### Electrolyte composition of the body fluids

Sodium is the major cation in plasma and interstitial fluid, and chloride is the major anion (Fig. 5-6). The major cation in intracellular fluid is potassium and the major anion is phosphate. Other ions are present in varying amounts in the different body fluids. Specific functions of these minerals will be discussed later in this chapter. Maintenance of the difference in the electrolyte concentration between the intracellular and extracellular fluids is vital for normal body function. As previously stated, they are separated by semipermeable membranes. These permit free exchange of water molecules but partially or completely prevent passage of dissolved particles, such as glucose or electrolytes. When there is a solution

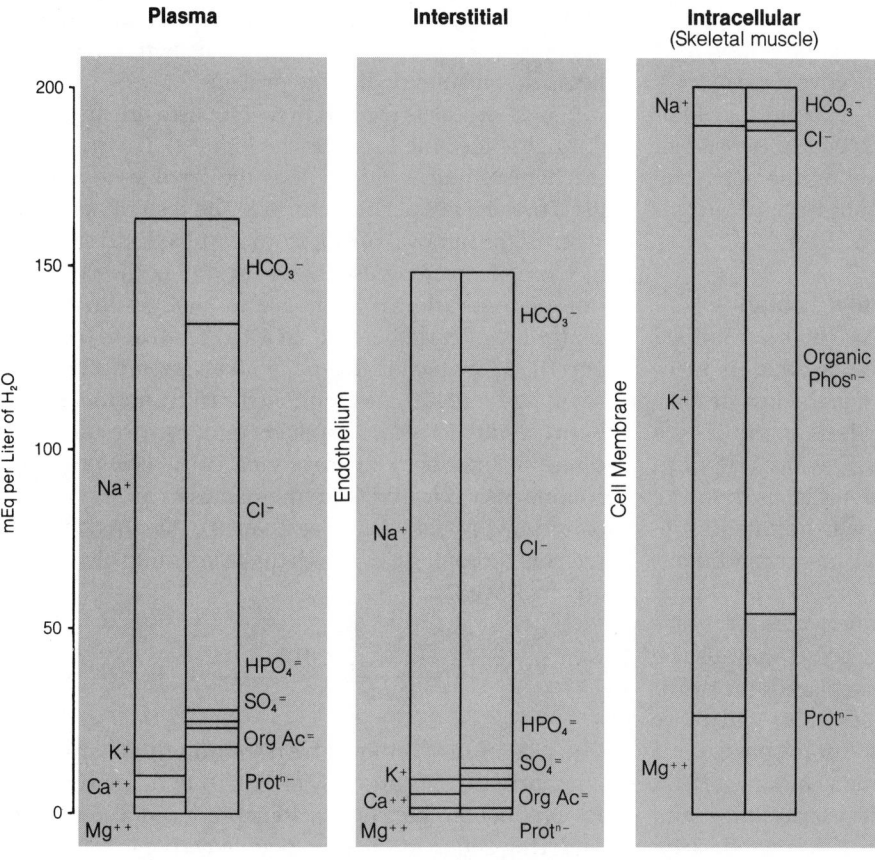

**Fig. 5-6.** Distribution and approximate composition of electrolytes in the major body fluid compartments. The main difference between plasma and interstitial fluid is their concentration of proteins, which normally cannot penetrate the capillary endothelium separating the two compartments. Maintenance of the striking differences between the intracellular and extracellular electrolytes and their concentration requires expenditure of energy by the cells. (Adapted from Valtin H: Renal Function: Mechanisms Preserving Fluid and Solute Balance in Health, p 20. Boston, Little, Brown and Company, 1973)

containing a relatively large number of dissolved particles on one side of a semipermeable membrane and a solution containing a relatively small number of dissolved particles on the other, the force of osmosis is brought into play. *Osmotic pressure* causes water to pass across the semipermeable membrane from the less concentrated to the more concentrated solution, until the concentration of dissolved particles on both sides is equal.

Even though the concentration of the individual electrolytes and protein differs between the intracellular and interstitial fluids, the total number of dissolved particles per liter of water is equal and, therefore, the two compartments are in osmotic equilibrium. Selective permeability through energy-requiring membrane transport systems prevents individual electrolytes from reaching equilibrium between the two compartments. Accordingly, sodium is concentrated in the extracellular space because it is expelled from the cell by the Na-K pump, which also brings potassium into the cell. A large portion of the body's basal energy expenditure is believed to be used in this process.[2] Normal activity of a membrane enzyme known as *Na-K ATPase* and an adequate supply of ATP appear to be essential for the maintenance of normal distribution of sodium and potassium between intracellular and extracellular fluids.[2,3] Because these two ions are the major regulators of the electrolyte concentration and, in turn, of the osmotic pressure in their respective com-

partments, any loss or gain in either electrolyte in one compartment disturbs the osmotic equilibrium and causes water to move into the compartment of higher osmotic pressure.

The capillary endothelium that separates plasma from interstitial fluids allows free passage of water, electrolytes, and other small molecules, but is not permeable to proteins. The differential distribution of protein in the two extracellular compartments is responsible for the small differences in the concentration of diffusible electrolytes in these fluids. This is attributed to the so-called *Gibbs-Donnan effect* of a nondiffusible ion upon the distribution of diffusible ions. Because electroneutrality must be maintained in each compartment, the plasma side of the membrane retains less anion ($Cl^-$) and more cation ($Na^+$) than the interstitial fluid because the cation must balance the negative charges of the proteins as well as other anions. At equilibrium the product of diffusible ions is equal in both sides, but their sums as well as the total number of particles (and osmolality) are higher in the compartment that contains the nondiffusible ions. As a result, a slightly higher osmolality is maintained in plasma compared with the interstitial and other body fluids.[3] If protein is lost from plasma, this equilibrium is disturbed, and water diffuses into the tissue space, resulting in *edema*, without a change in total body fluid volume. This situation may occur in severe protein deficiency and in some diseases of the kidneys (loss of protein in urine) or the liver (inadequate synthesis of plasma proteins), as is discussed in Chapters 32 and 33, respectively.

The Gibbs-Donnan effect between the intracellular and interstitial fluids is offset by the energy-dependent membrane transport systems, mainly by the active removal of $Na^+$ from the cell. As a result, isoosmolarity is maintained despite the Gibbs-Donnan effect.[3]

### Disturbances in water and electrolyte balance

Body fluid and electrolyte balance can be disturbed by excessive loss of water, electrolytes, or both. As mentioned earlier, severe loss of water over the loss of electrolytes results in intracellular dehydration, which the body attempts to correct by decreasing water output in the urine, and by the sensation of thirst (Fig. 5-5). Intake of water alone corrects the cellular dehydration and restores the urine volume. However, in many conditions, water loss is accompanied by loss of electrolytes. During excessive sweating due to high temperatures or heavy physical exertion, sodium and chloride losses may also be considerable. If only the lost water is replaced, the extracellular fluid becomes hypotonic, and water will move into the more concentrated intracellular space. This causes cellular overhydration, with many adverse effects on cellular function. Consequently, the extracellular fluid volume may diminish enough to cause decreased blood pressure, which, in turn, leads to other serious problems. For this reason, it may be necessary to replace salt along with water in order to restore both the volume and composition of body fluids. In illness associated with severe vomiting or diarrhea, losses of other electrolytes can also be serious enough to require replacement in order to restore body fluid and electrolyte balance and to prevent disturbances in acid-base balance.

## Acid-base balance

Electrolytes play an important part in maintaining the acid-base balance in the blood and throughout the tissues. The maintenance of this balance is a function of normal metabolism. The reaction of the blood is slightly alkaline ($p$H 7.3–7.45), varying only within narrow limits, regardless of the amount of acid products formed in metabolism. This equilibrium is maintained by a series of buffers in the blood and the tissue fluids. These buffers, which have a tendency to resist changes in their $p$H when treated with strong acids or bases, contain a weak acid or base and a salt of this acid or base. They have been likened to a chemical sponge because they can soak up or release anions or cations as needed to maintain the normal $p$H. Hence they serve as a first line defense against changes in $H^+$ concentration. The principal buffers in the regulation

of acid–base balance are the bicarbonate-carbonic acid system, the phosphate system, the hemoglobin-oxyhemoglobin system, and the proteins.

Acid products formed in metabolism are disposed of through either the lungs or the kidneys. The respiratory mechanism reacts quickly, but the renal system adapts itself over longer periods of time. The respiratory system controls the removal of $CO_2$ from the blood and can either increase or decrease its loss by regulating the depth and rate of respiration in response to changes in the concentration of carbonic acid ($H_2CO_3$) relative to bicarbonate ($HCO_3^-$), which is the major alkali reserve of the body (with $Na^+$ and $K^+$). As mentioned earlier, normal metabolism results in acidic products and, as a result, an increase in total body hydrogen ion concentration. $CO_2$ is continuously released from the tissues as an end product of oxidative metabolism (See Chap. 9). Dissolved in water, it forms carbonic acid, which dissociates into bicarbonate and hydrogen ion:

$$CO_2 + H_2O \underset{\text{Anhydrase}}{\overset{\text{Carbonic}}{\rightleftharpoons}} H_2CO_3 \rightleftharpoons HCO_3^- + H^+$$

The rate of $CO_2$ removal by respiration thus affects the equilibrium concentration of $H_2CO_3$ and, consequently, $H^+$ production. Carbonic acid is produced also from the buffering action of the bicarbonate-carbonic acid system to neutralize other acidic products of metabolism. Therefore, by its ability to regulate the concentration of $H_2CO_3$ in the system, the respiratory mechanism serves as a second line of defense to protect against a drop in the body $p$H. Similarly, reversal of these actions prevents a rise in $p$H if, for some reason, the alkalinity of body fluids is increased.

Although the combined action of the above two systems is essential in maintaining the neutrality of body fluids, they cannot continue to do so unless some of the hydrogen ion produced in normal metabolism is actually removed from the body, and the concentration of the bicarbonate ion used in the buffering action is restored. These adjustments are made by the kidneys, which act as the third and last line of defense in the maintenance of acid–base balance and involve some of the mineral cations and anions (see Fig. 32-1 and Chap. 32 for a description of renal anatomy and function). Sodium filtered through the glomeruli is actively reabsorbed by the proximal tubules and returned to the body fluids. Depending on the need to conserve alkali or acid reserves, either bicarbonate or chloride is returned with sodium to preserve electroneutrality; when hydrogen ion concentration is high, reabsorption of bicarbonate is increased. Two mechanisms in the distal kidney tubule result in actual removal of $H^+$ from the body and conservation of alkali reserves; they are also responsible for the slight acidity of normal urine and for the increased acidity observed in acidosis. The distal tubular cells secrete $H^+$ into the tubular lumen, where some of it exchanges with $Na^+$ in the conversion of filtered $Na_2HPO_4$ to $NaH_2PO_4$. The released $Na^+$ is reabsorbed with bicarbonate. Facing excess acidity, the tubular cells can also increase their production of ammonia ($NH_3$, from amino acids; see Chap. 9), which diffuses into the lumen and is converted to ammonium ion ($NH_4^+$). As a result, another $H^+$ is removed and, in addition, the $NH_4^+$ is excreted with acidic anions to conserve the basic cations that normally would be excreted (mainly $Na^+$ and $K^+$). In summary, the kidneys not only remove the excess acid from the body but also replenish the depleted alkali reserves, thereby restoring the buffering capacity of the body fluids.

## Foods as acid or base formers

Regardless of their food source, oxidation of carbohydrate, protein, and fat to form $CO_2$ and $H_2O$ results in acid production, as discussed above. In addition, the mineral content of foods contributes to both acid and base formation in the body. Some minerals are ingested as neutral salts, whereas others are present as complexes with organic substances and are released when the latter are metabolized. Depending on the balance between the base-forming and acid-forming elements in a particular food, the resulting mineral "ash" may be acidic, basic, or neutral. Of the acid-forming minerals, sulfur and phosphorus are high in proteins and lipoproteins and predominate in foods such as meat, eggs, and cereal products. Chlorine is also an acid-forming element but is ingested mostly as neutral salt, NaCl. Fruits and vegetables in general have more of the base-forming (sodium, potassium, calcium, and magnesium) than acid-forming elements, including fruits that taste acidic. Most of the organic acids found in fruits, such as citric acid (citrus fruit) and malic acid (apples), are present as salts with basic elements. When these acids are oxidized, the minerals are free to form neutral salts with acidic minerals or to neutralize other acidic products of metabolism. Even though milk as a high-protein food yields considerable amounts of sulfur and phosphorus, its high calcium content (with potassium) is more than enough to offset their acidity. The potential acidity or alkalinity of foods thus refers to the end products they will yield after being oxidized in the body and usually bears no relation to the taste. There are some exceptions, such as cranberries; their acid taste is due to benzoic acid, which is not oxidized in the body, and yields an acidic anion that must be neutralized by basic elements.

Ordinary mixed diets contain a reasonably good balance of basic and acidic factors, but, in general, diets high in protein tend to have a slight excess of acidic elements. However, the amount of hydrogen ion contributed by the acidic factors in foods is minor compared to that produced by normal metabolism and is not a contributor to disturbances in acid–base balance.

## Disturbances in acid-base balance

*Acidosis* is a result of conditions that would lead to a life-threatening decrease of the $pH$ of blood and other body fluids either through excess production or retention of acid or loss of base, were it not for the body's ability to compensate partially or completely for such changes. Corrective measures that are employed to treat acidosis depend on the cause and severity of the condition. Similarly, a condition with increased base or loss of acid is known as *alkalosis.* In general, the principal causes of disturbances in acid–base balance are considered to be either metabolic or respiratory in origin and are classified accordingly.

*Metabolic acidosis* is characterized by a decrease in bicarbonate and either a small or no change in carbonic acid. It is the most common type of acidosis that occurs in uncontrolled diabetes and in starvation (excess production of ketoacids from oxidation of fat; see Chap. 9), or in renal insufficiency (impaired excretion of $H^+$); it may also be caused by excess loss of base, for example, in the intestinal fluids lost in diarrhea or by drainage of fistulas. Both respiratory and renal compensatory mechanisms are employed by the body in an attempt to maintain $pH$ within the normal range compatible with life. Removal of the primary cause(s) and correction of acid–base balance require medical attention.

*Respiratory acidosis* is associated with an increased level of carbonic acid relative to bicarbonate; it results from hypoventilation caused by diseases that impair respiration. Renal compensation by increased reabsorption of sodium and bicarbonate and increased urinary excretion of chloride and hydrogen ion assists in returning $pH$ to normal.

*Metabolic alkalosis* is present when there is excess bicarbonate relative to carbonic acid. Ingestion of base as absorbable antacids and loss of chloride ion from gastric juice by vomiting or gastric suction (hypochloremic alkalosis) are common causes of metabolic alkalosis. Excessive loss of body potassium induced by certain diuretics also may lead to hypochloremic alkalosis. Replacement of both potassium and chloride is required to return pH to normal.[4] Efforts at renal compensation can lead to dehydration unless adequate amounts of sodium, potassium, chloride, and water are available.

*Respiratory alkalosis* is caused by hyperventilation, which leads to decreased carbonic acid concentration relative to bicarbonate. Renal compensation takes place through increased excretion of bicarbonate. The severity and treatment of respiratory alkalosis depend on the cause of hyperventilation.

## Sodium

Sodium is the most abundant cation in the extracellular fluid of the body. It acts with other electrolytes, especially potassium in the intracellular fluid, to regulate the osmotic pressure and maintain proper water balance within the body. Sodium is a major factor in maintaining acid–base equilibrium, in transmitting nerve impulses, and in relaxing muscle. Sodium is also required for glucose absorption and for the transport of other nutrients across cell membranes. One milliequivalent of sodium weighs 23 mg. An adult man (70 kg) has 2700 to 3000 mEq of sodium in his body. There is a concentration of 136 to 145 mEq per liter in the extracellular fluid and approximately 10 mEq per liter within the cells of the body. Bone contains 800 to 1000 mEq of sodium, of which about half is available if needed by the extracellular fluids.

The total content of body sodium, especially the concentration in the extracellular fluid, is under homeostatic control. One known regulator of sodium homeostasis is the hormone *aldosterone*, which is secreted by the adrenal gland and influences sodium reabsorption by the kidneys. Of the total sodium filtered through the glomeruli, over 99% is reabsorbed by the kidney tubules. A large proportion of this takes place in the proximal tubule, but the final adjustment is made by the distal tubular cells and the cells of the collecting ducts.[5] The regulation of sodium balance in the distal tubules includes its exchange with either $H^+$ or $K^+$ secreted by the tubular cells, depending on the needs for the maintenance of acid–base balance, as discussed earlier. When the need for sodium by the body increases, several mechanisms exist to alert the kidneys to this need (decreased arterial volume, decreased sodium at the distal tubular exchange site, hypokalemia). Specialized tissue of the renal cortex responds by releasing *renin* to the blood, where it initiates the conversion of angiotensinogen to *angiotensin II*, which, in turn, stimulates the production of aldosterone by the adrenal cortex. Aldosterone then increases sodium reabsorption by the distal parts of the nephron. The accompanying water retention helps to normalize the arterial volume, thereby suppressing further renin and aldosterone production.

The minimum requirement for sodium depends on the obligatory body losses in adults, but in infants and children it must also provide for the increase in body sodium content associated with growth. Normal sodium loss through urine, feces, and insensible water is estimated to be less than 200 mg per day in an adult. Additional variable losses may take place through sweating and must be covered by sodium intake. Except in cases of exceptional losses through profuse sweating due to stren-uous physical exertion in a hot environment or through vomiting or diarrhea, the daily sodium needs of most people are met generously by an intake of 50 mEq (1150 mg sodium; equivalent to 3 g as NaCl).[6] In the United States population this is well below the average daily intake, which is estimated to be between 100 mEq and 300 mEq (6–18 g NaCl).

Concern for the possible relationship between high sodium intake and hypertension prompted the Senate Select Committee on Nutrition and Human Needs to include a recommendation for reduction of salt intake as part of the Dietary Goals for the United States. Because they recognized that the restrictions in food selection and changes in dietary habits entailed in instituting their initial recommendation of 3 g of salt per day might be difficult, the Committee's revised goals propose that salt intake be limited to no more than 5 g per day.[7] The Food and Nutrition Board of the National Research Council also recommends a reduction in sodium intake by half of the usual intake, giving an estimated safe and adequate intake range of 50 mEq to 150 mEq sodium per day (3 g–9 g as NaCl).[5] Table 11-3 lists the suggested sodium intakes for all age groups.

Epidemiologic evidence from comparisons of usual salt intakes and the prevalence of hypertension in different populations show hypertension to be associated with high salt intakes, but direct evidence of a cause-effect relationship in humans is lacking. Also, studies comparing salt intakes of individuals with and without hypertension within a population have failed to detect significant differences.[8] It has been shown, however, that animals develop hypertension when fed high salt diets.[9] Genetic factors have been found to be important in determining susceptibility and resistance to salt-induced hypertension in the rat.[9] Because there is no known benefit from excessive salt consumption, it seems prudent for most people to reduce their salt intake, especially those with a family history of hypertension. The earlier in life the habit of low sodium intake is established, the more likely that it will have a protective effect in susceptible people.[10]

Sodium intake of persons with certain diseases may have to be restricted considerably below the levels discussed above. Such conditions and the planning of sodium-restricted diets are discussed in Chapters 31 (*Cardiovascular Disease*) and 32 (*Renal Disease*). Sodium content of various foods is given in Table 4, Part 4.

## Potassium

Potassium is found principally in the intracellular fluid where it plays an important role as a catalyst in energy metabolism and in the synthesis of glycogen and protein. Potassium ions maintain osmotic equilibrium with the sodium ions in the extracellular fluid. However, a small amount of potassium in the extracellular fluid is necessary for normal muscular activity, especially for the heart. Thirty nine mg of potassium equals 1 mEq. The average adult man has about 3200 mEq of potassium in his body, 125 mEq per liter within the cells and 3.5 to 5.0 mEq per liter in the plasma. Potassium levels in the body have been used to measure body composition. By estimating the amount of radioactive potassium-40 ($^{40}$K) in the body (whole body counter) a determination of the lean body mass can be made and compared with weight to determine body fat.

As is the case with sodium, the maintenance of potassium balance depends on the kidneys. Unlike that of sodium, potassium transport is bidirectional during the passage of the filtrate through the nephron. Although a major portion of filtered potassium is reabsorbed into the proximal tubule and the loop of Henle, it is both reabsorbed from the filtrate in the distal tubule and secreted into it, with net secretion in most conditions. Net reabsorption takes place in the collecting ducts.[11] Although the normal kidney can readily excrete excess potassium, its ability to conserve potassium is limited.[12] Under some conditions, however, the net transport in the distal tubule is reversed in favor of potassium reabsorption, and its reabsorption in the collecting tubule increased. Potassium excretion is decreased by low potassium intake, low sodium intake, acute acidosis, and adrenal insufficiency.[11] Conditions that increase potassium secretion in the distal tubule and its excretion include high sodium intake, increased level of aldosterone, and alkalosis.[11,12] As a result, regulation of body potassium is intricately linked to the maintenance of sodium homeostasis.

The minimum potassium requirement for adults has not been established but is amply met by the average American intake, estimated to range from 50 mEq to 150 mEq per day (2000 mg–6000 mg). In infants and growing children, the obligatory urinary, skin, and fecal losses plus the needs for growth add up to approximately 90 mg (2.3 mEq) per day.[6] Because of the possibility that high sodium to potassium ratios may be detrimental in individuals susceptible to hypertension and because of the influence of sodium intake on potassium excretion, the Food and Nutrition Board has concluded that the average current intake of potassium in a 1:1 ratio with sodium (on equivalent basis) is a safe and adequate intake for all age groups other than young infants. In early infancy, a higher intake ratio of potassium to sodium, such as that in human milk, is suggested.[6] Although potassium deficiency is most unlikely in the healthy person, medications, such as certain diuretics and adrenal cortical hormones, may cause potassium depletion if efforts are not made to replace potassium in the diet. As with sodium, potassium losses may also be increased with vomiting and diarrhea. Increasing the intake of potassium and decreasing the intake of sodium provide the best means of maintaining potassium balance when the loss is high. Foods that are high in potassium and low in sodium include fruits, fruit juices,

and vegetables. Values for the potassium content of individual foods are given in Table 1, Part 4. Hyperkalemia may develop in renal failure and requires restriction of potassium intake (see Chap. 32).

## Chloride

Chloride is the anion most commonly combined with sodium in the extracellular fluid and, to some extent, is also found with potassium in the cells. Unlike these bases, chlorine can pass freely between these two fluids through the cell membranes. Usually, movements of chloride between the body fluid compartments parallel those of sodium. An exception is the movement between plasma and erythrocytes, where chloride rapidly travels in and out of the cells in an exchange of bicarbonate, thereby enhancing the capacity of the red cells to carry $CO_2$ from the tissues to the lungs and aiding in the maintenance of acid–base balance. During digestion some of the chloride of the blood is used for the formation of hydrochloric acid in the gastric glands; it is secreted into the stomach, where it functions temporarily with the gastric enzymes and is then reabsorbed into the bloodstream along with other nutrients. Chloride intake and losses from the body also generally reflect those of sodium. The only time the body may be depleted of chloride in excess of sodium is after the loss of gastric contents due to vomiting or suctioning. Loss of chloride from the body fluids is replaced by bicarbonate to maintain electroneutrality, and the resulting alkalosis increases loss of body potassium. Chloride administration corrects both problems. Excess chloride is readily excreted by the kidneys and the skin, mostly as sodium chloride. The estimated safe and adequate intake of chloride is assumed to be the same as that of sodium and potassium on an equivalent basis (50–150 mEq for adults).[6] Human milk contains more chloride (11 mEq per liter) than sodium (7 mEq per liter) but less than potassium (13 mEq per liter). This results in a sodium + potassium to chloride ratio of close to 2:1, which is desirable for the regulation of acid–base balance, and is recommended for infant formulas by the Committee on Nutrition of the American Academy of Pediatrics.[13]

## Sulfur

Sulfur is part of the protein in every cell of the body and occurs in most food proteins. Sulfur intake is usually sufficient if protein is adequate. Sulfur occurs in a number of physiologically important organic compounds—in the amino acids methionine, cysteine and cystine; in insulin, glutathione, heparin, thiamin, biotin, and lipoic acid. Keratin (the protein of hair, fur, nails, and hoofs) is rich in sulfur; for this reason, the sulfur-containing amino acid requirement of hairy animals tends to be higher than that of humans. Sulfur has an important metabolic role in oxidation-reduction reactions because of the ready interconversion between disulfide (-S-S) and sulfhydryl (-SH) groups, as in the conversion of cystine to cysteine. The activity of many enzymes depends on the presence of intact sulfhydryl groups at their active sites. Disulfide bonds between cysteine residues of the polypeptide chains are important in the structure of many proteins.

Sulfates formed in the metabolism of the sulfur-containing amino acids have a role in the detoxification of phenols, indoxyls, and other compounds, which are excreted in the urine. They are also found as part of the sulfate mucopolysaccharides, chondroitin sulfate, and heparin.

## Study questions and activities

1. Identify the major fluid compartments of the body and the anions and cations that make up the electrolyte composition of each fluid. What forces are involved in the maintenance of body fluid composition?
2. How is water balance in the body maintained? If water in the body is not sufficient for metabolic needs, what makes a person aware of this particular need?
3. What happens when both water and electrolytes have been lost from the body, but only water is replaced?
4. What are the major mechanisms involved in the maintenance of acid–base balance in the body? How would you answer someone who said that she could not eat tomatoes "because they made her blood acid"? What determines whether a food is an acid-former or a base-former in the body?
5. Describe hypochloremic alkalosis, its causes and corrective treatment.
6. How is sodium homeostasis maintained in the body? Describe the effect of sodium on urinary excretion of potassium, and how this can be utilized to conserve potassium.
7. Why is there concern over excessive intake of salt and the ratio of dietary sodium to potassium? What are the recommended intakes and intake ratios for sodium, potassium, and chloride? What changes are required in their current intakes to achieve the recommended intake ratios?
8. What dietary factors contribute to sulfur intake? Why is sulfur needed by the body? Identify disulfide and sulfhydryl groups and their roles in metabolism.

## References

1. Review: Nutr Rev 19:23, 1961
2. Review: Nutr Rev 38:29, 1980
3. Valtin H: Renal Function: Mechanisms Preserving Fluid and Solute Balance in Health, pp 22–24. Boston, Little, Brown, 1973
4. Simopoulos AP, Bartter FC: Nutr Rev 38:201, 1980
5. Valtin H: Renal Function, pp 101–121
6. Food and Nutrition Board: Recommended Dietary Allowances, 9th rev ed. Washington, DC, NAS-NRC, 1980
7. Select Committee on Nutrition and Human Needs: Dietary Goals for the United States, 2nd ed. Washington, DC, United States Government Printing Office, 1977
8. Schlierf G et al: Am J Clin Nutr 33:872, 1980
9. Dahl KL: Am J Clin Nutr 25:231, 1972
10. American Academy of Pediatrics: Salt intake and eating patterns of infants and children in relation to blood pressure. Pediatrics 53:115, 1974
11. Valtin H: Renal Function, pp 197–209
12. Krehl WA: Nutr Today 1:20, June, 1966
13. American Academy of Pediatrics: Commentary on breast-feeding and infant formulas, including proposed standards for formulas. Pediatrics 57:278, 1976

## Supplementary readings

Armstrong B et al: Urinary sodium and blood pressure in vegetarians. Am J Clin Nutr 32:2472, 1979

Attschul AM, Grommet JK: Sodium intake and sodium sensitivity. Nutr Rev 38:393, 1980

Dahl LK: Salt and hypertension. Am J Clin Nutr 25:231, 1972

Dawber TR: Annual disclosure-Unproved hypothesis. N Engl J Med 299:452, 1978

Fregly MJ: Sodium and potassium. Ann Rev Nutr 1:69, 1981

Freis ED: Salt, volume and prevention of hypertension. Circulation 53:589, 1976

Krehl WA: The potassium depletion syndrome. Nutr Today 1:20, June, 1966

Lane HW et al: Effect of physical activity on human potassium metabolism in a hot and humid environment. Am J Clin Nutr 31:838, 1978

Masironi R, Shaper AG: Epidemiological studies of health effects of water from different sources. Ann Rev Nutr 1:375, 1981

Meneely GR, Battarbee HD: Sodium and potassium. Nutr Rev 34:225, 1976

Mickelsen O et al: Sodium and potassium intakes and excretions of normal men consuming sodium chloride or a 1:1 mixture of sodium and potassium chloride. Am J Clin Nutr 30:2033, 1977

Morgan T et al: Hypertension treated by salt restriction. Lancet 1:227, 1978

Review: Hypertension-salt poisoning. Lancet 1:1136, 1978

Review: Water and electrolytes in malnutrition. Nutr Rev 33:74, 1975

Robinson JR: Water, the indispensable nutrient. Nutr Today 5:16, Spring, 1970

Simopoulos AP, Bartter FC: The metabolic consequences of chloride deficiency. Nutr Rev 38:201, 1980

Schlierf G et al: Salt and hypertension: Data from the "Heidelberg Study." Am J Clin Nutr 33:872, 1980

*For further references see Bibliography in Part 4.*

# Mineral Metabolism

**6**

**CVD:** Cardiovascular Disease
**EDTA:** Ethylenediamine Tetraacetic Acid
**GRR:** Glucose Removal Rate
**GSH-Px:** Glutathione Peroxidase
**GTF:** Glucose Tolerance Factor
**MFP:** Meat, Fish, or Poultry
**NADH:** Reduced Niacin Coenzyme
**PTH:** Parathyroid Hormone
**RCR:** Relative Chromium Response
**RDA:** Recommended Daily Allowance
**TRF:** Thyrotropin-releasing Factor
**TSH:** Thyroid-stimulating Factor

## General aspects of mineral metabolism

Although mineral elements constitute only a small proportion (4%) of the body tissue, they are essential as structural components and in many vital processes. Some form hard tissues, such as bones and teeth; some are in the fluids and soft tissues. There are functions in which the balance of mineral ions is important—for example, for bone formation, the amount and the ratio of calcium and phosphorus, and for normal muscular activity, the ratio between potassium and calcium in the extracellular fluid. Electrolytes, of which sodium and potassium salts are the most important, are the major factors in the osmotic control of water metabolism as discussed in the preceding chapter. Other minerals may act as catalysts in enzyme systems or as integral parts of organic compounds in the body, such as iron in hemoglobin, iodine in thyroxine, cobalt in vitamin $B_{12}$, and sulfur in thiamin and biotin.

Plant life and animals, as well as bacteria and other one-celled organisms, all require proper concentrations of certain minerals to make life possible. In fact, changes in concentration of minerals, small in themselves, can be fatal to various forms of life. Common salt, which in dilute solution is necessary for most forms of animal life, becomes a preservative when foods are salted or kept in brine because the salt concentration kills bacteria. On the other hand, marine forms (fish and shellfish) quickly die when subjected to fresh water. In the human body, also, the maintenance of a normal concentration of minerals in body fluids is essential.

The mineral elements that the body requires are frequently classed as either macro- or micronutrients, depending on the amount of each that is needed in the diet. Calcium, phosphorus, potassium, sulfur, chlorine, sodium, and magnesium are considered macronutrients. Iron, iodine, fluorine, zinc, copper, chromium, selenium, cobalt, manganese, molybdenum, vanadium, tin, silicon, and nickel are often called micronutrients or trace elements. A comparison of the relative amounts of some of these minerals in the body is shown in Table 6-1. Cadmium, lead, mercury, arsenic, boron, lithium, aluminum, and other minerals may also be present in animal tissue as environmental contaminants, but at this time they have no known essential nutritional role.

### Mineral Content of Foods

In unrefined foods, minerals are present in various forms mixed or combined with proteins, fats, and carbohydrates. Processed or refined foods, such as fats, oils, sugar, and cornstarch, contain almost no minerals. The total mineral content of a food is determined by burning the organic or combustible part of a known amount of a food and weighing the resulting ash. The ash then is analyzed for individual mineral elements. Most foods have been analyzed for ten or more mineral elements, but in dietary practice the figures most commonly used are those for calcium, phosphorus, and iron and, for therapeutic purposes, sodium, potassium and magnesium (Tables 1 and 4, Part 4).

Minerals such as iodide, fluoride, copper, and other trace elements that are essential for life may be found abundantly in drinking water in certain areas or in foods grown in the soil of those areas, whereas in other parts of the country the same minerals are deficient in both soil and water. Still other mineral elements, such as sodium, potassium, chlorine, and sulfur—all necessary in human nutrition—are so universally present in foods that there is no need to worry about deficiencies.

Questions about the relative availability of mineral elements for physiologic processes continue to stimulate new investigations in this field. Fifty or more years ago, the opinion prevailed that the organic forms of minerals found in plant and animal foods were utilized better than the inorganic forms. However, modern research has disproved this theory. Today we are aware that many minerals occur in inorganic forms in natural foods and are absorbed from the digestive tract.

### Table 6-1. Mineral Composition of an Adult Human Body

| Element | Percent of Total Ash | g/70-kg Man |
|---|---|---|
| Calcium (Ca) | 39 | 1160 |
| Phosphorus (P) | 22 | 670 |
| Potassium (K) | 5 | 150 |
| Sulfur (S) | 4 | 112 |
| Chlorine (Cl) | 3 | 85 |
| Sodium (Na) | 2 | 63 |
| Magnesium (Mg) | 0.7 | 21 |
| Iron (Fe) | 0.15 | 4.5 |
| Zinc (Zn) | 0.007 | 2.0 |
| Iodine (I) | 0.0007 | 0.02 |

## Major minerals
### Calcium and phosphorus
Distribution and transport

Approximately 2% of the adult human body is calcium, and 1% is phosphorus (about 1200 g and 670 g in a 70-kg man, respectively); 99% of the calcium and 80% of the phosphorus in our bodies are found as constituents of bone and teeth, giving them strength and rigidity. Because of this common role and their many interactions in the body, calcium and phosphorus are considered together in most discussions. Yet it is important to recognize that their roles outside the skeleton are distinct and no less essential than their function in the bone.

In an adult, approximately 10 g of calcium are found in the extracellular fluids and soft tissues. In body fluids calcium exists in three forms: as ionized calcium ($Ca^{++}$), which is the physiologically active form; as a complex with organic or inorganic acids, such as calcium citrate, calcium phosphate, and calcium sulfate; and as protein-bound calcium. The first two forms are known as *diffusible* or *ultrafilterable* fractions because they can move from one fluid compartment to another and are filtered by the renal glomeruli, in contrast to the nondiffusible protein-bound fraction.

A relatively large proportion of phosphorus outside the bone is present in the soft tissues as organic phosphates. It is an important component of membrane lipoproteins, cellular nucleic acids, high-energy compounds, and other substances important in cellular metabolism. Soluble phosphate ions also contribute a sizable fraction of the intracellular anions.

About half of plasma phosphorus circulates as filterable phosphate ions ($HPO_4^=$ and $H_2PO_4^-$) and about one-third occurs as complexes with such cations as sodium, calcium, and magnesium; the remaining phosphorus is protein-bound.

### Functions of calcium and phosphorus
*Formation and maintenance of bone and tooth structure.* Bone is made up of a flexible, extremely strong organic matrix in addition to bone salts, which are deposited within the lattice-like framework of the matrix to make them hard and rigid. The bone matrix formed by the osteoblasts consists of protein collagen embedded in a gelatinous ground substance composed of mucopolysaccharides, such as chondroitin sulfate. The ground substance varies in consistency from a relatively thin fluid to a thick gel, which forms the interconnection with the tissue fluid that permits an exchange of ions and other elements in the blood. The bone salts or inorganic constituents of bone consist of small crystals of calcium phosphate in the form of hydroxyapatite ($3Ca_3(PO_4)_2 \cdot Ca(OH)_2$) and noncrystalline or amorphous calcium phosphate. Small amounts of magnesium, sodium, carbonate, citrate, chloride, and fluoride are also present in bone salts. The

hydroxyapatite crystals, although relatively stable in structure, are extremely small, which gives them a large surface area, and can rapidly exchange ions at their surface. The intercrystalline fraction is more soluble, and its elements can go back to the blood by the simple process of solution. During early life the amorphous material predominates, but it is replaced by the crystalline form in more mature bone. The size of the crystals increases with maturity as does the calcium to phosphorus ratio.[1] Bones contain blood and lymph vessels, nerves, and bone marrow. The nutrients needed for bone metabolism pass from the blood vessels into the interstitial fluid that surrounds the crystals, so that exchanges between the tissues and the blood are easily accomplished.

There is constant deposition and resorption of bone. In children bone deposition, controlled by the activity of the osteoblasts, bone-forming cells, is greater than the resorption controlled by the osteoclasts, bone-destroying cells. On the other hand, the skeletal changes frequently observed in old age occur when bone resorption dominates and there is a decrease in the absolute amount of bone (*osteoporosis*). In the healthy adult the two processes are equally balanced; both calcification, or *mineralization*, and demineralization depend on the level of calcium and phosphorus in the blood and extracellular fluids and on the normal functioning of the matrix cells. Approximately 600 mg to 700 mg of calcium enter and leave the bones each day.

Hormones influence these processes. The parathyroid hormone in conjunction with the vitamin D hormone, 1,25-$(OH)_2$D, controls the resorption of calcium from bone, and a thyroid hormone—calcitonin—inhibits calcium withdrawal from bone.

Bone, like other tissue, is in a state of dynamic equilibrium with the constituents of the plasma and other tissues. Calcium and phosphorus, when the food supply is abundant, can be stored in the trabeculae at the ends of the bones. From this storehouse these minerals are readily available to meet the needs of other tissues of the body when the dietary intake of calcium or phosphorus is inadequate. However, if calcium has not been stored in the trabeculae, calcium is withdrawn from the bone structure itself. Prolonged removal of calcium from bone naturally results in bones that are more easily bent or broken. When calcium phosphate is removed from bone, the remaining tissue is as flexible as cartilage; in fact, it is essentially the same as cartilage. Cartilage precedes bone in the development of the fetus and the young animal, and normally the calcium phosphate is deposited in it as growth and strain demand. The amount of calcium needed by the bones depends on the rate of skeletal development. The calcium content of the body increases from approximately 28 g at birth to about 1200 g at maturity. This is an average increase in body calcium of about 165 mg per day. However, the variation of calcium deposition throughout the growth period is extremely great, with maximum needs of 300 mg to 400 mg per day occurring in conjunction with the growth spurt in early adolescence. When nature's plan is thwarted by an inadequate supply of these minerals in food or by the body's inability to use them, growth may be retarded, or, as more often happens in young children, growth in size continues, but the new bone is abnormal in structure and poorly calcified. This may result in the bowed legs, enlarged ankles and wrists, prolapsed thorax, and other bone deformities characteristic of rickets.

Tooth structures, particularly dentin and enamel, are metabolically more stable than the bones. The calcium phosphate in the teeth occurs in the same form, hydroxyapatite crystals, as in the bones. The protein matrix in the enamel is keratin and in the dentin collagen. There is little turnover of calcium in the teeth.

The deciduous teeth begin to calcify in the fetus around the 20th week of pregnancy and continue almost until they erupt into the mouth. Calcification of the permanent teeth may commence anywhere from 3 months to 3 years. Wisdom teeth begin to erupt at around 10 years of age. Once formed, teeth do not require additional calcium because they cannot repair themselves after they have erupted.

However, poor tooth structure, reflected by increased susceptibility to dental caries, may be the result of inadequate calcium intake during the period of tooth formation.

***Body fluids and soft tissues.*** When compared with the amounts in bones and teeth, the concentrations of calcium and phosphorus in the blood are small, but their presence in normal amounts is essential for body function.

Bone calcium is in equilibrium with plasma calcium, which is maintained at a relatively constant level of approximately 10 mg calcium per dl (9–11 mg per dl) of blood. Plasma calcium levels are regulated by both the physical equilibrium between the plasma and the soluble bone salts (*noncrystalline form*) and by the mobilization of calcium from the less soluble bone salts (*crystalline form*) under the control of parathyroid hormone (PTH). Physical equilibrium tends to keep the plasma calcium level up to about 70% of the normal content, while the remainder is supplied by a feedback mechanism under control of the parathyroid glands. When the plasma calcium level falls below about 7 mg per dl, the parathyroid gland increases its secretion of parathyroid hormone, which acts on the osteoclasts in bone to break down bone tissue and release calcium and phosphate ions into the plasma; 1,25-$(OH)_2$D, magnesium ions and citrate also seem to be involved in the process of calcium mobilization. PTH also decreases the urinary excretion of calcium and increases the urinary excretion of phosphates, thereby preventing a rise in plasma phosphorus (3–4.5 mg per dl normal range) while the level of calcium is restored.

The major role of vitamin D in the maintenance of plasma levels and balance of calcium in the body is the promotion of intestinal absorption, which replenishes the calcium "pool" in the bone (see Chap. 7). Rise in plasma calcium, in turn, stimulates the release of calcitonin, which blocks bone resorption by osteoclasts, thereby re-

ducing the flow of calcium and phosphorus from the bone. High concentration of calcium in plasma also turns off the production of PTH and, secondarily, $1,25\text{-}(OH)_2D$, leading to increased urinary loss of calcium and decreased urinary loss of phosphorus. Because the levels of both calcium and phosphorus usually are inversely related,

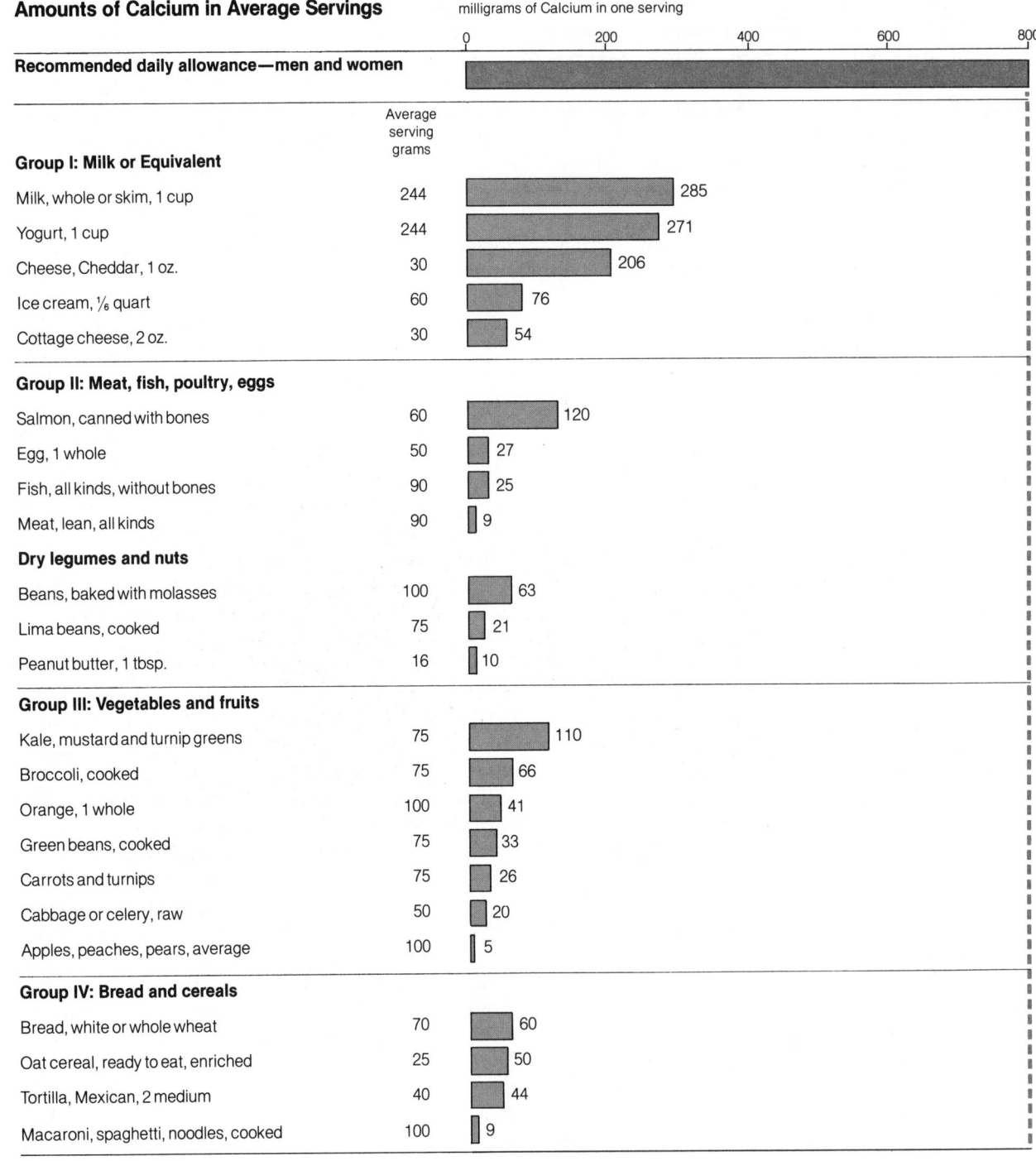

**Fig. 6-1.** Calcium in average servings of foods classified according to the four food groups.

these actions restore the normal levels of these minerals. Even though the hormonal responses are elicited primarily by changes in the level of plasma calcium, the opposite effects of PTH on the renal excretion of calcium and phosphorus are the major means for maintaining phosphorus homeostasis. Impairment of the excretion of phosphorus due to renal disease may result in elevation of plasma phosphorus and a drop in calcium level, which, in turn, stimulates the parathyroid gland, causing secondary hyperparathyroidism and associated problems (see Chap. 32).

A normal level of ionized calcium in the blood is necessary for blood clot formation. At least four vitamin K-dependent calcium-binding proteins function in the complex sequence that results in the conversion of soluble fibrinogen in the blood to insoluble fibrin (see Chap. 7). Ionized calcium in the body fluids also plays a vital role in the transmission of nerve impulses and in the maintenance of normal excitability of the heart, muscle, and nerve tissues. Ionized calcium is also involved in the differential permeability of the cell membranes, which is essential for the survival of the cells. Neuromuscular hyperirritability is characteristic of tetany, which occurs when the level of extracellular fluid calcium falls below normal. Calcium is an activator of several enzymes including ATPase, lipase, and certain proteolytic enzymes. The absorption of vitamin $B_{12}$ through the wall of the small intestine requires calcium.

Phosphorus is a necessary constituent of every cell in the body. It is part of the nucleic acids DNA (*deoxyribonucleic acid*) and RNA (*ribonucleic acid*), which determine the genetic code (see Chap. 9).

Phosphorus is part of the ATP (*adenosine triphosphate*)-ADP (*adenosine diphosphate*) energy-transporting systems in the cells (see Chap. 9) and is also a component of the phospholipids, which are involved in the transport of fats and fatty acids. Phosphates, as previously mentioned, also assist in maintaining the acid-base balance of the body.

## Food sources of calcium and phosphorus

It is apparent in Figure 6-1 that milk and milk products are the most important sources of calcium in readily available form. A few of the green, leafy vegetables used commonly in the Southern states are good sources of calcium, but others, such as spinach, chard, beet greens, and rhubarb, contain oxalic acid which forms insoluble calcium oxalate and thus may render the calcium unavailable. In most sections of the country greens are not used regularly enough or in sufficient quantity to be relied upon to replace milk, but they are important when milk is scarce or unobtainable. Meats and poultry are poor sources of calcium. Cereal products contribute little, except where breads are enriched with calcium or are made with a high percentage of milk solids. The pattern dietary of 1400 calories provides almost the recommended allowance of 800 mg (0.8 g), which is supplemented by the calcium of the foods added to make up the needed calories (see Table 6-2 and Chap. 11).

Phosphorus is more widely distributed than calcium and is more likely to be high than deficient in the average diet. Poultry, fish, meats, cereals, nuts, and legumes, as well as milk and milk products, are all good sources. Phosphate additives used in a wide variety of food products, such as carbonated beverages, processed meats and cheeses, dressings, and refrigerated bakery products, may contribute significantly to the total phosphorus intake of many Americans.[2] In the cooking of vegetables, there may be slight losses of calcium and phosphorus, especially if the cooking water is discarded.

## Table 6-2. Calcium, Phosphorus, Magnesium, and Iron in Pattern Dietary for 1 Day

| Food Group | Amount in g | Household Measure | Energy kcal | Calcium mg | Phosphorus mg | Magnesium mg | Iron mg |
|---|---|---|---|---|---|---|---|
| Milk or equivalent | 488 | 2 cups | 320 | 576 | 452 | 63 | 0.2 |
| Meat, fish, poultry or egg | 120 | 4 oz cooked | 376 | 13 | 212 | 104 | 3.3 |
| Vegetables: | | | | | | | |
| Potato, cooked | 100 | 1 medium | 65 | 6 | 48 | 22 | 0.5 |
| Green, leafy, and yellow | 75 | 1 serving | 21 | 44 | 28 | 29 | 0.9 |
| Other | 75 | 1 serving | 45 | 16 | 41 | 18 | 0.9 |
| Fruits: | | | | | | | |
| Citrus | 100 | 1 serving | 44 | 18 | 16 | 12 | 0.3 |
| Other | 100 | 1 serving | 85 | 10 | 21 | 16 | 0.8 |
| Bread, white, enriched | 100 | 4 slices | 270 | 84 | 97 | 20 | 2.5 |
| Cereal, whole grain or enriched | 30 | 1 oz dry or | | | | | |
| | 130 | 2/3 c cooked | 89 | 12 | 95 | 34 | 0.9 |
| Butter or margarine | 14 | 1 tbsp | 100 | 3 | 2 | 2 | |
| | | | 1415 | 782 | 1012 | 335 | 10.3 |

For basis of calculation, see Pattern Dietary in Chapter 11.

### Factors affecting absorption and retention

Not all of the calcium and phosphorus in foods is available to the body. Approximately 20% to 40% of the calcium and 70% of the phosphorus consumed by a person becomes available when it is absorbed from the intestinal tract into the bloodstream. The amounts absorbed, however, may be greatly increased during periods of rapid growth when mineral needs are high. People with limited intakes of calcium are also more efficient in their utilization of it than those with a more liberal intake. These factors help explain the following statement from the World Health Organization's (WHO) Report on Calcium Requirements. "In general, children and adults in most countries can grow normally and live healthily on a daily calcium intake between 300 mg and 1000 mg or, in the absence of nutritional disorders and if their vitamin D status is adequate, on even somewhat lower or higher intakes."[3]

Various factors, in addition to need and previous intake, influence the efficiency of calcium and phosphorus absorption. Adequate amounts of vitamin D (see Chap. 7), an acid *p*H in the upper part of the intestinal tract, and a normal motility of the gastrointestinal tract enhance the absorption of these minerals. Other dietary factors that appear to favor calcium absorption include some amino acids[2] and lactose.[4] On the other hand, large amounts of phytates (phosphorus compounds found in cereals) or oxalates, which can form insoluble compounds with calcium, may interfere with intestinal absorption. Even though these factors are not considered of practical significance when the intake of calcium is liberal,[5] they may need attention in some populations that obtain an important fraction of their total calcium intake from greens high in oxalates.[6] Steatorrhea due to impaired absorption of fat is associated with high loss of calcium in feces, believed to result from the formation of insoluble calcium salts with free fatty acids which are present in excessive amounts in the intestine.

Reports of increasing intake of phosphorus in relation to calcium[7] have heightened the interest of health professionals and researchers in the possible adverse effects that excess intake of phosphorus may have on metabolism of calcium. Recent research suggests that, contrary to previous assumption, increase in the intake of phosphorus within a range that is likely in human diets does not alter the intestinal availability of calcium significantly.[8-10] Of major concern, however, is the possibility of increased mobilization of calcium by bone resorption and its subsequent loss as endogenous fecal calcium, as observed in rats.[8] Induction of secondary hyperparathyroidism by a slight fall in serum calcium, which follows high phosphorus intake, appears to be involved.[4,9] The evidence in humans is only suggestive, and there are differences in interpretation of experimental results.[10,11]

The high protein intake typical of many Americans and other Westerners also may alter the retention of calcium. Even though protein may slightly enhance the intestinal absorption of calcium because of the specific effects of some amino acids,[2] this appears to be offset by the increased urinary excretion of calcium, which follows a high intake of protein.[12-15] A reduced rate of renal tubular reabsorption of calcium has been detected within a few hours after protein ingestion[14] and during high protein intake continued for 3 months.[13] Also, more calcium appears to be filtered due to an increase in the glomerular filtration rate.[13,15]

Still far from clear is the role of protein intake from mixed diets in determining the loss of body calcium. In a recent study in which varying intakes of meat were used to alter protein intake, slight calciuria was observed during the first few days on high meat diets, but the level of urine calcium soon returned to the level observed on the lower intakes of meat.[16] The authors suggested that the high intake of phosphorus from the high-meat diet actually may have protected against urinary loss of calcium. There is also disagreement whether the total loss of body calcium is affected by high protein intake, with negative balances being observed in some studies,[13] but not in others,[2,17] and whether adaptation to high protein intake occurs with time.[2,13,17]

Recent studies have demonstrated that decreasing the intake of protein reduces hypercalciuria in patients with urinary calculi more effectively than decreasing the intake of calcium,[18] which is part of the usual treatment (see Chap. 32).

Because of the observed reduction in calcium absorption with age and at least partial loss of the capacity to adapt to changes in calcium intake,[2] the possible roles that protein and phosphorus intakes may play in the varying degrees of bone loss associated with aging is of major concern and requires additional investigation.

In cases of parathyroid disturbances variations in calcium absorption and retention are even greater than under normal conditions. Hypercalcemia (high serum calcium) may occur in hyperparathyroidism, and hypocalcemia (serum calcium below normal) may result after removal of the parathyroid glands.

### Dietary requirements

The dietary requirements of calcium and phosphorus for children and adults have been investigated extensively. There is not, however, universal agreement among the experts on the interpretation of the findings.

Using balance studies to determine calcium and phosphorus requirements is a complicated procedure. As already mentioned, there are many factors that affect the amount of calcium absorbed and retained by the body. A person is said to be in equilibrium with respect to any nutrient if the intake approximately equals the output. The assumption that end products of metabolism appear in the urine and unabsorbed material in the feces does not hold for calcium and phosphorus. Some metabolized (endogenous) calcium and phosphorus may be excreted through the intestinal tract. Moreover, the evidence that humans can maintain calcium balance over a wide range of calcium intakes (the amount required to maintain this balance is largely determined by past dietary history) has made it impossible to determine the minimum requirement of this mineral. However, when balance studies have been conducted with groups of people accustomed to liberal intakes of calcium, their daily calcium losses through the various routes have been found to fall within relatively narrow ranges. As shown in Table 6-3, average daily losses derived from such studies were used initially by the Food and Nutrition Board as the bases for establishing the Recommended Dietary Allowance (RDA) of calcium for adult Americans as 800 mg (0.8 g) per day. The RDA for calcium has been continued at the same level through several revisions, including that of 1980.[5] The Food and Nutrition Board's Committee on Dietary Allowances acknowledged that many adults remain in calcium balance on intakes of 400 mg to 500 mg per day recommended as the "practical allowance" by the FAO/WHO Committee on Calcium Requirements,[3] and may adapt to intake levels as low as 200 mg to 400 mg per day. However, in defending its decision not to lower the adult RDA for calcium, the Committee cited "the possible effects of high dietary intakes of protein and phosphate on urinary excretion and enhanced bone resorption, respectively, along with the possibility of reduced calcium absorption with age" as arguments for recommending a liberal intake of calcium.

The calcium and phosphorus allowances during pregnancy and lactation are increased to 1200 mg per day to cover fetal needs and the calcium and phosphorus required for producing human milk. These amounts are comparable to the FAO/WHO Committee's suggestion of 1000 mg to 1200 mg each per day during these periods.

The calcium and phosphorus requirements for growth have been investigated in children of different ages by observing the level of intake at which maximum retention of calcium and phosphorus is attained. Growth of bone requires the storage of new calcium and phosphorus as well as replacement. The growth requirement varies with age, being highest in relation to weight in the infant, lower and fairly constant after the first year and until puberty, when there is a rise again during the period of rapid growth. The recommended allowances of calcium and phosphorus for children take into account different age needs. For ages 1 to 10 allowances of 800 mg per day of calcium and phosphorus are suggested; at preadolescence they should be increased to 1200 mg per day.

Except during infancy the calcium and phosphorus allowances are the same for all ages, although it is recognized that the intake of phosphorus is almost invariably

higher than that of calcium. A 2:1 ratio of calcium to phosphorus (as found in human milk) has been shown to result in maximum calcium absorption and retention in animals,[2] but the evidence for humans is less definitive.[5] However, it appears that the high phosphorus intake from cow's milk (Ca to P ratio 1.2:1) may be involved in the development of hypocalcemic tetany in some infants during the first week of life.[19] Because a higher Ca:P ratio may be beneficial and certainly is not harmful as is evident in breast-fed infants, a 1.5:1 ratio is recommended for the first year of life.[5]

In breast-fed infants the calcium and phosphorus needs are amply met from milk, and maintenance of the recommended Ca:P ratio is possible even when substantial amounts of other foods are added to the diet toward the end of the first year. However, because of the lower Ca:P ratio of cow's milk and most commercial infant formulas, which vary from 1.2 to 1.4:1, intakes with lower than the recommended Ca to P ratios are likely for a large number of infants.

For older children and adults, the requirements for calcium and phosphorus are most easily met by including 2 to 3 cups of milk a day or its equivalent in milk products. Avoiding excessive consumption of high-phosphorus low-calcium foods and beverages is essential if the recommended 1:1 ratio of these two minerals is to be maintained. Although a wide range of Ca to P ratios appears to be tolerated by adults as measured by calcium balance,[20] this is an area in which more research is needed.

During all periods of life, vitamin D, or sunshine, is essential for the most efficient absorption and utilization of these two minerals (see Chap. 7, *Fat-Soluble Vitamins*).

The relationship between calcium intake and *osteoporosis* needs special consideration. It is now recognized that a gradual reduction in bone mass occurs with age (*aging bone loss*) in a great majority of the population, usually beginning during the fifth decade and advancing faster in women than in men. There is evidence that the condition of the bones in later life is related to the amount of bone present in early adult life and not primarily re-

### Table 6-3. Bases for Calculating the Adult Recommended Dietary Allowance for Calcium

| | |
|---|---|
| Urinary calcium excretion | 175 mg/day |
| Endogenous fecal calcium excretion | 125 mg/day |
| Loss of calcium in sweat | 20 mg/day |
| Total calcium losses | 320 mg/day |
| Calcium absorbed from food          40% | |

$$\frac{320}{x} \times \frac{100}{40} = 800 \text{ mg/day}$$

| | |
|---|---|
| Recommended dietary allowance for adult | 800 mg/day |

(Data from Recommended Dietary Allowances. National Academy of Sciences/National Research Council Publ. No. 1146. Washington, DC, 1964)

lated to the calcium intake during adult life.[21] Both a decreased rate of bone formation and an accelerated rate of bone resorption probably contribute to the osteoporotic changes. Although it is not known why some people develop the disease, whereas other appear to be protected, it is becoming increasingly clear that multiple factors are involved, including nonnutritional factors, such as genetics, changes in the levels of hormones (estrogen, parathyroid hormone, calcitonin), and lack of physical activity.[2] Deftos and co-workers[22] recently reported that the level of circulating calcitonin decreased with age in both sexes. Release of calcitonin in response to infusion of calcium also diminished with age, more frequently in women than in men.

The role of nutritional factors in both the prevention and treatment of osteoporosis remains unclear and controversial. Beneficial effects of calcium supplementation on calcium balance[23] and in the prevention of bone loss[24] in postmenopausal women have been reported, but the long-term significance of such supplementation remains obscure. Such factors as the increase in urinary calcium loss due to a high intake of protein, the decreased absorption of calcium with advancing age (which may negatively affect a person's adaptability to low calcium intakes), and the bone loss that results in animals on a high intake of phosphorus would suggest that dietary modifications in susceptible people appear prudent. Because white women of small stature have the highest risk of developing osteoporosis, it has been suggested that they should consume liberal amounts of calcium and avoid excessive intake of phosphorus from the fifth decade on.[2,25]

Because of the apparent ability to adapt to a wide range of calcium intake, the existence of calcium deficiency due to inadequate dietary intake has been questioned in the past.[26] Recent studies, however, of school age children in South Africa have revealed hypocalcemia, hypocalciuria, elevated alkaline phosphatase concentrations, and in some cases, radiologically detectable bone defects, in association with low calcium intakes.[27,28] These changes are characteristic of vitamin D-deficiency rickets in younger children, but no evidence of vitamin D inadequacy has been found. Supplementation with calcium has resulted in rapid restoration of serum calcium to normal levels and in a gradual fall in the concentration of alkaline phosphatase.[28] Other recent reports have suggested calcium deficiency as a possible cause of rickets.[29,30] Hypophosphatemia due to inadequate phosphorus intake is unlikely but can develop from prolonged ingestion of nonabsorbable antacids.[31]

## Magnesium

Magnesium in the body (Table 6-1) is divided between the bone and other tissue; about 50% to 60% is combined with calcium and phosphorus in the structure of the bone, while most of the remainder is found in the cells of the body. The highest concentration occurs in muscles and red blood cells. Magnesium is second to potassium as the chief cation in all living cells. Extracellular fluid magnesium accounts for about 1% of the total body magnesium.

### Absorption, storage, and excretion of magnesium

The factors that control the intestinal absorption of magnesium are poorly understood. In humans, magnesium is absorbed mainly in the jejunum and the ileum and probably involves an active transport mechanism.[32] The level of magnesium intake influences its absorption; as intake increases, the percentage absorbed decreases.[33] There is also competition between magnesium and calcium for mucosal uptake; a high level of one decreases the absorption of the other. Other factors known to decrease magnesium absorption include high intake of phosphates, and steatorrhea. Substances that increase the mucosal uptake of water also enhance the absorption of magnesium.[32]

Renal excretion of magnesium is the major regulator of magnesium metabolism. The level of plasma magnesium is maintained relatively constant at about 1.7 mEq per liter (2–3 mg per dl normal range).[33] High intake of magnesium increases its urinary excretion and does not alter the plasma level. When the intake of magnesium is low, the urinary excretion falls to an almost undetectable level and, with a very low or prolonged low intake, the concentration of magnesium in plasma decreases. A sizable fraction of the magnesium in bone is adsorbed onto the hydroxyapatite crystals and appears to be available in magnesium deficiency by way of a physical equilibrium with the extracellular fluid magnesium. However, no specific mechanism for active mobilization of magnesium comparable to that of calcium is known to exist. The ability to mobilize bone magnesium decreases with age. Bone and extracellular fluid magnesium are not readily exchanged with the magnesium in the soft tissues. Although magnesium is found in the various fluids secreted into the intestine (bile, pancreatic juice, intestinal fluid) it appears to be reabsorbed efficiently; as a result, fecal magnesium represents mostly unabsorbed mineral. Magnesium in sweat can account for 10% to 25% of total magnesium loss during continuous exposure to high temperatures.[32,33]

### Functions of magnesium

Magnesium has a vital role in practically all major metabolic pathways of the body. It functions as an activator of enzymes (about 300 are known) involved in the hydrolysis and transfer of phosphate groups from ATP and other compounds containing high-energy phosphate bonds. For this reason, it is indispensable in the formation and use of ATP and, consequently, in the release of food energy and in the synthesis of new tissue and other essential substances required by the body. The use and storage of carbohydrate, fat, and protein in the body involve many reactions that are magnesium-dependent. For example, hexokinase catalyzed conversion of glucose to glucose-6-PO$_4$

$$glucose \xrightarrow[\underset{ATP \quad ADP}{Mg^{++}}]{hexokinase} glucose\text{-}6\text{-}PO_4$$

is the essential first step both in the release of energy from glucose and its storage as glycogen (see Fig. 9-9, Chap. 9). The magnesium dependency of the synthesis of both DNA and RNA provides another example of the biologic significance of magnesium. It is also an activator of alkaline phosphatase, an enzyme involved in calcium and phosphorus metabolism.

In addition to its metabolic functions, magnesium is involved in the binding of RNA to the ribosomes for protein synthesis, in the maintenance of the structural integrity of cellular membranes and macromolecules (such as DNA and RNA), and in neuromuscular transmission and activity.

### Magnesium deficiency

The intestinal absorption and the renal excretion of magnesium appear to be so well balanced in healthy people that magnesium deficiency rarely occurs as a result of low magnesium intake. However, magnesium depletion may occur in various conditions that either impair its intestinal absorption or increase its urinary excretion. Chronic diarrhea, steatorrhea, and other malabsorptive syndromes, chronic alcoholism, diabetes, prolonged fasting, and acute renal failure (with polyuria) are frequently associated with magnesium depletion. Hypomagnesemia in diabetics may be one of the risk factors in the development of diabetic retinopathy.[34] Magnesium depletion of iatrogenic origin may occur as a result of omitting magnesium in intravenous fluids or from extended periods of treatment with diuretics.

Magnesium deficiency leads to impairment of calcium and potassium homeostasis. Hypocalcemia and hypokalemia have been observed in both experimentally produced[35] and disease-related[36] magnesium deficiency. These disturbances seem to be at least partially caused by hypomagnesemia-induced changes in the production and function of the parathyroid hormone. Depression of serum magnesium initially may stimulate the parathyroid gland to produce more PTH, but as the deficiency becomes more severe, the sensitivity of the parathyroid gland to a decrease in serum calcium is impaired, and the level of PTH output is low in relation to the degree of hypocalcemia. In addition, a skeletal resistance to the action of PTH appears to develop. As a result, the mobilization of bone calcium, which is an essential mechanism for maintaining the level

of serum calcium, is impaired, and a hypocalcemic state persists. It should be noted that there are conflicting reports about the level and involvement of PTH in magnesium deficiency.[32,35]

The symptoms of magnesium deficiency are similar to the tetany seen when blood levels of calcium are reduced. There is hyperneuromuscular activity which, if untreated, results in convulsive seizures, as well as cardiac arrhythmia, or even cardiac arrest. Administration of magnesium is required to reverse the symptoms and to correct the secondary hypocalcemia and hypokalemia. Treatment with calcium without magnesium is ineffective and undesirable because in magnesium deficiency there is a tendency to deposit calcium in the soft tissues, especially the kidneys.[35]

The observed relationships between high levels of magnesium intake and the decreased incidence of calcium deposits in soft tissues[37] and the possible reduced susceptibility to cardiovascular disease await further research.

### Dietary requirements and food sources of magnesium

The recommended dietary allowances for magnesium are 350 mg per day for adult men and 300 mg per day for women. During pregnancy and lactation the recommended allowance is 450 mg per day. Allowances for infants and children are based on the magnesium content of human milk and cow's milk.

Magnesium is widely distributed in foods; it is a part of the chlorophyll in green vegetables and is also found in cocoa, nuts, cereal grains, meat, milk, and seafood. Table 4, Part 4, gives the magnesium content of various foods.

The recommended dietary allowance for the adult woman for magnesium (300 mg) is met by the pattern dietary of 1400 calories. The additional foods necessary to meet energy requirements further supplement the magnesium intake of the adult man (see Table 6-2 and Chap. 11). However, the magnesium content of the average American diet has been estimated to be only about 120 mg per 1000 kcal, which would make it difficult for those with low caloric requirements to meet the RDA for magnesium, especially during pregnancy.

Seelig,[38] in reviewing the published data on magnesium, has suggested that diets in Western countries, which contain less magnesium (less than 5 mg per kg per day) than oriental diets (more than 6 mg per kg per day), may be marginal in their magnesium content. There is also evidence that bone magnesium is not readily available for replacment in soft tissues when dietary magnesium is severely reduced. These two factors have contributed, no doubt, to the magnesium deficiencies observed in patients with certain clinical conditions where magnesium intake or absorption have been decreased or magnesium excretion has been increased, as previously discussed.

***Magnesium salts*** taken by mouth are both diuretic and laxative. The cathartic action is due to the slow absorption of magnesium from the intestines and the consequent drawing of water into the gut. Although the normal kidneys can readily excrete excess magnesium taken in the form of magnesium-containing drugs, a combination of long-term, high intake and impaired renal function may lead to hypermagnesemia, which adversely affects the functioning of nerves, muscle, and heart.

## Major trace elements

Many inorganic elements occur in animal tissues in extremely small quantities and are known as micronutrients or trace elements.

The essentiality of some micronutrients has been clearly established while that of others is under investigation. Mertz[39] has suggested a variety of criteria to determine essentiality, such as the presence of a trace mineral in healthy tissue. If the element also appears in the fetus and the newborn, an even better case is made for its nutritional need. Additional evidence is provided if the body maintains homeostatic control over the rate of its excretion or uptake into blood or tissues. Consistent changes in blood levels, tissue concentrations, or distribution within a metabolic pool as a result of physiologic activity further affirm its essentiality, as does the identification of the element in an enzyme or as the activator of an enzyme. Finally, animal studies provide the most conclusive evidence. If specific symptoms can be produced as a result of the total or partial absence of the element and then alleviated by its addition to the diet, the element can be considered essential.

As a result of changes in our food supply, there is currently some concern about the adequacy of trace elements in the American diet. The increased consumption of highly refined, processed, and fabricated foods can reduce the amount of a trace mineral present in the diet. The development of new varieties of foods and changes in fertilization practices, processing techniques, and equipment can also alter the concentration of trace minerals; the net effect of such changes is unknown.

The interrelationships among these elements also present problems in assessing needs. Because they occur together in varying amounts in the diet, their absorption from the intestinal tract may be dependent on their relative concentrations, which could affect their excretion and their tissue concentration as well. The interactions of the trace minerals might be synergistic or antagonistic; for this reason, the amount of any one element could depend on the amount of other essential or nonessential elements or other constituents in the diet.

### Iron

There is less than 5 g of iron in the body of a healthy adult, but its importance to our wellbeing is strikingly out of proportion to the quantitative requirement. In the body 60% to 70% of the iron is found in hemoglobin; iron stores in the liver, spleen, and bone marrow (as ferritin and hemosiderin) account for the next largest concentration of iron (30% to 35%). Small but essential amounts of iron are found in muscle myoglobin, in transport form (bound to protein-transferrin) in the blood serum, and in every cell as a constituent of heme enzymes (notably cytochromes, oxidase, peroxidase, and catalase) and other enzymes involved in cellular respiration (iron-containing flavoproteins and iron-sulphur proteins).

#### Hemoglobin synthesis

Iron is a necessary constituent of the hemoglobin of red blood cells. Hemoglobin is a conjugated protein composed of four iron-containing heme groups attached to four polypeptide chains, which make up the globin moiety. The heme is responsible for the characteristic color and the oxygen-carrying capacity of blood. Hemoglobin combines with oxygen in the lung capillaries to form oxyhemoglobin, which travels in the bloodstream to the tissues where the oxygen is released to take part in oxidative processes. Part of the carbon dioxide formed is carried back by the same hemoglobin, which drops its load in the lungs and starts out with a new supply of oxygen.

The synthesis of hemoglobin (approximately 800 g in the adult human) proceeds concomitantly with the maturation of the red blood cell in the bone marrow and lasts the "lifetime" of the cell—120 days. When the erythrocyte disintegrates, the reticuloendothelial cells, particularly those of the liver, spleen, and bone marrow, are responsible for the removal of the hemoglobin, the breakdown of the heme, and the release of the iron, which is then made available for reuse.

Hemoglobin synthesis depends on the presence of copper. The discovery of the catalytic action of copper in the use of iron for elaboration of hemoglobin was dramatic because it supplied the first proof that one inorganic element can function in the utilization of another; copper is not present in the hemoglobin molecule but functions in the mobilization of iron for use in the synthesis of heme. Adequate protein must also be available for synthesis of the globin fraction. Other dietary essentials, especially ascorbic acid, vitamin E, and vitamin $B_{12}$, influence the rate of destruction of the red blood cells.

#### Myoglobin

Myoglobin, found only in the muscle tissue, is related to blood hemoglobin in both structure and function. It is an oxygen carrier that serves as a reservoir of oxygen to the muscle cells and in the removal of carbon dioxide.

#### Cellular iron

Iron has an important role in cellular metabolism as an active component of various enzymes, especially those associated with the respiratory chain of the mitochondria (see Chap. 9). Nonheme iron is found in NADH dehydrogenase and succinate dehydrogenase, which are iron-flavoproteins of the respiratory chain. The cytochromes are the final carriers of electrons from flavoproteins to oxygen by alternate oxidation and reduction of the heme iron. This ready interconvertibility between reduced (ferrous, $Fe^{++}$) and oxidized (ferric, $Fe^{+++}$), forms of iron appears to be involved in all enzymatic functions of iron. Other iron enzymes include catalase, which is found in blood and liver and is one of the enzymes that destroy hydrogen peroxide ($H_2O_2$), aconitase of the citric acid cycle, and proline and lysine hydroxylases, which function in collagen synthesis.

### Iron absorption, transport, storage, and losses

Physiologic control of iron balance is primarily achieved by regulating iron absorption from the gastrointestinal tract. Significant amounts of iron are absorbed into the intestinal (duodenum) mucosal cells within 4 hours after ingestion. Body iron status and iron demand determine the magnitude of iron absorption under any given set of conditions, but the actual rate of uptake is influenced by the form and level of dietary iron and by the composition of the meal in which it is consumed. In healthy people with adequate iron stores and intake, iron is absorbed at a rate that tends to maintain the body iron content at a relatively constant level. A more liberal intake decreases the percentage of absorption, but more iron is absorbed than from a lower intake, and the amount of storage iron increases. In iron deficient people the rate of absorption may be two to three times that in healthy people. Gastric acidity is essential for solubilization of food iron and its conversion to an absorbable form. Although it has been generally assumed that only ferrous iron can be absorbed, definite proof still is lacking about the form in which iron enters and leaves the mucosal cell. Factors such as ascorbic acid, sugars, and amino acids both enhance reduction of ferric to ferrous iron and form low-molecular iron chelates, which increase the absorption of iron from neutral or slightly alkaline duodenal contents in which ferric iron would otherwise be poorly soluble. Although iron can be absorbed from the lower parts of the small intestine, the rate of absorption decreases as the alkalinity of the luminal contents increases. It has been suggested that the enhancement of iron absorption in iron deficiency and hemochromatosis (excessive amounts of iron deposited in the tissues) may be at least partially due to a reduced level of gastroferrin, an insoluble gastric iron-protein chelate, which presumably prevents iron absorption.[40] However, even the existence of gastroferrin has been questioned.[41] There may be other as yet unidentified gastric or intestinal substances that play a role in the control of iron absorption.

The mechanisms of iron uptake in the epithelial cells and its transport to the blood remain poorly understood. Once inside the mucosal cell some iron passes through rapidly, is released to the blood, and bound to a transport protein to form transferrin. Some iron combines with apoferritin to form ferritin, the storage form of iron, which may be available either for later release to the blood or retention in the mucosal cell. This iron is lost when the cell is sloughed off and excreted in the feces. Dietary iron occurs in two forms, as heme and nonheme or inorganic iron. Intestinal absorption of the heme iron found in the hemoglobin and the myoglobin of meat, fish, and poultry employs a mechanism different from that involved in the absorption of nonheme iron, but the details of the process are not known. Heme appears to be absorbed intact, followed by the release of iron within the mucosal cell. The absorption of heme iron is more efficient and less influenced by physiological and dietary factors than the absorption of nonheme iron.[42]

In healthy people, about one-third of the plasma iron-binding capacity (*apotransferrin*) is saturated (*transferrin*). Each transferrin molecule binds two atoms of iron in ferric form. In iron deficiency or when there are increased demands for iron (as in pregnancy), the total iron-binding capacity of plasma increases. When there is less iron, and more binding sites are available, the percentage of transferrin saturation is low. On the other hand, in hemochromatosis the iron-binding capacity is drastically reduced, and transferrin saturation is high.

The means by which the intestinal mucosa senses the body's iron status is not clear. According to current belief, transferrin in some way incorporates a signal of the body's iron status into the newly formed mucosal cells (renewed every 2–3 days), perhaps by the amount of iron that it brings to these new cells, and the mucosal cell then regulates both the uptake of iron from the lumen and its release to the blood.[41] This theory is consistent with the normal function of transferrin, which is to deliver iron not only to the bone marrow for hemoglobin synthesis, but to all other cells for their use and, in some instances, for storage. Transferrin receives its iron either from the intestinal absorption of dietary iron, from storage, or from hemoglobin breakdown and distributes it according to the needs of different tissues. Specific cell–surface receptors appear to be involved in the release of iron from transferrin to the cells.[41] Through reuse of the iron that is freed when the red cells disintegrate, body iron is conserved and continuously recycled. As a result, the actual daily use of iron by an individual far exceeds that supplied by the dietary intake for the same period, as is shown in Figure 6-2.

Iron is stored as two protein-iron complexes, ferritin and hemosiderin. The major storage sites include the parenchymal cells of the liver and the reticuloendothelial cells of the bone marrow, spleen, and liver. Hemosiderin is the more concentrated form of storage iron, and its proportion to ferritin increases at high levels of iron stores. Mobilization of the iron stores and the transfer of iron to transferrin during intestinal absorption and hemoglobin

## Iron Pathways in the Body

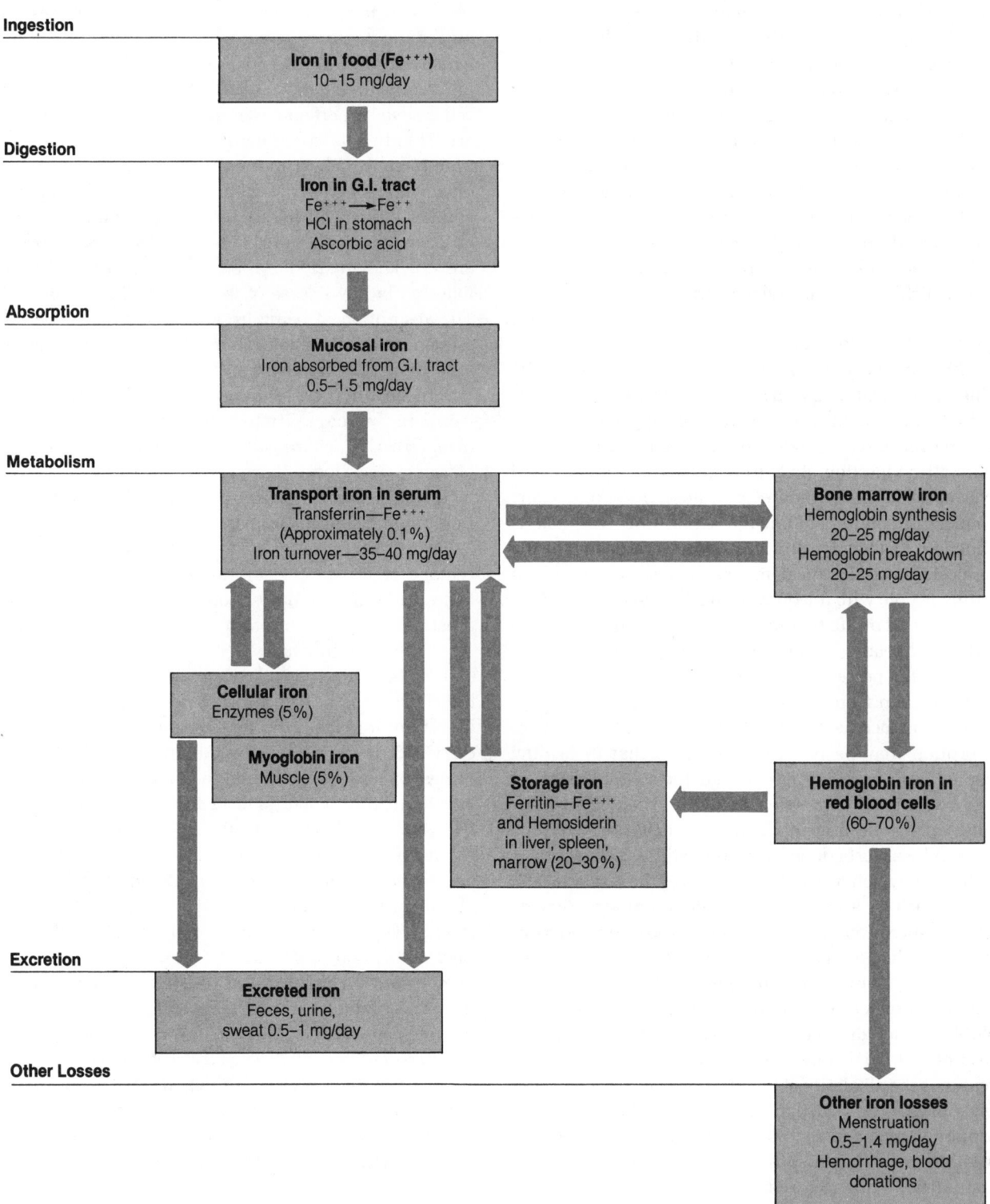

**Fig. 6-2.**   Schematic diagram of iron pathways in the body. Figures in parentheses indicate approximate percentage of total body iron in each compartment. Average amounts of iron consumed, absorbed, turned over in the body, and excreted per day are also included.

breakdown involve one or more changes in the oxidation state of iron (which must be in ferric form to combine with transferrin); these changes are facilitated by several other nutrients, including copper, ascorbic acid, and riboflavin.[43]

Small amounts of absorbed iron are lost daily. Most of this loss occurs in stools as sloughed mucosal cells and unabsorbed biliary iron. The remainder is lost by desquamation of skin and by urinary excretion (which is very low normally), with total losses amounting to 0.5 mg to 1.0 mg per day. The blood lost during menstruation by women of childbearing age causes an additional loss of iron, which, when averaged per day, varies from 0.5 mg to 1.4 mg. Major losses of iron also occur as a result of hemorrhage or blood donation.

### Food sources and bioavailability of iron

The best food sources of iron are found in the meat, fish, poultry, and egg group. Green, leafy vegetables, potatoes, dried fruits, and enriched bread and cereal products are the best plant sources. Milk and milk products are conspicuously low in iron (Fig. 6-3). Foods, such as molasses and raisins, popularly considered good sources of iron, are rich on a percentage basis, but small servings of these foods used infrequently do not constitute as important a source of food iron as some staple foods, for instance, whole grains or enriched breads and cereals (Fig. 6-4). The iron content of common foods is given in Table 1, Part 4.

It is now well recognized that the availabilities of iron from heme and nonheme sources are different and that the composition of the meal consumed with iron has a major influence on the absorption of nonheme iron.[42] On the average, about 40% of iron in meat, fish, and poultry is heme iron (hemoglobin and myoglobin). Although less influenced by the level of body iron stores than nonheme iron, the availability of heme iron varies from approximately 25% in people with 500-mg iron stores to about 35% in those with very low or no iron stores. The nonheme fraction of iron intake comes from the remainder of iron in meat, fish, and poultry, and all food iron from other sources, for example, eggs, grains, vegetables, and fruits, and the iron salts in supplements.

Studies have also indicated wide differences in the availability of iron from various compounds used for enrichment and supplementation. Iron is most available from ferrous sulfate and the ascorbate, fumarate, and citrate iron complexes. Iron is least available from iron phosphate, carbonate, and EDTA complexes. (Ethylenediamine tetraacetic acid is a chelating and sequestering agent that forms water-soluble complexes with many different cations in solutions.) The availability of iron from reduced or elemental iron is intermediate, depending on the size of the particle in the preparation.[44]

The common characteristic of all nonheme forms of iron is that their bioavailability is modified by the components of the foods ingested at the same time. For example, the absorption of nonheme iron from a single food can vary greatly, depending on the other foods with which it is consumed in a meal. The two dietary factors that are known to increase substantially the absorption of nonheme iron are ascorbic acid and an unknown "meat factor." In contrast to an "animal protein factor," this meat factor is present in beef, lamb, pork, chicken, liver, and fish, but not in milk, cheese, or eggs.[42]

Monsen and co-workers[42] have developed a method for the estimation of absorbable food iron based on the quantity of the enhancers present in each meal. As shown in Table 6-4, meals are classified as low, medium, and high availability meals, according to the percentage of absorption of nonheme iron that they provide. The values vary with the level of iron stores, but it is recommended that ordinarily, the level of absorption should be calculated with adequate iron stores (500 mg), although a large number of women are believed to have inadequate iron stores in contrast to high stores in men. It should be noted that the absorption of heme iron also varies with the level of iron stores, but not with the composition of the meal.

To calculate available iron from a day's intake, one must separate the heme and nonheme iron for each meal and snack, classify the level of iron availability (Table 6-4), then apply the appropriate factors to convert the total heme iron and nonheme iron of the meal or snack to available iron. Recently, a slightly simplified method of calculation was proposed by Monsen.[45] Instead of calculating the heme and nonheme iron, each meal or snack is separated into MFP iron (meat, fish, or poultry) and other iron. Combined factors for total available iron (heme + nonheme) are applied to the MFP iron. Assuming MFP iron to be 40% heme and 60% nonheme iron, the following combined factors can be used: 14%, 12.2%, and 11%, respectively, for high, medium, and low availability meals (with 500-mg body iron stores). The availability factors from Table 6-4 for the nonheme iron (8%, 5%, and 3%) are then used to calculate the other iron. See Table 6-5 for a sample calculation. Also see Table 15, Part 4.

There are also substances that decrease iron absorption when present in sufficient amounts. These include tannic acid in tea, phosvitin in egg yolk, and phytates in grains. Various calcium and phosphate salts, EDTA, and antacids also belong to this category. While there is some evidence that high fiber intake decreases the absorption of iron,[47] the impact of diets high in foods containing fiber on the bioavailability of iron is not defined well enough to assess its practical significance. Figure 6-5 demonstrates both the enhancing and suppressing effects of some individual foods when added to a standard continental breakfast.[46,47]

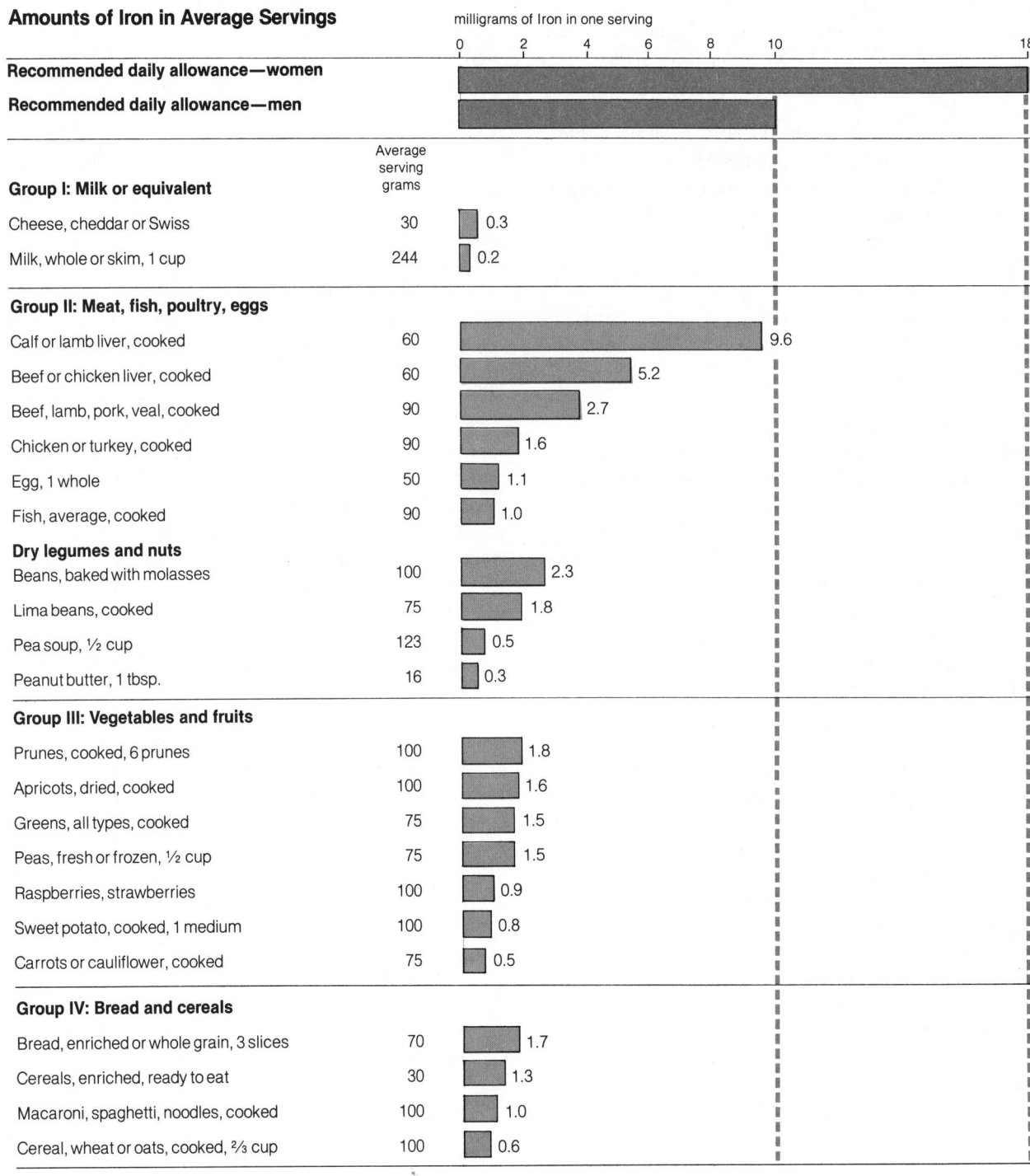

## Amounts of Iron in Average Servings

milligrams of Iron in one serving

| Food | Average serving grams | mg Iron |
|---|---|---|
| **Recommended daily allowance—women** | | 18 |
| **Recommended daily allowance—men** | | 10 |
| **Group I: Milk or equivalent** | | |
| Cheese, cheddar or Swiss | 30 | 0.3 |
| Milk, whole or skim, 1 cup | 244 | 0.2 |
| **Group II: Meat, fish, poultry, eggs** | | |
| Calf or lamb liver, cooked | 60 | 9.6 |
| Beef or chicken liver, cooked | 60 | 5.2 |
| Beef, lamb, pork, veal, cooked | 90 | 2.7 |
| Chicken or turkey, cooked | 90 | 1.6 |
| Egg, 1 whole | 50 | 1.1 |
| Fish, average, cooked | 90 | 1.0 |
| **Dry legumes and nuts** | | |
| Beans, baked with molasses | 100 | 2.3 |
| Lima beans, cooked | 75 | 1.8 |
| Pea soup, ½ cup | 123 | 0.5 |
| Peanut butter, 1 tbsp. | 16 | 0.3 |
| **Group III: Vegetables and fruits** | | |
| Prunes, cooked, 6 prunes | 100 | 1.8 |
| Apricots, dried, cooked | 100 | 1.6 |
| Greens, all types, cooked | 75 | 1.5 |
| Peas, fresh or frozen, ½ cup | 75 | 1.5 |
| Raspberries, strawberries | 100 | 0.9 |
| Sweet potato, cooked, 1 medium | 100 | 0.8 |
| Carrots or cauliflower, cooked | 75 | 0.5 |
| **Group IV: Bread and cereals** | | |
| Bread, enriched or whole grain, 3 slices | 70 | 1.7 |
| Cereals, enriched, ready to eat | 30 | 1.3 |
| Macaroni, spaghetti, noodles, cooked | 100 | 1.0 |
| Cereal, wheat or oats, cooked, ⅔ cup | 100 | 0.6 |

**Fig. 6-3.**   Iron in average servings of foods classified according to the four food groups.

### Dietary requirements for iron

Iron requirements are determined by the demands for tissue growth and hemoglobin accretion and by the need to replace iron lost in the urine, feces, and sweat and in the female in menstruation, pregnancy, and lactation.

The three periods of greatest demand for iron are during the first 2 years of life, adolescence, especially in girls, and the childbearing period. Due to individual variation in absorptive capacity, the differences among foods' availability of iron for absorption, and the ability of the body to

## Sources of Iron

**Percentage of Distribution**

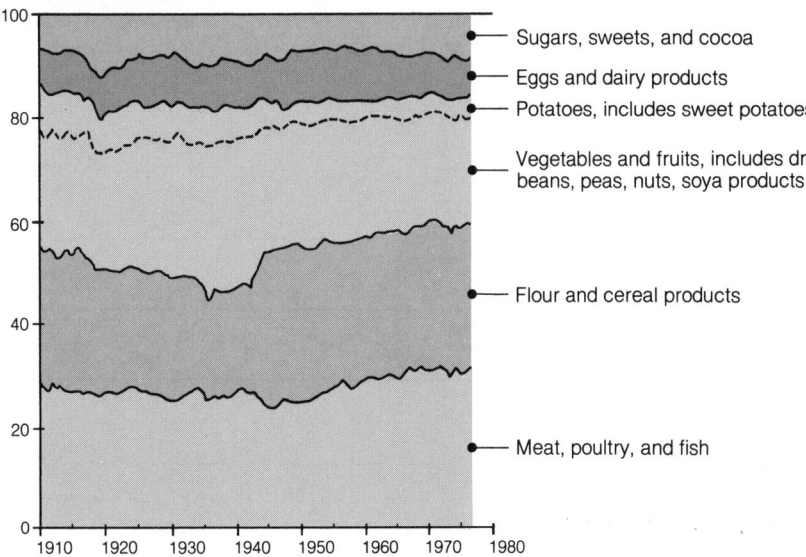

- Sugars, sweets, and cocoa
- Eggs and dairy products
- Potatoes, includes sweet potatoes
- Vegetables and fruits, includes dry beans, peas, nuts, soya products
- Flour and cereal products
- Meat, poultry, and fish

Per capita civilian food supply. 1977 preliminary data.

**Fig. 6-4.**   Sources of iron. (U.S. Department of Agriculture, Agricultural Research Service)

increase iron absorption during periods of deficiency, it is difficult to convert physiological requirements for iron into dietary allowances. Therefore, the United States' recommendations for iron set by the Food and Nutrition Board of the National Research Council and those set by the Joint FAO/WHO Expert Group differ although based on the same considerations.

The FAO/WHO Expert Group established the recommended level of absorbed iron for each age and sex group, then based their recommended, actual intakes on the percentage of animal food calories in the diet (Table 6-6).[48] It should be noted that, although it was recognized that the availability of iron was improved by the presence of animal foods in the diet, much of the current information was not available at the time these recommendations were established. As a result, the percentage of iron absorption from diets containing less than 10% of total calories from animal foods (including milk and eggs) was assumed to be 10%, which appears high on the basis of current information. On the other hand, the recommended intake of absorbable iron for the menstruating woman assumed a higher total iron loss (2.8 mg) than has been used by the Food and Nutrition Board of the National Research Council in establishing the RDA for American women (1.8 mg).[5] The recommended iron intakes for the United States' population (Table 6-7) still are based on an average absorption of 10% of total iron intake, but in its 1980 revision the Board recommended that calculation of absorbable iron, as discussed in the previous section, be used in the planning and evaluation of diets. For an ade-

quate diet the amount of absorbable iron multiplied by 10 should equal the RDA for iron.

***Adults.***   The recommended allowance is 10 mg (1.0 mg absorbed iron) per day for men and 18 mg for women. After menopause, the sex difference in the iron

### Table 6-4. Availability of Iron in Different Meals at Varying Levels of Storage Iron (Percentage of Absorption)

| | Iron Stores (mg) | | | |
| --- | --- | --- | --- | --- |
| | Women | | | Men |
| | 0 | 250 | 500 | 1000 |
| I. Heme iron | 35 | 28 | 23 | 15 |
| II. Nonheme iron | | | | |
| A. Low availability meal <30 g (1 oz)* meat, poultry, fish <25 mg ascorbic acid | 5 | 4 | 3 | 2 |
| B. Medium availability meal 30–90 g (1–3 oz) meat, poultry, fish *or* 25–75 mg ascorbic acid | 10 | 7 | 5 | 3 |
| C. High availability meal >90 g (3 oz) meat, poultry, fish *or* >75 mg ascorbic acid *or* 30–90 g (1–3 oz) meat, poultry, fish *plus* 25–75 mg ascorbic acid | 20 | 12 | 8 | 4 |

*Raw meat, poultry, or fish.

(Adapted from Monsen ER et al: Am J Clin Nutr 31:134, 1978)

## Table 6-5. Calculation of Available Iron from a Typical Day's Intake

| Time of Day | (1) Food/Beverage (in Meal/Snack Groupings) | (2) Wt. (g) | (3) MFP* Iron (mg) | (4) Other† Iron (mg) | (5) Ascorbic Acid (as served) (mg) | (6) MFP (g) | (7) Availability of Meal Iron — H | M | L | (8) Available MFP Iron (mg) | (9) Available Other Iron (mg) | (10) Total Available Iron (mg) |
|---|---|---|---|---|---|---|---|---|---|---|---|---|
| 7:30 a.m. | Oatmeal, 1 cup | 240 | | 1.4 | | | | | | | | |
| | Brown sugar, 1 T | 9 | | 0.3 | | | | | | | | |
| | Milk, 1 cup | 245 | | 0.1 | 2 | | | | | | | |
| | Orange juice, 6 oz | 187 | | 0.2 | 90 | | | | | | | |
| | Wheat toast, one slice | 21 | | 0.8 | | | | | | | | |
| | Honey, 1 T | 21 | | 0.1 | | | | | | | | |
| | SUBTOTALS | | 0 | 2.9 | 92 | 0 | ✔ | | | 0 | 0.23 | 0.23 |
| 10:30 a.m. | Coffee, 1 cup | 180 | | 0.2 | | | | | | | | |
| | SUBTOTALS | | 0 | 0.2 | 0 | 0 | | | ✔ | 0 | 0.01 | 0.01 |
| 1:00 p.m. | Tuna sandwich | | | | | | | | | | | |
| | tuna, 1-1/2 oz | 45 | 0.9 | | | 45 | | | | | | |
| | wheat bread, two slices | 50 | | 1.6 | | | | | | | | |
| | Carrot sticks | 50 | | 0.3 | 4 | | | | | | | |
| | Radishes | 50 | | 0.5 | 12 | | | | | | | |
| | Banana | 200 | | 1.0 | 14 | | | | | | | |
| | SUBTOTALS | | 0.9 | 3.4 | 30 | 45 | ✔ | | | 0.13 | 0.27 | 0.40 |
| 4:00 p.m. | Coffee | 180 | | 0.2 | | | | | | | | |
| | Peanuts | 10 | | 0.2 | | | | | | | | |
| | SUBTOTALS | | 0 | 0.4 | 0 | 0 | | | ✔ | 0 | 0.01 | 0.01 |
| 6:45 p.m. | Pork loin chop, lean with fat, 3 oz | 85 | 3.0 | | | 85 | | | | | | |
| | Baked potato, one | 202 | | 1.1 | 31 | | | | | | | |
| | Green peas, 1/2 c | 80 | | 1.5 | 10 | | | | | | | |
| | Tossed salad | 80 | | 1.6 | 6 | | | | | | | |
| | Applesauce, 2/3 c | 170 | | 0.9 | 2 | | | | | | | |
| | Ginger snaps, three | 21 | | 0.5 | | | | | | | | |
| | SUBTOTALS | | 3.0 | 5.6 | 49 | 85 | ✔ | | | 0.42 | 0.45 | 0.87 |
| 10:00 p.m. | Hot cocoa, 1 c | 250 | | 1.0 | 0.3 | | | | | | | |
| | SUBTOTALS | | 0 | 1.0 | 0.3 | 0 | | | ✔ | 0 | 0.03 | 0.03 |
| | TOTAL AVAILABLE IRON | | | | | | | | | | | 1.55 |

**Total Available Iron  = 1.6 mg**

*MFP: Meat, fish, or poultry.

†Other Iron: all food iron, except MFP IRON.

(USDA, Agricultural Research Service: Nutritive Value of American Foods in Common Units. Agriculture Handbook No. 456. Washington, DC, Superintendent of Documents, Nov. 1975. In Monsen ER: Food Nutr News 51:1, Mar-Apr, 1980)

requirement no longer exists. The basic pattern dietary of 1400 calories (Table 6-2) provides 10.3 mg of iron, which, therefore, meets the RDA for the adult man and postmenopausal woman. Although the additional foods chosen to supply extra energy increase the amount of iron slightly, they are not likely to meet the allowance of the menstruating woman. Because usual food patterns (5–6 mg iron per 1000 kcal) will not supply this amount of iron, many suggestions have been made to ensure an adequate intake of iron by women of childbearing age, adolescents, and children. They include supplementation with an iron compound, of which a variety are available; a return to iron cookware, which does not seem practical at the present time; and an increase in the use of whole grain flours. Increasing the levels of enrichment in cereal products has been proposed but has met with considerable opposition and postponement. The years of debates and hearings have resulted in a minor increase in the level of iron enrichment of bread and flour, from 11 mg to 12.5

mg per lb of bread and from 13 mg to 20 mg per lb of flour, effective July 1, 1981. The Board considers it impossible to meet the additional iron needs during pregnancy from the diet and recommends a 30-mg to 60-mg iron supplement per day. In order to replenish the iron stores, continuing supplementation for 2 to 3 months after delivery is advised.[5]

***Children.***   During the period of rapid growth, when an increase in red cells and hemoglobin is taking place, provision for new material, as well as replacement of old, requires a more liberal supply of iron. The anemias of infancy and childhood are evidence of the shortage that frequently occurs, although nature seems to have provided for the period of nursing. Milk is essentially low in iron, but a reserve of this mineral provided by the high hemoglobin level of the infant at birth is economically conserved for repeated utilization. The potential shortage of iron that may occur by the sixth or seventh month may be forestalled by the use of iron-fortified formulas and the introduction of fortified infant cereals and other suitable sources of iron into the infant's diet by his sixth month.

Recent research has demonstrated that the availability of iron from human milk is unusually high.[49,50] The factors responsible have not been identified. Despite the low iron content of human milk, breast-feeding has been estimated to be adequate to meet the iron needs during the first year of life because of the high bioavailability of this iron.[50] Addition of supplemental foods to the diet of the breast-fed infant, however, reduces the absorption of iron from human milk,[51,52] which argues against early introduction of solid foods when the supply of breast milk is adequate (see also Chap. 18).

### Iron Absorption

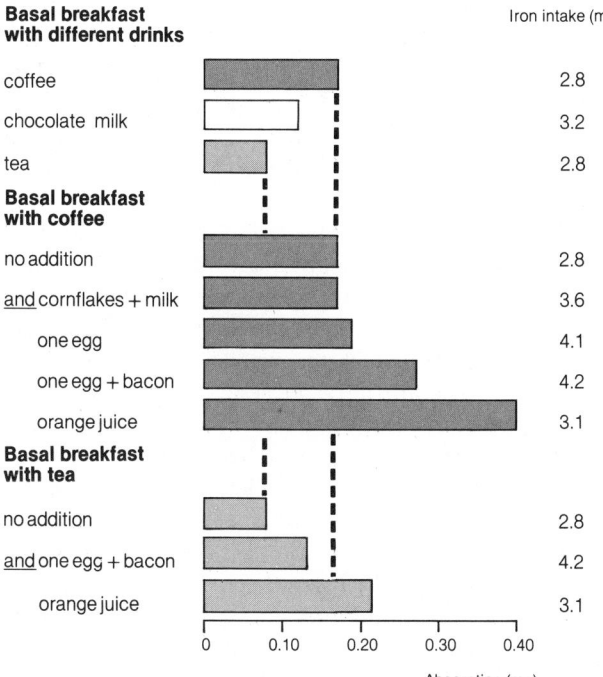

**Fig. 6-5.**   Absorption of iron from different breakfast meals. The values represent absorption in subjects having a 40% absorption from oral reference doses of ferrous ascorbate (3 mg Fe). The vertical dotted line represents the absorption of iron from a standard continental breakfast with coffee. Note that substitution of tea for coffee reduces the absorption of iron by more than 50%. Inclusion of an egg increases the total amount of iron absorbed slightly but not in proportion to the amount of iron added to the meal. Orange juice more than doubles the absorption of iron from the standard meal with coffee. The positive effect of orange juice is partially counteracted by the negative effect of tea. (Adapted from Rossander L et al: Am J Clin Nutr 32:2484, 1979)

### Table 6-6.  Joint FAO/WHO Expert Group Recommended Daily Intakes of Iron

| | | Recommended Intake According To Type of Diet | | |
|---|---|---|---|---|
| | *Absorbed Iron Required (mg)* | *Animal Foods Below 10% of Calories (mg)* | *Animal Foods 10%–25% of Calories (mg)* | *Animal Foods over 25% of Calories (mg)* |
| *Infants 0–4 months* | 0.5 | * | * | * |
| *5–12 months* | 1.0 | 10 | 7 | 5 |
| *Children 1–12 years* | 1.0 | 10 | 7 | 5 |
| *Boys 13–16 years* | 1.8 | 18 | 12 | 9 |
| *Girls 13–16 years* | 2.4 | 24 | 18 | 12 |
| *Menstruating women †* | 2.8 | 28 | 19 | 14 |
| *Men* | 0.9 | 9 | 6 | 5 |

*Breast feeding is assumed to be adequate.

†For nonmenstruating women the recommended intakes are the same as for men.

(From a joint FAO/WHO Expert Group Report: Requirements of ascorbic acid, vitamin D, vitamin B₁₂, folate, and iron. WHO Tech Rep Ser, No. 452, Geneva, World Health Organization, 1970)

***Adolescents.*** Few data are available for the requirements of this age group. The recommended allowance of 18 mg was estimated on the assumption that an adolescent's needs are at least as great as the adult woman's. Menstruation in adolescent girls means loss of hemoglobin and, consequently, an increased demand for all blood-building elements. Boys, who are growing rapidly at this age, also need iron for hemoglobin building.

Failure on the part of many people to meet these recommended allowances for iron was evident in the Ten State Nutrition Survey[53] and in the Health and Nutrition Examination Survey (HANES),[54] which reported a high incidence of iron-deficiency anemia in the population surveyed.

Adequacy of iron nutrition is assessed most frequently by measuring the level of hemoglobin or hematocrit of whole blood, because of the simplicity of these measurements. However, they are neither specific nor sensitive to iron deficiency. More specific methods of assessing iron status include determinations of plasma iron level (50–150 mcg per dl normal range) and transferrin saturation (20%–55% normal range), which decrease when iron stores are depleted and are affected before changes in hemoglobin level are detectable; the level of free erythrocyte protoporphyrin, which increases when sufficient iron is not available for heme formation; and plasma ferritin, which varies with body iron stores and provides a noninvasive method for estimating the level of iron stores.[55]

### Table 6-7. National Research Council's Recommended Daily Dietary Allowances for Iron

|  | Age Years | Iron mg |
|---|---|---|
| *Infants* | 0.0–0.5 | 10 |
|  | 0.5–1.0 | 15 |
| *Children* | 1–3 | 15 |
|  | 4–10 | 10 |
| *Men* | 11–18 | 18 |
|  | 19–51+ | 10 |
| *Women* | 11–50 | 18 |
|  | 51+ | 10 |
|  | Pregnant | * |
|  | Lactating | * |

*The increased requirement during pregnancy cannot be met by the iron content of habitual American diets nor by the existing iron stores of many women; therefore the use of 30–60 mg of supplemental iron is recommended. Iron needs during lactation are not substantially different from those of nonpregnant women, but continued supplementation of the mother for 2–3 months after parturition is advisable in order to replenish stores depleted by pregnancy.

(From National Research Council: Recommended Dietary Allowances. Washington, DC, 1980)

## Iodine

Iodine was one of the first micronutrients to be recognized as vital to nutrition, and it is still considered one of the most important.

Common goiter has been known since prehistoric times, but it was not recognized as a deficiency disease until the late 19th century. Baumann discovered iodine in the thyroid gland in 1895, and from then on iodine was used more or less as a preventive or curative treatment for endemic goiter. Before that time burnt sponge (a good source of iodine) had been a popular remedy.

Not until 20 years after Baumann's discovery was serious attention given to iodine as prophylaxis against goiter in large population groups. No doubt action was stimulated by the high incidence of goiter among draftees from certain states during World War I.

### Metabolism and function of iodine and thyroid activity

Before surveys were made of the iodine content of soil, it had been noted that the disease of common goiter was unevenly distributed over the United States and that it seemed to be most prevalent in the regions where there was the least iodine. This early suspicion was confirmed, and we now recognize that common goiter is primarily an iodine deficiency disease.

An essential constituent of the thyroid gland in humans and in animals, iodine in sufficient quantity must be supplied if that gland is to synthesize enough of the hormones thyroxine ($T_4$) and triiodothyronine ($T_3$) to function normally.

Dietary iodine is absorbed from the gastrointestinal tract as iodide ($I^-$) and is rapidly distributed throughout the extracellular fluid. Approximately one-third of the absorbed iodide is removed by the thyroid gland, and the remainder is excreted in the urine. There is no renal conservation of iodine in response to low intake, but the thyroid gland can recycle some of its own iodine supply and, if needed, the iodide released from other tissues from degradation of the thyroid hormones. Of the estimated 25 mg of iodine in an adult, 10 mg to 15 mg is found in the thyroid in *thyroglobulin*, an iodinated glycoprotein, which serves as a reserve of the thyroid hormones.

Iodide is taken up by an energy-dependent process into the epithelial cells that surround the colloid-filled follicles of the gland where it immediately enters the pathway of thyroid hormone synthesis. After undergoing an oxidative activation, iodide is incorporated into tyrosine residues of thyroglobulin to form *mono-* and *diiodotyrosine*, then these compounds are coupled to complete the synthesis of thyroxine and triiodothyronine. The iodinated thyroglobulin is stored in the follicular colloid and, when needed, the hormones are released through proteolytic degradation of thyroglobulin by lysosomal enzymes of the follicular cells. The remaining iodinated tyrosine residues undergo enzymatic deiodination, and the liberated iodide is reused for hormone synthesis. Thyroid activity is controlled by the thyroid-stimulating hormone (TSH) of the anterior pituitary. When the level of circulating thyroid hormones declines, a hypothalamic thyrotropin-releasing factor (TRF) stimulates the release of TSH, which, in turn, signals the thyroid gland to increase its activity, as is shown in Figure 6-6. When iodine supply is not adequate to maintain normal synthesis of thyroid hormones, continuous thyrotropic stimulation leads to both hypertrophy and hyperplasia of the follicular cells in an attempt to produce more hormone. The resulting enlargement of the thyroid gland is known as *simple goiter.*

$T_4$ and $T_3$ are transported in plasma by two specific transport proteins, *thyroxine-binding globulin* and *thyroxine-binding prealbumin*. This protein-bound iodine (PBI) appears to serve as a plasma reserve for the much smaller fractions of active $T_4$ and $T_3$, which circulate freely. The level of $T_3$ is small compared to that of $T_4$, but the latter is deiodinated by tissues to form both active $T_3$ and its inactive isomer, known as *reverse $T_3$*. Triiodothyronine is the more potent of the two hormones and may be the major functioning thyroid hormone in the tissues.

Iodine itself has no known metabolic function, but the effects of the thyroid hormones are many, although not well characterized. The thyroid hormones regulate the metabolic rate of the body through their effect on the oxidative reactions; hyper- and hypothyroidism are reflected in high or low basal metabolic rates, respectively (see Chap. 10). At high concentrations, the overall effects of thyroid hormones are catabolic, whereas in moderate concentration they are anabolic. They are essential for normal tissue growth and differentiation. Protein synthesis is facilitated both at the nuclear level by increased synthesis of RNA and at the ribosomal level by stimulation of the translation process. Administration of thyroxine also stimulates the intestinal absorption of glucose and lowers the level of cholesterol in the blood.

Severe thyroid hormone deficiency in adults can lead to *myxedema*, which is associated with distinct bodily and facial changes. Thyroid insufficiency during fetal development may cause *cretinism*, which is characterized by retarded physical and mental development.

## Natural food sources of iodine

The fact that goiter is not evenly distributed throughout the world or even within the United States indicates that some areas must provide natural protection through food or drinking water. People who live near the coasts and consume generous amounts of seafood get an adequate amount of iodine from these sources. In Japan, where seaweed as well as other seafoods in wide variety

**Regulation of thyroid hormone production**

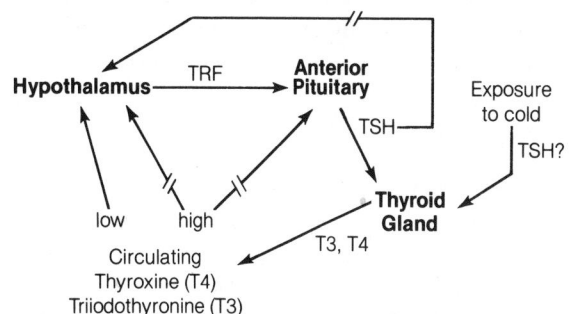

**Fig. 6-6.** Regulation of thyroid hormone production. Declining level of circulating hormones results in release of TRF (thyrotrophin-releasing factor or TSH-releasing factor) from the hypothalamus. TRF stimulates the production of TSH (thyroid-stimulating hormone) from the anterior pituitary. TSH increases thyroid activity, including $I^-$ uptake, hormone synthesis, and release. Exposure to cold also stimulates thyroid activity, but it is not known whether this is a direct action on the gland or is mediated by TSH. Note the negative feedback control by high levels of TSH, T4, and T3 as indicated by the broken arrows.

are popular, the iodine intake is estimated to be 0.5 mg to 1.0 mg per day. The incidence of goiter in Japan is the lowest of any country in the world.

The iodine content of milk, other dairy products, and eggs varies with the composition of the animals' feed. The amount of iodine in bread varies with the mixing process used. One slice of bread made by the continuous mix process will supply the daily iodine requirement, while one slice made by the batch process contains very little. It is not easily determined which process has been used for any individual slice of bread.

Because growing plants absorb iodine when it is present in the soil, plant foods vary widely in iodine content according to the soil in which they are grown. For example, plant foods grown near seacoasts and in our Southern states contain more iodine than those grown in the Great Lakes area or other regions where the surface soil is low in iodine. For this reason, it is impossible to list the iodine content of foods in tables of food composition or to estimate the amount in the pattern dietary. Urban markets today abound in foods grown in many different geographic regions, so there is less likely to be a severe iodine deficiency even in so-called goitrous regions. It is a very different situation where rural people confine their diet chiefly to home grown products in mountainous regions where the soil is notably low in iodine. It should also be noted that iodized salt is not used in many commercially prepared foods; for this reason the extensive use of these products with low or no iodine may contribute to the problem of goiter. Similarly, when salt is purchased in bulk, as it is in many institutions like schools and hospitals, it is usually not iodized. On the other hand, there is evidence that the intake of iodine in the United States is increasing, due to many indirect sources of iodine in the food chain.[5]

### Dietary allowances for iodine

The recommended dietary allowance set for iodine in 1980 is 150 mcg per day for adult men and women. An increase to 175 mcg per day for pregnancy and to 200 mcg per day during lactation is recommended. Because the need for iodine during growth is great, the recommendations for children are proportionately higher than those for adults (see Chap. 11). The recommended intake of adults is met by consumption of 2 g of iodized salt (74 mcg per g).

The importance of including the recommended level of iodine in infant formulas and other food products that are used as sole maintenance diets is stressed. Although daily iodine intake up to 1000 mcg is considered safe, there is some concern that chronically high intake, as from regular consumption of kelp (an iodine-rich seaweed) in some popular weight-reducing regimens, may be harmful to some people who are more sensitive to iodine than most of the population.[56] Ironically, goiter and even myxedema can be produced by chronically high iodine intake as well as by iodine deficiency.

### Goiter prophylaxis

The suggestion was made by Marine and Kimball that iodine might be administered to children in goitrous regions as a preventive measure. Consequently, as an experiment, iodine was administered to school children in Akron, Ohio, with remarkably successful results. By a similar project, in three cantons in Switzerland the incidence of goiter was diminished during 3 years from 87% to 13%. These demonstrations suffice to show that the body requirements for iodine, although they are exceedingly small, must be met in order to prevent goiter. Many sections of the country, notably the East Coast and the Southern states, as well as California on the West Coast, need pay little attention to this factor because iodine is indigenous. However, in the goitrous regions this is a problem requiring attention. Michigan has led the way in its solution by promoting education in goiter therapy as a public health measure.

***Administration of iodine*** as a prophylactic measure against goiter had to be planned as a public health activity so that it would reach all people in an area in safe but significant amounts. The use of tablets either at home or in school was impractical, and the addition of iodine to drinking water was too expensive. Common salt is used by nearly everyone in somewhat comparable amounts.

Therefore, a small percentage of an iodine compound was added to table salt to be marketed in goitrous regions, and an educational campaign was conducted to inform people why they should buy and use iodized salt.

This plan was adopted by Michigan in 1924, and all salt manufacturers in the state put on the market a table salt containing 0.02% of sodium iodide. Eleven years later the results of this plan adopted by the Michigan Department of Health far exceeded the hopes of those who instigated it. Endemic goiter or enlarged thyroid had become nearly extinct.[57] The decrease in the sale of iodized salt that has occurred since publicity on the subject has fallen off is paralleled by a slight increase in the number of goiters in school children. The discontinuance of iodized salt in one county in Michigan was followed by a marked rise in the incidence of goiter within 3 years. A 1959 to 1965 survey in Michigan found goiter in 6.6% of the 9000 people examined, and the incidence was higher in women than in men.[58]

In states where the use of iodized salt was not encouraged, the incidence of thyroid enlargement has remained fairly constant over the same period of years. The Ten-State Survey (1968–1970) did not identify iodine deficiency as a significant problem in the populations surveyed.

***Goitrogens,*** substances found in certain foods, possess antithyroid activity and, if consumed regularly in large quantities, can induce goiter, especially if the intake of iodine is low. Although the action of goitrogens cannot be prevented by iodine (they inhibit hormone synthesis), a liberal supply of iodine can provide some degree of protection against goitrogen-induced goiter, as does cooking foods which contain these substances. Common foods that contain one of the most potent goitrogens, *goitrin*, include Brussels sprouts, cauliflower, broccoli, rutabaga, and rape seed meal.[59]

## Zinc

Zinc occurs in animal and plant tissue in slightly smaller amounts than iron. The human body contains about 2 g of zinc, highly concentrated in the hair, skin, eyes, nails, and testes, but some is found in all human tissues and fluids and in all subcellular fractions. Because of their large mass, muscle and bone tissues contain about 90% of the total body zinc.

### Absorption, Transport, and Excretion

In the blood, the concentration of zinc is highest in the white cells, followed by that in the red cells and serum. The normal serum concentration averages about 100 mcg per dl and does not show any sex or age differences with the exception of the first 2 years of life during which there appear to be several highs and lows in the level of serum zinc until it finally stabilizes at about 2 years of age. Considerable diurnal variation has been observed at all ages. Approximately two-thirds of the serum zinc is in diffusible form, loosely bound to albumin which is in equilibrium with a small (2%) but active transport form present as Zn-amino acid complexes, mostly as Zn-cysteine and Zn-histidine. In this form zinc passes readily through the cell membranes and the blood–brain barrier.[60]

The maintenance of zinc homeostasis appears to be chiefly gastrointestinal.[61-63] With increasing intake, secretion of endogenous zinc into the intestine increases[64] and, although some is reabsorbed, fecal loss of endogenous zinc increases. Urinary excretion remains relatively stable at about 500 mcg per day within a wide range of intakes. Zinc loss in sweat is significant (approximately 115 mcg per dl) and can amount to 2 mg to 3 mg per day in extreme conditions.[60]

The intestinal absorption of zinc has been studied extensively during the past decade. Although much information has been gained, the details still remain uncertain and somewhat controversial. The absorption of zinc is concentrated in the duodenum, but some takes place throughout the GI tract.[60] The percentage of intake that is absorbed appears to vary highly (10%–90%; 20%–30% on the average), depending on the dose and presence of enhancing and inhibiting factors. A zinc-binding ligand believed to be responsible for the high efficiency of zinc absorption from human milk compared to cow's milk recently has been identified as *picolinic acid*, a metabolite of tryptophan.[64] Evans[64] has proposed that picolinic acid synthesized from tryptophan in a vitamin B-6-dependent pathway is secreted into the intestine in the pancreatic juice and participates in the absorption of dietary zinc by formation of Zn-dipicolinate, which then transports the metal through the epithelial membrane into the mucosal cell. Whether this ligand is further involved in the transport of zinc across the cell and in its release to the blood remains unclear. There is also evidence that an inducible protein ligand, metallothionein, is involved in regulating the passage of zinc through the mucosal cell, and that the body's zinc status influences the direction of movement of zinc from the mucosal cell.[61,63,65] Zinc-binding metallothionein has been demonstrated in other tissues, as well (liver, kidney), and although its role in zinc metabolism is uncertain, both detoxification and storage functions appear likely.[66]

It should be noted that there are other zinc-binding ligands in human milk, including citrate,[67] and that the physiologic function of picolinic acid remains to be confirmed.

Several lines of evidence support a role for picolinic acid in the intestinal absorption of zinc: zinc absorption is impaired by ligation of the pancreatic duct,[64] and it is increased by administration of either tryptophan or picolinic acid to rats on a low-protein diet.[68] Furthermore, Zn-dipicolinate has been found to be more effective than

zinc salts in treating *acrodermatitis enteropathica*, a rare hereditary zinc-deficiency syndrome in infants.[69] In breast-fed infants, the condition usually is not manifested until after weaning, and breast milk has been used to treat affected infants before the effectiveness of zinc supplementation was discovered in 1974. The specific defect in acrodermatitis enteropathica is still unknown, but impaired intestinal absorption of zinc appears to be involved.[64] (See Chap. 18.)

The presence of certain dietary factors in the intestinal lumen is known to enhance the absorption of zinc; these include the amino acids, histidine, cysteine, and methionine; vitamin C; and EDTA.[60] High concentrations of phytates, calcium, phosphorus, and cadmium decrease the absorption of zinc. The reduction in the bioavailability of zinc from soy protein appears to correlate with the concentration of phytate in soy protein.[70] There is an antagonistic relationship in the intestinal absorption of several trace elements, especially between zinc, copper, and iron.[71]

## Physiological functions and deficiency

When one considers the ubiquitous nature of zinc, it is not surprising that it appears to influence many body systems and functions, including growth, bone formation, brain development, behavior, reproduction, fetal development, sensory functions (taste, smell and, perhaps, vision), immune mechanisms, membrane stability, and wound healing. Although zinc-dependent enzymes participate in some fundamental metabolic reactions of the body, it is not obvious how the observed metabolic alterations are related to the pathology of zinc deficiency.

Some of the best known mammalian enzymes that contain zinc in their active site include pancreatic *carboxypeptidases*, which participate in the intestinal digestion of protein; *carbonic anhydrase*, which maintains a proper balance between carbon dioxide and the bicarbonate ion and thus affects $CO_2$ transport and exchange, the production of hydrochloric acid in the stomach, and the renal maintenance of acid–base balance (see Chap. 5); hepatic *alcohol dehydrogenase*, which is essential for the degradation of ethanol, and other similar dehydrogenases that oxidize alcohols, including *retinine reductase*, which converts retinol to retinal in the process of vision; *alkaline phosphatase*, which is a widely distributed nonspecific phosphate monoester hydrolase with a possible function in cellular phosphate transport and transfer as well as in bone mineralization; *superoxide dismutase* (also containing copper), which is a cytosomal enzyme that participates in the removal of highly reactive superoxide radicals and thus in the protection of cellular structures against oxidative damage (see Chap. 7, vitamin E). Numerous other enzymes are activated by zinc but also by other metals and, for this reason, may not represent primary metabolic functions of zinc.

The functions of zinc-dependent enzymes that participate in the synthesis and degradation of nucleic acids are not well defined at present, but probably represent the underlying mechanisms that are manifested in the observed effects of zinc in many systems. Dysfunctions in DNA and RNA metabolism and, subsequently, in protein metabolism, may result in impaired cell growth, differentiation, reproduction, and repair, depending on the specific nature and function of a particular tissue. Zinc may affect protein synthesis at more than one level and by several mechanisms, including the formation of polyribosomes and as part of an elongation factor.[72] In the synthesis of protein, individual proteins, such as collagen, may have further specific needs for zinc in the completion of their final structures.[60] Binding of zinc by DNA, RNA, and cellular membranes is believed to be essential for their structural and functional stability. The role of zinc in insulin action also appears to be related to the physical properties of the hormone-zinc complex. Although zinc-free insulin is active, the hypoglycemic action of zinc-insulin is more prolonged.[60] Numerous interactions between zinc and other hormones have been observed, but whether any of them represent primary functions of zinc remains to be established. Utilization of vitamin A is impaired in zinc deficiency. Evidence for zinc–vitamin A interactions is somewhat conflicting, but the need for zinc in the mobilization of liver vitamin A stores and in the utilization of vitamin A in vision is reasonably well established.[73] The possible role of zinc in the induction and growth of some types of cancer is of major interest and is under active investigation.[74,75]

Studies in the Middle East[76,77] first showed that zinc deficiency does occur in humans. The deficiency symptoms found in the population where zinc intake was presumed inadequate were dwarfism, hypogonadism, and iron deficiency anemia. Less severe states of zinc deficiency have since been observed in the United States. The accelerated rate of wound healing[78] and the improved sense of taste[79] observed after zinc supplements were administered indicate that zinc nutriture in the subjects studied was less than optimum. Marginal zinc deficiency was identified in a survey of children in Denver.[80] Of 150 apparently healthy children from middle income families, 8% displayed deficiency symptoms, which included low levels of zinc in the hair (below 70 mcg per g), impaired taste acuity, poor appetite, and suboptimal growth. When zinc intake was increased, the children showed improvement. The extent to which inadequate zinc nutrition might contribute to retarded growth of children is not known. Although several studies have shown a high incidence of low levels of plasma and hair zinc in growth-impaired children,[81,82] suggesting zinc deficiency as a possible cause of their poor growth, these measures of zinc status do not always correlate with growth in growth-retarded children.[83] Part of the problem undoubtedly can be attributed to genetic and other factors that affect growth and part to the inadequacy of the available measures of zinc status.[84] Although a progressive reduction in plasma zinc levels is observed in both naturally occurring and experimentally produced[85] zinc deficiency, a single determination of plasma zinc may be a poor measure of the body zinc status. In addition to diurnal variation, low zinc level can be associated with stress or disease-related hormone-mediated redistribution of zinc or with hypoalbuminemia or with a recent meal.[84] Lack of correlation between several measures of zinc status, such as plasma, hair, and saliva zinc, and taste acuity, also is common. As a result, it appears necessary to employ a battery of measures to assess adequately zinc nutriture. Only a response to zinc supplementation under carefully controlled conditions provides a definite diagnosis of zinc deficiency.

Low plasma zinc concentrations are common in acute and chronic infections, cirrhosis of the liver, chronic alcoholism, renal disease, protein-energy malnutrition, cardiovascular disease, pernicious anemia, sickle cell disease, some types of cancer, and in patients on extended parenteral feeding.[60] In chronic alcoholism greatly increased zinc excretion may occur even when serum levels are low and may result in zinc insufficiency.[60] Bone and muscle zinc do not appear to be easily mobilized; thus the available body zinc pool is limited, as is indicated by the rapid onset of symptoms from zinc deficient diets. Low calcium intake has been shown to alleviate the symptoms of zinc deficiency, presumably by increasing bone resorption, which makes bone zinc available to the body.[60]

### Requirement and food sources of zinc

In 1974 the Food and Nutrition Board set recommended dietary allowances for zinc for the first time. The average diet of the American adult had been estimated to contain approximately 10 mg to 15 mg of zinc, and metabolic studies indicated that this amount was adequate to maintain positive balance. Hence, the RDA for adult men and women was set at 15 mg per day. An additional 5 mg for pregnancy and 10 mg for lactation were recommended. Allowances were also established for adolescents (15 mg per day), children (10 mg per day), and infants (3 mg, 0–6 mo; 5 mg, 6 mo–1 yr) (see Chap. 11). No changes were made in the 1980 revision of the RDAs.

Animal products in general are important sources of zinc. Seafoods (especially oysters), meat, liver, eggs, and milk are good sources and contribute about 60% of total intake. Legumes and whole grain products, such as whole wheat bread, rye bread, oatmeal, and whole corn also contribute zinc to the diet (about 20% of total). Zinc from vegetable sources is less available to the body; for this reason, persons who consume primarily vegetable diets are at greater risk of zinc deficiency than those who include liberal amounts of animal foods. The zinc content of the pattern dietary has not been calculated because of the unavailability of adequate food analysis data for zinc. The USDA has published provisional tables on zinc in food (see Table 5, Part 4), which can be used until *Handbook 8* is completed.

There is some concern that the zinc content of the average American diet is not adequate to meet the adult allowance of the sizable segment of the population whose energy need is considerably below 3000 kcal per day. Two recent studies have concluded the average zinc intake to be between 4 mg and 5 mg per 1000 kcal, based on intakes from self-selected diets[86] and from a market basket survey.[87]

Although zinc toxicity appears to be relatively low, the Food and Nutrition Board warns against regular use of zinc supplements of more than 15 mg per day without medical supervision because a high intake of zinc may further impair a marginal copper status.

## Other essential trace elements
### Copper

The copper content of the adult human body averages 70 mg to 80 mg, of which about one-third is found in the liver and brain and the rest, in approximate order of decreasing concentration, in the heart, kidney, pancreas, spleen, lung, bone, and the skeletal muscle tissue.[43]

Copper-containing enzymes are involved in a number of reactions that affect a variety of tissues and body functions. Copper is required for mobilization of body iron, the production of normal erythrocytes, the synthesis of such specific tissue components as collagen, elastin, keratin, and phospholipids, the formation of the hair and skin pigment melanin, and the maintenance of cellular energy supply (ATP).[43,71]

The best known copper-enzymes include *ceruloplasmin*, also known as *ferroxidase I*, because of its enzymatic role in the oxidation of ferrous iron to the ferric form prior to its binding to transferrin. Other possible roles of ceruloplasmin include regulation of plasma and tissue levels of some biologically active amines, such as serotonin, epinephrine, and norepinephrine; it also serves as a specific source of copper for the cellular synthesis of *cytochrome c oxidase* (containing heme iron and copper). As the terminal enzyme in the respiratory chain, cytochrome c oxidase is involved in the production of cellular ATP. In copper deficiency, impaired phospholipid synthesis in some tissues is believed to be caused by an inadequate supply of ATP, due to low cytochrome oxidase activity. Consequently, processes such as myelinization of nerve cells may be defective. Copper deficiency also causes defects in the synthesis of connective tissue, presumably through reduced activity of *lysyl oxidase*, which functions in the formation of cross-links between the component peptide chains in collagen and elastin molecules. Forma-

tion of melanin pigment is reduced because of low *tyrosinase* activity. Other copper enzymes with less defined roles in the various manifestations of copper deficiency include the zinc-copper protein, *superoxide dismutase, dopamine beta hydroxylase, ascorbic acid oxidase*, and *delta-aminolevulinic acid oxidase*.[43,71]

Many cellular nonenzymatic copper-proteins have been detected, but their functions remain uncertain. A metallothionein-like protein present only in the livers of newborns is known as *hepatomitochondrocuprein* and appears to release its copper for the neonatal synthesis of ceruloplasmin, which is very low in plasma at birth.[43]

Intestinal absorption of copper is rapid and takes place primarily in the stomach and the duodenum. Some copper becomes complexed to amino acids and is believed to pass from the intestinal lumen to the blood through the active transport of amino acids. The major mechanism of copper absorption involves the delivery of copper to the absorptive surface by a copper-binding luminal protein, mucosal uptake and binding to metallothionein-like ligand(s), and release to the blood. Recent estimates suggest a 40% to 60% absorption of the intake, but variability is high, depending on the amount and form of ingested copper, and the presence of other competing and interfering dietary components. Of the other metals which interfere with copper by competing for mucosal metal-binding sites, zinc is of the greatest practical significance, especially when the intake of copper is low. Dietary cadmium, phytates, fiber, calcium carbonate, and ascorbic acid reduce the absorption of copper, as does the interaction between copper, molybdenum, and sulfate.[43]

Absorbed copper becomes loosely bound to plasma albumin and amino acids in the portal blood and is taken to the liver, which is the major site of copper metabolism and maintenance of copper homeostasis. Some copper passes in this form from the liver to the systemic blood and is readily available for cellular uptake by other tissues. This loosely bound "direct reacting" copper accounts for less than 10% of circulating plasma copper, but it has a rapid turnover and appears to serve as the major means for transport of copper. Over 90% of plasma copper is in ceruloplasmin. Average serum copper levels are higher in adult women (114.0±4.67 mcg Cu per dl) than in men (105.5±5.03 mcg Cu per dl). Serum copper levels also increase significantly in women both during pregnancy and when taking oral contraceptives. Elevated copper levels are found also in acute infections, leukemia, Hodgkin's disease, various anemias, hemochromatosis, myocardial infarction, and collagen diseases. Low serum copper levels are common in nephrosis, kwashiorkor, cystic fibrosis, celiac disease and other malabsorption syndromes, Wilson's disease, and Menkes' syndrome.[43]

The major route of copper excretion is in the bile. A considerable fraction of fecal copper is of endogenous biliary origin and copper from the desquamated mucosal cells. High copper intake does not significantly alter serum or urinary copper but increases biliary excretion. Urinary excretion of copper in normal people represents only 0.5% to 3% of intake, and sweat and menstrual losses are minor.[43]

On the basis of balance studies, the copper requirement of adults is estimated to be 1.5 mg to 2 mg per day.[88] Requirements for infants and children have been calculated between 0.05 mg and 0.1 mg per kilogram of body weight. The Food and Nutrition Board recommends 2 mg to 3 mg for adults and 0.08 mg per kilogram of body weight for infants and children as adequate and safe daily intakes of copper.

Copper intake is determined primarily by individual food selection. Crustaceans and shellfish, particularly oysters, and liver, kidney and brains, nuts, dried legumes, raisins, and cocoa are rich sources of copper. The amount of copper in green leafy vegetables, however, reflects to some degree the copper status of the soil. Copper contamination during processing, storage, and treatment of food also affects the total amount of copper ingested. Soft water contains more copper than hard water, and water from the tap contains more than reservoir water. However, the latter is a better source of copper than water taken directly from the stream.

Recent studies[89,90] suggest that daily copper intakes may be considerably lower (0.5 mg–2.0 mg per day) than the previously estimated average intake (2 mg–5 mg per day). There is also concern that a marginal copper intake in a diet with a high zinc to copper ratio may lead to copper deficiency. Evidence of elevated serum cholesterol levels in experimental animals made copper-deficient on diets low in copper and high in zinc has lead to postulation of mild copper deficiency as a possible etiological factor in atherosclerosis.[91] Although epidemiologic evidence relating the incidence of cardiovascular disease (CVD) to the dietary zinc to copper ratio has provided support for the hypothesis, more research is needed to clarify the possible role of copper nutrition in the development of CVD. Because copper is relatively nontoxic to man, toxicity from a dietary origin is unlikely, but the Food and Nutrition Board warns against long-term ingestion of amounts exceeding the recommended 2 mg to 3 mg range per day.

Although severe copper deficiencies of dietary origin are rare in humans, hypocupremia has been observed in protein-calorie malnutrition. Among malnourished children in Peru this was accompanied by anemia, neutropenia, and bone disease.[92] Some of the same symptoms have been observed in premature infants fed exclusively on modified cows' milk for 2 to 3 months and in infants after prolonged parenteral feeding.[93]

Menkes' "steely hair" or "kinky hair" syndrome is a severe congenital copper deficiency, which is inherited as a recessive X-linked trait. Progressive mental deterioration, defective keratinization of hair, low serum and liver copper levels, metaphyseal lesions, and degenerative changes in aortic elastin are characteristic features of the disease.

Although there appears to be a defect in the intestinal mucosal cell release of copper to the blood (uptake of copper to the mucosal cell is not affected), it is likely that transport or other defects are present elsewhere because early intravenous or intramuscular administration of copper has resulted in no inprovement in the disease (except in serum and liver copper levels), whereas response to copper in dietary deficiency is prompt.[43]

Wilson's disease is a recessive trait characterized by abnormally high tissue concentrations of copper, especially in the liver, brain, kidneys, and the cornea of the eye, and by very low serum copper level. Biliary excretion of copper appears impaired, and there may be an inability to synthesize ceruloplasmin. Recent research suggests that a defective metallothionein with an abnormally high affinity to copper may be the cause of the excessive storage of copper in the tissues. Early treatment with chelating agents to increase copper excretion is essential to prevent severe tissue damage from copper toxicity.[43]

### Manganese

Manganese plays essential roles in both plant and animal nutrition. Because of its presence in or activation of mammalian enzymes, it is presumed to be essential in humans.

The best known manganese metalloenzymes are *pyruvate carboxylase* and *superoxide dismutase.* The former functions in the biotin-dependent carboxylation of pyruvate to oxaloacetate, but it appears that when availability of manganese is limited, magnesium can replace manganese in this enzyme without appreciable change in its activity. The manganese-containing superoxide dismutase is assumed to have a role in the protection of mitochondria against oxidative damage, comparable to that of the zinc-copper enzyme in the cytoplasm.[94,95]

Manganese and other metals activate numerous enzymes in the pathways of carbohydrate, protein, lipid, and intermediary metabolism. That diverse metabolic alterations result from manganese deficiency in animals suggests that at least some of them represent physiologically important functions of manganese. Poor reproductive performance, growth retardation, congenital malformations in the young, defective bone and cartilage formation, impaired glucose tolerance, and delayed blood clotting are among the manifestations of manganese deficiency, but the actual expression varies with species, degree, and duration of the deficiency, and the stage of maturation of the animal. Many of the symptoms are believed to reflect the effects on mucopolysaccharide synthesis on the role of manganese in the activation of *glycosyltransferases.* A variety of mucopolysaccharides and glycoproteins are affected, ranging from those that form the organic matrix of cartilage to those involved in prothrombin formation for the clotting of blood. Manganese ions also influence the activity of *uricase* in urea synthesis and several enzymes in the pathways of cholesterol and fatty acid biosynthesis.[71] As one of the metal ions that bind to cellular macromolecules and membranes, manganese may play a role in the maintenance of their functional structures.[71]

Intestinal absorption of manganese generally is assumed to be low, and competing interactions have been demonstrated with iron and cobalt. High dietary calcium appears to reduce the availability of manganese, as is shown by increased fecal excretion and reduced retention in the liver. Absorbed manganese is taken to the liver in portal blood, possibly bound to an $\alpha_2$-macroglobulin. In the systemic circulation manganese is transported in a transferrin-like $\beta_1$-globulin designated as *trans-manganin*. Highly variable values have been reported as normal plasma manganese levels. Manganese levels are almost invariably highly elevated following a myocardial infarction. Plasma and liver mitochondrial manganese appears to be in equilibrium, and most of the body's manganese is in a dynamic, highly mobile state.[71]

The human body contains 10 mg to 20 mg of manganese, widely distributed throughout the tissues. It is found in high concentration in the mitochondria of cells and is also associated with melanocytes. Homeostatic control of manganese is regulated chiefly by its excretion in the bile; however, a regulatory role for intestinal absorption cannot be totally ruled out despite our limited knowledge of it. Two other routes of manganese excretion, which appear to become more important when the biliary route is blocked, include pancreatic juice and secretion by the mucosal cells from various segments of the small intestine.[71]

The minimum daily intake of manganese required to maintain balance in adults is not known, but 2.5 mg per day has been found adequate in balance studies. Because the estimated daily intake of 2 mg to 9 mg appears to be both adequate and safe, the Food and Nutrition Board recommends an average daily intake in the range of 2.5 mg to 5 mg for adults. Safe and adequate intakes for childhood and early adolescence are considered to be 0.08 mg and 0.06 mg per kilogram of body weight, respectively, with recommended daily total intake as follows: 1 mg to 1.5 mg for ages 1 to 3; 1.5 mg to 2 mg from 4 to 6 years; and 2 mg to 3 mg from 7 to 10 years of age. Manganese intake in infants fed exclusively either breast or cows' milk is low, but manganese deficiency in infants has never been reported. With the introduction of solid foods the intake of manganese increases appreciably. Daily intake of 0.5 mg to 0.7 mg is recommended for the first 6 months and 0.7 mg to 1 mg during the second half of the first year of life.

Nuts, whole grains, dried legumes, tea, and cloves are excellent sources of manganese. Fruits and vegetables are fair sources, depending on soil content. Blueberries tend to be the richest source in this group. Meat, fish, and dairy products are low in manganese.

Manganese deficiency has not been identified in humans, with the exception of one case in which impaired blood clotting was not corrected by vitamin K until manganese was also provided.[71]

A possible relationship between low intake of manganese and susceptibility to cancer has been proposed;[96] the significance of decreased activity of the manganese superoxide dismutase in tumor cells,[97] and the possible anticarcinogenic as well as carcinogenic effects of manganese are being investigated.[5] Association of low blood manganese levels to seizures has been postulated recently.[98]

## Fluorine

It has been recognized for some time that optimum quantities of fluorides are required for maximum resistance to dental caries. Only recently, however, has fluorine been identified as essential to animal growth. Rats raised in an isolated environment and fed very low levels of fluorine demonstrated an increase in growth when fluorine was added to their diets.[99]

Fluoride is deposited in both bones and teeth where it replaces the hydroxyl ion in hydroxyapatite $[Ca_3P_3O_8 \cdot Ca(OH)_2]$ and forms fluorapatite $[Ca_3P_2O_8 \cdot Ca(F)_2]$. The fluoride-containing teeth are more caries resistant and the bone less prone to resorption.

Although the principal protective effect against tooth decay is provided during the pre-eruptive phase of the teeth, further protection accrues to a continuous systemic or topical source of fluoride. Fluoride may also protect against periodontal disease and osteoporosis.

A total daily intake of 1.5 mg to 4 mg is recommended as adequate and safe for adults by the Food and Nutrition Board. An upper range of 2.5 mg was recommended for children and adolescents from 4 years on to prevent mottling of the teeth. Intakes from 0.1 mg to 1 mg were suggested during the first year of life and 0.5 mg to 1.5 mg during the subsequent 2 years. It was recognized that intakes within these ranges could not be met when the fluoride content of the water is substantially less than 1 mg per liter.

The fluoride content of foods varies widely according to where it is grown. However, this influence is reduced by the wide distribution of foods today. Dietary intake of fluoride from foods, exclusive of drinking water, varies not between low and high fluoride areas, but between areas of fluoridated and nonfluoridated water, averaging 2.63 mg $\pm$ 0.17 mg per day in the former compared to 0.91 mg $\pm$ 0.05 mg in the latter areas.[5,100] The difference is attributed to the contribution of fluoridated water in food preparation. Drinking water with 1 part per million (ppm) fluoride would add approximately 1 mg to 1.5 mg to the total intake, whereas only 0.1 mg to 0.6 mg would be obtained from water in the nonfluoridated areas. For this reason the total intake may vary from a low of approximately 1 mg per day to 4 mg per day, depending on the fluoride content of the water supply. The fluoride intake in the warm climates tends to be higher than in the colder regions because of the differences in the consumption of water, even by infants.[101]

Excess fluorine is recognized as the cause of mottled enamel in the permanent teeth of children in certain areas of the world. This condition is endemic in limited areas in the United States—for example, the Texas Panhandle and adjacent areas—and is commonly known as dental fluorosis. The mottling occurs when fluorine is present in the drinking water in excess of 1.5 ppm. In these same areas the low incidence of dental caries attracted attention. Subsequently, the relation of fluorine in local water supplies to the low incidence of dental caries has been well established. The question of finding a level of fluorine in drinking water low enough to eliminate mottled enamel but high enough to reduce the incidence of dental caries, had to be answered. It is now estimated that 1 ppm is about the critical level and that water supplies can be standardized by adding fluorine to bring the concentration up to 1 mg fluorine per liter of water.

If this amount is added to the water in a community, a reduction of 50% to 60% in dental caries in children may be anticipated. Large-scale experiments in several communities pointed the way to effective use of fluorine prophylaxis. Mass control of dental caries in children is possible and has been recommended by medical and public health authorities. Among the endorsers of fluoridation of water supplies naturally low in fluoride are the Food and Nutrition Committee of the NRC-NAS, The American Academy of Pediatrics Committee on Nutrition, the American Medical Association, the National Association of Dental Research, and the National Nutrition Consortium. Nevertheless, the advisability of fluoridation of the public water supply remains a controversial subject not only in the communities that are faced with a decision, but among the professionals as well.[102-104] (See further discussion of this subject in Chap. 21.)

There is also some evidence that fluoride is effective in the treatment of osteoporosis. Increased retention of calcium accompanied by a reduction in bone demineralization is observed in patients receiving fluoride salts.[105] In addition, the incidence of osteoporosis in women and aortic calcification in men is lower in areas where the drinking water has a high fluoride content.[106]

Fluoride appears to stimulate osteoblastic activity, thereby increasing bone mass. However, there is now concern about the breaking strength of the fluorotic bone which, even though dense, appears to be brittle. Negative

side-effects of continuous administration of relatively large doses of fluoride (up to 90 mg per day) include hypocalcemia and possible secondary hyperparathyroidism. It is hoped that combined fluoride-calcium therapy may prevent this problem.[2] However, it should be remembered that any treatment of osteoporosis remains exploratory until the cause of the disease is identified.

## Chromium

Chromium is associated with glucose metabolism, possibly as a cofactor for insulin.[107] An organic form of trivalent chromium, *glucose tolerance factor* (GTF), is believed to be the biologically active form of chromium. Present in high concentration in brewer's yeast, GTF appears to contain niacin, glycine, glutamic acid, and cysteine, but its structure continues to elude identification.[108]

Chromium is believed to function by facilitating the interaction of insulin with its cellular receptor sites, thereby enhancing its action in the peripheral tissues; the resulting increased cellular uptake of glucose is followed by metabolic changes that are associated with a high level of glucose, namely active synthesis of fatty acids and protein. There is some evidence to indicate that chromium influences protein and lipid metabolism independently of its effects on the utilization of glucose. A direct insulin-stimulated enhancement of the cellular uptake of certain amino acids and their incorporation into protein has been observed.[71]

The intestinal absorption and tissue distribution of different forms of chromium vary for reasons not yet understood. In general, less than 1% of inorganic chromium is absorbed compared to 10% to 25% of chromium from the brewer's yeast extracts, with an estimated 1% to 2% average availability from a varied diet. Intakes from Western diets have been estimated to vary from 50 mcg to 100 mcg per day, but much lower intakes are possible even from diets otherwise nutritionally adequate. Until more is known about the requirements and, especially, of the availability of dietary chromium, the Food and Nutrition Board recommends 50 mcg to 200 mcg per day as a safe and adequate intake of chromium by adults and adolescents, assuming an average availability of 1% to 2%. Comparable intakes for children were derived on the basis of estimated food intakes: 10 mcg to 40 mcg for the first and 20 mcg to 60 mcg for the second half of the first year; 20 mcg to 80 mcg from 1 to 3 years; and 30 mcg to 120 mcg from 4 to 6 years.[5]

Meats, cheeses, whole grains, and condiments are good sources of available chromium. It appears to be less available from the leafy vegetables and is very low from polished rice and refined flours and sugar. The chromium content of breast milk appears to be very low, with a reported mean of 0.39 mcg per liter for a group of healthy mothers.[109] The average daily intake of breast-fed infants has been found to be 0.27 mcg ±0.11 mcg. The authors suggest that the infant's needs during the first months of life may be met largely from fetal reserves, although a highly available form of chromium may also be obtained in human milk, as is the case with iron and zinc.

Newborn infants are known to have a low glucose removal rate (GRR), but chromium deficiency does not appear to be involved because supplementation with 250 mcg $CrCl_3$ during the first day of life does not influence the GRR during an intravenous glucose tolerance test performed on the following day.[110]

Existence of mild chromium deficiency in humans is suggested by demonstrations of chromium-responsive disturbances in glucose metabolism. In studies with human diabetic subjects, improved glucose tolerance tests (see Chap. 29) were reported following chromium supplementation for some subjects, whereas others did not respond.[108,111] Similar results (about 50% response) have been reported from chromium supplementation in the elderly. It is not known whether those who respond are chromium-deficient due to inadequate intake or have reduced ability to utilize dietary chromium for the formation of biologically active chromium. Chromium supplementation also has been reported to restore glucose tolerance in children suffering from kwashiorkor[112] or protein-energy malnutrition,[113] and in patients on extended parenteral nutrition.[114,115] Although decreased liver chromium and increased chromium absorption and urinary excretion by insulin-requiring diabetics have been reported,[108] a state of chromium deficiency has not been established definitely in any type of diabetic population. A relative chromium deficiency, even when it exists, is difficult to demonstrate due to a wide variation in the chromium content of body tissues and fluids among both healthy people and diabetics. Furthermore, there appear to be several seemingly independent body pools of chromium as indicated by lack of correlation among hair, plasma, red cell, or urine chromium in normal and diabetic men.[116]

Although the evidence is somewhat contradictory, administration of insulin or glucose appears to lead to a rapid increase in serum chromium level in healthy people but not in those with inadequate levels of available chromium.[111,117,118] A recent study suggests that serum chromium levels fall after a glucose load in subjects with inadequate chromium stores, and that the relative chromium response (RCR), that is, serum chromium level 1 hour after a glucose load/fasting serum chromium level × 100, is a useful indicator of chromium status.[118]

A possible relationship between chromium deficiency and cardiovascular disease has been postulated on the basis of limited epidemiologic and experimental evidence.[119] A recent study observed regression of cholesterol-induced atherosclerotic plaques in rabbit aortas after intraperitoneal administration of potassium chromate.[120] Although these findings are interesting, much remains to be learned about chromium metabolism in humans and of the possible consequences of inadequate chromium intake.

## Selenium

A biochemical role for selenium was demonstrated in 1973 when it was identified as a constituent of the metalloenzyme, glutathione peroxidase (GSH-Px).[121] The function of selenium is apparently complementary to the antioxidant effect of vitamin E (see Chap. 7) in protecting the integrity of cellular membranes. By reducing peroxides, GSH-Px decreases the formation of highly reactive free radicals and thereby provides an essential link in the body's protective mechanism against oxidative damage (see Fig. 7-10). It is not known whether the antioxidant activity of GSH-Px is responsible for all the possible functions of selenium.

Selenium is found in all tissues, with high concentrations in the liver, kidney, and heart and very low concentrations in the adipose tissue. Selenium occurs in proteins as seleno-analogs of sulfur amino acids (selenomethionine and selenocysteine) or else bound to proteins and, to a lesser extent, as smaller organic compounds. GSH-Px contains four atoms of selenium, presumably as selenocysteine, one molecule in each of the four peptide chains that make up the enzyme. Selenium also has been detected in many other highly purified proteins of diverse functions, for example cytochrome c, hemoglobin, myoglobin, myosin, and ribonucleoproteins, but it is not known what functions, if any, selenium has in these proteins.[72]

Intestinal absorption, tissue distribution, and retention of selenium are not well understood and appear to vary with the amounts and chemical forms of the ingested element. They are further influenced by the intake of other minerals, such as sulfur, mercury, arsenic, and cadmium. Absorption is generally efficient (44%–80%); selenium from plant sources may be more available than selenium from either animal products or from selenates and selenites, and it is poorly absorbed as elemental selenium or selenides.[71]

Selenium is excreted mainly in the urine and feces but on high intakes, substantial amounts may be lost in the breath. The urinary excretion correlates positively with the dietary intake and blood level of selenium. Excretion increases during catabolic stress, such as surgery. Plasma selenium concentration responds to dietary changes more rapidly than erythrocyte selenium and is considered a sensitive index to short-term changes in selenium status, whereas erythrocyte selenium and the GSH-Px activity are more indicative of long-term selenium nutrition.[122]

On the basis of current information, the Food and Nutrition Board suggested a range of 50 mcg to 200 mcg per day as adequate and safe intake of selenium by adults. Recommendations for other age groups were derived from this range on the basis of expected food consumption (see Table 11-3, Chap. 11). American diets balanced in the major nutrients provide selenium intakes within this range.

Seafoods, kidney, liver, and meat are good sources of selenium and vary less than grains, which are more directly influenced by the selenium content of the soil. Fruits and vegetables in general are low in selenium. However, the selenium content of plant foods can be significantly enhanced when grown in selenium-rich soils.

Selenium toxicity due to high dietary intake has not been seen in humans, but selenosis is a well-known problem with livestock consuming herbage from the seleniferous areas of the world.

A case of human selenium deficiency in a patient on total parenteral nutrition (TPN) in New Zealand has been reported.[123] The patient developed general muscle soreness and thigh muscle pain severe enough to make her unable to walk. The plasma selenium concentration was the lowest ever reported in humans and comparable to the levels found in selenium-deficient animals. A daily supplement of 100 mcg selenium as selenomethionine completely restored her mobility and removed all discomfort after 1 week of treatment. Low blood selenium levels without clinical symptoms were found also in other patients on TPN. Occurrence of muscular aches and pains has been described by a local physician as an endemic problem affecting 40% to 50% of the population in a low-selenium region of New Zealand,[123] but trials of selenium supplementation have been inconclusive, with similar frequencies of response in the supplemented and placebo groups.[124]

Recent reports from the Chinese Academy of Sciences provide evidence to suggest that the cardiac muscle in humans may be affected by selenium deficiency. Selenium supplementation with 150 mcg to 300 mcg (as sodium selenite) per week from 1974 through 1977 dramatically decreased the incidence of Keshan cardiomyopathy (with cardiac failure) among children given the supplement compared with children living in the same region who received a placebo. However, a similar dose of selenite was ineffective in a child with established cardiomyopathy whose plasma, and hair selenium levels were very low.[125] Epidemiologic evidence of a relationship between low selenium intake and different forms of cardiovascular disease is inconclusive at this time.

Both epidemiologic and experimental evidence suggest that high intake of selenium during the period of tooth development may increase the incidence of dental caries.[71]

Another area of interest and vital concern is the possible cancer-protecting effect of selenium. Some epidemiologic studies have shown a higher than normal incidence of certain cancers that affect the gastrointestinal tract in geographic regions of low selenium content, and others have found significant negative correlations of the dietary selenium intakes and blood selenium levels with the occurrence of specific cancers. Lower than normal blood selenium levels in cancer patients have been reported in some studies but not in others. Although anticarcinogenic effects of selenium have been observed in animals, the evidence to link low selenium status to development of any type of cancer in humans is still far from conclusive.[74,122] It has been suggested that the selenium status of patients with carcinoma most likely is related to their general nutritional status, and when low, is probably a consequence rather than a causal factor of their disease.[126,127]

## Molybdenum

Naturally occurring molybdenum deficiency has never been identified in humans or any animal species. Nevertheless, this element is considered to be an essential nutrient within the broad definition of essentiality because it is found in all body tissues and fluids and is a constitutent of at least three important mammalian enzymes, *xanthine oxidase*, *aldehyde oxidase*, and *sulfite oxidase*. Both xanthine and aldehyde oxidases are complex metalloflavoproteins, which in addition to molybdenum also contain iron and the riboflavin coenzyme, FAD, all of which are essential for the activity of the enzyme. The physiological significance of molybdenum is supported by the fact that lack of liver sulfite oxidase activity due to a genetic defect identified in one child was associated with severe physical and neurologic abnormalities and resulted in early death.[71]

Molybdenum is readily absorbed from normal diets, but the level of dietary sulfate or its metabolic precursors (sulfur-containing amino acids) can significantly alter the absorption and retention of molybdenum. High sulfate concentration is believed to block the transport of molybdenum through cell membranes, thereby reducing its intestinal absorption and renal tubular reabsorption, the latter resulting in increased urinary excretion of molybdenum. As was mentioned earlier in this chapter, the interaction between molybdenum and copper and among molybdenum, sulfate, and copper can significantly influence the utilization of copper. Research in humans has shown that increasing molybdenum intake from sorghum within a relatively low range significantly increased urinary losses of copper and probably its mobilization from the tissues, but did not alter the fecal loss.[128] Copper is presumed to become biologically unavailable through formation of insoluble complexes with molybdate or sulfate.[71]

Because molybdenum deficiency has never been observed, human requirements for molybdenum appear to be satisfied even from the most restrictive diets. Estimates from a limited number of studies suggest that molybdenum balance is maintained by most adults on daily intakes between 50 mcg and 100 mcg.[5] Early estimates indicated daily intakes between 100 mcg and 460 mcg, with an average of approximately 350 mcg, but recent studies indicate that the actual intakes are considerably lower. Calculated on the basis of a market basket analysis and the estimated food consumption (USDA consumption surveys), the daily molybdenum intakes were found to vary from 120 mcg to 240 mcg, depending on the age, sex, and income.[129] Regional differences in the molybdenum content of individual foods were minor. A daily intake from 150 mcg to 500 mcg was recommended by the Food and Nutrition Board as safe and adequate for adults. Because of their high molybdenum content grains and legumes are major contributors to the dietary intake of molybdenum, as are meats and poultry, which are consumed regularly in relatively large amounts.

Daily intakes of 10 mg to 15 mg of molybdenum by people living in a high selenium environment in the USSR are suspected of being causally related to the high incidence of a gout-like syndrome in this population.[5]

### Cobalt

Cobalt is a component of vitamin $B_{12}$, a nutritional factor necessary for the formation of red blood cells. Because humans and monogastric animals cannot utilize dietary cobalt to synthesize vitamin $B_{12}$, the nutritional requirement of cobalt is restricted to the body's need for this vitamin (see Chap. 8). Cobalt in relatively large doses is a nonspecific stimulant of erythropoiesis and to a limited extent has been used in the treatment of some types of anemias. Overdose in animals produces polycythemia, that is, excessive concentration of red cells, but the toxicity of cobalt both in humans and animals appears to be relatively low. A possible interaction between low levels of cobalt and iodine in the environment in relation to thyroid function and the incidence of goiter requires further investigation.[71]

## Recently identified essential trace elements

Nickel, tin, vanadium, and silicon have been identified as essential trace elements in laboratory animals raised in all-plastic isolated environments protected from metallic contamination. With the exception of tin, deficiencies for each of these elements have been confirmed in at least two animal species.[71] There is now evidence to suggest that silicon is required for connective tissue metabolism, probably as a constituent of mucopolysaccharides.[130] If confirmed, this function would make silicon essential for many vital body systems. Reduced bone collagen matrix appears to be the cause of abnormal skull development and other bone defects observed in chicks fed diets low in silicon.[131] Although widely ranging effects of vanadium and nickel have been reported, it is not possible to identify any specific physiological or biochemical functions for either trace element at this time. Whereas the contamination of foods and environment from tin, nickel, or vanadium is not considered a health hazard, *silicosis* is a serious respiratory disease affecting miners who inhale large amounts of silica particles. Formation of malignant tumors also is associated with inhalation of particles of silica and asbestos (silicates of complex composition).[71]

### Toxicity of other trace elements

Many trace elements, including several of those now established as essential nutrients for humans and animals, initially were investigated because of their toxicity to some form of animal life. One of the contributions that research of trace elements has made is the reaffirmation of the concept that nutrients essential for normal body function at lower levels of intake provide no further benefit or may even be toxic at higher levels of intake.

Although the biologic significance of many other trace elements known to be present in tissues remains uncertain, there is increasing public health concern about increasing environmental exposure to some of the more toxic elements, such as lead, cadmium, mercury, and arsenic.

*Lead* enters the body from air, food, and water, but home environment may contribute additional contamination. Lead paint on walls, woodwork, and toys, lead glazes on ceramics, and pewter containers may all contribute to the total lead intake and to the possibility of lead poisoning. Children between the ages of 1 and 6 years have been the main victims of lead poisoning, chiefly from the ingestion of flaking paint (pica) from old houses and apartments.[132] Of the children who survive lead poisoning, many are left permanently retarded or with neurologic handicaps.

Food is the major source of *cadmium* for most people; heavy smokers can receive significant amounts of cadmium from smoke inhalation. Intestinal absorption of cadmium is low (3%–8% of intake) compared with inhaled cadmium (10%–40%), but there is a gradual accumulation of cadmium in the tissues with age because its excretion is very slow.[71] Cadmium bound to metallothionein has been detected in both the liver and the kidney, but the significance of this compound in the body remains unclear, as mentioned in connection with several other trace minerals. Although evidence of cadmium requirement for growth in the rat has been reported,[133] further confirmation and elucidation of its possible physiological function is needed.

Studies by Schroeder on trace metals implicated cadmium in the development of hypertension in the rat, but proof of the relationship between cadmium and human hypertension is lacking. An extreme manifestation of chronic cadmium poisoning was seen in Japan, caused by

## Table 6-8. Summary of Mineral Elements in Nutrition

| Element | Rich Sources | Dietary Allowance for Adults | Function in the Body | Elimination |
|---|---|---|---|---|
| Calcium | Milk, cheese, some green vegetables | 0.8 g daily, 1.2 g in pregnancy and lactation | Bone and tooth formation; coagulation of blood. Regulates muscle contractibility including heartbeat; activates enzymes. | Urine and feces; some in sweat |
| Phosphorus | Milk, poultry, fish, meats, cheese, nuts, cereals, legumes | 0.8 g daily, 1.2 g in pregnancy and lactation | Bone and tooth formation; forms high-energy phosphate compounds for muscular and tissue cell activity; constituent of DNA, RNA, phospholipids, and buffer systems. | Urine and feces |
| Magnesium | Nuts, cereals, legumes, green vegetables, milk, meat | Women, 300 mg; men, 350 mg; 450 in pregnancy and lactation | Constituent of bone; enzyme activator for energy producing systems; regulates muscles and nerves. | Feces and urine; some in sweat |
| Iron | Liver, meat, legumes, whole or enriched grains, potatoes, egg yolk, green vegetables, dried fruits | Women, 18 mg; men, 10 mg; 30–60 mg supplement during pregnancy and for 2–3 mo after parturition recommended | Constituent of hemoglobin, myoglobin, and cellular enzymes. | Feces, small amounts in urine and sweat; menstruation blood loss |
| Iodine | Seafoods, water and plant life in nongoitrous regions; sodium iodide in iodized salt | 150 mcg daily; 175 mcg in pregnancy; 200 mcg in lactation | Necessary for formation of thyroid hormones. | Urine |
| Zinc | Seafoods, meat, liver, eggs, milk | 15 mg daily; 20 mg in pregnancy; 25 mg during lactation | Constituent of carbonic anhydrase and other metalloenzymes; growth; sexual maturation; wound healing; taste acuity. | Urine and feces; some sweat and dermal losses |
| Copper | Liver, nuts, legumes | Estimated safe and adequate intake 2.0–3.0 mg | Aids in utilization of iron in hemoglobin synthesis; constituent of many enzymes; electron transfer; connective tissue metabolism; phospholipid synthesis. | Chiefly in feces—bile |
| Manganese | Nuts, whole grains, legumes, tea, cloves | Estimated safe and adequate intake 2.5–5.0 mg | Synthesis of mucopolysaccharides, glucose utilization; constituent or activator of several enzymes. | Chiefly in feces—bile |
| Fluorine | Fluoridated water | Estimated safe and adequate intake 1.5–4.0 mg | Resistance to dental caries. | Urine, feces, and sweat |
| Chromium | Brewer's yeast, some animal products, whole grains | Estimated safe and adequate intake 0.05–0.2 mg | Glucose metabolism; cofactor for insulin. | Feces and urine |
| Selenium | Seafoods, kidney, liver | Estimated safe and adequate intake 0.05–0.2 mg | Cellular antioxidant as constituent of enzyme glutathione peroxidase. | Urine and feces; some in breath |
| Molybdenum | Whole grains and legumes | Estimated safe and adequate intake 0.15–0.5 mg | Constituent of several enzymes (purine and sulfur metabolism). | Urine and feces |

The information summarized here is given in more detail in text.

excessive ingestion of cadmium from foods contaminated by industrial pollution. *Itai-Itai disease*, as this form of cadmium poisoning was called, resulted when a sensitive population, low in both calcium and vitamin D, consumed rice and drinking water from a river that had been polluted. The disease was characterized by multiple painful fractures as a result of severe osteomalacia.

Of the many forms of *mercury*, methylmercury found chiefly in fish is the most toxic. Mercury from industrial sources dumped into water can be changed into methylmercury and consumed by the fish. If fish with high mercury levels are in turn consumed by humans, mercury poisoning, such as occurred in Minimata, Japan, can result. In this tragic incident of mercury poisoning from industrial pollution, most of the survivors were left with permanent neurologic damage.

*Arsenic* is another trace mineral that can be toxic in relatively small amounts. It is found in seafood and in the human body. It accumulates in hair and nails. The levels in food can be increased as a result of industrial contamination and from the use of arsenicals as insecticides and as additives to animal feeds. The minimum level of chronic exposure to arsenic that leads to toxicity is not well established, due to high variation in individual susceptibility and in the toxicity of different chemical forms of arsenic. Other trace minerals appear to be harmless in the amounts and forms found in foods. It is also important to emphasize that the safe level of an individual trace element can be affected by the amount of other trace minerals present in the environment. For example, zinc, copper, selenium, and calcium all appear to increase tolerance levels for cadmium. Indiscriminate ingestion of any mineral supplements is inadvisable due to the complexity of the possible interactions in the body.

## Study questions and activities

1. Explain the function of calcium in bones and teeth. What happens in growth if calcium and phosphorus are inadequate in the diet? Why are these two minerals usually discussed together?
2. Identify the major factors that control the plasma calcium concentration. Why does low calcium intake influence bone calcium more than plasma calcium?
3. How do plasma calcium and phosphorus concentrations relate to each other? What is the major mechanism for maintaining phosphorus homeostasis?
4. What is the significance of dietary Ca:P ratio? What is the recommended ratio for infants? For adults?
5. Milk is the single best source of calcium in the diet. See if you can write a diet that meets the calcium allowance for the adult, allowing cheese but omitting milk. Repeat, omitting both cheese and milk. Calculate the amounts of phosphorus and the Ca:P ratios in both these diets and compare with the recommended dietary allowance for the adult.
6. How does magnesium deficiency influence calcium and potassium utilization? Identify conditions that may lead to magnesium deficiency.
7. Identify the major physiological and dietary factors that influence the intestinal absorption of iron. How can meal planning serve to maximize the availability of dietary iron?
8. Compare the dietary intake of iron with the daily use of iron by the body and explain the difference. Why do men generally have larger iron stores and smaller iron requirements than women?
9. Identify the high-risk populations in regard to iron deficiency anemia. When is iron supplementation recommended and why?
10. Why is iodine deficiency most likely to occur in certain regions of the world? What has been the main contributor to the reduction in the incidence of goiter in the United States and other Western countries? Why is iodine supplementation sometimes ineffective in preventing goiter?
11. What are the manifestations of zinc deficiency in humans? What have been identified as the probable causes of zinc deficiency in the Middle East?
12. How does the zinc content of the average American diet compare with the recommended dietary allowance of zinc for adults?
13. How does copper influence the utilization of iron? Identify other physiological functions postulated for copper. Why is there some concern over the dietary ratio of zinc to copper?
14. Why is fluoride considered as an essential trace element for humans? How is this nutrient supplied to the body?
15. Identify the proposed biologically active form of chromium in the body. What specific population groups have been reported to respond to chromium supplementation?
16. Identify a common biochemical function for zinc, copper, and manganese.
17. How does molybdenum affect the utilization of copper?
18. What is the biologically active form of cobalt?
19. Identify four trace elements that are of more concern because of their toxicity than because of their nutritional significance.

## References

1. Posner AS: In Barzel DS (ed): Osteoporosis, pp 101–113. New York, Grune & Stratton, 1970
2. Draper HH, Bell RR: In Draper HH (ed): Advances in Nutritional Research, Vol 2, pp 79–106. New York, Plenum Press, 1979
3. FAO/WHO Expert Committee on Calcium Requirements: WHO Chron 16:251, 1962
4. Schaafsma G, Visser R: J Nutr 110:1101, 1980
5. Food and Nutrition Board: Recommended Dietary Allowances, 9th rev ed. Washington, DC, NAS-NRC, 1980
6. Pingle U, Ramasastri BV: Br J Nutr 39:119, 1978
7. Page L, Friend B: BioScience 28:192, 1978
8. Draper HH et al: J Nutr 102:1133, 1972
9. Sie T-L et al: J Nutr 104:1195, 1974
10. Spencer H et al: J Nutr 108:447, 1978
11. Bell RR et al: J Nutr 107:42, 1977
12. Linkswiler HM: In Hegsted DM et al (eds): Present Knowledge of Nutrition, 4th ed, pp 232–239. New York, Nutrition Foundation, 1976

13. Allen LH et al: Am J Clin Nutr 32:741, 1979
14. Allen LH et al: J Nutr 109:1345, 1979
15. Younghee K, Linkswiler HM: J Nutr 109:1399, 1979
16. Spencer H et al: Am J Clin Nutr 31:2167, 1978
17. Schwartz R et al: Am J Clin Nutr 26:519, 1973
18. Nutr Rev 38:9, 1980
19. Mizrahi A et al: N Engl J Med 278:1163, 1968
20. Spencer H et al: J Nutr 86:125, 1965
21. Newton-John HF, Morgan DB: Lancet 1:232, 1968
22. Deftos LJ et al: N Engl J Med 302:1351, 1980
23. Heaney RP: Am J Clin Nutr 30:1603, 1977
24. Recker RR et al: Ann Intern Med 87:649, 1977
25. Avioli LV: In Avioli LV, Krane SM (eds): Metabolic Bone Disease, pp 307–385. New York, Academic Press, 1977
26. Walker ARP: Am J Clin Nutr 25:518, 1972
27. Pettifor JM et al: J Pediatr 92:320, 1978
28. Pettifor JM et al: Am J Clin Nutr 32:2477, 1979
29. Maltz HE et al: Pediatrics 46:865, 1970
30. Kooh SW et al: N Engl J Med 297:1264, 1977
31. Lotz M et al: N Engl J Med 278:409, 1968
32. Ebel H, Günther T: J Clin Chem Clin Biochem 18:257, 1980
33. Aikawa JK: World Rev Nutr Diet 28:112, 1978
34. McNair P et al: Diabetes 27:1075, 1978
35. Shils ME: In Goodhart RS, Shils ME (eds): Modern Nutrition in Health and Disease, 6th ed, pp 310–323. Philadelphia, Lea & Febiger, 1980
36. Nutr Rev 37:6, 1979
37. Hamuro Y et al: J Nutr 100:404, 1970
38. Seelig MS: Am J Clin Nutr 14:342, 1964
39. Mertz W: Fed Proc 29:1482, 1970
40. Multany JS: Biochemistry 9:3970, 1970
41. Beutler E: In Goodhart and Shils, Modern Nutrition, pp 324–354
42. Monsen ER et al: Am J Clin Nutr 31:134, 1978
43. Mason KE: J Nutr 109:1979, 1979
44. Fritz J: Measures to increase iron in food and diets. Proceedings of a Food and Nutrition Board workshop. Washington, DC, NRC-NAS, 1970
45. Monsen ER: Food Nutr News 51:1, Mar-Apr, 1980
46. Rossander L et al: Am J Clin Nutr 32:2484, 1979
47. Kelsay JL: Am J Clin Nutr 31:142, 1978
48. FAO/WHO Expert Committee: Requirements of ascorbic acid, vitamin D, vitamin B$_{12}$, folate and iron. WHO Tech Rep Ser, no. 1452. Geneva, World Health Organization, 1970
49. Saarinen UM et al: J Pediatr 91:36, 1977
50. McMillan JA et al: Pediatrics 58:686, 1976
51. Saarinen UM, Siimes MA: Pediatr Res 13:143, 1979
52. Oski F, Landaw SA: Am J Clin Nutr 134:459, 1980
53. Ten-State Nutrition Survey, 1968–70. DHEW Publ. No. 72-8132, Washington, DC, 1972
54. Hemoglobin and Selected Iron-Related Findings of Persons 1–74 Years of Age: U.S., 1971–74. Advance Data—Vital and Health Statistics, DHEW (PHS) Jan 26, 1979
55. Dallman PR et al: Am J Clin Nutr 33:86, 1980
56. Medical News: Kelp diets can produce myxedema in iodide-sensitive individuals. JAMA 233:9, 1975
57. McClure RD: JAMA 109:783, 1937
58. Matovinovic J et al: JAMA 192:234, 1965
59. Strong FM: In Hegsted et al, Present Knowledge of Nutrition, pp 516–527
60. Subcommittee on Zinc, Committee on Medical and Biologic Effects of Environmental Pollutants: Zinc. Baltimore, NRC, Division of Medical Sciences, Assembly of Life Sciences, University Park Press, 1979
61. Cousins RJ: Am J Clin Nutr 32:339, 1979
62. Weigand E, Kirchgessnes M: J Nutr 110:469, 1980
63. Smith KT, Cousins RJ: J Nutr 110:316, 1980
64. Evans GW: Nutr Rev 38:137, 1980
65. Starcher BC et al: J Nutr 110:1391, 1980
66. Hsu JM: World Rev Nutr Diet 33:42, 1979
67. Hurley LS, Lönnerdal B: Nutr Rev 38:295, 1980
68. Evans GW, Johnson EC: J Nutr 110:1076, 1980
69. Nutr Rev 38:148, 1980
70. Nutr Rev 37:365, 1979
71. Underwood EJ: Trace Elements in Human and Animal Nutrition, 4th ed. New York, Academic Press, 1977
72. Li T-K, Vallee BL: In Goodhart and Shils, Modern Nutrition, pp 408–441
73. Solomons NW, Russell RM: Am J Clin Nutr 33:2031, 1980
74. Schrauzer GN: In Draper, Advances in Nutritional Research, pp 219–244
75. Nutr Rev 38:131, 1980
76. Prasad AS et al: Am J Clin Nutr 12:437, 1963
77. Reinhold JB et al: Am J Clin Nutr 18:294, 1966
78. Pories WJ et al: Lancet 1:121, 1967
79. Henkin RH et al: JAMA 217:434, 1971
80. Hambidge KM et al: Pediatr Res 6:868, 1972
81. Buzina R et al: Am J Clin Nutr 33:2262, 1980
82. Hambidge KM et al: Am J Clin Nutr 29:734, 1976
83. Chase HP et al: Am J Clin Nutr 33:2346, 1980
84. Solomons NW: Am J Clin Nutr 32:856, 1979
85. Nutr Rev 37:76, 1979
86. Holden JM et al: Am J Clin Nutr 75:23, 1979
87. Harland BE et al: J Am Diet Assoc 77:16, 1980
88. Klevay LM et al: Am J Clin Nutr 33:45, 1980
89. Klevay LM: Nutr Rep Int 11:237, 1975
90. Milne DB et al: J Am Diet Assoc 76:41, 1980
91. Klevay LM: Am J Clin Nutr 26:1060, 1973
92. Cordano A et al: Pediatrics 34:324, 1968
93. Al-Rashid RA, Spangler J: N Engl J Med 285:841, 1971
94. Paynter DI: J Nutr 110:447, 1980
95. deRosa G et al: J Nutr 110:795, 1980
96. Marjanen H, Soini S: Ann Agric Fenn 11:391, 1972
97. Oberley LW, Buettner GR: Cancer Res 39:1141, 1979
98. Miller JA: Science News 112:171, 1977
99. Schwarz K, Milne DB: Bioinorganic Chem 1:331, 1972
100. Singer L et al: Am J Clin Nutr 33:328, 1980
101. Ophaug RH et al: Am J Clin Nutr 33:324, 1980
102. Richmond VL: J Nutr Educ 11:62, 1979
103. Farkas CS: J Nutr Educ 11:162, 1979
104. Waldbott GL: J Nutr Educ 12:145, 1980
105. Bernstein DS et al: J Clin Invest 42:916, 1963
106. Bernstein DS et al: JAMA 198:439, 1966
107. Schwarz K, Mertz W: Arch Biochem Biophys 85:292, 1959
108. Doisy RJ et al: In Prasad AS (ed): Trace Elements in Human Health and Disease, Vol 2, pp 79–104. New York, Academic Press, 1976
109. Kumpulainen J, Vuori E: Am J Clin Nutr 33:2299, 1980
110. Saner G et al: Am J Clin Nutr 33:232, 1980
111. Glinsmann WH et al: Science 152:1243, 1966
112. Hopkins LL Jr et al: Am J Clin Nutr 21:203, 1968

113. Gürson CT, Saner G: Am J Clin Nutr 24:1313, 1971
114. Jeejeebhoy KN et al: Am J Clin Nutr 30:531, 1977
115. Jacobson S, Wester PO: Br J Nutr 37:107, 1977
116. Rabinowitz MB et al: Metabolism 29:355, 1980
117. Davidson IWF, Burt RL: Am J Obstet Gynecol 116:601, 1973
118. Liu VJK, Morris JS: Am J Clin Nutr 31:972, 1978
119. Schroeder HA et al: J Chronic Dis 23:123, 1970
120. Abraham AS et al: Am J Clin Nutr 33:2294, 1980
121. Rotruck JT et al: Science 179:588, 1973
122. Thomson CD, Robinson MF: Am J Clin Nutr 33:303, 1980
123. van Rij AM et al: Am J Clin Nutr 32:2076, 1979
124. Robinson MF et al: Br J Nutr 39:589, 1978
125. Nutr Rev 38:278, 1980
126. Broghamer WL et al: Cancer 37:1384, 1976
127. Robinson MF et al: Am J Clin Nutr 32:1477, 1979
128. Deosthale YC, Gopalan C: Br J Nutr 31:351, 1974
129. Tsongas TA, et al: Am J Clin Nutr 33:1103, 1980
130. Nutr Rev 38:194, 1980
131. Carlisle EM: J Nutr 110:352, 1980
132. Lin-Fu JS: Lead Poisoning in Children. DHEW Publ. No. (PHS) 2108. Washington, DC, 1970
133. Schwarz K, Spallholz J: Fed Proc 35:255, 1976

## Supplementary readings

### Calcium, phosphorus, and magnesium

Allen LH et al: Reduction of renal calcium reabsorption in man by consumption of dietary protein. J Nutr 109:1345, 1979

Allen LH et al: Protein-induced hypercalciuria: A longer term study. Am J Clin Nutr 32:741, 1979

Lee CJ et al: Effects of supplementation of the diets with calcium and calcium-rich foods on bone density of elderly females with osteoporosis. Am J Clin Nutr 34:819, 1981

Pettifor JM et al: Calcium deficiency in rural black children in South Africa—A comparison between rural and urban communities. Am J Clin Nutr 32:2477, 1979

Review: Clinical signs of magnesium deficiency. Nutr Rev 37:6, 1979

Rude RK, Singer FR: Magnesium deficiency and excess. Ann Rev Med 32:245, 1981

### Iron and copper

Dallman PR et al: Iron deficiency in infancy and childhood. Am J Clin Nutr 33:86, 1980

Hallberg L: Bioavailability of dietary iron in man. Ann Rev Nutr 1:123, 1981

Klevay LM et al: The human requirement for copper. I. Healthy men fed conventional American diets. Am J Clin Nutr 33:45, 1980

Mason KE: A conspectus of research on copper metabolism and requirements of man. J Nutr 109:1979, 1979

Monsen ER et al: Estimation of available dietary iron. Am J Clin Nutr 31:134, 1978

Rossander L et al: Absorption of iron from breakfast meals. Am J Clin Nutr 32:2484, 1979

### Zinc

Buzina R et al: Zinc nutrition and taste acuity in school children with impaired growth. Am J Clin Nutr 33:2262, 1980

Case study: Picolinic acid in the treatment of disorders requiring zinc supplementation. Nutr Rev 38:148, 1980

Chase HP et al: Low vitamin A and zinc concentrations in Mexican-American migrant children with growth retardation. Am J Clin Nutr 33:2346, 1980

Evans GW: Normal and abnormal zinc absorption in man and animals: The tryptophan connection. Nutr Rev 38:137, 1980

Duchateau J et al: Influence of oral zinc supplementation on the lymphocyte response to mitogens of normal subjects. Am J Clin Nutr 34:88, 1981

Holden JM et al: Zinc and copper in self-selected diets. J Am Diet Assoc 75:23, 1979

Review: Experimental zinc deficiency in humans. Nutr Rev 37:76, 1979

Review: Host zinc nutrition and Ehrlich ascites tumor growth. Nutr Rev 38:131, 1980

Review: Phytate and zinc bioavailability. Nutr Rev 37:365, 1979

Review: Zinc and immunocompetence. Nutr Rev 38:288, 1980

Solomons NW: On the assessment of zinc and copper nutrition. Am J Clin Nutr 32:856, 1979

Solomons NW, Russell RM: The interaction of vitamin A and zinc: Implications for human nutrition. Am J Clin Nutr 33:2031, 1980

### Fluoride

Ophaug RH et al: Estimated fluoride intake of 6-month-old infants in four dietary regions of the United States. Am J Clin Nutr 33:324, 1980

Richmond VL: Health effects associated with water fluoridation. J Nutr Educ 11:62, 1979

Schamschula RG, Barmes DE: Fluoride and health: dental caries, osteoporosis and cardiovascular disease. Ann Rev Nutr 1:427, 1981

Singer L et al: Fluoride intake of young male adults in the United States. Am J Clin Nutr 33:328, 1980

### Selenium

Sunde RA, Hoekstra WG: Structure, synthesis and function of glutathione peroxidase. Nutr Rev 38:265, 1980

Thomson CD, Robinson MF: Selenium in human health and disease with emphasis on those aspects peculiar to New Zealand. Am J Clin Nutr 33:303, 1980

van Rij AM et al: Selenium deficiency in total parenteral nutrition. Am J Clin Nutr 32:2076, 1979

### Miscellaneous

Abraham AS et al: The effect of chromium on established atherosclerotic plaques in rabbits. Am J Clin Nutr 33:2294, 1980

Harland BE et al: Calcium, phosphorus, iron, iodine, and zinc in the "total diet". J Am Diet Assoc 77:16, 1980

Milne DB et al: Trace mineral intake of enlisted military personnel. J Am Diet Assoc 76:41, 1980

Review: Prevention of Keshan cardiomyopathy by sodium selenite. Nutr Rev 38:278, 1980

Review: Silicon and bone formation. Nutr Rev 38:194, 1980

Stowe HD et al: Vitamin A–iodine interrelationships. J Nutr 110:1947, 1980

Tsongas TA et al: Molybdenum in the diet: An estimate of average daily intake in the United States. Am J Clin Nutr 33:1103, 1980

*For further references see Bibliography in Part 4.*

# Fat-soluble Vitamins

# 7

**CaBP:** Calcium-binding Protein
**CRABP:** Cellular Retinoic Acid-binding
  Protein
**CRBP:** Cellular Retinol-binding Protein
**GSH:** Reduced Glutathione
**IU:** International Units
**LBW:** Low Birth Weight
**PA:** Prealbumin
**RBP:** Retinol-binding Protein
**RE:** Retinol Equivalents
**TXA$_2$:** Thromboxane

## General Discussion of All Vitamins

The term, *vitamine*, meaning a vital amine, was proposed by Funk in 1911 to designate a new food constituent necessary for life, which he thought he had identified chemically. Other terminology was proposed as new factors were discovered, but the word *vitamin*, with the final "e" dropped to avoid any chemical significance, met with popular favor.

At first the individual vitamins were named by letter or according to their curative or preventive properties, but present opinion favors names descriptive of the substance itself. As a vitamin's chemical structure is discovered, it is named appropriately, if it is not already a recognized compound. However, the lettered nomenclature may still be used to some extent, especially in popular discussions. From time to time new vitamins are postulated and are added to the accepted list after extensive research.

When a supposedly single vitamin proved to be more than one chemically and physiologically unrelated compound, the term, *complex*, was incorporated for additional identification, as for the B complex.

Sometimes it is convenient to group the vitamins according to solubility. Vitamins A, D, E, and K are fat-soluble. Two water-soluble groups are recognized—those having vitamin C activity and the large group known as the vitamin B complex.

## Definitions

*Vitamins* are potent organic compounds that occur in low concentrations in foods; they perform specific and vital functions in the cells and the tissues of the body. They cannot be synthesized by the organism, and their absence or inadequate utilization results in specific deficiency diseases. They differ from each other in physiologic function, in chemical structure, and in distribution in food.

As more knowledge of the vitamins has been gained, their classification according to function has been modified. Certain fat-soluble vitamins (*i.e.*, vitamins A and D) are now classified by many authorities as hormones.

Other vitamins (*i.e.*, B complex) may be classified according to their function as biologic catalysts or co-enzymes in the many varied enzyme systems of the body.

A brief review of enzyme terminology is appropriate before specific functions of the various vitamins are discussed. Enzymes consist of at least two parts: the cofactor portion or the prosthetic group, and the protein portion. The specific amino acids that compose the protein part of the enzyme are determined by the genetic code (see Chap. 9), and this portion is often referred to as the *apoenzyme*. Either mineral ions (such as $Ca^{++}$, $Mg^{++}$, $Zn^{++}$) or vitamins or, in many instances, both, make up the cofactor portion of the complete enzyme (*holoenzyme*). The vitamin portion of the enzyme is usually called the *coenzyme* and the mineral, the *activator*; for this reason, the term coenzyme is applied to certain vitamins.

There are also terms that apply to vitamins in general. Different chemical forms of a vitamin, which have the same biologic activity, are sometimes referred to as *vitamers* (*e.g.*, pyridoxal, pyridoxine, and pyridoxamine are vitamers of vitamin $B_6$). A *provitamin*, or *precursor*, is a compound structurally related to a vitamin, which the body can convert to a vitamin active compound. The word, *avitaminosis* literally means without vitamins, although it is generally used with a letter following (*e.g.*, avitaminosis A) to indicate the specific deficiency of that factor. The word, *deficiency*, may be used to indicate varying degrees of shortage—mild, moderate, severe, or complete. The possibility of an excess intake of certain vitamins has been postulated, and in some instances a large excess has proved to be harmful; such a condition is termed *hypervitaminosis*. Early stages of vitamin deficiencies, which show no clinical symptoms but may be detected by biochemical evaluation, are called *marginal*.

## History

A few physicians early recognized the connection between food habits and the incidence of certain diseases. Beri-beri was described in the 7th century and scurvy in the 13th, but it was not until centuries later that certain foods were recommended as protective. The first vitamins were discovered as "accessory factors" in foods proven to be curative of specific deficiency diseases. In other words, vitamins were first recognized by their absence rather than by their presence.

In the early years of the 20th century, workers in Germany, the Netherlands, Great Britain, and the United States were beginning to use animals for nutrition experiments. A number of investigators showed that purified rations containing only protein, fat, carbohydrate, and minerals would not support growth. They observed that natural foods provided some substances other than the basal constituents that were essential for normal growth and wellbeing. These workers initiated the search for "accessory food factors," later called vitamins. Since then our knowledge of vitamins has grown rapidly.

There are still, however, wide gaps in our understanding of the total vitamin story. For instance, although we can recognize a specific vitamin deficiency and cure it with appropriate amounts of the vitamin, the actual roles of certain vitamins in metabolic processes remain to be defined.

## Vitamin units and assay methods

Feeding tests on animals at first offered the only device for testing foods for their vitamin content. This type of procedure, called the bio-assay method, may be used as the basis of comparison for the standardization of newer chemical or microbiologic methods of assay. After the chemists succeed in concentrating, identifying, and synthesizing a vitamin, its amount is expressed in metric weights of the pure crystalline substance.

The International Units (IU) as originally defined by a League of Nations committee are still used in most tables of food composition to express the contents of vitamins A, D, and E. All others are given in milligrams (mg) or micrograms (mcg), whichever is appropriate. The FAO/WHO Expert Committee on Vitamin Requirements has suggested that vitamin A and D values also be given in micrograms (mcg).[1,2] The 1980 revision of the Recommended Dietary Allowances gives all recommendations in metric units and explains the conversion factors for each vitamin in the text.[3] These will be discussed for individual vitamins later in this chapter.

## Vitamin content of foods

Determination of the specific vitamin activity of natural foods becomes an increasingly difficult task as the number and the complexity of vitamins increase. Table 1, Part 4, gives figures for many of the vitamins in foods. Vitamin losses in the cooking and storage of food will be mentioned more specifically under each vitamin, but, in general, certain principles of vitamin conservation are worth noting. Fat-soluble vitamins (A, D, E, K) are not easily lost by ordinary cooking methods, and they do not dissolve out in the cooking water. Water-soluble vitamins (B complex and C) are dissolved easily in cooking water, and a portion of the vitamins actually may be destroyed by heating; therefore, the best procedure for conserving vitamins is, in general, cooking food only until tender in as little water as possible. Vitamin losses due to storage of vegetables tend to parallel the degree of wilting; such losses are progressive in the long storage of fresh fruits and vegetables.

## The Fat-Soluble Group

The four vitamins A, D, E, and K that are all soluble in fat and fat solvents are known as the fat-soluble group. Absorption from the intestinal tract follows the same path as the fats; thus, any condition that interferes with fat absorption may result in poor absorption of these vitamins. They can all be stored in the body to some extent, mostly in the liver, and as a consequence, manifestation of deficiencies is likely to be slower than it is for most of the water-soluble group. In several instances, vitamin activity is not confined to a single substance, and several related substances produce a similar effect on the body.

## Vitamin A
### History

Vitamin A was the first fat-soluble vitamin to be recognized. This occurred in 1913 when two groups of workers—McCollum and Davis, at the University of Wisconsin, and Osborne and Mendel, at Yale—demonstrated independently that rats fail to grow normally on diets deficient in natural fats. At about the time growth ceased, the eyes became inflamed and apparently infected. This characteristic eye disease, known as *xerophthalmia*, was relieved in a few days by the addition to the diet of a little butter fat or cod-liver oil, which contained the protective or curative factor known as vitamin A.

### Nomenclature

Today we recognize a group of structurally related compounds that have vitamin A activity. Those found in animal products are colorless or only slightly pigmented; the most common of these *preformed vitamins* are vitamin $A_1$ alcohol, or *retinol*, and vitamin $A_2$, 3-dehydroretinol. Other forms that have specific physiologic reactions include vitamin A aldehyde, *retinal*, and vitamin A acid, *retinoic acid*. The term *retinoid* includes the natural forms of vitamin A as well as its synthetic derivatives with or without biologic activity.

Vitamin A can occur in different isomeric forms determined by the configuration of the double bonds in the side chain. The all-trans retinol is the most common naturally occurring form and possesses the highest biologic activity. It can be converted in the body to 11-cis-retinal, which is the functional form of vitamin A in vision. The exact chemical form or forms in which vitamin A performs its other functions in the body are not known.

A number of forms of *provitamin A* are found in the yellow carotenoid plant pigments. *Beta-carotene* ($\beta$-carotene) has the highest biologic activity of the carotenes, yielding two molecules of vitamin A per molecule of beta-carotene (Fig. 7-1).

Some animal products, such as cream and butter, may contain both preformed vitamin A and carotene, because some of the provitamin may remain unchanged. Dietary preformed vitamin A consists mainly of retinyl esters (long chain fatty acid esterified at the side chain of retinol).

Although vitamin A values in most food composition tables are given as International Units, the Report of the Joint FAO/WHO Expert Group on Requirements of Vitamin A, Thiamin, Riboflavin, and Niacin, 1967, urges that this practice be changed and that units of weight be used.[1] This will necessitate that tables of food composition report separately the amounts of retinol, $\beta$-carotene, and other mixed carotenoids in individual foods. The 1974 revision of the Recommended Dietary Allowances introduces the term, *retinol equivalents*, (RE), which is used to express the vitamin A allowances in the 1980 revision.[3]

International Units can be converted to micrograms as follows:[1]

> 1 IU (or USP unit) of vitamin A
> = 0.3 mcg retinol
> = 0.344 mcg retinyl acetate
> = 0.6 mcg $\beta$-carotene
> = 1.2 mcg other mixed carotenes with vitamin A activity

Vitamin A values can be converted to retinol equivalents as follows:[3]

> 1 retinol equivalent of vitamin A
> = 1 mcg retinol
> = 6 mcg $\beta$-carotene
> = 12 mcg other provitamin A carotenoids
> = 3.33 IU retinol
> = 10 IU $\beta$-carotene

To calculate the retinol equivalents in a diet or foodstuff, one of the following equations should be used:[3]

a. If retinol and $\beta$-carotene are given in mcg, then:

$$\text{mcg retinol} + \frac{\text{mcg } \beta\text{-carotene}}{6} = \text{retinol equivalents}$$

**Example:**

A diet contains 500 mcg retinol and 1800 mcg $\beta$-carotene.

$$500 + \frac{1800}{6} = 800 \text{ retinol equivalents}$$

b. If both are given in IU, then:

$$\frac{\text{IU of retinol}}{3.33} + \frac{\text{IU of } \beta\text{-carotene}}{10} = \text{retinol equivalents}$$

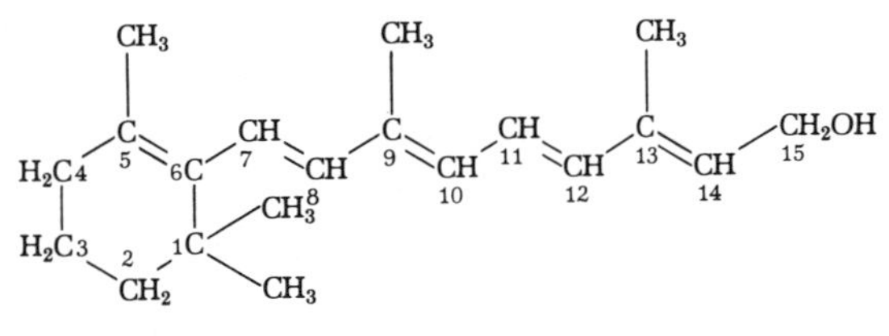

Retinol (vitamin $A_1$)

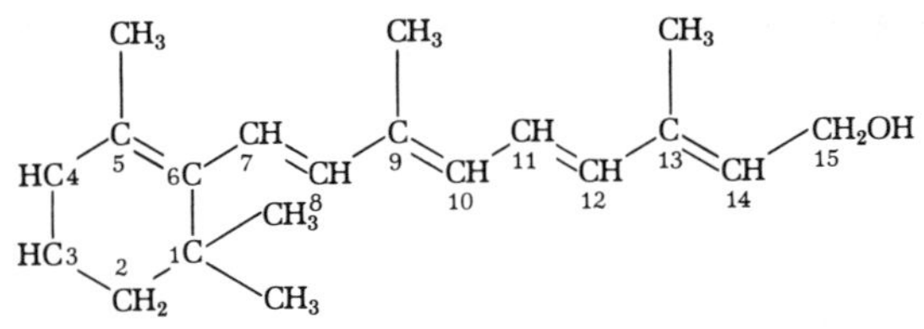

3-dehydroretinol (vitamin $A_2$)

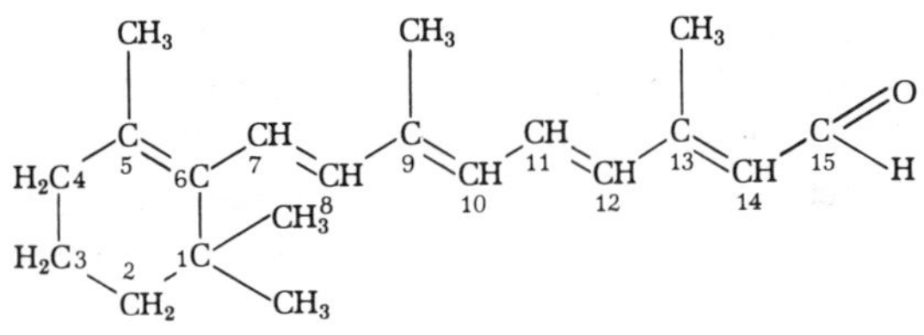

Retinal

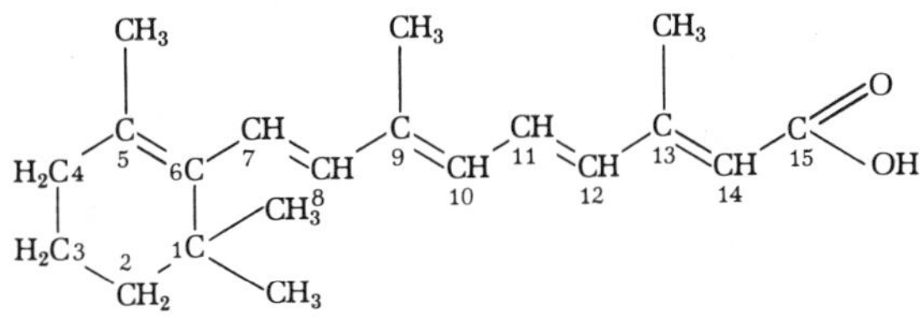

Retinoic acid

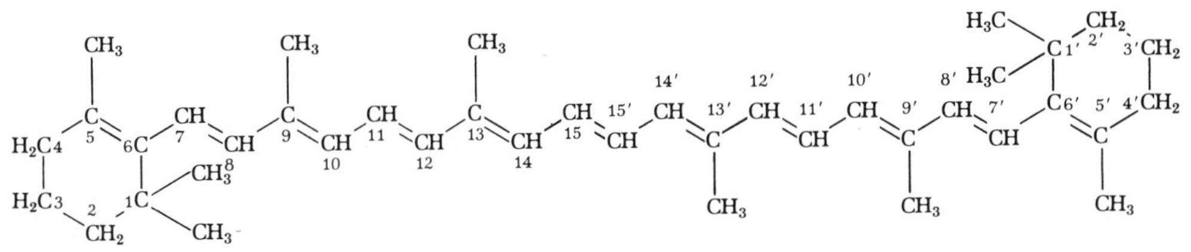

Beta-carotene

**Fig. 7-1.** Compounds with vitamin A activity.

Example:

A diet contains 1666 IU of retinol and 3000 IU of $\beta$-carotene.

$$\frac{1666}{3.33} + \frac{3000}{10} = 800 \text{ retinol equivalents}$$

c. If $\beta$-carotene and other provitamin A carotenoids are given in mcg then:

$$\frac{\text{mcg } \beta\text{-carotene}}{6} + \frac{\text{mcg other carotenoids}}{12} = \text{retinol equivalents}$$

Example:

A 100-g sample of sweet potatoes contains 2400 IU $\beta$-carotene and 480 IU of other provitamin A carotenoids.

$$\frac{2400}{6} + \frac{480}{12} = 440 \text{ retinol equivalents}$$

This approach to evaluating the vitamin A content of foods is recommended because, as will be discussed later, the vitamin A requirement depends on the proportion of vitamin A (retinol) to provitamin A (carotene) in the diet.

## Absorption, transport, metabolism, storage, and excretion of vitamin A and carotene

### Vitamin A

Dietary vitamin A (*i.e.*, retinyl esters) is hydrolyzed in the gastrointestinal tract into retinol and is absorbed in this form across the mucosal cell membrane into the cell, where it recombines with a fatty acid, usually palmitate or stearate. The retinyl ester then travels in the chylomicrons by way of the lymphatic system and blood-stream to the liver, where it is stored (Fig. 7-2).

Liver stores of vitamin A (retinyl esters) are hydrolyzed by enzymes to free retinol, which is transported by a retinol-binding protein (RBP) complex to the tissues of the body wherever a metabolic requirement exists. The liver stores can maintain the blood at relatively constant vitamin A levels even when the diet is deficient. For this reason, vitamin A deficiencies may not develop for long periods of time, depending on the reserve stores in the liver and the ability of the body to mobilize these reserves of vitamin A.

RBP is a relatively small protein synthesized in the liver and released in response to the need for vitamin A transport. In plasma it forms a complex with another larger protein known as prealbumin (PA), which also transports plasma thyroxine. This larger complex is believed to protect retinol from oxidative destruction and to reduce the removal and catabolism of retinol and RBP by the kidneys.[4] In vitamin A deficiency RBP accumulates in the liver and is rapidly released upon administration of vitamin A.[5]

Protein deficiency can interfere with vitamin A mobilization from the liver reserves.[6] With inadequate protein (and energy) intake the concentration of several plasma proteins synthesized in the liver decreases; RBP and PA are among the first ones affected.[7,8] Because of their rapid response to changes in protein-energy status, the plasma concentration of RBP and PA has been recommended as a means of detecting subclinical malnutrition and of monitoring the effectiveness of dietary treatment.[7]

Plasma levels of vitamin A, RBP, and PA are also low in liver disease (see Chap. 33) and in children with protein-energy malnutrition.[4] When such children are treated with a diet adequate in protein and energy, their plasma vitamin A, RBP, and PA levels increase, suggesting that low plasma levels of vitamin A were due to protein deficiency rather than lack of vitamin A. However, in most severely malnourished children the liver reserves of vitamin A are minimal, and, unless vitamin A is provided with protein and energy, an acute vitamin A deficiency may develop as their vitamin A requirement is suddenly increased with the restoration of rapid growth.[9]

It is estimated that the liver may contain as much as 95% of the vitamin A of the entire body, with small amounts in adipose tissue, lungs, and kidneys. Infants and young animals probably have low reserves of vitamin A at birth but, if they are well-fed, they store it rapidly. The liver gradually acquires, over a period of years, an increasing reserve of vitamin A, which normally reaches its peak in adult life. The function of this reserve is chiefly to take care of temporary shortages or increased requirements. Obviously, an intake above the minimum requirement must be maintained most of the time if such a reserve is to be built up. Reserve stores of vitamin A are evident even in young animals.

### Carotene

In the present of fat and bile acids carotene is absorbed into the intestinal wall, where some is converted to vitamin A (Fig. 7-2). The carotene that is not converted is absorbed into the lymph and carried to the blood-

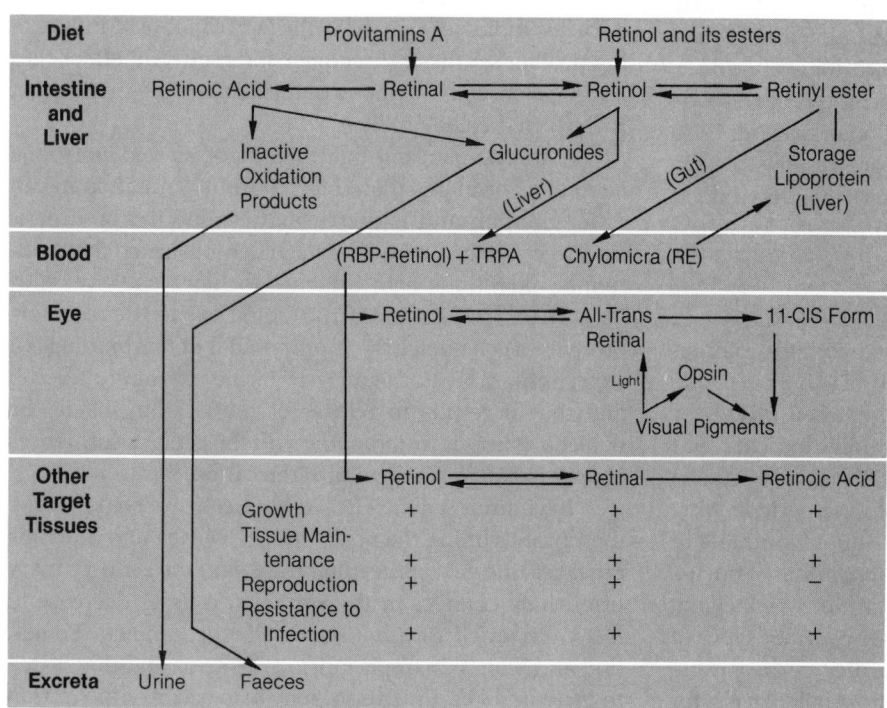

**Fig. 7-2.** Metabolic and functional relationships between different forms of vitamin A. RBP, plasma retinol-binding protein; TRPA, tryptophan-rich prealbumin; RE, retinyl ester. Ability to support specific functions in the target tissues by the different forms of vitamin A is indicated by a + sign. (Vitamin A Deficiency and Xerophthalmia, WHO Tech. Rep. Ser. No. 590, p 15. Geneva, World Health Organization, 1976)

stream. Some carotene may be converted to vitamin A in the liver, and some is stored in adipose tissue. According to the report of the FAO/WHO committee on vitamin requirements and the Food and Nutrition Board, approximately one-third of the carotene in food is available to the body. Moreover, the amount of available carotene that is then converted to vitamin A varies considerably, but, in general, only about half is used this way. As a result, in the human the utilization efficiency of carotene is 1/6; in other terms, 1 mcg of $\beta$-carotene would have the same biologic activity as 0.167 mcg of vitamin A alcohol, retinol. Other carotenoids have about 1/2 the biologic activity of $\beta$-carotene (1 mcg other carotenoids = 0.0833 mcg retinol).

Inadequate protein intakes decrease the absorption, transport, and metabolism of carotenes.

## Functions of vitamin A

### Constituents of visual pigments

The best-defined function of vitamin A is its role in the visual process. Vitamin A aldehyde, 11-*cis*-retinal, combines with the protein opsin, to form rhodopsin, or visual purple, in the rods of the retina of the eye, which are responsible for vision in dim light (scotopic vision). When light strikes the eye, the rhodopsin is bleached to yield the original protein opsin and retinal. The retinal is converted to retinol and, although most of it is reconverted to retinal to combine again with opsin, some is lost and must be replaced. Adaptation to dim light depends on the completion of the cycle. When bright light causes excessive bleaching of the visual purple, the eyes' ability to regenerate it appears to be directly related to the amount of vitamin A available. The "dark adaptation" test, which measures the eyes' ability to recover visual acuity in dim light, has been used as a means of determining vitamin A status. Insufficient vitamin A for the synthesis of rhodopsin results in night blindness, or *nyctalopia* (see Fig. 7-2).

The cones of the retina, which are responsible for vision in bright light (photopic vision), also contain a light-sensitive vitamin A-protein complex, iodopsin (a photo-sensitive violet pigment).

### Maintenance of epithelial tissue

Vitamin A has long been associated with the maintenance of normal epithelial tissue, but it is only recently that some metabolic explanations have been found for this function of vitamin A. Animal studies indicate that during cell differentiation the basal cells of the epithelia have two alternative pathways open to them, depending on the availability of vitamin A. If adequate amounts of the vitamin are present they form columnar, mucus-secreting goblet cells, whereas, if vitamin A is lacking, they keratinize. The effect of vitamin A on other types of epithelial tissue can be explained further by proposing that different tissues have varying threshold levels for vitamin A.

Wolf and DeLuca[10] suggest four types of epithelial tissue with different threshold levels for each. The lowest threshold is indicated for the simple columnar epithelium lining the gastrointestinal tract. During differentiation in the presence of vitamin A these basal cells form mucus-secreting goblet cells. Squamous cells are formed in vitamin A deficiency. Next in order of threshold levels are the epithelial cells lining the trachea; these also normally consist of simple columnar cells, but in the absence of vitamin A they differentiate into stratified squamous tissue. The corneal epithelium is an example of stratified squamous tissue, which has a still higher threshold for the vitamin, but in a state of vitamin A deficiency produces keratin. Finally, the highest threshold level of vitamin A is proposed for the cells of the epidermis; normally they produce some keratin, but lacking vitamin A, they produce increased amounts.

When the same level of circulating vitamin A is available to these tissues, it must either possess different "potencies" in different cells, or its entry to the cells must be regulated. The second possibility is supported by the recent demonstration that the plasma retinol carrier, RBP, attaches to a specific cell-surface receptor of the target cell and releases retinol inside the cell.[5,11] It remains to be established whether the cell-surface receptors actually regulate the entry of retinol to the cells. Another specific protein, cellular retinol-binding protein (CRBP), binds the vitamin inside the cell and, presumably, delivers it to its cellular site of action.[12] The existence of a cellular retinoic acid-binding protein (CRABP) distinct from CRBP has also been demonstrated.[12]

Although the mechanism for the role of vitamin A in modifying cell differentiation has not been identified, evidence indicates that "vitamin A is capable of influencing protein synthesis directly or indirectly, an effect that results in observable fine structural differences in many of the affected cells."[13]

A mechanism similar to that of steroid hormone action has been postulated for vitamin A function in cell differentiation and is increasingly supported by experimental evidence. It now has been demonstrated that both retinol and retinoic acid, attached to their respective cellular carriers (CRBP and CRABP), bind to specific receptor-proteins of cell nuclei.[14] It is proposed that this binding is a step comparable to the delivery of the vitamin to the cell and that it results in release of the vitamin inside the nucleus, where its interaction with the genome influences its expression, leading to differentiation.[14]

In vitamin A deficiency, it has been observed that the membranes lining the nose, throat, trachea and other air passages, the gastrointestinal tract, and the genitourinary tract show changes in the epithelial cells. A decrease in taste and smell thresholds has also been noted. Rough, dry, and scaly skin, especially on the arms and thighs due to increased keratinization, may also occur with vitamin A deficiency.

Whenever these tissue changes occur, the natural mechanism for protection against bacterial invasion is impaired, and the tissue may easily become infected. Clinical observations show that normal mucous membranes lining nose, throat, sinuses, and ear passages are the best defense against infections and that adequate vitamin A is an important factor in maintaining the normal functions of these membranes. Renal calculi may also be related to the keratinization of the urinary tract.

Damage to the epithelial layer of the eye is one of the most important clinical signs of vitamin A deficiency in humans, particularly children (see Chap. 21). There is a drying and thickening of the conjunctiva, the tear ducts fail to secrete, and keratinization results, with the epithelial cells of the cornea becoming opaque and sloughing off. Infection and permanent blindness may follow if vitamin A is not administered. It should be noted that this function of vitamin A in the eye is distinct from its function in the visual process.

### Maintenance of bone growth

Bones also depend on vitamin A for normal growth and development, and this function of the vitamin is thought by several investigators to relate to cell changes that occur during differentiation. Hayes[13] suggests that when vitamin A is deficient, periosteal progenitor cells in bones and the fibroblasts in collagen have priority in synthesizing collagen fibers and ground substances at the expense of the remodeling osteoclasts and fibroclasts. Evidence of this defect is seen in the crippling that occurs in young rats fed a vitamin A deficient diet.

The nerve damage that frequently appears in vitamin A deficiency may be traced to the compression of growing tissue in a skeleton that ceases to grow rather than as a direct result of vitamin A deficiency.

### Growth and reproduction

Failure to grow is noted in vitamin A deficiency, as it is in many other nutrient deficiencies, before any other symptoms appear. The need for vitamin A for normal growth appears associated with protein utilization, weight gain, and perhaps cell mitosis,[13] although simple organisms, which grow by cell division, do not require vitamin A.

Vitamin A is essential to normal reproduction in rats, pigs, and other animals. Studies have shown that for successful reproduction and lactation the diet must furnish more vitamin A than is needed for good growth. Female rats on a minimal supply of vitamin A intake may show no outward signs of vitamin A deficiency yet are not able to bear or rear vigorous young. With an outright deficiency there is interference with the normal estrus cycle in the female and a testicular degeneration in the male rat. These symptoms appear related to cell changes, which occur during differentiation. Sows deprived of adequate vitamin A may give birth to litters of pigs with defective eyes or without eyeballs. This finding was one of the first evidences that prenatal malnutrition may cause abnormalities in the fetus.

### Other roles

Vitamin A is believed to be essential for the maintenance of normal cellular membrane structure and function. Both vitamin A deficiency and excess appear to cause membrane instability.[5] The synthesis of a number of specific glycoproteins in different tissues appears to be influenced by the availability of vitamin A.[15,16] Transfer of mannose to glycoproteins of the intestinal mucosa and other tissues is believed to involve formation of mannosylretinylphosphate as an intermediate from which the mannose residue is transferred to a protein acceptor.[16,17]

Mild anemia has been associated with vitamin A deficiency, both in human population surveys and in experimentally-produced human and animal deficiencies.[18,19] On the basis of animal studies, impaired mobilization of iron stores from the liver has been proposed as the cause of the anemia.[19]

The role of vitamin A and its derivatives (retinoids) in the prevention of certain types of cancers of epithelial origin has been under investigation for several years.[20] A number of synthetic derivatives of vitamin A and its two naturally occurring metabolites, retinoic acid and 5,6-epoxyretinoic acid, appear to have anti-tumor activity in experimental animals by inhibiting tumor promotion, a phase following tumor initiation by a carcinogen.[20,21] Whether vitamin A nutritional status plays a role in the development or prevention of certain cancers in humans is still uncertain.

The homeostasis of the thyroid hormones appears to be disturbed by vitamin A deficiency. An effect on the brain's thyroid hormone receptors through glycoprotein synthesis has been postulated.[22]

## Interconversions and active forms

Retinol and retinal are easily interconvertible in the body, and both can be supplied by the retinyl esters from the diet or liver reserves. Retinoic acid is formed in the tissues by oxidation of retinal, but this reaction is not reversible. Neither retinal nor retinoic acid is stored in the body, and their circulating levels are very low compared to retinol.[23] Retinal (11-cis) is known to be the active form in the visual process, but the active form or forms in the other functions of vitamin A are not known. The fact that some cells have both CRBP and CRABP suggests that both may be capable of performing the same functions in these cells, or that perhaps both are needed. It is also possible that they undergo further activation; retinoic acid is known to be converted to 5,6-epoxyretinoic acid in some tissues, but whether this represents further activation or catabolism remains to be established.[23] Retinol can provide the active forms for all tissues, whereas retinoic acid for only some; it cannot supply retinal for the visual pigments, and it has only partial activity in the reproductive tissues, which also appear to have sex and species differences.[24] However, the acid can support growth and differentiation of the epithelial tissues; it is actually more active than retinol in these functions and, therefore, may be the active form.[23]

## Metabolism and excretion

Vitamin A and other fat-soluble vitamins (except vitamin K) differ from the water-soluble vitamins in that the body has an almost unlimited capacity to store them but only a limited capacity to excrete them. The major route of vitamin A excretion from the body is through bile into the intestine, where some may be reabsorbed and some is lost in the feces. Most of the biliary vitamin A is in the form of retinoyl-glucuronides. In addition to glucuronides, a large number of different oxidation products of retinoic acid are found in the urine; nevertheless, urinary excretion of vitamin A metabolites represents a very small daily loss of the vitamin.[23] The possible significance of vitamin A metabolism in regard to its physiological functions is being actively investigated. Figure 7-2 summarizes the metabolic and functional relationships between the different forms of vitamin A.

## Dietary requirement for vitamin A

Human requirements for vitamin A are based on studies of two kinds: nutritional status studies on various population groups throughout the world and controlled depletion experiments carried out on humans and other animals. Field studies have indicated that in countries where the vitamin A intake is 3000 IU to 9000 IU (900 mcg–2700 mcg RE), per person per day, vitamin A deficiency is rarely seen, whereas, in other countries, on intakes of 1000 IU to 2500 IU (300 mcg–750 mcg RE), vitamin A deficiency is known to occur in the population. Research has shown that varying doses of vitamin A are required to relieve different symptoms: 150 mcg of retinol per day reversed the changes in the eye; 300 mcg per day of retinol resulted in normal balance as well as normal taste and smell thresholds; however, 600 mcg per day of retinol were required to clear the skin lesions. Blood levels also returned to the normal range when a 600-mcg dose was given. Twice the amount of pure beta-carotene compared to retinol was necessary to correct the symptoms.[25] The overall vitamin A requirement found in this study agreed fairly well with the earlier estimates from population studies and the now classic human experiments conducted under the auspices of the British Medical Research Council,[26] which have influenced the recommended allowances of vitamin A established by the United States National Research Council's Food and Nutrition Board. As a result, there has been very litte change in the vitamin A allowances over the years.

The 1980 recommended allowance of 1000 mcg RE (5000 IU vitamin A) for an adult man is in excess of the minimum to allow some reserve of vitamin A to be stored in the body. The allowance for the adult woman is 800 mcg RE (4000 IU vitamin A) or 80% of the male allowance because of the usually smaller body size of women. The allowances assume that the American diet provides half of the total vitamin A activity as retinol and half as provitamin A carotenoids. When calculated as International Units, this is 2500 IU as retinol and 2500 IU as provitamin A or a total of 5000 IU. In terms of retinol equivalents (RE), it is 750 mcg retinol (1 RE = 3.33 IU retinol) and 250 retinol equivalents as beta-carotene (1 RE = 10 IU $\beta$-carotene) for a total of 1000 RE.[3]

Allowances for infants are based on the amount of retinol in human milk, about 49 mcg per 100 ml. An infant consuming 850 ml of breast milk would receive approximately 420 mcg RE of retinol; this amount is set as the recommendation for infants from birth to 6 months. It is reduced to 400 mcg RE for infants 6 months to 1 year of age. Because no definite information is available regarding the actual requirements of children and adolescents, these recommendations have been interpolated from the infant and the male adult allowances and are based on body weight and growth needs. The female allowance increases to 1000 mcg RE during pregnancy and 1200 mcg RE during lactation.

The FAO/WHO committee on vitamin requirements have adopted a recommended intake of 750 mcg (2500 IU) of retinol per day for the normal adult.[1] No additional recommendation for pregnancy was made, provided that the usual diet supplies the recommended adult intake. To cover the vitamin A secreted in milk, 1200 mcg (4000 IU) of retinol was recommended during lactation. Recommendations for infants are based on the amount of vitamin A in breast milk. Suggested levels for children range from 300 mcg (1000 IU) for the 6 month child to 750 mcg (2500 IU) for the older adolescent.

Because carotene, which is less efficiently utilized (1/6) than retinol, is often the major source of vitamin A in the diet, the recommended intake of vitamin A is modified depending on the percent of vitamin A supplied by carotene.

Figure 7-3 illustrates the percentage of vitamin A supplied by various food groups in different countries throughout the world. Note the wide variation in sources of this vitamin. (For complete table of vitamin A allowances for all age and sex categories, see Chap. 11.)

## Hypervitaminosis A

An overdose of vitamin A may cause serious injury to health. It is most likely to happen when children are given too much of a high-potency supplement. Because water-miscible preparations are better utilized than oily preparations, they are more toxic when intake levels are equal.[27] The symptoms of hypervitaminosis A are loss of appetite,

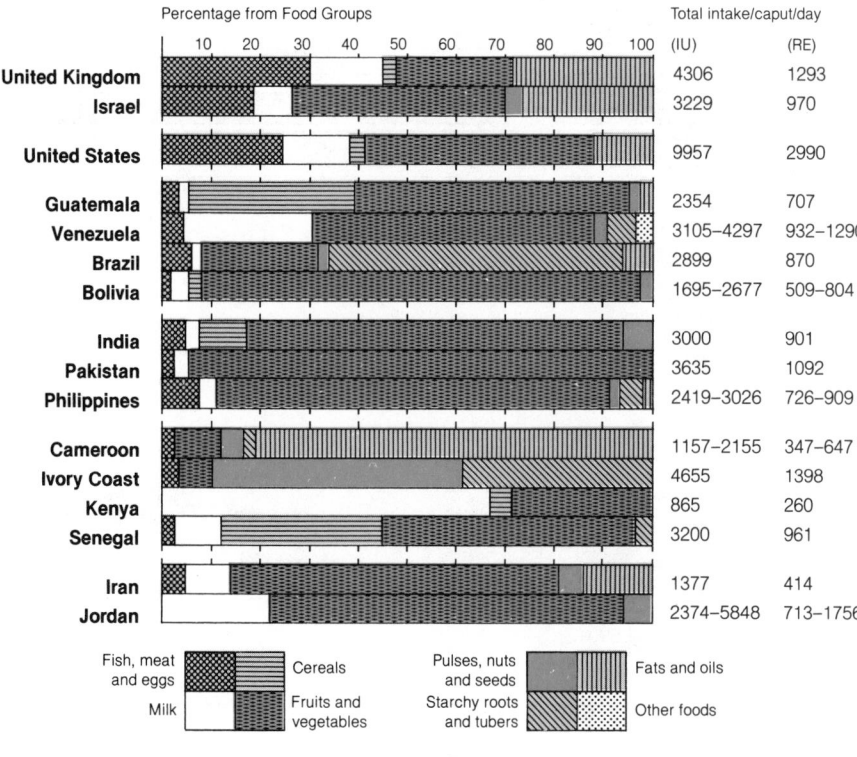

Percentage from Food Groups

Total intake/caput/day

| | (IU) | (RE) |
|---|---|---|
| United Kingdom | 4306 | 1293 |
| Israel | 3229 | 970 |
| United States | 9957 | 2990 |
| Guatemala | 2354 | 707 |
| Venezuela | 3105–4297 | 932–1290 |
| Brazil | 2899 | 870 |
| Bolivia | 1695–2677 | 509–804 |
| India | 3000 | 901 |
| Pakistan | 3635 | 1092 |
| Philippines | 2419–3026 | 726–909 |
| Cameroon | 1157–2155 | 347–647 |
| Ivory Coast | 4655 | 1398 |
| Kenya | 865 | 260 |
| Senegal | 3200 | 961 |
| Iran | 1377 | 414 |
| Jordan | 2374–5848 | 713–1756 |

Fish, meat and eggs; Cereals; Pulses, nuts and seeds; Fats and oils; Milk; Fruits and vegetables; Starchy roots and tubers; Other foods

**Fig. 7-3.** Sources of vitamin A in the diets of population groups surveyed in some countries. (Report of a Joint FAO/WHO Expert Group: Requirements of Vitamin A, Thiamine, Riboflavin, and Niacin. FAO Nutrition Meetings Report Series No. 4, Rome).

abnormal skin pigmentation, loss of hair, dry skin (with itching), pain in the long bones, and increased fragility of the bones in general. Regular supplementation of more than 3000 RE (10,000 IU) of retinol above that consumed in the diet should be carefully supervised by a physician.[3] In adults, regular daily ingestion of more than 7500 RE (25,000 IU) is not advisable.[3]

In three cases of adolescent girls reported by Morrice and Havener,[28] massive doses of 90,000 and 200,000 IU of vitamin A caused symptoms of brain tumor (pseudotumor cerebri), along with most of the syndrome described above.

It now appears that vitamin A toxicity develops when the capacity of the liver to store the vitamin is exceeded. Normally, retinyl esters are mobilized from the liver as retinol bound to RBP, and only a small fraction of total circulating vitamin A is in the ester form. In hypervitaminosis the proportion of total plasma vitamin A as retinyl ester found in association with the low-density lipoproteins is greatly increased. This nonspecifically bound vitamin is believed to be toxic to cellular membranes due to its surface-active properties.[5,29]

Carotene in large doses is not toxic but usually causes a yellow coloration of the skin which disappears when the carotene is discontinued.

## Food sources

The richest natural sources of vitamin A are the fish-liver oils, which are usually classed as food supplements rather than as foods. They vary according to the species

and the season when caught, but commercial brands are well standardized for our convenience.

All animal livers are good sources of vitamin A, but they are not as rich as fish liver. All milk products that include milk fat, such as whole milk, butter, cream, or full cream cheese, are rich in vitamin A. The milk of cows on green pasture is usually higher in vitamin A than is the milk of stall-fed animals.

Because margarines, lowfat and dried skim milk products and many ready-to-eat breakfast cereals are now fortified with vitamin A, they contribute a significant amount to the total vitamin A intake in the United States and other countries where these products are used.

Carotene is abundant in carrots, from which it derives its name, but it is also present in even higher concentration in certain green, leafy vegetables and grasses in which the color of the chlorophyll masks the yellow of the carotene. In certain species, such as corn, there is more carotene—hence, more vitamin-A activity—in yellow varieties than in white. There are African countries where red palm oil is used extensively and contributes greatly to the carotene intake.

Animal foods that contain mostly preformed vitamin A seem to be more efficient sources of this factor for humans than are the precursors found in plants. However, the ample supply of carotenes in plant foods may well contribute a large share of the vitamin A requirement. Cooking, puréeing, or mashing of vegetables ruptures the cell membranes and makes the carotene more available. Figure 7-4 shows the relative vitamin A values of some common foods in the four food groups.

## Vitamin A Values in Average Servings

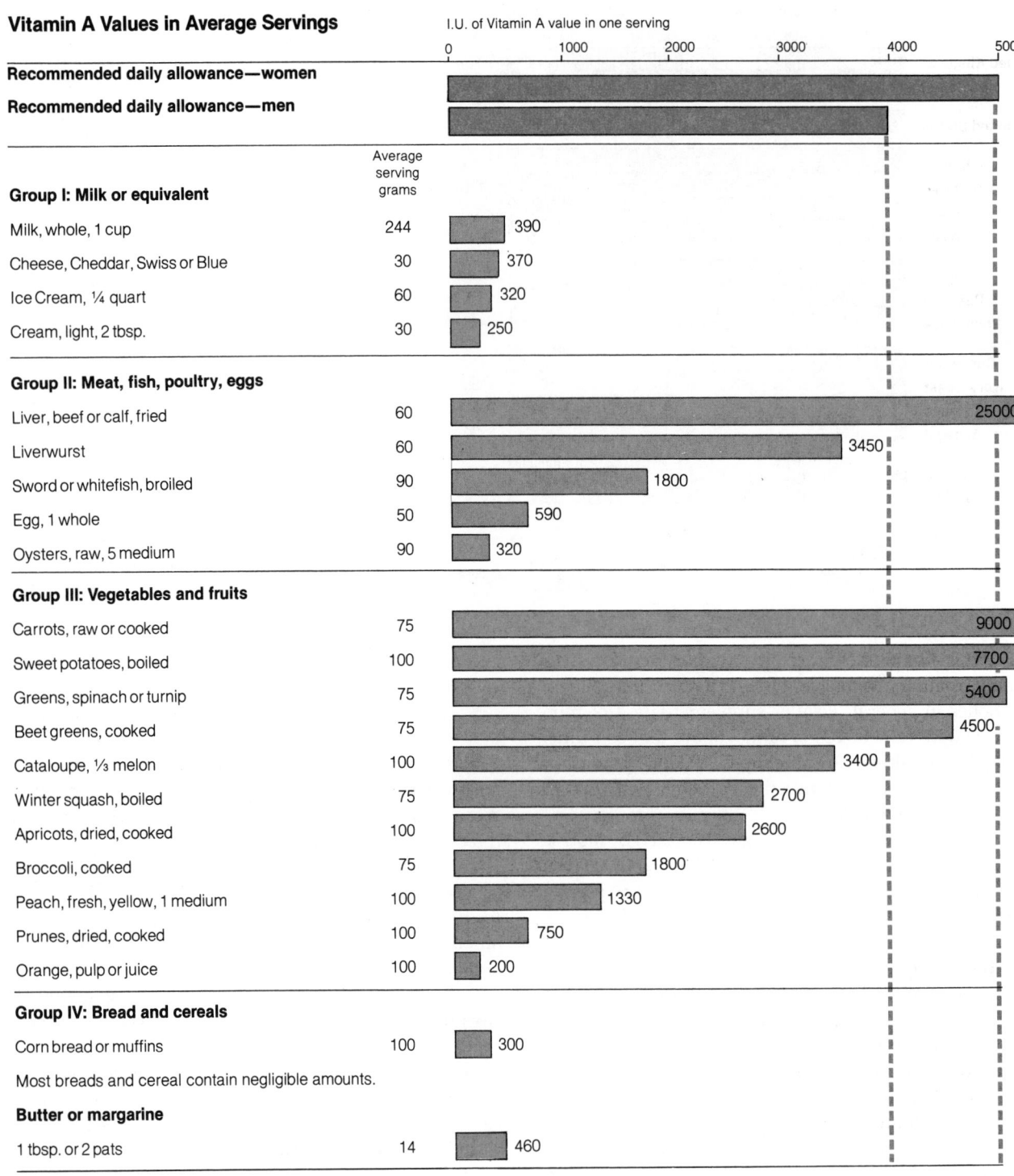

**I.U. of Vitamin A value in one serving**

| | Average serving grams | I.U. of Vitamin A value in one serving |
|---|---|---|
| **Recommended daily allowance—women** | | 5000 |
| **Recommended daily allowance—men** | | 4000 |
| **Group I: Milk or equivalent** | | |
| Milk, whole, 1 cup | 244 | 390 |
| Cheese, Cheddar, Swiss or Blue | 30 | 370 |
| Ice Cream, ¼ quart | 60 | 320 |
| Cream, light, 2 tbsp. | 30 | 250 |
| **Group II: Meat, fish, poultry, eggs** | | |
| Liver, beef or calf, fried | 60 | 25000 |
| Liverwurst | 60 | 3450 |
| Sword or whitefish, broiled | 90 | 1800 |
| Egg, 1 whole | 50 | 590 |
| Oysters, raw, 5 medium | 90 | 320 |
| **Group III: Vegetables and fruits** | | |
| Carrots, raw or cooked | 75 | 9000 |
| Sweet potatoes, boiled | 100 | 7700 |
| Greens, spinach or turnip | 75 | 5400 |
| Beet greens, cooked | 75 | 4500 |
| Cataloupe, ⅓ melon | 100 | 3400 |
| Winter squash, boiled | 75 | 2700 |
| Apricots, dried, cooked | 100 | 2600 |
| Broccoli, cooked | 75 | 1800 |
| Peach, fresh, yellow, 1 medium | 100 | 1330 |
| Prunes, dried, cooked | 100 | 750 |
| Orange, pulp or juice | 100 | 200 |
| **Group IV: Bread and cereals** | | |
| Corn bread or muffins | 100 | 300 |
| Most breads and cereal contain negligible amounts. | | |
| **Butter or margarine** | | |
| 1 tbsp. or 2 pats | 14 | 460 |

**Fig. 7-4.**   Vitamin A value in average servings of foods classified according to the four food groups.

## Vitamin D

### History

Rickets has been known as a deficiency disease of infants for several centuries. Renaissance painters often depicted children with rachitic deformities, signs so common that they were considered normal. The history of rickets as a deficiency disease is much older than our knowledge of how to prevent it. In the early 19th century cod-liver oil was a well-known folk remedy in Holland; somewhat later it was accepted as a therapeutic agent for rickets by physicians in Holland, France, and Germany. During the latter part of the 19th century cod-liver oil lost favor with the medical profession because physicians could not explain its action. It was not used extensively for many years until the period of World War I, when active research on the prevention and the treatment of rickets was inaugurated.

Early workers recognized that normal bone growth apparently was controlled by some substance in natural fats. This unknown factor was credited with some control over the metabolism of calcium and phosphorus.

Research on the chemical nature of vitamin D was initiated in 1924, when Steenbock and Hess demonstrated independently that antirachitic activity could be induced in foods containing certain fat-soluble substances by exposure to ultraviolet light. This discovery of the activation of fat-like substances by ultraviolet rays permitted the manufacture of a concentrated vitamin D preparation, such as viosterol, long before the pure crystalline vitamin D, calciferol, was isolated in 1935.

## Nomenclature

The two major compounds with vitamin D activity—considered until recently to be responsible for the functions of this vitamin—are *cholecalciferol*, vitamin $D_3$, and *ergocalciferol*, vitamin $D_2$ (Fig. 7-5). Each can be formed from a naturally occurring precursor (provitamin) by irradiation with ultraviolet light—$D_3$ from 7-dehydrocholesterol found in the skin and other animal tissues and $D_2$ from ergosterol found in lower forms of plants. Although both appear to be equally active in man and have been shown to undergo similar metabolic conversions,[30] the discussion that follows refers to cholecalciferol ($D_3$); this is the form available to humans as a result of exposure to sunlight, and it has been used in most of the studies that have resulted in our present knowledge of vitamin D metabolism and function.

Vitamin D is now considered a *prohormone* and is converted in the body to at least one active hormone, 1,25-dihydroxycholecalciferol (1,25-$(OH)_2D_3$), which performs the known physiologic functions of vitamin D. Sev-

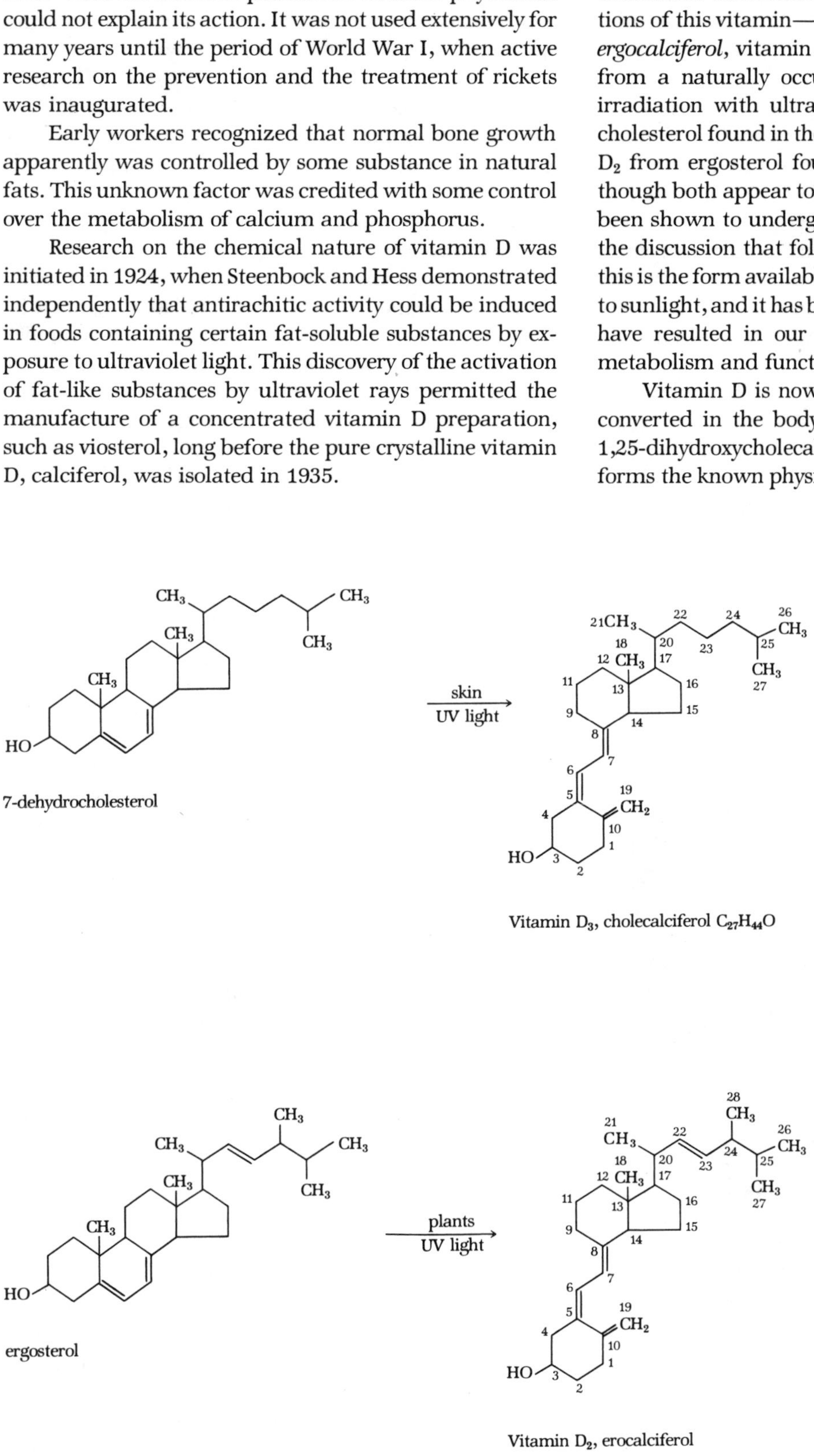

Vitamin $D_3$, cholecalciferol $C_{27}H_{44}O$

Vitamin $D_2$, erocalciferol

**Fig. 7-5.** Compounds with vitamin D activity and their precursors.

eral other vitamin D metabolites have been discovered (as is discussed in the following section), but their biologic significance remains mostly unknown at present, with the exception of 25-hydroxycholecalciferol, which is the immediate precursor of $1,25\text{-}(OH)_2D_3$.

### Measurement of vitamin D

Until very recently, vitamin D activity has been expressed in International Units (IU). One IU is equal to the activity of 0.025 mcg of pure crystalline cholecalciferol; thus 2.5 mcg equals 100 IU. It is important to know this relationship; for although IU is still used in the food composition tables and also on the labels of foods fortified with vitamin D, the 1980 recommended dietary allowances[3] as well as the WHO/FAO recommended intakes[2] are given in micrograms.

Criteria used for judging the severity of experimental rickets are roentgenograms (x-rays) showing the total mineral content of bone and the calcification of the metaphyses (the growing portion) of the long bones. The last observation has resulted in the development of a standardized line test on rats, which is employed for routine assays of vitamin D preparations. Rats are fed on a rickets-producing diet until a definite stage of early rickets occurs; the source of vitamin D (the product to be tested) is then fed, and the animals are sacrificed on the eleventh day. Longitudinal sections of certain bones are stained in silver nitrate solution, which darkens only the calcified areas.

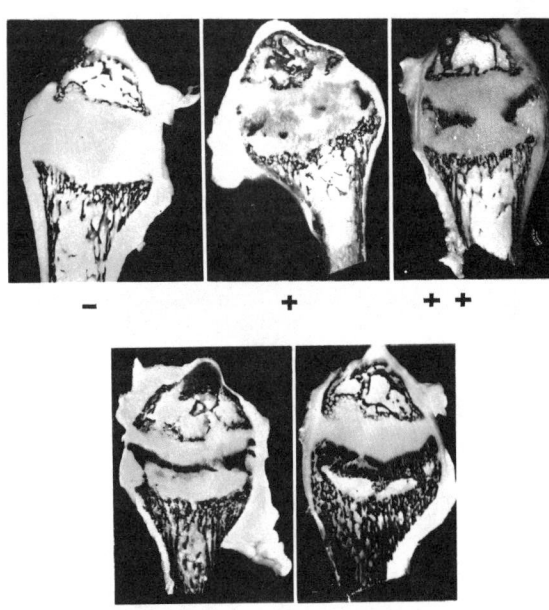

**Fig. 7-6.** Progressive degrees of recalcification or healing of rachitic bones due to graded doses of vitamin D. The increasing extent of the dark areas, where the white band appeared in the first photo, indicates mineral deposits. Photo marked + + + + represents one Steenbock or 2.7 U.S.P. units of vitamin D. (Wisconsin Alumni Research Foundation)

Figure 7-6 shows the progressive degrees in recalcification, or healing, that take place in rachitic bone when graded doses of vitamin D are administered. Other promising methods have been developed, which shorten the time and the expense of vitamin D assays.

In spite of advances in the investigation of vitamin D—long recognized as necessary for the normal calcification of bones—many questions remain to be answered in regard to the mechanisms of the action of this vitamin.

### Absorption, transport, metabolism, storage, and excretion

Vitamin D is absorbed in the presence of bile, probably from the jejunum and is transported like vitamin A in the lymph chylomicrons to the bloodstream. It is rapidly taken up by the liver, where it is hydroxylated to 25-hydroxycholecalciferol ($25\text{-}OH\text{-}D_3$). $D_3$ formed in the skin or injected as an alcohol solution also is removed by the liver.[31] Released from the liver, $25\text{-}OH\text{-}D_3$ undergoes another hydroxylation in the kidney to form $1\text{-}25\text{-}(OH)_2D_3$, which is the active hormone in the vitamin D endocrine system.[32] A number of other metabolites have been identified in the kidney, liver, and intestine, but, although they may show some vitamin D activity, their functional significance is unknown (Fig. 7-7). Of these, $24,25\text{-}(OH)_2D_3$, formed from $25\text{-}OH\text{-}D_3$ in the kidney and the intestine, has received most attention because it is found in relatively large amounts in the plasma, and its production appears to be governed by the regulatory system that controls the production of $1,25\text{-}(OH)_2D_3$.[32] Recent research provides strong evidence against a specific requirement for 24-hydroxylation for activity in bone mineralization as has been proposed.[32] Therefore, the presently known conversions of vitamin $D_3$ obligatory for its known functions are as follows:

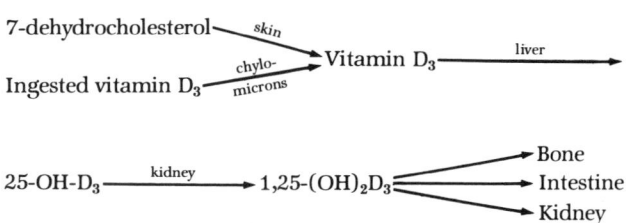

Vitamin $D_3$ and its metabolites are transported in the plasma bound to an $\alpha$-globulin that has not been well characterized.[31] The major circulating form of vitamin D is $25\text{-}OH\text{-}D_3$, as is shown in Table 7-1.

Although administration of vitamin D results in an initial uptake by the liver and in increased formation of $25\text{-}OH\text{-}D_3$, the excess vitamin appears to be stored mostly in the adipose tissue. Considerable amounts are also found in the liver and other tissues.[31] The major route of vitamin D excretion is through the bile; some metabolites are found also in the urine, but as is the case with vitamin A, daily loss of vitamin D by urinary excretion is small.[33]

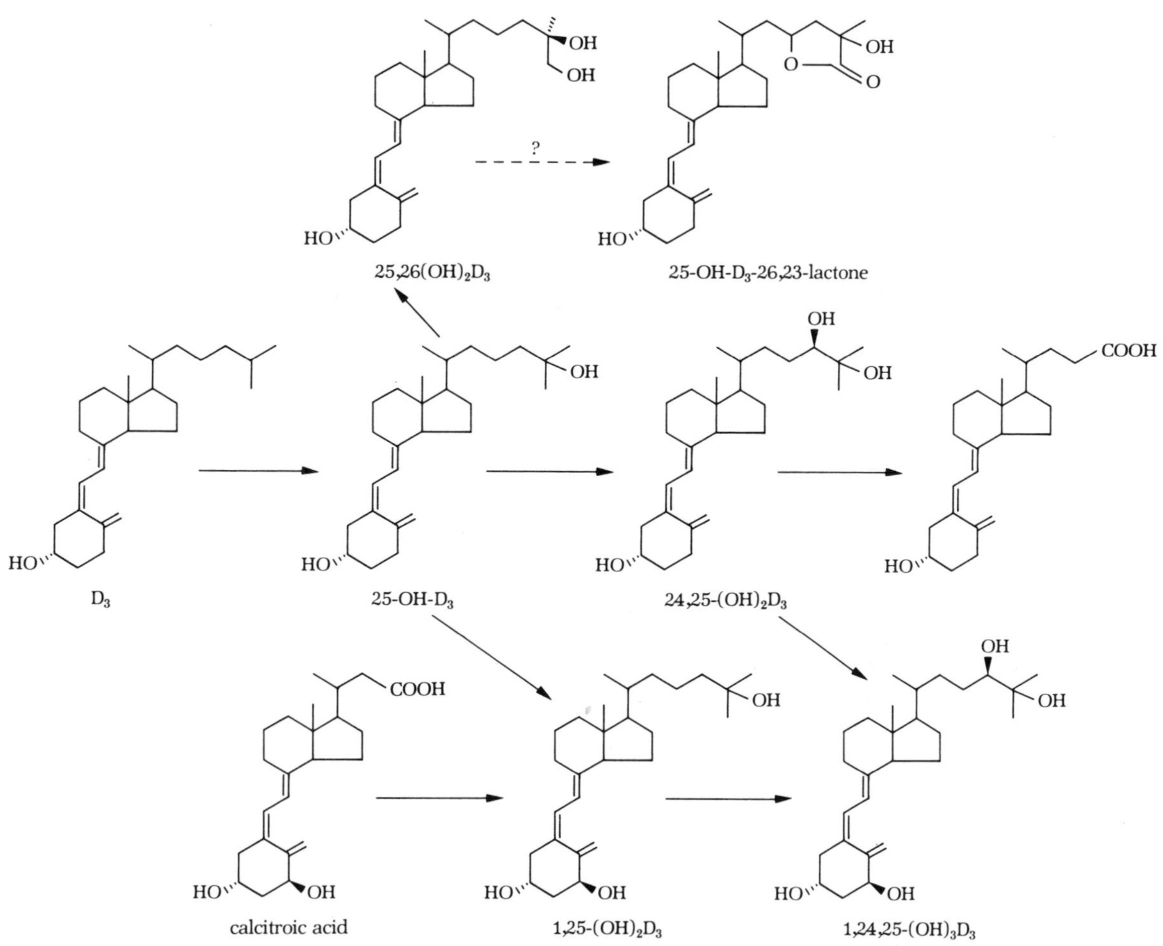

**Fig. 7-7.** Metabolism of Vitamin $D_3$. (From DeLuca HF: Nutr Rev 38:169, 1980)

## Functions

Current research on the action of vitamin D is rapidly unfolding its relationship to calcium and phosphorus metabolism. The major function of vitamin D presently known is to elevate the concentration of plasma calcium and phosphorus to levels that allow normal bone mineralization and prevent the tetany of hypocalcemia (see Chap. 6).[32] To accomplish this, vitamin D acts at a number of different sites.

### Absorption of calcium and phosphorus from the intestinal tract

Elevation of plasma calcium from dietary intake involves vitamin D-stimulated active transport of calcium from the intestinal lumen to the bloodstream against a concentration gradient. This process takes place throughout the intestine including the colon, but is most active in the duodenum.[32] The function of $1,25\text{-}(OH)_2D_3$ in the enhancement of calcium transport includes multiple actions, which are not well understood. Carried by blood to the intestine, $1,25\text{-}(OH)_2D_3$ binds to a cytosomal receptor of the mucosal cell and is translocated to the nucleus, where its interaction with the genome is presumed to

initiate protein synthesis that includes a specific calcium-binding protein (CaBP). Although $1,25\text{-}(OH)_2D_3$ stimulates both the entry of calcium into the epithelial cell at the brushborder and its exit to the serosa through the basolateral membrane of the cell, only the latter process requires new protein synthesis. Stimulation of calcium uptake by $1,25\text{-}(OH)_2D_3$ at the brushborder is rapid and precedes the vitamin D-induced production of CaBP, which is followed by enhancement of calcium exit from the cell. The function of CaBP remains uncertain, but it may entail transfer of calcium from its intracellular transport vehicles (mitochondria or membrane vesicles) to the basolateral cation pump for extrusion from the cell. Al-

### Table 7-1. Plasma Levels of Vitamin D and Its Metabolites

| Compound | Concentration | Reference |
|----------|---------------|-----------|
| Vitamin D | 1–2  ng/ml | 31 |
| 25-OH-D | 20–40 ng/ml | 32 |
| $1,25\text{-}(OH)_2D$ | 30–40 pg/ml | 32 |
| $24,25\text{-}(OH)_2D$ | 1 ng/ml | 33 |

though the mechanism of this calcium release is not certain, experimental evidence supports an ATPase-dependent exit of calcium in exchange for entering sodium.[30,34]

Other observations after administration of 1,25-$(OH)_2D_3$ include stimulation of adenyl cyclase (and an increase in cAMP) and an increase in alkaline phosphatase.[30,34] No direct role for alkaline phosphatase in the absorption of calcium is indicated, and it has been suggested that perhaps it hydrolyzes organic complexes of calcium and phosphorus at the brushborder, thereby increasing their availability for absorption.[34] The role of cAMP is also uncertain, but some evidence suggests that it may in someway aid the entry of calcium into the mucosal cell[30,34] and may, perhaps, act as a mediator of the trophic action of 1,25-$(OH)_2D_3$ on the intestine[34]; this "second messenger" role of cAMP is well known in the action of several other hormones (see Chap. 9).

It should be noted that some calcium absorption takes place by mechanisms independent of vitamin D. The amount of calcium absorbed without vitamin D under most circumstances is not adequate to satisfy the calcium requirement, as is evident from the development of rickets in children and osteomalacia in adults. It has been long recognized that the rate of intestinal absorption of calcium is responsive to the body's need for calcium and adapts to the level of calcium intake. This adaptation is dependent on the availability of 1,25-$(OH)_2D_3$ and is mediated by the parathyroid hormone (PTH).[30] However, it appears that under conditions of high calcium need, such as pregnancy and lactation, other adaptive mechanisms may also be functioning.[32]

Intestinal absorption of phosphorus also involves at least two mechanisms, both of which are stimulated by vitamin D.[32] Because the vitamin D-dependent active absorption of calcium results in increased absorption of phosphorus as an accompanying anion, the effect on phosphorus absorption is secondary. Phosphorus is also transported by an active transport process that is stimulated by vitamin D, requires sodium, but does not result in transport of calcium.[32,35]

## Mobilization of calcium and phosphorus from the bone

The normal level of plasma calcium and phosphorus is maintained within relatively narrow limits of concentration. When intestinal absorption is not taking place, bone serves as a reserve for calcium and phosphorus. The primary factor in the mobilization of these minerals from the bone fluid compartment is PTH, but the presence of 1,25-$(OH)_2D_3$ appears to be required for the process.[32] It should be noted that while this mechanism is essential in the maintenance of calcium and phosphorus homeostasis, it cannot be drawn upon continuously without replacement by dietary intake.

## Renal reabsorption of calcium and phosphorus

The third site for the control of plasma calcium and phosphorus levels is the kidney. When the plasma levels of these minerals are low the kidneys can increase their reabsorption, thereby reducing loss of them from the body. Vitamin D has been shown to stimulate the reabsorption of calcium in the distal tubules, but its role in phosphorus reabsorption is still controversial; the latest evidence does not support a vitamin D function in renal reabsorption of phosphorus.[32]

## Other functions

It has long been suspected that vitamin D is required in the actual process of bone mineralization in addition to its function in providing supersaturation levels of calcium and phosphorus. Despite many attempts, direct proof for such function is still lacking. Vitamin D (1,25-$(OH)_2D_3$) appears to increase muscle strength in rachitic children and in patients with renal osteodystrophy.[30] There is no information at present about how this effect might be brought about. Although uptake of radioactive 1,25-$(OH)_2D_3$ by tissues other than the previously known target tissues has been demonstrated recently, muscle was not among them.[32] A search for possible new functions of vitamin D has led to a recent demonstration that 1,25-$(OH)_2D_3$ enhances the accumulation of 7-dehydrocholesterol in the skin in the rat, thereby increasing the substrate for the production of its prohormone, vitamin $D_3$.[32]

## Regulation of vitamin D metabolism and function

Metabolism of vitamin D is intricately linked to the endocrine control of calcium and phosphorus homeostasis and involves the parathyroid and thyroid glands (see Chap. 6, *Calcium and Phosphorus*). The primary site of control of vitamin D metabolism appears to be the renal synthesis of 1,25-$(OH)_2D_3$, which responds to changes in the body's need for calcium and phosphorus. Hypocalcemia stimulates the parathyroid gland to release PTH, which, in turn, increases the activity of renal 1-hydroxylase (25-hydroxycholecalciferol-1-hydroxylase) and, consequently, the level of circulating 1,25-$(OH)_2D_3$.[32,36] However, the most immediate effect is the mobilization of calcium from the bone by PTH with the existing 1,25-$(OH)_2D_3$. Both also cause increased reabsorption of calcium by the kidneys, but independently and at different sites. These two mechanisms are responsible for restoring the plasma calcium and plasma phosphorus levels. The specific effects of PTH on phosphorus are discussed in Chapter 6. The elevation of 1,25-$(OH)_2D_3$ eventually increases the intestinal absorption of calcium and phosphorus, but this action is more important in replenishing the bone minerals to maintain calcium and phosphorus balance than in the short-term control of plasma levels.[33]

When the plasma calcium reaches a normal level, the production of PTH decreases and results in the suppression of 1-hydroxylase in the kidney. Suppression of this enzyme by its product 1,25-$(OH)_2D_3$ has been observed, but as with some other factors, it may not have a direct effect on the enzyme as much as a secondary one due to reduced PTH.[36] In hypercalcemia, calcitonin is released by the thyroid gland, blocking further mobilization of bone minerals. High plasma calcium concentration turns off the production of PTH and, secondarily, 1,25-$(OH)_2D_3$, thereby reducing calcium flow from all three sites.

Hypophosphatemia also increases the level of 1,25-$(OH)_2D_3$ as part of the changes initiated to restore plasma phosphorus level, but the magnitude of the response is much smaller than that produced by hypocalcemia.[32]

There is also evidence that other hormones play a role in the regulation of vitamin D metabolism. Prolactin, growth hormone,[37] and insulin have been reported to stimulate formation of 1,25-$(OH)_2D_3$.[33] Whether these hormones affect vitamin D metabolism directly or indirectly remains uncertain.

Concentration of 1,25-$(OH)_2D_3$ in the plasma is much lower than that of 25-OH-$D_3$ (Table 7-1), and its half life is only 5 to 8 hours compared with 15 to 30 days for 25-OH-$D_3$. Although the synthesis of 25-OH-$D_3$ increases, following administration of vitamin $D_3$, the increased supply of substrate does not affect the rate of the renal production of 1,25-$(OH)_2D_3$.[36] Consequently, the hepatic 25-hydroxylase does not appear to be part of the regulatory system that controls the level of active vitamin D in the body. The physiological significance and control of the 24-hydroxylation of 25-OH-$D_3$ and 1,25-$(OH)_2D_3$ remain to be clarified.

## Human requirements

Because vitamin D may be supplied either by ingesting it in foods or supplements or by exposure to certain wavelengths of sunlight, its requirement has been difficult to determine.

In infants 100 IU (2.5 mcg) of vitamin D per day prevents rickets and provides for adequate calcium absorption, normal bone mineralization, and a satisfactory growth rate. However, because increased growth and better calcium absorption resulted from feeding 300 IU to 400 IU (7.5 mcg–10.0 mcg) daily, the National Research Council's Food and Nutrition Board and the Joint FAO/WHO Expert Committee recommend 10 mcg (400 IU) of vitamin D per day for infants and young children, birth through 6 years of age. These recommendations apply to both formula-fed and breast-fed infants. The premature infant who is growing rapidly and is usually not exposed to sunlight for a considerable length of time is more prone to develop rickets than the full term infant; for this reason he should be assured an adequate amount of vitamin D.

Because there is little information regarding vitamin D requirements in older children and adolescents and because rickets is practically nonexistent in this age group, the Joint FAO/WHO Expert Committee has reduced their recommendation to 2.5 mcg (100 IU) per day for children over 6 years and adults.

The Food and Nutrition Board, however, recognizing the same situation, recommends a daily intake of 10 mcg (400 IU) of vitamin D from birth through age 18, 7.5 mcg (300 IU) during years 19 to 22, and 5 mcg (200 IU) for adults over the age of 22 years.[3] Although adults are expected to meet their requirement through exposure to sunlight under most conditions, certain circumstances and customs may necessitate a dietary source of vitamin D. During pregnancy and lactation, 10 mcg (400 IU) daily are recommended by both the Food and Nutrition Board and by the Joint FAO/WHO Expert Committee.

## Sources of vitamin D

### Sunshine

The low incidence of rickets in tropical climates suggested that sunshine might play a role in its prevention. Even after it had been demonstrated conclusively that the ultraviolet light from sunshine aided in the healing of rickets, it was difficult to understand the connection between this effect of light and the similar effect of vitamin D from such sources as cod-liver oil. Eventually, the puzzle was solved when it was discovered that vitamin D activity could be produced by irradiation. The amount of ultraviolet light in sunlight varies with the season and the locality, as does the total amount of sunlight. These rays are also filtered out by fog, smoke and ordinary window glass. It is obvious that an adequate natural source of ultraviolet light is impossible in northern climates during the winter months. For this reason, some other source of vitamin D is needed.

Similarly, the pigments in the skin that protect against overproduction of vitamin D in dark-skinned peoples living in the tropics also reduce the effectiveness of the smaller amount of irradiation in temperate climates. As a result, the incidence of rickets is higher in dark-skinned babies living in temperate zones than in either light-skinned babies in this zone or dark-skinned infants in the tropics.

### Foods and supplements

The natural distribution of vitamin D in common foods is limited to small, often insignificant amounts in fatty tissue, cream, butter, eggs, and liver. Consequently, we have come to depend on fortified foods, fish-liver oil, or concentrates for preventive and therapeutic use.

Because it was necessary to decide on one food, commonly used by children, that would be fortified with a standard amount of vitamin D, the Council on Foods and Nutrition of the American Medical Association made the following decision:

> Of all the common foods available, milk is the most suitable as a carrier of added vitamin D. Vitamin D is concerned with the utilization of calcium and phosphorus, of which milk is an excellent source.[38]

Vitamin D milk now on the market is produced by adding a vitamin D concentrate to homogenized milk; the present standard of 10 mcg (400 IU) per quart means that a quart of milk provides a day's requirement of vitamin D. All brands of evaporated milk also have vitamin D added, and strong recommendations to fortify nonfat milk solids with vitamins A and D have also been made by the American Medical Association.[39] Indiscriminate fortification of a variety of other foods with vitamin D does not seem to be either necessary or desirable.

Among the numerous fish-liver oils investigated there is a wide range of potency. This seems to vary with the season of the catch and the oil content of the livers. The highest-potency oil is often yielded from fish that give the

lowest amount of oil. Concentrates are made from the natural fish-liver oils or by irradiating pure ergosterol and cholesterol. Such preparations are labeled with the exact units per dose or per capsule and are prescribed accordingly. A protective dose to meet the daily requirement is considerably lower than what may be prescribed as a curative dose.

In a study of the consumption of vitamin D by children (birth–18 years) the average daily intake for all age groups was above 400 IU. Fortified milk supplied the largest amount of vitamin D, the percentage increasing with age. Vitamin preparations were more important in the infant and preschool groups than with older children. Fortified foods contributed to intakes of vitamin D over the recommended dietary allowance, particularly in the school age group (Fig. 7-8).[40]

It is becoming evident that changing social, cultural, and environmental conditions are contributing to the re-emergence of rickets as a nutritional problem in the Western countries.[41] The staff of the Children's Hospital in Philadelphia has diagnosed 24 cases of rickets in black children between the ages of 4 months and 5 years, from 1974 to 1978. Many cases involved severely restricted vegetarian diets, and many of the infants were breast-fed, with no vitamin supplements. None of the mothers had received supplements during pregnancy or lactation. Other cases of rickets involving children of white vegetarians also have been reported.[41]

## Stability

Vitamin D in foods and in food concentrates is remarkably stable to heating, aging, and storage. Vitamin D milk that is warmed for the baby is still a reliable source of this factor.

## Medical uses of vitamin D compounds

With the discovery of the metabolic activation of vitamin D prior to its function in the body it became evident that some of the disorders that did not respond well to vitamin D might benefit from one of its metabolites. Subsequent chemical synthesis of these compounds and their analogs has allowed some clinical testing of their usefulness. Treatment with $1,25\text{-}(OH)_2D_3$ has been found effective in some patients with renal osteodystrophy associated with chronic renal failure (see Chap. 32).[30] The circulating level of this metabolite in these patients is hardly detectable, but because of the greatly reduced kidney function, other complicating metabolic imbalances are present, which make the condition difficult to manage. Other conditions that appear to benefit from $1,25\text{-}(OH)_2D_3$ include hypoparathyroidism, vitamin D-dependent rickets, a rare genetic disease due to a defect in 1-hydroxylase, and hypophosphatemic vitamin D-resistant rickets. The latter condition requires daily phosphate supplementation along with vitamin D because a defect in

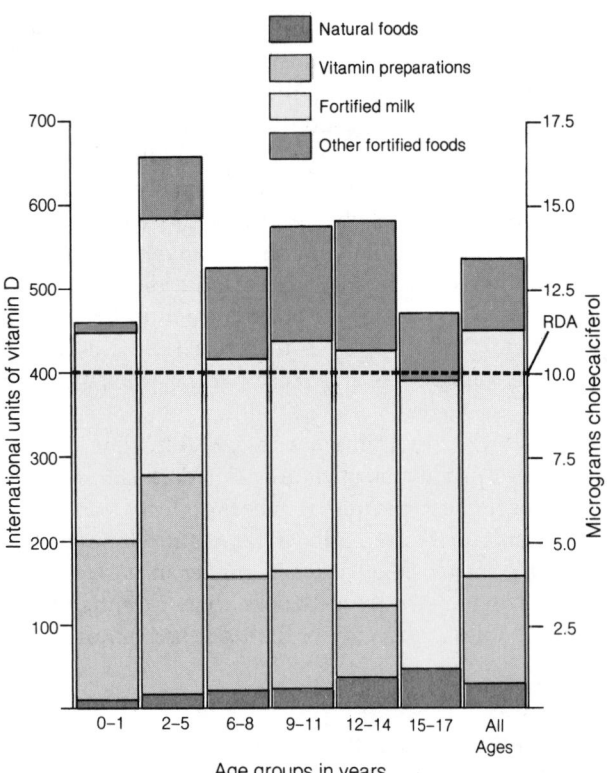

**Fig. 7-8.**   Average daily intakes of vitamin D by age groups and sources. (Adapted from Dale AE, Lowenberg ME: J Pediatr 70:954, 1967)

renal phosphate transport is the primary lesion that causes hypophosphatemia.[33] These conditions have been treated with massive doses of vitamin D or its synthetic analog, dihydrotachysterol. The former probably acts after conversion to 25-OH-$D_3$, which in large doses is known to substitute for 1,25-(OH)$_2D_3$ in the target tissues.[30] Dihydrotachysterol also is active in large doses without 1-hydroxylation.[31]

Administration of 1,25-(OH)$_2D_3$ to postmenopausal osteoporotic women has been shown to increase intestinal calcium absorption and to improve calcium balance.[30] Good discussions of metabolic defects involving vitamin D can be found in recent reviews.[30,31,33]

## Hypervitaminosis D

Excessive intake of vitamin D is toxic. Usually, toxicity is not manifest except after huge doses, which result in calcification of soft tissues due to persistent hypercalcemia. Cases of vitamin D toxicity occur "because of unjustified and indiscriminate medical use of the vitamin, lack of appreciation of its toxicity, and the self-administration of highly concentrated preparations."[42] The maximum safe level of vitamin D for infants has yet to be precisely established, although intakes of 40 mcg (1600 IU)—four times the recommended dietary allowance—have not interfered with the rate of growth in either length or weight of infants.[43] However, evidence that certain infants may be more sensitive to the toxic effects of vitamin D and may develop hypercalcemia on intakes of 50 mcg (2000 IU) has caused considerable concern regarding the infant's total intake of this vitamin.[44] It is particularly important that the mother recognize the need for vitamin D, but, even more important, that she be aware of the harmful effects of overdosage. This means, of course, that the physician and the mother should know of the sources of vitamin D in the diet as well as in supplements.

In adults, hypercalcemia has been accompanied by such symptoms as anorexia, nausea, weight loss, polyuria, constipation, and azotemia. Similar symptoms are seen in infants, and, in certain rare severe forms, mental retardation also occurs.

Vitamin D toxicity symptoms are associated with high plasma levels of 25-OH-$D_3$, but normal or even below normal levels of 1,25-(OH)$_2D_3$.[33] Because 25-OH-$D_3$ is known to substitute for 1,25-(OH)$_2D_3$ at the tissue receptor sites when present in large amounts, it is possible that its action in the bone and intestine is responsible for the excessive calcium load brought to the system.[33] Because of the potential danger of high intakes and because there is no known benefit from intake levels above the recommended dietary allowances, the Food and Nutrition Board has stressed the importance of maintaining a daily intake close to the recommended levels for both children and adults.[3] When a special need for vitamin D therapy is indicated, therapy should be carefully supervised by a physician, and the plasma calcium levels should be monitored continually. Treatment of vitamin D toxicity involves withdrawal of the vitamin supplement, reduction of calcium intake, and administration of a furosemide diuretic.[33] Glucocorticoid therapy may be required to normalize plasma calcium.[33,42]

# Vitamin E
## History

The existence of a dietary factor essential for reproduction in the rat was recognized in the early 1920s by Evans; Sure named it vitamin E, or antisterility factor. In rats, on which much of the experimental work was done, the males and the females are affected differently. Vitamin E deficiency leads to destruction of germ cells in the testes of the male and thus to permanent sterility. In a vitamin E deficient female mated with a normal male, ovulation and implantation of the ovum may take place normally, but about halfway through the gestation period resorption of the developing fetus occurs, and no young are born. With less severe vitamin E deficiency, which may permit the birth of a weakling litter, the chances of survival are poor because this same deficiency seems to interfere with lactation or, later, with growth of the young.

Vitamin E has turned out to be perhaps the most elusive of the nutritional factors discovered so far. In experimental animals a large number of different deficiency symptoms and distinct deficiency diseases were demonstrated, depending on the species. Furthermore, it was later discovered that some of these conditions could be either totally or partially prevented by factors other than vitamin E, for example, selenium, various compounds with antioxidant activity, and sulfur-amino acids. It was also discovered that high intake of polyunsaturated fatty acids increased the severity of some but not all of these syndromes. It now appears that although the manifestations in different species vary, the same body systems are involved—the reproductive system, the musculature, the nervous, and the vascular systems.

Even more perplexing has been the fact that no clinical evidence of vitamin E deficiency could be produced in humans. Evidence has failed to indicate that vitamin E is a significant factor in reproduction or muscular dystrophy, the first two conditions that were extensively studied in connection with the effects of vitamin E in humans. Even though the role of vitamin E in human nutrition is still not well defined, there is no question that it is an essential nutrient for human health.

## Nomenclature

Eight naturally occurring compounds have vitamin E activity. They are fat-soluble alcohols of high molecular weight, closely related in structure, called *tocopherols* and *tocotrienols.* They all have the same basic ring structure but vary in number and location of methyl substitutions (Fig. 7-9). All tocopherols have a saturated phytyl side chain, whereas the side chain of tocotrienols possesses the three double bonds indicated by its name. Alpha-tocopherol (α-tocopherol) is the most active form (Fig. 7-9). It deteriorates on exposure to light and decomposes upon irradiation with ultraviolet light. Contact with lead and iron hastens destruction. Tocopherols, because they are readily oxidized themselves, have antioxidant properties and prevent deterioration of certain foods by oxidation. This characteristic probably exerts a protective action on vitamin A.

As with vitamins A and D, vitamin E activity was initially expressed in IU but the current preference is to give the individual compounds as milligrams (mg) and the total vitamin E activity as *mg d-α-tocopherol equivalents.* The IU was established as the biologic activity of 1 mg of dl-α-tocopheryl acetate. The biopotencies of the other available α-tocopherol compounds expressed as IU are as follows:

> 1 mg d-α-tocopherol (naturally occurring form) = 1.49 IU
> 1 mg d-α-tocopheryl acetate (natural) = 1.36 IU
> 1 mg dl-α-tocopherol (synthetic) = 1.1 IU

The other tocopherols (β, γ, and δ) and the tocotrienols (α, β, γ, and δ) have varied biologic activities from 1% to 50% of that of α-tocopherol. However, in mixed diets some may be present in amounts several times that of α-tocopherol, thereby contributing significantly to the total vitamin E activity. Only limited analytical data are available on the total vitamin E content of foods and, except for α-tocopherol, even less on the food values of individual tocopherols and tocotrienols. A compilation of the vitamin E content of foods has been published recently[45] (Table 6, Part 4).

For the purpose of estimating the total vitamin E activity of mixed diets from limited information, the Food and Nutrition Board has recommended the following procedure.[3] If only α-tocopherol is reported (in mg), the value should be multiplied by 1.2 to account for the estimated 20% higher total activity due to the other tocopherols

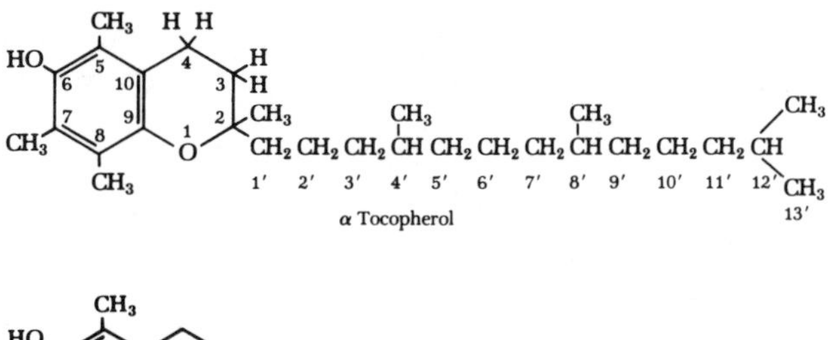

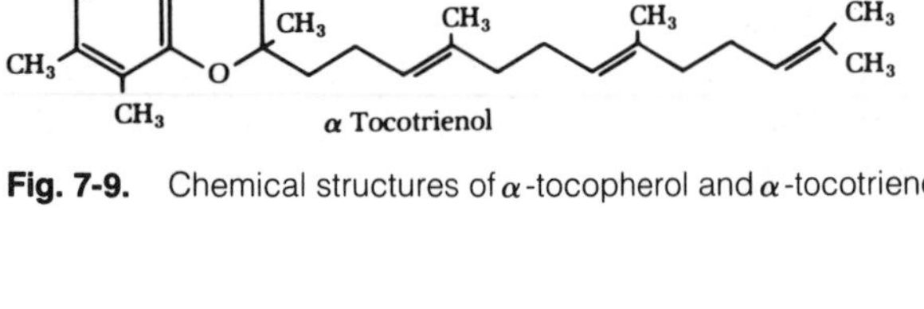

present. When separate values are available, they can be converted to α-tocopherol equivalents by multiplying mg β-tocopherol by 0.5, mg α-tocopherol by 0.1, and mg α-tocotrienol by 0.3. Added to the reported α-tocopherol value, the total vitamin E activity is obtained as milligrams α-tocopherol equivalents.

### Absorption, transport, storage, and excretion

The intestinal absorption of vitamin E follows the pattern for fat and other fat-soluble nutrients, reaching the blood through the lymph chylomicrons. The percentage of dietary vitamin E absorbed appears to be relatively constant over a narrow range of normal dietary intakes[46] and to decrease with increasing dose from high intakes of α-tocopherol.[46,47] However, there are great differences in the actual efficiency of vitamin E absorption observed in different studies, the reported values ranging from less than 30% to over 90%.[46-48]

Transported by the lipoproteins, the total plasma tocopherol concentration shows a positive correlation with plasma total lipids over a wide range of lipid concentrations, in both children[49,50] and adults.[50,51] Normal plasma tocopherol values in adults range from 0.5 mg to 1.6 mg per dl.[52] Values below 0.5 mg per dl have been considered deficient for all ages, as they appear to be associated with increased peroxide-induced erythrocyte hemolysis *in vitro,* another measure of vitamin E adequacy.[53] An alternate and, according to some investigators, preferred measure of vitamin E adequacy is the ratio of plasma tocopherols (mg) to total lipids (g); a ratio of 0.8 or greater is considered normal.[50] Whereas plasma tocopherol levels of infants and children may be lower than in adults,[49,50,54] their normal tocopherol to total lipid ratios appear to be above 0.8.[49,50]

Newborn infants tend to have low plasma levels of vitamin E (approximately one-third the adult level) due not only to lower concentrations of blood lipids in the newborn but also to limited transfer of the vitamin across the placenta. Plasma levels begin to rise after birth, more rapidly in the breast-fed infant, and reach normal concentrations by about one month of age. Low birth weight (LBW) infants have even lower levels of vitamin E at birth.[3] However, recent findings suggest that an appreciable number of children between 4 months and 13 years of age have plasma tocopherol levels below 0.5 mg per dl, with normal erythrocyte hemolysis test results.[49,55] It is not known at present below what plasma tocopherol level increased erythrocyte hemolysis becomes evident in this age group.

Vitamin E is readily taken up from plasma lipoproteins by the erythrocytes and other body tissues. Their vitamin E levels reflect the average intake of the vitamin over a period of time.[56] It appears to be concentrated in the phospholipids of the cellular and subcellular membranes in all tissues, and the excess is stored in the adipose

**Fig. 7-9.** Chemical structures of α-tocopherol and α-tocotrienol.

tissue fat as free tocopherol.[47] The major route of $\alpha$-tocopherol excretion is through the bile into feces as unaltered vitamin; its oxidation products are $\alpha$-tocoquinone and $\alpha$-tocohydroquinone, the latter mainly in the form of glucuronides.[47,57] Some oxidation products are also found in the urine.[57]

## Functions and physiological significance of vitamin E in humans

Although there is little disagreement among investigators about the general protective role of vitamin E in the cellular and subcellular membrane structures, there is little agreement about the mechanism by which the specific function of vitamin E as an essential nutrient is carried out. Three major theories have been advanced. Tappel[58] makes a strong case for the *lipid antioxidant* theory, which suggests that vitamin E is a physiological antioxidant protecting the polyunsaturated fatty acids and other easily oxidizable essential components of the body structure and function against peroxidative damage by internal and external insults. According to the *respiratory chain* hypothesis, vitamin E has a specific catalytic role in electron transport through the mitochondrial respiratory chain.[59] The *genetic regulation* hypothesis postulates that vitamin E exerts control over the transfer of genetic information in the cells.[60]

Although many arguments have been raised against the antioxidant theory,[61] evidence has accumulated to indicate that vitamin E is part of a multilevel cellular defense system that protects susceptible structures against oxidative damage by lipid peroxidation.[47,58] It is now believed that lipid peroxidation is initiated by a hydroxyl-free radical ($\cdot OH$), which is produced from a reaction between superoxide ($O_2^-$) and hydrogen peroxide ($H_2O_2$), both products of normal cellular metabolism.[47] In an unprotected cell these free radicals attack membrane lipids at the double bonds of the polyunsaturated fatty acids and form lipid peroxide radicals, which propagate chain reactions along the membrane and form lipid hydroperoxides at each double bond left behind. Unless stabilized, further oxidative degradation of these hydroperoxides results in damage to the membrane.

In a normal cell, first line defense is provided by sequential reactions that remove $O_2^-$ and $H_2O_2$, thereby reducing the substrates available for free radical formation. As discussed in Chapter 6, the joint action of superoxide dismutases (zinc-, copper- and manganese-containing enzymes in the mitochondria and cytoplasm, respectively) and the selenium-containing glutathione peroxidase (GSH-Px) results in the reduction of $O_2^-$ and $H_2O_2$ to water (Fig. 7-10). Reduced glutathione (GSH), a cysteine-containing tripeptide, is the source of reducing equivalents in the degradation of $H_2O_2$ and must be continuously replenished (reaction I-3).

The second line of defense is provided at the membrane site of peroxidation by vitamin E and GSH-Px. Vitamin E molecules, stationed among the membrane lipids, reduce the advancing peroxide radicals within their

I. Removal of superoxide and hydrogen peroxide

1. $2O_2^- + 2 H^+ \xrightarrow[\text{dismutase}]{\text{Superoxide}} H_2O_2 + O_2$

2. $H_2O_2 + 2 GSH \xrightarrow[\text{peroxidase}]{\text{Glutathione}} GSSG + H_2O$

3. $GSSG + NADPH + H^+ \xrightarrow[\text{reductase}]{\text{Glutathione}} 2 GSH + NADP$

II. Reduction of lipid peroxide radicals and hydroperoxides

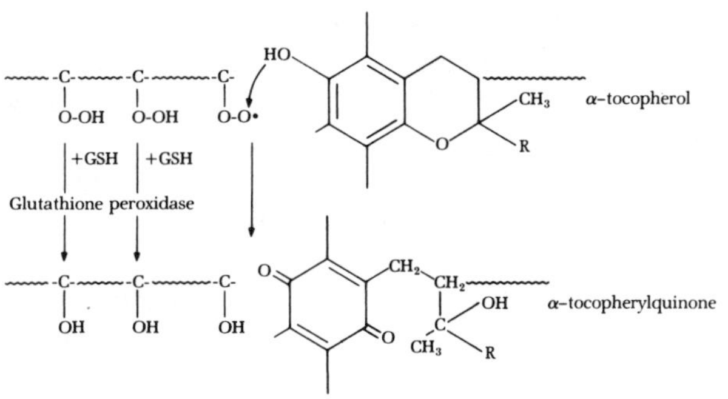

**Fig. 7-10.** Role of vitamin E in the cellular defense against lipid peroxidation. See text for details.

reach and stop the chain reactions. GSH-Px reduces the hydroperoxides as they are formed and, by formation of hydroxy fatty acids, stabilizes the membrane against autoxidative degradation. Scott and co-workers[47] have demonstrated that protection against *in vitro* peroxidation of mitochondrial and microsomal lipids is dependent on the presence of vitamin E in the membranes and GSH-Px in the soluble cell fraction and required GSH.

It has not been possible to measure lipid peroxidation *in vivo* until the recent introduction of a new experimental technique that employs the measurement of volatile oxidation products of polyunsaturated fatty acid (PUFA) in the expired air collected from intact animals (ethane and pentane gases from linolenic and linoleic acids, respectively). With this method several investigators[62] have demonstrated *in vivo* lipid peroxidation in rats fed diets deficient in vitamin E, selenium, and sulfur-containing amino acids, and observed variable protective effects from supplementation with each individually or in combinations. Feeding cod-liver oil or corn oil in place of lard greatly increased lipid peroxidation when measured by this method. In rats fed cod-liver oil, selenium supplementation reduced ethane production by half, while vitamin E supplementation reduced it to almost zero.

Although specific catalytic or hormone-like functions proposed for vitamin E have not been ruled out by these findings, it is possible that the effects of vitamin E observed in numerous enzyme systems or individual enzymes are the result of alterations in membrane structure and permeability which in turn are intricately linked to the normal functioning of the major systems that are responsible for cellular metabolism.

There is strong agreement among the investigators that the need for vitamin E is related to the amount of polyunsaturated fatty acids in the tissues. Red blood cells from subjects on low vitamin E and high polyunsaturated fatty acid dietary intakes have less resistance to hemolysis in the presence of hydrogen peroxide than those from subjects on higher vitamin E and lower PUFA intakes. Although the clinical significance is not clear, this test is one of the measurements used to determine the vitamin E status of individuals. Vitamin E deficiencies in man are very rare; however, considerable interest has been shown in this area because of the relationship of vitamin E to PUFA and the present trend toward increasing PUFA in the diets of large segments of the population.

There are some special conditions in which inadequate vitamin E status may develop. This has been most clearly demonstrated in premature infants, who have low plasma vitamin E levels because of its poor transfer across the placenta; immaturity of the intestine reduces the absorption of dietary vitamin E. As a result, vitamin E deficiency syndrome characterized by hemolytic anemia, edema, and skin lesions may develop, especially if the infant is fed a formula high in PUFA.[63] Effectiveness of oral vitamin E supplementation increases with gestational age; supplementation with iron alone has been shown to aggravate the anemia by acting as a pro-oxidant and by further reducing the absorption of vitamin E[64] (see Chap. 35).

Vitamin E supplementation in premature infants also has been reported to decrease the incidence of retrolental fibroplasia [65] and chronic bronchopulmonary dysplasia.[66] Adequate vitamin E status may be important in protecting the lungs against oxidative damage in patients receiving pure $O_2$[47] and against damage by air pollutants, such as ozone ($O_3$) and nitrous oxide ($NO_2$).[58]

In a long-term experiment to study vitamin E deficiency in humans, low plasma tocopherol levels, increased susceptibility of erythrocytes to peroxide-induced hemolysis, and slightly decreased erythrocyte survival time were the only changes observed in male subjects ingesting approximately 3 mg $\alpha$-tocopherol per day over 6 years.[67] Supplementation with vitamin E showed a small but significant increase in reticulocytes. Decreased erythrocyte survival time and correction by vitamin E also has been reported in patients with cystic fibrosis and other conditions in which low plasma vitamin levels are found secondary to intestinal malabsorption.[65] Inefficient erythropoiesis has been observed in vitamin E-deficient monkeys, which also had anemia and decreased erythrocyte survival.[68] Treatment with $\alpha$-tocopherol acetate corrected all abnormalities. It appears that anemia in vitamin E deficiency may result from the combined effects of increased hemolysis and inefficient erythropoiesis.

The hematopoietic effect of vitamin E on children with protein-calorie malnutrition is not clear because different workers report varying results from the administration of this vitamin.

Increased creatinuria, presumed to reflect muscle breakdown, has been observed in both children and adults with cystic fibrosis and in premature infants; reduction in creatinuria followed vitamin E supplementation.[66]

## Human requirement

The recommended dietary allowances of vitamin E for adults are based on the vitamin E content of the average American diet, assumed to be adequate as no biochemical or clinical evidence exists to indicate inadequate vitamin E intakes by healthy people ingesting balanced diets.[3] Even though the daily intakes may vary considerably, the average over several days should fall between 7 mg and 13 mg d-$\alpha$-tocopherol equivalents (10–20 IU) from diets supplying 1800 kcal to 3000 kcal. The recommended allowance for boys and men is 10 mg $\alpha$-TE (15 IU), beginning at 15 years and 8 mg $\alpha$-TE (12 IU) for girls and women, beginning at 11 years. Because requirements for vitamin E in the body tissues are related to their PUFA content, the Food and Nutrition Board has stressed that these recommendations "should be considered as average adequate intakes in balanced diets in the United States, but the adequacy of these intakes will vary if the PUFA content of the diet deviates significantly from that which is customary."[3] For this reason, these allowances are not expected to meet the needs of practically everyone as are the allowances for other vitamins. People with a high degree of polyunsaturation in their tissue lipids are also likely to have high vitamin E intakes, comparable to their requirements, because diets high in PUFA that result in high tissue polyunsaturation are also high in vitamin E. The allowance for infants (3–4 mg $\alpha$-TE) is based on the vitamin E content of human milk, 1.3 to 3.3 mg $\alpha$-TE per liter. Vitamin E allowances for children increase with increasing body weight. The adult female allowance for vitamin E is increased to 10 mg $\alpha$-TE (15 IU) during pregnancy and to 11 mg $\alpha$-TE during lactation.

The Food and Nutrition Committee of the American Academy of Pediatrics[69] recommends that the formulas for LBW infants provide 0.5 mg (0.7 IU) of vitamin E per 100 kcal and at least 0.7 mg (1.0 IU) per gram of linoleic acid because of the impaired utilization of vitamin E, related to the reduced fat absorption, in these infants. They also recommend a daily oral supplement of 3.3 mg (5 IU) of water-soluble $\alpha$-tocopherol.

## Food sources

Wheat germ and wheat-germ oil afford the richest source of this factor, but it is so widely distributed in common foods that it is actually difficult to obtain a food mixture for experimental purposes that is deficient in vitamin E.

The vitamin E content of vegetable oils and fats has been reported to vary according to source of the plant, time of harvest, stability after harvest, refining procedure, and commercial hydrogenation procedures.[70]

Animal foods are relatively poor sources of vitamin E although depot fat and liver contain moderate amounts. Some tocopherol is removed from oils in the purification process. When chlorine dioxide is used to bleach flour, tocopherol is lost.

Table 7-2 lists some common representative food sources of vitamin E. Additional foods are included in Table 6, Part 4.

There have been many misleading claims but very little experimental evidence that supplementation of the diet with pharmacologic doses of vitamin E cures or prevents human abnormalities, such as sterility, lack of virility, abnormal termination of pregnancy, heart disease, muscle weakness, cancer, ulcers, skin disorders, or burns. Although there is no medical justification for megavitamin therapy in large population groups with such disorders, there is increasing evidence that pharmacological doses of vitamin E may have some beneficial

effects in a few specific conditions, including intermittent claudication and some hereditary enzyme deficiencies.[65,71] The evidence for such medical uses of vitamin E has been discussed in recent reviews.[47,65] Recently, megadoses of vitamin E have been shown to increase the vi-

### Table 7-2. Comparison of Some Representative Foods as Sources of Vitamin E

| Food | Total Vitamin E | Alpha Tocopherol | Total Active Tocopherols* |
|---|---|---|---|
| | *mg/100 g of Food* | | |
| *Oils* | | | |
| coconut | 3.58 | 0.35 | 0.78 |
| cod liver, commercial | 21.96 | 21.96 | 21.96 |
| corn, refined | 83.17 | 14.26 | 21.10 |
| cottonseed, refined | 65.24 | 35.26 | 38.26 |
| olive | 12.64 | 11.92 | 11.99 |
| palm, refined | 35.53 | 18.32 | 21.82 |
| peanut, refined | 25.00 | 11.62 | 12.92 |
| rapeseed, refined | 44.81 | 17.65 | 20.35 |
| safflower seed, refined | 38.10 | 34.05 | 34.40 |
| sesame seed, refined | 29.07 | 1.38 | 4.07 |
| soybean, refined | 93.74 | 10.99 | 17.43 |
| sunflower seed, refined | 63.62 | 59.50 | 59.85 |
| wheat germ | 254.58 | 149.44 | 183.00 |
| wrasse liver, non-commercial | 250.67 | 250.67 | 250.67 |
| | | | |
| *Other foods* | | | |
| almond, raw | 24.48 | 23.96 | 24.01 |
| bean | | | |
|   kidney, dry | 2.08 | tr | 0.21 |
|   soy, dry | 20.43 | 0.85 | 2.03 |
| beef, skeletal muscle, raw | 0.43 | 0.41 | 0.41 |
| bread, white, U.S. | 1.19 | 0.12 | 0.20 |
| butter, U.S. | 1.58 | 1.58 | 1.58 |
| carrot, raw | 0.51 | 0.44 | 0.46 |
| corn, fresh | 7.78 | 1.20 | 1.86 |
| eggs, whole large, raw | 1.06 | 0.70 | 0.74 |
| herring, light muscle, frozen | 2.00 | 2.00 | 2.00 |
| infant formulas | | | |
|   milk-fat based, unfortified | 0.04 | 0.03 | 0.03 |
|   soybean-oil based, unfortified | 1.94 | 0.46 | 0.59 |
| margarine, soybean and cottonseed oils—stick | 45.49 | 11.15 | 13.87 |
| milk | | | |
|   cow, commercial | 0.09 | 0.06 | 0.06 |
|   human | 0.99 | 0.88 | 0.90 |
| peanut, raw | 16.37 | 8.33 | 9.13 |
| pecan, raw | 19.86 | 1.24 | 3.10 |
| spinach, raw | 3.00 | 1.88 | 1.90 |
| tomato, raw | 0.49 | 0.34 | 0.35 |
| walnut, English, raw | 19.62 | 0.84 | 2.63 |
| wheat germ | 27.56 | 14.07 | 17.38 |

*Expressed as alpha-tocopherol.

(From McLaughlin PJ, Weihrauch JL: J Am Diet Assoc 75:647, 1979)

tamin K requirement of young rats about tenfold and that its major metabolite, tocopheryl quinone, is a competitive inhibitor of vitamin K-dependent $\gamma$-carboxylation (see vitamin K, p. 125).[72] This anti-vitamin K activity and its reported inhibition of platelet aggregation has been suggested to explain the claims that vitamin E has beneficial effects in some patients with undesirable blood clotting.[65,73] The effect of vitamin E on platelet aggregation could involve the production of thromboxane (TXA$_2$; see Chap. 3), a potent initiator of platelet aggregation synthesized from arachidonic acid (and related to prostaglandins). The conversion of arachidonic acid to endoperoxides, thromboxane precursors, depends on hydroperoxide activation of cyclo-oxygenase (see Fig. 3-3).[74] Vitamin E has been shown to reduce the sharp rise in hydroperoxides usually associated with platelet aggregation.[65]

Fortunately, vitamin E appears to be relatively nontoxic in comparison with vitamins A and D. However, just as the lack of a specific disease syndrome in vitamin E deficiency does not indicate that there is no need for vitamin E, the lack of symptoms from ingestion of large doses of vitamin E does not guarantee the absence of undesirable effects, especially from long-term ingestion.

# Vitamin K
## History

In 1935 Dam recognized a severe deficiency disease in newly hatched chicks fed on a ration adequate in protein, minerals, and all known vitamins. Hemorrhage apparently was due to a fall in prothrombin, the clotting agent in the blood; normal clotting time was restored by administering hog-liver fat or by feeding alfalfa. The antihemorrhagic factor found in these materials Dam called vitamin K—Koagulation Vitamin.

This discovery and the identification, isolation, and synthesis of compounds with vitamin K activity have

Vitamin K$_1$, phylloquinone

Vitamin K$_2$ series, menaquinone-n

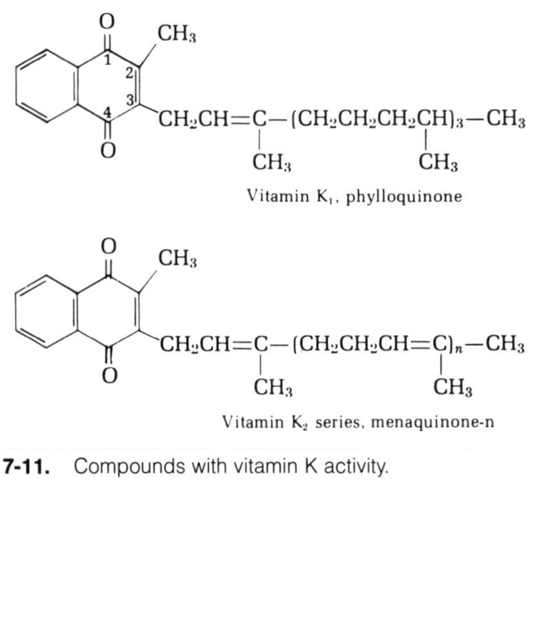

**Fig. 7-11.** Compounds with vitamin K activity.

made possible extensive clinical use of this vitamin for the control and the prevention of hemorrhages due to vitamin K deficiency.

## Nomenclature

Vitamin K is a generic term for the structurally related compounds that exhibit antihemorrhagic activity, including the parent compound, *menadione*, and the two major naturally occurring forms, *phylloquinone* or vitamin K$_1$ synthesized by the plants and *menaquinone-n* or vitamin K$_2$, a family of compounds of microbial origin (Fig. 7-11). The naming of menaquinones depends on the number of isoprenyl units present in the sidechain; bacterial menaquinones with a range from 7 to 13 isoprenyl units have been identified. Menadione, formerly known as vitamin K$_3$, is activated in the body to menaquinone-4.

The various forms of vitamin K are resistant to heat, but are labile to alkali, strong acids, light, and certain oxidizing agents.

Vitamin K can be measured in micrograms of the pure synthetic compound, and the vitamin K activity of other substances can be expressed in similar terms. One method of assay uses young chicks and is based on the minimum dose that will maintain the normal coagulation time of the blood at the end of one month. The vitamin K content in foods also is measured by a chick bioassay. The level of prothrombin maintained by the test material in vitamin K deficient chicks is compared to the levels maintained by known amounts of phylloquinone.

## Absorption, transport, synthesis, and tissue distribution

Ingested vitamin K is absorbed by the intestines in much the same way as dietary fat. The absorption of vitamin K seems to be dependent on the presence of bile and pancreatic juice, and the percentage (10%–80%) absorbed depends on the vehicle used for its administration. It is carried first in the lymph chylomicrons, then transferred to the beta-lipoproteins. A series of studies in the rat has revealed that both the site and mechanism of vitamin K absorption appear to depend on the form in which it is ingested.[75] Whereas phylloquinone is absorbed mainly from the proximal intestine by an energy-requiring process, menadione and menaquinones are absorbed from the lower intestine and colon by a passive process. This is consistent with the assumption that synthesis of menaquinones by the intestinal bacteria (located in the lower GI tract) contributes significantly to the vitamin K requirement of man. Just as the concentration of fat and bile salts affects the rate of passive diffusion of these compounds, the low concentration of conjugated bile salts in the lower segment of the intestine probably limits the absorption of vitamin K from bacterial synthesis. Presence

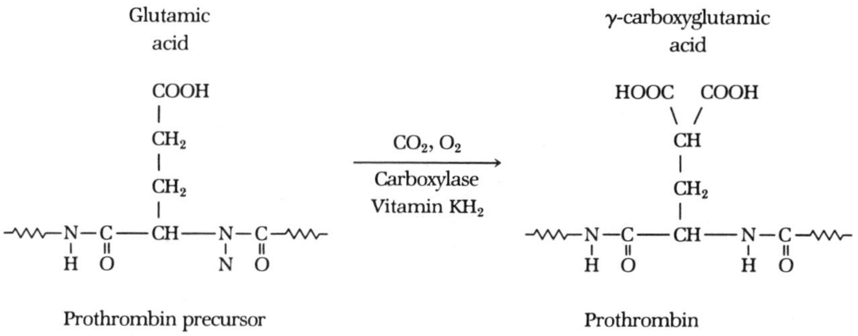

Glutamic
acid

γ-carboxyglutamic
acid

COOH
|
CH₂
|
CH₂
|
—ⱳ—N—C—CH—N—C—ⱳ—
      |  ‖       |  ‖
      H  O      N  O

$CO_2, O_2$
————————→
Carboxylase
Vitamin $KH_2$

HOOC  COOH
   \   /
    CH
    |
    CH₂
    |
—ⱳ—N—C—CH—N—C—ⱳ—
      |  ‖       |  ‖
      H  O      H  O

Prothrombin precursor

Prothrombin

**Fig. 7-12.** Vitamin K-dependent γ-carboxylation of glutamic acid residues in prothrombin synthesis.

of a high concentration of vitamin A in the intestine also appears to inhibit the absorption of vitamin K.[75]

The tissue distribution, retention, and route of excretion following vitamin K administration also vary with the form administered. In contrast to the other fat-soluble vitamins, vitamin K is not stored in the body to any appreciable extent.[75] Menadione is taken up rapidly and distributed widely in the tissues, but it is not retained long; 24 hours after administration, urinary metabolites accounted for 70% of the dose, and some was also excreted in the bile.[75] Phylloquinone is initially concentrated in the liver but is later distributed to other tissues and excreted; its half life in the liver is less than 24 hours. It is excreted mainly in the bile, both as unaltered vitamin and as glucuronide conjugates.[75,76] Administration of warfarin, a vitamin K antagonist, appears to change its excretion pattern by increasing the more polar urinary metabolites and decreasing the biliary excretion.[77] Menadione excretion is not affected by warfarin.[75]

## Physiologic function and metabolism of vitamin K

Vitamin K is essential in blood coagulation for the maintenance of normal prothrombin time through its effect on factor II (prothrombin), factor VII (proconvertin), factor IX (Christmas factor), and factor X (Stuart-

Prower factor). These four vitamin K-dependent factors are present in the extrinsic (activated by injury) and intrinsic (activated by platelets) coagulation systems and in the common pathway leading to clot formation by conversion of fibrinogen to fibrin.

The complex puzzle of the stage at which vitamin K regulates the synthesis of these proteins has been solved recently with the discovery of vitamin K-dependent γ-carboxylation of selected glutamic acid residues of the prothrombin precursor peptide. This means that the role of vitamin K is not in the synthesis of the actual polypeptide chain but in the post-translational activation of the precursor,[75] as shown in Figure 7-12.

This microsomal reaction requires $CO_2$, $O_2$, and vitamin K in its hydroquinone form.[78] The microsomal carboxylase activity is closely associated with a dehydrogenase required for this conversion and also with two other enzymes that allow regeneration of vitamin K from its hydroquinone[79] (see Fig. 7-13). There is considerable evidence to suggest that the vitamin K-epoxide cycle is obligatory for the vitamin K-dependent carboxylation of prothrombin, but definite proof is still lacking. Not only are the two activites found in the same subcellular location and have a common intermediate, vitamin K hydroquinone, but the conditions that stimulate or inhibit

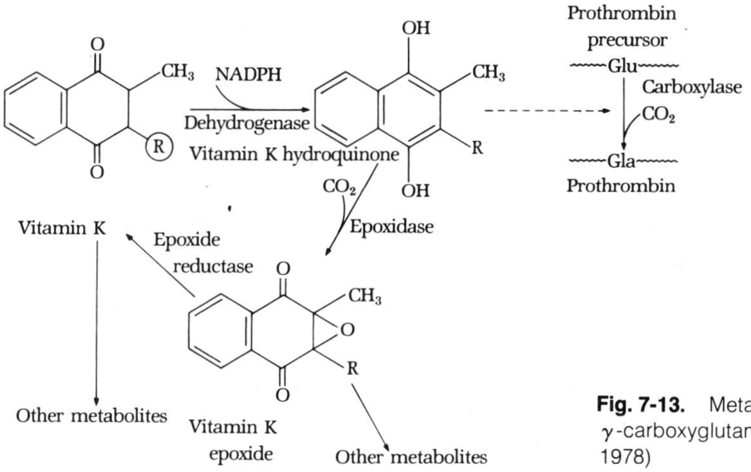

**Fig. 7-13.** Metabolism of vitamin K and its relationship to the formation of γ-carboxyglutamic acid (Gla). (Adapted from Bell RG: Feder Proc 37:2599, 1978)

prothrombin formation affect similarly the epoxidation.[79] There is no doubt, however, that vitamin K epoxide is a major metabolite of vitamin K produced not only in the liver, but in several extrahepatic tissues as well.[77]

The synthesis of the other clotting factors has not been studied to the same extent as that of prothrombin, but γ-carboxylation of glutamate appears to be part of their activation also.[75]

Soon after the discovery of the hepatic γ-carboxylation of prothrombin it became evident that vitamin K may have other physiological functions than blood clotting. Several other proteins have been identified that contain γ-glutamate, and all appear to require vitamin K for this reaction—a protein in the bone, known as osteocalcin; two proteins in the plasma, designated plasma proteins C and S; a protein in normal kidney cortex. In addition, and

of most interest, vitamin K is also found in association with pathologic calcifications, such as hard atheromatous plaques and renal calculi.[80] Although the functions of these proteins are not known, they all bind calcium and appear connected in some way to calcium metabolism, both normal and abnormal.[80,81] The synthesis of osteocalcin appears to be stimulated by 1,25-(OH)$_2$D and may be involved in the mobilization of calcium from bone.[82]

Dicumarol and warfarin (coumarin compounds) are used in anticoagulation therapy to prevent thrombus formation and act as vitamin K antagonists. Their presence in the liver stops prothrombin synthesis and reduces the levels of all vitamin K-dependent clotting factors.

As mentioned earlier in this chapter, vitamin E in megadose concentrations also appears to act as a vitamin

## Table 7-3. Summary of Fat-Soluble Vitamins

|  | *A* | *D* | *E* | *K* |
|---|---|---|---|---|
| Active compounds | Retinol (A$_1$)<br>3-dehydroretinol (A$_2$)<br>Retinal<br>Retinoic acid<br>Carotenoids | Cholecalciferol (D$_3$)<br>Ergocalciferol (D$_2$)<br>25-OH-D<br>1,25-(OH)$_2$D | Tocopherols<br>(α, β, δ, and so on)<br>Tocotrienols | Phylloquinone (K$_1$)<br>Menaquinone (K$_2$)<br>Menadione |
| Important food sources | Liver<br>Egg yolk<br>Butter, cream<br>Fortified milk and milk<br>  products<br>Fortified margarine<br>Fortified breakfast cereals<br>Green and yellow<br>  vegetables<br>Apricots<br>Cantaloupe | Fortified milk<br>Fortified breakfast<br>  cereals<br>Small amounts in:<br>  Butter<br>  Egg yolk<br>  Liver<br>  Salmon<br>  Sardines<br>  Tuna fish | Wheat germ<br>Leafy vegetables<br>Vegetable oils<br>Egg yolk<br>Legumes<br>Peanuts<br>Margarine | Cabbage<br>Cauliflower<br>Spinach<br>Other leafy vegetables<br>Beef liver<br>Vegetable oils |
| Stability to cooking, drying, light, and so on | Gradual destruction by<br>  exposure to air, heat,<br>  and drying; more rapid<br>  at high temperatures | Stable to heating and<br>  storage<br>Destroyed by excess<br>  ultraviolet irradiation | Stable to methods of<br>  food processing<br>Destroyed by oxidation<br>  and UV irradiation | Stable to heat and<br>  exposure to air<br>Destroyed by light and<br>  strong acids, alkalis,<br>  and oxidizing agents |
| Function | Maintains function of<br>  epithelial cells, mucous<br>  membranes, skin, bone;<br>  constituent of visual<br>  pigments | Calcium and<br>  phosphorus<br>  absorption and<br>  utilization in bone<br>  growth | Protects cell structures | Necessary in formation<br>  of four factors<br>  essential for clotting<br>  of blood |
| Deficiency: signs and symptoms | Night blindness<br>Glare blindness<br>Rough, dry skin<br>Dry mucous membranes<br>Xerophthalmia | Rickets<br>Soft bones<br>Bowed legs<br>Poor teeth<br>Skeletal deformities | Increased hemolysis of<br>  red blood cells<br>Creatinuria<br>Anemia, edema, and<br>  skin lesions in infants | Low concentration of<br>  clotting factors<br>Increased clotting time<br>Hemorrhagic disease of<br>  newborn |
| Adult recommended dietary allowance | Male 1000 RE<br>  (5000 IU)<br>Female 800 RE<br>  (4000 IU) | 19–22 years 7.5 mcg<br>  (300 IU)<br>Adults after 22 years<br>  5 mcg (200 IU) | Male 10 mg α-TE<br>  (15 IU)<br>Female 8 mg α-TE<br>  (12 IU) | 70–140 mcg estimated<br>  safe and adequate<br>  intake |

K-antagonist, probably through formation of tocopheryl quinone, which bears a structural resemblance to vitamin K.[73] Alpha-tocopheryl quinone has been shown to inhibit the microsomal carboxylation of peptide-bound glutamate.[72] Administration of vitamin E potentiates the effect of warfarin and may result in bleeding if taken regularly without adjusting the dose of the anticoagulant.[73]

### Human requirement

Studies of liver stores of vitamin K indicate that approximately 50% of the vitamin comes from the diet and 50% from bacterial synthesis in the intestines. The total daily requirement, which has been postulated as approximately 2 mcg per kilogram is met by a diet supplying 1 mcg per kilogram. Because the average diet in the United States contains 300 mcg to 500 mcg of vitamin K per day, there is little danger of inadequate intake under normal conditions. No recommended dietary allowance has been established, but the Food and Nutrition Board has estimated that 70 mcg to 140 mcg per day represents an adequate and safe range of intake for adults.[3] A deficiency state would most likely be caused by a failure to absorb or utilize the vitamin. Low vitamin K intakes plus antibiotic therapy (*neomycin*), which reduces the bacterial synthesis, may result in lowered levels of the vitamin K-dependent coagulation factors. The use of mineral oil in reducing diets or as a laxative interferes with the absorption of vitamin K as well as other fat-soluble vitamins and for this reason this is not recommended.

Infants have special requirements for vitamin K because of limited placental transfer of the vitamin and because the gut of the newborn is sterile and cannot synthesize the vitamin. As a result, some infants require vitamin K administration to prevent hemorrhage. It may be given in a water-soluble or fat-soluble form, usually intramuscularly.[3] The Committee on Nutrition of the American Academy of Pediatrics[83] has recommended that all infant formulas contain a minimum of 4 mcg of vitamin K per 100 kcal, which is the level supplied by the commonly used milk-based formulas, and appears to be adequate for healthy infants.

### Toxicity of vitamin K

Menadione in large doses can be toxic. It is believed to combine with sulfhydryl groups in the tissues (intact sulfhydryl groups are essential for the activity of many enzymes and for many other cellular functions).[3] Reported symptoms of vitamin K toxicity include liver damage, hypoprothrombinemia, petechial hemorrhages, renal tubule degeneration, and, in premature infants, hemolytic anemia.[84]

In 1963 the Food and Drug Administration recommended the removal of menadione from all food supplements. Vitamins $K_1$ and $K_2$ are still permitted in carefully regulated amounts.

### Food sources

Although vitamin K is found in relatively low concentrations in most foods, it is so widely distributed that it is almost impossible to ingest a diet that does not supply an adequate level of vitamin K. It appears abundantly in cauliflower, broccoli, cabbage, spinach, beef liver, soybeans and, to a lesser extent, in wheat and oats. Animal products contain little vitamin K; however, cow's milk is a better source than human milk.

## Study questions and activities

1. How was the term vitamin arrived at? Can you define a vitamin as distinct from any other food nutrient?
2. Why are vitamins A and D referred to as hormones?
3. Describe the function of each of the fat-soluble vitamins and good food sources for each, if there are any.
4. Does the depth of yellow color in butter or egg yolks indicate the vitamin A potency? Why, or why not?
5. For each of the fat-soluble vitamins, list the unit in which its current recommended dietary allowance or safe level of intake is given.
6. Make the following conversions: 10,000 IU of $\beta$-carotene to mcg RE; 1200 mcg of other carotenoids to mcg RE; 1000 IU of vitamin D to mcg vitamin D; 10 mg $\alpha$-tocopherol from a mixed diet to mg $\alpha$-TE; 10 mg $\beta$-tocopherol + 30 mg $\gamma$-tocopherol + 10 mg of $\alpha$-tocotrienol to mg $\alpha$-TE.
7. Identify RBP, CRBP, and CRABP and describe their proposed roles in the physiological functions of vitamin A.
8. Describe two functions for vitamin A in the eye and identify the chemical forms that can support these functions.
9. How is vitamin A assumed to produce toxic effects in the body?
10. Show the conversions which 7-dehydrocholesterol in the skin must undergo to be active in the absorption of dietary calcium. Identify the site of each reaction.
11. Describe how the thyroid and parathyroid glands are involved in the regulation of vitamin D metabolism.
12. Explain why the plasma tocopherol concentration sometimes is expressed as a ratio to plasma total lipids?
13. Why are LBW infants more susceptible to developing a vitamin E deficiency than are the full term infants?
14. How is the enzyme glutathione peroxidase related to the function of vitamin E in the body? How is glutathione (GSH) related to the sulfur amino acids?
15. Why is it difficult to establish a single recommended dietary allowance for vitamin E for any age group? How does the current RDA for vitamin E differ from the RDAs for the other vitamins?
16. What is believed to be the major source of menaquinones in the human body? Why is development of

vitamin K deficiency unlikely in normal individuals? Under what conditions may vitamin K deficiency develop in humans?

## References

1. Joint FAO/WHO Expert Group: Requirements of vitamin A, thiamine, riboflavin and niacin. WHO Tech Rep Ser, no. 362. Geneva, World Health Organization, 1967
2. Joint FAO/WHO Expert Group: Requirements of ascorbic acid, vitamin D, vitamin $B_{12}$, folate, and iron. WHO Tech Rep Ser, no. 452. Geneva, World Health Organization, 1970
3. Food and Nutrition Board: Recommended Dietary Allowances, 9th rev ed. Washington, DC, NAS-NRC, 1980
4. Smith JE, Goodman DS: In Hegsted DM et al (eds): Present Knowledge of Nutrition, 4th ed, p 64. New York, Nutrition Foundation, 1976
5. Smith JA, Goodman DS: Fed Proc 38:2504, 1979
6. Venkataswamy G et al: Am J Clin Nutr 30:1968, 1977
7. Shetty PS et al: Lancet II:230, 1979
8. Smith FR et al: Am J Clin Nutr 28:732, 1975
9. Smith FR et al: Am J Clin Nutr 26:982, 1973
10. Wolf G, DeLuca L: In DeLuca HF, Suttie JW (eds): The Fat-Soluble Vitamins, p 257. Madison, University of Wisconsin Press, 1969
11. Nutr Rev 35:220, 1977
12. Chytil F, Ong DE: Fed Proc 38:2510, 1979
13. Hayes KC: Nutr Rev 29:3, 1971
14. Nutr Rev 38:23, 1980
15. Nutr Rev 35:97, 1977
16. Wolf G et al: Fed Proc 38:2540, 1979
17. DeLuca LM et al: Fed Proc 38:2535, 1979
18. Hodges RE et al: Am J Clin Nutr 31:876, 1978
19. Nutr Rev 37:38, 1979
20. Nutr Rev 37:153, 1979
21. Sporn MB, Newton DL: Fed Proc 38:2528, 1979
22. Nutr Rev 37:90, 1979
23. DeLuca HF: Fed Proc 38:2519, 1979
24. Nutr Rev 35:305, 1977
25. Hodges RE, Kolder H: Summary of proceedings. Workshop on biochemical and clinical criteria for determining human vitamin A nutriture, pp 10–16. Washington, DC, NAS, 1971
26. Hume EM, Krebs HA: Vitamin A requirement of human adults. Report of the Vitamin A Subcommittee of the Accessory Food Factors Committee. British Medical Research Council Special Report, Ser. No. 264. London, HM Stationary Office, 1949
27. Körner WF, Völlm J: Int J Vitam Nutr Res 45:363, 1975
28. Morrice F Jr, Havener WH: JAMA 173:1802, 1960
29. Nutr Rev 34:119, 1976
30. DeLuca HF: Nutr Rev 37:161, 1979
31. DeLuca HF: Vitamin D Metabolism and Function. Monographs on Endocrinology, pp 1–60. New York, Springer-Verlag, 1979
32. DeLuca HF: Nutr Rev 38:169, 1980
33. DeLuca HF: In DeLuca HF (ed): The Fat-Soluble Vitamins. Handbook of Lipid Research, Vol 2, pp 69–121. New York, Plenum Press, 1978
34. Bikle DD et al: Am J Clin Nutr 32:2322, 1979
35. Brickman AS et al: Am J Clin Nutr 30:1064, 1977
36. Frazer DR: Physiol Rev 60:551, 1980
37. Nutr Rev 37:57, 1979
38. Council on Food and Nutrition: A.M.A., Decision. JAMA 159:1018, 1955
39. Council on Food and Nutrition: A.M.A., Statement. JAMA 159:1018, 1955
40. Dale AE, Lowenberg ME: J Pediatr 70:954, 1967
41. Nutr Rev 38:116, 1980
42. Fomon SJ et al: J Nutr 88:345, 1966
43. Nutr Rev 19:158, 1961
44. American Academy of Pediatrics: The relation between infantile hypercalcemia and vitamin D—Public health implications in North America. Pediatrics 40:1050, 1967
45. McLaughlin PJ, Weihrauch JL: J Am Diet Assoc 75:647, 1979
46. Losowsky MS et al: Ann NY Acad Sci 203:212, 1972
47. Scott ML: In DeLuca: Fat-Soluble Vitamins, Handbook of Lipid Research, pp 133–197
48. Bieri JG: In Hegsted et al, Present Knowledge of Nutrition, pp 98–106
49. Farrell PM et al: Am J Clin Nutr 31:1720, 1978
50. Horwitt MK et al: Ann NY Acad Sci 203:223, 1972
51. Farrell PM, Bieri JG: Am J Clin Nutr 28:1381, 1975
52. Bieri JG, Farrell PM: Vitam Horm 34:31, 1976
53. Sauberlich HE et al: Laboratory Tests for the Assessment of Nutritional Status, p 77. Cleveland, CRC Press, 1974
54. Ogunmegan AO: Am J Clin Nutr 32:2269, 1979
55. McWhirter WR: Acta Paediatr Scand 64:446, 1975
56. Bieri JG: Ann NY Acad Sci 203:181, 1972
57. Draper HH, Csallany AS: Fed Proc 28:1690, 1969
58. Tappel AL: Nutr Today 8:4, July-Aug, 1973
59. Schwartz K: Ann NY Acad Sci 203:43, 1972
60. Olson RE: Food Nutr News 44:5, Feb-Mar, 1973
61. Green J: Ann NY Acad Sci 203:29, 1972
62. Nutr Rev 36:84, 1978
63. Hussan H et al: Am J Clin Nutr 19:147, 1966
64. Gross S, Melhorn DK: Ann NY Acad Sci 203:141, 1972
65. Horwitt MK: Nutr Rev 38:105, 1980
66. Nutr Rev 37:11, 1979
67. Horwitt MK et al: Am J Clin Nutr 4:408, 1956
68. Fitch CD et al: Am J Clin Nutr 33:1251, 1980
69. American Academy of Pediatrics: Nutritional needs of low-birth-weight infants. Pediatrics 60:519, 1977
70. Herting DE, Drury E-JE: J Nutr 81:335, 1963
71. Nutr Rev 38:120, 1980
72. Olson RE, Jones JP: Fed Proc 38:710, 1979
73. Horwitt MK: Am J Clin Nutr 29:569, 1976
74. Lands WEM: Ann Rev Physiol 41:633, 1979
75. Suttie JW: In DeLuca, Fat-Soluble Vitamins, Handbook of Lipid Research, pp 221–265
76. Olson RE: In Goodhart RS, Shils ME (eds): Modern Nutrition in Health and Disease, 6th ed, pp 170–179. Philadelphia, Lea & Febiger, 1980
77. Bell RG: Fed Proc 37:2599, 1978
78. Olson RE et al: Fed Proc 37:2610, 1978
79. Suttie JW et al: Fed Proc 37:2605, 1978
80. Lian JB et al: Fed Proc 37:2615, 1978
81. Nelsestuen GL: Fed Proc 37:2621, 1978
82. Nutr Rev 39:282, 1981

83. American Academy of Pediatrics: Commentary on breast-feeding and infant formulas, including proposed standards for formulas. Pediatrics 57:278, 1976
84. Smith AM Jr, Custer RP: JAMA 173:502, 1960

## Supplementary readings

Bikle DD, Morrissey RL, Zolock DT: The mechanism of action of vitamin D in the intestine. Am J Clin Nutr 32:2322, 1979

DeLuca HF: The vitamin D system in the regulation of calcium and phosphorus metabolism. Nutr Rev 37:161, 1979

DeLuca HF: Some new concepts emanating from a study of the metabolism and function of vitamin D. Nutr Rev 38:169, 1980

DeLuca HF: Recent advances in the metabolism of vitamin D. Ann Rev Physiol 43:199, 1981

Farrell PM et al: Plasma tocopherol-lipid relationships in a normal population of children as compared to healthy adults. Am J Clin Nutr 31:1720, 1978

Fitch CD et al: Abnormal erythropoiesis in vitamin E-deficient monkeys. Am J Clin Nutr 33:1251, 1980

Hodges RE et al: Hematopoietic studies in vitamin A deficiency. Am J Clin Nutr 31:876, 1978

Horwitt KM: Therapeutic uses of vitamin E in medicine. Nutr Rev 38:105, 1980

Massry SG: Requirements of vitamin D metabolites in patients with renal disease. Am J Clin Nutr 33:1530, 1980

Review: Osteocalcin: A vitamin K-dependent calcium binding protein. Nutr Rev 37:54, 1979

Review: The function of vitamin E as an antioxidant as revealed by a new method for measuring lipid peroxidation. Nutr Rev 36:38, 1978

Review: Vitamin A deficiency anemia. Nutr Rev 37:38, 1979

Review: Vitamin D metabolism in the rickets of very-low-birth-weight, premature infants. Nutr Rev 39:234, 1981

*For further references see Bibliography in Part 4.*

# Water-soluble Vitamins

## 8

**ACP:** Acyl Carrier Protein
**CAC:** Citric Acid Cycle
**dU:** Deoxyuridine
**dUMP:** Deoxyuridine Monophosphate
**FAD:** Flavin Adenine Dinucleotide
**FIGLU:** Formiminoglutamic Acid
**FMN:** Flavin Mononucleotide
**GABA:** Gamma Aminobutyric Acid
**HMS:** Hexose Monophosphate Shunt
**IF:** Intrinsic Factor
**NAD:** Nicotinamide Adenine Dinucleotide
**NE:** Niacin Equivalent
**OAA:** Oxaloacetate
**OCA:** Oral Contraceptive Agents
**PALP:** Pyridoxal-5-phosphate
**PGA:** Pteroylglutaminic Acid
**PL:** Pyridoxal
**PM:** Pyridoxamine
**PMP:** Pyridoxamine Phosphate
**PN:** Pyridoxine
**PNP:** Pyridoxine Phosphate
**PPS:** Pteroylpolyglutamate Synthetase
**SGOT:** Serum Glutamate Oxaloacetate
    Transaminase
**TC:** Transcobalamin
**THFA:** Tetrahydrofolic Acid
**TMP:** Thiamin Monophosphate
**TPP:** Thiamin Pyrophosphate

## Ascorbic acid

The history of scurvy as a deficiency disease in humans is discussed in Chapter 21. Experimental scurvy was first accidentally induced in guinea pigs in 1907 by Holst and Frölich in Norway; these animals, unlike rats, chickens, dogs, and other domestic animals, develop characteristic hemorrhages around the joints, teeth, and other bony structures very similar to the symptoms of scurvy in humans (Fig. 8-1). The antiscorbutic food factor was named vitamin C in 1919 by Drummond, as it was clear that its properties and distribution in foods were very different from the antiberiberi and growth factors earlier designated as *water-soluble B* and *fat-soluble A*. Humans, the primates, guinea pigs, some fish, and a few other exotic species do not possess the ability to synthesize vitamin C and must rely totally on the vitamin C ingested with their food.

By 1932 the isolation of vitamin C in pure crystalline form had been accomplished independently by two groups of workers. The chemical structure was identified and the product synthesized in physiologically active form soon afterwards; in 1938 *ascorbic acid* was officially accepted as the chemical name for vitamin C. It occurs naturally in foods in two forms, the reduced form (usually designated as *ascorbic acid*) and the oxidized form, (*dehydroascorbic acid*). Both are physiologically active, and both are found in body tissues. Further oxidation of dehydroascorbic acid to diketogulonic acid results in irreversible inactivation of the vitamin. Figure 8-2 shows the chemical structures and interconversions of these compounds. The ascorbic acid in fruits and vegetables and the synthetic form are equally well utilized.

### Functions of ascorbic acid

Vitamin C appears to have a variety of roles in the life processes, but to date its specific functions at the biochemical level are not fully understood. Its major form, L-ascorbic acid, is a powerful reducing agent and apparently functions in that capacity in a variety of *hydroxyla-*

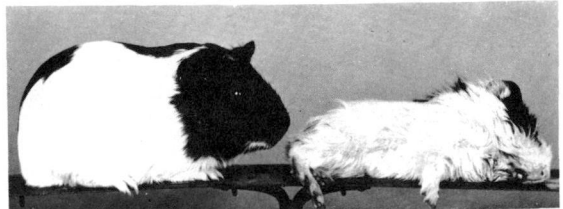

**Fig. 8-1.** Scurvy results from vitamin C deficiency. Guinea pigs are used for experiments in vitamin C because they need a food source with this factor, just as humans do. (*Left*) Normal guinea pig. (*Right*) Scorbutic guinea pig. (Nutrition Laboratory, Battle Creek Sanitarium)

tion reactions, which are known to be impaired in vitamin C deficiency.

Perhaps the most significant, and certainly best characterized, are the hydroxylations required in the synthesis of *collagen.* Collagen is a fibrous protein made up of three polypeptide chains coiled together to form a helix. These peptides have an unusual amino acid composition, consisting mainly of glycine, hydroxyproline and hydroxylysine. The last two amino acids are not found in other proteins. The hydroxylations of proline and lysine take place after they have been incorporated into the polypeptides and are essential for normal physical structure of the completed protein molecule. These reactions are performed by enzymes *prolyl hydroxylase* and *lysyl hydroxylase;* the roles of ascorbic acid and other cofactors (iron, $O_2$, and alphaketoglutarate) in the reaction have been characterized recently.[1–3] Reduced iron ($Fe^{++}$) participates in the reaction and is oxidized in the process ($Fe^{+++}$). Ascorbic acid apparently serves as a specific, nonreplaceable reducing agent to regenerate $Fe^{++}$ and is itself converted to dehydroascorbic acid.

Collagen fibers give rigidity to the amorphous ground substance of connective tissue that fills the space between the cellular and circulatory components of tissues and aids in holding them together. It also is a major component in the organic matrix of bone and teeth and in the scar tissue formed during healing of wounds and bone fractures. Defects in these systems underlie many of the

pathologic lesions of scurvy (see Chap. 21). The widespread bleeding has been attributed to defects in the basement membrane and intercellular cement of the capillaries. However, Hodges has questioned this conclusion after his group was unable to detect such defects by electron microscopic examination of tissues from patients with evidence of hemorrhaging due to vitamin C deficiency.[4]

Other hydroxylations that are known to utilize the same cofactors include the conversion of thymine to hydroxymethyluracil, and two steps in the biosynthesis of carnitine, which functions in fatty acid metabolism.[1] Ascorbic acid-dependent hydroxylations also take place in the synthesis of at least two neurotransmitters, *serotonin* (5-OH-tryptamine) from tryptophan and *norepinephrine* from tyrosine;[4] the exact role of ascorbic acid in these hydroxylations has not been established, but reduction of required enzyme cofactors is likely ($Cu^+$ is required in norepinephrine formation). Para-OH-phenylpyruvate oxidase is another enzyme in tyrosine metabolism that is stimulated by ascorbic acid. The activity of this enzyme develops late in fetal life and may be low in some premature infants. The resulting *transient tyrosinemia* is corrected by ascorbic acid supplementation (usually 100 mg per day).[5] Regulation by ascorbate of the biosynthesis of tyrosine hydroxylase, another enzyme in the pathway of epinephrine synthesis, has been reported,[6] but this proposed role of ascorbic acid needs confirmation.

Intestinal absorption of iron is enhanced by the presence of ascorbic acid in the lumen[7] (see Chap. 6, *Iron*). Mobilization of iron stores in guinea pigs from the spleen appears to be impaired in vitamin C deficiency, causing depletion of hepatic iron stores.[8] However, evidence regarding mobilization and redistribution of iron stores in vitamin C deficiency is equivocal.[9]

Because the two forms of ascorbic acid are readily interconvertible, they are believed to participate in other cellular functions, such as regulation of oxidation-reduction potential and transfer of hydrogen in the various electron transport systems; involvement of ascorbic acid in microsomal drug metabolism has been reported.[10] The reduced form may also function as a cellular antioxidant

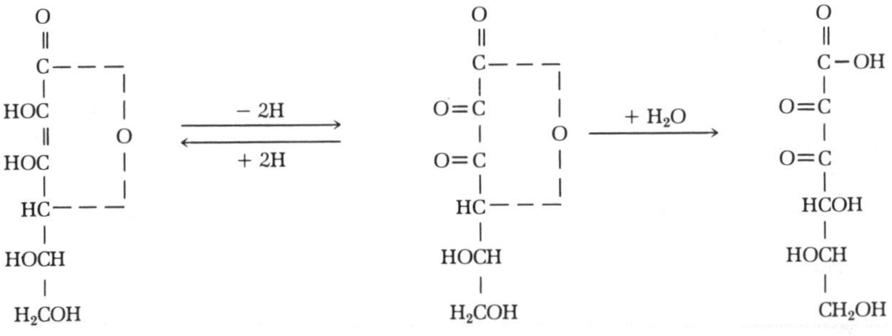

**Fig. 8-2.** Structural formulas and interconversion of the two forms of vitamin C and their inactivation by oxidation.

L-Ascorbic acid
(reduced form)

L-Dehydroascorbic acid
(oxidized form)

Diketogulonic
acid (inactive)

that protects other easily oxidizable substances, such as vitamins A and E, and the active forms of folic acid.[4]

Clinical observation of a number of infections accompanied by fever shows a decreased blood level of ascorbic acid, indicating either increased need for this vitamin or increased destruction of it. It appears, however, that a suboptimal intake of vitamin C is not a predisposing cause of any of these diseases. It has also been observed that the normally high concentration of ascorbic acid in the adrenal cortex is depleted whenever the gland is stimulated by hormones or certain toxins. The role of ascorbic acid in the adrenal gland remains unclear. One suggestion is that its presence in high concentration prevents the release of cortical hormones and that its depletion upon stimulation of the gland is necessary for normal hormonal response to various stresses.[5]

Administration of large doses of ascorbic acid appears to protect an individual exposed to very low environmental temperatures. However, the controversy involving the use of large doses of ascorbic acid to prevent and cure the common cold[11] has not been resolved. Anderson,[12] in reporting the results of a large double-blind Canadian study, stated that vitamin C in large amounts appeared to have some pharmacologic effects not related to its vitamin function at nutritional levels.

Disturbances in protein and lipid metabolism have been observed in scurvy.[13] Loss of nitrogen in the urine was increased and the plasma albumin to globulin ratio lowered. The level of plasma cholesterol appeared to be reduced and increased during repletion of tissue ascorbic acid. However, the role of ascorbic acid in cholesterol metabolism is controversial. Its participation in the removal of cholesterol from the tissues to the liver[14] and in the conversion of cholesterol to bile acids[15,16] has been proposed. It has been suggested that water-soluble cholesterol sulfate is formed by an ascorbic acid metabolite, ascorbic acid sulfate, to facilitate the removal of cholesterol from the enterohepatic circulation.[17] Such mechanisms have been linked to the reported hypocholesterolemic role of large doses of ascorbic acid in hypercholesterolemic subjects,[18] but other attempts to demonstrate such effects have failed to support these claims.[12,19] Even more controversial and unproven to date are the claims[20] for the effectiveness of ascorbic acid in the prevention and treatment of cancer and other diseases.

## Utilization of ascorbic acid

Active absorption of ascorbic acid has been demonstrated in the jejunum and ileum in humans.[21,22] Uptake of ascorbic acid into the mucosal cell depends on the presence of sodium in the lumen. A membrane sodium carrier also binds ascorbic acid and, while sodium enters the cell by facilitated diffusion, ascorbic acid is carried along regardless of its intracellular concentration. Energy

is required in the expulsion of sodium to the serosal fluid to maintain its normally low intracellular concentration and, as a result, for the absorption to continue. In the absence of sodium, absorption of ascorbate proceeds at a slow rate by simple diffusion. The mechanism of ascorbate absorption resembles that of actively absorbed sugars and amino acids but is not shared by them.[23] The efficiency of absorption decreases with increased intakes. From single doses of up to 100 mg 80% to 90% is absorbed compared with about 55% from a dose of 1000 mg (1 g), about 35% from 4 g, and less than 20% from doses exceeding 10 g.[4,24,25] Secretion of water into the gut with high intakes of ascorbic acid appears to be responsible for the diarrhea that is frequently associated with ingestion of megadoses of vitamin C.[22] The amount of ascorbic acid in different tissues varies; adrenal and pituitary tissue, brain, pancreas, kidney, liver, and spleen have relatively high concentrations; blood cells contain more than blood serum. The level of circulating ascorbic acid responds to changes in the intake of the vitamin. It also reflects the adequacy of tissue reserves, but this level cannot be used to estimate the body pool size because correlation between blood ascorbate level and the body pool size is not very good.[13] Nevertheless, the level of plasma ascorbic acid is used most commonly to assess vitamin C status because the assay is relatively simple. Use of radioactive ascorbic acid to label the tissue reserves permits calculation of excretion rates and the body pool size. Such studies have shown that at low levels of intake, very little of the unaltered vitamin is excreted in the urine.[13,26] As intake increases, the proportion of vitamin to metabolites increases, accounting for almost 90% of total excretion from a daily intake of 2 g in contrast to only about 7% from 30 mg.[26] It appears, therefore, that most of the ascorbic acid utilized by the body is excreted as metabolites, whereas the "excess" intake is excreted unaltered. It is not known whether any of the metabolites of vitamin C are produced during performance of its function or whether they represent nonfunctional metabolism in the tissues. One metabolite, ascorbic acid sulfate, has antiscorbutic action in some fish but not in guinea pigs or humans.[27]

The body pool of ascorbate in healthy adult men approximates 1500 mg on an average daily intake of 45 mg to 75 mg.[26,28] When no ascorbic acid is ingested, about 3% (2.2%–4.1%) of the reserves are depleted daily;[13,28] as a result, 45 mg (34 mg–61.5 mg) of absorbed ascorbic acid per day would be needed to maintain the body pool at that level. Clinical symptoms of scurvy appear in 30 to 45 days when the body pool drops below 300 mg.[13]

Higher intakes (200 mg) have been shown to increase the total body pool to 2300 mg to 2800 mg.[29] Such intakes maintain the maximum plasma concentration, which in most people is between 1.1 mg and 1.4 mg per dl, depending on the renal threshold. No benefits are known to accrue from maintenance of maximum tissue reserves.

Table 8-1 shows approximate ranges for blood ascorbic acid levels and body pool sizes that correspond to different levels of intake.

## Human requirement

Elaborate studies have been made to determine human requirements for ascorbic acid at different ages, under different conditions of environment, during physical exertion, in fevers, and in infections. The amount necessary to prevent frank symptoms of scurvy in humans is far less (10 mg) than that recommended for an optimum state of health.

In the 1980 edition of the *Recommended Dietary Allowances*,[30] the Food and Nutrition Board increased the recommended intake for adults to 60 mg per day from the 45 mg recommended in 1974. This intake level was calculated to maintain an average ascorbate body pool of 1500 mg at a daily catabolic rate of 3% to 4% and 85% efficiency of absorption. Daily intake of 35 mg was recommended for infants during the first year of life. This amount would be obtained by a breast-fed infant who consumed 850 ml of milk per day. However, 100 mg per day was recommended for the newborn during the first week of life to protect against transient tyrosinemia, which is especially common in premature infants. During pregnancy and lactation, daily intakes of 80 mg and 100 mg, respectively, were recommended.

The joint FAO/WHO Expert Committee set somewhat lower recommendations: 30 mg for adults (men and women over 13 years), 50 mg during pregnancy and lactation, and 20 mg for infants and children up to 13 years old.[31]

These intakes in adults are usually associated with plasma ascorbate levels of ⩾ 0.4 mg per dl and normal

## Table 8-1. Ascorbic Acid Nutritional Status in Humans

| | Dietary Intake mg | Serum or Plasma Concentration mg/dl | Whole Blood Concentration mg/dl | Buffy Coat* Concentration mcg/10⁸ Cells | Body Pool Size mg |
|---|---|---|---|---|---|
| *Well-nourished†* | >45 | >0.60 | >1.0 | >16 | 1500 |
| *Adequate†* | 30–44 | 0.40–0.59 | 0.60–0.99 | 11–15 | 600–1499 |
| *Low* | 10–29 | 0.20–0.39 | 0.30–0.59 | 2–10 | 300–599 |
| *Deficient* | <10 | <0.20 | <0.30 | <2 | 0–299 |

*White blood cells and platelets.

†These represent approximate ranges, not absolute values. This table is offered only as a guide to interpret current values.

(Adapted from Hodges RE, Ascorbic acid. In Goodhart RS, Shils ME (eds): Modern Nutrition in Health and Disease, 6th ed. Philadelphia, Lea & Febiger, 1980)

health. It should be noted that these recommendations were established more than a decade ago. Significant new information about ascorbic acid metabolism has since become available. Considering the possible but quantitatively unknown effects of individual variation, emotional and environmental stress, age, smoking, and oral contraceptive agents and other drugs, the Food and Nutrition Board concluded that higher intake levels were desirable and easily attainable from the average diet in the United States.

## Pharmacologic intakes of vitamin C

In previous sections reference has been made to pharmacologic doses of ascorbic acid. Fortunately it is relatively nontoxic, considering the recent use of megadoses of ascorbic acid for colds, and the infrequency of reports of adverse reactions to these doses. However, some adverse effects have been reported.[32] Gastrointestinal disturbances, including nausea, cramps, and, especially, diarrhea are most frequent.[33] Increased excretion of uric acid,[34] impaired bactericidal activity of leukocytes,[35] and absorption of excessive amounts of food iron[36] are undesirable effects that have been demonstrated under well-controlled experimental conditions. There is also evidence that prolonged high intakes of ascorbic acid may affect the body's catabolic and excretory systems, leading to a higher than normal need for the vitamin, which persists after the intake of large doses is discontinued. Not only have such effects been reported in adults, but rebound scurvy has been observed in infants whose mothers were consuming large amounts of vitamin C during pregnancy.[33]

After reviewing the current evidence of the effects of high intakes of ascorbic acid on the common cold and other diseases, the Food and Nutrition Board concluded that the demonstrated benefits are minor and do not justify recommending routine intake of pharmacologic doses of ascorbic acid.

## Food sources

It is obvious from the bar chart (Fig. 8-3) that the commonly used fruits and vegetables of Group 3 are the richest sources of ascorbic acid, with citrus fruits, strawberries, cantaloupe, and a number of raw, leafy vegetables topping the list. Canned or frozen citrus juice may be the cheapest source of vitamin C when fresh citrus fruit is scarce or expensive and may be cheaper than tomato juice because it takes three times as much tomato as citrus juice to supply the same amounts of vitamin C.

Many factors affect the ascorbic acid content of fruits and vegetables; variety, maturity, length of storage, part of the plant, seasonal and geographical factors are all influential. As plants mature they generally have less ascorbic acid; the sprouts of beans or grains, however, do contain vitamin C. Exposure to sunlight also tends to

### Amounts of Ascorbic Acid in Average Servings

milligrams of Ascorbic Acid in one serving

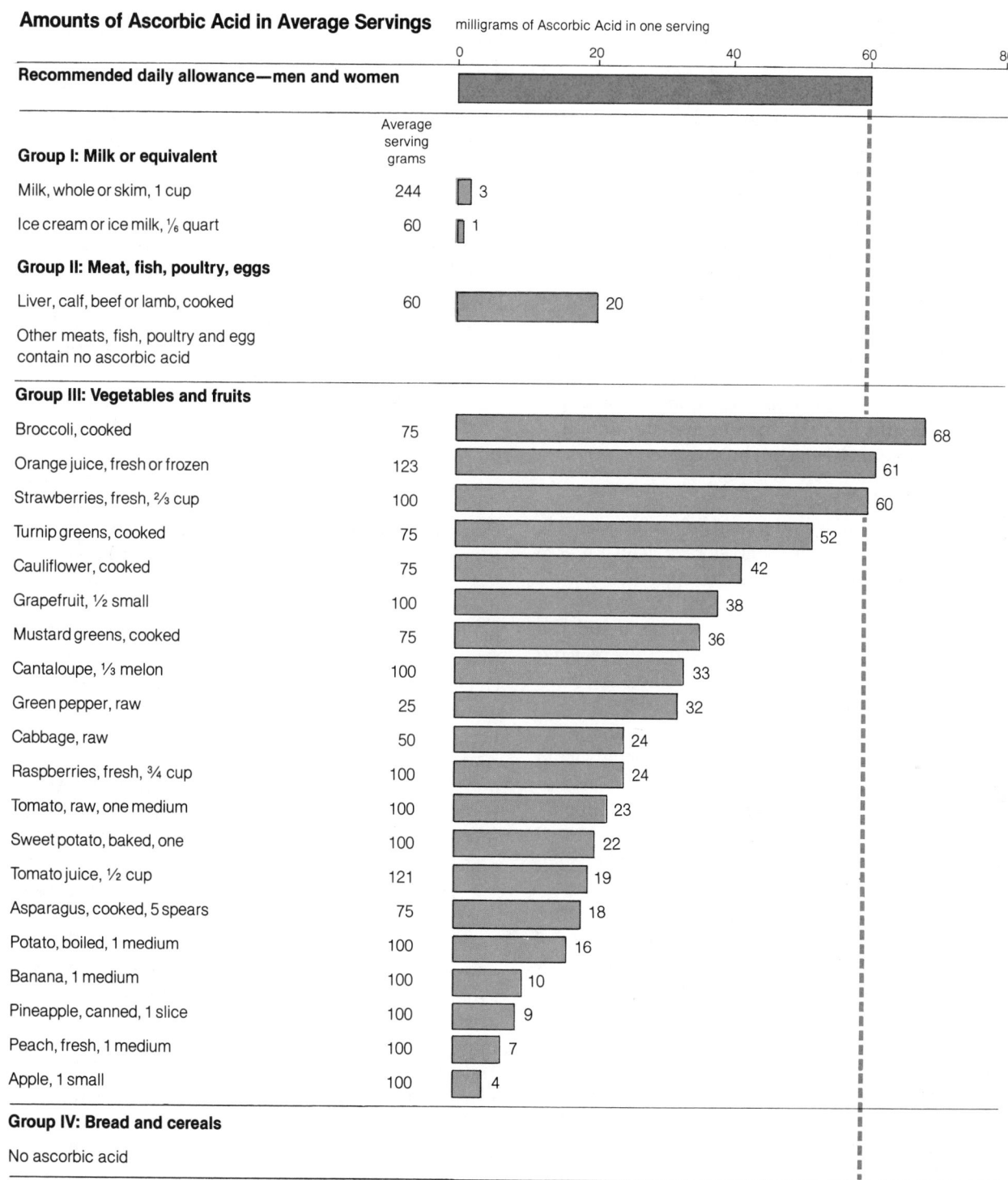

**Fig. 8-3.**   Ascorbic acid in average servings of foods classified according to the four food groups.

increase the plant's ascorbic acid content. Food value tables give average representative amounts, whereas any individual food may vary considerably from this value.[37] From analyses of the ascorbic acid content of such foods as potatoes, cabbage, and broccoli purchased during the winter in northern Vermont, the authors[38] conclude "that certain vegetables, as purchased during the winter months, provide dependable quantities of total ascorbic acid, even though they have been subjected to transportation, storage, and handling."

In some countries indigenous fruits high in vitamin C are overlooked, even though they are readily available. For example, in Puerto Rico the acerola (*azarole*, or West Indian cherry) has the highest ascorbic acid content of any known food.[39] Only after attention had been called to it, did the acerola become popular in that country. In Great Britain during World War II rosehip and black-currant syrups or jams served to supplement the meager supply of vitamin C from garden vegetables. Even before the war, in northern Russia an extract of pine needles rich in vitamin C was being added to berry juice as a health beverage for school children. In another part of northern Europe raw turnip juice saved the lives of many infants who otherwise would have died of scurvy. Depending on diet, human milk may contain more ascorbic acid than average cow's milk and considerably more than is found in pasteurized milk, thereby affecting the amount and the timing of additional sources needed in an infant's diet.

### Stability in Foods

Of all the vitamins, ascorbic acid is the most unstable under heat, oxidation, drying, and storage, which makes it one of the most difficult nutrients to supply in adequate amounts to troops or civil populations in wartime. In World War II the American army rations included a lemon powder fortified with ascorbic acid; if the men did not drink lemonade, as was frequently the case, their ration was deficient in vitamin C.

Alkalinity, even to a slight degree, is distinctly destructive to this vitamin; therefore, baking soda should never be added to food in cooking. Acid fruits and vegetables lose much less ascorbic acid when heated than nonacid foods. Vitamin C is extremely soluble in water and dissolves out of some vegetables during the first few minutes of the cooking process.

To reduce as much as possible the loss of ascorbic acid in cooking vegetables, the least possible amount of cooking water, shortest cooking time (water should be boiling when vegetable is added), and least chopping or cutting is recommended. Studies have shown that baked, boiled, or steamed potatoes retain a large proportion of their vitamin C if cooked whole. Fresh fruits and, especially, vegetables lose vitamin C activity rapidly when stored at room temperature and somewhat less rapidly at refrigerator temperatures. Experts advise not to shell peas, cut beans, or peel vegetables until ready to cook. Quick freezing of fruits and vegetables destroys little if any of this factor. To retain a maximum of the ascorbic acid, frozen fruits should be used promptly after thawing, and frozen vegetables should be plunged directly into boiling water for immediate cooking.

## The vitamin B complex

Discovery of thiamin as an essential food factor for prevention of the disease, *beriberi*, began the fascinating advances in nutrition research, which during the first half of the 20th century led to the identification of all currently known vitamins. Descriptions of beriberi by the Chinese date back to about 2600 B.C., and some of the earliest attempts to treat the disease were reported from Japan and the Philippines. A medical officer in the Japanese Navy, Takaki, is credited with the recognition of the causal relationship of diet to this disease. In the 1880s Takaki, alarmed by the high incidence of beriberi among the Japanese sailors, compared their diets with that of the British Navy, which did not have this problem. Convinced that the higher protein content in the diets of the British prevented beriberi, he revised the Japanese ration to include more meat, vegetables, and "condensed" milk, and less rice. The new diet was tested on a special training ship which returned from a 287-day voyage with a report of only a few cases of beriberi and no deaths. The men who developed the disease had refused to eat the meat and milk.

The next significant milestone in the history of thiamin, and of nutrition in general, was achieved by two Dutch physicians who worked in the Dutch East Indies, the present Indonesia. In 1897 Eijkman noted that poultry fed table scraps of polished rice from the prison hospital developed polyneuritic symptoms similar to those of his patients suffering from beriberi. Brown rice or addition of rice polishings to the diet cured the condition in the chickens. Eijkman suggested that polished rice contained a "toxic factor," which was "neutralized" by the polishings. A few years later Grijn concluded that natural foods contained an unknown food factor that prevented beriberi and that this factor was lacking in polished rice. After he had produced polyneuritis in birds on a diet consisting mostly of starch, he showed that they could be cured by other foods as well as by rice polishings.

Following these discoveries many workers began to observe a variety of symptoms due to deficiencies among peoples with different dietary patterns, and in animals fed diets of different compositions. It thus became evident that foods contain a number of the so-called accessory factors, later called *vitamines* by Funk. The first important breakthrough toward the eventual separation and identification of individual vitamins came in 1916 when McCollum and Davis recognized that milk contained at least two factors required for growth—one in the milk fat named *fat-soluble A* and another in the liquid portion of milk designated as *water-soluble B*. This established the practice of using the alphabet to name newly discovered vitamins before their chemical structures were known.

The search for the identity of the water-soluble antiberiberi factor soon led to another major discovery. Several independent research groups observed that the antiberiberi activity of their partially purified preparations was destroyed by heating, although its growth-promoting activity remained. The antiberiberi factor became known as $B_1$ and the heat-stable factor as $B_2$. This was the beginning of distinctions in a group of vitamins, which have been referred to as the *vitamin B complex*. The group includes eight distinct vitamins, which are discussed individually in the following sections.

## Thiamin

The intense research efforts that followed eventually led to the isolation of crystalline antiberiberi factor in 1926 by Jansen and Donath, who called it *aneurine*. Its chemical structure was identified 10 years later by Williams and Cline, who also accomplished the chemical synthesis of thiamin hydrochloride and showed it to be identical with the natural vitamin (Fig. 8-4).

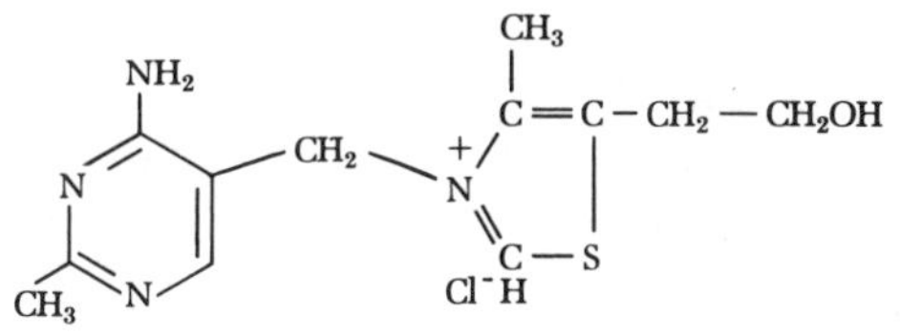

### Functions of Thiamin

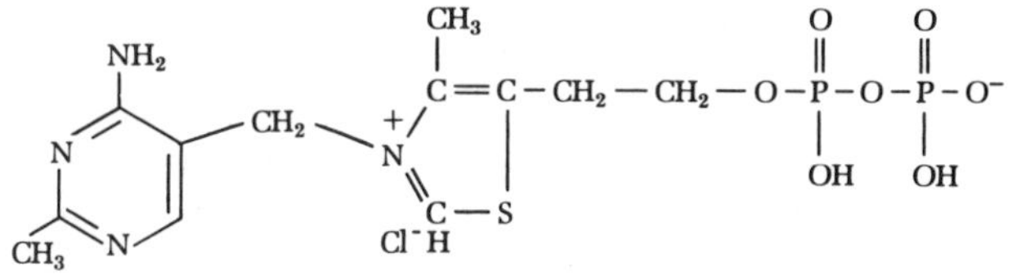

The known biochemical functions of thiamin require its conversion to thiamin pyrophosphate (TPP), which serves as a coenzyme in a number of metabolic reactions. TPP is known also as *cocarboxylase* because one of its major functions involves an *oxidative decarboxylation* (removal of $CO_2$) of alpha-ketoacids, of which *pyruvate* and *alpha-ketoglutarate* are most significant. Catabolism of the branched-chain amino acids involves a similar reaction.

Oxidative decarboxylation of pyruvate to acetyl coenzyme A (CoA) is a key reaction for further oxidation of carbohydrate and some amino acid substrates in the citric acid cycle (CAC) and for storage of excess carbohydrate as fat; this is discussed in Chapter 9 (see Fig. 9-9). Formation of succinyl CoA from alpha-ketoglutarate takes place in the common pathway of energy metabolism in the CAC, thereby influencing the release of energy from proteins and also fats (Fig. 9-7). Oxidative decarboxylation is a complex reaction with many steps, which in addition to TPP requires lipoic acid and the coenzymes of three other B-vitamins—pantothenic acid (CoA), riboflavin (FAD), and niacin (NAD)—thereby demonstrating the interdependent roles of several of the B-vitamins in energy metabolism.

In thiamin deficiency pyruvic and alpha-ketoglutaric acids tend to accumulate in the body, and their levels in blood have been measured as a means of determining thiamin nutriture. However, more specific measures of thiamin status are now used more frequently.

TPP also participates in *transketolations*, which involve the transfer of 2-carbon units (including a keto group) between several intermediates of the hexose monophosphate shunt (HMS), an alternate pathway of glucose metabolism. Active in red blood cells, and in liver, kidney, and other tissues, this pathway is important in providing 5-carbon sugars for the synthesis of various ribonucleotides, including those found in DNA and RNA. Normal functioning of the HMS also produces the reduced form of the niacin coenzyme, NADP, which is needed in several synthetic pathways, such as fatty acid, cholesterol, and steroid syntheses.

Thiamin

Thiamin pyrophosphate (TPP)

**Fig. 8-4.** Structures of thiamin hydrochloride and its coenzyme.

Measurement of the erythrocyte transketolase activity, which reflects the availability of TPP in the tissues, has become a widely used method in the assessment of thiamin nutriture. Addition of exogenous TPP to a red cell hemolysate from a thiamin-deficient individual stimulates the activity of this enzyme by more than 25% under standardized conditions, whereas less than 15% stimulation is seen with a hemolysate from an individual with adequate endogenous TPP.

Thiamin deficiency generally affects the neural, cardiac, and gastrointestinal functions, and the symptoms in mild deficiency are nonspecific. Loss of appetite, constipation, irritability, and fatigue are all symptoms that have been associated with low thiamin intakes. Changes in the central nervous system affecting peripheral nerves, eye–hand coordination, and mental ability are found among chronic alcoholics who have inadequate intakes of thiamin. The various forms and symptoms of beriberi and the Wernicke-Korsakoff syndrome are discussed in Chapter 21.

There is no well-defined relationship between the biochemical abnormalities and the clinical manifestations that result from thiamin deficiency. Although failure to provide sufficient energy (ATP) to the cell, failure to produce a compound essential to the neuromuscular transmission (acetylcholine), and accumulation of "toxic metabolites" have been implicated in the nerve and muscle disease seen in thiamin deficiency, none of them adequately explains all the experimental observations and the specificity of thiamin in these conditions.[40,41]

Research has demonstrated impaired synthesis of both fatty acids and cholesterol in certain types of brain cells cultured in a thiamin-deficient medium.[42] It appears that the synthesis of the key enzymes that control fatty acid production is impaired in the absence of thiamin and can be restored by its addition to the culture medium. The mechanism by which thiamin regulates the production of these enzymes remains to be established as does the possible role of these biochemical defects in the manifestations of thiamin deficiency.

Rare genetic disorders causing various degrees of thiamin dependency have been reported. In children two cases of megaloblastic anemia have been identified which responded to large doses of thiamin but not to any of the other vitamins normally associated with this type of anemia.[41] The metabolic defect has not been identified. Recently, a transketolase with lower than normal affinity to TPP has been discovered in cultured fibroblasts from four patients with the Wernicke-Korsakoff syndrome associated with a history of alcoholism.[43] These patients appear to require much more thiamin for normal functioning of this enzyme than is required by healthy people. The possible role of this enzyme in the development of the Wernicke-Korsakoff syndrome remains to be determined. Rare cases of branched-chain ketoaciduria (see maple syrup urine disease in Chap. 36) appear to involve an alpha-ketoacid decarboxylase with reduced affinity for TPP and respond to large doses of thiamin, whereas most cases of this disease do not.[44]

### Utilization of thiamin

Intestinal absorption of thiamin takes place throughout the upper intestine but appears to be most effective in the jejunum. Recent research has demonstrated that the mechanism of thiamin absorption depends on the level of intake.[45,46] From physiologic doses thiamin is absorbed by an active, probably carrier-mediated mechanism. Presence of sodium and unimpaired Na-K ATPase function are necessary for the release of thiamin from the mucosal cell to the serosa. Both the entry into and the exit from the mucosal cell take place as thiamin—TPP is hydrolyzed in the intestinal lumen prior to its uptake into the mucosa. Although phosphorylation to mono- and pyrophosphate forms takes place within the mucosal cell, followed by dephosphorylation before exit from the cell, these reactions are not considered essential for absorption of thiamin. Passive diffusion is insignificant as a mechanism of thiamin absorption from normal dietary intakes but becomes the major means of thiamin absorption at high levels of intake.[46]

The active intestinal transport of thiamin is not shared by other vitamins but is subject to inhibition by other factors. Thiamin absorption is decreased in folate deficiency[47] and in chronic alcoholism, probably due to secondary folate deficiency. The mechanism by which folate deficiency affects thiamin absorption is not known, but it is evident before significant structural alterations in the mucosa are detected. Alcohol also has a direct effect on thiamin absorption by interfering with its release from the mucosal cell, presumably through inhibition of the Na-K ATPase activity.[46] This effect is observed only in the presence of alcohol and is not detected with large doses of thiamin. Thus it appears that thiamin absorption in alcoholics may be reduced by two mechanisms—the direct effect by alcohol and a secondary effect due to folate deficiency. Because severe thiamin deficiency is very costly in terms of human suffering and the institutional care that is required for affected individuals, fortification of alcoholic beverages with thiamin has been proposed recently.[48]

Thiamin is found in the tissues mostly as TPP, but some free thiamin and its mono- (TMP) and triphosphate (TTP) forms are also present. Thiamin cannot be stored to any extent in the animal body, although certain tissues—heart, brain, liver, and kidney—tend to have higher concentrations than others. Because these amounts decrease quickly when thiamin is not supplied, an adequate daily intake is important. On low intake, urinary excretion of thiamin decreases. When intake is increased, a proportional increase in urinary excretion is observed, thereby providing another measure of the adequacy of thiamin intake. Appreciable amounts of various thiamin metabolites are also found in the urine.

Although some thiamin may be synthesized by bacterial action in the large intestine of humans, it is believed that very little is absorbed.

### Human requirement

Because thiamin functions primarily in terms of energy metabolism, the recommended allowances suggested by both the joint FAO/WHO Expert Committee[49] and the National Research Council's Food and Nutrition Board[30] are based on calorie levels. However, the FAO/WHO Expert Committee set the recommendation at 0.4 mg per 1000 kcal, whereas the Food and Nutrition Board recommends 0.5 mg per 1000 kcal. This latter figure indicates 1.4 mg for the average man and 1.0 mg for the woman. An increase of 0.4 mg over the allowance recommended for the nonpregnant woman is suggested for the pregnant woman and 0.5 mg for the nursing mother. Recommendations for infants and children are the same as those for adults, 0.5 mg of thiamin per 1000 kcal (see Chap. 11).

### Food sources

Thiamin is widely distributed in a large variety of animal and vegetable tissues, but there are few foods in which it occurs in abundance. This is strikingly emphasized in Figure 8-5, which shows the thiamin content of average servings of some common foods. Obviously, several servings of even the better sources of thiamin are needed to meet the recommended allowance. Therefore, enrichment of bread and cereals was instigated to make it

## Amounts of Thiamin in Average Servings

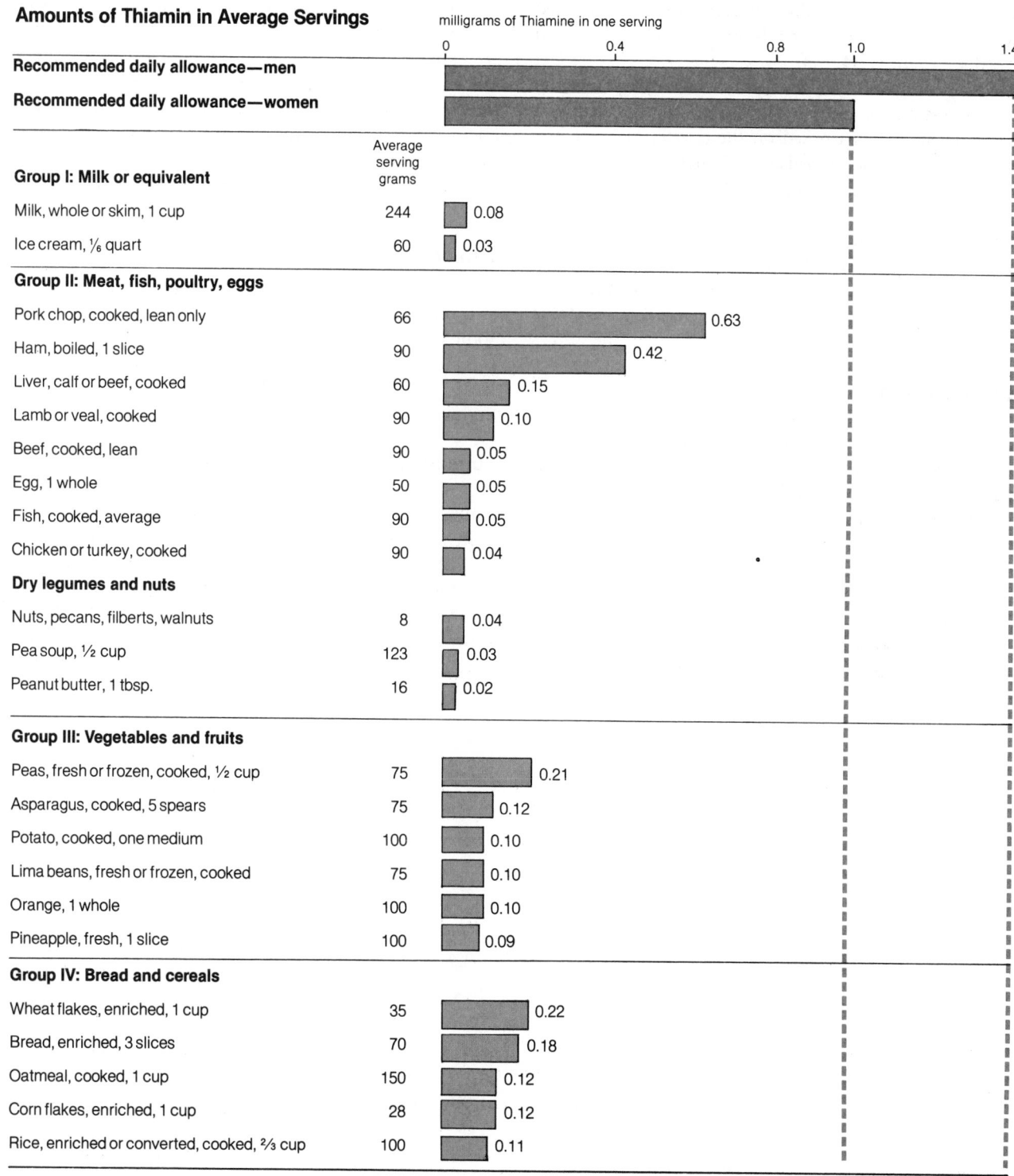

milligrams of Thiamine in one serving

| | Average serving grams | mg Thiamine |
|---|---|---|
| **Recommended daily allowance—men** | | |
| **Recommended daily allowance—women** | | |
| **Group I: Milk or equivalent** | | |
| Milk, whole or skim, 1 cup | 244 | 0.08 |
| Ice cream, ⅙ quart | 60 | 0.03 |
| **Group II: Meat, fish, poultry, eggs** | | |
| Pork chop, cooked, lean only | 66 | 0.63 |
| Ham, boiled, 1 slice | 90 | 0.42 |
| Liver, calf or beef, cooked | 60 | 0.15 |
| Lamb or veal, cooked | 90 | 0.10 |
| Beef, cooked, lean | 90 | 0.05 |
| Egg, 1 whole | 50 | 0.05 |
| Fish, cooked, average | 90 | 0.05 |
| Chicken or turkey, cooked | 90 | 0.04 |
| **Dry legumes and nuts** | | |
| Nuts, pecans, filberts, walnuts | 8 | 0.04 |
| Pea soup, ½ cup | 123 | 0.03 |
| Peanut butter, 1 tbsp. | 16 | 0.02 |
| **Group III: Vegetables and fruits** | | |
| Peas, fresh or frozen, cooked, ½ cup | 75 | 0.21 |
| Asparagus, cooked, 5 spears | 75 | 0.12 |
| Potato, cooked, one medium | 100 | 0.10 |
| Lima beans, fresh or frozen, cooked | 75 | 0.10 |
| Orange, 1 whole | 100 | 0.10 |
| Pineapple, fresh, 1 slice | 100 | 0.09 |
| **Group IV: Bread and cereals** | | |
| Wheat flakes, enriched, 1 cup | 35 | 0.22 |
| Bread, enriched, 3 slices | 70 | 0.18 |
| Oatmeal, cooked, 1 cup | 150 | 0.12 |
| Corn flakes, enriched, 1 cup | 28 | 0.12 |
| Rice, enriched or converted, cooked, ⅔ cup | 100 | 0.11 |

**Fig. 8-5.**   Thiamin in average servings of foods classified according to the four food groups.

easier for the average person to meet his requirement economically. Because bread constitutes about one-fifth of the calories in the average American diet and only a very small fraction of the bread consumed in this country is made from whole wheat, the enrichment of white flour and bread with thiamin, riboflavin, niacin, and iron was a logical step. On the basis of the average per capita consumption of flour and bread in the United States, as much as 35% of the daily thiamin requirement is now supplied by these foods. For more details about enriched flour and bread see Chapter 11.

Rice enrichment has been practiced for years in some of the rice-eating countries. The Rice Research Institute in the Philippines has worked on the development of improved strains of rice and also on methods of enrichment. Much of the rice used in Japan is enriched.

Dry yeast and wheat germ are the richest natural sources of thiamin, but they are eaten only in relatively small amounts. Except for pork, which is outstanding, muscle meats contain less than the organs, such as liver, heart, and kidney. Fruits in general are poor sources of this vitamin.

### Stability in foods

The losses of thiamin in cooking depend on several factors, such as type of food, method of preparation, temperature, length of cooking, and the acidity or alkalinity of the cooking medium. Research indicates that on the whole fresh vegetables retain thiamin well during cooking. From a trace to 15% is dissolved in the cooking water, and up to 22% may be destroyed by cooking. If the cooking water is discarded, thiamin losses may be from 20% to 35%.

In acid foods this vitamin is quite stable, but its activity is destroyed rapidly by sulfite, a fact which may explain the loss of thiamin in dried fruits, such as apricots and peaches treated with sulfur.

Thiamin is well retained in cereals, as they are generally cooked slowly and at a moderate temperature, and the cooking water is not discarded. Baked products lose about 15% of their original thiamin. Generally, the losses in cooking meat are greater than in cooking other foods, ranging from 25% to 50% of the raw value.

## Riboflavin

The second member of the B complex—riboflavin—was recognized in the 1920s when it became evident that some growth-promoting properties of vitamin B were retained after heat had destroyed the antiberiberi activity. In 1932 the vitamin was identified as part of an enzyme and was synthesized in 1935.

### Functions

Riboflavin functions as a part of a group of enzymes, called *flavoproteins*, which are involved in the metabolism of carbohydrates, fats, and proteins. The metabolically active forms of riboflavin include riboflavin-5'-phosphate, also known as riboflavin mononucleotide (FMN) and flavin adenine dinucleotide (FAD), which is shown in Figure 8-6. The ring structure of the riboflavin part of the coenzymes can alternate between oxidized

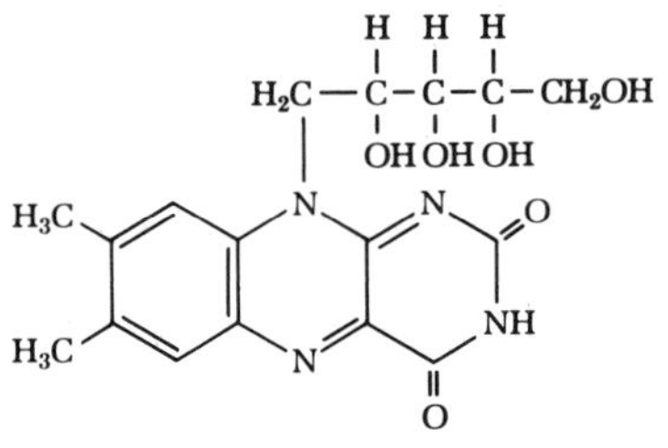

Riboflavin

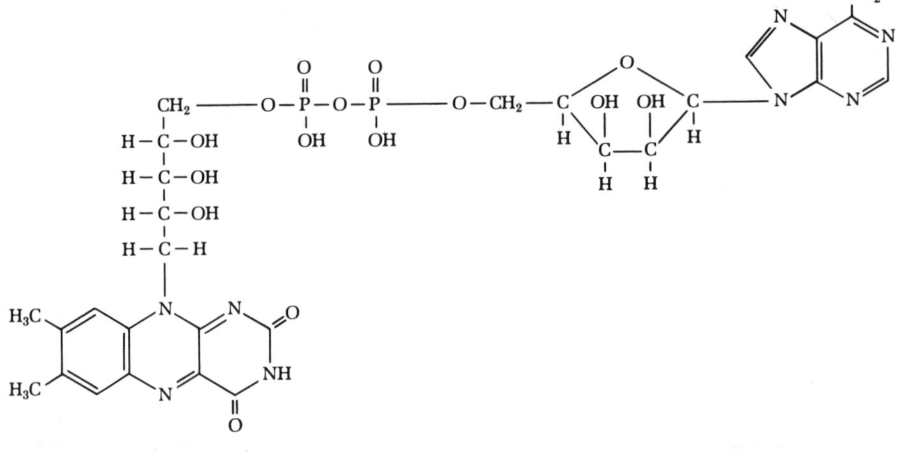

**Fig. 8-6.** Structural formulas of riboflavin and one of its coenzyme forms.

Flavin adenine dinucleotide (FAD)

(FMN, FAD) and reduced forms (FMNH$_2$, FADH$_2$) and is responsible for their role as hydrogen carriers in a variety of metabolic reactions, too numerous to mention. In general, flavoprotein dehydrogenases initiate the transfer of hydrogen from the oxidation of specific substrates to oxygen in the process of cellular respiration that results in the formation of ATP (see Chap. 9). For example, FAD-dependent oxidations are involved in the decarboxylation of pyruvate and other alpha-ketoacids (reoxidation of lipoic acid), conversion of succinate to fumarate in the CAC, and $\beta$-oxidation of fatty acids. FMN is found in the flavoprotein that transfers hydrogen from reduced niacin-coenzyme, NADH, to the next acceptor in the mitochondrial electron transport chain. Examples of riboflavin enzymes not involved in energy metabolism include xanthine oxidase, L-amino acid oxidase, pyridoxine-5'-phosphate oxidase, and glutathione reductase. *In vitro* stimulation by FAD of the erythrocyte glutathione reductase activity has become a widely used measure of riboflavin status.[50]

Riboflavin is essential for normal growth and tissue maintenance. Deficiency of riboflavin damages some types of tissues more than others. Fissures on the lips and at the corners of the mouth (cheilosis) and scaly, sometimes greasy dermatitis around the nose are characteristic of riboflavin deficiency in humans. Anemia has been observed in some studies,[51] and a reduction in erythrocyte survival time has been reported recently.[52]

Riboflavin also plays an important role in the health of the eye. Ocular symptoms appear on a low riboflavin diet and may precede all other manifestations. Eye strain and fatigue, itching and burning, sensitivity to light, and frontal headaches are the most frequent complaints. Cataracts have been observed in rats, mice, chickens, and monkeys after prolonged deficiency of riboflavin. Riboflavin deficiency has also been shown to lead to adrenal cortex dysfunction in humans.[53] In humans, riboflavin deficiency is apt to occur along with a deficiency of other members of the B complex. In experimental animals, maternal riboflavin deficiency causes congenital malformations in the offspring.

### Utilization of riboflavin

Little is known about the mechanism of intestinal absorption of riboflavin from normal levels of dietary intake in humans. Absorption of doses from 5 mg to 30 mg has been found to be much greater when the riboflavin is ingested with food than when given on an empty stomach.[54] Bile also appears to stimulate riboflavin absorption.[55] Phosphorylated forms of riboflavin are dephosphorylated prior to the mucosal uptake and rephosphorylated within the cell. Active absorption against the concentration gradient has been demonstrated in the rat from low luminal concentrations of the vitamin, but not from high concentrations.[45]

Most of the tissue riboflavin is found in flavoproteins as FAD (70%–90%) and the remainder as FMN and free riboflavin. FMN is an intermediate in the synthesis of FAD.[56] On low riboflavin intakes the tissues appear to conserve FAD at the expense of the other forms, and very little riboflavin is excreted in the urine. The tissues have a limited capacity to retain riboflavin and on increasing intakes, urinary excretion of riboflavin increases. The level of urinary excretion of riboflavin is used as a measure of riboflavin status. However, negative nitrogen balance due to insufficient protein intake or other causes is associated with increased loss of riboflavin in the urine and can result in erroneous interpretation of excretion data.[57]

Utilization of riboflavin and, accordingly, riboflavin status, also are influenced by hormones. Both thyroid and adrenal hormones are known to affect the conversion of riboflavin to its coenzyme forms.[58] The use of oral contraceptive agents (OCA) is associated with an increased frequency of marginal riboflavin status in women of low socioeconomic status,[59] but no effects have been observed in presumably well-nourished OCA users.[60,61] Biochemical evidence of riboflavin deficiency has been found in newborn infants with hyperbilirubinemia who are treated with phototherapy.[62] Because it is light-sensitive, riboflavin is presumed to decompose during the treatment.

### Human requirement

The Food and Nutrition Board of the National Research Council[30] has set the recommended dietary allowance for riboflavin at 0.6 mg per 1000 kcal or 1.6 mg for the average man aged 23 to 50 years and 1.2 mg for the average woman aged 23 to 50 years. An increment of 0.3 mg per day for pregnancy and 0.5 mg per day for lactation is suggested. The recommended dietary allowance for infants and children is also 0.6 mg per 1000 kcal. The actual recommendation for each age and sex group is given in Chapter 11.

The Joint FAO/WHO Expert Committee set the riboflavin recommendation at 0.55 mg per 1000 kcal for all age groups.[49]

### Food sources

Riboflavin is widely distributed in animal and vegetable foods but only in small amounts in most of them. Organ meats, milk, and green leafy vegetables are the outstanding food sources. This is strikingly emphasized in Figure 8-7, which shows the riboflavin content of average servings of some common foods and the contribution they make toward the day's requirement.

The average person is not likely to get an optimum amount of riboflavin unless he consumes a generous amount of milk. The addition of riboflavin in the enrichment of flour and bread has helped to raise the average intake.

## Amounts of Riboflavin in Average Servings

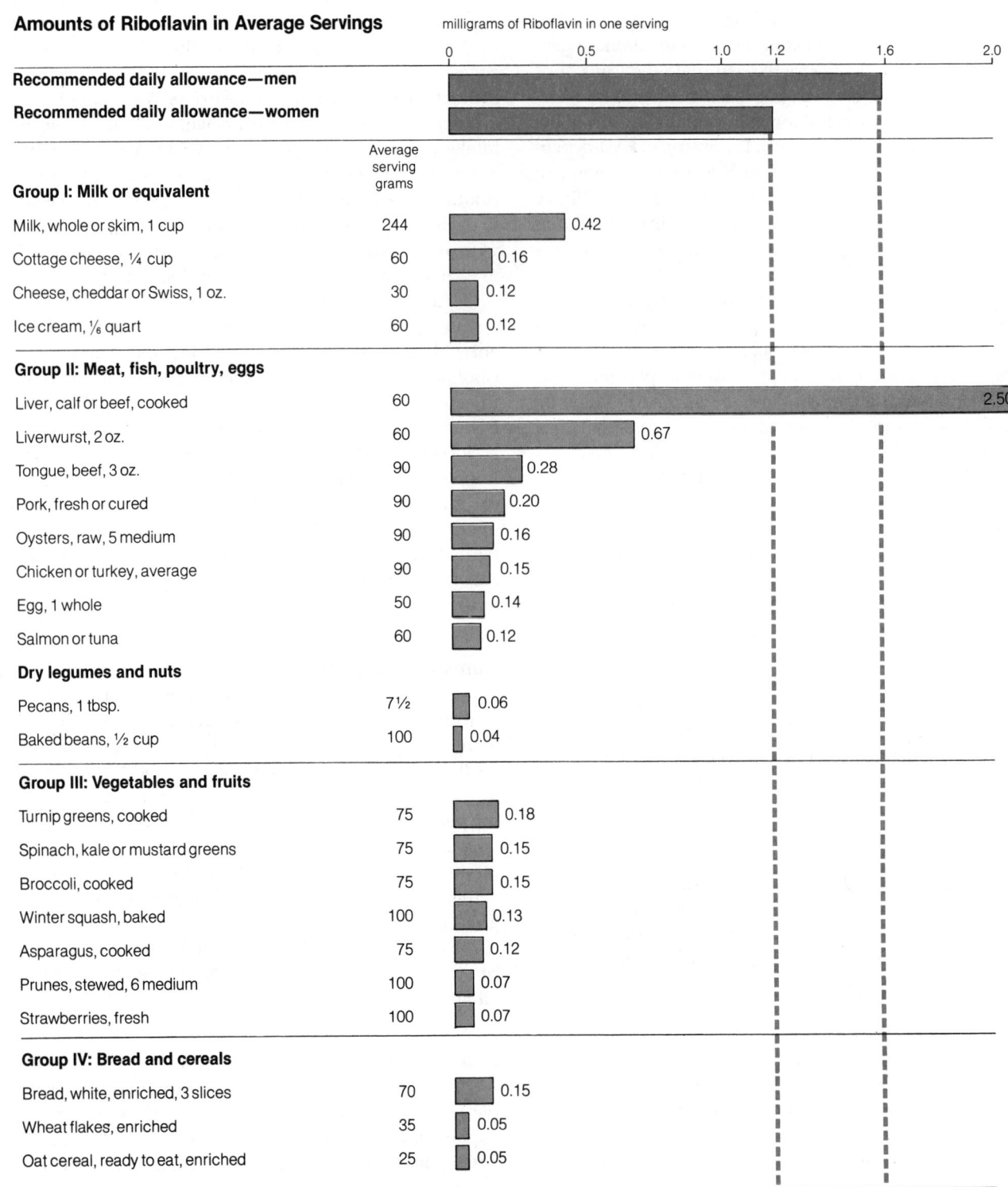

milligrams of Riboflavin in one serving

| | Average serving grams | Riboflavin (mg) |
|---|---|---|
| **Recommended daily allowance—men** | | 1.6 |
| **Recommended daily allowance—women** | | 1.2 |
| **Group I: Milk or equivalent** | | |
| Milk, whole or skim, 1 cup | 244 | 0.42 |
| Cottage cheese, ¼ cup | 60 | 0.16 |
| Cheese, cheddar or Swiss, 1 oz. | 30 | 0.12 |
| Ice cream, ⅛ quart | 60 | 0.12 |
| **Group II: Meat, fish, poultry, eggs** | | |
| Liver, calf or beef, cooked | 60 | 2.50 |
| Liverwurst, 2 oz. | 60 | 0.67 |
| Tongue, beef, 3 oz. | 90 | 0.28 |
| Pork, fresh or cured | 90 | 0.20 |
| Oysters, raw, 5 medium | 90 | 0.16 |
| Chicken or turkey, average | 90 | 0.15 |
| Egg, 1 whole | 50 | 0.14 |
| Salmon or tuna | 60 | 0.12 |
| **Dry legumes and nuts** | | |
| Pecans, 1 tbsp. | 7½ | 0.06 |
| Baked beans, ½ cup | 100 | 0.04 |
| **Group III: Vegetables and fruits** | | |
| Turnip greens, cooked | 75 | 0.18 |
| Spinach, kale or mustard greens | 75 | 0.15 |
| Broccoli, cooked | 75 | 0.15 |
| Winter squash, baked | 100 | 0.13 |
| Asparagus, cooked | 75 | 0.12 |
| Prunes, stewed, 6 medium | 100 | 0.07 |
| Strawberries, fresh | 100 | 0.07 |
| **Group IV: Bread and cereals** | | |
| Bread, white, enriched, 3 slices | 70 | 0.15 |
| Wheat flakes, enriched | 35 | 0.05 |
| Oat cereal, ready to eat, enriched | 25 | 0.05 |

**Fig. 8-7.**  Riboflavin in average servings of foods classified according to the four food groups.

## Stability in foods

Riboflavin is stable to ordinary cooking processes but unstable in alkaline solutions. It is stable in milk—an important source—if the milk is distributed in cartons or dark bottles or otherwise protected from light. One-half or more of the riboflavin in milk may be lost in 2 hours if exposed to light.

## Niacin

When Elvehjem reported the spectacular cure of blacktongue in dogs by means of nicotinic acid, now known as niacin, the logical supposition was that a niacin deficiency might be the cause of pellagra in humans. Later, Spies, and others demonstrated that most of the classic symptoms of pellagra were relieved by the administration of niacin. However, most persons suffering from pellagra have multiple deficiencies, and it has been found that certain symptoms formerly associated with the disease are not relieved until thiamin and riboflavin are supplied along with niacin. Earlier concepts that related pellagra to a protein deficiency have been clarified by the discovery that one of the amino acids—tryptophan—is a precursor from which niacin may be synthesized in the animal body. Human pellegra is discussed in Chapter 21.

Nicotinic acid had long been known as a simple organic compound, but its physiologic properties were not realized until it was isolated from potent liver concentrates by Elvehjem and associates in 1937.

Two forms of niacin—nicotinic acid and nicotinamide (Fig. 8-8)—have antipellagra activity. Therapeutic doses of nicotinic acid may cause temporary flushing or hot flashes, but nicotinamide does not produce this reaction.

## Functions

Niacin, like thiamin and riboflavin, also functions as a coenzyme in energy metabolism. In its amide form, niacin is part of the coenzymes NAD (nicotinamide adenine dinucleotide) and NADP (nicotinamide adenine dinucleotide phosphate), which serve as hydrogen carriers in numerous reactions catalyzed by substrate-specific dehydrogenases. $NAD^+$ is required in all the major metabolic pathways that result in oxidative breakdown of hexoses, amino acids, and fatty acids, including glycolysis, oxidative decarboxylation of pyruvate, citric acid cycle, deamination of amino acids, and $\beta$-oxidation of fatty acids (see Chap. 9). It also participates in the oxidation of a variety of other biologic substances, such as ethanol and retinol (vitamin A). $NADP^+$ can substitute for $NAD^+$ in some of these reactions, and it is the active form in two reactions of the hexose monophosphate shunt. The resulting reduced coenzymes either channel hydrogen to the mitochondrial electron transport chain (from $NADH+H^+$ to FMN) to produce ATP, or they are used as specific reducing agents in a variety of reactions, such as the conversion of pyruvate to lactate. Reduced NADP ($NADPH+H^+$) is required for the synthesis of fatty acids, cholesterol, and steroid hormones. Hence niacin is essential in every cell and tissue of the body.

In niacin deficiency, some tissues are affected more than others, especially the skin, the gastrointestinal tract, and the nervous system (see *Pellagra* in Chap. 21). Early signs of niacin deficiency are nonspecific and include lassitude, anorexia, weakness, mild digestive disturbances, and such emotional changes as anxiety, irritability, and depression.

Large doses of nicotinic acid (100 to 200 times the recommended allowance) administered orally have resulted in the lowering of serum cholesterol and beta-lipoprotein levels. The mechanism of this action is not understood, and the amide form is ineffective. Undesirable effects of large doses of nicotinic acid on the metabolism of the heart muscle have been observed. In human subjects, intravenously administered nicotinic acid caused the depletion of cardiac muscle glycogen and endogenous lipid because the use of free fatty acids from the blood as an energy source was inhibited.[63] In addition, Winter and Boyer have reported a case history in which large doses of nicotinamide (3 g to 9 g) taken in the treatment of schizophrenia caused liver toxicity. Consequently this vitamin is not an innocuous therapeutic agent.[64]

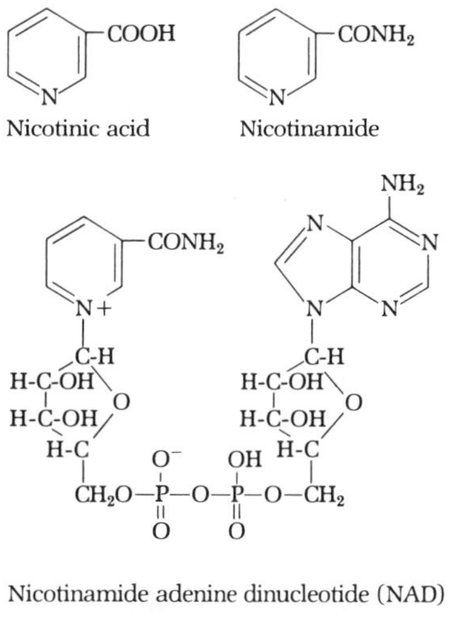

Nicotinic acid     Nicotinamide

Nicotinamide adenine dinucleotide (NAD)

**Fig. 8-8.** Structural formulas of niacin and one of its coenzyme forms.

## Relationship of tryptophan to niacin

The amino acid tryptophan can be converted to niacin in the body. Research studies have indicated that approximately 60 mg of tryptophan are equivalent to 1 mg of niacin. Animal and vegetable proteins contain about 1.4% and 1% of tryptophan, respectively. Table 8-2 illustrates how an approximate amount of niacin can be calculated from protein. Total niacin equals the preformed niacin plus the niacin available from protein. The accepted ratio of 60:1 is not applicable under a variety of conditions. The conversion is less efficient on very low intakes of niacin and tryptophan[65] and is increased during pregnancy[66,67] and in the users of oral contraceptive agents.[67] Estrogen apparently raises the level of corticosteroids, which, in turn, stimulates tryptophan oxygenase, the first enzyme in the pathway.[67] Earlier suggestions that amino acid imbalance caused by high intake of leucine impairs the utilization of dietary tryptophan as a source of niacin[68] were not confirmed in a metabolic study in adult men.[69]

## Utilization of niacin

Little is known about the bioavailability of niacin from foods and the intraluminal factors that might affect its absorption. The mechanism for the transport of niacin across the intestinal mucosa has not been established in humans. In the rat, both the acid and amide forms of niacin are absorbed by sodium-mediated facilitated diffusion at low concentrations and by passive diffusion at high concentrations.[70] Some nicotinic acid is converted to nicotinamide during passage through the mucosa. Neither form is transported against a concentration gradient.[70,71]

Only nicotinic acid and nicotinamide can pass in and out of the cells of the body tissues; each cell is capable of synthesizing the coenzymes for its own use. Catabolism of tryptophan produces quinolinic acid which is then converted to NAD without formation of free nicotinamide. Nicotinamide released from the breakdown of NAD can be reused within the cell or returned to the circulation and utilized where needed.[72] However, an appreciable amount of nicotinamide is metabolized to $N^1$-methylnicotinamide and 2-pyridone ($N^1$-methyl-2-pyridone-5-carboxamine), which are the two major metabolites of niacin excreted in the urine. Some niacin is also excreted, but the amount is not influenced by the intake or tissue reserves, whereas the excretion levels of the two metabolites reflect the body's niacin status and the adequacy of niacin intake. Although the urinary excretion of $N^1$-methylnicotinamide has been used most widely in the nutrition status surveys, the ratio of 2-pyridone to $N^1$-methylnicotinamide is currently considered the best available measure of niacin nutriture. On low intake the excretion of 2-pyridone declines faster than $N^1$-methylnicotinamide and is undetectable by the time clinical symptoms of niacin deficiency appear. The level of $N^1$-methylnicotinamide declines more gradually, reaching a minimum at about the time when clinical signs become evident.[73]

## Human requirement

Early studies indicated that 4.4 niacin equivalents per 1000 kcal per day were adequate to prevent pellagra in adult men. To provide a margin of safety, both the Food and Nutrition Board[30] and the Joint FAO/WHO Expert Committee[49] have established the recommended dietary allowance for niacin at 6.6 mg per 1000 kcal for all age groups. Depending on calorie intake, the 1980 NRC-RDA for adult men is from 16 mg to 19 mg niacin equivalent (NE) daily and for adult women 13 mg to 14 mg NE daily. An increase of 2 mg and 5 mg, respectively, above the allowance for the nonpregnant women is recommended during pregnancy and lactation by the Food and Nutrition Board. Infants and children follow the same recommendations as adults.

NE is equal to 1 mg of niacin or 60 mg of dietary tryptophan.

## Food sources

In general, meat, poultry, and fish are better sources of niacin than plant products, as emphasized in Figure 8-9, showing average servings. The use of meat drippings is recommended, because niacin in easily dissolved out of foods in cooking. Whole grain and enriched products also make a contribution. A bound form of niacin, that is, niacytin, in wheat, corn, and rye bran is practically unavailable to humans,[74] unless released by the method of preparation, for example, lime-treated corn. Fruits and vegetables (other than mushrooms and legumes) are insignificant sources of niacin. Milk and eggs are poor sources of preformed niacin but good sources of its precursor, tryptophan. The average American diet is estimated to contain 8 mg to 17 mg niacin and 500 mg to 1000 mg or more of tryptophan, with a total of 16 mg to 34 mg of niacin equivalents.

## Table 8-2. Approximate Calculation of Niacin from Tryptophan

| | |
|---|---|
| Dietary protein | 60 g |
| Tryptophan content 1% (approx.) | 0.01 |
| Tryptophan | 0.60 g or 600 mg |
| 60 mg of tryptophan = 1 mg of niacin | $600 \div 60 = 10$ |
| Niacin converted from tryptophan | 10 mg |

## Vitamin $B_6$

Pyridoxine was identified in 1938 as a separate fraction of the B complex. Subsequently, vitamin $B_6$ proved to be a complex of three closely related chemical compounds—*pyridoxine* (PN), *pyridoxal* (PL), and *pyridoxamine* (PM) (Fig. 8-10)—all of which are active physiolog-

## Amounts of Niacin in Average Servings

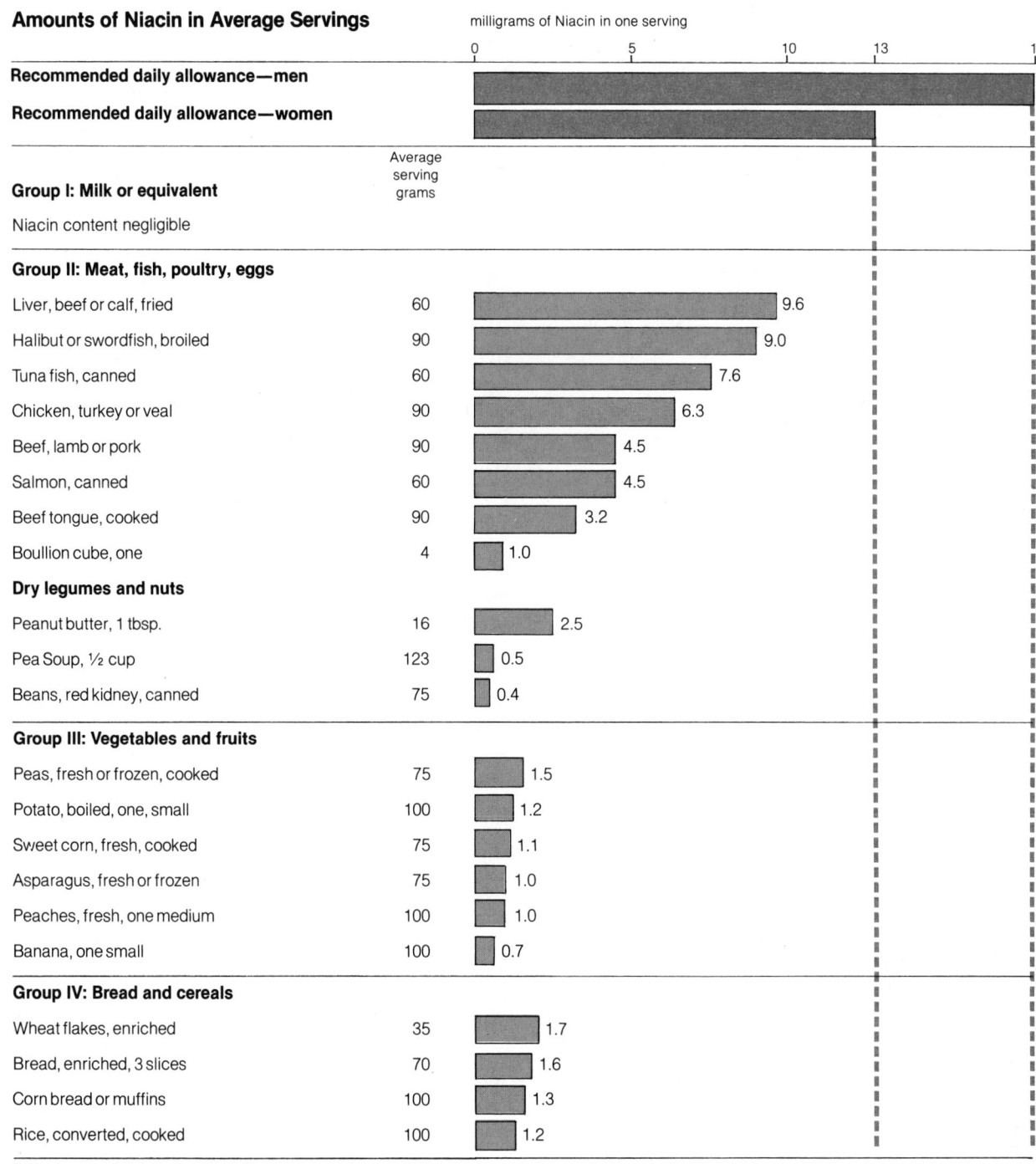

milligrams of Niacin in one serving

| | Average serving grams | mg Niacin |
|---|---|---|
| **Recommended daily allowance—men** | | 18 |
| **Recommended daily allowance—women** | | 13 |
| **Group I: Milk or equivalent** | | |
| Niacin content negligible | | |
| **Group II: Meat, fish, poultry, eggs** | | |
| Liver, beef or calf, fried | 60 | 9.6 |
| Halibut or swordfish, broiled | 90 | 9.0 |
| Tuna fish, canned | 60 | 7.6 |
| Chicken, turkey or veal | 90 | 6.3 |
| Beef, lamb or pork | 90 | 4.5 |
| Salmon, canned | 60 | 4.5 |
| Beef tongue, cooked | 90 | 3.2 |
| Boullion cube, one | 4 | 1.0 |
| **Dry legumes and nuts** | | |
| Peanut butter, 1 tbsp. | 16 | 2.5 |
| Pea Soup, ½ cup | 123 | 0.5 |
| Beans, red kidney, canned | 75 | 0.4 |
| **Group III: Vegetables and fruits** | | |
| Peas, fresh or frozen, cooked | 75 | 1.5 |
| Potato, boiled, one, small | 100 | 1.2 |
| Sweet corn, fresh, cooked | 75 | 1.1 |
| Asparagus, fresh or frozen | 75 | 1.0 |
| Peaches, fresh, one medium | 100 | 1.0 |
| Banana, one small | 100 | 0.7 |
| **Group IV: Bread and cereals** | | |
| Wheat flakes, enriched | 35 | 1.7 |
| Bread, enriched, 3 slices | 70 | 1.6 |
| Corn bread or muffins | 100 | 1.3 |
| Rice, converted, cooked | 100 | 1.2 |

**Note:** Average diet contains enough tryptophan to increase the niacin value about a third.

**Fig. 8-9.**  Niacin in average servings of foods classified according to the four food groups.

ically. The need for this factor was first demonstrated in rats, but it is now established that it is required by most animals. A deficiency is associated with a peculiar type of anemia in some species and extreme muscular weakness, dermatitis, and nervous disorders in others. Vitamin $B_6$ can be synthesized by intestinal organisms in the rat, but whether or not this is true in humans has not been established.

The need for and the function of vitamin $B_6$ in humans has been demonstrated conclusively in both adults and infants. The accidental destruction of this factor in a canned-milk formula resulted in the occurrence of ner-

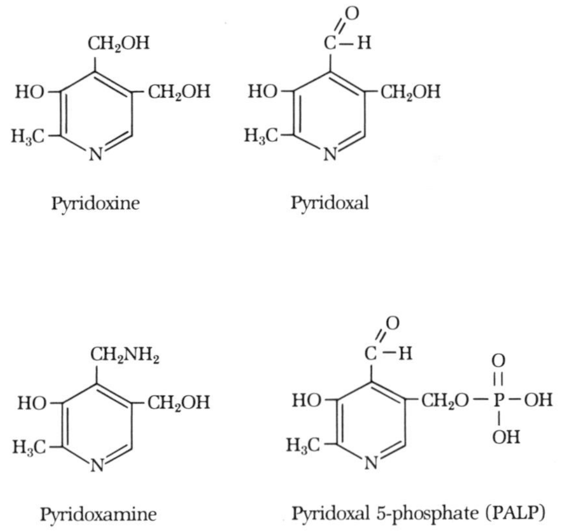

**Fig. 8-10.** Structural formulas of B$_6$-vitamers and pyridoxal phosphate (PALP).

vous irritability and convulsive seizures in young infants.[75] Rapid recovery followed injection of the vitamin, proving conclusively that the symptoms noted were the result of a deficiency.

### Functions of vitamin B$_6$

The metabolic significance of the B$_6$ vitamers depends on their conversion to pyridoxal-5-phosphate (PALP), which functions as a coenzyme in numerous biochemical reactions, most of which in some way involve amino acids. PALP-dependent *aminotransferases* (transaminases) carry the amino group (NH$_2$) from one amino

### Table 8-3. Inherited Conditions of Vitamin B$_6$ Dependency

| Condition | Metabolic Defect |
|---|---|
| Convulsive seizures in infants | Reduced synthesis of γ-amino butyric acid (GABA) due to abnormal glutamic acid decarboxylase |
| Vitamin B$_6$-responsive chronic anemia | Impaired synthesis of heme due to reduced formation of its δ-amino-levulinic acid precursor |
| Xanthurenic aciduria | Decreased conversion of hydroxy-kynurenine to hydroxyanthranilic acid due to low activity of kynureninase (in tryptophan metabolism) |
| Cystathioninuria | Decreased cleavage of cystathionine to cysteine and homoserine due to deficiency of cystathionase (in methionine metabolism) |
| Homocystinuria | Impaired conversion of homocysteine and serine to cystathionine due to absence of or defect in the enzyme cystathione synthetase (in methionine metabolism) |

acid to an acceptor keto acid to produce a different amino and keto acid, in a process called *transamination* (see Chap. 9). Transamination is the first step in the utilization of most amino acids for energy, and also in the synthesis of nonessential amino acids. Aminotransferases are mostly cellular enzymes, but small amounts of some are normally present in the blood serum. Elevation in serum aminotransferase activity is associated with recent tissue damage. Aspartate aminotransferase (also known as serum glutamate oxaloacetate transaminase or SGOT) is especially active in the cardiac muscle. Its activity in serum rises sharply following myocardial infarction and is widely used as a diagnostic test to confirm infarction. In liver damage, elevation of serum alanine aminotransferase (serum glutamate pyruvate transaminase or SGPT) generally is more pronounced than that of SGOT. Both of these aminotransferases are found in the blood cells, and their activity in the erythrocytes has been employed as a measure of vitamin B$_6$ status, especially in metabolic research.

PALP-containing enzymes are also involved in *decarboxylation* and *transulfuration* (removal of CO$_2$ and H$_2$S groups) of amino acids. Chemical changes in the central nervous system, that is, formation of *serotonin* from tryptophan and gamma aminobutyric acid (GABA) from glutamic acid, require vitamin B$_6$-dependent decarboxylases, as does formation of *norepinephrine* from tyrosine (through dopa and dopamine).[76] Several PALP-dependent enzymes are involved in the metabolic pathways of sulfur-containing amino acids, which result in the conversion of methionine to cysteine and cysteine to taurine. Two of these enzymes are affected in genetic B$_6$-dependency syndromes in which defective enzyme proteins are unable to function with physiologic levels of PALP; however, they respond to pharmacologic doses of the vitamin, varying from 10 mg to 1000 mg, in contrast to a normal requirement of approximately 2 mg.[77] Table 8-3 lists the most common B$_6$-dependency syndromes and the specific enzymes involved.[44]

Several other reactions in the metabolism of tryptophan require PALP, including its conversion to niacin (NAD). In B$_6$ deficiency, formation of niacin is reduced, and more tryptophan is metabolized by alternate pathways, which are normally insignificant. If a large dose of tryptophan (tryptophan load test) is administered to a person with a vitamin B$_6$ deficiency, various intermediate and alternate products—including xanthurenic acid—accumulate in the urine. Excretion of xanthurenic acid after a tryptophan load is, therefore, an indirect measure of vitamin B$_6$ status, which is used for clinical and research purposes.

Vitamin B$_6$ is required also for the formation of delta-amino-levulinic acid in the synthesis of heme and in the metabolism of folic acid.[78] A significant fraction of vitamin B$_6$ in tissues, especially the liver and muscle, is found in phosphorylase, the enzyme that initiates the mobilization of glycogen stores by formation of glucose-1-phosphate. Presence of PALP appears to be essential for the activity of the enzyme, but its exact catalytic function in the reaction is not known. Because administration of excess vitamin $B_6$ increases the level of phosphorylase parallel to the increase in tissue $B_6$ retention, phosphorylase, in turn, may serve as a tissue reservoir of vitamin $B_6$.[79] Recent research[80] indicates that PALP also may serve as a modulator of steroid hormone action by reacting with the activated hormone-receptor complex to inhibit its binding to DNA and cell nuclei.

Cellular uptake of amino acids is impaired in vitamin $B_6$ deficiency. Results from recent studies suggest that the defect in amino acid transport is related to the reduced levels of growth hormone and, perhaps, insulin, instead of the direct effect by the lack of vitamin $B_6$.[81] The mechanism by which vitamin $B_6$ influences the secretion of these hormones is not known.

Several drugs act as vitamin $B_6$ antagonists. These include isoniazid and cycloserine, which may be used in tuberculosis therapy, and penicillamine, which is used as a copper-chelator in Wilson's disease (see Chap. 33). Desoxypyridoxine has been used in the production of experimental vitamin $B_6$ deficiency.[78]

Inadequate intake of vitamin $B_6$ by infants may result in growth retardation or weight loss, vomiting and abdominal stress, hyperirritability, convulsive seizures, and anemia.[82] Vitamin $B_6$ deficiency in adults may cause personality changes, such as depression and confusion, abnormal changes in electroencephalograms, convulsions, seborrheic dermatitis, and oral lesions resembling those caused by riboflavin and niacin deficiency.[83] Biochemical alterations usually precede the clinical manifestations.

### Utilization of vitamin $B_6$

Several studies have indicated that the intestinal absorption of the three $B_6$-vitamers is equally efficient and takes place by passive diffusion over a wide range of luminal concentrations.[84,85] A recent human study suggests, however, that the absorption of PM is either slower than that of PL or PN, or it is metabolized differently from PL or PN, or both.[93] The phosphorylated forms are hydrolyzed prior to absorption; however, some may be absorbed intact.[87,88] Even though the free vitamers are phosphorylated in the mucosal cell, the rate of phosphorylation apparently does not affect the rate of transport of the vitamin from the lumen to the serosa.[84,88] Despite an increased mucosal activity of pyridoxal kinase in children with acute celiac disease,[89] the net absorption of vitamin $B_6$ is reduced.[90] The availability of vitamin $B_6$ from foods is highly variable; little is known about the possible influence on the absorption of vitamin $B_6$ by other food components. The effects on bioavailability of vitamin $B_6$ by food processing and storage also vary and probably depend on the composition of food and the conditions of processing and storage.[85]

Cellular uptake of vitamin $B_6$ in tissues occurs most rapidly as the free vitamers, but each form can be phosphorylated by the cell. The phosphorylated forms of pyridoxine (PNP) and pyridoxamine (PMP) can be converted to PALP to provide the cells with the active coenzyme form of the vitamin. Although PMP can activate some enzymes, most depend on PALP.[91]

Both the free bases and the phosphorylated forms of pyridoxal and pyridoxamine are found in the blood, but no pyridoxine or its phosphate have been detected.[91] The plasma and erythrocyte levels of pyridoxal and PALP are influenced by dietary intake of the vitamin and have been used in research studies to assess the nutritional status and requirements of vitamin $B_6$.

Vitamin $B_6$ is excreted in the urine in the form of free and phosphorylated vitamers and as 4-pyridoxic acid, the major metabolite of the vitamin. The excretion levels of total vitamin $B_6$ and 4-pyridoxic acid reflect the adequacy of intake and provide another means of assessing vitamin $B_6$ nutriture.

### Human requirements

Studies have shown that the human requirement of vitamin $B_6$ for adults is related to the level of protein intake and is amply satisfied at the level of 0.02 mg per gram of protein.[92,93] On this basis the Food and Nutrition Board[30] set the recommended dietary allowances for adults at 2.0 mg per day for women and 2.2 mg per day for men. These levels would permit protein intakes of 100 g by women and 110 g by men. The vitamin $B_6$ requirement is high in pregnancy, due to the increased need of protein, increased catabolism of tryptophan as a result of hormonal influence, and the active transport of the vitamin to fetal blood by the placenta. Thus an allowance of 2.6 mg per day is recommended during pregnancy; the allowance for lactating women is 2.5 mg. A complete list of the recommended dietary allowances for each age and sex group is given in Chapter 11.

Although the vitamin $B_6$ requirement of some but not all users of oral contraceptive agents may be slightly higher than that of nonusers,[94] the Food and Nutrition Board concluded that current evidence does not justify routine supplementation by all users. Biochemical evidence of marginal vitamin $B_6$ status has been observed in the elderly[95] and in chronic alcoholics,[96] but whether these groups have a higher vitamin $B_6$ requirement than the rest of the population has not been established.

### Food sources

Of the animal foods, pork and the glandular meats are the richest, with lamb and veal relatively better than fish or beef muscle. Considerable losses of vitamin $B_6$ occur during cooking. Milk and eggs are only fair sources.

Of the plant foods, legumes, potatoes, oatmeal, wheat germ, and bananas are the richest, with cabbages, carrots, and other vegetables providing fair amounts. Current information on the vitamin $B_6$ content of foods and on its bioavailability is limited.

## Folacin (folic acid)

Folic acid was recognized as a dietary essential for chicks in 1938 and was later shown to be a requirement of other animals. It was first used clinically in 1945 by Spies, who showed it to be effective in the treatment of macrocytic anemias of pregnancy and tropical sprue, and these findings have since been confirmed.

Folic acid (pteroylglutamic acid, PGA) is not found as such in foods or in the human body, but it is converted to the active forms by the body. It is the parent compound that is common in the structure of the different forms that perform the metabolic functions of folacin (Fig. 8-11). Folacin occurs in foods chiefly as one of the polyglutamate derivatives of tetrahydrofolic acid (THFA), methyl tetrahydrofolic acid ($N^5$ methyl THFA).

## Functions

The major role of the enzymatically active forms of folacin is in the transfer of 1-carbon unit to various compounds in the synthesis of the purines and pyrimidines of DNA and RNA, and in amino acid interconversions.[97]

Some of the folacin-requiring reactions use THFA, which serves as an *acceptor* of a 1-carbon unit from the substrate (as in the conversion of serine to glycine). The resulting THFA derivatives then serve as *donors* of 1-carbon units in other reactions, such as the synthesis of the nucleotide thymidylate ($N^{5,10}$-methylene THFA), which is part of the DNA structure. Similarly, $N^{5,10}$-methenyl THFA and $N^{10}$-formyl THFA contribute a carbon to the ring structure of purine bases.

The amino acid, histidine, requires THFA for its complete utilization. When it is not available, the intermediary product, formiminoglutamic acid (FIGLU), is excreted in the urine. FIGLU excretion levels can then be used to determine folacin nutritional status. However, increased excretion of FIGLU is only an indirect, nonspecific indication of a possible folacin deficiency.

Because the major function of folacin is in DNA and RNA synthesis and indirectly affects protein synthesis, the manifestations of folacin deficiency are most pronounced in rapidly growing tissues or in tissues with rapid cell turnover. Folacin deficiency in humans results in megaloblastic anemia, glossitis, and gastrointestinal disturbances. Because of the interdependence of vitamins $B_{12}$,

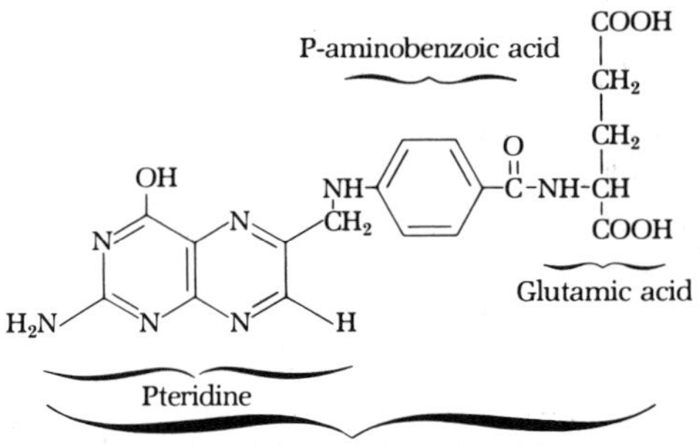

Folic acid (Pteroylglutamic acid)

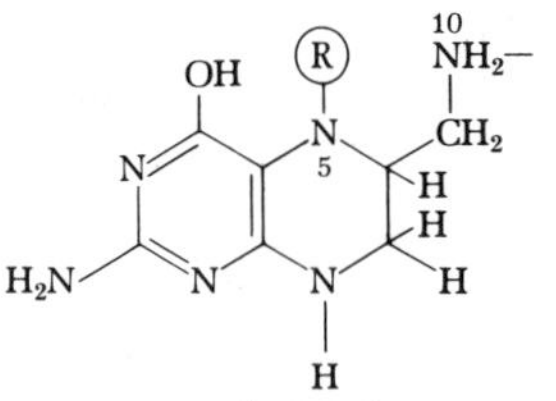

| R-group | Name of Compound |
|---------|------------------|
| -H | Tetrahydrofolic acid (THFA) |
| -CHO | $N^5$-formyl-THFA |
| -CH = NH | $N^5$-formimino-THFA |
| >$CH_2$ | $N^{5,10}$-methylene-THFA |
| -$CH_3$ | $N^5$-methyl-THFA |

Tetrahydro form

**Fig. 8-11.** Compounds with folacin (folate) activity. Folic acid is the stable oxidized form usually present in pharmaceutical preparations; it is reduced in the body, first to dihydro- and then to tetrahydro form (THFA). THFA is an active coenzyme and a precursor of the other coenzyme forms, some of which are shown. Each coenzyme represents an addition of a one-carbon unit in place of hydrogen in the $N^5$ position of THFA, or links $N^5$ and $N^{10}$.

$B_6$, ascorbic acid, and folacin, the anemia found in these deficiency diseases may be similar and may respond to treatment with one or several of these nutrients. It should be pointed out, however, that even though the anemia in pernicious anemia may be relieved by folic acid, only vitamin $B_{12}$ cures the neurologic symptoms.

## Utilization of folacin

Folates may be absorbed along the entire length of the small intestine; however, there is evidence that the jejunum is the primary site for absorption.

Much of the vitamin occurs in the diet in the form of polyglutamates. Before it can be absorbed, excess glutamates must be removed from the side chain of the molecule by folate conjugases found in intestinal mucosa. The activity of the brushborder conjugase appears to be critical in the hydrolysis of pteroylpolyglutamates.[98] Thus the absorption of food folates appears to be controlled by the conjugase activity, which may, in turn, be affected by conjugase inhibitors in food, for example, yeast. Zinc deficiency reduces the absorption of the polyglutamate but not the monoglutamate forms of folacin, suggesting a role in the conjugase activity.[99] The mucosal uptake of the monoglytamyl forms probably involves a specific carrier; inability to absorb folates is known as a genetic defect.[99] Folate uptake is stimulated by presence of glucose, but no energy requirement for the process has been established. The maximum cellular uptake also depends on a very narrow intraluminal $pH$, close to 6.0, and is decreased by both acidification and alkalinization of the intestinal contents. Intracellular metabolism results in the release of methyl THFA and some THFA to the serosal fluid.[99,100] Decreased mucosal uptake of pteroylmonoglutamate has been demonstrated in patients with untreated sprue.[98]

The chief form of folacin in plasma is methyl-THFA, which is loosely bound to proteins, mainly albumin, and serves as a source of folacin to bone marrow cells, reticulocytes, and other cells. Inside the cell it is either first demethylated to THFA, which can be converted to all active forms of folate, or it is directly used in polyglutamate synthesis by the pteroylpolyglutamate synthetase (PPS). Conversion to polyglutamate form is believed to be essential to the various coenzyme functions of folacin and probably also for tissue retention, although some of the cellular vitamin exists as monoglutamate. It is still uncertain whether the PPS can use methyl-THFA as a substrate or requires THFA or another specific form of folate as substrate for polyglutamate formation. Vitamin $B_{12}$ is known to be essential for the demethylation of $N^5$-methyl-THFA to THFA. It has been postulated that in vitamin $B_{12}$ deficiency, the active pool of THFA is reduced due to an inability to demethylate methyl-THFA. This, in turn, would result in secondary cellular deficiency of folacin due to trapping of the vitamin in the methylated form—known as the *methyl trap* theory of the folacin-$B_{12}$ interrelationship.[97] Whatever the mechanism, tissue folacin concentration (the polyglutamate form) is reduced in vitamin $B_{12}$ deficiency, but the serum folacin level is normal or elevated. In folate deficiency both erythrocyte and serum vitamin levels are reduced, whereas only the erythrocyte folacin is low in vitamin $B_{12}$ deficiency; this fact is used as part of the differential diagnosis in patients with megaloblastic anemia.

Serum and erythrocyte folate levels are used most frequently to assess folacin nutriture. Normal serum levels of folacin range from 7 to 16 nanograms (1 ng = $10^{-9}$ g) per ml of serum. A new test for clinical use has been introduced recently, known as the *deoxyuridine (dU) suppression test*.[101] It is based on the fact that with adequate folacin, synthesis of thymidylic acid takes place mainly by the $N^{5,10}$-methylene-THFA-dependent conversion of deoxyuridine monophosphate (dUMP) to thymidylic acid. With inadequate THFA, recycling of "salvaged" thymidine (from thymidylate degradation) by direct incorporation into thymidylate increases. This salvage pathway is inhibited by an ample supply of thymidylate formed from dUMP. In the test, the effect of added dU on the incorporation of radioactive thymidine into thymidylate and DNA by bone marrow or peripheral lymphocytes is measured *in vitro*. In cells from people with adequate folacin and vitamin $B_{12}$ status, the added dU is converted to thymidylate, thereby suppressing the direct incorporation of thymidine. Failure of dU to suppress thymidine incorporation indicates inadequacy of the active coenzyme. If the cause is folacin deficiency, incubation of the cells with folate but not with vitamin $B_{12}$ results in suppression. In $B_{12}$-deficient cells, partial response may be obtained with folate, but complete suppression is produced only when vitamin $B_{12}$ also is added. Studies of the test suggest that use of peripheral lymphocytes, which have a long life span, permits diagnosis even after the hematologic symptoms have been corrected, up to 2 to 3 months after therapy. The test may be especially useful in patients whose diagnosis of megaloblastic anemia is complicated by presence of iron deficiency.[101]

The liver appears to play a major role in the metabolism and excretion of folacin and may be responsible for the utilization of some forms of the vitamin. When folic acid (stable oxidized form found in pharmaceutical preparations) is administered orally, it is readily reduced to THFA then methylated in the mucosal cell. When administered intravenously, the same functions are performed by the liver, which rapidly removes folic acid from the circulation; intravenously administered methyl-THFA is removed by other tissues as well. Considerable amounts of THFA are secreted by the liver into the bile, as both methyl- and other derivatives. A significant portion is believed to be reabsorbed, thus participating in the enterohepatic circulation of folate. Normal enterohepatic circulation of folate appears to be essential for the maintenance of the serum folate level, which falls rapidly if the enterohepatic circulation is disturbed by cannulation of the bile duct.[102]

Ingestion of alcohol also is associated with a rapid fall in serum folate.[103] Recent research suggests that this may result from interference by ethanol with the transfer of nonmethyl folate to the bile by the liver, thereby altering the enterohepatic circulation of folate.[102,103] Reduced serum level, in turn, interferes with the delivery of folate to the bone marrow and other tissues. However, other effects of acute ingestion of alcohol may contribute to the folate deficiency commonly observed in alcoholics after binge drinking. These include reduced intake, malabsorption and, perhaps, creation of the "methyl trap" in the liver. Oxidation of ethanol increases the hepatic NADH:NAD ratio, which could result in increased reduction of $N^5N^{10}$-methylene-THFA to methyl-THFA by the NADH-dependent reductase.[103,104] In addition, chronic alcohol consumption appears to result in intestinal malabsorption and in decreased capacity by the liver to retain folates.[103]

Small amounts of folate also are excreted in the urine, mainly as methyl-THFA. Ascorbic acid is believed to be essential in maintaining an active pool of reduced folates in the body. A person with scurvy was found to excrete mostly $N^{10}$-formyl folic acid in the urine prior to treatment with ascorbic acid and $N^5$-methyl THFA after treatment.[105]

### Human requirement

The adult recommended dietary allowance for folacin is 400 mcg per day. Due to the increased needs of the fetus, the allowance for pregnancy was set at 800 mcg per day; 500 mcg is the RDA for lactation. The infant allowance is 35 mcg per day for the first 6 months and 45 mcg during the second half of the first year, at which time it is increased to 100 mcg per day until 4 years of age. The recommendation for folic acid from 4 to 6 years is 200 mcg per day; from 7 to 10 years it is 300 mcg per day. The adult recommendation (400 mcg) starts at 11 years of age and is continued throughout life for both sexes. Use of a folacin supplement is recommended during pregnancy to provide for the increased need.[30]

Folate deficiency has been reported in women using oral contraceptive agents. However, the incidence appears to be relatively low, considering the large number of women using these drugs.[106] Although several mechanisms have been implicated as causes of impaired folate utilization when oral contraceptive agents are used (see

Chap. 19, p. 338), the evidence for all of them remains equivocal. Similarly, increased folate requirement has not been conclusively demonstrated in persons treated with anticonvulsant drugs.[106] Patients receiving anticonvulsant therapy have significantly lower levels of folic acid in serum and cerebrospinal fluid than healthy people. Administration of folic acid to these patients causes the serum level of the anticonvulsant drug to fall.[107] In daily doses up to 15 mg, folic acid does not seem to interfere with the control of seizures, but it does have a convulsant effect at very high concentrations.[108] In addition to pregnancy, increased need for folate has been clearly demonstrated only in hemolytic anemias and alcohol intoxication.[106] The actual amount of folacin in foods that is available for absorption has not been well established (see Food Sources). Therefore, the NRC-RDA has included a large margin of safety for this nutrient.

Because more than 100 mcg of folic acid per day may prevent anemia but not cure the neurologic symptoms of pernicious anemia, vitamin preparations that contain more than 100 mcg of folic acid cannot be sold without prescription.

### Food sources

The presence of this group of factors in green leaves was the basis for the name folacin (*folium*, meaning *leaf*). In addition to their presence in green leaves, these factors are found in liver, meats and fish, nuts, legumes, and whole grains.

The availability of folacin from foodstuffs varies. In one study the percentage of folate absorbed ranged from 92% for frozen lima beans to 25% in lettuce. Only 31% of the folate in orange juice was absorbed compared to 82% from bananas. A mean availability of about 50% was found in a recent study of several common foods.[109]

Many of the folates in food are easily destroyed by storing, cooking, and other processing. Because of the destruction of folic acid activity in dried milk, it has been suggested that ascorbic acid be added as a preservative to the milk before processing.[110] The protective effect of ascorbic acid against folate destruction in cow's milk during boiling has been reported recently.[111] When pasteurized milk was boiled for 1 minute, two-thirds of total folate was destroyed; this was prevented by addition of 1 mg per milliliter of ascorbic acid. Evidence was presented to indicate that the lower blood folacin levels seen in infants who were fed cow's milk formulas compared to breast-fed infants are due to destruction of folate during formula preparation.

## Vitamin B₁₂

Pernicious anemia was a fatal disease until 1926 when Minot and Murphy demonstrated that treatment with large amounts of liver could reverse the symptoms and prevent recurrence. The cause of the disease was uncovered by Castle and co-workers who demonstrated in 1929 that normal gastric secretion contains an *intrinsic factor* (IF) that is essential for the absorption of the *antipernicious anemia principle* or *extrinsic factor* from liver and other animal products. Patients with pernicious anemia lack the gastric IF. The active substance in liver was isolated in 1948 simultaneously by two groups, one in England and the other in the United States. It was found to be identical to the extrinsic factor and the antipernicious anemia principle.

Hodgkin, the 1964 Nobel Prize winner in chemistry, and her co-workers delineated the structural formula of the vitamin (Fig. 8-12). The structure of vitamin $B_{12}$ was established as an extremely complex nitrogenous compound containing two major portions, the corrin nucleus (which includes cobalt) and the attached nucleotide. Active forms of this vitamin are cyanocobalamin (vitamin $B_{12}$), a stable form present in pharmaceutical preparations but not found naturally, hydroxocobalamin (vitamin $B_{12a}$), aquacobalamin (vitamin $B_{12b}$), and nitritocobalamin (vitamin $B_{12c}$) (Fig. 8-12). Cobalt, long known as a trace element essential for some animals, had never before been found in a natural organic compound.

The predominant forms of vitamin $B_{12}$ found in blood and other tissues are its two known coenzyme forms, 5'-deoxyadenosylcobalamin (adenosylcobalamin) and methylcobalamin, and hydroxocobalamin.[30]

Vitamin $B_{12}$ is remarkably potent. It has a biologic activity 11,000 times that of a standard liver concentrate formerly used in the treatment of pernicious anemia. Consequently, $B_{12}$ appears to be one of the most potent biologically active substances known. It has been administered therapeutically in doses from 6 to 150 mcg. Comparative results with folic acid in other types of anemia require doses from 20,000 to 50,000 mcg.

### Functions of vitamin $B_{12}$

Each of the vitamin $B_{12}$ coenzymes is known to participate in one major metabolic reaction. Methylcobalamin is required for the transmethylation of homocysteine to methionine. Methyl-THFA serves as a cosubstrate in the reaction by donating the methyl group to vitamin $B_{12}$, which then transfers it to homocysteine. Thus this reaction regenerates the cellular pool of THFA, as discussed earlier. This metabolic function makes vitamin $B_{12}$ essential for DNA synthesis, which requires an ade-

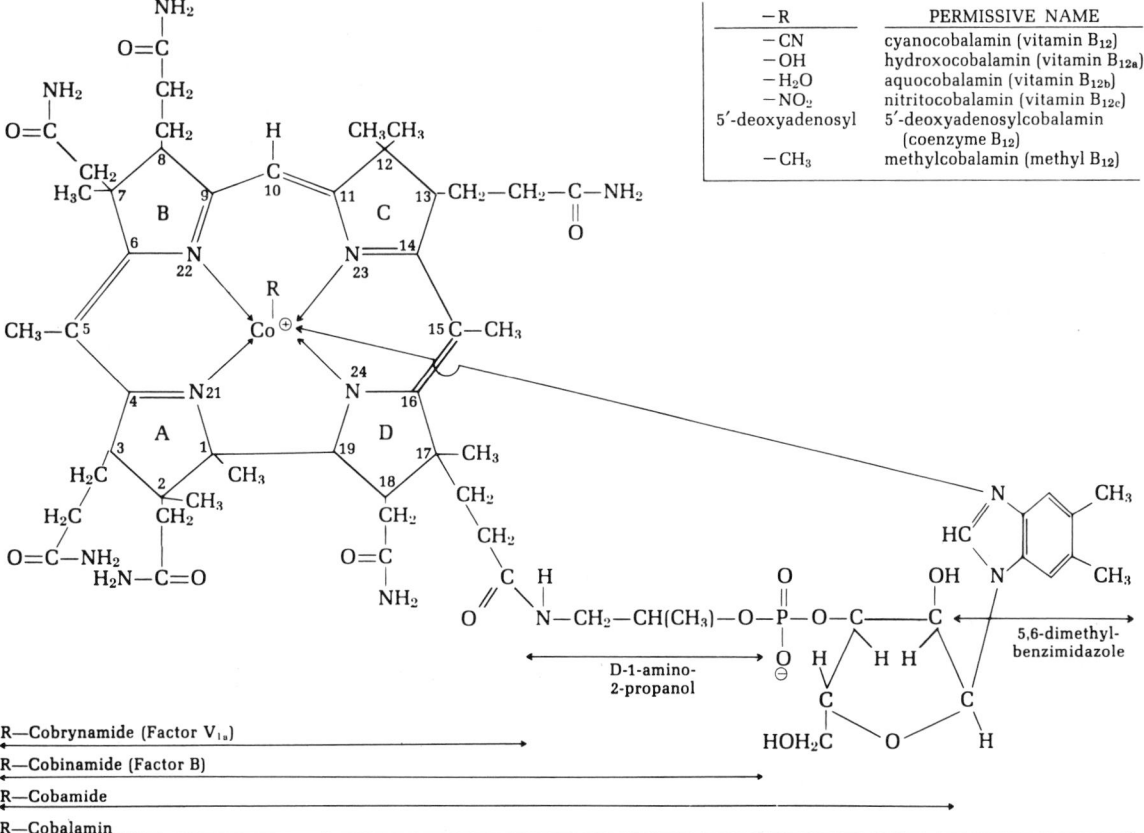

| —R | PERMISSIVE NAME |
|---|---|
| —CN | cyanocobalamin (vitamin $B_{12}$) |
| —OH | hydroxocobalamin (vitamin $B_{12a}$) |
| —$H_2O$ | aquocobalamin (vitamin $B_{12b}$) |
| —$NO_2$ | nitritocobalamin (vitamin $B_{12c}$) |
| 5'-deoxyadenosyl | 5'-deoxyadenosylcobalamin (coenzyme $B_{12}$) |
| —$CH_3$ | methylcobalamin (methyl $B_{12}$) |

**Fig. 8-12.** Structural formula of vitamin $B_{12}$ (cyanocobalamin). The numbering system for the corrin nucleus is made to correspond to that of the porphin nucleus by omitting the number 20. (Modified from Brown and Reynolds, Biogenesis of water-soluble vitamins. Ann Rev Biochem 32:419, 1963, by Herbert V: Folic acid and vitamin $B_{12}$. In Goodhart RS, Shils ME (eds): *Modern Nutrition in Health and Disease*, 5th ed. Philadelphia, Lea & Febiger, 1973)

quate supply of thymidylic acid. With inadequate regeneration of THFA in $B_{12}$ deficiency, $N^{5,10}$-methylene-THFA is not available for normal production of thymidylate and, as a result, DNA (Fig. 8-13). Cell duplication and differentiation are impaired, and megaloblastosis develops in tissues that depend on continuous cell duplication. Therefore, the hematologic manifestations of vitamin $B_{12}$-deficiency anemia are believed to be caused by secondary cellular deficiency of folate and can be relieved by relatively large doses of folate. However, treatment with vitamin $B_{12}$ is essential when $B_{12}$ deficiency is the primary cause of megaloblastic anemia because folacin cannot replace $B_{12}$ in either the homocysteine to methionine conversion, which also is important in the regulation of the methyl-transfer capacity of the cell, or in its other functions.

Vitamin $B_{12}$ deficiency is associated with impaired folacin transport and storage in the cells, resulting in reduced concentration of the polyglutamyl forms of folate. It has been suggested that both the release of methyl-THFA inside the cell and its use for pteroylpolyglutamate synthesis require its $B_{12}$-dependent demethylation.[97]

Adenosylcobalamin (also known as coenzyme $B_{12}$) is required for the conversion of methylmalonyl CoA to succinyl CoA by methylmalonyl-CoA-isomerase in a reaction that involves both isomerization and hydrogen transfer. This reaction is essential in the utilization of the carbon skeletons from the catabolism of amino acids, methionine and isoleucine (propionyl CoA), valine (methylmalonyl CoA), and of odd chain fatty acids (propionyl CoA). Oxidation of succinyl CoA in the citric acid cycle permits their complete oxidation to $CO_2$ (propionyl CoA $\rightarrow$ methylmalonyl CoA $\rightarrow$ succinyl CoA $\rightarrow$ CAC), thereby involving vitamin $B_{12}$ in intermediary metabolism.

Although the role of vitamin $B_{12}$ in the methylmalonate-succinate conversion has been linked to the function of this vitamin in the nervous system, the exact biochemi-cal defect that causes the neural damage in $B_{12}$ deficiency remains unknown. Myelin synthesis appears to be impaired, resulting in insidious degeneration of peripheral and central nervous systems, usually starting with the former.[108] The presence of high concentrations of odd carbon number straight and branched chain fatty acids ($C_{15}$ and $C_{17}$) and their increased synthesis from propionic acid has been demonstrated in nerve samples from pernicious anemia patients.[112]

Methylmalonic acid is barely detectable in the urine of healthy people, but it is excreted in large amounts in vitamin $B_{12}$ deficiency and by people with inherited methylmalonic aciduria. More than one mutation apparently can cause this condition, and only some respond to large doses of vitamin $B_{12}$. Defective synthesis of adenosylcobalamin is suspected to be the cause in the responsive cases. A combined homocystinuria and methylmalonic aciduria also exists and is believed to involve defective synthesis of both $B_{12}$ coenzymes.[44]

Utilization of other amino acids also may be altered in vitamin $B_{12}$ deficiency (reduced protein synthesis related to DNA levels), resulting in the elevation of several amino acids in blood and urine. Increased availability of tyrosine is suspected as a cause of hyperpigmentation (increased melanin synthesis from tyrosine) in some patients with pernicious anemia or folate deficiency. In pernicious anemia, decreased inhibition of tyrosinase by reduced levels of glutathione (GSH) may also contribute to the increased production of melanin.[113]

### Utilization of vitamin $B_{12}$

Because vitamin $B_{12}$ has the largest and, probably, the most complicated molecule of any of the water-soluble nutrients, it is not surprising that its deficiency is caused more frequently by problems of absorption than by dietary inadequacy. Of equal interest is the fact that its active absorption requires the presence in the gastric secretions of an even larger molecule, a glycoprotein called

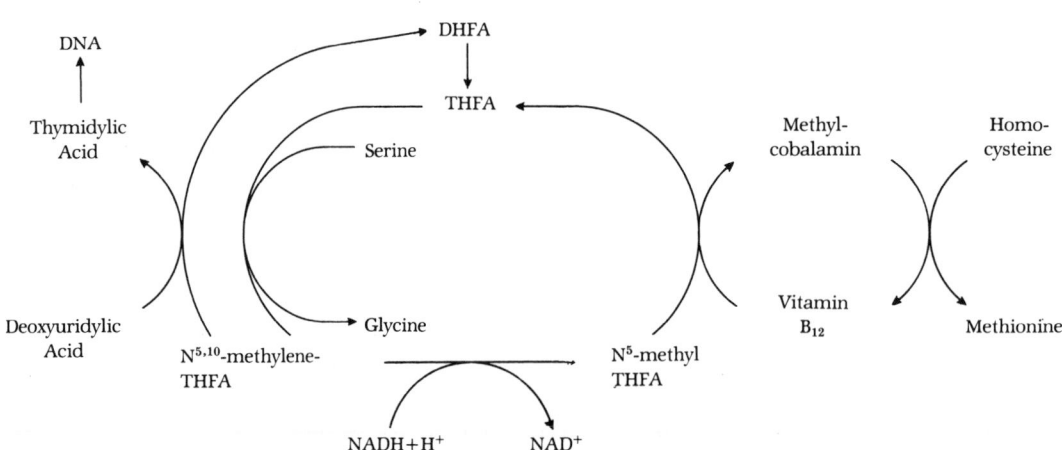

**Fig. 8-13.** A simplified scheme of the folacin and vitamin $B_{12}$ interrelationship.

*Castle's intrinsic factor* (IF), which is produced by the parietal cells of the gastric mucosa. The $B_{12}$-IF complex forms in the stomach and passes through the upper part of the small intestine to the ileum, where the IF attaches itself to the epithelial cells specific to this area of the gut and thereby facilitates the transfer of vitamin $B_{12}$ into the ileal epithelium. Calcium and luminal $p$H above 6 are also necessary for this transfer. Because the IF is not found in lymph or plasma, it is presumed to remain in the intestinal tract.[108]

The $B_{12}$-IF complex is stable against proteolytic degradation in the intestine, whereas gastric and intestinal hydrolysis of food proteins that bind $B_{12}$ is essential for its release before it forms a complex with the IF and thereby makes the vitamin available to the body.

Passive absorption by simple diffusion can account for a limited amount (1% to 3%) of absorption. This is inadequate from normal dietary intake of vitamin $B_{12}$, but in the absence of IF, permits the effective oral administration of large doses of vitamin $B_{12}$. However, intramuscular administration of the vitamin is the more common mode of treatment.

When cobalamin is released into the bloodstream, it is attached to another protein (transcobalamin II) and carried to the various tissues. Protein-bound vitamin $B_{12}$ not immediately needed is stored in the liver (mainly as adenosylcobalamin), which is capable of storing relatively large amounts of this nutrient. As the quantity of the vitamin increases in the diet, the percentage absorbed decreases.

The major form of vitamin $B_{12}$ in serum is methylcobalamin. Normal serum levels of vitamin $B_{12}$ range from 200 to 700 picograms (1 pg = $10^{-12}$ g) per ml.

In addition to transcobalamin II (TCII), at least two other serum proteins bind vitamin $B_{12}$, known as TCI and TCIII. Most of the total $B_{12}$-binding capacity is as TCII, which is believed to be the source of $B_{12}$ to the tissues. Cellular uptake of $B_{12}$ from TCII requires a receptor mechanism similar to the ileal uptake of the vitamin and is calcium and $p$H dependent. The functions of the other transcobalamins are not known; $B_{12}$ bound to TCI has a long turnover time and, therefore, has been suggested to represent a circulating storage form of the vitamin. Both TCI and TCII are glycoproteins and are also known as R-proteins or cobalophilins, whereas TCII contains only amino acids.[114]

The storage of vitamin $B_{12}$ in the liver, its enterohepatic circulation, and lack of significant catabolism in the body contribute to the efficient utilization of this vitamin in healthy people. Deficiency symptoms can take from 5 to 10 years to develop after total removal of the vitamin from the diet (for example, by adoption of a strict vegetarian diet). Some of the biliary vitamin is lost in the feces, and some is also excreted in the urine. The total excretion seems to be proportional to the total vitamin $B_{12}$ content of the body; as the result of low intake and tissue reserves, excretion is reduced. Consequently, a wide range of intakes can maintain adequate tissue levels of the vitamin to support normal function.[30]

### Human requirement

The Food and Nutrition Board recommends 3 mcg vitamin $B_{12}$ per day for adults. The allowance during pregnancy and lactation is 4 mcg per day (see Chap. 11 for a complete list of recommendations for each age and sex category).

The Joint FAO/WHO Expert Group recommends 2 mcg per day for the adult (over 10 years of age). This allowance is increased to 3 mcg for the pregnant woman and 2.5 mcg for the nursing mother.

Pernicious anemia patients who have been treated to replenish their stores can meet their body needs with 1 mcg to 1.5 mcg $B_{12}$ daily, given intramuscularly, or a larger dose given intramuscularly once a month.

### Food sources

In surveys of typical diets the remarkable difference between diets adequate and poor in the vitamin $B_{12}$ content emphasizes the importance of the contribution made by meats and other animal products to the $B_{12}$ intake. Dietary deficiencies of vitamin $B_{12}$ have been found among vegans when no animal foods are consumed.

A severe case of congenital vitamin $B_{12}$ deficiency has been reported recently in a breast-fed infant whose mother had adhered to a strict vegetarian diet for 8 years.[115]

Seafoods, meats, eggs, and dairy products are all good sources of vitamin $B_{12}$. Foods of vegetable origin do not contain vitamin $B_{12}$ unless it is added in enrichment. Contributions by bacterial contamination of food and water and, perhaps, by limited synthesis in the small intestine, may be responsible for the rarity of vitamin $B_{12}$ deficiency in vegetarians in developing countries.[116]

## Pantothenic acid

Pantothenic acid (Fig. 8-14) is another of the vitamin B complex group first recognized as a growth factor in yeast in 1933. After the complete synthesis of pantothenic acid was accomplished in 1940, it was found to be essential for rats, dogs, pigs, pigeons, and chicks. A deficiency has been reported to cause emaciation, loss of hair, gray-

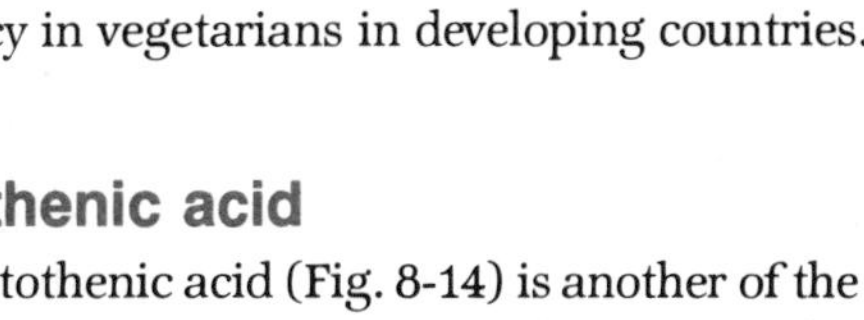

**Fig. 8-14.**  Structural formula of pantothenic acid.

ing of hair in dark animals, ulcers of the intestinal tract, and damage to several internal organs. Spontaneous deficiency of pantothenic acid in humans has not been reported. However, it was suspected of being one of the multiple deficiencies in the prisoners of World War II held in the Far East. They experienced a burning sensation on the soles of the feet—known as the *burning-feet syndrome*—which improved after pantothenic acid treatment in some but required other B-vitamins for complete reversal in others.

### Functions

Pantothenic acid is a part of coenzyme A (CoA), which plays a basic role in metabolism—in the release of energy from carbohydrates, fats, and proteins, and also in the synthesis of fatty acids, sterols, and steroid hormones (see Chap. 9). Acetyl CoA or *active acetate* is formed in the oxidative decarboxylation of pyruvic acid, $\beta$-oxidation of fatty acids, and degradation of some amino acids. It can then be oxidized completely in the citric acid cycle, or it can transfer the acetyl-group to various acceptors in the synthesis of the substances mentioned above. Pantothenic acid is also essential for the formation of porphyrin (for heme synthesis) and acetylcholine (a neurotransmitter) and in the acetylation of certain drugs before excretion (sulfonamides). Other important thioesters of CoA that participate in the intermediary metabolism include succinyl CoA, propionyl CoA, and malonyl CoA. Coenzyme A also acts as a carrier of acyl groups that are intermediates in fatty acid oxidation and in the incorporation of fatty acids to triglycerides and other lipids.

In addition to CoA, pantothenic acid is found in the 4′-phosphopantetheine of the acyl carrier protein (ACP), which serves as a cofactor in fatty acid synthesis by the fatty acid synthetase complex. Acyl carrier protein binds the growing acyl group during the stepwise addition of 2-carbon units.

In contrast to other vitamins, pantothenic acid does not constitute the functional part of CoA or ACP; the sulfhydryl group of pantetheine participates in the thioester formation with the organic acid substrates.

Pantothenic acid deficiency has been produced experimentally in humans either by a combination of deficient diet and an antagonist,[117] omega methyl pantothenic acid, or by feeding a semisynthetic diet almost free of pantothenic acid.[118] Similar symptoms were reported in both studies, including vomiting and general malaise, abdominal soreness and cramps, weakness and cramping of the legs, tenderness in the heels, and insomnia.

In a recent study[119] of patients with ulcerative or granulomatous colitis, a markedly reduced coenzyme A activity was observed in the colonal mucosa. Impaired synthesis of CoA was suggested because the total con-centration of pantothenic acid in affected mucosa was normal. Whether this biochemical defect is the result of or a causative factor in the disease is not known.

### Human requirement

A definite dietary requirement for pantothenic acid has not been established. In a survey by Chung and co-workers,[120] it was found that the pantothenic acid content of high-cost diets averaged 16.3 mg per day and for the poorest diets, 6.0 mg per day. These workers estimated that the average American diet provides from 10 mg to 20 mg per day. However, more recent studies suggest that the actual intakes may be considerably lower. In a group of teenage girls, some of whom were pregnant or postpartum, the estimated daily intake ranged from 1.1 mg to 7.2 mg.[121] The Food and Nutrition Board recommends from 4 mg to 7 mg as safe and adequate daily intakes for adults.[30] See Table 11-3 in Chapter 11 for the recommendations for other age groups.

### Food sources

The word *pantothenic*, meaning widespread, indicates that the distribution of this vitamin is extensive. Walsh and co-workers[122] determined the pantothenic acid content of 75 processed and cooked foods. Of them, about one-third contained 2 mg or more per 1000 kcal. This group included chicken, beef, liverwurst, potatoes, oat cereals, tomato products, and whole grain cereals. About one-half of the pantothenic acid is lost in the milling of grains, which constitute an important, if not a rich, source of this factor in the average diet. Fruits are relatively poor sources of this vitamin.

## Biotin

Biotin (Fig. 8-15), another member of the vitamin B complex, was first isolated in 1936 as a growth essential for yeast cells. Previous to this date many workers had described factors called by various names but having similar antidermatitis properties in experimental animals. These several factors proved to be identical and are now known as biotin. Investigations have shown that a biotin deficiency can be produced in rats, rabbits, and monkeys by feeding them a substance called *avidin* found in raw egg white. Avidin is known as an antivitamin because it binds biotin, making it unavailable for absorption. A few cases of biotin deficiency have been recognized in humans when their diets have included large amounts of raw egg white. A biotin-responsive seborrheic dermatitis develops in some infants, usually during the first 6 months of life.[123]

Intestinal microorganisms can synthesize biotin, but the extent to which this biotin is available to humans remains uncertain.

## Functions of biotin

Unlike other B-vitamins, biotin itself functions as a coenzyme and is covalently bound to the enzyme proteins.

Biotin plays an essential role as a coenzyme in $CO_2$ *fixation;* fatty acid synthesis, for instance, requires a biotin-containing enzyme, acetyl-CoA carboxylase, to form malonyl coenzyme A from acetyl coenzyme A.

There are several other biotin-dependent carboxylases that are important in human metabolism. Pyruvate carboxylase converts pyruvate to oxaloacetate (OAA), a critical reaction in gluconeogenesis. Production of OAA also permits continuous feeding of acetyl CoA into the citric acid cycle and, when not needed for energy production, the citrate formed from OAA and acetyl CoA transfers the two carbons of acetyl CoA to the cytosol for fatty acid synthesis (acetyl CoA cannot penetrate the mitochondrial membrane and is regenerated from citrate in the cytosol). Propionyl CoA from the catabolism of methionine, isoleucine, and odd chain fatty acids must first be converted to methylmalonyl CoA by methylmalonyl CoA carboxylase before it is further utilized in the citric acid cycle, by means of succinyl CoA. Similarly, $\beta$-methylcrotonyl CoA carboxylase is essential in the catabolism of leucine.

Biotin deficiency in animals is associated with a number of metabolic alterations that cannot be directly attributed to its known enzymatic functions.[124] Protein synthesis is reduced and appears to reflect the effect on the formation of soluble RNA. Both fasting hypoglycemia and impaired glucose tolerance have been observed in the rat. Hypercholesterolemia has been associated with biotin deficiency in humans.[125] Metabolic interrelationships of biotin with vitamin $B_{12}$, folacin, and ascorbic acid have been reported but require further elucidation.[126]

Biotin deficiency results in lassitude, anorexia, depression, malaise, muscle pain, nausea, anemia, hypercholesterolemia, and changes in the electrocardiogram. Biotin-responsive genetic conditions, which involve one or several defective carboxylase(s), have been identified in recent years.[123,127]

## Human requirement and food sources

Because the combined urinary and fecal losses of biotin usually exceed the daily intake, much of the fecal biotin is assumed to be of microbial origin. The obligatory urinary loss has been estimated to be less than 50 mcg per day; excretion increases at higher levels of intake. As the contribution by the intestinal synthesis is unknown, and the availability of biotin from foods is highly variable, no recommended allowance has been established. However, estimates of daily intakes suggest that 100 mcg is more than adequate for adults; thus the Food and Nutrition Board recommends a daily intake of 100 mcg to 200 mcg as safe and adequate. Recommendations for infants and children are estimated on the basis of 50 mcg per 1000 kcal.

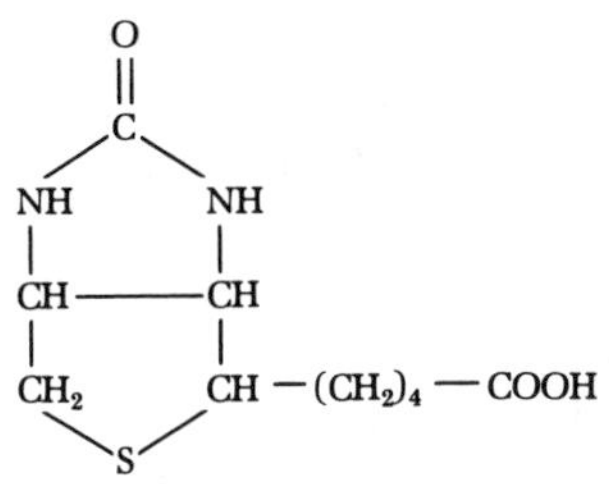

**Fig. 8-15.** Structural formula of biotin.

Few foods have been analyzed for this factor. It is abundant in liver and other organs, in mushrooms, and in peanuts. Lesser amounts occur in milk, eggs, and certain vegetables and fruits.

## Other food factors

### Para-aminobenzoic acid

Para-aminobenzoic acid (PABA) is a moiety of pteroylmonoglutamic acid (PGA), one of the forms of folic acid, and is no longer considered a vitamin.

### Inositol

Inositol was first considered to be a vitamin in 1940, but there is no evidence today that humans cannot synthesize all that is needed by the body.

### Choline

The classification of this nitrogenous compound as a vitamin is questioned by some. It is a structural component of body cells rather than a catalyst. It also is a precursor of the neurotransmitter, acetylcholine. Choline occurs in foods as well as in the body in relatively large amounts and has never been associated with a deficiency disease in humans. The body can make choline from methionine, an amino acid, with the aid of vitamin $B_{12}$ and folacin. The action of choline, betaine or methionine in the prevention of so-called fatty livers is known as *lipotropic* (fat moving); all three compounds serve as methyl-group donors in the body. Choline is distributed widely in plant and animal tissues, and a deficiency is not likely in the average diet.

### Carnitine

Carnitine is another nitrogenous compound found in tissues and foods which, like choline, has a definite biologic function in the body. Carnitine appears to accept the acyl-groups of long chain fatty acids from acyl CoA and (as acyl carnitine) translocates them through the mitochondrial membranes to the matrix where they can be oxidized. Carnitine is not considered a vitamin, because it can be synthesized in the body and therefore no dietary requirement for it exists. The possible role of carnitine in various disorders of lipid metabolism is under investigation.

### Bioflavonoids

Bioflavonoids are a group of widely distributed phenolic compounds that exhibit some biologic activity in higher animals. They appear to have both antioxidant and metal-chelating properties. However, there is no evidence that they have any biologic function in the body and have not been shown to be required by any species. Therefore, they are not vitamins despite being designated as *vitamin P* in the older literature.

## Vitamins in dietary pattern for one day

The contribution made by the dietary pattern (see Table 8-4) to the five vitamins for which we have specific recommendations and appropriate food composition tables is given in the accompanying table. Since the dietary pattern provides only 1400 calories, the foods chosen to supplement this provide additional vitamins to bring the totals up to recommended allowances.

## Antivitamins or vitamin antagonists

Research in the chemical structure of vitamins has led logically to more understanding about their characteristic reactions. Some are destroyed by oxidation or light

### Table 8-4. Vitamins in Dietary Pattern for 1 Day

| Food Group | Amount In g | Household Measure | Energy kcal | Vitamin A IU | Thiamin mg | Riboflavin mg | Niacin mg | Ascorbic Acid mg |
|---|---|---|---|---|---|---|---|---|
| Milk or equivalent | 488 | 2 c | 320 | 700 | 0.16 | 0.84 | 0.3 | 5 |
| Meat, fish, poultry, egg | 120 | 4 oz cooked | 376 | 280 | 0.14 | 0.23 | 6.1 | |
| Vegetables: | | | | | | | | |
| Potato | 100 | 1 medium | 65 | | 0.09 | 0.03 | 1.2 | 16 |
| Green or yellow | 75 | 1 serving | 21 | 4700 | 0.05 | 0.10 | 0.5 | 25 |
| Other | 75 | 1 serving | 45 | 300 | 0.08 | 0.06 | 0.6 | 12 |
| Fruits: | | | | | | | | |
| Citrus | 100 | 1 serving | 44 | 140 | 0.06 | 0.02 | 0.3 | 43 |
| Other | 100 | 1 serving | 85 | 365 | 0.03 | 0.04 | 0.5 | 4 |
| Bread, white enriched | 100 | 4 slices | 270 | | 0.25 | 0.21 | 2.4 | |
| Cereal, whole grain or enriched | 30 | 1 oz dry or | | | | | | |
| | 130 | 2/3 c cooked | 89 | | 0.08 | 0.03 | 0.7 | |
| Butter or margarine | 14 | 1 tbsp. | 100 | 460 | | | | |
| | | Totals | 1415 | 6945 | 0.94 | 1.56 | 12.6 | 105 |

For basis of calculation, see Pattern Dietary in Chapter 11.

### Table 8-5. Water-soluble Vitamins

| | Ascorbic Acid | Thiamin | Riboflavin | Niacin |
|---|---|---|---|---|
| *Important food sources* | Citrus fruits<br>Strawberries<br>Cantaloupe<br>Tomatoes<br>Sweet peppers<br>Cabbage<br>Potatoes<br>Kale, parsley<br>Turnip greens | Pork<br>Liver<br>Organ meats<br>Whole grains<br>Enriched cereal<br>  products<br>Nuts<br>Legumes<br>Potatoes | Liver, milk<br>Meat, eggs<br>Enriched cereal<br>  products<br>Green, leafy vegetables | Liver, poultry<br>Meat, fish<br>Whole grains<br>Enriched cereal<br>  products<br>Legumes<br>Mushrooms |
| *Stability to cooking, drying, light, and so forth* | Unstable to heat and oxidation, except in acids<br>Destroyed by drying and aging | Unstable to heat and oxidation | Stable to heat in cooking, to acids and oxidation<br>Unstable to light | Stable to heat, light, and oxidation, acid and alkali |
| *Essential function* | Formation of collagen, cellular oxidation, and reduction | Energy metabolism; coenzyme form TPP (cocarboxylase) | Carbohydrate, fat and protein metabolism; coenzyme forms FMN and FAD | Carbohydrate, fat and protein metabolism; coenzyme forms NAD and NADP |

**Table 8-5. Water-soluble Vitamins** *(Continued)*

|  | *Ascorbic Acid* | *Thiamin* | *Riboflavin* | *Niacin* |
|---|---|---|---|---|
| *Deficiency manifest as* | Scurvy<br>Sore mouth<br>Sore and bleeding<br>gums<br>Weak-walled capillaries | Beriberi<br>Poor appetite<br>Fatigue<br>Constipation | Eye sensitivity<br>Cheilosis (humans) | Pellagra<br>Dermatitis<br>Nervous depression<br>Diarrhea |
| *Recommended Dietary Allowance* | Men and women 60 mg | Men and women 0.5<br>mg/1000 kcal | Men and women 0.6<br>mg/1000 kcal | Men and women 6.6<br>mg NE/1000 kcal |

|  | *Vitamin $B_6$* | *Folacin* | *Vitamin $B_{12}$* | *Pantothenic Acid* | *Biotin* |
|---|---|---|---|---|---|
| *Important food sources* | Pork<br>Organ meats<br>Legumes, seeds<br>Grains<br>Potatoes<br>Bananas | Green leafy<br>vegetables<br>Liver and organ<br>meats<br>Milk<br>Eggs | Liver and other<br>organ meats,<br>milk, eggs | Liver<br>Organ meats<br>Eggs, peanuts<br>Legumes<br>Mushrooms<br>Salmon, whole<br>grains | Liver<br>Organ meats<br>Peanuts<br>Mushrooms |
| *Stability to cooking, drying, light, and so forth* | Stable to heat,<br>light, and<br>oxidation | Unstable to heat<br>and oxidation | Stable during<br>normal cooking | Unstable to acid,<br>alkali, heat, and<br>certains salts | |
| *Essential function* | Metabolism of<br>amino acids—<br>coenzyme form<br>PALP | Growth<br>Blood formation<br>Synthesis DNA,<br>RNA<br>Choline<br>Amino acid<br>interconversions | Blood formation,<br>choline syn-<br>thesis, amino<br>acid metabo-<br>lism; mainte-<br>nance of ner-<br>vous system | Carbohydrate, fat<br>and protein me-<br>tabolism, con-<br>stituent of co-<br>enzyme A and<br>acyl carrier<br>protein | Carboxylation re-<br>actions; fatty<br>acid synthesis,<br>gluconeogenesis,<br>amino acid<br>catabolism |
| *Deficiency manifest as* | Convulsions<br>Anemia<br>Renal calculi | Megaloblastic<br>anemia<br>Glossitis<br>Diarrhea | Macrocytic ane-<br>mias, sprue and<br>pernicious<br>anemia | General malaise<br>Abdominal sore-<br>ness and<br>cramps<br>Weakness and<br>cramping of<br>legs<br>Tenderness in the<br>heels<br>Insomnia | Lassitude<br>Anorexia<br>Depression<br>Anemia |
| *Recommended Dietary Allowance* | Men 2.2 mg and<br>women 2 mg | Men and women<br>400 mcg | Men and women<br>3 mcg | Safe and ade-<br>quate intake,<br>men and<br>women 4–7 mg | Safe and ade-<br>quate intake,<br>men and<br>women,<br>100–200 mcg |

or are inactivated by reaction with other compounds. Any substance that prevents the absorption or metabolic functioning of a vitamin in the body is called an antivitamin or a vitamin antagonist; for example, avidin is an antagonist to biotin.

One type of antagonist is a compound so similar in chemical structure to the vitamin that it starts to react like the true vitamin but cannot finish the reaction, thereby blocking the space where the real vitamin could function.

An interesting example of this type of reaction is a folic acid antagonist, which has been used clinically in the treatment of malignant growths. The theory is that rapidly dividing cells may need more folic acid than normal cells, and, therefore, an antagonist might inhibit growth of the abnormal cells. Unfortunately, the folic acid antagonist inhibits growth in normal as well as in abnormal cells.

Antibiotics and, possibly, some of the sulfa drugs

used in the treatment of infections may be vitamin antagonists. Normally, bacteria in the intestinal tract have the ability to synthesize certain vitamins. When a sulfa drug or an antibiotic is given orally, it may make some of the intestinal bacteria incapable of vitamin synthesis, thereby inhibiting growth. Conversely, in other animals antibiotics seem to stimulate growth by changing the balance of the intestinal microorganisms.

## Study questions and activities

1. From a historical point of view, which deficiency diseases were first recognized as such?
2. List properties and food sources of ascorbic acid.
3. Identify the functions of ascorbic acid in connective tissue, formation of neurotransmitters, and metabolism of tyrosine.
4. Compare the minimum ascorbic acid requirement for prevention of scurvy with the current RDA for adults. Describe the differences in blood and tissue levels and in urinary excretion of ascorbic acid at these two levels of intake.
5. What are some of the undesirable effects that have been observed in people consuming pharmacologic doses of ascorbic acid?
6. How many B vitamins are recognized today? Which ones are listed in the Recommended Dietary Allowances?
7. Which B vitamins function in the release of energy from carbohydrates, fats, and proteins? Name the coenzyme forms of each of these vitamins.
8. What methods may be used to assess the nutritional status of a person with respect to thiamin?
9. What single food is the best source of riboflavin in the diet? What kind of diet may result in vitamin $B_{12}$ deficiency?
10. Discuss the functions of vitamin $B_6$ in relation to protein metabolism.
11. Which vitamins are likely to be reduced in foods under the following treatment:

    (A) Bottled milk exposed to sunlight
    (B) Cabbage kept overnight after shredding
    (C) Vegetables to which baking soda has been added in cooking
    (D) Potatoes peeled and allowed to soak 2 to 3 hours before cooking

12. Which vitamins are preventive and curative of macrocytic anemias?
13. What is meant by a vitamin dependency? Identify the vitamins for which such conditions have been discovered.
14. What is meant by an antivitamin, and how is the vitamin activity destroyed or prevented?

## References

1. Nutr Rev 37:26, 1979
2. Puistola U et al: Biochim Biophys Acta 611:40, 1980
3. Puistola U et al: Biochim Biophys Acta 611:51, 1980
4. Hodges RE: In Goodhart RS, Shils ME (eds): Modern Nutrition in Health and Disease, 6th ed, pp 259–273. Philadelphia, Lea & Febiger, 1980
5. Passmore R: Nutr Today 12:6, Mar-Apr, 1977
6. Nutr Rev 31:93, 1973
7. Monsen ER et al: Am J Clin Nutr 31:134, 1978
8. Smith CH, Bidlack WR: Biochem Med 24:43, 1980
9. Lipschitz DA et al: Br J Haematol 20:155, 1971
10. Zannoni VG, Sato PH: Ann NY Acad Sci 258:119, 1975
11. Pauling L: Vitamin C and the Common Cold. San Francisco, WH Freeman, 1970
12. Anderson TW: Nutr Today 12:6, Jan-Feb, 1977
13. Hodges RE et al: Am J Clin Nutr 24:432, 1971
14. Zaitsev VF et al: Fed Proc (Transl Suppl) 24:971, 1965
15. Ginter E: Ann NY Acad Sci 258:410, 1975
16. Harris WS et al: Am J Clin Nutr 32:1837, 1979
17. Mumma RO, Verlangieri AJ: Fed Proc 30:370, 1971
18. Ginter E et al: Int J Vitam Nutr Res 47:123, 1977
19. Peterson VE et al: Am J Clin Nutr 28:584, 1975
20. Cameron E et al: Cancer Res 39:663, 1979
21. Stevenson NR: Gastroenterology 67:952, 1974
22. Nelson EW: J Clin Pharmacol 18:325, 1978
23. Rose RC: Annu Rev Physiol 42:157, 1980
24. Mayersohn M: Eur J Pharmacol 19:140, 1972
25. Kallner A et al: Int J Vitam Nutr Res 47:383, 1977
26. Kallner A et al: Am J Clin Nutr 32:530, 1979
27. Machlin LJ et al: Am J Clin Nutr 29:825, 1976
28. Baker EM et al: Am J Clin Nutr 24:444, 1971
29. Baker EM et al: Am J Clin Nutr 19:371, 1966
30. Food and Nutrition Board: Recommended Dietary Allowances, 9th rev ed. Washington, DC, NAS-NRC, 1980
31. Joint FAO/WHO Expert Committee: Requirements of ascorbic acid, vitamin D, vitamin $B_{12}$, folate, and iron. WHO Tech Rep Ser no 452. Geneva, World Health Organization, 1970
32. Nutr Rev 34:236, 1976
33. Barness LA: Ann NY Acad Sci 258:523, 1975
34. Stein HG et al: Ann Intern Med 84:385, 1976
35. Shilotri PG, Bhat KS: Am J Clin Nutr 30:1077, 1977
36. Cook JD, Monsen ER: Am J Clin Nutr 30:235, 1977
37. Merrill AL: J Am Diet Assoc 44:264, 1964
38. Livak JK, Morse EH: J Am Diet Assoc 41:111, 1962
39. delCampello A, Asenjo CF: J Agriculture 61:161, 1957
40. Schenker S et al: Am J Clin Nutr 33:2719, 1980
41. Nutr Rev 38:374, 1980
42. Nutr Rev 37:24, 1979
43. Nutr Rev 37:226, 1979
44. Scriver CR: Metabolism 22:1319, 1973
45. Meinen M et al: Nutr Metab (Suppl 1) 21:264, 1977
46. Hoyumpa AM: Am J Clin Nutr 33:2750, 1980
47. Howard L et al: J Nutr 104:1024, 1974
48. Centerwall BS, Criqui MH: N Engl J Med 299:285, 1978
49. Joint FAO/WHO Expert Group: Requirements of vitamin A, thiamine, riboflavin and niacin. WHO Tech Rep Ser, no 362. Geneva, World Health Organization, 1967

50. Nichoalds GE et al: Clin Chem 20:624, 1974
51. Lane M et al: J Clin Invest 43:357, 1964
52. Powers HJ et al: Proc Nutr Soc 39:17A, Feb, 1980
53. Fry H, Kondi A: Vitam Horm 28:653, 1968
54. Levy G, Hewitt RR: Am J Clin Nutr 24:401, 1971
55. Mayersohn M et al: J Nutr 98:288, 1969
56. Rivlin RS: N Engl J Med 283:463, 1970
57. Pollack H, Bookman JJ: J Lab Clin Med 38:561, 1951
58. Rivlin RS: Nutr Rev 37:241, 1979
59. Newman LJ et al: Am J Clin Nutr 31:249, 1978
60. Guggenheim K, Segal S: Int J Vitam Nutr Res 47:234, 1977
61. Carrigan PJ et al: Am J Clin Nutr 32:2047, 1979
62. Gromisch DS et al: J Pediatr 90:118, 1977
63. Lassers BW et al: J Appl Physiol 33:72, 1972
64. Winter SL, Boyer JL: N Engl J Med 289:1180, 1973
65. Nutr Rev 32:76, 1974
66. Wertz AW et al: J Nutr 64:339, 1958
67. Horwitt MK et al: Am J Clin Nutr 28:403, 1975
68. Gopalan C, JayaRao KS: Vitam Horm 33:505, 1975
69. Patterson JI et al: Am J Clin Nutr 33:2157, 1980
70. Sadoogh-Abasian F, Evered DF: Biochim Biophys Acta 598:385, 1980
71. Henderson LM, Gross CJ: J Nutr 109:646, 1979
72. Dietrich LS: Am J Clin Nutr 24:800, 1971
73. Darby WJ et al: Nutr Rev 33:289, 1975
74. Kodicek E: Bibl Nutr Dieta 23:86, 1976
75. Coursin DB: JAMA 154:406, 1954
76. Ebabi M: In Human Vitamin $B_6$ Requirements, pp 129–161. Washington, DC, National Academy of Sciences, 1978
77. Sturman JA: In Human Vitamin $B_6$ Requirements, pp 37–60.
78. Gershoff S: In Hegsted DM et al (eds): Present Knowledge of Nutrition, pp 149–161. New York, Nutrition Foundation, 1976
79. Nutr Rev 36:55, 1978
80. Nutr Rev 38:350, 1980
81. Nutr Rev 37:300, 1979
82. Snyderman SE et al: Am J Clin Nutr 1:200, 1953
83. Sauberlich HE, Canham JE: In Goodhart RS, Shils ME (eds): Modern Nutrition in Health and Disease, 6th ed, pp 216–229. Philadelphia, Lea & Febiger, 1980
84. Middleton HM: Gastroenterology 76:43, 1979
85. Gregory JF, Kirk JR: Nutr Rev 39:1, 1981
86. Wozenski JR et al: J Nutr 110:275, 1980
87. Middleton HM: J Nutr 109:975, 1979
88. Mehansho H et al: J Nutr 109:1542, 1979
89. Reinken L et al: Am J Clin Nutr 29:750, 1976
90. Reinken L, Zieglauer H: J Nutr 108:1562, 1978
91. Shane B: In Human Vitamin $B_6$ Requirements, pp 111–128
92. Linkswiler HM: In Human Vitamin $B_6$ Requirements, pp 279–290
93. Donald AD: In Human Vitamin $B_6$ Requirements, pp 226–237
94. Bosse TR, Donald EA: Am J Clin Nutr 32:1015, 1979
95. Driskell JA: In Human Vitamin $B_6$ Requirements, pp 252–256
96. Li TK: In Human Vitamin $B_6$ Requirements, pp 210–225
97. Herbert V, Das KC: Vitam Horm 34:1, 1976
98. Halsted CH: Annu Rev Med 31:79, 1980
99. Halsted CH: Am J Clin Nutr 32:846, 1979
100. Cooper BA: In Folic Acid: Biochemistry and Physiology in Relation to the Human Nutrition Requirement, pp 188–197. Washington, DC, National Academy of Sciences, 1977
101. Nutr Rev 37:77, 1979
102. Nutr Rev 38:220, 1980
103. Halsted CH: Am J Clin Nutr 33:2736, 1980
104. Nutr Rev 38:223, 1980
105. Stokes PL et al: Am J Clin Nutr 28:126, 1975
106. Lindenbaum J: In Folic Acid, pp 256–291
107. Nutr Rev 32:70, 1974
108. Herbert V et al: In Goodhart and Shils, Modern Nutrition, pp 229–259
109. Babu S, Srikantia SG: Am J Clin Nutr 29:376, 1976
110. Ghitis J: Am J Clin Nutr 18:452, 1966
111. Ek J, Magnus E: Am J Clin Nutr 33:1220, 1980
112. Nutr Rev 32:204, 1974
113. Nutr Rev 37:137, 1979
114. Jacob E et al: Physiol Rev 60:918, 1980
115. Higginbottom MC et al: N Engl J Med 299:317, 1978
116. Nutr Rev 38:274, 1980
117. Hodges RE et al: J Clin Invest 39:1421, 1959
118. Fry PC et al: J Nutr Sci Vitaminol 22:339, 1976
119. Ellestad Soyed JJ et al: Am J Clin Nutr 29:1333, 1976
120. Chung ASM et al: Am J Clin Nutr 9:573, 1961
121. Cohenour SH, Calloway DH: Am J Clin Nutr 25:512, 1972
122. Walsh JH et al: J Am Diet Assoc 78:140, 1981
123. Bonjour JP: Int J Vitam Nutr Res 47:107, 1977
124. Murthy PNA, Mistry SP: Prog Food Nutr Sci 2:405, 1977
125. Scott D: Acta Med Scand 162:69, 1958
126. Bridgers WF: Nutr Rev 25:65, 1967
127. Cowan MJ et al: Lancet II:115, 1979

## Supplementary readings
### Ascorbic acid

Anderson TA: New horizons for vitamin C. Nutr Today 12:6, Jan-Feb, 1977
Kallner A et al: Steady-state turnover and body pool of ascorbic acid in man. Am J Clin Nutr 32:530, 1979
Kallner A et al: On the requirement of ascorbic acid in man: steady state turnover and body pool size in smokers. Am J Clin Nutr 34:1347, 1981
Passmore R: How vitamin C deficiency injures the body. Nutr Today 12:6, Mar-Apr, 1977
Report: How vitamin C really works . . . or does it? Nutr Today 14:6, Sept-Oct, 1980
Review: The role of ascorbic acid in the hydroxylation of peptide-bound proline. Nutr Rev 37:26, 1979

### Thiamin

Hoyumpa AM Jr et al: Effect of thiamin deficiency and acute ethanol ingestion on jejunal glucose transport in rats. Am J Clin Nutr 34:14, 1981
Peterson DR et al: Erythrocyte transketolase activity and sudden infant death. Am J Clin Nutr 34:65, 1981
Review: A biochemical abnormality of transketolase in patients with Wernicke-Korsakoff syndrome. Nutr Rev 37:226, 1979
Review: Role of thiamine in regulation of fatty acid and cholesterol biosynthesis in cultured brain cells. Nutr Rev 37:24, 1979

Review: Thiamine-responsive megaloblastic anemia. Nutr Rev 38:374, 1980

Sauberlich HE et al: Thiamin requirement of the adult human. Am J Clin Nutr 32:2237, 1979

## Riboflavin and niacin

Bates CJ et al: Riboflavin status of Gambian pregnant and lactating women and its implications for Recommended Dietary Allowances. Am J Clin Nutr 34:928, 1981

Carrigan PJ: Riboflavin nutritional status and absorption in oral contraceptive users and nonusers. Am J Clin Nutr 32:2047, 1979

Darby WJ et al: Niacin. Nutr Rev 33:289, 1975

Lopez R et al: Riboflavin deficiency in an adolescent population in New York City. Am J Clin Nutr 33:1283, 1980

Patterson JI et al: Excretion of tryptophan-niacin metabolites by young men: Effects of tryptophan, leucine and vitamin $B_6$ intakes. Am J Clin Nutr 33:2157, 1980

Rivlin RS: Hormones, drugs and riboflavin. Nutr Rev 37:241, 1979

## Vitamin $B_6$

Bosse TR, Donald EA: The vitamin $B_6$ requirement in oral contraceptive users. I. Assessment by pyridoxal level and transferase activity in erythrocytes. Am J Clin Nutr 32:1015, 1979

Donald EA, Bosse TR: The vitamin $B_6$ requirement in oral contraceptive users. II. Assessment by tryptophan metabolites, vitamin $B_6$ and pyridoxic acid levels in urine. Am J Clin Nutr 32:1024, 1979

Gregory JF, Kirk JR: The bioavailability of vitamin $B_6$ in foods. Nutr Rev 39:1, 1981

Review: The function of vitamin $B_6$ coenzyme in the activation and nuclear binding of steroid receptors. Nutr Rev 38:350, 1980

Review: The role of growth hormone in the action of vitamin $B_6$ on cellular transfer of amino acids. Nutr Rev 37:30, 1979

Wozenski JR et al: The metabolism of small doses of vitamin $B_6$ in men. J Nutr 110:275, 1980

## Folacin and Vitamin $B_{12}$

Ek J, Magnus E: Plasma and red cell folacin in cow's milk-fed infants and children during the first 2 years of life: The significance of boiling pasteurized cow's milk. Am J Clin Nutr 33:1220, 1980

Halsted CH: Folate deficiency in alcoholism. Am J Clin Nutr 33:2736, 1980

Halsted CH: Intestinal absorption and malabsorption of folates. Annu Rev Med 31:79, 1980

Halsted CH: The intestinal absorption of folates. Am J Clin Nutr 32:846, 1979

Review: Alcohol and enterohepatic circulation of folate. Nutr Rev 38:220, 1980

Review: Contribution of the microflora of the small intestine to the vitamin $B_{12}$ nutriture of man. Nutr Rev 38:274, 1980

Review: Vitamin $B_{12}$ deficiency in the breast-fed infant of a strict vegetarian. Nutr Rev 37:142, 1979

Review: Zinc and intestinal absorption of folates. Nutr Rev 37:221, 1979

Tamura T et al: Human milk folate and folate status in lactating mothers and their infants. Am J Clin Nutr 33:193, 1980

## Biotin and pantothenic acid

Bonjour JP: Biotin in man's nutrition and therapy—A review. Int J Vitam Nutr Res 47:107, 1977

Walsh JH et al: Pantothenic acid content of 75 processed and cooked foods. J Am Diet Assoc 78:140, 1981

## Other

Herbert V: The vitamin craze. Arch Intern Med 140:173, 1980

Kishi H et al: Thiamin and pyridoxine requirements during intravenous hyperalimentation. Am J Clin Nutr 32:332, 1979

Lewis CM et al: Effect of oral contraceptive agents on thiamin, riboflavin and pantothenic acid status in young women. Am J Clin Nutr 33:832, 1980

Tarr JB et al: Availability of vitamin $B_6$ and pantothenate in an average American diet in man. Am J Clin Nutr 34:1328, 1981

*For further references see Bibliography in Part 4.*

# Nutrient Utilization: Digestion, Absorption, and Metabolism

**9**

**CMC:** Critical Micellar Concentration
**GDP:** Guanosinediphosphate
**GTP:** Guanosinetriphosphate
**IDL:** Intermediate Density Lipoproteins
**LCAT:** Lecithin-cholesterol
 Acyltransferase
**LCT:** Long-chain Triglycerides
**LES:** Lower Esophageal Sphincter
**MCT:** Medium-chain Triglycerides
**NEFA:** Nonesterified Fatty Acids
**PHLA:** Postheparin Lipolytic Activity
**SCT:** Short-chain Triglycerides

Ingestion of food initiates a multitude of physical and chemical processes that allow the body to utilize food nutrients for maintenance of body temperature and functioning of its vital organ systems, for making new tissue for growth or repair, and for performing work. These processes are generally known as digestion, absorption, and metabolism of nutrients.

Although it is customary to study separately each of these phases of nutrient utilization, one should understand that they all go on simultaneously and are highly interdependent; on the level of the individual molecule, however, they are sequential for a specific location and time. To illustrate, while some molecules of starch are being degraded by the digestive enzymes in the intestinal lumen, the digestion products (glucose) of other molecules ingested in the same meal are being absorbed into the epithelial cells of the mucosa. Still others are being metabolized in the mucosal cell to provide energy for continuous absorption, and some have already reached the liver and are being used to replenish the glycogen stores of this organ. Yet others may have been removed from the blood by other tissues and are being oxidized to provide energy for work in the muscle or converted to fat in the adipose tissue.

## Digestive-Absorptive Processes

Because the organs and the processes of digestion and absorption may have already been studied in anatomy, physiology, and chemistry courses, this section focuses primarily on the nutrients that form the substrates, the specific enzymes involved in the hydrolysis reactions, the products that are formed by the digestive process, and the mechanisms of absorption. One should remember, however, that foods are eaten in a variety of forms and combinations; cooking and other processing methods may, therefore, begin the breakdown of complex compounds, such as starch and collagen (protein), before foods are ingested.

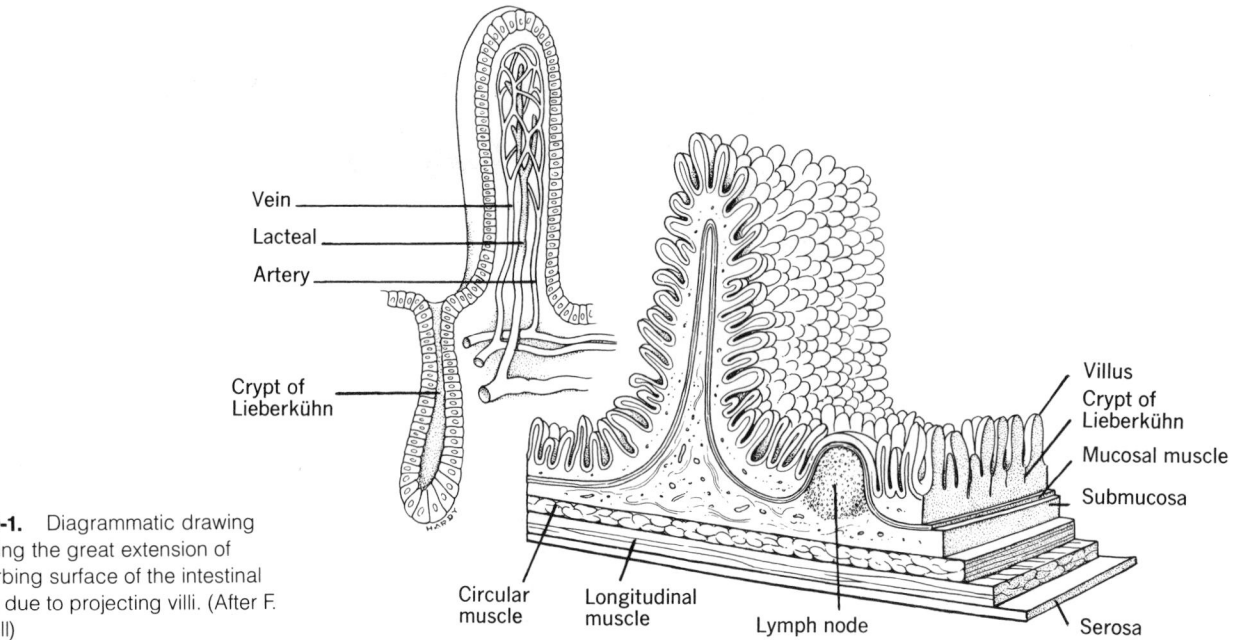

**Fig. 9-1.** Diagrammatic drawing showing the great extension of absorbing surface of the intestinal lining due to projecting villi. (After F. P. Mall)

Although the general aspects of digestion and absorption are discussed separately, they are considered together for individual nutrients. It is useful to visualize the process as a whole and to focus on the transformations that take place in three sequential sites of the gastrointestinal tract: in the lumen (*luminal phase*), in the lipoprotein membrane of the microvilli (*brushborder phase*), and in the epithelial cell (*intracellular phase*). For a review of the structure of the gastrointestinal tract see Figures 9-1 and 9-2.

## Digestion

The two major and interrelated processes of digestion—that is, the mechanical and the chemical—proceed simultaneously. In the first category are the muscular contractions of the walls of the gastrointestinal tract, which move the food in solution (*chyme*), making contact possible between the food and the digestive enzymes. The second—chemical digestion—is the process of hydrolysis by which carbohydrates, fats, and proteins are divided into simpler units, which can be absorbed through the walls of the small intestine. Table 9-1 summarizes briefly the chemical digestion of carbohydrates, fats, and proteins. They are discussed in more detail later. Each enzyme involved in the process is specific for the substrate—for example, pepsin (gastric protease) acts only on protein and is capable of breaking them down only as far as polypeptides.

In addition to the enzymes listed in Table 9-1, there are other chemical substances that affect digestion. The

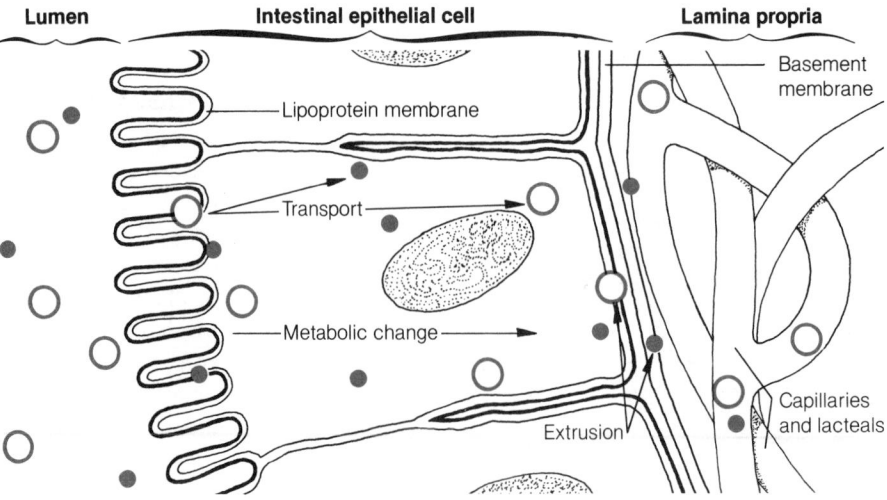

**Fig. 9-2.** Diagrammatic drawing, showing the process of absorption of nutrients from the lumen through the intestinal epithelial cell into the blood and lymph vessels of the lamina propria. (Ingelfinger FJ: Gastrointestinal absorption. Nutrition Today 2:3, 1967)

stomach secretes *hydrochloric acid* (HCl), which activates the gastric protease pepsinogen to pepsin, creates the proper acidity for the digestion of protein, acts as a bactericidal agent, and increases the solubility of certain minerals, such as iron and calcium. Gastric secretions also contain *mucin*, which protects the lining of the stomach from the HCl both by neutralizing the strongly acid contents and by forming a protective covering on the gastric epithelium.

*Bile* is produced by the liver and stored in the gallbladder, which releases it into the duodenum through the common bile duct, as a result of hormonal action initiated by the presence of fat (see Table 9-2). Bile plays an important role in the digestion and absorption of fat through emulsification, which provides a larger surface for lipase action, and through solubilization of digestion products, which allows them easier access to the absorptive surface at the epithelial brushborder. These processes are performed mainly by bile salts, but the phospholipids present in bile also participate. The solubilization function of bile salts is critical for the absorption of water-insoluble nutrients (fat-soluble vitamins, cholesterol) and digestion products (fatty acids and monoglycerides). The absorptive surface of the microvilli is surrounded by a thin layer of water (0.01 mm–1.0 mm), which is not mixed by peristalsis and muscular contractions. In order to be absorbed, nutrients must diffuse through this "unstirred water layer." Whereas the small, water-soluble molecules cross this barrier rapidly, the rate of diffusion is very slow for large and water-insoluble molecules. By providing them transport "vehicles" through micelle formation, bile facilitates the diffusion of fat-soluble substances through the "unstirred water layer." Micelles are aggregates of molecules that are hydrophilic on the outside (due to polar regions of bile salt and phospholipid molecules) and hold their passengers in the hydrophobic center. Even though the rate of diffusion of the micelles is slow, their slowness is overcome by the large load of the nutrients delivered to the absorptive surface by each micelle.

Bile acids (cholic and chenodeoxycholic acid) are synthesized from cholesterol and combine with the amino acids glycine or taurine in the liver to form conjugated bile acids before being secreted into the gallbladder. At the pH of the bile and intestines, they form highly soluble salts with $Na^+$ or $K^+$ and participate in the digestive process mainly as conjugated bile salts. Some deconjugation by intestinal bacteria may take place, but normally this occurs in the lower part of the intestines after they have already participated in the digestion and absorption of fat (p. 172).

## Table 9-1. Digestion of Carbohydrates, Fats, and Proteins

| Source of enzyme | Enzyme | + | Substrate | → Products |
|---|---|---|---|---|
| Mouth<br>Salivary glands | Salivary amylase<br>(ptyalin) | | Starch | → Dextrins and maltose |
| Stomach<br>Gastric mucosa | Gastric protease<br>pepsin<br>rennin | | Proteins<br>Casein | → Polypeptides, amino acids, oligopeptides<br>→ Insoluble casein |
| | Gastric lipase | | Short chain<br>and medium<br>chain triglycerides | → Fatty acids and diglycerides |
| Small Intestine<br>Pancreas | Pancreatic proteases<br>trypsin<br>chymotrypsin<br>carboxypeptidases | | Proteins and<br>polypeptides | → Smaller polypeptides and<br>amino acids |
| | Pancreatic lipase<br>(steapsin) | | Tri- and<br>diglycerides | → Monoglycerides, fatty<br>acids and glycerol |
| | Pancreatic amylase<br>(amylopsin) | | Amylose and<br>amylopectin | → Maltose, oligosaccharides and<br>α-limit dextrins |
| Intestinal mucosa<br>Brushborder | Intestinal peptidases<br>aminopeptidases<br>dipeptidases | | Polypeptides<br>Oligopeptides<br>Dipeptides | → Small peptides and<br>amino acids |
| | Intestinal saccharidases<br>sucrase—α-dextrinase (isomaltase)<br>glucoamylase (maltase) | | Sucrose and<br>α-limit dextrins<br>Oligosaccharides—<br>Maltose | → Glucose and fructose<br>→ Glucose<br><br>→ Glucose |
| | lactase | | Lactose | → Glucose and galactose |

## Regulation of gastrointestinal function

The mechanical and chemical processes of digestion are controlled by an extremely complex regulatory system that is only partially understood at present. The occurrence of digestive events in a sequential, coordinated manner is controlled by a regulatory network that is currently believed to involve several different but apparently overlapping functions performed by the endocrine, paracrine, and neurocrine systems. Each system uses chemical messengers that are derived from amino acids, mostly peptides and monoamines. The three systems differ mainly in the mechanism by which the messenger is delivered to the target cells.[1]

In addition to containing enzyme-secreting glands, the walls of the gastrointestinal tract are highly innervated, and the mucosal lining consists of a mixture of many cell types with different structural features related to their principal function, either absorptive, secretory, or regulatory. Although absorptive cells predominate in the lining of the small intestine, other types of cells are dispersed among them, with access to stimuli from the components of the intestinal lumen and neural and hor-

### Table 9-2. Gastrointestinal Peptides and Other Regulatory Substances

| Substance | Source | Stimulus | Action |
|---|---|---|---|
| Gastrin | Specialized cells in the antropyloric mucosa | Peptides and amino acids in the stomach<br>Vagal excitation<br>Gastric distention | Stimulates HCl and pepsin secretion<br>Trophic action on gastric mucosa |
| Secretin | Duodenal and jejunal mucosa | Acid chyme in the duodenum (*p*H 4.5 or below) | Stimulates pancreatic and biliary bicarbonate secretion<br>Augments the action of CCK on pancreatic enzyme production and cell growth<br>Inhibits gastric acid secretion, gastrin release, and motility |
| Cholecystokinin (CCK) or cholecystokinin-pancreozymin (CCK-PZ) | Mucosa of the small intestine | Peptides, amino acids, and fat in the duodenum | Stimulates pancreatic enzyme secretion and gallbladder contraction to release bile<br>Stimulates growth of pancreatic exocrine cells<br>Inhibits gastric emptying<br>Stimulates intestinal motility |
| Gastric inhibitory peptide (GIP) | Duodenal and jejunal mucosa | Peptides, amino acids, fats, and glucose in the duodenum | Inhibits gastric acid production and motility<br>Stimulates insulin release from the pancreas |
| Vasoactive intestinal peptide (VIP) | Neurons throughout the intestine | Not known | Stimulates pancreatic enzyme secretion and pancreatic and intestinal bicarbonate secretion<br>Inhibits gastric acid and pepsin production |
| Motilin | Duodenal and jejunal mucosa | Alkaline *p*H in the duodenum | Stimulates gastric and intestinal motility |
| Pancreatic polypeptide (PP) | Specialized cells in the pancreas | Ingestion of a meal—vagal cholinergic stimulation | Inhibits basal and secretin-stimulated secretion of trypsin |
| Somatostatin | Specialized antropyloric, intestinal, and pancreatic cells | Intragastric and intraduodenal HCl<br>Amino acids and fat? | Inhibits gastric HCl production and the release of all circulating GI hormones (to varying extent)<br>Inhibits action of motilin |
| Histamine | Gastric mucosa | Not known<br>Specific stimulants in foods? | Stimulates gastric HCl production |
| Acetylcholine | Gastric neurons | Sight and smell of foods<br>Mastication of food (sham feeding)<br>Distention of the stomach | Stimulates HCl production<br>May cause release of gastrin |

Same or similar substances are found and/or function elsewhere in the body; only sources and functions related to the GI tract are listed. (Grossman MI: Annu Rev Physiol 41:27, 1979; Soll AH, Walsh JH: Annu Rev Physiol 41:35, 1979; Jones RS, Meyers WC: Annu Rev Physiol 41:67, 1979, and Clin Gastroenterol 9:483-798, Sept, 1980)

monal stimuli. Endocrine cells are found throughout the intestinal tract but are especially concentrated in the antrum of the stomach, duodenum, and the upper small intestine. Like the absorptive cells, the luminal side of the endocrine cells may have microvilli, which sense the luminal stimuli. These cells have secretory granules, which contain the peptide hormone specific to the cell type; some may also contain a biogenic amine, such as histamine or serotonin. Under the influence of specific stimuli, the endocrine cells release the hormone to the blood, thereby sending messages through the systemic circulation to the target cells, which have specific receptors for a particular hormone.[2]

The cells of the paracrine system employ similar messengers, but their action is restricted to target cells within the reach of the messenger by diffusion through the intercellular space. It appears that the reach of paracrine cells may be extended by the presence in some cells of cytoplasmic extensions (resembling the processes of the neurons), which can deliver their messenger past several nontarget cells.[2] The paracrine regulation is local and resembles the neurocrine-mediated regulatory action, which also is restricted to a short distance covered by the synaptic cleft. The three regulatory systems may have joint or separate target cells. In the former instance, separate receptor sites are involved. However, for reasons not understood, the effects of the messengers delivered by the different systems are interdependent and frequently result in potentiation of the regulatory response. Overlapping between the systems is indicated also by the fact that some cells may release both an endocrine and a paracrine messenger or that the same substance may be produced by more than one system. As a result, many of these regulatory agents are not hormones according to the strict definition of the term.[1,2]

The complexity and interdependence of the regulatory actions of the neuro-, endo- and paracrine systems are best demonstrated by their roles in gastric acid production. The three best understood stimulants of gastric hydrochloric acid production are acetylcholine (neurocrine), gastrin (endocrine), and histamine (paracrine), each of which acts at a different receptor site of the parietal cells. However, the combined effect of the three exceeds the secretory response expected from their individual potencies. Furthermore, agents that are specific inhibitors of certain stimulants *in vitro* may be nonspecific *in vivo*. For example, anticholinergic agents not only inhibit the effects of cholinergic stimulants but also reduce the secretory response to gastrin. Cimetidine, which is a specific blocker of $H_2$ receptors involved in histamine-stimulated acid production (regular antihistaminic agents block $H_1$ receptors), also inhibits gastrin action, and its inhibition is further augmented by simultaneous administration of anticholinergic agents. This general action makes cimetidine a useful therapeutic agent for prevention of excessive gastric acid production (see Chap. 26).[3]

The production of other digestive juices and gastrointestinal motility also are regulated by multiple mechanisms, and the functions of the various agents are overlapping. Table 9-2 summarizes the functions and stimuli of the currently known major gastrointestinal peptides and other regulatory substances. It should be noted that effects produced *in vitro* by a high concentration of a substance may not represent the physiological role of the subtance. Also, as indicated in Table 9-2, many substances previously considered to function only in the GI tract may have regulatory roles elsewhere in the body as well.

## Digestibility

There is strong popular conviction but not very much basic knowledge about the "digestibility" of specific foods and their effect on the physiology of the gastrointestinal tract. Foods are said to be "hard to digest" or, conversely, "easy to digest." They are classed as "irritating" or "gasforming." Or they possess a quality described as "bland." Most of these terms may be traced to reported experiences of individuals who have gastrointestinal disorders, to incorrectly interpreted results of early studies of gastrointestinal function, and perhaps, most frequently, to long usage.

"Digestibility" of a food has been equated with the rate at which it leaves the stomach. Because fat remains longest in the stomach, it is thought to be more "difficult to digest" than protein and carbohydrate foods. Fried foods are said to be "irritating" to the gastrointestinal tract, although there is little evidence to support this statement.

When foods are ingested together in a meal the picture becomes even more complex. Our knowledge about the effects of individual foods on the physiology of the gastrointestinal tract when consumed in mixed diets is very scarce. It is obvious also that the factors mentioned above are not related to the true digestibility of foods. In professional usage the term *digestibility* refers to the proportion of the food that becomes available to the body as absorbed nutrients; the indigestible portion is excreted in the feces.

Under normal conditions the bulk of the indigestible residue consists of cellulose, pectins, and other complex carbohydrates found in foods of plant origin, which cannot be degraded by the digestive enzymes in humans. The amount of bulk in the diet has received a lot of attention in recent years, as it may have a role in the development of some disorders of the colon which are common today in the Western world (see Chaps. 2 and 26 for more information).

Some of the protein, fat, and carbohydrate of foods is also passed in the feces. In normal, healthy people the average proportions of the major dietary nutrients digested (and absorbed) are: 98% for carbohydrate, 95% for fat, and 92% for protein. It is in this connection that the word digestibility is most meaningful and widely used by professionals. It is often expressed as a *coefficient of digestibility*, which would be 0.98, 0.95, and 0.92 for carbohydrate, fat, and protein, respectively. The coefficients of digestibility for nutrients vary with each person and with the food source, especially with protein. For example, the proteins of egg, milk, and meat have a coefficient of digestibility of 0.97, whereas those for plant products range from 0.89 for flour to 0.65 for most vegetables.

The amounts of nutrients lost in the feces can be greatly increased in disease states. For example, a deficiency in intestinal lactase activity results in fecal loss of milk sugar lactose and is responsible for milk intolerance in some individuals. Other disease conditions may be less specific and cause general malabsorption of nutrients. The various gastrointestinal disorders that influence digestion and absorption are discussed in Chapter 26.

Some foods are also said to cause "indigestion and heartburn." Although sensitivity to specific foods has been demonstrated in some individuals with symptomatic esophagitis, the same foods have had no effect in others.[4] The mechanism causing diet-induced heartburn remains unknown. Although several recent studies have suggested that heartburn is associated with acid reflux caused by lowering of the pressure of the lower esophageal sphincter (LES) by the offending food, other investigations have not supported this conclusion. Of the foods and beverages commonly associated with heartburn, fat, chocolate, and alcohol have been shown to reduce LES pressure, but orange juice and tomato products showed no sustained effect.[5,6] The results with coffee have been inconsistent; both a reduction[7] and an increase[8] in LES pressure have been reported. Price and co-workers[4] found that sensitivity to orange juice, tomato juice, and coffee was not related to their acidity because it remained even after the foods were neutralized. There was also variability among susceptible people about the specific foods to which they were sensitive. Therefore, it is not possible to attribute any common characteristics to the foods that cause heartburn in some people.

## Absorption

### Sites of absorption

Absorption consists primarily of the transfer of nutrients from the lumen of the small intestine through the intestinal epithelium into the *lamina propria*, where the nutrients enter the blood and lymph vessels. Although limited amounts of water, alcohol, simple salts, and glucose are absorbed through the gastric mucosa, the small intestine is by far the more important organ for absorption. The most active absorptive area in the small intestine is the lower part of the duodenum and the first part of the jejunum.

### Structure of intestinal wall

The inner lining, or mucosa, of the small intestine is gathered into folds and covered by a mass of fingerlike projections (*villi*), which increase its surface area tremendously (Fig. 9-1). The epithelial cells that cover them have a so-called brushborder consisting of thousands of tiny rodlets, or *microvilli*, which further increase the surface area available for absorption.

A complex membrane made up of protein and lipid defines the outside edge of the microvilli. The exact molecular organization of this membrane is still not well understood, but it is believed to consist of a bimolecular layer of lipid in the center, covered or intermixed with protein. This membrane has a major role in the digestion and absorption of nutrients. The single layer of epithelial cells lining the lumen rests on a connective tissue structure (lamina propria) that contains blood and lymph vessels (see schematic Fig. 9-2).

For normal absorption to occur, the substrate—for instance, glucose—must enter the intestinal epithelial cell through the lipoprotein membranes and make its way across the cell, where it sometimes undergoes a chemical change. Then the substrate, glucose in this case, not only must leave on the opposite side of the cell but must pass through two additional layers of tissue before it finally enters a blood vessel. If the substrate were a fat-soluble nutrient, such as a long chain monoglyceride, the process would be similar, except that it would undergo a series of changes in the mucosal cell and enter a lacteal or lymph vessel rather than a blood capillary. Figure 9-2 schematically represents nutrients in the process of absorption.

### Mechanisms of absorption

The nutrients presented for absorption at the mucosal brushborder vary widely in molecular size, solubility, and other properties. Due to the unique nature of the lipoprotein membrane of the microvilli, several mechanisms are necessary to ensure passage into the cell of all nutrients regardless of their size and solubility. Also, as was pointed out, the nutrients encounter several different barriers while passing from the luminal to the serosal side (lamina propria) of the epithelial cell and finally into the blood or lymph vessels. Therefore, more than one mechanism is likely to be involved in the total absorption process for any one nutrient.

When a solute passes "downhill" from a higher to a lower concentration, it is said to move along its concentration gradient; the process does not require expenditure of energy and is known as *passive transport*. In the same manner osmotic pressure differences and electrical gradients across the membranes also can determine the direction of the movement of water and ions, respectively, by passive mechanisms.

During intestinal absorption many nutrients are transported "uphill," against the gradient; this can be accomplished only by expenditure of energy, and the process is known as *active transport.*

Several nutrients are known to be absorbed by both active and passive mechanisms. Furthermore, it is likely that in active absorption only one step, such as entrance into or exit from the mucosal cell, requires energy.

### Passive transport

At least three major types of passive transport across cellular membranes are recognized:

1. *Diffusion through pores.* It is postulated that passage of water and very small water-soluble molecules takes place through *pores* or water-filled channels in the membrane. The transport by this route can proceed in either direction depending on the gradient. In addition to solubility, the size of the molecule is the major limiting factor; both monosaccharides and amino acids are too large to enter the pores.
2. *Diffusion through membrane.* Instead of molecular size, solubility within the membrane is the major limiting factor. This mechanism is believed to be of importance in the absorption of monoglycerides, fatty acids, and other substances that are lipid in nature.
3. *Carrier-mediated (facilitated) diffusion.* Water-soluble compounds that cannot pass through the pores can cross the membrane through carrier-mediated processes. These carriers, located in the lipoprotein membrane, interact with the substances to be transported and facilitate their passage, probably by rendering them temporarily membrane-soluble. Some carriers may be involved with two or more compounds, such as glucose and galactose. These sugars then compete for the available carriers. Because the number of carriers is also probably limited, carrier transport slows down or ceases as vehicles become unavailable. This passive carrier-mediated diffusion continues only until there is a balance between the solutes on both sides of the barrier.

### Active transport

In order to achieve continued absorption when there is a greater concentration in the cell or in the blood than in the lumen, a nutrient must be actively transported or pumped across the membrane barrier. These "pumps," which probably involve carriers, require energy to operate, but they do permit a very large and rapid transfer into the body of such nutrients as glucose, galactose, many amino acids, sodium, and several vitamins and minerals.

### Pinocytosis

This is an amoeba-like action of the epithelial cell membrane in which a food particle or a macromolecule is encompassed and thereby brought into the cell. It may account for occasional absorption of large molecules, such as those of a protein or a fat. It is unlikely that this mechanism plays an important role in the normal absorption of any nutrient. However, pinocytosis is believed to be functioning during the later stages of fetal life and in the prenatal period, enabling nursing infants to absorb antibodies from breast milk. Similarly, artificially fed infants appear to absorb foreign antigens and antibodies from their feedings.[9] Extrusion of these macromolecules from the epithelial cell employs the same process in reverse.

## Carbohydrates

Carbohydrate (starch) digestion begins in the mouth by the action of salivary amylases, which are capable of degrading starch to maltose and $\alpha$-limit dextrins. The significance of salivary digestion is limited by the usually short stay and incomplete mastication of food in the mouth. By the time the food is well mixed with the gastric juice in the stomach, the action of salivary amylase is inhibited by the low $p$H of the medium.

The small intestine is the major site of carbohydrate digestion and absorption. In the luminal phase pancreatic amylases continue the degradation of starch where the salivary action ends, yielding maltose, maltotriose and other oligosaccharides (up to 9 glucose units), and $\alpha$-limit dextrins (1,6 linkages at the branching points). No free glucose or isomaltose is formed in the lumen.[10]

The final stages of carbohydrate digestion take place by membrane-bound enzymes on the luminal side of the lipoprotein membrane of the mucosal cell (the brush-border phase). The brushborder exhibits multiple enzyme activity, which results in the hydrolytic breakdown of di- and oligosaccharides. As a result, the digestion of starch is completed by production of glucose from $\alpha$-limit dextrins by $\alpha$-dextrinase (previously called isomaltase) and from maltose and oligosaccharides by glucoamylase (maltase). The common dietary disaccharides, sucrose and lactose, are also hydrolyzed by the mucosal disaccharidases, sucrase and lactase, respectively. Sucrase activity is actually part of a hybrid molecule, which also hydrolyzes the 1,6 linkages of $\alpha$-limit dextrins and, for this reason, is referred to as sucrase-$\alpha$-dextrinase. Sucrase activity is known to respond to changes in the intake of sucrose.[10] Figure 9-3 summarizes the major aspects of carbohydrate digestion and absorption.

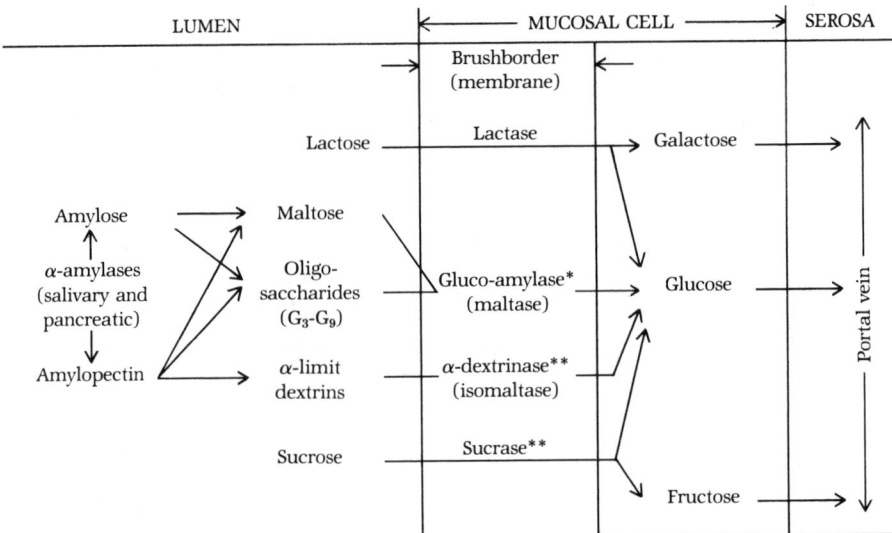

**Fig. 9-3.** Summary of the digestion and absorption of carbohydrates. Carbohydrate digestion in the intestinal lumen is incomplete and is finished by the membrane-bound oligosaccharidases. Only monosaccharides are believed to enter the mucosal cell. The action of $\alpha$-amylases on starch yields oligosaccharides, including maltose and maltotriose, from both the amylose and amylopectin fractions; the branching points of the amylopectin molecules produce $\alpha$-limit dextrins. These products, along with ingested disaccharides, lactose and sucrose, are further hydrolyzed into monosaccharides by their respective oligo- or disaccharidases, which are found in the membranes of the brushborder. After their passage through the mucosal cell the monosaccharides enter the capillaries of the portal venous system. (Adapted from Gray GM: Fed Proc 26:1415, 1967)

*Glucoamylase is an $\alpha$-glucosidase which removes one glucose unit at a time from the nonreducing end of linear oligosaccharides with 1,4 $\alpha$-linkage;

**Sucrase-$\alpha$-dextrinase is a hybrid molecule with two enzyme activities—one hydrolyzes sucrose and the other the 1,6 branching points of $\alpha$-limit dextrins (also known as isomaltase).

Only monosaccharides can enter the mucosal cell and, subsequently, the blood. Deficient mucosal disaccharidase activity is the cause of a group of malabsorption syndromes discussed in Chapters 26 and 35.

The membrane digestion is closely integrated with the absorption of the resulting monosaccharides. Only lactase activity limits the rate of the absorption of lactose. From other substrates, monosaccharides are produced at a rate greater than the mucosal uptake, and some diffuse to the intestinal contents, from which they are absorbed later at a site distal to the site of their production.[10]

Glucose and galactose are believed to share a common carrier system for the uptake into the mucosal cell. Although some of this transport is passive during the peak period of their production, the bulk of these sugars is absorbed by a process linked to the transport of $Na^+$. The exact nature of this process is still unsettled despite the many models that have been proposed for the system.

The most widely accepted theory[11] suggests that glucose and galactose are transported together with sodium by a carrier, which facilitates the diffusion of sodium into the cell along the concentration gradient. The monosaccharide is bound to the same carrier and, because of this coupling, can be transported into the cell against its concentration gradient. The monosaccharides can then exit by diffusion downhill, and enter the portal vein. According to this theory, the step that requires energy in the absorption of glucose and galactose is the expulsion of sodium from the cell.

Fructose absorption proceeds at a slower rate than that of glucose and galactose and has been assumed to be by a passive mechanism, although the rate is relatively high when compared to passive transport of other sugars. Existence of a separate specific mechanism for fructose transport is suggested by studies on sugar absorption in a patient with the rare defect known as *glucose-galactose malabsorption*[12] (see Chap. 35). An adult diagnosed as having this condition showed only minimal absorption of glucose and galactose (believed to be by passive diffusion). The rate of fructose absorption was normal, about four times that of glucose and galactose, suggesting a mechanism of facilitated diffusion.

After leaving the mucosal cell all monosaccharides enter the capillaries of the portal venous system and are carried to the liver, where fructose and galactose are readily converted to glucose.

## Proteins

Unlike other digestive enzymes, those with proteolytic activity are generally secreted in an inactive form. As a result, the gastric initiation of protein breakdown by pepsins depends on activation of pepsinogen (the inactive form of pepsin) by HCl or by small amounts of pepsin itself. The mixture of polypeptides (known as *proteoses, peptones,* and *oligopeptides*) produced by gastric digestion is further degraded by pancreatic proteases (see Table 9-1), which principally function in the lumen of the small intestine. Trypsin, secreted as trypsinogen, is activated by intestinal enterokinase or by trypsin itself, depending on the *p*H of the medium. Trypsin also converts chymotrypsinogen to its active form. Both of these enzymes are endopeptidases and can degrade either intact proteins or polypeptides into smaller units, the major difference in their action being the specificity of the peptide bonds cleaved by each. Appreciable amounts of intact protein enter the intestine daily from the intestinal secretions and desquamated epithelial cells and are digested along with the dietary proteins. Thus gastric digestion is not essential for the use of protein in the body.

Though much of protein degradation by pancreatic proteases takes place in the lumen of the digestive tract, some polypeptide hydrolysis is also believed to occur at the brushborder by adsorbed enzymes. Pancreatic juice also contains exopeptidases, mostly carboxypeptidases, which split off amino acids from the carboxyterminus of peptides.[13]

The digestive process in the intestinal lumen produces a mixture of amino acids and oligopeptides that may be very complex, as one can envision from the many possible amino acid sequences that occur in proteins. Further cleavage of oligopeptides into dipeptides and amino acids results from the action of intestinal peptidases located on the brushborder.[13,14] Though only free amino acids are found in the portal blood after protein ingestion, a significant proportion of protein is believed to leave the lumen as small peptides, which are then hydrolyzed by mucosal peptidases either in the brushborder or intracellularly.[15] Present experimental evidence favors both sites, as shown in the scheme of protein absorption proposed by Matthews (Fig. 9-4).

Dipeptides appear to be hydrolyzed mostly intracellularly, whereas membrane hydrolysis predominates for tetra- and larger oligopeptides, and extensive hydrolysis of tripeptides takes place at both sites.[13]

The transport mechanisms for amino acids, and more recently for peptides, have been the subject of intensive study. According to presently available evidence the

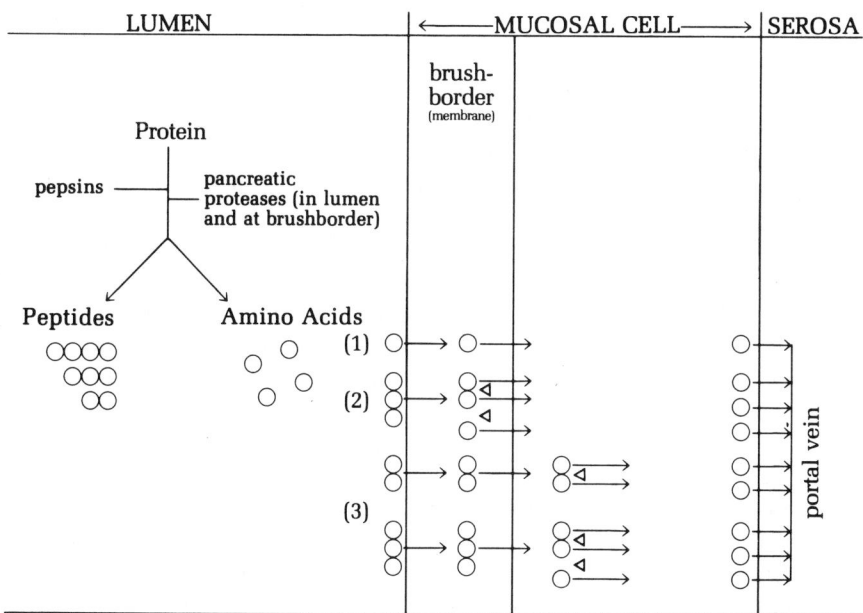

**Fig. 9-4.** Schematic description of protein absorption. Protein absorption may proceed by several mechanisms. (1) Amino acids produced in the lumen are absorbed through the mucosal cell into the portal vein by several different mechanisms, depending on the structure of the amino acid. (2) Membrane hydrolysis of small peptides upon passage into the mucosal cell; amino acids pass through the cell and enter the portal vein. (3) Small peptides enter the cell and are hydrolyzed by intracellular peptidases, followed by passage though the cell and into the portal vein. The uptake of small peptides and amino acids into the mucosal cell is believed to involve separate transport systems. Although only free amino acids can enter the capillaries of the portal venous system, their absorption from di- and tripeptides is more rapid than from the equivalent amino acid mixtures. (Adapted from Matthews DM: J Clin Path 24 (Suppl 5): 29, 1971)

transport of free amino acids from the lumen to the portal capillaries is accomplished by carrier-mediated processes that seem to be sodium- and energy-dependent for most amino acids. Several distinct transport mechanisms seem to exist, each of which is active with a group of amino acids with similar properties. It is also likely that individual amino acids may use more than one transport system.

Competition between amino acids of the same transport group has been demonstrated. This competition is avoided if the same amino acids are present as small peptides.[15] These observations suggest the existence of separate transport systems for uptake of peptides and amino acids into the epithelial cell. Other lines of evidence also support this view.[13]

Contrary to a view long held, the absorption of amino acids from di- and tripeptides is more rapid than that from the equivalent amino acid mixtures.[15] Similarly, in some diseases involving severely impaired absorption of free amino acids due to a defective transport system (Hartnup disease, cystinuria) the same amino acids can be absorbed when they are part of small peptides.[15] The capacity to absorb peptides independently of amino acid absorption explains the relatively good nutritional status and freedom from intestinal disturbances of patients with defective amino acid transport.

Because various pathologic conditions appear to affect peptide absorption less than amino acid absorption, the use of a mixture of peptides may be most beneficial in the treatment of protein deficits in patients with problems of maldigestion or malabsorption from diverse causes.[15]

In contrast to the pancreatic exopeptidases, the mucosal enzymes are aminopeptidases. Studies have shown that mucosal peptidase activity responds to changes in the level of dietary protein, due mainly to the adaptive response of the brushborder enzymes.[16]

## Fats and other lipids

Of the dietary lipids, 90% to 95% are triglycerides, generally known as fats. Small amounts of di- and monoglycerides, cholesterol, and phospholipids are also ingested. Digestion, absorption, and transport of fat in the body present special problems because of the insolubility of fat in the intestinal contents and other body fluids. Depending on the length of the carbon chain of the constituent fatty acids, there are also differences in the *solubility* of triglyceride molecules and, therefore, in the ways that the body handles them.

The bulk of fat in a normal diet consists of so-called long chain triglycerides (LCT) with fatty acid length from 14 carbons up (including some 12 carbon fatty acids). Medium chain triglycerides (MCT, predominantly 8–10 carbon fatty acids) are of little significance except in therapeutic diets consumed by patients with certain mal-

absorption syndromes. (See Chap. 26.) Short chain triglycerides (SCT, less than 8 carbons) are used in a manner similar to MCT and are found mainly in milk fat.

Although differences exist in the rate of absorption of triglycerides with different fatty acid composition (chain length and saturation), it is rapid enough in healthy people to allow 95% to 99% absorption with intakes up to 250 g per day.[17]

Because of the completeness of fat absorption in healthy adults, comparative studies of the absorption rates of dietary fats have been conducted mainly in disease states with reduced overall fat absorption or in premature infants whose capacity to handle dietary fat is also limited. It is evident from such studies that the melting point of fat influences the rate at which it is absorbed. For this reason, very hard fats, those with a large proportion of completely saturated long chain fatty acids, are absorbed less readily than liquid oils with a high content of unsaturated or short chain fatty acids.[17] The effect of triglyceride composition on the overall rate of fat absorption can probably be attributed to differences both in the rate of hydrolysis and in the rate of absorption of the end products, although the mechanisms involved are not known. As was mentioned earlier, these differences are of little significance in healthy people but may be very important in determining the extent of steatorrhea present in certain malabsorption syndromes (see Chaps. 26 and 35).

## Long chain triglycerides (LCT)

The mechanical and chemical actions of the stomach release the food fat from the protein and carbohydrate. Fat enters the duodenum in a coarse, unstable emulsion. Two digestive juices essential for normal lipolysis of fat are secreted into the upper duodenum, bile and the pancreatic juice. The mechanical action of the intestine and the emulsifying capacity of the bile salts and phospholipids of the bile allow formation of a finely divided stable emulsion. The emulsified fat droplets consist mainly of triglycerides and of lesser amounts of diglycerides and fatty acids. They form what is known as the *oil phase*, which is dispersed in the bulk of the intestinal contents, the *water phase*.

The enzymatic hydrolysis of triglycerides takes place at the oil–water interphase by pancreatic lipase (glycerol ester hydrolase) present in the water phase. The finer the emulsion, the larger the surface area available for the enzyme action; an ample supply of lipase is normally available, making the accessibility to the substrate molecules the determining factor for the rate of lipolysis.[17] Pancreatic juice also contains a peptide molecule known as *colipase*. Colipase increases the activity of pancreatic lipase, probably by strengthening its binding to the substrate. The role of colipase appears to be especially important in the presence of a high concentration of bile salts which, although essential for the emulsification of dietary fat, also weaken or prevent the binding of lipase to its substrate at the water–oil interface and thereby inhibit triglyceride hydrolysis. This inhibition is prevented by colipase.[18]

The intestinal digestion of long chain triglycerides consists of two essential steps: hydrolysis and solubilization of the end products. The pancreatic lipase releases the fatty acids esterified at carbons 1 and 3 of the triglyceride glycerol (also known as $\alpha$-positions). The resulting free fatty acids and 2-monoglycerides (remaining fatty acid in $\beta$-position) are solubilized and removed from the site of hydrolysis through formation of micelles with conjugated bile salts. Small amounts of other lipids are also found in these micelles, including cholesterol, phospholipids, and the fat-soluble vitamins. Though the micelles are aggregates of molecules, they are much smaller than the emulsified triglyceride droplets, and they form a clear dispersion in the aqueous medium in the lumen (water phase). The major luminal events of LCT digestion and absorption are summarized in Figure 9-5.

Micelle formation allows the monoglycerides and fatty acids to make close contact with the absorptive surfaces of the epithelial brushborder by facilitating their diffusion through the unstirred water layer. The minimun level of bile salts required to accomplish complete solubilization of the insoluble monoglycerides and fatty acids is known as the critical micellar concentration (CMC) of bile

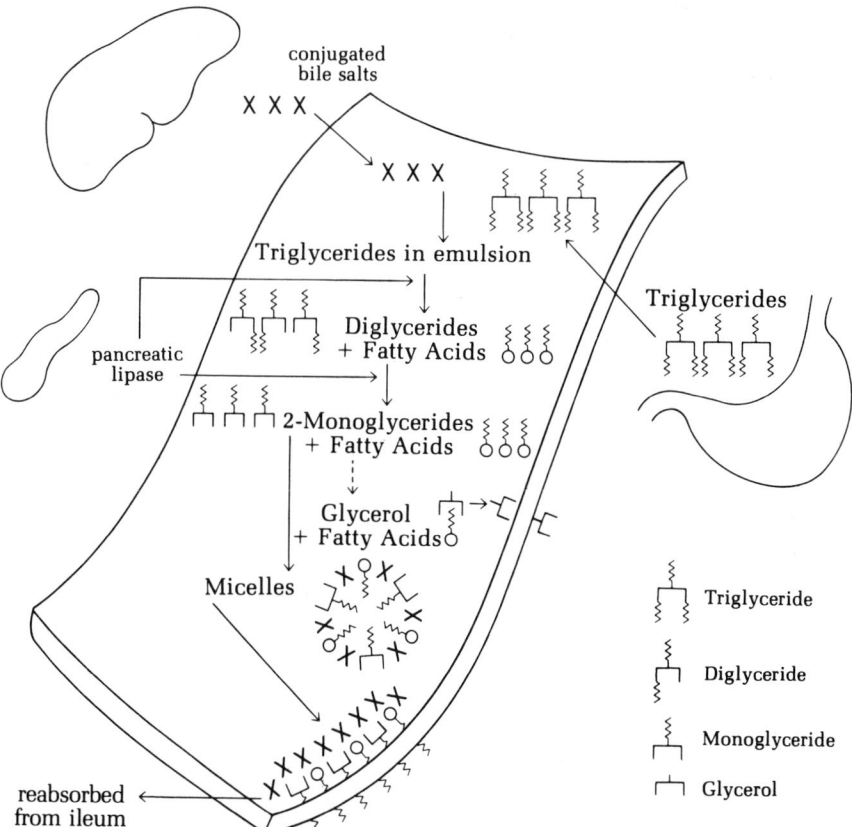

**Fig. 9-5.** Schematic representation of the luminal phase of digestion and absorption of long chain triglycerides (LCT). Triglycerides emulsified with conjugated bile salts are hydrolyzed into 2-monoglycerides by the pancreatic lipase. The resulting monoglycerides and fatty acids are solubilized by formation of mixed micelles with bile salts. Further hydrolysis of the micellar monoglyceride occurs but is limited. At the brushborders of the intestinal villi the micellar fatty acids and monoglycerides are absorbed into the mucosal cells, whereas the bile salts pass further along the intestine until they are reabsorbed from the ileum. The absorption of fatty acids and monoglycerides is normally completed by the time the chyme reaches the midjejunum. Some of the bile salts are deconjugated by the bacteria found in the lower intestine before being reabsorbed. After passage through the mucosal cell into the portal vein, the bile salts are carried back to the liver where they are reconjugated and, along with the newly synthesized bile salts, are secreted into the gallbladder, ready to be released to the intestine again. This recycling is known as the enterohepatic circulation of bile salts. See Fig. 9-6 for the intracellular phase of LCT absorption. (Redrawn from Isselbacher KJ: Fed Proc 26:1420, 1967)

salts. Below this level some of the end products of hydrolysis remain in the oil phase, and the entire process of digestion and absorption is slowed down.[14]

LCTs are absorbed into the epithelial cell as monoglycerides, fatty acids, and glycerol. Glycerol is produced by limited hydrolysis of micellar monoglycerides, probably by intestinal lipase(s). About two-thirds to three-fourths of the dietary LCTs are absorbed as monoglycerides.[17] The exact mechanism by which they enter the epithelial cell is not known, but the available evidence points to passive diffusion across the lipoprotein membrane.

At the site of absorption the bile salts separate from the rest of the micellar components and move farther down the intestinal lumen to the ileum, where about 95% are reabsorbed. They pass through the mucosal cell and into the capillaries of the portal system, which carries them back to the liver. If the bile salts are deconjugated in the intestine (by bacteria) before reabsorption, they are reconjugated in the liver and, along with the newly synthesized bile salts, are secreted into the gallbladder ready to be released once more into the duodenum as needed. This recycling is known as the *enterohepatic circulation* of bile salts.

The small fraction of bile salts lost daily in the feces is replaced by synthesis from cholesterol in the liver. This activity represents the major means of cholesterol removal from the body and can be increased by administration of certain drugs, such as cholestyramine, which binds the bile salts, preventing their reabsorption and thereby increasing the conversion of cholesterol into bile acids in the liver. The net result is a reduction in blood cholesterol of hypercholesterolemic people (Chap. 30).[19]

The intracelluar phase in the absorption of LCT is of major importance (Fig. 9-6). The entering fatty acids and monoglycerides become mixed with those already present

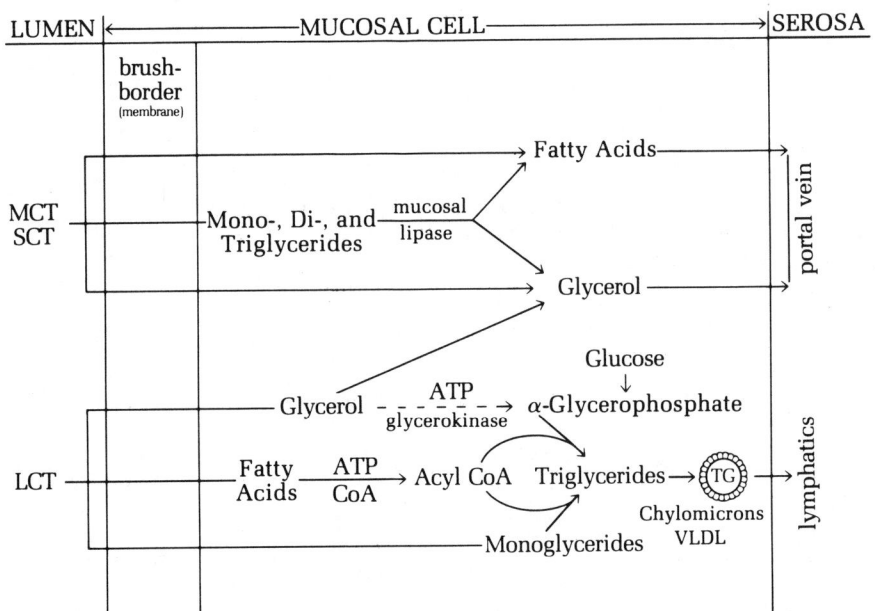

**Fig. 9-6.**  Intracellular transformations in triglyceride absorption. Long chain triglycerides (LCT) enter the mucosal cell as monoglycerides, fatty acids, and glycerol. Monoglycerides are reconverted to triglycerides (TG) by addition of two activated fatty acids (acyl CoA). Another pathway for the reesterification of fatty acids involves addition of two acyl CoAs to "activated" glycerol, $\alpha$-glycerophosphate, removal of phosphate to form a diglyceride, and addition of another acyl CoA to complete the triglyceride molecule. Metabolism of glucose provides most of the $\alpha$-glycerophosphate for TG synthesis due to limited glycerokinase activity in the mucosal cell. The newly synthesized triglycerides are "packaged" into chylomicrons and, to a lesser extent, the very low-density lipoproteins (VLDL), which leave the cell and enter the lymphatics. These, in turn, empty into the left subclavian vein through the thoracic duct.

Medium chain and short chain triglycerides (MCT, SCT) may enter the mucosal cell intact, partially hydrolyzed (di- and monoglycerides), and as fatty acids and glycerol. The glycerides undergo intracellular lipolysis and leave the mucosal cell as fatty acids and glycerol. They enter the portal vein, which carries them directly to the liver. Some medium chain fatty acids may be reesterified to TG.

For this reason, the portal route is the major one for the transport of fatty acids with less than 12 carbons and the lymphatic system for fatty acids with more than 12 carbons. The 12-carbon fatty acid, lauric acid, is between the long chain and the medium chain fatty acids and enters the circulation through both the portal route and the lymphatic system.

in the cell and lose their "identity." They also must undergo reconversion into triglycerides before leaving the cell. The major pathway involves the direct acylation of the monoglycerides, and its activity responds to the changes in the dietary intake of fat.[18]

The newly synthesized triglycerides are "packaged" into lipoprotein particles known as *chylomicrons*. The core of these particles consists of triglyceride and some cholesterol. They are covered with a protein-phospholipid "wrapping," which allows them to be dispersed in water. The Golgi complex of the mucosal cell appears to be the site for the completion of chylomicrons before their release.[18] Some of this dietary or exogenous triglyceride is incorporated into very low density lipoproteins (VLDL) by the epithelial cells, although this blood lipoprotein fraction is mainly known as the carrier of endogenous triglycerides synthesized in the liver (see p. 186).

Both lipoprotein particles are then released from the cells and enter the lacteals, the small vessels of the lymphatic system in the lamina propria. The contents of the lymph reach the left subclavian vein through the thoracic duct and, from there, the various sites of utilization in the body.

## Medium chain triglycerides (MCT)

The digestion and absorption of medium chain and short chain triglycerides are similar; therefore, the discussion in this section pertains to both, although only MCTs are referred to.

Gastric lipase, which has practically no activity in digesting LCT, can initiate the breakdown of MCT.[20] Though gastric lipolysis is considered insignificant in the digestion of fat in general, it may be important when a sizable proportion of total fat intake is in the form of MCT, as is recommended for certain therapeutic diets and in the digestion of milk fat.[21]

In the intestinal lumen, MCTs are rapidly hydrolyzed into monoglycerides and fatty acids by the pancreatic lipase. In contrast to the long chain monoglycerides, a considerable proportion of medium chain monoglycerides normally undergoes further hydrolysis to glycerol and fatty acids before absorption.[22]

Both intact MCTs and their digestion products are readily dispersed in the aqueous intestinal contents; as a result, although the presence of bile salts stimulates their digestion and absorption, these processes proceed relatively rapidly, even in bile-deficiency states in which ingestion of LCT causes severe steatorrhea.[17]

Uptake into the mucosal cell can also proceed at any stage of digestion; even intact MCTs can enter the cell when luminal hydrolysis is incomplete, as in patients with pancreatic insufficiency. Once they are inside the mucosal cell, the hydrolysis of these glycerides (mono-, di-, and triglycerides) is completed by intracellular lipases, which have little activity with long chain glycerides. This intra-cellular lipolysis is followed by rapid removal of the fatty acids from the cell. Unlike the LCT fatty acids, which are absorbed into the lymphatics, the bulk of the MCT fatty acids are directly absorbed into the portal circulation and carried to the liver, where they are readily metabolized.[23] The intracellular transformations of LCT and MCT during absorption are compared in Figure 9-6.

Lauric acid (12 carbons), found especially in coconut oil, is usually classified as a medium chain fatty acid. In intestinal absorption, it seems to be on the borderline between the long chain and medium chain fatty acids. Although some lauric acid enters the circulation through the portal route, a considerable proportion is reesterified and enters the lymph in chylomicrons. To some extent the same is true with other fatty acids below and above lauric acid in chain length, but proportionally the portal route is the major one for fatty acids with fewer than 12 carbons and the lymphatic system for those with more than 12 carbons.

The therapeutic value of MCT preparations is based on their special behavior in digestion, absorption, and transportation. Their major use is in digestive disorders (see Chap. 26), but more recently they have proven beneficial in the rare disorders of lipid transport in which chylomicron removal from the blood is defective (see Chap. 30).

## Cholesterol

Cholesterol is an essential component of all animal cells and, therefore, is ingested in foods of animal origin. The average daily intake in a typical American diet is estimated to be 600 mg to 800 mg, but undoubtedly higher as well as lower intakes are common. Some cholesterol is also secreted into the intestinal tract in bile and becomes mixed with the dietary cholesterol. It exists either free or esterified with fatty acids (see Chap. 3), but the latter are cleaved in the intestine by pancreatic cholesterol ester hydrolase before absorption. The amount of cholesterol present in the intestines is small compared to the triglycerides and their digestion products, and it is easily solubilized within the bile salt-lipid micelles from which it is absorbed. It is well known that both dietary fat and bile stimulate cholesterol absorption.[24] In addition to facilitating the solubilization of cholesterol, bile salts are required to activate the pancreatic cholesteryl ester hydrolase. Only free cholesterol is believed to be absorbed into the mucosal cell.[17]

Further mixing of dietary with endogenous cholesterol occurs in the mucosal cell, which actively synthesizes this compound. Some intracellular reesterification of free cholesterol also takes place, and both free and esterified cholesterol are incorporated into chylomicrons (60%–80% esterified) and the VLDL.

The extent to which dietary cholesterol is absorbed in humans seems to be variable, and the information available is somewhat contradictory, especially about the effect of the level of dietary cholesterol on the percentage and absolute amount of cholesterol that reaches the blood.

The results of several studies support the view that within the common range of cholesterol intake in American diets the amount of cholesterol absorbed is directly proportional to the dietary intake.[25-27] The percentage of ingested cholesterol absorbed seemed to average 40% to 50% of the intake. In a number of studies, cholesterol absorption in patients with diagnosed hypercholesterolemia has been found to be normal.[25,27]

It is generally agreed that with high cholesterol intakes there is a gradual decrease in the percentage absorbed,[17] but the total absorption still increases with intake. The amount and type of triglycerides ingested simultaneously also influences cholesterol absorption.[24]

### Phospholipids

Phospholipids are found in foods of both animal and plant origin although in relatively small amounts. The main dietary phospholipid is lecithin (see Chap. 3) and, like cholesterol, it becomes mixed with endogenous lecithin both in the intestinal lumen (from bile) and inside the mucosal cell (synthesized).

Before absorption, lecithin and other gylcerophospholipids are hydrolyzed to lysophospholipids by pancreatic phospholipase $A_2$, which removes the fatty acid in the 2-position of the glycerophosphatides.[18] Lysolecithin and other lysophosphatides participate in micelle formation in the intestine and are absorbed by passive diffusion like the other lipid digestion products. Lysophospholipids undergo extensive breakdown and resynthesis in the mucosal cell. Some parts of the molecule may be found in triglycerides or in other phospholipids manufactured in the cell. Phospholipids are important structural components of the triglyceride-transporting chylomicrons and other lipoproteins and are actively synthesized in the mucosal cell.

### Metabolism

When the nutrients in the bloodstream pass through the cellular membranes of the body, they enter into the metabolic processes of the cell. Metabolism may be defined as a process by which the cells convert nutrients from food into useful energy, which can be utilized for performance of work as well as for synthesis of new compounds vital for cellular structure and function. The process by which nutrient molecules are degraded, with concurrent release of energy and subsequent elimination of waste products, is generally known as *catabolism*, whereas *anabolism* refers to the synthesis of new compounds. The anabolic processes depend on energy from the catabolic processes, both proceeding simultaneously.

Some may be linked together through common intermediates. Metabolism is an ongoing process in every cell of the body, requiring a continuous supply of nutrients.

Wide variations exist among groups of people and individuals in their daily intake of foods. Some people have meals at stated times; others cannot or do not. Fortunately, mechanisms exist that allow a steady flow of nutrients to the cells to continue for limited periods of time, even though no food is ingested.

In the period immediately following ingestion of food, the levels of most nutrients in the blood rise due to absorption from the intestine. The rate of absorption varies with the nutrient, the quantity ingested, and the person, but in general the peak level for carbohydrate (glucose) is reached in 1 hour and for fat (chylomicron triglycerides) in 4 to 6 hours. At the same time the uptake of nutrients by the tissues also is rapid and eventually exceeds the rate of flow from the intestine, resulting in a gradual decline in the blood nutrients to fasting levels. In most people fasting levels for triglycerides are attained in 8 to 12 hours and for glucose in 2 to 3 hours.

The rate of protein (amino acid) absorption falls somewhere between those of carbohydrate and fat. However, the changes in the amino acid concentration and pattern in the blood are relatively small after protein ingestion because the absorbed amino acids pass through the liver, which removes a large proportion of them and controls their release to the general circulation.[28]

Upon reaching the cells, some of these nutrients enter the catabolic pathways to supply energy for immediate needs. Aside from small functional needs, the remaining nutrients are converted to various storage forms from which they can be recalled later when needed.

Glucose is converted to glycogen to replenish the tissue stores, but due to the body's limited ability to store gycogen, the remaining glucose is converted to fat and stored as triglyceride, mostly in the adipose tissue and, to a lesser extent, in the liver and muscle. Excess dietary fatty acids also are stored as triglyceride. Protein synthesis in the tissues is high after ingestion of a balanced mixture of amino acids; the excess is either oxidized to provide energy or first converted to glucose or fat.

### Biologic oxidation of foodstuffs

Liberation of food energy in the body is not a process of instant combustion as in the bomb calorimeter. It is a slow, gradual redistribution of energy of the original molecules into intermediates of lower energy value with concomitant release of both heat and usable energy (as ATP) from the oxidative and other energy-yielding reactions of the metabolic pathways.

Biologic oxidations include all reactions in which electrons are removed from an atom or ion that is part of the substrate; in some oxidations, the electron loss is accompanied by an addition of oxygen to or removal of hydrogen from the substance being oxidized. Oxidation of one substance (loss of electrons) always results in the reduction of another substance (gain of electrons, which may be accompanied by loss of oxygen or gain of hydrogen); oxygen is commonly referred to as an oxidizing agent or electron acceptor. Although oxygen may serve as an electron (hydrogen) acceptor in biologic reactions, with the formation of water ($H_2O$) or hydrogen peroxide ($H_2O_2$), most of the intermediary steps in the oxidation of foodstuffs initially involve other electron or hydrogen acceptors. The two major ones are the coenzymes, nicotinamide adenine dinucleotide ($NAD^+$) and flavin adenine dinucleotide (FAD). Both are required for the initial breakdown of glucose, amino acids, and fatty acids as well as the final oxidative cycle of energy production, the citric acid cycle, where the carbons of these nutrients become oxidized to $CO_2$. The resulting reduced coenzymes, often referred to as "reducing equivalents" ($NADH + H^+$ and $FADH_2$), are either used in the synthesis of new compounds (in energy-requiring reductive steps) or reoxidized by the enzymes of the *respiratory chain*. Oxygen serves as the final hydrogen acceptor in this stepwise electron transfer, which is accompanied by capture of energy as ATP in the so-called *oxidative* or *respiratory chain phosphorylation*. This oxidative phosphorylation at the respiratory chain level is the major means of ATP production in the body.

A sizable fraction of total ATP formation takes place directly at the *substrate level*, linked to the cleavage of a high-energy bond, as seen in the conversion of 1,3-diphosphoglyceric acid to 3-phosphoglyceric acid in the glycolytic breakdown of glucose:

$$1,3\text{-diphosphoglyceric acid} \xrightarrow[\phantom{x}]{\text{ADP} \quad \text{ATP}} 3\text{-phosphoglyceric acid}$$

The quantitative aspects of ATP production from oxidative metabolism are discussed in the following sections.

## Common pathways in energy production

The following sections discuss the major metabolic pathways involved in energy production from and storage of food nutrients and their role in the maintenance of metabolic homeostasis in the body. Even though it is customary to denote certain metabolic pathways as catabolic, they may also have important anabolic functions because the intermediates may serve as substrates for biosynthetic pathways or as required intermediates for another catabolic pathway. Accordingly, one should keep in mind that although the emphasis in the discussion of the various metabolic pathways is on the end products formed and on the connections between the pathways, there are many other directions in which some of the intermediates can be diverted, depending on the body's needs.

Food energy becomes available to the body cells primarily in the form of glucose, fatty acids, and amino acids carried in the blood. Although the initial catabolism of these nutrients takes place through pathways that are specific for each nutrient, only a fraction of their potential energy is released in these reactions. The end products, such as pyruvate produced from glucose, still hold the major portion of their total energy value, which becomes available only through complete oxidation into $CO_2$ and $H_2O$ in the common pathways of intermediary metabolism.

Understanding the central role of the common pathways and the energy-conserving mechanism of biologic oxidations is helpful for visualizing the role of the individual pathways in the whole metabolic process of the cell. For this reason, the common pathways are discussed first.

The common pathways involved in energy production are located in the mitochondria, which rightfully are known as the "powerhouses" of the cell. Figure 9-7 outlines the sequence of transformations through which complete oxidation of the energy-yielding nutrients is accomplished.

### The citric acid cycle (CAC, Krebs Cycle)

This oxidative cycle serves as a "melting pot" for the products of carbohydrate, fat, and protein metabolism after initial catabolism in separate pathways. Even though it is sometimes considered as a pathway of glucose oxidation because of the carbohydrate nature of its intermediates, the citric acid cycle does not discriminate on the basis of the origin of its substrates. Furthermore, the catabolism of several amino acids also provides intermediates for the cycle, as indicated in Figure 9-7.

The key compound that channels the carbons of glucose, amino acids, and fatty acids into the cycle is acetyl CoA (or "active" acetate). The condensation of acetyl CoA with oxaloacetic acid initiates the series of reactions that result in the oxidation of the two acetate carbons into $CO_2$, with regeneration of CoA and oxaloacetic acid (OAA). Even though OAA is not used up in the cycle, its supply can become limiting for the oxidation of acetyl CoA because there are other uses for OAA, as is shown in the subsequent sections. OAA is produced from carboxylation of pyruvate by a biotin-dependent pyruvate carboxylase and is plentiful when carbohydrates are actively metabolized. Catabolism of certain amino acids also replenishes the supply of the CAC intermediates and is especially important when the supply of carbohydrates is limited.

The energy generated in the oxidative steps (dehydrogenations) of the cycle is utilized in the concomitant reduction of coenzymes $NAD^+$ (nicotinamide adenine dinucleotide) and FAD (flavin adenine dinucleotide) and

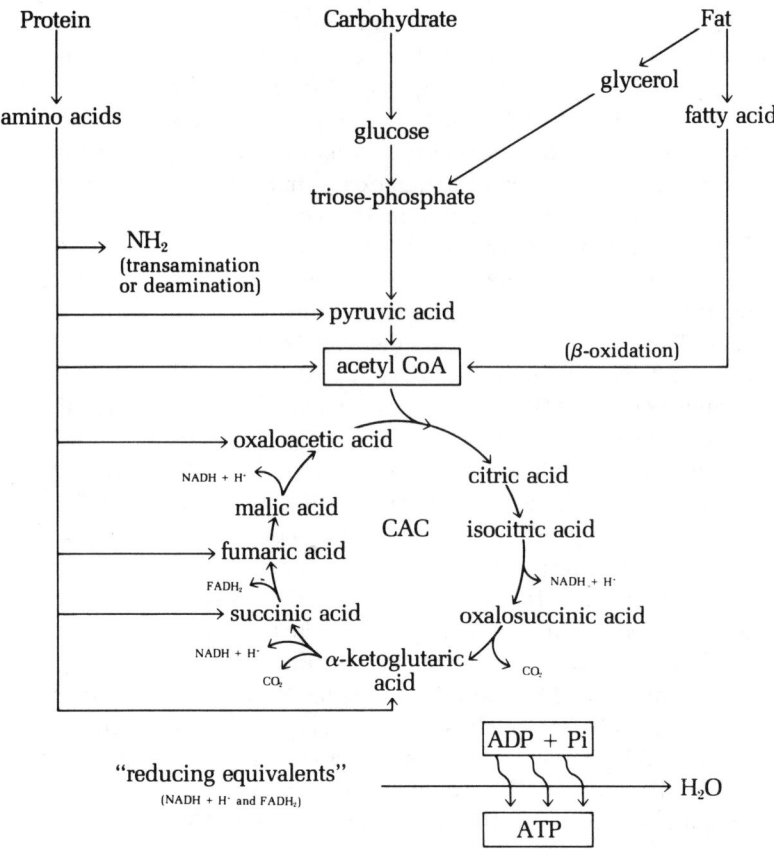

Respiratory chain linked production of ATP (oxidative phosphorylation)

**Fig. 9-7.** The common pathway in energy production. Carbohydrate, fat, and the carbon skeletons from some amino acids* are first converted to acetyl CoA, which then channels the two-carbon units into the citric acid cycle (CAC) where they are oxidized into $CO_2$. Initial catabolism of other amino acids† provides several intermediates for this cycle. Oxidation of substrates in the cycle is accompanied by simultaneous reduction of coenzymes NAD (nicotinamide adenine dinucleotide) and FAD (flavin adenine dinucleotide) which then are reoxidized by the enzymes of the respiratory chain, with ultimate formation of $H_2O$. The energy released by the respiratory chain oxidations is "trapped" as ATP (adenosine triphosphate), three per each NADH + $H^+$ and two per each $FADH_2$ oxidized. (Pi = inorganic phosphate.) In addition to the high energy bonds generated by the phosphorylation of ADP (adenosine diphosphate) to ATP (adenosine triphosphate), as shown in the illustration, another high energy bond is generated in the CAC by the substrate-linked phosphorylation of GDP (guanosine diphosphate) to GTP (guanosine triphosphate), not shown in the illustration. As a result, the net yield from the oxidation of each 2-carbon unit of acetyl CoA is 12 high energy bonds.

*(alanine, cysteine, glycine, isoleucine, leucine, lysine, phenylalanine, serine, tryptophan, tyrosine)

†(arginine, aspartate, glutamate, histidine, proline, OH proline, methionine, threonine, valine, isoleucine, lysine, phenylalanine, tyrosine, tryptophan)

thereby conserved as "reducing equivalents" (NADH + $H^+$ and $FADH_2$). This energy can then be reclaimed by reoxidation of the coenzymes in the respiratory chain, or it may be directly used in synthetic reactions involving reductive steps specific for these coenzymes.

### Electron transport and oxidative phosphorylation

Reoxidation of the "reducing equivalents" is accomplished by the enzymes of the electron transport or respiratory chain, which are located in close proximity and linked to those of the citric acid cycle in the mitochondria. As discussed earlier, the oxidation-reduction steps of the respiratory chain result in transport of the "reducing equivalents" (hydrogens or electrons) from substrates to oxygen with production of $H_2O$ (see Fig. 9-8). The liberated energy is "captured" for the synthesis of the high-energy bonds of adenosine triphosphate (ATP) from adenosine diphosphate (ADP) and inorganic phosphate in a process known as *respiratory chain*, or oxidative phosphorylation.

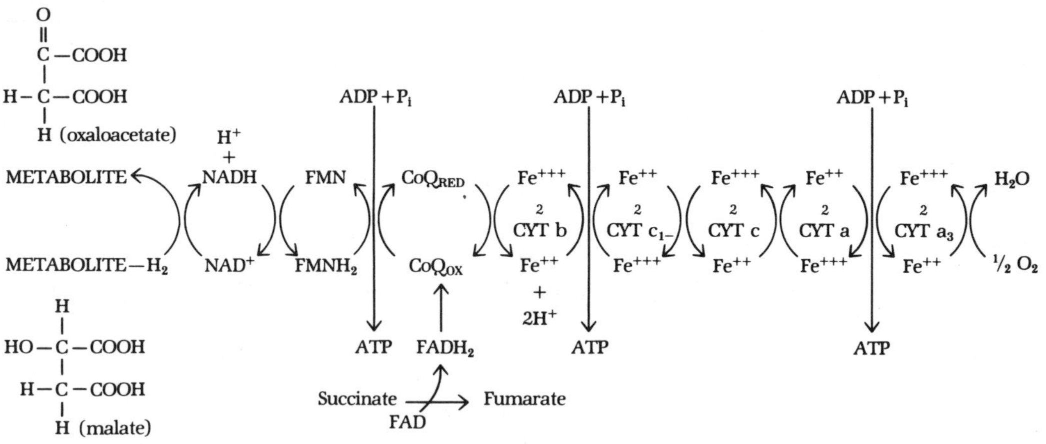

**Fig. 9-8.** Oxidative phosphorylation at the respiratory chain level. Consider the oxidation of malate (metabolite-$H_2$) to oxaloacetic acid (metabolite) in the citric acid cycle as an example. Malate dehydrogenase requires coenzyme $NAD^+$, which is reduced $NADH + H^+$ when malate is oxidized to oxaloacetate. NADH dehydrogenase then channels the electrons from NADH to the respiratory chain, initiating a sequence of electron transfers through the components of the chain with $O_2$ as the final acceptor. At certain points of the chain, the liberated energy is captured in the formation of ATP from ADP (adenosine diphosphate) and inorganic phosphate ($P_i$). Oxidation of some substrates is linked to the respiratory chain through flavoprotein dehydrogenases (FAD or FMN as coenzyme) at the level of CoQ, resulting in two instead of three ATPs per pair of electrons. Oxidation of succinate is an example (see Fig. 9-7).

The oxidation of each molecule of NADH yields three molecules of ATP, whereas only two ATPs are recovered from each $FADH_2$ (Fig. 9-8). In addition, one high-energy bond is generated directly in the citric acid cycle by the substrate-linked phosphorylation of guanosinediphosphate (GDP) to guanosinetriphosphate (GTP). As a result, the net yield from the oxidation of each 2-carbon unit of acetyl CoA is 12 high-energy bonds (see Figs. 9-8 and 9-9).

## Carbohydrates

Every tissue in the body is capable of removing glucose from the circulation and utilizing it for production of energy. Differences exist among tissues in the essentiality of glucose as a source of energy and the metabolic pathways through which it is liberated. As mentioned before, the tissues of the central nervous system (CNS) and the formed elements of the blood are most dependent on a continuous supply of glucose, although adaptation to oxidation of ketone bodies (products of incomplete fatty acid oxidation) is known to take place in the CNS during limited availability of glucose (prolonged fasting). Some glucose is always needed, however, and the body has means for storing it when a surplus is available and for mobilizing these stores or converting other substances to glucose when the supply is limited.

### Pathways of carbohydrate metabolism

Uptake of glucose into the cells is the limiting step in its utilization in many tissues, including muscle, heart, and adipose tissue. Insulin is essential for glucose entrance to these tissues, whereas the process is independent of insulin in the liver and CNS.

Equally important and possibly related to glucose uptake is its phosphorylation to glucose-6-phosphate by *hexokinases* before it can enter the metabolic pathways of the cell. This reaction is practically irreversible in most tissues. Once glucose-6-phosphate is formed, it must enter the metabolic pathways and cannot be returned to the blood except from the liver and kidney, where another enzyme, *glucose-6-phosphatase*, can release free glucose. Glucose-6-phosphate serves as a link between the major pathways of glucose metabolism, which are shown in Figure 9-9.

In contrast to the extrahepatic tissues, insulin regulates the metabolism of glucose in the liver after its uptake by affecting the activities of hexokinase and other hepatic enzymes.

### Glycolysis

Glycolysis is a pathway of glucose catabolism which, under most conditions, is a necessary preliminary step for the release of all the energy biologically available in the glucose molecule. It results in the conversion of glucose-6-phosphate (either from glucose or glycogen breakdown) to two molecules of pyruvate or lactate, depending on the tissue and oxygen supply to the cell. The reactions that make up the pathway are outlined in Fig. 9-9. The energy yield of the pathway depends on the end product. Some ATP is produced directly in the pathway by substrate level phosphorylations regardless of the availability of oxygen.

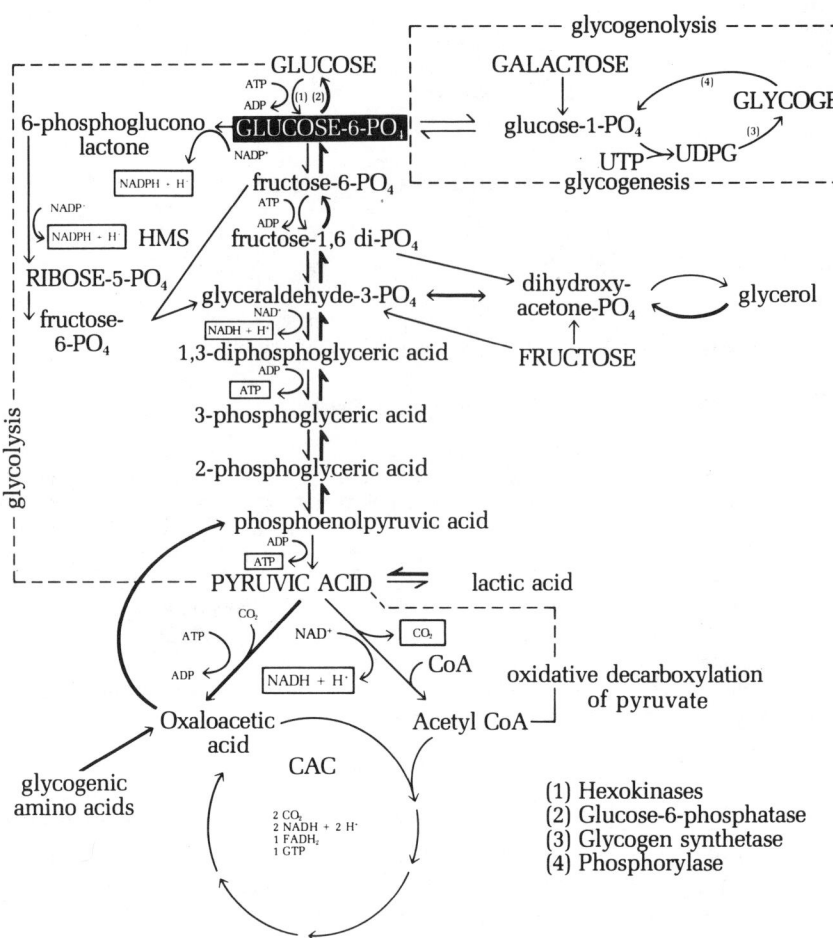

**Fig. 9-9.** Major pathways of carbohydrate metabolism. Note the key position of glucose-6-$PO_4$. Some reactions and intermediates have been deleted in order to emphasize the energy-yielding steps and the points of connection between different pathways. Heavy arrows indicate reactions involved in GLUCONEOGENESIS. Separated arrows point to individual reactions or segments of pathways where different enzymes are required for each direction. GLYCOLYSIS is the breakdown of glucose-6-phosphate to 2 molecules of pyruvate or lactate if oxygen is limited. OXIDATIVE DECARBOXYLATION of pyruvate into acetyl CoA links carbohydrate catabolism to the CAC. CAC (citric acid cycle) is the common pathway for the products of carbohydrate, fat and protein metabolism after initial catabolism in separate pathways. The condensation of acetyl CoA with oxaloacetic acid initiates the series of reactions, which result in the oxidation of the 2 acetate carbons into $CO_2$ with regeneration of CoA and oxaloacetic acid. GLYCOGENOLYSIS is the breakdown of glycogen to glucose or, in the absence of glucose-6-phosphatase, to pyruvate or lactate. GLYCOGENESIS is the synthesis of excess glucose-6-phosphate to glycogen, mostly by the liver and muscle. GLUCONEOGENESIS is the formation of glucose or glycogen from noncarbohydrate sources in the liver or to a lesser degree in the kidneys. HMS (hexose monophosphate shunt) is an alternative pathway for the utilization of glucose-6-phosphate in certain tissues including liver, adipose, and erythrocytes.

The other energy-releasing reactions involve concurrent reduction of $NAD^+$, which under aerobic conditions is reoxidized, with generation of ATP.

During the periods of limited oxygen supply, such as in the muscle during vigorous exercise, pyruvate is reduced to lactate by *lactic dehydrogenase*, using the reduced NAD as the coenzyme. Although this reduces the net supply of ATP, it can serve as an important source of energy for muscle by resupplying oxidized NAD for continuing the breakdown of glucose and ATP production (from glycolysis), which would otherwise cease due to an inability to oxidize further pyruvate and NADH.

When oxygen becomes available again, lactate can be reoxidized to pyruvate and metabolized further through the CAC. In the skeletal muscle, conversion of lactate back to pyruvate is limited. Instead, it is released into the blood and removed by the liver for reoxidation and subsequent conversion to glucose (see gluconeogenesis below). Released to the blood, this glucose becomes available to the muscle again. This recycling of glucose carbons between liver and muscle is known as the *lactic acid* or *Cori cycle*. Some pyruvate is also converted to alanine in the muscle and recycled in the same manner as lactate (both cycles are shown in Fig. 9-10).

### Oxidative decarboxylation of pyruvate

Oxidative decarboxylation of pyruvate into acetyl CoA (Fig. 9-9) under aerobic conditions links carbohydrate catabolism to the common pathway (CAC) and allows a release of the remaining energy from glucose. Decarboxylation of pyruvate involves a complex sequence of reactions in which lipoic acid and four vitamins—thiamin, pantothenic acid, riboflavin, and niacin—are required as coenzymes (TPP, CoA, FAD, NAD$^+$). Thiamin deficiency may be associated with elevated blood pyruvate levels due to an impairment in its conversion to acetyl CoA. The energy generated by this reaction is conserved as reduced NAD, with ultimate formation of ATP.

Pyruvate is produced in the cytosol but can enter the mitochondria for decarboxylation to acetyl CoA and subsequent oxidation in the CAC.

### Glycogenolysis

Glycogenolysis results in the breakdown of glycogen and is often considered as part of glycolysis, because in many tissues the end product is pyruvate or lactate instead of glucose as a result of lack of glucose-6-phosphatase. In the liver, glycogenolysis releases glucose into the blood, allowing maintenance of blood glucose from glycogen stores during the postabsorptive state. In certain inherited metabolic diseases, the glycogen storage diseases, either the synthesis of glycogen or its breakdown to glucose in the liver is defective. Consequently, individuals affected with one of these conditions show a tendency to severe hypoglycemia as well as other abnormalities. By frequent feeding of small meals containing glucose (starch) these hypoglycemic periods can be prevented.

### Glycogenesis

Glycogenesis is an anabolic pathway that converts excess glucose-6-phosphate to glycogen, which serves as a short-term storage form of carbohydrate energy. Because of the large proportion of muscle, most of the body's quantity of glycogen is found in the muscle, where it is stored during periods of high supply and utilized for the maintenance of metabolic intermediates when the supply of glucose from the blood diminishes. The liver has the highest concentration of glycogen; small amounts are found in other tissues, including adipose tissue. Although in essence the reversal of glycogenolysis, the last step in the glycogen synthesis is catalyzed by *glycogen synthetase*, whereas *phosphorylase* initiates glycogen breakdown. Both of these enzymes occur in both active and inactive states and, therefore, are important sites of metabolic control by hormones (see p. 193).

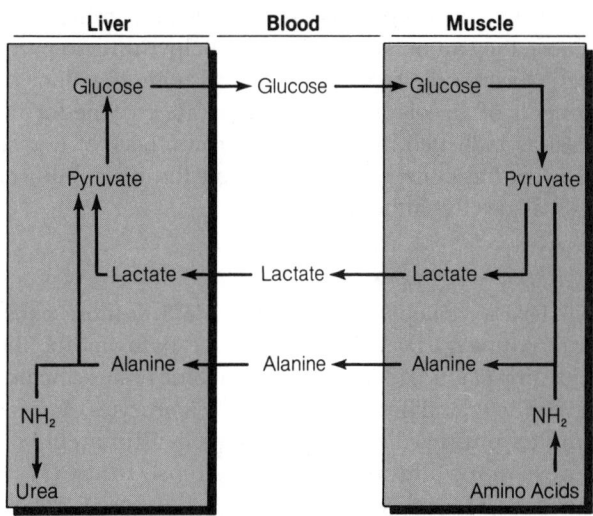

**Fig. 9-10.** The relationship between the metabolism of muscle and liver during gluconeogenesis. Note the parallelism of the lactic acid (Cori) cycle and the alanine cycle. The latter represents the major pathway by which the amino groups from muscle amino acids are conveyed to the liver for conversion to urea. (Redrawn from Bondy PK, Felig P: Disorders of carbohydrate metabolism. In Bondy PK, Rosenberg LE (eds): Duncan's Diseases of Metabolism, 7th ed, p 228. Philadelphia, WB Saunders, 1974)

### Gluconeogenesis

Gluconeogenesis refers to the formation of glucose or glycogen from noncarbohydrate sources and takes place primarily in the liver but also to a lesser extent in the kidneys. During active gluconeogenesis (in normal fasting individuals or during periods of inadequate supply of insulin in diabetics) the substrates are amino acids and lactate, primarily from the muscle, and glycerol from the adipose tissue. Only the amino acids provide new carbons for net synthesis of glucose; lactate and glycerol are products of glucose metabolism in these tissues and represent recycling of glucose carbons between the liver and the peripheral tissues. As they cannot be further used in their respective tissues under the conditions of their release, gluconeogenesis from lactate and glycerol clears the blood of these metabolites as well as provides a continuous supply of glucose for the minimal needs of the body during periods of fasting. In poorly controlled diabetics, gluconeogenesis is high even in the fed state, and contributes to hyperglycemia. Because of insulin insufficiency, catabolic conditions exist in both the muscle (protein) and the adipose tissue (triglycerides), flooding the liver with gluconeogenetic substrates. Administration of insulin reverses the process by decreasing the catabolic and increasing the anabolic reactions in the extrahepatic tissues. Insulin also decreases hepatic gluconeogenesis by depressing the key gluconeogenetic enzymes.

Essentially, gluconeogenesis is the reversal of glycolysis. As evident from Figure 9-9, oxaloacetate plays a key role in gluconeogenesis from lactate and amino acids because the reaction from phosphoenolpyruvate to pyruvate is practically irreversible. Several other reactions or segments of glycolysis require a separate enzyme for reversal as indicated by separated arrows. Lack of one or several of these enzymes is responsible for the inability of most tissues to synthesize glucose.

### Hexose monophosphate shunt

Hexose monophosphate shunt (HMS, pentose phosphate pathway) provides an alternate pathway for the utilization of glucose-6-phosphate in some tissues, including the liver, adipose tissue, and erythrocytes. It is a complex multicyclic pathway, which ultimately can achieve complete oxidation of glucose into $CO_2$ (3 glucose-6-$PO_4$ + 6 $NADP^+ \rightarrow 3CO_2$ + 2 glucose-6-$PO_4$ + glyceraldehyde-3-$PO_4$ + 6 NADPH + $6H^+$). Probably less than 10% of total glucose oxidation in the body takes place through this cycle, but it may play a more important role in the energy production in some tissues, such as erythrocytes. NADP (nicotinamide adenine dinucleotide phosphate) acts as a hydrogen acceptor in the dehydrogenation (oxidation) reactions of HMS, and 5-carbon sugars are produced as intermediates. Consequently, production of pentoses for nucleotide and nucleic acid synthesis and reduced NADP for fatty acid synthesis (p. 189) are considered two major functions of the pathway. *Transketolase*, one of the enzymes involved in the shunt, requires thiamin pyrophosphate (TPP) as the coenzyme. Measurement of erythrocyte transketolase activity with and without addition of TPP has become a useful measure in the diagnosis of thiamin deficiency.

There are other pathways that use glucose for the synthesis of many essential body components, but they account for a minor fraction of glucose utilization in comparison to the major pathways summarized in Figure 9-9.

### Utilization of galactose and fructose

Ingestion of galactose presents no problem in healthy people. In the liver it is readily converted to uridine-diphosphoglucose (UDP-glu), which can be incorporated into glycogen or converted to glucose-1-phosphate, which can then be metabolized in the pathways discussed for glucose.

1. galactose + ATP $\xrightarrow[\text{galactokinase}]{}$

   galactose-1-phosphate $\xrightarrow[\substack{\text{galactose-1-phosphate} \\ \text{uridyl transferase}}]{\text{UDP-glu}}$

   UDP-gal + glucose-1-phosphate

2. $$\text{UDP-gal} \xleftrightarrow{\quad} \text{UDP-glu} \nearrow \text{glycogen} \\ \searrow \text{glucose-1-phosphate}$$

In a congenital disorder known as *galactosemia* (see Chap. 36) the ability to metabolize galactose is impaired due to deficiency of the enzyme *gal-1-$PO_4$ uridyl transferase* required for the conversion of galactose-1-phosphate to UDP-galactose. Consequently, galactose-1-phosphate accumulates in many tissues.

The major initial step in utilization of fructose in humans is considered to be its conversion to fructose-1-phosphate by *fructokinase*. Neither the cellular entry of fructose nor the activity of fructokinase is affected by insulin.[29] Fructose-1-phosphate enters the glycolytic pathway after it is split into two 3-carbon units by an *aldolase*; the 3-carbon units also can be converted to glucose and fatty acids, and, as a result, fructose can be stored as glycogen and triglycerides.

fructose + ATP $\xrightarrow[\text{fructokinase}]{}$ fructose-1-phosphate $\xrightarrow[\text{aldolase}]{}$

glyceraldehyde + dihydroxyacetonephosphate

Because of the differences in the utilization of glucose and fructose, there has been considerable interest in the use of fructose as a sweetener in diabetic diets. Studies[29] have shown that ingestion of fructose results in lower postprandial glucose and insulin levels in both normal and noninsulin-dependent diabetic subjects than ingestion of sucrose or glucose. It also appears that less exogenous insulin may be required to maintain normal postprandial blood glucose levels in insulin-dependent diabetics after a meal containing fructose than after a meal containing sucrose. However, in poorly controlled diabetes, inadequate availability of insulin is associated with increased production of glucose and decreased conversion of fructose to glycogen and triglycerides, with resultant hyperglycemia. Because of inadequate information about possible beneficial or adverse effects from the long-term use of fructose by diabetics, its inclusion in the diabetic diets is not recommended (see Chap. 29). Hereditary deficiency of aldolase activity leads to a condition known as *fructose intolerance* (or fructosemia).

## Proteins and amino acids
### Amino acid "pools"

The amino acids of the circulating blood and interstitial fluid constitute an *extracellular* amino acid "pool," which is available to all cells for protein synthesis and other special needs. This "pool" represents a mixture of amino acids absorbed from the intestine and of those released from the *intracellular* "pools" of the tissues as a result of protein breakdown. Figure 9-11 depicts the interrelationships between the free amino acids and proteins in the major compartments of the body.

Except for a fluctuation observed during a 24-hour period, the average levels of individual amino acids in the plasma remain relatively constant under normal conditions. Flow of amino acids from intestinal absorption into the blood is balanced by the rapid removal by the tissues, especially by the liver. The cellular uptake of amino acids is accomplished by active transport, allowing for a rise in intracellular concentration of free amino acids, which then serve as the immediate supply for cellular needs. The intracellular free amino acid pool far exceeds in size the extracellular pool, which mainly serves a transport function. Factors that influence the cellular uptake and utilization of amino acids also regulate the extracellular amino acid pool. For example, administration of insulin, which increases amino acid uptake and protein synthesis in the tissues, causes a decrease in the plasma amino acids, whereas adrenal glucocorticoids increase protein breakdown in a fasting state and, subsequently, plasma amino acid levels.

### Protein turnover

Under the conditions of adequate protein intake, the body proteins in an adult are in a state of dynamic equilibrium undergoing constant breakdown of the old and synthesis of the new without an appreciable change in total body protein content. The turnover (rate of renewal) of individual proteins and tissues varies widely. The epithelial cells of the intestinal mucosa are renewed in less than 2 days, whereas the red blood cells circulate about 120 days. Of the individual proteins, serum albumin has a relatively rapid turnover, whereas the collagen of the bone matrix is replaced very slowly. The total protein renewal during any specific day represents a much higher demand for amino acids than is supplied in the diet. The balance is maintained by the recycling of endogenous amino acids from the breakdown of body proteins and the synthesis of nonessential amino acids.

### Protein reserves

There are no protein stores in the body comparable to those of fat and carbohydrate; however, some body proteins are more labile than others; that is, they are called upon to supply the amino acids required for vital cellular functions when dietary supply is inadequate. Although these proteins represent functional or structural components of the cells, instead of a special storage form, they serve as body protein reserves that can be depleted and repleted, depending on the availability of and need for amino acids. The proteins of the liver are the most labile, whereas those of the brain are spared to the end. It has been estimated that people can lose about 25% of their total body protein without a serious loss of function or threat to life.

### Plasma and serum proteins

Plasma is the liquid portion of circulating blood. The total protein content of the plasma is about 7 g to 7.5 g per dl. Clotting of blood removes the plasma protein, *fibrinogen*, which forms insoluble *fibrin* during the process of clot formation. All the other plasma proteins remain in the serum, a clear liquid that separates from the blood when the blood clots. Serum contains two major protein fractions, *albumins* and *globulins*, the latter being

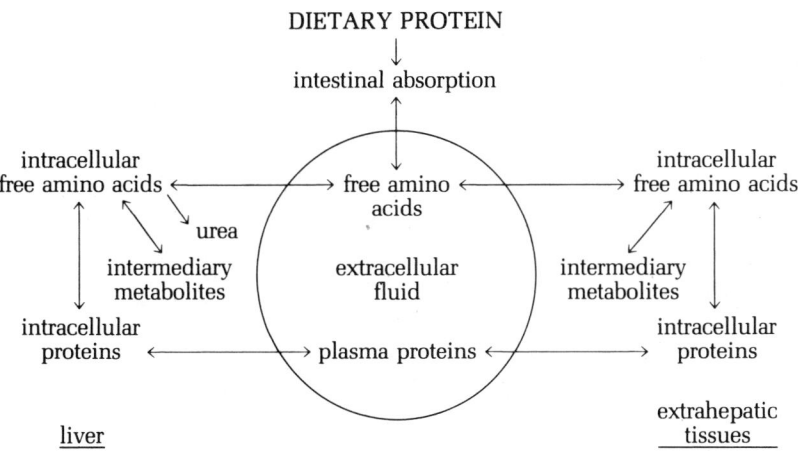

**Fig. 9-11.** Interrelations between amino acids and proteins in the major compartments of the body. The amino acids of the blood and interstitial fluid make up an extracellular amino acid pool which is available to all cells for protein synthesis and other special needs. Flow of amino acids from intestinal absorption into the blood is balanced by the rapid removal by the tissues, especially by the liver. The intracellular pool is much greater than the extracellular pool, which mainly serves a transport function. (From Felig P: Disorders of carbohydrate metabolism. In Bondy PK, Rosenberg LE (eds): Duncan's Diseases of Metabolism, 8th ed. Philadelphia, WB Saunders, 1980)

a complex mixture of simple and conjugated proteins, including glycoproteins and lipoproteins. The circulating antibodies, also known as immunoglobulins, are found in the gamma globulin fraction.

Fibrinogen is only a minor fraction of the total plasma proteins, with a normal range of 0.2 g to 0.4 g per dl. The level of plasma albumin is susceptible to nutritional influences and is often used as a measure of protein nutrition, as is the level of total plasma proteins. Other plasma transport proteins, such as transferrin, retinol-binding protein and thyroxine-binding prealbumin, also respond to changes in protein and energy intakes and may be used to assess protein-energy status in clinical situations.[30]

With the exception of gamma globulins, the serum proteins are synthesized in the liver and, consequently, low plasma protein levels are characteristic of chronic liver disease (cirrhosis). The cells of the reticuloendothelial system are believed to be the source of gamma globulins.

The albumin to globulin ratio (A:G) is altered in many disease states. Tissue destruction, inflammation, or infection is usually associated with an increase in the globulin and decrease in the albumin fraction, both of which contribute to a decrease in the A:G ratio.

### Amino acids in intermediary metabolism

When the protein intake is inadequate in total quantity or the proportion of essential amino acids required for protein synthesis, or if there is a deficit in the energy supply, the catabolism of amino acids exceeds their incorporation into tissue proteins, and a state of negative nitrogen balance results (see Chap. 4). Amino acid catabolism is also a means of using the energy from extra amino acids ingested in a high-protein diet.

In view of the number of different amino acids and the diversity of their structure, one can appreciate the great number of metabolic pathways involved in their breakdown as well as in the synthesis of nonessential ones. Again, the catabolism of one amino acid may represent the biosynthesis of another (phenylalanine→tyrosine→further degradation) and a clear line cannot be drawn between the catabolic and anabolic reactions. Discussion of the metabolism of each individual amino acid is beyond the purpose and scope of this book. Rather, the emphasis will be placed on those reactions of the amino acids that are common to most and are essential initial steps in linking protein to the common energy-yielding pathways of intermediary metabolism. In brief, the catabolism of amino acids is essentially concerned with the separation of the amino groups from the carbon skeleton and the subsequent fate of these two components.

The *carbon compounds* derived from the breakdown of individual amino acids are shown in Table 9-3 (no reactions shown). Depending on the metabolic state of the body, they may be directly oxidized into $CO_2$ and $H_2O$ with the production of ATP, or they may be first converted to glucose or fatty acids for later use or storage when excessive calories are ingested. Some may also be reincorporated into nonessential amino acids. The important fact is that once the amino group has been removed, the resulting carbon compounds enter the common "pool" of metabolic intermediates and are further handled as the products of carbohydrate or fat catabolism. It has become

### Table 9-3. Intermediary Metabolites Resulting from the Catabolism of Amino Acids (Carbon Skeletons)

| Amino Acid | Product of Catabolism | Metabolic Fate |
|---|---|---|
| Alanine | pyruvate | glycogenic |
| Arginine | α-ketoglutarate | glycogenic |
| Aspartate | fumarate | glycogenic |
| Cysteine | pyruvate | glycogenic |
| Glutamate | α-ketoglutarate | glycogenic |
| Glycine → serine | pyruvate | glycogenic |
| Histidine → glutamate | α-ketoglutarate, β-ketoglutarate | glycogenic |
| Proline ⎫ OH-proline ⎭ glutamate | α-ketoglutarate | glycogenic |
| Methionine | succinyl CoA | glycogenic |
| Serine | pyruvate | glycogenic |
| Threonine | succinyl CoA | glycogenic |
| Valine | succinyl CoA | glycogenic |
| Isoleucine | acetyl CoA, succinyl CoA | glycogenic and ketogenic |
| Lysine | α-ketoglutarate, acetyl CoA, acetoacetyl CoA | glycogenic and ketogenic |
| Phenylalanine → tyrosine | fumarate, acetyl CoA | glycogenic and ketogenic |
| Tryptophan | succinyl CoA, acetyl CoA | glycogenic and ketogenic |
| Leucine | acetyl CoA, acetoacetate | ketogenic |

a common practice to denote as *glycogenic* those amino acids that can contribute to the net synthesis of glucose, because of the nature of the carbon compounds they yield (pyruvate or intermediates of the citric acid cycle, which can be converted to glucose). Because acetyl CoA and acetoacetyl CoA are precursors of ketone bodies (and fatty acids—see p. 189) but cannot supply carbons for glucose synthesis, the amino acid yielding these compounds are know as *ketogenic*. As shown in Table 9-3, only leucine is purely ketogenic, and several others have both glycogenic and ketogenic potential.

The *amino nitrogen* is eventually excreted in the urine, mainly as urea, but small amounts are also excreted as creatinine, uric acid, and ammonia.

## Deamination of amino acids

The first step in the degradation of most amino acids is the removal of the $\alpha$-amino group. Two distinct reactions that accomplish this task are known to occur in mammalian cells. *Transamination* is the most common mechanism for amino acid deamination and involves the transfer of the amino group from one amino acid to a keto acid, with the formation of a new amino acid and a keto acid. Vitamin $B_6$ in the form of pyridoxal phosphate is required as the coenzyme in transaminations. *Oxidative deamination* with liberation of ammonia is another reaction for the conversion of amino acids to the corresponding keto acids.

Although most amino acids can participate in the transaminations, some play a more important role in total amino acid metabolism than others. The transaminases (amino transferases) are specific for one pair of amino and keto acids but nonspecific for the other. In the muscle, alanine amino transferase activity seems to be especially important. When amino acids are released from the muscle, alanine accounts for a much higher proportion of the total amino acids than it represents in muscle proteins. Synthesis by transamination of pyruvate seems to be responsible.

$$\text{amino acid} + \text{pyruvate} \overset{\substack{\text{alanine}\\\text{transaminase}}}{\rightleftharpoons} \text{keto acid} + \text{alanine}$$

Alanine is removed from blood by the liver, where pyruvate is regenerated by another transamination. The pyruvate carbons are reconverted to glucose (gluconeogenesis) and released again into the circulation. This *glucose-alanine cycle* (Figure 9-10) serves as a nontoxic carrier of nitrogen from muscle amino acid catabolism to the liver for urea synthesis.[31]

Formation of glutamate by transamination of $\alpha$-ketoglutarate is another important reaction in the sequence leading to final elimination of amino nitrogen from the body.

$$\text{amino acid} + \alpha\text{-ketoglutarate} \overset{\substack{\text{glutamate}\\\text{transaminase}}}{\rightleftharpoons} \text{keto acid} + \text{glutamate}$$

Glutamate transaminase can use alanine as well as other amino acids as substrates. Glutamate thus formed can be oxidatively deaminated with release of ammonia.

$$\text{glutamate} \overset{\substack{\text{glutamate}\\\text{dehydrogenase}}}{\rightleftharpoons} \alpha\text{-ketoglutarate} + NH_3$$

The enzyme for this deamination is very active in the liver and is believed to function in conjunction with the synthesis of carbamyl phosphate, which is the key intermediate in the conversion of ammonia to urea. Thus a series of transaminations that ultimately concentrate the amino nitrogen as glutamate prevents excessive formation of free ammonia, which is highly toxic to the central nervous system.

Deamination reactions are reversible; they synthesize amino acids from the corresponding keto acids and a nitrogen supply. The discovery that nitrogenous products from body protein catabolism could be utilized for this purpose has led to the introduction of new approaches to the treatment of the so-called nitrogen-accumulation diseases (chronic uremia and advanced liver disease).

It has now been well documented that in uremic patients, protein catabolism can be reduced and nitrogen balance maintained, with concurrent decline in the blood urea nitrogen (BUN) level, by limiting the dietary nitrogen intake to a mixture of essential amino acids[32] or to a small quantity of protein of high biologic value.[33] Presumably, nitrogenous waste products are utilized for synthesis of nonessential amino acids (see Chap. 32).

Research indicates that, with the possible exceptions of lysine and threonine, even the essential amino acids could be synthesized from endogenous nitrogen when the precursor keto acids are fed.[34] It was hoped that restricting nitrogen intake to small amounts of lysine and threonine would further improve the control of urea and ammonia production in both renal[35] and hepatic[36] nitrogen-accumulation problems. The results have been variable, with both beneficial effects[37,38] and lack of effects[39] reported in uremic patients. More research is needed to clarify fully the metabolic changes that are produced by the keto acids[40] and to appraise their role in the overall dietary management of disease.[41]

## Urea synthesis

Ammonia formed by the oxidative deamination of the amino acids normally is rapidly removed by conversion to less toxic excretory products, the major one in humans being urea. Only liver is capable of urea synthesis. The nitrogen is channeled to the cycle through carbamyl

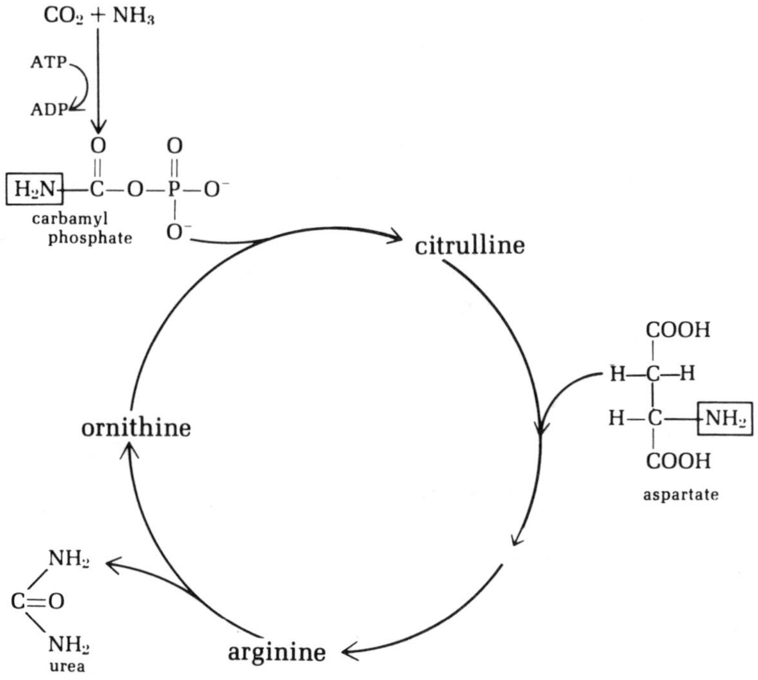

CO$_2$ + NH$_3$

ATP

ADP

O    O
‖    ‖
H$_2$N—C—O—P—O$^-$
         |
         O$^-$
carbamyl
phosphate

citrulline

COOH
|
H—C—H
|
H—C—NH$_2$
|
COOH

aspartate

ornithine

NH$_2$
|
C=O
|
NH$_2$
urea

arginine

**Fig. 9-12.** Formation of urea by the Krebs-Henseleit cycle.

phosphate and aspartate (Fig. 9-12). Energy is required for the functioning of this cycle, which can also serve as a mechanism for synthesis of the amino acid arginine.

It should be noted that the formation of carbamyl phosphate utilizes not only ammonia but also CO$_2$, another metabolic waste product. In addition to urea synthesis, carbamyl phosphate is used for the synthesis of the pyrimidine bases, which are further incorporated into nucleic acids.

When liver function is severely impaired, as in advanced cirrhosis, the urea formation is inadequate, and toxic levels of ammonia accumulate in the tissues unless protein intake is restricted (see Chap. 33).

### Glutamine synthesis

Another means of detoxifying and transporting ammonia produced in the cells is by the synthesis of glutamine, as shown below.

$$\text{glutamic acid} + \text{NH}_3 \underset{\text{glutaminase}}{\overset{\substack{\text{glutamine}\\\text{synthetase}}}{\rightleftharpoons}} \text{glutamine}$$

The reaction is reversible but requires a separate enzyme. Glutamine synthesis and breakdown are especially important in the kidneys where they function in the maintenance of the acid–base balance and in the conservation of cations. In metabolic acidosis glutaminase releases ammonia from glutamine. It is secreted into the tubules where it is converted to the ammonium ion (NH$_4^+$) and excreted in the urine as ammonium salts. In addition to removing excess H$^+$ from the body, excretion of the ammonium ion conserves K$^+$ and Na$^+$, which otherwise would be excreted with the acidic anions.

Glutamine released from the muscle also is taken up by the intestinal tissue where it is converted back to glutamate and alanine (from pyruvate). Alanine is released to the portal circulation and removed by the liver; following deamination, the carbons are used in gluconeogenesis, and the nitrogen is converted to urea.[28]

The fact that glutamine levels of the blood are generally high in comparison with levels of other amino acids supports its postulated role in the transport of ammonia from the tissues.

### Other uses of amino acids

In addition to their role in protein synthesis, energy production, and gluconeogenesis, many amino acids serve as precursors for synthesis of other biologically important compounds. *Glycine* is used for the biosynthesis of purines (nucleic acids), porphyrin (heme), creatine (Fig. 9-13), glutathione,* and conjugated bile salts (p. 163). *Phenylalanine* is converted to *tyrosine* as a first step in its catabolism. When the enzyme, phenylalanine hydroxylase, required for this conversion, is missing, a condition known as *phenylketonuria* results (Chap. 36). Several other enzymatic defects involving the metabolism of phenylalanine and tyrosine are also known. Tyrosine serves as a direct precursor of the hormones, *epinephrine, norepinephrine,* and *thyroxine,* and of *melanin* pigment, found in the skin and hair. *Tryptophan* catabolism may involve several alternate pathways. Formation of 5-hydroxytryptophan followed by decarboxylation yields 5-hydroxytryptamine, or *serotonin,* a potent vasoconstrictor and a

---

* A tripeptide, composed of glutamic acid, cysteine, and glycine, which serves as an activator of many enzymes.

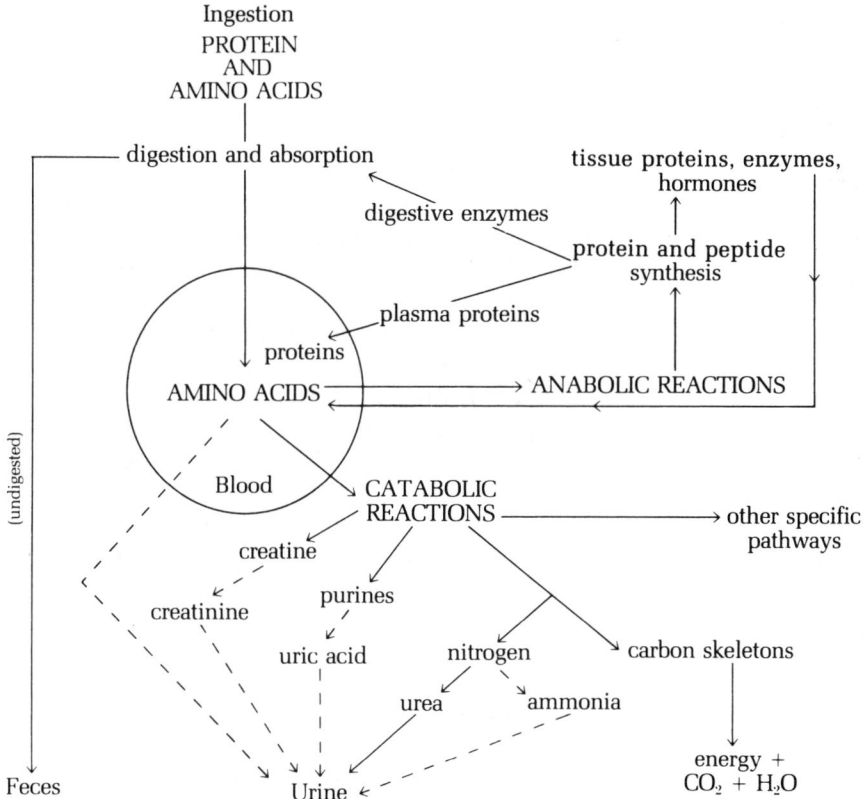

**Fig. 9-13.** General metabolic interrelations of amino acids and proteins. Ingested protein reaches the blood as amino acids. From this extracellular amino acid pool (including the interstitial fluid), they are actively removed by the tissues and concentrated in their intracellular pools, where they become mixed with the amino acids released from the cellular breakdown of protein. In fed state, the incorporation of amino acids into proteins is faster than their release, resulting in net increase of tissue protein. During periods of fasting or inadequate protein intake, the breakdown of protein in the tissues is high, leading to an increased release of amino acids into the extracellular pool. Under such conditions amino acid catabolism in the tissues is high. The carbon skeletons are utilized for energy production and the nitrogen is excreted in the urine, mainly as urea.

stimulator of smooth muscle contraction. Serotonin is formed in the brain, but its function in that tissue remains unknown. Tryptophan can also be converted to nicotinic acid (niacin—see Chap. 8). *Histidine* decarboxylation yields *histamine*, another physiologically active amine. Histamine stimulates the production of HCl by the gastric mucosa and is also a powerful vasodilator. It may be used in treating various allergies.

*Glutamic acid* decarboxylation produces *γ-amino-butyric acid* (GABA) which acts as a regulator in the tissues of the central nervous system. *Methionine* can be activated by ATP to form S-adenosyl methionine, which functions as a donor of methyl ($CH_3$) groups in various transmethylation reactions, including the synthesis of choline and creatine.

**Protein synthesis**

The ability to produce the many different kinds of proteins needed by the body is determined by the pattern for protein synthesis, which is carried in the DNA (deoxy-

ribonucleic acid) of the cell's nucleus. Because this pattern is genetically determined, the various diseases that result from enzyme deficiencies are often referred to as "inborn errors of metabolism" (Chap. 36). For each protein a set of directions is carried on a specific segment, a gene, of the very long DNA molecule.

The DNA itself does not leave the nucleus, but in a process called *transcription* its message is copied to a specific type of RNA (ribonucleic acid—messenger-RNA, or m-RNA), which carries the information to the site of protein synthesis. Each of these messenger-RNAs binds several ribosomes (particles composed of so-called ribosomal RNA and protein and located in the endoplasmic reticulum of the cell) into a polysome, which then serves as a template or pattern for the assembly of amino acids into a protein.

Another type of RNA, transfer-RNA (also known as t-RNA or soluble RNA) not only recognizes a specific amino acid in the cytoplasm, but, after carrying it to the site of protein synthesis, interprets the code carried in the messenger-RNA (*translation*) and delivers the amino acid to its proper place in the sequence required to form a specific protein. The actual assembly of a protein molecule on the polysome also requires initiation, chain elongation, and termination factors. The synthesis of the different types of RNA takes place in the cell nucleus and is subject to hormonal regulation.

Because the cells of the body are constantly manufacturing a wide variety of proteins, the need for a regular supply of the essential amino acids becomes obvious.

The general metabolic interrelations of amino acids and proteins from ingestion to excretion are summarized in Figure 9-13.

## Fats and other lipids

### Blood lipids and lipoproteins

Oxidation of fat—obtained through intestinal absorption and, during fasting, from adipose tissue—accounts for a sizable fraction of total energy production. It is no wonder then that the transport of lipids in the blood plays an important role in energy metabolism. The major forms of lipid found in normal plasma or serum are triglycerides, cholesterol, phospholipids, and free or non-esterified fatty acids (FFA, NEFA). Their origin and lipoprotein carriers are shown in Figure 9-14 (see also Chap. 3 for composition of the different lipoproteins).

### Chylomicrons

Chylomicrons contain most of the triglycerides of nonfasting plasma and transport exogenous triglycerides and cholesterol from the intestinal mucosa, where they are formed during absorption of fat, to the other body tissues for utilization. They are the largest and least dense of the blood lipoproteins, and their presence gives a milky appearance to the serum. Consequently, their removal by the tissues is often referred to as *clearing*. After ingestion of a fat-containing meal, the chylomicron concentration in the blood reaches its peak in about 4 hours and normally is cleared by 8 to 10 hours, varying from person to person and depending on the amount of fat ingested. If chylomicrons are present in plasma after a 12-hour fast, defective clearance is suspected, as is seen in a rare familial defect known as type I *hyperlipoproteinemia* (see Chap. 30).

Removal of chylomicron triglycerides by the tissues involves hydrolysis into fatty acids by *lipoprotein lipase* followed by cellular uptake of the fatty acids. Lipoprotein lipase is a membrane-bound enzyme, which is believed to be present either at the cell surface or in the walls of the blood capillaries supplying the tissues. It is released and activated by administration of heparin, a natural anticoagulant found in the body. Measurement of postheparin lipolytic activity (PHLA) is a common test for lipoprotein lipase activity.

Adipose tissue is the major site of chylomicron triglyceride uptake, although other tissues are known to have lipoprotein lipase activity. The chylomicron remnants are rapidly removed by the liver.

### The very low-density lipoproteins

The very low-density lipoproteins (VLDL, prebeta lipoproteins) are synthesized mainly in the liver but also to a lesser extent in the intestine and transport endogenous triglycerides. Most of the fasting blood triglyceride is accounted for by this lipoprotein fraction. Because of the much larger amounts carried in the chylomicrons, determination of total triglycerides in nonfasting plasma has little value; the nonfasting level varies with the amount and time of fat ingestion. A high level of VLDL is usually responsible for elevation of serum triglycerides in the fasting state. The fatty acids found in the VLDL triglycerides represent two main sources: nonesterified fatty acids (NEFA) from adipose tissue triglyceride breakdown and biosynthesis in the liver from nonlipid precursors, mainly glucose.

The dietary components that most consistently influence the level of circulating VLDL are total calories and carbohydrates.[42] Weight gain is usually associated with an elevation and weight loss with a reduction in VLDL triglycerides in the blood. Ingestion of a very high carbohydrate diet (about 75% of total calories) causes transient elevation of VLDL in most individuals, whereas even normal carbohydrate intake has the same effect in so-called carbohydrate sensitivity.[43] The cause for this sensitivity is not known. Although there is some evidence that the simple sugars, especially fructose and sucrose, may have a greater effect than complex carbohydrates in elevating the VLDL levels in the rat, this does not appear to be true in humans.[24,43] It should be emphasized that the populations that generally ingest a high carbohydrate (starch) diet show low average VLDL and total triglyceride levels.

The VLDL triglycerides are also cleared from the blood by the action of lipoprotein lipase, as discussed in connection with chylomicrons.

### The intermediate-density lipoproteins

The intermediate-density lipoproteins (IDL, broad beta lipoproteins) represent an intermediate in the breakdown of the VLDL and usually are not considered a separate lipoprotein class. They normally have a rapid turnover (2 hr–6 hr) but are found to accumulate in people affected by a genetic hyperlipoproteinemia known as Type III (see Chap. 30).[44]

### The low-density lipoproteins

The low-density lipoproteins (LDL, beta lipoproteins) originate in the liver but are believed to be formed from the VLDL remnants (IDL) after further removal of lipid and protein rather than by *de novo* synthesis. This lipoprotein fraction is a normal component of fasting plasma, accounting for about 65% to 75% of total serum cholesterol, and is usually elevated in people with hypercholesterolemia (see Chap. 30). Of the dietary factors, high cholesterol and saturated fat intake are most likely to be associated with an elevation in the level of LDL. These lipoproteins are believed to carry cholesterol to the peripheral tissues, where their degradation is followed by release of unesterified cholesterol for cellular use. Excess cholesterol, either from LDL or cellular synthesis, is released to the cell surface, where it may be incorporated into HDL.[45]

### The high-density lipoproteins

The high-density lipoproteins (HDL, alpha lipoproteins) consist mostly of proteins, phospholipids, and cholesterol, and their function in the body is still uncertain. The initial particles are formed mainly in the liver, but their formation is completed in the circulation, where they may remove free cholesterol from the cell membranes. Esterification of this cholesterol by the lecithin-cholesterol acyltransferase (LCAT) uses HDL lecithin, which is converted to lysolecithin in the process. Some of the esterified cholesterol may be transferred to the VLDL and some taken to the liver for degradation (by conversion to bile acids) or excretion (in bile). Thus HDL may function to transfer cholesterol from the extrahepatic tissues to the liver.[45] High concentration of HDL is associated with a reduced risk of cardiovascular disease, whereas high concentration of LDL is one of the major risk factors in the development of atherosclerosis.[46-48] HDL concentration is not altered by changes in the diet but is known to be increased by estrogens (level is higher in young women than in men), by physical activity, and by moderate intake of alcohol.[45]

### The nonesterified fatty acids

The nonesterified fatty acids (NEFA) are released as a result of adipose tissue lipolysis and circulate bound to serum albumin. They constitute the most metabolically active fraction of blood lipids, although their concentration at any one time is very low. Their release from the adipose tissue is followed by a rapid uptake by other tissues, allowing a large quantity of fatty acids to pass through the blood in this form daily. Under the conditions of excessive adipose tissue lipolysis, such as in uncontrolled diabetes or after administration of lipolytic hormones, the uptake and utilization of fatty acids by the liver are increased. Consequent stimulation of VLDL synthesis can lead to hyperglyceridemia, which is secondary to adipose tissue fat mobilization.

### Blood lipid levels

It is obvious that the total level of individual blood lipids represents the sum total found in the different lipoprotein fractions. In recent years their possible role in

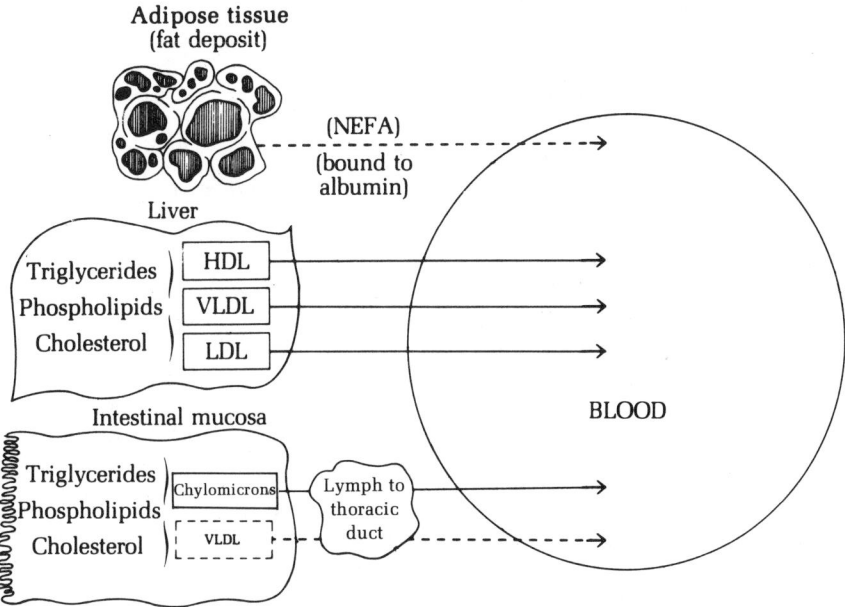

**Fig. 9-14.** Simplified schematic representation of sources of plasma lipids. The major forms of lipid found in the blood are triglycerides, cholesterol, phospholipids and nonesterified fatty acids (NEFA). Their origins, adipose tissue, liver and intestinal mucosa, are shown with their lipoprotein carriers. (HDL = high-density lipoprotein or alpha lipoprotein; VLDL = very low-density lipoprotein or prebeta lipoprotein; LDL = low-density lipoprotein or beta lipoprotein) (Redrawn from Lipids . . . in Brief, 2nd ed., with permission of Ayerst Laboratories)

the development of cardiovascular disease has generated great interest in the blood lipid levels, not only among professionals but the public as well. Fasting levels of both cholesterol and triglyceride are relatively constant in any one person, but wide variations exist within any population and in the average levels among populations. As is true with body weight, the average blood lipid levels tend to increase with age. The desirability of this change is being questioned. Sex differences are also evident, men generally showing higher blood lipid levels than women during the first 5 decades of life. One may speak about "normal" values, but these usually refer to averages or common ranges, which include a sizable proportion of the apparently healthy population. Such a range for serum triglycerides in an adult is 50 to 150 mg per dl, and for cholesterol, 150 to 250 mg per dl. Although we do not know what the optimum levels are from the standpoint of health, there is a considerable body of experimental evidence showing that a relatively small risk of cardiovascular disease is associated with cholesterol levels of 200 mg per dl or below and with triglyceride levels of 125 mg per dl or below. It should be emphasized that these levels do not represent cutoff points with a high risk above and a

low risk below; the blood lipid levels, especially cholesterol, have a continuous relationship to the risk of cardiovascular disease (CVD). A more detailed discussion of blood lipids and CVD in relation to diet is found in Chapter 30.

### Release of energy from fats

About 90% of the total energy value of fat is held in the fatty acids and the remainder in the glycerol moiety of the triglyceride molecules.

#### Oxidation of fatty acids

In order for the energy of fatty acids to be used, they must first be activated by formation of acyl CoA, which then can undergo a series of *β-oxidations*. Each of these results in a release of one 2-carbon unit as acetyl CoA and acyl CoA, which is 2 carbons shorter than the original fatty acid. A schematic representation of oxidation of palmitic acid (C16:0) is shown in Figure 9-15.

The initial activation of long chain fatty acids is extramitochondrial; they cannot penetrate the mitochondrial membranes to reach the oxidizing enzymes without facilitation by *carnitine* (β-hydroxy-γ-trimethylammo-

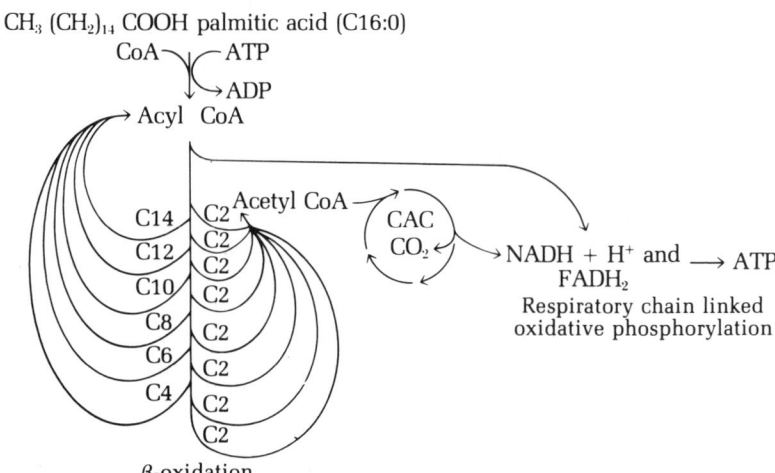

**Fig. 9-15.** Schematic representation of energy production from fatty acids, using palmitic acid as an example. Palmitic acid (C:16) undergoes β-oxidation seven times, yielding 8 acetyl CoAs (two from the last cycle). Each turn of the cycle results in reduction of one FAD and one NAD, which are equivalent to 5 ATPs when reoxidized. With one ATP consumed in the activation, the total yield from β-oxidation of palmitate is 34 ATPs ($7 \times 5 - 1 = 34$). Further oxidation of each acetyl CoA in the citric acid cycle (CAC) liberates the remaining energy through the respiratory chain linked oxidative phosphorylation; 12 ATPs for each acetyl CoA, with a total production of 96 ATPs ($8 \times 12$). The energy value of a mole of ATP is estimated to be 7.6 kcal. and the combustion of a mole of palmitate in a calorimeter yields 2340 kcal. Therefore, the efficiency of the biologic oxidation of palmitate is 42%.

$$\left( \frac{130 \times 7.6}{2340} \times 100 \right)$$

Most fatty acids contain an even number of carbons and thus yield only acetyl CoA as a result of β-oxidation. Odd numbered fatty acids follow the same system but the final cycle (not shown) yields 1 acetyl CoA and 1 propionyl CoA. Propionyl CoA is converted to succinyl CoA and enters the CAC, thus contributing substrate to gluconeogenesis.

nium butyrate). Carnitine acyl transferase transfers the acyl group from CoA to carnitine present in the membranes. The resulting acyl carnitine penetrates the membranes and, once inside mitochondria, the acyl group is transferred back to CoA.

Just as was true with glycolysis in catabolism of glucose, β-oxidation releases only a small portion (about one-quarter) of total energy available in the fatty acid molecule. The remainder is held in acetyl CoA and released upon its oxidation by the CAC. Most of the common fatty acids contain an even number of carbons and yield only acetyl CoA as a result of β-oxidation. Odd-numbered fatty acids can be oxidized in the same system, but the final cycle yields one acetyl CoA and one propionyl CoA. Propionyl CoA is converted to succinyl CoA, which is part of the CAC; therefore, the fatty acids with uneven carbon numbers contribute substrates to gluconeogenesis, whereas the even-numbered fatty acids do not.

### Fate of glycerol

The glycerol portion of the triglyceride molecule is also glycogenic, as was discussed earlier. It can also be metabolized through glycolysis without first being converted to glucose (see Fig. 9-9). The first step in the metabolism of glycerol is its conversion to α-glycerophosphate by *glycerokinase*. Because of the low activity of this enzyme in most tissues, liver is the major site of glycerol metabolism. Alpha-glycerophosphate can also be reincorporated into triglycerides, but under the conditions of high glycerol production from triglyceride breakdown, gluconeogenesis in the liver is the principal route of glycerol metabolism.

### Lipid synthesis
### Triglyceride synthesis

Triglyceride synthesis and deposition in the adipose tissue result in the storage of excess energy in the body regardless of the form in which it is ingested.

Liver, adipose tissue, and intestinal mucosa are the major sites of triglyceride synthesis. Each can activate fatty acids to acyl CoA, from which they are esterified with glycerol, starting with α-glycerophosphate. Although adequate glycerokinase activity is present in the liver, the major source of α-glycerophosphate for triglyceride synthesis in all tissues is glucose metabolism. Triglyceride synthesis is stimulated in the fed state when availability of glucose is high. It is low during fasting, the oxidation of fatty acids for energy being favored over their incorporation into triglyceride.

### De novo synthesis of fatty acids

De novo synthesis of fatty acids involves building the carbon chain from 2-carbon units, starting with one acetyl CoA as a primer and proceeding through successive additions by means of malonyl CoA, which is formed from acetyl CoA by the addition of $CO_2$. In the transfer of the 2-carbon units from malonyl CoA, the $CO_2$ is released again. Because of the need for malonyl CoA as an "active" intermediate in fatty acid synthesis, the pathway is often referred to as the malonyl CoA pathway. Two B-vitamins are required in fatty acid synthesis: biotin, which participates in the formation of malonyl CoA (as well as in other carboxylations), and niacin in the form of reduced NADP, which is required in the reductions following each 2-carbon addition. The major source of acetyl CoA for fatty acid synthesis is glucose, but excess dietary amino acids may also provide it. Therefore, fatty acid synthesis from acetyl CoA is stimulated by high caloric intake, and it represents one of the major steps in the conversion of excess energy into adipose tissue triglycerides.

The actual incorporation of the 2-carbon units into a fatty acid is a complex sequence of reactions which, as part of the multienzyme fatty acid synthetase complex, involves a pantothenic acid containing acyl carrier protein to which the substrates are transferred from CoA. Just as in the oxidation of fatty acids, the location of the substrate (acetyl CoA) and the enzyme (fatty acid synthetase) in different cellular compartments requires additional reactions to bring the two together. Acetyl CoA used for fatty acid synthesis is mainly produced from pyruvate in the mitochondria (by oxidative decarboxylation), whereas the fatty acid synthetase complex is present in the cytosol. Because acetyl CoA cannot leave the mitochondrion, it condenses with oxaloacetate to form citrate (see Fig. 9-7), which then is transported to the cytosol and cleaved to regenerate acetyl CoA and OAA. Fatty acid synthesis provides a good example of the regulation of a metabolic pathway by the availability of its substrates and products, and, ultimately, by food intake. Figure 9-16 shows a highly simplified scheme of the major conversions involved in lipogenesis and their regulation.

*Chain elongation* of existing fatty acids provides a means of increasing the chain length by addition of 2-carbon units until a desired length is reached. This mechanism does not produce a net increase in fatty acid, but it allows the body to alter its fatty acid composition according to its need.

*Desaturation* of fatty acids (formation of a double bond) is another means of altering the fatty acids available to satisfy the needs of the body. For example, the monounsaturated oleic acid (C18:1) is formed from stearic acid (C18:0). Polyunsaturated fatty acids are also synthesized from existing unsaturated fatty acids. Linoleic acid (C18:2) is converted to arachidonic acid (C20:4) by initial desaturation (removal of two hydrogens) and addition of a 2-carbon unit, followed by another desaturation. Because of the specificity of the enzyme system for locations at which the desaturation can take place, the structure of the unsaturated precursor deter-

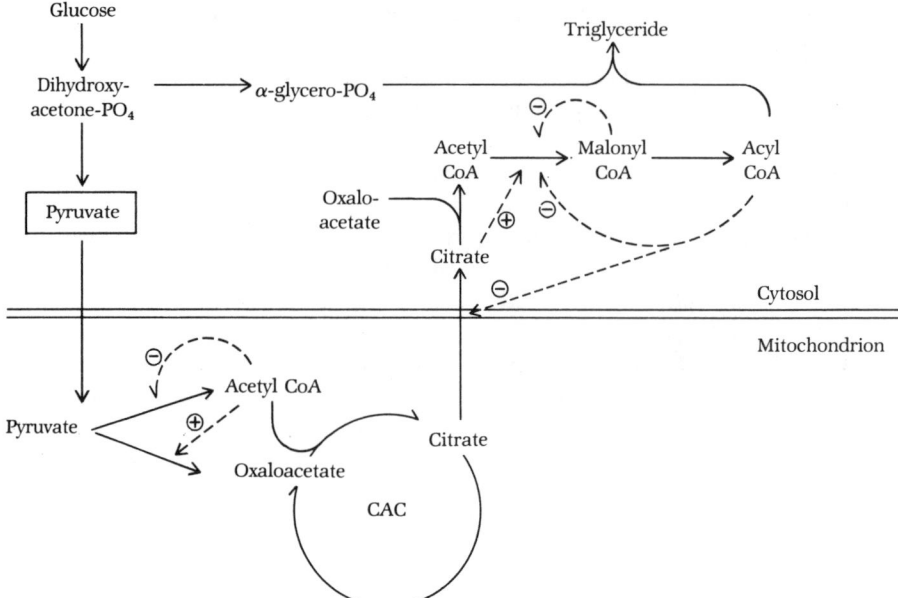

**Fig. 9-16.** Simplified presentation of lipogenesis. Fatty acid synthesis is high in fed state when more glucose is available than is needed. Pyruvate produced from glycolysis is converted to acetyl CoA and oxaloacetate in the mitochondria. Excess citrate is transported to the cytosol where it is cleaved to regenerate oxaloacetate and acetyl CoA to provide substrate for fatty acid synthesis. The broken arrows identify the major steps that are regulated by the availability of substrate or accumulation of products. High rate of triglyceride synthesis in fed state prevents the powerful feedback inhibition that free fatty acids have on lipogenesis from glucose. High level of circulating free fatty acids during fasting and on high-fat diets practically shuts off lipogenesis from glucose. Acetyl CoA stimulates the conversion of pyruvate to OAA needed for its further metabolism.

mines the location of the new double bonds. Linoleic acid cannot be synthesized because no precursor is available in the body.

### Cholesterol synthesis

Cholesterol, a structural component in all cellular membranes, can be synthesized in all tissues. Biosynthesis from acetyl CoA in the liver and, possibly, in the intestine contributes to the circulating (serum) cholesterol, as does dietary intake.[49] Cholesterol ingestion exerts a negative feedback control on hepatic but not on intestinal cholesterol production.[49] Unfortunately, this mechanism is not adequate to prevent elevation of serum cholesterol induced by high influx of dietary cholesterol. With increased cholesterol intake, the maximal suppression of synthesis observed in whites in the United States is about 25% compared to a cholesterol-free diet, whereas 36% supression has been reported for Alaskan Eskimos and 50% for African Masai.[50] On the other hand, because of the incompleteness of this feedback mechanism, decreasing dietary cholesterol intake to below 300 mg per day results in a fall of serum cholesterol despite the stimulation in hepatic cholesterol production. As previously mentioned, the major mechanism for cholesterol degradation is its conversion into bile acids in the liver.

## Metabolic interrelationships among carbohydrate, protein, and fat in the major tissues of the body

Adipose tissue, liver, and muscle are the three major tissues that maintain the metabolic homeostasis in the body, despite the differences in their individual functions and metabolic machinery. The major factors that determine the metabolic state of these tissues are the availability of glucose and the level of insulin relative to other hormones that oppose its actions.

### Adipose tissue

Instead of being a static storage area for energy, the adipose tissue is metabolically very active and exerts a profound influence on the metabolic balance of the body. Like the proteins of muscle, the adipose tissue triglycerides are in a dynamic equilibrium, with continuous breakdown and resynthesis taking place without any appreciable change in the total fat content. During the normal course of a 24-hour day there are periods when the triglyceride synthesis exceeds the breakdown and vice versa.

In the fed state when the supply of glucose is plentiful, its utilization in all metabolic pathways in the adipose tissue is high. Under these conditions triglyceride synthesis is favored over breakdown in several ways. First, glucose oxidation in the CAC provides a large proportion of the energy needs, thereby minimizing fatty acid oxidation and directing fatty acids to triglyceride synthesis. Second, the ample supply of glucose also provides adequate amounts of $\alpha$-glycerophosphate for fatty acid re-esterification. Due to low glycerokinase activity, the glycerol released from triglyceride breakdown cannot be reused in the adipose tissue. It is released into the blood and metabolized in the liver. Third, the high rate of glucose breakdown also provides more acetyl CoA than is needed for immediate energy needs, the excess providing substrate for fatty acid synthesis. This lipogenesis serves as a means of storing carbohydrate and protein energy for the periods when intestinal absorption is not delivering nutrients to the body. The same mechanism is responsible for weight gain if more triglyceride is stored than is mobilized to supply the daily energy needs. Finally, oxidation of glucose in the hexose monophosphate shunt yields reduced NADP (nicotinamide adenine dinucleotide phosphate), which is required for fatty acid synthesis from acetyl CoA.

In the postabsorptive state (fasting) the supply of glucose to adipose cells is low, and its utilization in all pathways is reduced. Even though a high proportion of the available glucose reverts to production of $\alpha$-glycerophosphate, it is not sufficient for the triglyceride synthesis to keep up with its breakdown, and fatty acids are released into the blood as NEFA. This fat mobilization is a normal mechanism for supplying the body tissues with a source of energy when blood glucose is low. Some of the NEFA is directly removed by muscle and other tissues, whereas some is first resynthesized into VLDL triglycerides in the liver. The latter activity especially occurs when excessive mobilization of fat takes place, leading to secondary hyperglyceridemia.

Insulin has a major influence on the metabolism of adipose tissue. A high level of circulating insulin such as that found in the normal fed state facilitates the uptake of glucose and, secondarily, favors triglyceride synthesis. Insulin also has a direct influence on the adipose tissue triglyceride storage. The first step in lipolysis (TG→DG) is catalyzed by an enzyme known as *hormone-sensitive lipase*. Insulin inhibits the activity of this enzyme, whereas several other hormones stimulate its lipolytic activity. Figure 9-17 shows the interrelationships of the major metabolic pathways in the adipose tissue and the hormonal influence on fat mobilization.

In the fed state the influence of insulin prevails over the lipolytic action of the opposing hormones, and fat storage takes place. When insulin activity is low (fasting), lipolysis is favored and adipose tissue fat is mobilized according to the needs of the body, in a controlled fashion. In conditions of hormonal imbalance, such as insulin insufficiency in untreated diabetes, fat mobilization continues uncontrolled. Although the blood glucose level is very high due to its inability to enter adipose and muscle cells without adequate insulin, the "message" to the adipose cell is to mobilize the energy stores. Lack of $\alpha$-glycerophosphate in the cell reduces the capacity for re-esterification of fatty acids and they are released into the blood.

## Muscle

Both glucose and fatty acids are normally oxidized in the muscle, the proportion of each at any one time depending on the metabolic state of the body and its nutrient supply. When glucose is plentiful its uptake is high, and it is converted to glycogen as well as used for energy production along with fatty acids. The amino acid uptake is also high, stimulated by the relatively high level of circulating insulin, and active protein synthesis takes place.

When blood glucose and insulin levels drop in the postabsorptive state, fatty acid uptake and oxidation increase with corresponding decrease in glucose uptake and utilization. This reciprocal relationship between glucose and fatty acid utilization in the muscle and adipose tissue has been attributed to the existence of a so-called glucose-fatty acid cycle proposed by Randle and co-workers.[51] According to this concept the high levels of NEFA and their oxidation products suppress the uptake and catabolism of glucose during carbohydrate deprivation, and, conversely, ingestion of carbohydrate with consequent increase in insulin level promptly reduces fatty acid release from the adipose tissue.

During the early postabsorptive period glycogenolysis provides intermediates for the CAC to allow complete oxidation of fatty acids. When fasting continues, glycogen stores become depleted, and protein breakdown increases, releasing amino acids into the blood. As with fat mobilization in adipose tissue, the protein catabolism in muscle is under control and represents a normal response to provide substrates for gluconeogenesis in the liver, allowing maintenance of a blood glucose level that satisfies the minimal needs of the body. In untreated diabetes mellitus the amino acid mobilization is excessive, resulting in wasting of body tissues.

## Liver

The liver plays a central role in the many homeostatic mechanisms of the body. When the flow of glucose from intestinal absorption is high, the glycogen stores of the liver are being filled, lipogenesis from glucose-derived acetyl CoA is active, and amino acids are incorporated into proteins. Glycogenolysis, lipolysis, and gluconeogenesis are minimal. Hormonal balance and substrate levels again exert a controlling influence in these metabolic events. The activity of insulin is high relative to the hormones, which oppose its actions, and anabolism prevails.

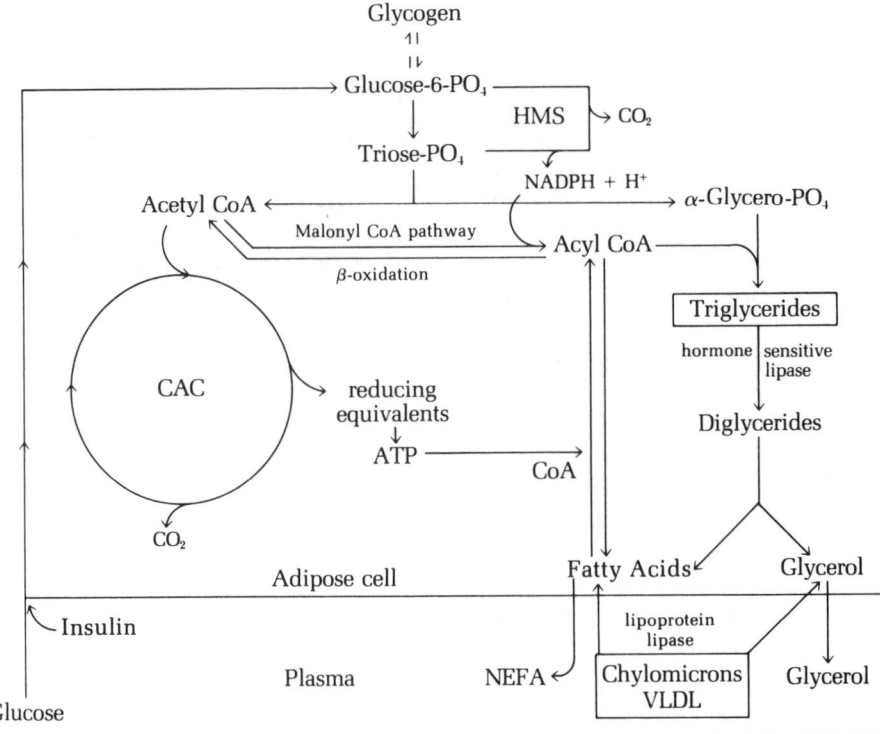

**Fig. 9-17.** The major metabolic pathways of the adipose tissue. Hormone-sensitive lipase is activated by several hormones including epinephrine, norepinephrine, glucagon, ACTH (adrenocorticotropic hormone), and TSH (thyroid-stimulating hormone), whereas insulin inhibits it. In fed state, the uptake of fatty acids from chylomicron triglycerides by the adipose tissue is high. The level of insulin is also high, resulting in low lipolytic activity and increased uptake and utilization of glucose by the adipose tissue. Under such conditions, glucose not only provides energy, but also supplies precursors for fatty acid and triglyceride synthesis (acetyl CoA, NADPH + H$^+$, and $\alpha$-glycerophosphate). Therefore, the synthesis of triglycerides exceeds the breakdown, and storage of energy as adipose tissue triglycerides takes place. In fasting state the level of insulin and the availability of glucose and fatty acids to the adipose tissue are low. Triglyceride breakdown is stimulated by the action of the lipolytic hormones and fatty acids (as NEFA) and glycerol are released into the blood. Thus adipose tissue fat is mobilized to provide energy to the body during the periods when nutrients are not supplied by ingestion of food. (HMS = hexose monophosphate shunt; CAC = citric acid cycle; NADP = nicotinamide adenine dinucleotide phosphate; CoA = coenzyme A; ATP = adenosine triphosphate; NEFA = nonesterified fatty acids; VLDL = very low density lipoproteins)

When the blood glucose and insulin levels fall in the postabsorptive state, glycogenolysis increases and glucose is released into the circulation. With the reduction of glycogen stores, amino acid uptake and conversion to glucose increase. Glucose breakdown by glycolysis diminishes whereas the fatty acid uptake and $\beta$-oxidation accelerate. All of these adjustments contribute to maintenance of blood glucose levels and provide a continuous supply of glucose to the tissues that most depend on it. Figure 9-18 summarizes the balance of glucose and glucose precursors in postabsorptive humans.

### Ketosis

When fat mobilization from adipose tissue is high, $\beta$-oxidation of fatty acids in the liver produces more acetyl CoA than can be oxidized in the CAC or used for synthetic purposes. The high concentration of fatty acids and low relative insulin activity seem to inhibit both the activity of the CAC and the conversion of acetyl CoA into fatty acids as well as the conversion of the latter to triglycerides.

Under such conditions a high proportion of acetyl CoA is converted to acetoacetate, which is further converted to $\beta$-hydroxybutyrate and acetone, all of which are known as *ketone bodies* and are released into the blood. Ketone bodies are normal metabolites, which are usually oxidized by the extrahepatic tissues at a rate comparable to their production in the liver. When the production is excessive, as in prolonged fasting and in untreated diabetes, the ketone bodies accumulate in the blood (ketonemia) and spill into the urine (ketonuria), a condition known as *ketosis*. Decreased utilization of ketone bodies appears to be a contributing factor in the ketonemia during fasting.[52] Ketoacidosis is a result of severe ketosis with concurrent loss of base from the body, leading to a drop in blood *p*H. Carbohydrate metabolism in the cells seems to be necessary for clearance of ketone bodies from the blood. Mild ketosis, observed when dietary carbohydrate is restricted to a very low level (as advocated for some reducing diets), is promptly reversed by increasing carbohydrate intake. Administration of insulin to a diabetic has a comparable effect. The antiketogenic effects of insulin and carbohydrate are due more to a decreased production of acetyl CoA from β-oxidation of fatty acids than to an increased utilization of ketone bodies.[53]

### Hormonal regulation of metabolism

It is obvious from the preceding discussions that the balance between the catabolic and anabolic reactions in the body tissues is influenced by hormones. Detailed discussion of the actions of individual hormones is beyond the purpose of this book. Only the major directions of such hormonal control are summarized in order to emphasize the complex integration of the many mechanisms and tissues that are involved in the maintenence of metabolic balance in the body.

*Insulin* is probably the only hormone that has an anabolic effect in each of its target tissues and influences the metabolism of each of the body fuels. Table 9-4 summarizes the metabolic activity of carbohydrate, protein, and fat in normal fed and fasting states, which are characterized by high and low insulin activity, respectively.

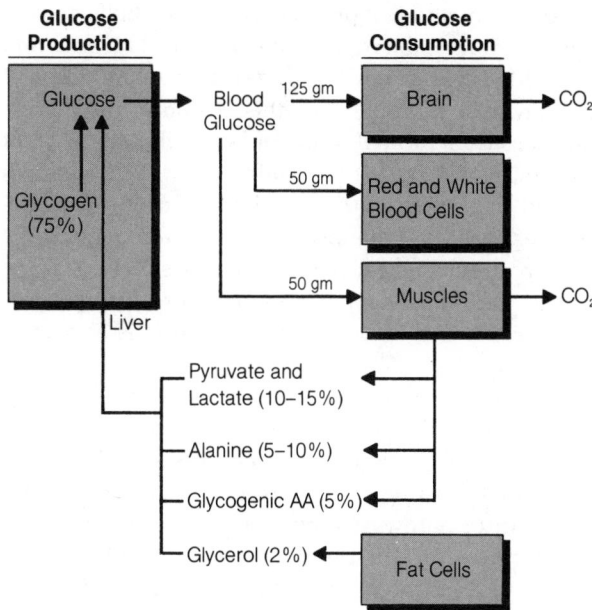

**Fig. 9-18.** Balance of glucose and glucose precursors in postabsorptive man. The brain is the prime site of glucose consumption. Most of the glucose released by the liver is derived by glycogenolysis. As fasting progresses, gluconeogenesis replaces glycogenolysis as the predominant mode of glucose formation. Numbers in parentheses represent proportion of glucose output attributable to uptake of various precursors in postabsorptive state. (Redrawn from Felig P: Metabolism 22:179, 1973. By permission)

**Table 9-4. Metabolic Activity of the Body Fuels in Normal Fed (High-Insulin) and Fasting (Low-Insulin) States**

| Metabolic Fuels | Metabolic State | Liver | Adipose cells | Muscle |
|---|---|---|---|---|
| Carbohydrate | Fed | ↑ glycogen synthesis<br>↑ glycolysis<br>↓ gluconeogenesis | ↑ glucose uptake<br>↑ glucose metabolism | ↑ glucose uptake<br>↑ gycolysis<br>↑ glycogen synthesis |
| | Fasted | ↑ glycogenolysis<br>↓ glycolysis<br>↑ gluconeogenesis<br>↑ glucose release | ↓ glucose uptake<br>↓ glucose metabolism | ↓ glucose uptake<br>↓ glycolysis<br>↑ glycogenolysis |
| Fat | Fed | ↑ fatty acid synthesis<br>↓ β-oxidation<br>↑ triglyceride synthesis | ↑ fatty acid uptake<br>↑ triglyceride synthesis<br>↑ fatty acid synthesis<br>↓ lipolysis | ↓ fatty acid uptake<br>↓ fatty acid oxidation |
| | Fasted | ↓ lipogenesis<br>↑ fatty acid uptake<br>↑ β-oxidation<br>↑ ketogenesis | ↓ triglyceride synthesis<br>↑ lipolysis<br>↑ fatty acid release | ↑ fatty acid uptake<br>↑ fatty acid oxidation |
| Protein | Fed | ↓ amino acid catabolism | | ↑ amino acid uptake<br>↑ protein synthesis |
| | Fasted | ↑ amino acid uptake<br>↑ amino acid catabolism | | ↑ proteolysis<br>↑ amino acid release |

As was mentioned previously, the metabolic activity at any one time is the result of the hormonal balance and availability of various substrates rather than the action of any individual hormone. For this reason all of the activities listed in Table 9-4 cannot be attributed to direct effects of insulin or lack of insulin. Many of the changes observed in fasting are due to the action of other hormones as well as to the decrease in insulin action. The direction of metabolic changes in diabetes mellitus is the same as that in fasting, but even at the low fasting levels insulin exerts a metabolic control, which is absent in diabetes.

A review of Table 9-4 indicates that glycolysis, glycogenesis, and lipogenesis are increased in the fed state, and glycogenolysis, gluconeogenesis, and lipolysis are low. In the fasting state, the reverse is true. As a result, the first three pathways (and insulin) use the energy of dietary nutrients for the body's needs and storage, whereas the last three satisfy the body's needs from its endogenous sources.

Although many of the individual reactions that are subject to hormonal control are known, the mechanisms by which these agents act are not understood in some instances. It has become evident in recent years that the metabolic actions of several hormones are mediated by a widely distributed substance, cyclic adenosine monophosphate (cAMP), designated as a *second messenger*. Hormones, the *first messengers*, control the level of cAMP by influencing either its synthesis or breakdown in their target cells. As a result, the "lipolytic" hormones (Fig. 9-17) elevate the level of cAMP in the adipose cells and other tissues, whereas insulin seems to decrease its concentration in the same tissues. In the adipose tissue a high concentration of cAMP activates the hormone-sensitive lipase, thereby increasing triglyceride breakdown. Conversely, lipolytic activity is reduced by low levels of cAMP.

*Glucagon.* In the liver the synthesis and breakdown of glycogen are controlled by cAMP. Of the hormones "antagonistic" to insulin, glucagon has probably the most powerful effect on the level of this metabolic regulator in the liver.[53] Glucagon is secreted in response to low levels of blood glucose. It increases the synthesis of cAMP, which at high levels increases glycogenolysis by activating the enzyme, phosphorylase. It also inactivates glycogen synthetase, thereby preventing storage of glucose as glycogen, and stimulates gluconeogenesis. All of these actions increase the release of glucose into the blood.

*Epinephrine* also influences blood glucose through the cAMP-mediated mechanisms comparable to those of glucagon, but it is less potent in the liver. It is a powerful stimulus to muscle glycogenolysis and adipose tissue lipolysis, again through activation of phosphorylase and hormone-sensitive lipase, respectively, by increased concentrations of cAMP. Involvement of cAMP in the regulation of protein synthesis and breakdown in muscle is likely, but the site of such control is not known for certain.

*Adrenal glucocorticoids* are known to increase protein catabolism and interfere with protein synthesis in the peripheral tissues. They also stimulate gluconeogenesis in the liver. The proteolytic effect of glucocorticoids is evident in fasting but not in nonfasting muscle.[54]

## Study questions and activities

1. Identify the structural features of the intestinal mucosa which play a major role in the digestive-absorptive processes.
2. What is the main difference between active and passive absorption mechanisms?
3. Differentiate between simple and facilitated diffusion.
4. Identify the differences in the luminal phase of LCT and MCT digestion.
5. Identify the differences in the intracellular phase of digestion and absorption of LCT and MCT.
6. Describe the enterohepatic circulation of bile salts.
7. What is the role of bile salts in the digestion and absorption of LCT?
8. Describe the role of the epithelial brushborder in the digestion and absorption of carbohydrates and proteins.
9. What is the role of acetyl CoA in the production of energy in the body? In storing excess food energy?
10. What is the role of $\beta$-oxidation in the production of energy from fat?
11. List in sequence the metabolic pathways involved in the complete oxidation of glucose to produce $CO_2$, $H_2O$, and ATP.
12. Describe the roles of the Cori cycle and the glucose-alanine cycle in the skeletal muscle.
13. How is the level of blood glucose maintained in different metabolic stages (fed, fasting, and starvation)?
14. Describe how excess food energy is converted to adipose tissue fat regardless of the form in which it is ingested.
15. What are the dietary factors that most consistently influence the level of plasma VLDL? LDL? Chylomicrons?
16. Differentiate between the m-RNA, t-RNA, and ribosomal RNA as they relate to protein synthesis.
17. Compare the metabolic effects of insulin in the adipose tissue, liver, and muscle.

## References

1. Grossman MI: Annu Rev Physiol 41:27, 1979
2. Larsson L-I: Clin Gastroenterol 9:485, Sept, 1980
3. Soll AH, Walsh JH: Annu Rev Physiol 41:35, 1979
4. Price SF et al: Gastroenterology 75:240, 1978
5. Babka JC, Castell DO: Am J Dig Dis 18:391, 1973
6. Castell DO: Ann Intern Med 83:390, 1975
7. Thomas FB et al: Clin Res 24:537A, 1976
8. Cohen S, Booth GH: N Engl J Med 293:897, 1975
9. Lecce JG: Environ Health Perspect 33:57, 1979

10. Gray GM: N Engl J Med 292:1225, 1975
11. Crane RK: Fed Proc 24:1000, 1965
12. Phillips SI, McGill DB: Am J Dig Dis 18:1017, 1973
13. Sleisenger MH, Kim YS: N Engl J Med 300:659, 1979
14. Peters TJ, Donlon J, Fottrell PF: In Burland WL, Samual PD (eds): Transport Across the Intestine, p 153. Baltimore, Williams & Wilkins, 1972
15. Matthews DM: Proc Nutr Soc 31:171, 1972
16. Nicholson JA et al: J Clin Invest 54:890, 1974
17. Holt PR, Clark BS: J Am Diet Assoc 60:491, 1972
18. Friedman HI, Nylund B: Am J Clin Nutr 33:1108, 1980
19. McIntyre N, Isselbacher KJ: Am J Clin Nutr 26:647, 1973
20. Cohen M et al: Gastroenterology 60:1, 1971
21. Olivecrona T, Hernell O: Bibl Nutr Dieta 22:50, 1975
22. Ockner RKF et al: J Clin Invest 48:2367, 1969
23. Kalser M: Adv Intern Med 17:301, 1973
24. Boyd GS: In Vergroesen AJ (ed): The Role of Fats in Human Nutrition, pp 353–380. New York, Academic Press, 1975
25. Kudchodkar BJ, Sodhi HS, Horlick L: Metabolism 22:155, 1973
26. Mattson FH, Erickson BA, Kligman AM: Am J Clin Nutr 25:589, 1972
27. Connor WE, Lin DS: J Clin Invest 53:1062, 1974
28. Munro HN, Crim MC: In Goodhart RS, Shils ME (eds): Modern Nutrition in Health and Disease, 6th ed, pp 51–98. Philadelphia, Lea & Febiger, 1980
29. Crapo PA, Olefsky JM: Nutr Today 15:10, July-Aug, 1980
30. Shetty PS et al: Lancet II: 230, 1979
31. Felig P: Metabolism 22:179, 1973
32. Giordano C: J Lab Clin Med 62:231, 1963
33. Giovannetti S, Maggiore A: Lancet 1:1000, 1964
34. Close JH: N Engl J Med 290:663, 1974
35. Walser M, Coulter AW, Dighe S: J Clin Invest 52:678, 1973
36. Madrey WC, Chura CM, Coulter AW: Gastroenterology 5:553, 1973
37. Walser M: Am J Clin Nutr 33:1629, 1980
38. Frohling PT et al: Am J Clin Nutr 33:1667, 1980
39. Hecking E et al: Am J Clin Nutr 33:1678, 1980
40. Mitch WE: Am J Clin Nutr 33:1642, 1980
41. Giordano C: Am J Clin Nutr 33:1649, 1980
42. Albrink MJ: J Am Diet Assoc 62:626, 1973
43. Bierman EL: Am J Clin Nutr 33:2712, 1980
44. Ernst N, Levy RI: In Goodhart and Shils, Modern Nutrition, pp 1045–1070
45. Dairy Council Digest 50:31, Nov-Dec, 1979
46. Miller GJ, Miller NE: Lancet I:16, 1975
47. Castelli WP et al: Circulation 55:767, 1977
48. Gordon T et al: JAMA 238:497, 1977
49. Dietschy J, Wilson J: N Engl J Med 282:41, 1979
50. Ho KJ et al: Am J Clin Nutr 25:737, 1972
51. Randle PJ et al: Ann NY Acad Sci 131:324, 1965
52. Balasse EO: Metabolism 28:41, 1979
53. Cahill GF Jr: In Fajans SS, Sussman KE (eds): Diabetes Mellitus: Diagnosis and Treatment, Vol III, p 57. New York, American Diabetes Association, 1970
54. Goldberg AL et al: Fed Proc 39:31, 1980

## Supplementary readings

Cholesterol metabolism. Dairy Council Digest 50:31, 1979

Crapo PA, Olefsky JM: Fructose—Its characteristics, physiology and metabolism. Nutr Today 15:10, July-Aug, 1980

de Kalbermatten N et al: Comparison of glucose, fructose, sorbitol, and xylitol utilization in humans during insulin suppression. Metabolism 29:62, 1980

Frazer GE et al: The effect of various vegetable supplements on serum cholesterol. Am J Clin Nutr 34:1272, 1981

Friedman HI, Nylund B: Intestinal fat digestion, absorption and transport: A review. Am J Clin Nutr 33:1108, 1980

Gray GM: Carbohydrate digestion and absorption: Role of the small intestine. N Engl J Med 292:1225, 1975

Grossman MI: Neural and hormonal regulation of gastrointestinal function: An overview. Annu Rev Physiol 41:27, 1979

Hinkle PC, McCarty RE: How cells make ATP. Sci Am 238:104, Mar, 1978

Milson JP et al: Factors affecting plasma amino acid concentrations in control subjects. Metabolism 28:313, 1979

Mitch WE: Metabolism and metabolic effects of ketoacids. Am J Clin Nutr 33:1642, 1980

Sleisenger MH, Kim YS: Protein digestion and absorption. N Engl J Med 300:659, 1979

van Raaij JMA et al: Effects of casein versus soy protein diets on serum cholesterol and lipoproteins in young healthy volunteers. Am J Clin Nutr 34:1261, 1981

*For further references see Bibliography in Part 4.*

# Energy Metabolism

## 10

Energy Value of Foods
Measurement of Energy Expenditure
Rate of Energy Expenditure
Total Energy Requirements

Solar energy is the power that makes life on earth possible. However, only a fraction of all the sun's energy can be adapted or stored for future use. Even the most efficient devices presently available that are constructed for harnessing solar energy are less efficient by far than plants. In the process known as *photosynthesis*, plants use light energy to convert carbon dioxide and other inorganic substances into organic compounds, which they need for growth and maintenance (Chap. 2). The chemical energy, which either directly or indirectly drives all processes of life, is held in the high-energy bonds of adenosine triphosphate (ATP), which is universal in all forms of life. Because plants can derive ATP from light energy (by a process known as *photophosphorylation*), they can produce and store excess carbohydrate (mostly as starch) instead of metabolizing it for energy as animals do. In this way, the stored energy of plants becomes the potential energy of humans and animals. They, in turn, convert it through their metabolic processes to a usable form (ATP) to sustain their life processes.

The practice of raising animals for food is an inefficient way of using plant energy. First, the animal body can capture in usable form (ATP) only about 40% of the total energy liberated from the oxidation of foodstuffs; the rest is released as heat. Second, a large proportion of the energy that is conserved is used for performance of work, with heat again as a by-product. Only the portions of energy that are used in the synthesis of new tissue during growth of the animal and that are deposited as fat represent storage energy. A great deal of this is lost to humans when only selected parts of the carcass are used as food.

### Conservation of energy

Like inanimate matter, humans and other living creatures obey the fundamental law of conservation of energy—they can neither create nor destroy it but only transform it from one form to another. As a result, when no change is occurring in the energy stores of the body—no growth, weight gain, or weight loss—most of the

**BMR:** Basal Metabolic Rate
**RMR:** Resting Metabolic Rate
**SDA:** Specific Dynamic Action

energy consumed as food is accounted for as heat, either released directly in metabolic reactions or as a by-product of work performed by the body. A minor fraction is lost as unoxidized nutrients or metabolites in urine and feces, through the skin and, occasionally, the lungs (alcohol, acetone).

Energy is expended whenever the body performs any function, small or large. It does not matter whether the action is voluntary, such as walking, sitting, and the various acts involved in the performance of one's daily work, or involuntary, such as respiration, digestion, the circulation of blood, the maintenance of muscular tone, the transmission of nerve impulses, and the transport of nutrients across the membranes. Only that fraction of food energy that is captured in chemical form in the high-energy bonds of ATP can support these functions; the portion liberated as heat is useless to the body, with the exception of the small amount needed for the maintenance of body temperature.

If more energy is required for these functions than is provided for by the daily food intake, the energy reserves, primarily adipose tissue fat, are used. This is dramatically illustrated by the loss of body fat in starvation. Similarly, excess food intake leads to obesity (see Chap. 28).

### Units of energy

As the various forms of energy are quantitatively interchangeable, a single unit can be used to express a quantity of energy regardless of the form in which it is expended. In the past, the energy value of foods as well as the energy exchanges of the body have been expressed in terms of the calorie, which is a unit of heat. One kilocalorie, the unit used by nutritionists, is the amount of heat required to raise the temperature of 1 kg of water 1°C (15°C–16°C). In recent years, attempts have been made to replace the calorie with the *joule*,* the internationally accepted unit for all forms of energy in the metric system.

Adoption of the joule in place of the calorie was recommended by the VII International Congress of Nutrition in Prague (1969) and by the American Institute of Nutrition (1970). Both groups suggested that a gradual change be made in the literature, with initial inclusion of the conversion factor whenever either unit is mentioned.[1]

One kilocalorie is equivalent to 4.184 kilojoules (kJ). Because tables of food composition still list energy content of foods as kilocalories, this factor can be used when conversion is necessary or appropriate.†

Acceptance of the joule as a unit of energy in nutrition has been slower than was, perhaps, anticipated by its proponents. Review of literature a decade after the original recommendation shows that the kilocalorie is still preferred by many scientists, whereas others continue to use both units. The 1980 revision of the Recommended Dietary Allowances lists the recommended intakes in both units, but only the kilocalorie is used in the text.[2] Continuing the use of the kilocalorie as the measure of the energy content of foods certainly seems prudent at this time. The term *calorie* has attained a definite meaning in the mind of the public. It, therefore, provides a tangible reference point to the professionals in discussing the nutritional value of foods and planning of adequate diets.

The recommended energy allowances are at best approximations and are usually rounded to the closest 50 kcal and, with the joule, to the closest 100 kJ. For example, an allowance of 2000 kcal equals 8368 kJ but is rounded to 8400 kJ, equalling 8.4 MJ (megajoule).

## Energy value of foods

The total energy value of food nutrients can be determined by measuring the amount of heat produced by complete oxidation (combustion) of a known quantity of food in a *bomb calorimeter*, shown in Fig. 10-1. The apparatus is thoroughly insulated against loss of heat, and the amount of heat produced is measured by the change in temperature of a measured volume of water.

### Physiologic energy values

The energy values of nutrients determined by the bomb calorimeter must be modified to take into account the losses in the feces and urine due to incomplete absorption and oxidation in the body. Table 10-1 shows the total and the physiologic energy values of the major nutrients as determined by Atwater over 75 years ago. Whereas carbohydrate and fat are completely oxidized to $CO_2$ and $H_2O$ in the body as in the calorimeter, protein metabolism is incomplete. The nitrogen of amino acids is eliminated from the body in organic forms, which still contain some energy, urea being the main end product (see Fig. 9-12).

From the energy value of feces of subjects consuming typical mixed diets, Atwater estimated that, on an average, 92% of protein, 95% of fat, and 99% of carbohydrate is absorbed. The nitrogenous compounds excreted in urine were found to contain unused energy equivalent to 1.25 kcal per gram of protein oxidized in the body. Based on these estimates, the commonly used *Atwater factors* for protein, carbohydrate, and fat (4, 4, and 9 kcal per g, respectively) were derived. As there are slight differences in the energy contents of protein, carbohydrate, and fat from different foods, these factors are approximations only. However, they have been verified as adequate for computation of the energy content of customary American diets from the protein, carbohydrate and fat content of the foods.[3,4]

---

*One joule is equal to the energy expended when 1 kg is moved a distance of 1 m by a force of 1 newton.

†1000 kcal = 4184 kJ = 4.184 MJ; 1 kJ = 0.239 kcal; 1000 kJ = 1 MJ = 239 kcal.

The energy values of foods found in tables of food composition, such as the *Agriculture Handbook No. 8*[5] and *Home and Garden Bulletin No. 72*,[6] were determined by this procedure, but more specific modified factors were employed for different types of foods on the basis of more recent information.

It should be recognized that if accurate values for energy contents of specific foods are required, the use of food composition tables is not adequate due to the wide variability in the carbohydrate, protein, and fat content of different samples of the same food, especially of animal products, such as meats. Careful laboratory analysis of the composition of representative food samples is essential to calculate their energy values accurately.

## Measurement of energy expenditure

Though the oxidation of the energy-yielding nutrients in the body yields the same end products ($CO_2$, $H_2O$) as would occur through burning in a bomb calorimeter, the two processes are very different. In contrast to the rapid release of energy as heat in the bomb calorimeter, the slow liberation of energy in the biologic oxidations (see Chap. 9) allows about 40% of the total energy to be conserved as chemical energy of ATP, which serves as the power supply for the body's functions. However, because heat is also a by-product of all energy expended as work, production of heat can serve as a measure of energy expenditure by the body.

### Direct calorimetry

Direct calorimetry involves measurement of the amount of heat released as a result of energy expended by the body. Much of the information on the rates of energy expenditure by man was obtained from the early studies of Atwater and Benedict.[7] They employed a chamber calorimeter where the heat given off by the subject was absorbed by the water in the coils surrounding the well insulated chamber, much like the bomb calorimeter.

Although direct calorimetry seems simple in theory, it is quite complicated and expensive in practice. With development of the simpler, indirect measures of body energy exchanges, relatively few whole-body calorimeters have been constructed and used over the years. However, because many questions remain about regulation of human energy balance in extreme conditions, such as obesity and cachexia, there appears to be a renewed interest in direct calorimetry, indicated by a number of recent reports describing the principles and capabilities of newly designed human calorimeters.[8-10]

Technological advances since the development of the Atwater-Benedict calorimeter have permitted a number of different principles to be used in the accurate measure of heat given off by the subject while engaged in a variety of activities. Whereas most of the human calorimeters are

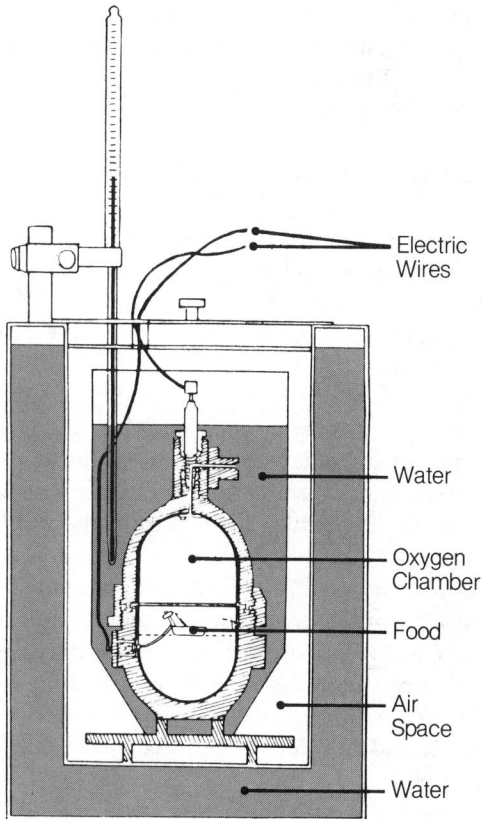

**Fig. 10-1.** Diagram of the parts of a bomb calorimeter. The water in the inner chamber changes in temperature when the food is burned. The water in the outer chamber acts with the intervening air space as insulation.

Electric Wires

Water

Oxygen Chamber

Food

Air Space

Water

room-like chambers equipped for sleeping, eating, exercise, and even for watching TV and telephoning,[9] a water-cooled insulated garment has been developed by Webb and associates.[8]

### Indirect calorimetry

The methods of indirect calorimetry have been widely used in the study of energy expenditure. They involve the measurement of oxygen consumption with or without concurrent collection of $CO_2$ produced by a subject breathing into one of several types of respiration apparatus.

The amount of $O_2$ consumed in oxidation of a food in either a calorimeter or a human body is directly related to

### Table 10-1. Heat of Combustion and the Biologically Available Energy (kcal/g)

| | *Heat of Combustion* | *Loss in Urine* | *% Absorption* | *Atwater Factor* |
|---|---|---|---|---|
| Protein | 5.6 | 1.25 | 92 | 4 |
| Carbohydrate | 4.1 | | 99 | 4 |
| Fat | 9.4 | | 95 | 9 |
| Alcohol | 7.1 | tr | 100 | 7 |

the amount of energy liberated as heat. For example, no matter how glucose is oxidized, the total amount of $O_2$ required and energy produced can be represented as follows:

$$C_6H_{12}O_2 + 6O_2 \rightarrow 6CO_2 + 6H_2O + \text{heat (664 kcal/mole)}$$

Similar equations could be used to express the oxidation of fatty acids, such as palmitic acid:

$$C_{16}H_{32}O_2 + 23O_2 \rightarrow 16CO_2 + 16H_2O + \text{heat (2340 kcal/mole)}$$

The quantity of energy produced when 1 liter of $O_2$ is consumed in the oxidation of glucose or a fatty acid can be calculated. Such values are relatively close to experimentally determined values for dietary carbohydrates and fats.

Due to the variable and unknown structure of dietary proteins, the oxidation of protein cannot be expressed by a simple equation. However, the experimentally determined energy equivalency of $O_2$ in oxidation of protein (4.600 kcal per liter $O_2$) has been found to lie close to that of starch and fat (5.047 and 4.686 kcal per liter $O_2$, respectively).[11]

Because the mixed carbohydrates and fats of the diet also differ from pure glucose or a single fatty acid, and because the body metabolizes a mixture of nutrients at the same time, an average of the three experimentally determined values (4.8 kcal per liter $O_2$) is often used as a good approximation in calculations of energy expenditure from the measured $O_2$ consumption.

As with direct calorimeters, a number of different systems have been devised for the collection and analysis of the respiratory gases. Unlike earlier ones, those currently in use allow the subjects to be mobile during the measurements. This has permitted estimation of energy costs of many individual activities. The major limitation of respirometers is the restricted time span that they can be used continuously, due to discomfort to the subject, who must wear a mouthpiece or a mask, or with some respirometers, a limited capacity for gas storage.

Most direct calorimeters are also equipped for simultaneous measurement of gas exchanges, allowing comparison of the two methods. The equivalency of direct measurement of heat produced in a calorimeter and of calculated heat production obtained by indirect calorimetry was convincingly demonstrated by the early studies of Atwater and Benedict.[7] Later studies have shown greater differences between the results obtained by the two methods, especially in short-term experiments. Even in 24-hour measurements the results from the two methods appear to compare best when obtained in resting conditions and when the energy intake during the measurement period closely approximates the expenditure.[12] Further research is needed to identify the causes for these discrepancies.

Estimation of energy expenditure from the heart rate provides another indirect measure.[13] The method requires calibration of the heart rate of each subject against a measure of energy expenditure, such as $O_2$ consumption, over a wide range of expenditure levels. Heart rate is then measured continuously while the subjects go about their normal activities. The accuracy of the method appears to be greatest at moderate levels of activity and poorest in resting conditions, when assessed by a whole-body calorimeter.[14] The heart rate method has been used recently to estimate the nonresting component of total energy expenditure of a group of schoolchildren.[15]

## Respiratory quotient

The amount of oxygen consumed in relation to the carbon dioxide produced by the oxidation of different foodstuffs varies with the oxygen content of the nutrient. Carbohydrates have higher oxygen content than fats (see the equations above) and, therefore, require less $O_2$ in the conversion to $CO_2$. The ratio of the volume of carbon dioxide produced to the oxygen consumed is known as the *respiratory quotient* (RQ). It is 1.0 for carbohydrate, 0.70 for fat, and about 0.8 for protein. When the mixture of the three energy-yielding nutrients is being metabolized, the value lies somewhere between 0.70 and 1.0, depending on the proportion of each. For an average mixed diet, the RQ has been found to be about 0.85. It is lowered during fasting and in uncontrolled diabetes; both are associated with decreased glucose and increased fatty acid oxidation. Low RQs also are found in subjects on ketogenic diets, such as the protein sparing modified fast sometimes employed for weight reduction (see Chap. 28). Oxidation of fatty acids mobilized from the adipose tissue is assumed to be the major source of energy on such regimens. In studying substrate utilization in such subjects, RQs below 0.70 have been observed in some subjects.[16] It was suggested that production of ketone bodies by the liver at a rate exceeding their oxidation by extrahepatic tissues could account for the low values. Because conversion of fatty acids to ketone bodies consumes $O_2$ but produces no $CO_2$, the RQ for the fraction of fatty acids incompletely oxidized would be zero.

## Metabolic mixture

By measuring the urinary nitrogen excretion in addition to the $O_2$ consumption and the $CO_2$ production, one can calculate the amount of carbohydrate, fat, and protein oxidized in a given period. This is known as the *metabolic mixture* and allows the total energy consumption to be calculated more precisely. Details of such calculations can be found elsewhere.[17]

## Energy balance

Maintenance of one's body weight over a period of time is considered indicative of energy balance, that is, when the energy intake equals the energy output. Similarly, weight gain and weight loss result from positive and negative energy balances, respectively. Short-term changes in body weights frequently result from fluctuations in fluid balance rather than energy balance (Chaps. 5 and 28). Therefore, studies concerned with the effects of different dietary regimens on energy balance must include not only careful measurements of caloric intake, energy expenditure, and weight changes, but several measures of body composition as well. Such experiments, even though laborious and complicated by varying degrees of methodological inaccuracies, provide more objective comparisons of the efficiency of energy utilization than do body weights alone.

The principles of energy conservation dictate that energy intake must be accounted for by the sum of the energy losses in urine and feces, metabolic expenditure (measured by direct or indirect calorimetry), and changes in the body energy stores and body temperature. In general, changes in the excretory losses and body temperature are minor; metabolic expenditure, including direct heat production and work, and energy storage are the major variables.

The composition of weight change is estimated from the changes in body composition during the experimental period. For such calculations, the energy cost of weight gain or loss has been assumed to be equal to the energy content of the tissue, which is about 6000 kcal per kilogram of adipose tissue and 2500 kcal per kilogram of lean body tissue.[18] However, weight losses and gains actually observed usually have been lower than what is predicted from the energy excess or deficit. One of the factors contributing to lower than expected weight loss is a progressive decrease in the BMR during deficient energy intake,[19,20] resulting in increased efficiency of energy utilization. Similarly, the efficiency of energy utilization decreases when the intake is above maintenance requirements.[20,21]

At least two factors appear to contribute to the decreased efficiency of energy utilization during overfeeding. First, it has recently been demonstrated in rats and pigs that deposition of energy as protein and fat during normal growth requires considerably more energy than the energy value of the deposited tissue, with approximate efficiencies of 75% for fat and 45% for protein storage.[22] Second, it has been proposed that some of the excess energy intake during overfeeding is dissipated as heat and referred to as dietary-induced thermogenesis, or *luxuskonsumption*.[23]

Although increased thermogenesis following overfeeding has been observed by several investigators,[20,23,24] others have failed to detect such an effect.[25-27] Similarly, attempts to demonstrate a subnormal thermogenic response to ingestion of food by obese individuals, compared to lean people have yielded equivocal results.[28,29] Reasons for these discrepancies are not obvious, but procedural differences such as duration and magnitude of overfeeding, composition of diets, and timing and frequency of measurements of energy expenditure may be responsible. It appears that weight gain from excess calories provided as fat approximates more closely the predicted weight gain than when excess calories are provided in a mixed diet.[21] The measurements of energy expenditure are frequently made in the morning. Some recent studies suggest that the metabolic rate during rest[30] and exercise[29,30] increases during the day, perhaps as a result of accumulating thermogenic effects of meals enhanced by the physical activity during the day. Therefore, studies employing 24-hour simultaneous measurements of energy expenditure by direct and indirect calorimetry are essential to clarify some of these inconsistencies in the efficiency of energy utilization during over- and underfeeding and the possible mechanisms involved in changes in energy efficiency.

## Rate of energy expenditure

The energy requirement of a person consists of two major components of expenditure: the energy expended for growth and maintenance and the energy expended in physical activity. The total energy requirement is determined by a number of inherent and environmental factors, which influence either or both components of energy expenditure and which are not totally independent variables.

### Basal and resting metabolism

The energy expended for the maintenance of the basal activities of the body is relatively constant and includes:

1. Maintenance of muscle tone and body temperature
2. Circulation
3. Respiration
4. Other glandular and cellular activities, including those related to growth

It is customary to determine energy expenditure for these basal activities under standard conditions—the subject is lying down, awake, at complete rest; the test is taken at least 14 hours after the last meal and several hours after any vigorous exercise.

The most convenient time to comply with these conditions is in the morning before breakfast. The rate of metabolism determined under these "standard" conditions is known as the *basal metabolic rate* (BMR). It is quite constant for subjects of the same sex, age, and body composition. Therefore, marked variations in the basal rate of metabolism are an indication of disease.

Formerly, the basal metabolism test was used extensively as a means of diagnosis, particularly in cases of hyperthyroidism, hypothyroidism, myxedema, and other endocrine disturbances that may alter the metabolic rate. Because the thyroid hormones have the greatest effect on the metabolic rate, the various thyroid function tests have gained wide acceptance in clinical diagnosis. The measurements of total serum tyroxine ($T_4$) and of triiodothyronine ($T_3$) have largely replaced the former widely employed measurement of protein-bound iodine (PBI), which is difficult to interpret because falsely high values are frequently encountered due to iodide contamination.[31] Uptake of [131]I by the thyroid gland is another thyroid function test that is still frequently used. All thyroid function tests are subject to misinterpretation unless interferences are eliminated by careful selection of appropriate methods and combinations of available tests.

Because of the specific conditions associated with the measurement of the BMR, the so-called resting metabolic rate (RMR) is frequently used for practical purposes. It refers to the metabolic rate at rest and under conditions of thermal neutrality. "It includes the specific dynamic action of meals, and is an average minimal metabolism for the night and the periods of the day when there is no exercise and no exposure to cold."[2]

## Factors influencing the rate of energy expenditure

The maintenance component of the total energy expenditure is quite constant for an adult. There are normal variations in the metabolism of different people, the causes of which lie within the body itself—the size, the shape, and the composition of the body, the person's age, and the activity of certain internal glands. It is generally accepted that a variation of from 10% to 15% either way from the accepted metabolic rate (all variables considered) is within normal limits.

### Body size and composition

These factors influence the energy requirements by affecting both the resting metabolism and the amount of energy expended in the movements of the body. The resting metabolic rate is related to the proportion of actively metabolizing cell mass to the total body mass. The latter is influenced by the size of the body skeleton and the amount of adipose tissue, both of which are low in metabolic activity compared to that of the organ and skeletal muscle tissues. Therefore, when expressed as kcal/kg/hr, the BMR (and RMR) is quite constant for people varying in size but with similar proportions of these three body compartments, but it varies with extreme departures from the average. For example, an athlete is likely to have a higher BMR (kcal per kg per hr) than a sedentary person, who, in turn, would have a higher rate than an obese person. Table 10-2 shows the basal metabolic rates of adults with the recommended weights for heights.

In addition to body weight, the surface area has customarily been used as a measure of body size in studies comparing the metabolic rates of individuals or of groups of varying size, age, and sex distribution. The body surface area can be easily determined from weight and height by using nomograms developed from actual measurements of body surface areas of people of different heights and weights. Despite its long usage, the expression of metabolic rate in terms of surface area does not fully eliminate the variability caused by marked departures in body shape and composition. For example, grossly obese individuals tend to show lower than normal metabolic rates and women lower rates than men (who have proportionately less fat). Both differences are eliminated if the *fat-free mass* * is used as the basis of expressing the metabolic rate.

With continuous improvements in the methods and standards for estimating total body fatness, fat-free body mass (sometimes referred to as *lean body mass*) is likely to be used more widely. This allows more accurate assessment of the factors that alter the apparent metabolic rate but may or may not actually influence the cellular metabolic activity.

### Age and growth

Normal variations in resting metabolic rate result from age and growth. The relative rate is highest during the first and second years of life and decreases after that, although it is still high through puberty in both boys and girls.

Although the energy requirements of children as well as of adults are usually given in terms of weight (and sex), age may be more appropriate for young children in populations where malnourishment is common, to allow them to catch up in both height and weight. For older children with irreversible stunting, energy allowances based on desirable height and weight for age could lead to obesity.

The recommended energy allowances for children up to 10 years of age are the same for both sexes, but they are higher for boys than for girls after 11 years due to the differences in growth rates and the changes in body composition that are taking place during puberty, as well as changing activity patterns.[2] Spady[15] has recently suggested that the requirements for girls may be less than those for boys before age 10, as he found that both the resting and total energy expenditures of girls ($9.5 \pm 0.7$ yr) were lower than those of boys ($9.7 \pm 1.0$ yr), even when expressed on the basis of lean body mass. Because of the small number of children involved and the methods used to estimate the various components of total energy expenditure, these results need verifying.

During adult life there is a steady decrease in energy expenditure. The basal and resting metabolic rates fall due to the decrease in active cell mass, which is compensated by an increase in total body fat. This reduction in resting metabolic rate is estimated to be about 2% per each decade after age 21.[2] From age 40 to 60, physical activity both at work and during leisure time is likely to be reduced with advancing age. Further decreases in both

---

*Fat-free body weight = body weight − total body fat.

**Table 10-2.  The Basal Metabolic Rates of Adults with Recommended Weights for Heights**

| Height | | Men | | | Women | | |
| --- | --- | --- | --- | --- | --- | --- | --- |
| | | Median Weight | | BMR | Median Weight | | BMR |
| in | cm | lb | kg | kcal/day | lb | kg | kcal/day |
| 60 | 152 | | | | 109 ± 9 | 50 ± 4 | 1399 |
| 62 | 158 | | | | 115 ± 9 | 52 ± 4 | 1429 |
| 64 | 163 | 133 ± 11 | 60 ± 5 | 1630 | 122 ± 10 | 56 ± 5 | 1487 |
| 66 | 168 | 142 ± 12 | 64 ± 5 | 1690 | 129 ± 10 | 59 ± 5 | 1530 |
| 68 | 173 | 151 ± 14 | 69 ± 6 | 1775 | 136 ± 10 | 62 ± 5 | 1572 |
| 70 | 178 | 159 ± 14 | 72 ± 6 | 1815 | 144 ± 11 | 66 ± 5 | 1626 |
| 72 | 183 | 167 ± 15 | 76 ± 7 | 1870 | 152 ± 12 | 69 ± 5 | 1666 |
| 74 | 188 | 175 ± 15 | 80 ± 7 | 1933 | | | |
| 76 | 193 | 182 ± 16 | 83 ± 7 | 1983 | | | |

(From Food and Nutrition Board: Recommended Dietary Allowances, 8th rev. Washington, DC, National Academy of Sciences/National Research Council, 1974)

categories are likely after age 60, but such changes become more unpredictable due to a variable degree of disease and disability.

## Physical activity

The major determinant of variation in the rate of energy expenditure among people of the same sex, age, and body size, and composition is physical activity. Although one's occupation is an important contributor to the total energy cost of physical activity, increasing leisure time activities are becoming equally important, especially in the developed countries where the shortened workdays allow equal time for occupational and recreational activities.

Nevertheless, the Joint FAO/WHO Expert Committee on Energy and Protein Requirements concluded that "studies of both food intake and energy expenditure in groups of people show that by far the most important intergroup variable is the energy expenditure in the physical activity required by occupation." A rough classification of occupations into four activity categories proposed by the committee is shown in Table 10-3. It was recognized that considerable variation may occur in the amount of physical work involved in any one occupation, such as farming, due to differences in the degree of mechanization.

In the highly industrialized nations, such as the United States, where most occupations fall into the light or moderate activity categories, grouping of activities—both occupational and recreational—according to the estimated energy cost has provided a useful tool for estimating the total energy requirements of both groups and individuals (Table 10-4).

## Diseases

Infections or fevers raise the BMR in proportion to the elevation of the body temperature, approximately 7% for each degree Fahrenheit rise in temperature.

## Endocrine glands

Secretions of certain endocrine glands, such as the thyroid, the adrenals, and the pituitary affect metabolism. The secretion of the thyroid gland has the most marked effect. Hyperthyroidism is that condition in which the metabolism is accelerated by increased production of the thyroid hormones, whereas hypothyroidism is characterized by a decrease that results in subnormal metabolism. At least part of the increased energy expenditure in hyperthyroidism is attributed to increased activity of the sodium pump ($Na^+$, $K^+$ ATPase),[32] which is respon-

## Table 10-3.  Classification of Occupations According to the Extent of Physical Activity Involved

*Light Activity*
**Men:** Office workers, most professional men (such as lawyers, doctors, accountants, teachers, architects, and so on), shop workers, unemployed men
**Women:** Office workers, housewives in houses with mechanical household appliances, teachers, and most other professional women

*Moderately Active*
**Men:** Most men in light industry, students, building workers (excluding heavy laborers), many farm workers, soldiers not on active service, fishermen
**Women:** Light industry, housewives without mechanical household appliances, students, department store workers

*Very Active*
**Men:** Some agricultural workers, unskilled laborers, forestry workers, army recruits and soldiers on active service, mine workers, steel workers
**Women:** Some farm workers (especially peasant agriculture), dancers, athletes

*Exceptionally Active*
**Men:** Lumberjacks, blacksmiths, rickshaw-pullers
**Women:** Construction workers

(From Report of a Joint FAO/WHO Committee: Energy and protein requirements. WHO Tech Rep Ser, no. 522. Geneva, World Health Organization, 1973)

sible for the maintenance of normal gradients of sodium and potassium ions between the intracellular and extracellular fluids (see Chap. 5). Epinephrine (adrenalin), a secretion of the adrenal medulla, causes a temporary increase in the BMR. Those pituitary hormones that stimulate thyroid and adrenal secretions also affect the metabolic rate.

### The state of nutrition

In order to conserve energy during severe starvation or prolonged undernutrition, the body adapts by decreasing its metabolic rate, possible by as much as 50%. In a recent study in East Java, Edmunson[19] found that the average BMR of a group of farmers whose energy intake averaged about 2400 kcal per day was about twice the rate of another group of comparable body size with an average energy intake of about 1500 kcal per day. Work by Rhao and Khan in India suggests that in children, malnutrition must be severe before the BMR is significantly depressed.[33]

They compared children with either kwashiorkor or marasmus with controls from the same socioeconomic group who showed no clinical signs of protein-calorie malnutrition. The BMR of the children suffering from kwashiorkor or marasmus was significantly reduced when compared to that of the controls and increased progressively with treatment. The BMR of the control group was similar to that of healthy American children, although the control group showed weight deficits ranging from 17% to 35%.

### Climate

The effect of climate on both the resting metabolic rate and the energy expended in standard tasks has also been studied. Although a lower than normal basal metabolic rate has been observed in inhabitants of some tropical communities, this finding does not seem to apply uniformly. The energy expended in standard tasks is believed to be the same within a wide temperature range, above 14°C but is about 5% higher in mean temperatures below this level.[2] Total energy requirement may be increased by an additional 2% to 5% due to the weight of extra clothing.[2]

The total energy expenditure also may be increased during heavy work at high temperatures due to the additional expenditure needed for the maintenance of thermal balance in such extreme conditions.[2]

The human body has several ways of protecting itself against temperature changes. Exposure to cold initiates shivering, which consists of a series of rapid muscular contractions set up involuntarily by the body to increase heat production in order to make up for the rapid heat loss. Upon continuing exposure, nonshivering thermogenesis develops. Of course, increased heat production means increased energy expenditure.

The metabolic processes of the body under normal conditions and average daily activity produce enough heat to increase the body temperature by about 2° F an hour if no heat is lost. However, nature has provided for a carefully controlled heat loss through perspiration, which may vary as climate and environment dictate.

Although these involuntary processes are important in the control of body temperature, they are not adequate to protect the body against extreme climatic conditions. Adjustments in clothing, housing, and level of activity are normal means of responding to changes in thermal needs.

Because of the variable and unpredictable nature of both the involuntary and voluntary adjustments to climatic changes, the Third FAO/WHO Committee on Caloric Requirements considered that "there was no quantifiable basis for correcting the resting and exercise energy requirements according to the climate."[34] They emphasized, however, the need to adjust the activity category to take into account climatic effects on the physical activity pattern and its contribution to the total energy expenditure. A similar approach was maintained in the 1980 revision of the energy allowances for the population of the United States by the Food and Nutrition Board of the National Research Council.

### Table 10-4. Examples of Daily Activities of Individuals in Light Occupations and Average Energy Expenditure in Each Category

| | Average Energy Expenditure, kcal/kg/hr | |
| Activity Category | Men | Women |
| --- | --- | --- |
| *Very Light* Seated and standing activities, painting trades, auto and truck driving, laboratory work, typing, playing musical instruments, sewing, ironing | 1.5 | 1.3 |
| *Light* Walking on level, 2.5–3 mph, tailoring, pressing, garage work, electrical trades, carpentry, restaurant trades, cannery workers, washing clothes, shopping with light load, golf, sailing, table tennis, volleyball | 2.9 | 2.6 |
| *Moderate* Walking 3.5–4 mph, plastering, weeding and hoeing, loading and stacking bales, scrubbing floors, shopping with heavy load, cycling, skiing, tennis, dancing | 4.3 | 4.1 |
| *Heavy* Walking with load uphill, tree felling, working with pick and shovel, basketball, swimming, climbing, football | 8.4 | 8.0 |

(Adapted from Food and Nutrition Board: Recommended Dietary Allowances, 8th rev. Washington, DC, National Academy of Sciences/National Research Council, 1974)

## Thermogenic effect of food (Specific Dynamic Action)

Ingestion of food is known to increase the metabolic rate above that in fasting resting conditions (BMR). This effect has been called the Specific Dynamic Action (SDA) of food, but the cause for the increased metabolic rate is still not clear. The long held concept that the increased rate of $O_2$ consumption following a meal is dependent on the type of food ingested (hence, "specific")—with protein having the highest effect (up to 30%) and carbohydrate the lowest (5%)—has recently been challenged. On the basis of a carefully controlled study with normal adults, Garrow and Hawes concluded that there was a similar increase in metabolic rate after a meal of a given caloric content, no matter whether protein, carbohydrate, or fat was the source.[35] These results have been confirmed by Pittet and co-workers[36] by using either glucose, amino acids, or both.

There is evidence that exercise enhances the thermogenic effect of a large meal (about 1000 kcal or more)[23,37] but may have no effect at lower caloric intakes.[38] In a recent study, caffeine and regular coffee consumed with a meal were found to increase the thermogenic effect of the meal when compared to a meal with decaffeinated coffee.[39] This effect was associated with increased oxidation of fat in comparison to the premeal period. Similarly, coffee was found to increase the metabolic rate of fasting normal and obese subjects during the 3-hour period measured. This increase was accompanied by increased fatty acid oxidation in normal but not in obese subjects.

It is evident that the thermogenic effect of a meal may be influenced by a number of factors. However, there is no indication that the overall cost of this energy expenditure in normal individuals exceeds the usually estimated 10% of the total energy intake during a 24-hour period.

## Total energy requirements

It should be obvious from the previous discussion that there is no single, easily quantifiable variable from which the total energy requirements can be accurately determined. Even the energy expenditure of each person varies from day to day according to the time spent in different activities. A student studying for final exams may feel that he is working very hard, yet his energy expenditure may be considerably less than that during a regular school day when he is attending classes in different buildings on the campus and perhaps spending some time in recreational activities, such as playing tennis.

Individual variation in the amount of energy spent in a given task or activity may also be considerable. Thus energy requirements calculated from the number of hours spent in various activities are only average estimates based on a typical pattern in each activity category. For many people the actual energy expenditure may be higher or lower than the average.

## Energy allowances

Because of the many factors that influence the energy requirements of people and the undesirable consequences of excess energy intakes, allowances for the various categories cannot be established "to ensure that the needs of nearly all in the population are met,"[21] as for other nutrients. To emphasize this difference the 1980 edition of the Recommended Dietary Allowances did not tabulate the energy allowances with those of the other nutrients. The energy allowances are said to be

> . . . estimates of the average needs of population groups, not recommended intakes for individuals. These needs vary from person to person and are not easily predictable without detailed information about physical characteristics and activity of the individual. Hence, *average* energy needs for each age and sex group are provided as guidelines . . .[2]

The values were estimated for the average adult man and woman assumed to be engaged in light occupations, with a typical activity pattern consisting of 8 hours of sleeping/reclining, 12 hours of very light, 3 hours of light, and 1 hour of moderate activity. By using the energy costs shown in Table 10-4 and estimating the energy expenditure of sleep to be 90% of the BMR (Table 10-2), the daily allowance of 2700 kcal for the reference man (70 kg) and 2000 kcal for the reference woman (55 kg) was obtained. Adjustments can be made for differences in body size and activity patterns by using the appropriate values from these tables. For moderately active adults, the energy requirement is estimated to be about 1.7 times the basal energy expenditure for men and 1.6 times that for women.[2] Using the BMR value for a 72-kg man (Table 10-2), an energy need of about 3100 kcal is obtained, which is 400 kcal more than that for the reference man (70 kg) with light activity pattern. In estimating energy requirements in clinical practice, the basal energy expenditure (BEE), as determined from the Harris-Benedict equation (see Chap. 23), is used frequently in place of the BMR; the BEE formula takes into consideration the effect of age on metabolic rate.

A quick estimate of energy needs of sedentary people can be made as follows:

- Basal needs = 1 kcal per kg per hr
- Weight in kg $\times$ 24 = BMR for 1 day
- Add 50% of BMR for activity to estimate the total energy need.

It has been recognized that for many people the recommended levels are too high for a sedentary life.[2] For persons who are overweight or underweight, caloric requirements should be estimated according to the desired weight for height instead of actual weight (Table 10-2). On the basis of the small known decline in the BMR with age and the assumed decline in physical activity, the energy allowances between 51 and 75 years of age were set at 90% of these for the young adults and a further reduction to 75% to 80% was suggested for those beyond 75 years.[2]

Although many people seem to be able to adjust their food intake to their energy expenditure without any special effort, this regulatory mechanism does not work as well at very low levels of energy expenditure, as a result leading to obesity.[2] Instead of reduction of energy intake, the Food and Nutrition Board recommends increasing energy output through increased activity by people whose daily energy expenditure is below 1800 kcal. It is very difficult to maintain adequate intake of essential minerals and vitamins with low caloric intake due to the relatively low nutrient density of the average American diet, which is high in fat and sugar, providing a lot of "empty calories."

The reader should consult Chapters 18 and 19 for a discussion of the energy needs of infants and adolescents and Chapter 17 for those of pregnant and lactating women. Energy allowances for all age groups are shown in Table 11-1.

## Study questions and activities

1. What are the two units of energy presently used to express the energy value of foods? How can you convert one unit to the other?
2. Why are the physiologic fuel values of foods different from their heat of combustion?
3. Milk has the percentage composition of 3.5 g of protein, 4 g of fat, and 5 g of carbohydrate per 100 g. Calculate the caloric value of a glass of milk weighing 240 g.
4. How does the biologic oxidation of the energy nutrients differ from their combustion in a bomb calorimeter?
5. How can the energy expenditure of an individual be estimated from the measurement of $O_2$ consumption?
6. What is the RQ? Why is it low during fasting?
7. What is meant by a metabolic mixture?
8. Differentiate between the BMR and RMR.
9. What are the major factors that determine the total energy requirements of an individual?
10. Estimate the energy requirements of a moderately active 50-kg woman by the quick method. Now use Tables 10-2 and 10-4 to calculate her energy needs more carefully, using the typical activity pattern described in the text.

## References

1. Ames SR: J Am Diet Assoc 57:415, 1976
2. Food and Nutrition Board: Recommended Dietary Allowances, 9th rev ed. Washington, DC, NAS-NRC, 1980
3. Bernstein LM et al: United States Army Medical Nutrition Laboratory Department No. 168. Denver, Fitzsimmons Army Hospital, 1955
4. Southgate BAT, Durnin JVGA: Br J Nutr 24:517, 1970
5. Watt BK, Merrill LA: Composition of Foods: Raw, Processed, and Prepared. Agriculture Handbook No. 8. Washington, DC, USDA, 1963
6. Nutritive Value of Foods. Home and Garden Bulletin No. 72. Washington, DC, USDA, United States Government Printing Office, 1981
7. Atwater AO, Benedict FG: USDA Office of Experiment Stations Bulletin No. 136. Washington, DC, United States Government Printing Office, 1903
8. Webb P et al: J Appl Physiol 32:412, 1972
9. Dauncey MJ et al: Br J Nutr 39:557, 1978
10. Tschegg E et al: Metabolism 28:764, 1979
11. Zuntz N: T Flug Arch Ges Physiol 68:191, 1897
12. Webb P et al: Am J Clin Nutr 33:1287, 1980
13. Andrews RB: Am J Clin Nutr 24:1139, 1971
14. Dauncey MJ, James WPT: Br J Nutr 42:1, 1979
15. Spady DW: Am J Clin Nutr 33:766, 1980
16. Schutz Y, Ravussin E: Am J Clin Nutr 33:1317, 1980
17. Passmore R, Draper MH: In Albanese AA (ed): Newer Methods in Nutritional Biochemistry, p 41. New York, Academic Press, 1965
18. Webb P: Am J Clin Nutr 33:1299, 1980
19. Edmunson W: Ecol Food Nutr 8:189, 1979
20. Apfelbaum M et al: Am J Clin Nutr 24:1405, 1971
21. Sims EAH et al: Rec Prog Horm Res 29:457, 1973
22. Pullar JD, Webster AJF: Br J Nutr 37:355, 1977
23. Miller DS et al: Am J Clin Nutr 20:1223, 1967
24. Dauncey MJ: Br J Nutr 43:267, 1980
25. Hanson JS: J Appl Physiol 35:587, 1973
26. Whipp BJ et al: Am J Clin Nutr 26:1284, 1973
27. Norgan NG, Durnin JVGA: Am J Clin Nutr 33:978, 1980
28. Kaplan ML, Leveille GA: Am J Clin Nutr 29:1108, 1976
29. Glick Z et al: Am J Clin Nutr 30:1026, 1977
30. Zahorska-Markiewicz B: Nutr Metab 24:238, 1980
31. MacMurry JF Jr: Postgrad Med 57:52, 1975
32. Ismail-Beigi F, Edelman IS: J Gen Physiol 57:710, 1971
33. Rao KSJ, Khan L: Am J Clin Nutr 27:892, 1974
34. Joint FAO/WHO Committee: Energy and protein requirements. WHO Tech Rep Ser, no 522. Geneva, World Health Organization, 1973
35. Garrow JS, Hawes SF: Br J Nutr 27:211, 1972
36. Pittet PH et al: Br J Nutr 31:343, 1974
37. Bray GA et al: Am J Clin Nutr 27:254, 1974
38. Swindells YE: Br J Nutr 27:65, 1972
39. Acheson KJ et al: Am J Clin Nutr 33:989, 1980

## Supplementary readings

Acheson KJ et al: The measurement of daily energy expenditure—An evaluation of some techniques. Am J Clin Nutr 33:1155, 1980

Acheson KJ et al: The measurement of food and energy intake in man—An evaluation of some techniques. Am J Clin Nutr 33:1147, 1980

Cunningham JJ: A reanalysis of the factors influencing basal metabolic rate in normal adults. Am J Clin Nutr 33:2372, 1980

Dauncey MJ: Influence of mild cold on 24-hour energy expenditure, resting metabolism and diet-induced thermogenesis. Br J Nutr 45:257, 1981

Mahalko JR, Johnson LK: Accuracy of prediction of long-term energy needs. J Am Diet Assoc 77:557, 1980

Norgan NG, Durnin JVGA: The effect of overfeeding on the body weight, body composition, and energy metabolism of young women. Am J Clin Nutr 33:978, 1980

Pullar JD, Webster JF: The energy cost of fat and protein deposition in the rat. Br J Nutr 37:355, 1977

Review: Energy balance throughout the life cycle. Dairy Council Digest 51:19, July-Aug, 1980

Rothwell NJ, Stock MJ: Regulation of energy balance. Annu Rev Nutr 1:235, 1981

Spady DW: Total energy expenditure of healthy free ranging school children. Am J Clin Nutr 33:766, 1980

Tschegg E et al: An isothermic gradient-free, whole-body calorimeter for long-term investigations of energy balance in man. Metabolism 28:764, 1979

Webb P: The measurement of energy exchange in man: An analysis. Am J Clin Nutr 33:1299, 1980

Webb P, Annis JF, Troutman SJ: Energy balance in man measured by direct and indirect calorimetry. Am J Clin Nutr 33:1287, 1980

*For further references see Bibliography in Part 4.*

# Meeting Nutritional Norms

## 11

**MDR:** Minimum Daily Requirement
**NAS-NRC:** National Academy of
  Sciences-National Research Council
**RDA:** Recommended Dietary Allowances
**US-RDA:** United States Recommended
  Daily Allowances

## Interpretation and use of recommended dietary allowances

In the discussion in preceding chapters of the various nutrients needed for health, references have frequently been made to the Recommended Dietary Allowances. These represent the establishment of a nutritional norm for planning and assessing dietary intake.

When the Food and Nutrition Board was appointed by the National Academy of Sciences-National Research Council (NAS-NRC) in 1940, it undertook as one of its most important projects the establishment of a set of figures for human needs in terms of specific nutrients. As a result of long and careful consideration, Recommended Dietary Allowances (RDA) were first published in 1943. Since then, they have been revised many times as new research data have become available. Their use has also expanded. They are used as a guide for planning and procuring food supplies for population groups; for interpreting food consumption records; for establishing standards for public assistance programs; for evaluating the adequacy of food supplies in meeting national nutritional needs; for developing nutrition education programs; for the development of new products for industry; and for establishing guidelines for nutritional labeling of foods.[1]

### Allowances in contrast to requirements

The 1980 (9th) edition of the Recommended Dietary Allowances describes the process and some of the problems involved in determining the allowances.

The *ideal* method in developing an allowance would be to determine the average requirement of a healthy and representative segment of each age group for the nutrient under consideration, then to assess statistically the variability among the individuals within the group, and finally to calculate the amount by which the average requirement must be increased to meet the needs of nearly all healthy individuals. Unfortunately, experiments on man are costly; they must be of long duration; certain types of experiments are not possible for ethical reasons; and, even under the best conditions, only a small number of subjects can be studied in a single experiment. Thus requirement estimates often must be derived from limited information.

In practice, estimates of nutrient requirements are determined by a number of techniques: (1) collection of data on nutrient intake from the food supply of apparently normal, healthy people, (2) review of epidemiological observations when clinical consequences of nutrient deficiencies are found to be correctable by dietary improvement, (3) biochemical measurements that assess degree of tissue saturation or adequacy of molecular function in relation to nutrient intake, (4) nutrient balance studies that measure nutritional status in relation to intake, (5) studies of subjects maintained on diets containing marginally low or deficient levels of a nutrient, followed by correction of the deficit with measured amounts of that nutrient (such studies are undertaken in humans only when the risk is minimal), and (6) in some few instances, extrapolation from animal experiments in which deficiencies have been produced by the exclusion of a single nutrient from the diet. The estimation of precise nutrient requirement by some of these techniques individually may be equivocal. However, with the corroborative evidence arising from application of several reinforcing procedures, the requirements, and hence the allowances, may be stated with greater confidence.

Estimation of the recommended allowances follows essentially four steps:

1. Estimating the average requirement of a population for a given nutrient and the variability of requirement within that population
2. Increasing the average requirement by an amount sufficient to meet the needs of nearly all members of a population
3. Increasing the allowance to account for inefficient utilization by the body of the nutrients as consumed (poor absorption, poor conversion of precursor to active forms, etc.)
4. Using judgment in interpreting and extrapolating allowances when information on requirements is limited

There is not always agreement on the basis for determining when the requirement has been met. The requirement for a nutrient is the minimum intake that will maintain normal function and health. The requirement for infants and children may be equated with the amount that will maintain a satisfactory rate of growth; for an adult, with the amount that will maintain body weight and prevent depletion of the nutrient from the body, as judged by balance studies or maintenance of acceptable blood and tissue concentrations. For certain nutrients, the requirements may be assessed as the amount that will just prevent failure of a specific function or the development of specific deficiency signs—an amount that may differ greatly from that required to maintain maximum body stores. Thus there are differences of opinion about the criteria that should be used to establish requirements.

Following a review of the scientific evidence of nutrient requirements judged by the Committee on Dietary Allowances to be most reliable, a logical approach in setting a recommended allowance for nutrients other than energy is to select a value above the average requirement by an amount that includes the range of variability observed. However, for some nutrients there is inadequate information about the variability of individual requirements and judgments must be made.

Since allowances other than that for energy are recommended amounts of nutrients that must be consumed in order to ensure that the requirements of most people are met, it is necessary to take into account any factor that influences the efficiency of nutrient utilization in setting these allowances. For some nutrients, a part of the requirement may be met by a precursor that is converted to the essential nutrient within the body. Some carotenes, for example, are precursors of vitamin A; therefore, when carotenes are included as a vitamin A source, allowance is made for efficiency of conversion of these precursors. For some nutrients, requirements are expressed in terms of a single constituent, whereas the requirement is actually for a composite of several constituents that may differ in efficiency of utilization. Protein intake, for example, is estimated in terms of nitrogen, not of specific amino acids; therefore, possible inefficient utilization of the mixture of amino acids in the protein ingested is taken into account in developing protein allowances. For some nutrients, absorption is incomplete; allowance must, therefore, be made for failure of a portion of the ingested nutrient to gain entrance to the body. For example, only a part of the iron in foods is absorbed, and this is considered in establishing the recommended allowances. Since the importance of each of these factors differs from nutrient to nutrient, the degree to which the recommended allowance exceeds the average requirement is not uniform but varies with individual nutrients. . . .

With limited information about requirements, about the variability of requirements, and about factors that influence the utilization of ingested nutrients, allowances for many nutrients cannot be estimated directly from the available scientific knowledge; judgment must be invoked in interpreting and extrapolating from the available information.

It is necessary to recognize these problems in order to understand why recommendations for nutrient allowances may differ from country to country and why the allowances for some nutrients exceed the presumed requirement by a much greater proportion than those for others. On the whole, those who accept responsibility for estimating allowances tend to select the higher of alternate levels when there is little evidence that small surpluses of nutrients are detrimental; on the other hand, consistent uncompensated deficits, even small ones, will lead to deficiencies over a long period of time.[1]

The Recommended Dietary Allowances are defined in the 1980 (9th) edition as follows:

Recommended Dietary Allowances (RDA) are the levels of intake of essential nutrients considered . . . to be adequate to meet the known nutritional needs of practically all healthy persons.

RDA are recommendations for the average daily amounts of nutrients that population groups should consume over a period of time. RDA should not be confused with requirements for a specific individual. Differences in the nutrient requirements of individuals are ordinarily unknown. Therefore, RDA (except for energy) are estimated to exceed the requirements of most individuals and thereby to ensure that the needs of nearly all in the population are met. Intakes below the recommended allowances for a nutrient are not necessarily inadequate, but the risk of having an inadequate intake increases to the extent that intake is less than the level recommended as safe.

RDA are recommendations established for healthy populations. Special needs for nutrients arising from such problems as premature birth, inherited metabolic disorders, infections, chronic diseases and the use of medications require special dietary and therapeutic measures. These conditions are not covered by the RDA.[1]

The RDA (Tables 11-1–11-3) are expressed in nutrients rather than in specific foods because these particular recommendations can be attained from a variety of different food patterns. The Committee on Dietary Allowances also points out that, to ensure that possibly unrecognized nutritional needs are met, RDA should be provided from a wide selection of foods rather than by supplementation or extensive fortification of single foods. One should also remember that the allowances are not minimum requirements; failure to achieve these intake levels should not be interpreted as malnutrition unless additional nutritional status information (physical, biochemical, or clinical assessment) is available and is also indicative of deficiencies. Convincing evidence is also lacking that any special health benefits result from a greatly excessive intake of any one nutrient or combination of nutrients.

The Dietary Standards for Canada[2] and the recommended intakes set by Joint FAO/WHO Expert Groups[3-7] (Chap. 21, Table 21-8) also represent nutritional norms, which according to Dr. J. A. Campbell of Canada are similar to RDA in "philosophy, derivation, and use of allowances. Differences in individual figures are related largely to the degree of ignorance in relating minimum requirements to recommended levels for optimal health."[8] Many other countries have also established appropriate standards in attempts to improve national dietary intakes.

## Energy allowances

The body requires food energy for metabolic processes, physical growth including pregnancy, lactation, and maintenance of body temperature. Energy needs vary greatly with the size and activity of each person. The energy allowances were established as the "average needs of people in each category."[1] The recommendations for average adults (man, 70 kg, 178 cm; woman, 55 kg, 163 cm) engaged in light occupations were set for three age groups—23 to 50 years, 51 to 75 years, and over age 75 (Table 11-1). They are presumed to live in an environment with a mean temperature of 20°C (70°F). Adjustments must be made when the characteristics of an individual population group differ from the size, activity, or climate defined above (see Chap. 10, *Energy Metabolism*).

The energy allowances set for infants during the first year of life are based on the general pattern of intake recorded for thriving infants. Energy allowances (kilocalories per kilogram) decrease gradually throughout infancy, childhood, and adult life. Age groups, except for the first year, are given in 3- or 4-year intervals up to age 23. The allowances for children are listed separately for the sexes after age 10, when differences in growth rate between boys and girls occur. Allowances are based on needs for the middle years in each age group and for light activity. Allowances for pregnancy and lactation are also included.

Although the recommended allowances are given in kilocalories (kcal), they may be converted to kilojoules (kJ) as follows: 1 kcal equals 4.2 kJ.*

Carbohydrate, fat, and protein provide sources of energy. Alcohol may also contribute calories to the diet. No specific recommendations were made for the proportion of calories to be derived from different sources. However, guidelines were suggested for "individual consideration, especially by people suspected or known to be in the high-risk category for certain diseases."[1]

> Total fat intake, particularly in diets below 2000 kcal, should be reduced so fat is not more than 35% of dietary energy. . . . There should be greater reduction in fats containing predominately saturated fatty acids, . . . an upper limit of 10% of dietary energy as polyunsaturated fatty acid is advisable.

> Intake of refined sugar should be reduced and complex carbohydrates maintained or even increased . . .

> For many individuals a reduction in alcohol consumption would also assist in achieving proper caloric balance.[1]

Warnings that surplus intake is stored as fat and if continued leads to obesity and is harmful to health are given in this edition, which emphasizes that the recommendations for energy are strictly estimates of average needs of population groups and not recommended intakes for individuals.[1]

Adjustment of caloric needs to size and activities, however, is not simple. Dictates of appetite and maintenance of body weight help. For extreme degrees of activity, such as heavy physical work, the allowance may be increased as much as 50%; for sedentary people it may be reduced by 25%. For example, a large teenage boy, active in athletics, may require 3600 calories, whereas his grandmother, aged 70, cannot use more than 1200 calories (one-third as many) without gaining weight.

---

*This figure is used for convenience in clinical work and is rounded from the 4.184 listed in Chap. 10.

**Table 11-1. Mean Heights and Weights and Recommended Energy Intake**

| Category | Age (Years) | Weight (kg) | Weight (lb) | Height (cm) | Height (in) | Energy Needs (with Range) (kcal) | Energy Needs (with Range) (mJ) |
|---|---|---|---|---|---|---|---|
| *Infants* | 0.0–0.5 | 6 | 13 | 60 | 24 | kg × 115 (95–145) | kg × 0.48 |
| | 0.5–1.0 | 9 | 20 | 71 | 28 | kg × 105 (80–135) | kg × 0.44 |
| *Children* | 1–3 | 13 | 29 | 90 | 35 | 1300 ( 900–1800) | 5.5 |
| | 4–6 | 20 | 44 | 112 | 44 | 1700 (1300–2300) | 7.1 |
| | 7–10 | 28 | 62 | 132 | 52 | 2400 (1650–3300) | 10.1 |
| *Males* | 11–14 | 45 | 99 | 157 | 62 | 2700 (2000–3700) | 11.3 |
| | 15–18 | 66 | 145 | 176 | 69 | 2800 (2100–3900) | 11.8 |
| | 19–22 | 70 | 154 | 177 | 70 | 2900 (2500–3300) | 12.2 |
| | 23–50 | 70 | 154 | 178 | 70 | 2700 (2300–3100) | 11.3 |
| | 51–75 | 70 | 154 | 178 | 70 | 2400 (2000–2800) | 10.1 |
| | 76+ | 70 | 154 | 178 | 70 | 2050 (1650–2450) | 8.6 |
| *Females* | 11–14 | 46 | 101 | 157 | 62 | 2200 (1500–3000) | 9.2 |
| | 15–18 | 55 | 120 | 163 | 64 | 2100 (1200–3000) | 8.8 |
| | 19–22 | 55 | 120 | 163 | 64 | 2100 (1700–2500) | 8.8 |
| | 23–50 | 55 | 120 | 163 | 64 | 2000 (1600–2400) | 8.4 |
| | 51–75 | 55 | 120 | 163 | 64 | 1800 (1400–2200) | 7.6 |
| | 76+ | 55 | 120 | 163 | 64 | 1600 (1200–2000) | 6.7 |
| *Pregnancy* | | | | | | +300 | |
| | | | | | | +500 | |

See Food and Nutrition Board's Recommended Dietary Allowances, 9th rev ed. Washington, DC, NAS-NRC, 1980 for the sources and explanation of the figures for heights and weights shown in this table.

The energy allowances for the young adults are for men and women doing light work. The allowances for the two older groups represent mean energy needs over these age spans, allowing for a 2% decrease in basal (resting) metabolic rate per decade and a reduction in activity of 200 kcal/day for men and women between 51 and 75 years, 500 kcal for men over 75 years, and 400 kcal for women over 75. The customary range of daily energy output is shown for adults in parentheses, and is based on a variation in energy needs of ± 400 kcal at any one age, emphasizing the wide range of energy intakes appropriate for any group of people.

Energy allowances for children through age 18 are based on median energy intakes of children of these ages followed in longitudinal growth studies. The values in parentheses are 10th and 90th percentiles of energy intake, to indicate the range of energy consumption among children of these ages.

## Recommended allowances for other nutrients

The specific (Table 11-2) nutrients included in the 1980 RDA[17] and the quantities of each for the several categories of persons were based upon the consensus of authorities at the time the table was published. Because nutritional requirements differ according to age, sex, body size, physiological state, and genetic makeup, broad age-sex groups have been used for the table of RDA. The accompanying text includes additional information for adjusting the allowances to suit special population groups (see Chaps. 5–8).

## Estimated safe and adequate intakes

For the first time, in the 1980 edition of the Recommended Dietary Allowances, the Committee on Dietary Allowances has established estimated safe and adequate intakes for an additional 12 nutrients. Because the scientific data on which these values are based are less complete than the data for the nutrients for which RDA were established, they are given in ranges and for fewer, more generalized age categories (Table 11-3). The Committee has stated their justification for establishing these recommendations.

Perhaps the most persuasive argument for establishing estimated safe and adequate intakes is the increased availability of formulated foods, food analogs, and vitamin and mineral supplements, which may increase the risk of deficiency or of toxicity. Guidelines are needed for manufacturers that formulate these products and for the public that consumes them. As more information becomes available, estimated intakes will be further refined and may be included for additional nutrients.[1]

## Other considerations

Intakes of some nutrients exceed the RDA standard when the diet just provides the recommended quantities of others that are in low concentration in the food supply. For example, animal products that are naturally high in protein are important sources of several trace nutrients; to meet the allowances for some of the trace nutrients, it may be necessary to exceed the allowances for protein and other nutrients.

The recommended allowance values in the tables are for nutrients in foods that are consumed, and consideration should be given to prior losses due to storage, waste, and cooking. Provision should be made for these losses in planning practical dietaries.

## Table 11-2. Food and Nutrition Board, National Academy of Sciences/National Research Council Recommended Dietary Allowances (Revised 1980) Designed for the Maintenance of Good Nutrition of Practically All Healthy People in the United States

| | Age (Years) | Weight (kg) | Weight (lbs) | Height (cm) | Height (in) | Protein (g) | Fat-Soluble Vitamins | | | Water-Soluble Vitamins | | | | | | | Minerals | | | | | |
|---|---|---|---|---|---|---|---|---|---|---|---|---|---|---|---|---|---|---|---|---|---|---|
| | | | | | | | Vitamin A (μg RE)* | Vitamin D (μg)† | Vitamin E (mg α TE)‡ | Vitamin C (mg) | Thiamin (mg) | Riboflavin (mg) | Niacin (mg NE)§ | Vitamin B6 (mg) | Folacin (μg)∥ | Vitamin B12 (μg) | Calcium (mg) | Phosphorus (mg) | Magnesium (mg) | Iron (mg) | Zinc (mg) | Iodine (μg) |
| **Infants** | 0.0–0.5 | 6 | 13 | 60 | 24 | kg × 2.2 | 420 | 10 | 3 | 35 | 0.3 | 0.4 | 6 | 0.3 | 30 | 0.5# | 360 | 240 | 50 | 10 | 3 | 40 |
| | 0.5–1.0 | 9 | 20 | 71 | 28 | kg × 2.0 | 400 | 10 | 4 | 35 | 0.5 | 0.6 | 8 | 0.6 | 45 | 1.5 | 540 | 360 | 70 | 15 | 5 | 50 |
| **Children** | 1–3 | 13 | 29 | 90 | 35 | 23 | 400 | 10 | 5 | 45 | 0.7 | 0.8 | 9 | 0.9 | 100 | 2.0 | 800 | 800 | 150 | 15 | 10 | 70 |
| | 4–6 | 20 | 44 | 112 | 44 | 30 | 500 | 10 | 6 | 45 | 0.9 | 1.0 | 11 | 1.3 | 200 | 2.5 | 800 | 800 | 200 | 10 | 10 | 90 |
| | 7–10 | 28 | 62 | 132 | 52 | 34 | 700 | 10 | 7 | 45 | 1.2 | 1.4 | 16 | 1.6 | 300 | 3.0 | 800 | 800 | 250 | 10 | 10 | 120 |
| **Males** | 11–14 | 45 | 99 | 157 | 62 | 45 | 1000 | 10 | 8 | 50 | 1.4 | 1.6 | 18 | 1.8 | 400 | 3.0 | 1200 | 1200 | 350 | 18 | 15 | 150 |
| | 15–18 | 66 | 145 | 176 | 69 | 56 | 1000 | 10 | 10 | 60 | 1.4 | 1.7 | 18 | 2.0 | 400 | 3.0 | 1200 | 1200 | 400 | 18 | 15 | 150 |
| | 19–22 | 70 | 154 | 177 | 70 | 56 | 1000 | 7.5 | 10 | 60 | 1.5 | 1.7 | 19 | 2.2 | 400 | 3.0 | 800 | 800 | 350 | 10 | 15 | 150 |
| | 23–50 | 70 | 154 | 178 | 70 | 56 | 1000 | 5 | 10 | 60 | 1.4 | 1.6 | 18 | 2.2 | 400 | 3.0 | 800 | 800 | 350 | 10 | 15 | 150 |
| | 51+ | 70 | 154 | 178 | 70 | 56 | 1000 | 5 | 10 | 60 | 1.2 | 1.4 | 16 | 2.2 | 400 | 3.0 | 800 | 800 | 350 | 10 | 15 | 150 |
| **Females** | 11–14 | 46 | 101 | 157 | 62 | 46 | 800 | 10 | 8 | 50 | 1.1 | 1.3 | 15 | 1.8 | 400 | 3.0 | 1200 | 1200 | 300 | 18 | 15 | 150 |
| | 15–18 | 55 | 120 | 163 | 64 | 46 | 800 | 10 | 8 | 60 | 1.1 | 1.3 | 14 | 2.0 | 400 | 3.0 | 1200 | 1200 | 300 | 18 | 15 | 150 |
| | 19–22 | 55 | 120 | 163 | 64 | 44 | 800 | 7.5 | 8 | 60 | 1.1 | 1.3 | 14 | 2.0 | 400 | 3.0 | 800 | 800 | 300 | 18 | 15 | 150 |
| | 23–50 | 55 | 120 | 163 | 64 | 44 | 800 | 5 | 8 | 60 | 1.0 | 1.2 | 13 | 2.0 | 400 | 3.0 | 800 | 800 | 300 | 18 | 15 | 150 |
| | 51+ | 55 | 120 | 163 | 64 | 44 | 800 | 5 | 8 | 60 | 1.0 | 1.2 | 13 | 2.0 | 400 | 3.0 | 800 | 800 | 300 | 10 | 15 | 150 |
| **Pregnant** | | | | | | +30 | +200 | +5 | +2 | +20 | +0.4 | +0.3 | +2 | +0.6 | +400 | +1.0 | +400 | +400 | +150 | ** | +5 | +25 |
| **Lactating** | | | | | | +20 | +400 | +5 | +3 | +40 | +0.5 | +0.5 | +5 | +0.5 | +100 | +1.0 | +400 | +400 | +150 | ** | +10 | +50 |

*Retinol equivalents. 1 retinol equivalent = 1 μg retinol or 6 μg β carotene. See Chapter 7 for calculation of vitamin A activity of diets as retinol equivalents.

†As cholecalciferol. 10 μg cholecalciferol = 400 IU vitamin D.

‡α-tocopherol equivalents. 1 mg d-α-tocopherol = 1 α TE. See Chapter 7 for variation in allowances and calculation of vitamin E activity of the diet as α-tocopherol equivalents.

§1 NE (niacin equivalent) is equal to 1 mg of niacin or 60 mg of dietary tryptophan.

∥The folacin allowances refer to dietary sources as determined by *Lactobacillus casei* assay after treatment with enzymes ("conjugases") to make polyglutamyl forms of the vitamin available to the test organism.

#The RDA for vitamin B12 in infants is based on average concentration of the vitamin in human milk. The allowances after weaning are based on energy intake (as recommended by the American Academy of Pediatrics) and consideration of other factors such as intestinal absorption.

**The increased requirement during pregnancy cannot be met by the iron content of habitual American diets nor by the existing iron stores of many women; therefore the use of 30–60 mg of supplemental iron is recommended. Iron needs during lactation are not substantially different from those of nonpregnant women, but continued supplementation of the mother for 2–3 months after parturition is advisable in order to replenish stores depleted by pregnancy.

(The allowances are intended to provide for individual variations among most normal persons as they live in the United States under usual environmental stresses. Diets should be based on a variety of common foods in order to provide other nutrients for which human requirements have been less well defined. See Table 11-1 for heights and weights and recommended energy intakes.)

**Table 11-3.  Estimated Safe and Adequate Daily Dietary Intakes of Selected Vitamins and Minerals**

| | Vitamins | | | Trace Elements* | | | | | | Electrolytes | | |
| --- | --- | --- | --- | --- | --- | --- | --- | --- | --- | --- | --- | --- |
| Age (Years) | Vitamin K (µg) | Biotin (µg) | Pantothenic Acid (mg) | Copper (mg) | Manganese (mg) | Fluoride (mg) | Chromium (mg) | Selenium (mg) | Molybdenum (mg) | Sodium (mg) | Potassium (mg) | Chloride (mg) |
| **Infants** | | | | | | | | | | | | |
| 0–0.5 | 12 | 35 | 2 | 0.5–0.7 | 0.5–0.7 | 0.1–0.5 | 0.01–0.04 | 0.01–0.04 | 0.03–0.06 | 115–350 | 350–925 | 275–700 |
| 0.5–1 | 10–20 | 50 | 3 | 0.7–1.0 | 0.7–1.0 | 0.2–1.0 | 0.02–0.06 | 0.02–0.06 | 0.04–0.08 | 250–750 | 425–1275 | 400–1200 |
| **Children and Adolescents** | | | | | | | | | | | | |
| 1–3 | 15–30 | 65 | 3 | 1.0–1.5 | 1.0–1.5 | 0.5–1.5 | 0.02–0.08 | 0.02–0.08 | 0.05–0.1 | 325–975 | 550–1650 | 500–1500 |
| 4–6 | 20–40 | 85 | 3–4 | 1.5–2.0 | 1.5–2.0 | 1.0–2.5 | 0.03–0.12 | 0.03–0.12 | 0.06–0.15 | 450–1350 | 775–2325 | 700–2100 |
| 7–10 | 30–60 | 120 | 4–5 | 2.0–2.5 | 2.0–3.0 | 1.5–2.5 | 0.05–0.2 | 0.05–0.2 | 0.1–0.3 | 600–1800 | 1000–3000 | 925–2775 |
| 11+ | 50–100 | 100–200 | 4–7 | 2.0–3.0 | 2.5–5.0 | 1.5–2.5 | 0.05–0.2 | 0.05–0.2 | 0.15–0.5 | 900–2700 | 1525–4575 | 1400–4200 |
| **Adults** | 70–140 | 100–200 | 4–7 | 2.0–3.0 | 2.5–5.0 | 1.5–4.0 | 0.05–0.2 | 0.05–0.2 | 0.15–0.5 | 1100–3300 | 1875–5625 | 1700–5100 |

*Because the toxic levels for many trace elements may be only several times usual intakes, the upper levels for the trace elements given in this table should not be habitually exceeded.

(Because there is less information on which to base allowances, these figures are not given in the main table of the RDA and are provided here in the form of ranges of recommended intakes.)

When the table of allowances is used to calculate the needs of population groups, the total estimate should take into account the composition of the population, that is, the age and sex categories. In planning meals the RDA can be assessed for a week's food supply rather than for a single meal or a single day's meals. Emergency conditions may necessitate some modification in the interpretation of recommendations. It then becomes desirable to raise the food allowances of as many people as possible to maintenance levels. Rationing at such times should give special attention to the most vulnerable groups.

## Nutrient allowances per 1000 kilocalories

To maintain appropriate weight in the adult and to support optimum growth in children and adolescents, a person's food intake must closely reflect energy requirements. Similarly, the foods consumed to meet energy needs must also fulfill each person's recommended allowances for all other nutrients. Thus the concept of nutrient density has been suggested as a basis for presenting the RDA. Hansen and Wyse[9] converted the RDA for each nutrient into an allowance per 1000 calories by dividing each RDA by the average calorie allowance and then multiplying by 1000. In an attempt to establish a single-valued allowance for each nutrient, they reviewed the nutrients for constants. Thiamin, riboflavin, niacin, and vitamin E allowances per 1000 calories were constant. They suggested that the single-valued allowances for the other nutrients should reflect the allowances for those people whose nutrient to calorie needs are the greatest. The single-valued nutrient allowances per 1000 kcal in Table 11-4 are therefore based on the nutrient per 1000 kcal needed by persons with the lowest energy requirements in as much as it is most difficult for them to meet the allowances for other nutrients. Because in many situations it would be helpful to have guidelines for fat and carbohydrate as well as protein, Hansen and Wyse set an arbitrary standard of 35% of total calories as fat and the remaining as carbohydrate (protein equals 10% of total calories, Table 11-4). The allowances for fatty acids are based on a P:S ratio of 0:7. The fluoride allowance is based on the amount of that mineral found in fluoridated water supplies and, for this reason, is stated as mg per liter of water rather than per 1000 kcal.

The use of a single-valued allowance for nutrient density as a guide for menu planning recognizes the fact that because many family members share a common table, the needs of the members with the highest requirements per energy unit can be satisfied. Such a single-valued allowance is also appropriate when planning and procuring food supplies for a general population group. If a person must drastically reduce his caloric intake, it is necessary to select foods having a higher nutrient density. A diet prescription for 1000 kcal would require approx-

imately doubling the allowance suggested per 1000 kcal. For the nutrition counselor planning diets for a group of people of specific age and sex, their more specific allowance would be a more appropriate frame of reference, calculated as follows:

$$\frac{\text{RDA for specific nutrient}}{\text{Average caloric allowance}} = 1000$$

The usefulness of this method of applying RDA to nutrition counseling is increased by expressing the nutrient composition of an individual food in terms of its nutrient density, or Index of Nutritional Quality (INQ).[10] Milk supplies 54 g of protein per 1000 kcal, whereas the suggested allowance for protein is 25 g per 1000 kcal. Thus the INQ (54/25) for milk protein is 2.2. The density of the other nutrients can be similarly determined. Using the INQ concept, the computer has been employed to represent the nutrient content of a food by a bar graph of the

### Table 11-4. Single-Value Nutrient Allowances Per 1000 Kilocalories

| Nutrient | Amount |
| --- | --- |
| Vitamin A | 400 mcg RE |
| Vitamin D | 4 mcg |
| Vitamin E | 4 mg TE |
| Vitamin C | 30 mg |
| Thiamin | 0.5 mg |
| Riboflavin | 0.6 mg |
| Niacin | 7 mg NE |
| Vitamin B$_6$ | 1.0 mg |
| Folacin | 200 mcg |
| Vitamin B$_{12}$ | 1.5 mcg |
| Vitamin K | 30 mcg |
| Biotin | 50 mcg |
| Pantothenic acid | 2 mg |
| Calcium | 450 mg |
| Phosphorus | 450 mg |
| Magnesium | 150 mg |
| Iron | 8 mg |
| Zinc | 8 mg |
| Iodine | 75 mcg |
| Copper | 1 mg |
| Manganese | 1.5 mg |
| Fluoride | 1 mg/l H$_2$O |
| Chromium | 0.03 mg |
| Selenium | 0.035 mg |
| Molybdenum | 0.08 mg |
| Sodium | 1500 mg |
| Potassium | 2500 mg |
| Chloride | 1500 mg |
| Protein | 25 g |
| Carbohydrate | 137.5 g |
| Fat | 39 g |
| Oleic acid | 12.25 g |
| Linoleic acid | 10 g |
| Saturated fatty acids | 14.25 g |

*double*

(Adapted from Hansen RG, Wyse BW: Expression of nutrient allowances per 1000 kilocalories. J Am Diet Assoc 76:223, 1980)

percentage of the daily requirements satisfied by a given portion. This is referred to as the nutrient profile.[11] Nutrient profiles can be used as a tool to evaluate and improve the nutritional quality of diets. The INQ has been suggested as one method of evaluating the nutritional quality of individual foods.[12] Wyse and Hansen have also published nutrient density food profiles of the individual Exchange Lists for Meal Planning.[13]

## United States recommended daily allowances (US-RDA)

The United States Recommended Daily Allowances (US-RDA), as distinct from the RDA established by the National Research Council, are a set of standards developed by the Food and Drug Administration for use in regulating nutrition labeling (see Chap. 15). They replace the Minimum Daily Requirements (MDR), which were formerly used by the FDA for nutrient labeling. Although these new standards are derived from the NRC-RDA, they are based on a very few broad categories. The values for adults and children over the age of 4 were taken from the highest value for each nutrient given in the 1968 NRC-RDA tables for men and nonpregnant, nonlactating females 4 or more years of age except for calcium, phosphorus, biotin, pantothenic acid, copper, and zinc. Separate US-RDA values were established for infants (not more than 12 mo of age), children (under 4 yr old), and pregnant or lactating women. More and more foods have nutrition information on the label; the US-RDA is the reference standard for the values presented.

## Daily food guide

The recommended allowances for nutrients for most people can be obtained from a well chosen variety of ordinary foods including those in our markets that are commonly fortified or enriched with vitamins and minerals. The Daily Food Guide (Fig. 11-1), prepared by nutritionists in the United States Department of Agriculture, presents one way to select food.[14] With this aid almost anyone can get the nutrients needed from common, easily available foods.

Most foods contain more than one nutrient, but no single food contains all the nutrients in the amounts needed. The Daily Food Guide suggests the kinds that together supply nutrients in the amounts needed. In using the Guide one selects the main part of the diet from the four broad food groups. To this one adds other foods as desired to make meals appealing and satisfying. The additional foods should add enough calories to meet energy needs, which will vary widely for different members of the family.

Because it is possible, however, to obtain the recommended dietary allowance of nutrients in many different diet patterns due to the wide variety of foods yielding similar nutrients, anyone attempting to evaluate or teach nutrition should be conscious of this fact and avoid any tendency to use stereotyped diet yardsticks for judging individual diets.

If a patient's calcium intake is being estimated and only his milk intake is scrutinized, an entirely erroneous evaluation may be made. It is possible for some people to get enough calcium from the daily use of cheese, fish,

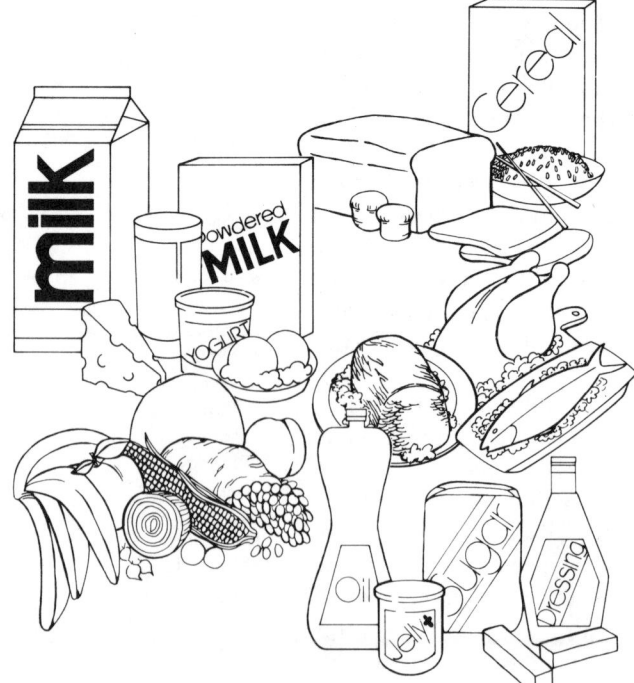

**Milk Group**
Some milk for everyone
Children under 9 . . . 2 to 3 cups
Children 9 to 12 . . . 3 or more cups
Teenagers . . . 4 or more cups
Adults . . . 2 or more cups

**Vegetable Fruit Group**
4 or more servings
Include—
A citrus fruit or other fruit or vegetable important for vitamin C
A dark-green or deep-yellow vegetable for vitamin A—at least every other day
Other vegetables and fruits, including potatoes

**Bread Cereal Group**
4 or more servings
Whole grain, enriched, or restored

**Meat Group**
2 or more servings
Beef, veal, pork, lamb, poultry, fish, eggs
As alternatives—dry beans, dry peas, nuts

**Other Foods**
To round out meals and meet energy needs, most everyone will use some foods not specified in the Four Food Groups. Such foods include breads, cereals, flours, sugars, butter, margarine, other fats. These often are ingredients in a recipe or added to other foods during preparation or at table. Try to include some vegetable oils among the fats used.

**Fig. 11-1.** Food for Fitness: A Daily Food Guide. (Modified from Leaflet 424, U.S. Department of Agriculture, Institute of Home Economics)

legumes, and leafy vegetables, even though the more usual pattern would be from the use of milk. For this reason, although nutrition guides such as the Four Food Groups are valuable, their limitations when applied to an individual must be recognized.

## Pattern dietary

The accompanying pattern dietary (Table 11-5) planned according to the Daily Food Guide provides only about 1400 calories—less than needed by an active person—but meets or approaches the recommended allowances for all nutrients for an adult man. Supplementary foods such as extra milk for children will help meet the calcium level recommended for them. In general, the foods added to meet energy needs of individual people will provide additional nutrients as well as contribute to taste and satisfaction of meals.

The iron provided in the sample dietary is low for women, compared to the 18 mg recommended. This

amount of iron is impossible to obtain unless a special effort is made to include iron-rich foods. It is suggested that women might use slightly more meat, poultry, or fish and try to include some type of liver in the diet at least once a week. Iron availability is improved if some meat and ascorbic acid is included in each meal. Iron supplements may still be needed. The level of the B vitamins, which appears to be slightly low for men and boys, can be raised to the RDA when calories are increased to meet their needs.

In Chapter 22 it is noticed that hospital diets are also based upon this pattern dietary, modified as required to meet specific needs.

## Food composition tables as a tool for assessing dietary practices

The basic tool for the assessment of dietary practices is the knowledge of the proximate energy and nutrient composition of foods—calories, protein, fat, carbohy-

## Table 11-5. Evaluation of a Pattern Dietary for Its Nutritive Content

| Food Group | Amount in g | Household Measure | Energy (kcal) | Pro-tein (g) | Fat (g) | Carbo-hydrate (g) | Cal-cium (mg) | Phos-phorus (mg) | Magne-sium (mg) | Iron (mg) | A (IU) | Thia-min (mg) | Ribo-flavin (mg) | Niacin (mg NE) | Ascorbic Acid (mg) |
|---|---|---|---|---|---|---|---|---|---|---|---|---|---|---|---|
| Milk or equivalent* | 488 | 2 c (1 pint) | 320 | 17 | 17 | 24 | 576 | 452 | 63 | 0.2 | 700 | 0.16 | 0.84 | 0.3 | 5 |
| Meat, fish, poultry, or egg† | 120 | 4 oz, cooked | 376 | 30 | 31 | | 13 | 212 | 104 | 3.3 | 280 | 0.14 | 0.23 | 6.1 | |
| Vegetables: | | | | | | | | | | | | | | | |
| Potato, cooked | 100 | 1 medium | 65 | 2 | | 15 | 6 | 48 | 22 | 0.5 | | 0.09 | 0.03 | 1.2 | 16 |
| Deep green or yellow, cooked‡ | 75 | ½ c | 21 | 2 | | 6 | 44 | 28 | 29 | 0.9 | 4700 | 0.05 | 0.10 | 0.5 | 25 |
| Other, raw or cooked§ | 75 | ½ c | 45 | 2 | | 10 | 16 | 41 | 18 | 0.9 | 300 | 0.08 | 0.06 | 0.6 | 12 |
| Fruits: | | | | | | | | | | | | | | | |
| Citrus‖ | 100 | 1 serving | 44 | 1 | | 10 | 18 | 16 | 12 | 0.3 | 140 | 0.06 | 0.02 | 0.3 | 43 |
| Other# | 100 | 1 serving | 85 | | | 22 | 10 | 21 | 16 | 0.8 | 365 | 0.03 | 0.04 | 0.5 | 4 |
| Bread, white, enriched | 100 | 4 slices | 270 | 9 | 3 | 50 | 84 | 97 | 20 | 2.5 | | 0.25 | 0.21 | 2.4 | |
| Cereal, whole grain or enriched** | 130 / 30 | ⅔ c cooked or 1 oz dry | 89 | 3 | 1 | 18 | 12 | 95 | 34 | 0.9 | | 0.08 | 0.03 | 0.7 | |
| Butter or margarine | 14 | 1 tbsp | 100 | | 11 | | 3 | 2 | 2 | | 460 | | | | |
| Totals | | | 1415 | 66 | 63 | 155 | 782 | 1012 | 335 | 10.3 | 6945 | 0.94 | 1.56 | 12.6†† | 105 |
| Compare with recommended allowances‡‡ | | | | | | | | | | | | | | | |
| Men (70 kg, 23–50 yrs old) | | | 2700 | 56 | | | 800 | 800 | 350 | 10.0 | 5000§§ | 1.40 | 1.60 | 18 | 60 |
| Women (55 kg, 23–50 yrs old) | | | 2000 | 44 | | | 800 | 800 | 300 | 18.0 | 4000‖‖ | 1.00 | 1.20 | 13 | 60 |

*Milk equivalents means evaporated milk and dried milk in amounts equivalent to fluid milk in nutritive content; cheese, if water-soluble minerals and vitamins have not been lost in whey; and food items made with milk.

†Evaluation based on the use of 700 g of beef (chuck, cooked), 200 g of pork (medium fat, roasted), 200 g of chicken (roaster, cooked, roasted), and 100 g of fish (halibut, cooked, broiled) per 10-day period, and egg occasionally.

‡Evaluation based on figures for cooked broccoli, carrots, spinach, and squash (all varieties).

§Evaluation based on figures for raw tomatoes and lettuce, and cooked peas, beets, lima beans, and fresh corn.

‖Evaluation based on figures for whole orange and grapefruit, and orange and grapefruit juices.

#Evaluation based on figures for banana, apple, unsweetened cooked prunes, and sweetened canned peaches.

**Evaluation based on figures for shredded wheat biscuit and oatmeal.

††The average diet in the United States, which contains a generous amount of protein, provides enough tryptophan to increase the niacin value by about one-third.

‡‡From the National Research Council Recommended Dietary Allowances, revised 1980.

§§5000 IU equals 1000 RE.

‖‖4000 IU equals 800 RE.

(From Composition of Foods. Handbook No. 8. USDA, revised 1963)

drate, minerals, and vitamins. The nutrients in foods are discussed in previous chapters, and an extensive table of the nutrient composition of common foods is found in Table 1, Part 4. In this section the derivation of food composition tables, commonly used tables, average servings, and the limitations of food tables are discussed.

## Food composition tables

Food composition tables give the proximate energy, protein, fat, and carbohydrate values and the mineral and vitamin contents of a defined amount of food, usually 100 g. The household measure that approximates the gram weight may or may not be stated. Today the values for energy are given in kilocalories. However, it is possible that the joule instead of the calorie may be used in future tables (4.2 kJ = 1 kcal). In all tables the values for minerals are given in milligrams with the exception of certain trace elements, such as fluorine, iodine, chromium, molybdenum, and selenium, which are stated in micrograms. Calcium may be given in grams. Values are given in International Units (IU) for vitamins A, D, and E, although recently retinol equivalents have been introduced for vitamin A, mcg of cholecalciferol for vitamin D, and mg d-$\alpha$-tocopherol equivalents for vitamin E (see Chap. 7). Values for other vitamins (1 mg = 0.001 g) are expressed as milligram ($10^{-3}$ g), microgram ($10^{-6}$ g), nanogram ($10^{-9}$ g), or picogram ($10^{-12}$ g).

When figures from more than one food composition table are used to estimate the nutrient content of a meal or a day's food intake, care must be taken to see that the units of measurement are the same in each table. If not, it is necessary to convert the units from one table to correspond to those of the other. For example, Table 1 in Part 4 gives the thiamin values in mg, whereas another commonly used table gives thiamin in mcg (1 mg = 1000 mcg).[15]

The term *proximate analysis* refers to those values in food composition tables for water, protein, lipids, carbohydrates, and ash. The term, proximate, is used because the figures may reflect substances that are unrelated chemically as well as the substance itself. For example, protein values are calculated from the total nitrogen in a food. Some of this nitrogen may come from nonprotein substances, such as purine bases. Carbohydrate figures reflect total carbohydrate by difference, that is, the difference between the total amount of water, protein, lipid, and ash and the total weight of the food. The carbohydrate figure includes pentoses and fiber in addition to mono-, di-, and polysaccharides, unless otherwise indicated. Crude fiber content may be determined by a routine procedure and subtracted from total carbohydrate to give an estimate of the amount of carbohydrate in foods that the body can convert to simple sugars.

In general, the figures given in food composition tables are representative values and apply to food as it is usually produced and marketed for year-round and countrywide use by the consumer. The values are derived from the research carried out in various food technology laboratories in universities, in the United States Department of Agriculture, and in industries throughout the country. The methods used for determining nutrient composition are usually those accepted by the Association of Official Agricultural Chemists. Although they are generally regarded as highly reproducible, they are not necessarily totally accurate in reflecting the amount of nutrient available. For instance, studies analyzing carotene values in yellow and green vegetables indicate losses of vitamin A activity of the carotenes in these vegetables when cooked or canned, which is not apparent when the usual laboratory procedures for determining this nutrient are followed.[16]

The value given for each nutrient in a food composition table represents an average (sometimes a weighted average) for the total number of samples of the particular food for which analyses were available. The figures for some nutrients were derived from the analysis of many samples, whereas others were derived from a limited number of analyses. In any case, the actual amount of a nutrient in any specific sample of a food may vary more or less widely from the average. Average values for ascorbic acid in tomato juice ranged only from 12.5 to 16.0 mg per deciliter over a 10-year period, whereas, in a single year individual samples ranged from 3.2 to 21.7 mg per deciliter.[17] Also, averages do not tell, for example, that half the ascorbic acid in potatoes is lost after several months' storage and that an additional amount is lost in cooking and reheating.

The representative values for such plant foods as cereal grain, fruits, and vegetables reflect variability in samples due to variety (genetics), maturity, part of the plant (such as leaves, flowers, stems, or roots), seasonal or geographical differences, length and type of storage, or other factors. Also, new methods or modifications of old methods of food processing may affect nutrient composition. At this time there are limited data on the mineral and vitamin contents of raw and prepared meats and poultry and on the nutrient values of baked products, such as sweet rolls, doughnuts and pizza, new varieties of tomatoes, which can be mechanically harvested, and a number of convenience foods.[18]

A statement made by research workers in the USDA when introducing a *Provisional Table on the Zinc Content of Foods* indicates some of the problems related to food tables.

> Values in the table . . . have been derived from data obtained by an exhaustive search of published literature and unpublished sources of information. . . . The table is called "provisional" because many of the values are derived from a limited number of analyses. It is not yet possible, from the data base available, to determine the extent to which fac-

tors such as variety, season, geographic location and fertilization may affect zinc content of some foods. The data reported here are considered by the authors to be the current best estimates for zinc content of foods as presently marketed.[19]

## Commonly used food composition tables

### Composition of foods: raw, processed, and prepared, USDA Handbook No. 8

Since its original publication in 1950, *USDA Handbook No. 8* has been the most widely used food composition table. It was revised in 1963 and has been undergoing a major change that will update and expand the handbook; both versions of the handbook are used by nutrition counselors and are described in the following paragraphs.

### Handbook No. 8, 1963 edition

This edition of *Handbook No. 8* contains five tables: Table 1, *Composition of Foods, 100 Grams, Edible Portion*; Table 2, *Nutrients in the Edible Portion of 1 Pound of Food as Purchased*; Table 3, *Selected Fatty Acids in Foods*; Table 4, *Cholesterol Content of Foods*; and Table 5, *Magnesium Content of Foods*. Tables 1 and 2 give a description of each food item and figures for the water, food energy, protein, fat, carbohydrate, ash, calcium, phosphorus, iron, sodium, potassium, vitamin A, thiamin, riboflavin, niacin, and ascorbic acid content of foods by alphabetical listing. No brand names are used to describe foods. Table 2 also gives the percentage of refuse per pound of the food as purchased. Table 3 gives the total fat, total saturated fatty acids, and the unsaturated fatty acids (oleic C18:1, linoleic C18:2) in 100 g, edible portion, and in the edible portion of 1 lb of food as purchased. Arachidonic (C20:4) acid is not listed because very little of this fatty acid occurs naturally in foods.

The items in Tables 1, 2, and 3 have been numbered uniformly. For example, item no. 410 in all three tables refers to *biscuits, baking powder, baked from home recipe*. Whenever the figures in *Handbook No. 8* are used to estimate the nutrient composition of a food or an intake, the item number as well as the nutrient values should be recorded on the analysis form in order to verify the figures easily.

Whenever Table 1 in *Handbook No. 8* is used to identify the nutrient content of a food in other than a 100-g portion, the appropriate calculations must be carried out. For example, the values for the 100-g portion of milk in Table 1 is multiplied by 2.4 to derive the figures for 240 g (one 8-oz cup). To derive the figures for 5 g of butter (1 tsp) the values for 100 g of butter are multiplied by 0.05.

When only the household measure of a food is known, such as ½ cup string beans, this measure must be converted to grams in order to calculate its nutritive value from Table 1 in *Handbook No. 8*. Fabietti[20] has offered a

method for converting volume to weight, or the serving of food can be weighed on a gram scale to determine its gram weight.

It is strongly recommended that anyone using *Handbook No. 8* carefully study the introduction and the information in Appendices A, B, and C and have a worksheet that reflects the format of Table 1 in order to record conveniently the nutritive values of food intakes and for filling in patients' charts when appropriate.

### Handbook No. 8, 1976 edition

The latest revision is being published in sections, each of which contains a table of nutrient data for a major food group. To facilitate continual and rapid updating, the handbook is prepared in looseleaf form, and each page contains the nutrient profile for a single food item, given on a 100-g food basis, in two common measures and in the edible portion, one pound as purchased. Values are listed for refuse, energy, proximate composition—water, protein, lipid, carbohydrate, and ash; nine minerals (calcium, iron, magnesium, phosphorus, potassium, sodium, zinc, copper, and manganese); nine vitamins (ascorbic acid, thiamin, riboflavin, niacin, pantothenic acid, vitamin $B_6$, folacin, vitamin $B_{12}$ and vitamin A); individual fatty acids, total saturated, monounsaturated, and polyunsaturated fatty acids; cholesterol, total phytosterols, and eighteen amino acids. The standard error of the values and the number of samples on which the values are based are also included.

### Nutritive value of American foods, USDA Handbook No. 456

The figures in *USDA Handbook 456* are calculated from the 1963 edition of *Handbook No. 8* with a limited amount of updating for some nutrients. It includes values for all the nutrients listed in the 1963 edition, except fiber and ash, in terms of specified volume measurements or units of food. The weight of food in grams corresponding to the various measures is also given for each item.

### Nutritive value of foods, Home and Garden Bulletin No. 72 (1981)

This Bulletin published by the USDA for consumers contains food values for over 730 foods based on average servings or common household units. The figures are derived from *Handbook No. 8*, 1963 edition, with some changes to reflect different food marketing and processing techniques. *Home and Garden Bulletin No. 72 (1981)* is given in Table 1, Part 4.

### Food values of portions commonly used[15]

This food composition table, now in its 13th edition, is commonly referred to as Bowes and Church because Anna dePlanter Bowes, a nutritionist, and Dr. C. F. Church were the authors of the first edition, published in

1937. The nutrient values given in this table have been derived from *Agriculture Handbook No. 8*, 1963 edition, other USDA food tables, and other resources as listed in the bibliography. This publication differs from *Agriculture Handbook No. 8* in that the food items are listed by groups, for example, breads, cereals and cereal products; the household measure as well as the gram weights (not necessarily 100 g) are given; brand names are used for some items; and, in addition to total protein, the quantities of the eight essential amino acids are given.

### Food industry tables

Some food processors make available tables of the food composition, and in some instances, the ingredients in their products. Some of these tables contain nutrient values derived from *Agriculture Handbook No. 8*, whereas others are figures from the analyses of the product done in the company's laboratory by food technologists. The institution of nutrition labeling by the United States Food and Drug Administration (see Chap. 15) has resulted in more tables that report actual analyses of products by brand name.

### Nutrient data bank

In 1973 the USDA, in cooperation with other government agencies and the food industry, initiated the establishment of a computerized Nutrient Data Bank. Food research laboratories have been given a form for submitting food composition data to the Nutrient Data Research Center. This system should make available in the future much more extensive information regarding nutrient composition of foods.

### Other computer nutrient data bases

Since 1959 the USDA has had available punched cards for computer-stored nutrient data bases. However, the great impetus for use of computerized nutrient data bases did not occur until after 1963 when the USDA provided both punched cards and magnetic tape of all the data included in that revision of *Handbook No. 8*. As each section of the new *Handbook No. 8* series is published, machine-readable tapes are also made available.

A number of institutions have developed extensive nutrient data banks for their specific purposes. In addition to the data from the USDA, they have acquired analysis from a variety of other sources, such as food manufacturers and other research laboratories.[21]

### Average servings

An average serving of a food is used in nutrition to describe the amount of food in a household measure by weight or volume or in a common unit that can be readily identified, such as 3 oz of cooked meat; $\frac{1}{2}$ pint or one 8-oz cup of milk; $\frac{1}{2}$ cup of cooked carrots, or one slice of bread. An average serving may or may not be a 100-g serving. One-half cup of carrots is approximately 100 g, whereas 8

oz of milk is 240 g, almost two and one-half times 100 g. In dietetics, $\frac{1}{2}$ cup refers to one-half of a standard 8-oz measuring cup; 1 tablespoon (tbsp) or 1 teaspoon (tsp) refers to standard measuring spoons.

Nutrition labeling regulations (see Chap. 15) require *serving size* to appear on each label as the basis for the nutrient content information. There have been many discussions among nutritionists, food technologists, and consumer specialists about what constitutes an average serving. The serving size used on the nutrition information panel is frequently larger than nutrition counselors suggest for "average-size servings."

### Limitations of food composition tables

Because the figures in food composition tables are representative of the energy and nutrient content of a food, it must be remembered that when one calculates the nutritional value of a day's food intake, of a diet plan, or of a recipe, the result will be an *estimation* of the energy and nutrient composition, not the exact composition. If the intake of food for any period is reported accurately by a person, or the intake is accurately observed and recorded, the analysis of energy, protein, fat, and carbohydrate in the intake, derived from commonly used food composition tables, will be reasonably accurate.

The variation of the fat composition of meat and convenience foods may result in an overestimation or underestimation of fat in an intake, with the result that the energy composition of the actual intake may vary as much as 10% to 15% from the estimation. The mineral and vitamin values in any food composition table are probably the least valid figures when used to estimate intakes. These nutrients in foods vary naturally, especially in fresh fruits and vegetables, and if these foods are processed or cooked, it must be remembered that certain vitamins, and, to some extent, minerals, are soluble in water, and that some vitamins can be destroyed by heat.

Therefore, in reports of the energy and nutrient intake of a person for any period of time, the figures recorded should reflect the limitation of the method, that is, the use of food composition tables. For example, recording a day's energy intake for one person calculated from a food composition table as 1832.8 kcal suggests a degree of accuracy that cannot be achieved by this method. A more appropriate recording in this situation would be 1835 kcal, or 1825 kcal to 1850 kcal.

This is not to imply that food composition tables are of little or no value; rather, they must be used appropriately within the limitations inherent in the method.

## Some generalizations about the nutrient composition of foods

The complexity of food composition tables may "turn off" the uninitiated. The nutrition educator cannot carry a food composition table or textbook with her at all times, although she should have one readily accessible. The Daily Food Guide (Fig. 11-1) can be used to assess a specific person's usual food intake, but this guide may not be adequate in all situations. Life-styles vary in our society, and food practices that differ from the Food Guide can supply adequate nutrient intakes. Some generalizations about food composition are offered in this section to assist the counselor in answering questions on the spot about food or in coping with the assessment of intake in the person whose food practices are "different."

## Energy

Fat and carbohydrates are the major sources of energy in the American diet today. In 1979, the USDA estimated that 3500 calories per person per day were available for civilian consumption.[23] Of these calories, 18% came from fats and oils, including butter and margarine and 17% from sugars and other sweeteners. Even at this level of consumption these two food groups do not contribute significantly to the intake of other nutrients, such as vitamins and minerals. For this reason, the term *empty calories* is frequently applied to fats and sugars.

At the same time, the USDA estimated that flour and cereals represented 19% of the calories available for civilian consumption, and potatoes and sweet potatoes represented 3%. In addition to calories from carbohydrates, these two groups of food can contribute very significant amounts of protein, iron, and the B vitamins to a person's daily nutrient intake. At 3% of the energy intake, potatoes contributed 15% of the 120 mg of ascorbic acid available per capita for civilian consumption in 1979.

Fat is the nutrient that most directly affects the energy value of a food and, therefore, a person's daily energy intake. One g of fat yields 9 kcal. In addition to fats, oils, butter, and margarine, varying amounts of fat occur naturally in foods. The variation in the amount of fat in meat is illustrated in Table 11-6. Note that if one consumes 100 g ($3\frac{1}{3}$ oz) of broiled steak, including both the lean and fat portions, he consumes significantly more calories than if he consumes 100 g of the cooked, lean portion only (387 kcal vs. 200 kcal).

The energy value of any portion of meat can be reduced by trimming off the visible fat around or between the muscle mass. However, the fat between the meat fibers of the muscle mass cannot be removed by trimming, and only partially by cooking, nor can the lipid layer of the cell membranes of meat be removed by trimming or cooking. Therefore, any portion of commonly used meats contains some fat. Chicken, turkey, and certain lean fish (commonly classified as dry fish) have considerably less fat than red meat per 100 g (see Table 11-6).

An example of the effect on the energy value of a food from which practically all the naturally occurring fat can be removed is shown in Table 11-7. Eight oz (1 cup) of skim milk contains approximately one-half the calories of a cup of whole milk (85 kcal vs. 150 kcal), whereas the energy value of 1 cup of partially skimmed milk reflects only a moderate reduction of total fat, compared with whole milk (120 kcal vs. 150 kcal).

The effect of the addition of fat to a food during preparation is illustrated in Table 11-8. Note that a potato is not a "high" calorie food *per se*, but the addition of fat during preparation markedly increases its energy value (65 kcal for 100-g boiled potato vs. 274 kcal for 100-g french fried potato).

Gravy served with mashed potatoes may or may not be a significant source of additional calories. One cup of gravy made with 2 tbsp flour and pan drippings from which *all* fat has been removed contains approximately 60 kcal, whereas 1 cup of gravy made with 2 tbsp flour and pan drippings from which the fat has *not* been removed may contain as much as 500 kcal. Therefore, $\frac{1}{4}$ cup of the gravy (an average serving) *without* fat contains 15 kcal, whereas $\frac{1}{4}$ cup *with* fat may contain as much as 125 kcal.

### Table 11-6. Energy, Protein, and Fat in 100 Grams of Selected Meat, Fish, and Poultry

| Food (100 g, $3\frac{1}{2}$ oz) | Energy (kcal) | Protein (g) | Fat (g) |
|---|---|---|---|
| Chicken, light meat, without skin | 166 | 32 | 3 |
| Cod, broiled | 170 | 29 | 5 |
| Beef, steak broiled | | | |
| lean and fat | 387 | 23 | 32 |
| lean | 200 | 32 | 8 |
| Pork, roast loin and shoulder | | | |
| lean and fat | 373 | 23 | 31 |
| lean | 283 | 29 | 13 |

(From Composition of Foods. Handbook No. 8. USDA, revised 1963)

### Table 11-7. Energy and Fat in 1 Cup of Whole Milk, Skimmed Milk, and Partially Skimmed Milk

| Food | Weight (g) | Energy (kcal) | Fat (g) |
|---|---|---|---|
| Milk, whole | 244 (1 c) | 150 | 8 |
| Milk, skim | 245 (1 c) | 85 | tr |
| Milk, partly skimmed* | 244 (1 c) | 120 | 5 |

*2% nonfat milk solids added.

(See Part 4, Table 1)

### Table 11-8. Energy and Fat in 100 Grams of Boiled, Mashed, and French-Fried Potatoes

| Food (100 g) | Energy (kcal) | Fat (g) |
|---|---|---|
| Boiled* ($\frac{1}{2}$ c) | 65 | tr |
| Mashed† ($\frac{1}{2}$ c) | 94 | 4 |
| French-fried (20 pc) | 274 | 13 |

*Pared before cooking.

†Milk and table fat added.

(From Composition of Foods. Handbook No. 8. USDA, revised 1963)

Another variation in energy value that can occur during food preparation is illustrated in Table 11-9. The two samples of veal cutlet, breaded and fried, differ in value by approximately 100 kcal (203 kcal vs. 294 kcal). Standel and co-workers reported that samples A and B came from two different restaurants, and it appeared that restaurant B used more bread, which, in turn, absorbed more fat during the frying process as reflected in the quantity of fat and carbohydrate in sample B.[24]

The energy value of a food can vary due to the carbohydrate content. Carbohydate yields 4 kcal per g. The energy value of fruits and vegetables varies directly with the water and carbohydrate content, as illustrated in Table 11-10. In general, certain fruits and the flowers, leaves, and stems of vegetables have a proportionately high water and low carbohydrate content, whereas certain fruits and seeds, tubers, and roots have less water and

more carbohydrate. Fruits and vegetables, including cooked potatoes, vary from approximately 5% to 20% in carbohydrate content. Dry cereal grains, such as oatmeal, are approximately 8% water and 75% carbohydrate. However, since cereal grains must be hydrated in order to be digested, the average serving of cooked cereal ($^1/_2$ cup or 100 g) is approximately 83% water and 15% carbohydrate.

The addition of sugar to fruits and the addition of sugar or fats to flavor cooked vegetables increases the energy content of these foods per serving. The energy value of precooked cereals can be modified significantly by the addition of sugar during processing. For example, 1 cup of plain cornflakes, without added sugar, contains approximately 95 kcal, whereas the same amount of flakes sugar-coated during production contains approximately 155 kcal.[25]

Sugar and fats combined with flour in desserts account for the energy value of these foods. This is illustrated in Table 11-11. Snack foods are an increasingly important source of energy in the diets of both children and adults.

The energy value of any person's food intake is directly dependent on the size of the portions of food consumed either at a meal or as a snack. If a person usually consumes a 200-g serving of lean steak, not 100 g as in Table 11-6, then the energy value of the serving will be 400, not 200, kcal. Similarly, one-quarter of a 9-in apple pie contains 605 kcal, not the 345 kcal for one-seventh of a 9-in apple pie as in Table 11-11.

### Table 11-9. Energy, Protein, Fat, and Carbohydrate in Two Samples of Veal Cutlet Breaded and Fried

| Food (100 g) | Energy (kcal) | Protein (g) | Fat (g) | Carbohydrate (g) |
|---|---|---|---|---|
| Sample A | 203 | 26.9 | 9.1 | 3.4 |
| Sample B | 294 | 12.9 | 18.8 | 18.4 |

(Standal BR et al: J Am Diet Assoc 56:392, 1970)

### Table 11-10. Water, Energy, and Carbohydrate in 100 Grams of Selected Fruits and Vegetables

| Food (100 g) | Water (Percent) | Energy (kcal) | Carbohydrate (g) |
|---|---|---|---|
| Broccoli, cooked | 91 | 26 | 5 |
| Tomatoes, raw | 94 | 22 | 5 |
| Pears, raw | 83 | 61 | 15 |
| Potato, cooked | 83 | 65 | 15 |
| Banana, raw | 76 | 85 | 22 |
| Corn, fresh, on cob | 74 | 91 | 21 |

(From Composition of Foods. Handbook No. 8. USDA, revised 1963)

### Table 11-11. Energy, Fat, and Carbohydrate in Average Servings of Selected Desserts

| Food | Weight (g) | Energy (kcal) | Fat (g) | Carbohydrate (g) |
|---|---|---|---|---|
| Brownies, with nuts, home recipe | 20 (one bar) | 95 | 6 | 10 |
| Ice cream | 66 ($^1/_2$ c) | 135 | 7 | 16 |
| Chocolate cake (with frosting) | 69 (one piece) | 235 | 8 | 40 |
| Apple pie | 135 ($^1/_7$ of pie) | 345 | 15 | 51 |

(See Part 4, Table 1)

### Protein

In 1979, the USDA reported that of the 104 g of protein available per person per day for civilian consumption, 42% was provided by meat, fish, and poultry; 22% by dairy products; 18% by flours and cereals; 5% by eggs; and 6% by dry beans and peas, nuts, and soya flour. Approximately 69% of the protein available for civilian consumption was from meat, eggs, and dairy products, which provide protein of high biologic value.

Meat, fish, and poultry vary from 20% to 30% protein (20 g–30 g in 100 g of food). The remainder is water (both in and around the cells), fat, undigestible connective tissue, minerals, and vitamins. Eggs are approximately 13% protein, and milk 3.5% protein.

In the United States, cereal grains, dried beans, or peas, nuts, or soya products are not considered significant sources of protein, even though these foods are used widely around the world and are listed as an alternate for meat in the Daily Guide published by the USDA. Cereals and dried beans or peas are usually classified as starchy (carbohydrate) foods. However, in situations where either money for purchasing food is limited or a person prefers to use cereals and dried peas or beans, these foods can make a significant contribution to the adequacy of the intake of protein and to the intakes of iron, thiamin, riboflavin, and niacin, especially if the cereals are whole grain or enriched.

## Vitamins

Milk, meat, fish and poultry, eggs, and whole or enriched grain products (cereals, breads, and flours) are the significant sources of the B vitamins. Consumed in the amounts recommended in the Daily Food Guide, these foods supply from one-half to two-thirds of the recommended dietary allowances for these nutrients. The recommended servings of fruits and vegetables supply an adequate intake of vitamin C. However, if instead of citrus fruit and tomatoes, liberal servings of fresh potatoes and other fresh vegetables and fruits are consumed daily, the diet will contain adequate amounts of vitamin C.

The fat-soluble vitamins require special attention. An adequate intake of vitamin A can be derived from dark green and deep yellow fruits and vegetables, milk fats, and fortified margarine. As a group, the fat-soluble vitamins require fat for absorption.

## Minerals

The evidence presently available indicates that adequate iron intake is a problem, especially for infants 6 to 18 months of age, toddlers 1 to 3 years, adolescent girls, and women of childbearing age. The most significant food source of iron—liver—is not a popular food and, for this reason, not a widely acceptable solution to the problem. Also, because the liver is only 1.5% of the dressed weight of a steer, it will probably never be available in quantities large enough to solve the problem.

In 1979, the USDA reported that approximately 18.5 mg of iron per person per day was available for civilian consumption. Meat, fish and poultry, and eggs contributed 34% of the available iron, whereas flour and cereal grains contributed 29% due partly to the iron enrichment of flour and cereal products. Fruits, vegetables including potatoes, dry beans and peas, nuts, and soya flour contributed 26% of the available iron.

The percentage of iron absorbed from food is influenced not only by the form of iron in the specific food but also by other constituents of the diets. This problem is under intensive study and has resulted in a suggested formula for the determination of the availability of iron in the diet (see Chap. 6).

The major source of calcium in the American diet is milk and the milk products, with the exceptions of butter, cream cheese, and cottage cheese. The Daily Food Guide recommends 2 or more cups of milk for an adult. This amount of milk contains 582 mg of calcium—a significant contribution to the 800 mg recommended by the National Research Council. The usual selection of foods from the other groups in the Daily Food Guide contributes 200 mg to 300 mg of calcium per day (see Table 11-5).

The addition of milk products, specifically milk solids, to bread and a variety of processed foods can contribute significantly to a person's daily intake of calcium. The adolescent boy who eats ten slices of bread made with 4% nonfat dry milk is consuming 210 mg of calcium. Also, in areas where monocalcium phosphate baking powder is used daily to make hot breads, such as biscuits and cornbread, these foods can be significant sources of calcium.

Phosphorus is widely distributed in foods from both animal and plant sources.

## Convenience foods

Convenience foods have entered the retail market in volume in the past 15 years, and the information needed to compare the nutritive values of these products with comparable products made in the home is not readily available.

Table 11-12 shows the calorie and nutrient variation in only one product—macaroni and cheese. For two of the items in the table, brand B-1 and brand B-2, all of the data are not available. Brand A is a canned product; B-1 is a dry mix; and B-2 and C are frozen products. Note that the convenience-packaged products vary significantly in energy, protein, and calcium content from the product made from a commonly used home recipe.

Table 11-13 illustrates the variation in a product depending on whether enriched or unenriched flour is used. The nutrient composition of the homemade cookies was calculated from a recipe using enriched flour. From

**Table 11-12. Nutrient Composition of Homemade and Convenience-Packaged Macaroni and Cheese**

| Food | Weight (g) | Household Measure | Energy (kcal) | Protein (g) | Fat (g) | Carbohydrate (g) | Calcium (mg) | Iron (mg) | Vitamin A (IU) | Thiamin (mg) | Riboflavin (mg) | Niacin (mg) |
|---|---|---|---|---|---|---|---|---|---|---|---|---|
| Homemade* | 100 | ½ c | 215 | 8 | 11 | 20 | 181 | 0.9 | 430 | 0.10 | 0.20 | 0.9 |
| Brand A† | 100 | ½ c | 97 | 3.7 | 4.2 | 11.0 | 56 | 0.6 | 230 | 0.09 | 0.09 | 1.2 |
| Brand B-1‡ | 100 | ½ c | 179 | 5.8 | 7.1 | 23.0 | 81 | NA‖ | NA | NA | NA | NA |
| Brand B-2‡ | 100 | ½ c | 170 | 7.8 | 8.4 | 15.5 | 224 | NA | NA | NA | NA | NA |
| Brand C§ | 100 | ½ c | 134 | 5.9 | 6.0 | 13.9 | 127 | 0.4 | 237 | 0.03 | 0.11 | 0.32 |

*See Part 4, Table 1. Values calculated from a recipe.

†Canned.

‡Same manufacturer: B-1 dry mix; B-2 frozen.

§Frozen.

‖NA—Figures not available.

(Figures courtesy Preschool Nutrition Survey; Owen GM et al: Preschool Nutrition Survey. Pediatrics (Suppl) 53: Apr, 1974)

the nutrient values provided by the manufacturer for the chilled cookie dough to be baked in the home, it appears that unenriched flour was used in this convenience product. The energy values are similar.

## Foods fortified or enriched to help meet nutritional norms

About 60 years ago nutritionists began to investigate how certain nutritional limitations in our food supplies could be corrected. The first large-scale experiment was the addition of iodine to salt to prevent goiter. This program was so successful that iodized salt is available in most markets today (see Chap. 6).

In the 1930s the fortification of homogenized milk with vitamin D was started in an attempt to prevent rickets in infants. Today most of the homogenized milk in our markets is fortified with 400 IU of vitamin D per quart. Much of the dry, skimmed milk is also fortified with vitamins A and D (see Chap. 7).

In the 1940s the increased use of margarines prompted the addition of vitamin A to make the content equivalent to average butter. Today all margarines in our markets are fortified with 15,000 IU of vitamin A per pound. Some margarines also have 2000 IU of vitamin D per pound added.

During World War II, the enrichment of bread and flour with iron, thiamin, riboflavin, and niacin was initiated when it was realized that repeated attempts to persuade people to use whole grains were unsuccessful. The modification of natural grains by milling had produced a more acceptable flour—whiter and with better keeping qualities, but had reduced the vitamin and mineral content. Now the practice of enriching milled grains and breads has expanded to include not only wheat, but also corn and rice and ready-to-eat breakfast cereals. Some macaroni, spaghetti, and noodle products are also enriched. Dry infant cereals have relatively large amounts of iron as well as certain B-complex vitamins added to them. Enrichment of white flour and bread is now mandatory in most states and in Puerto Rico, and enrichment of cornmeal is common in Southern states. Actually, most of the bread and all-purpose flour sold in the United States today is enriched, although this is not mandatory in all states. However, many of the prepared foods, such as packaged mixes, frozen baked products, refrigerated doughs, and crackers are made from nonenriched flour.

Although the indiscriminate fortification of foods has been discouraged, a number of other food products have had vitamins and minerals added to them in varying amounts. Careful consideration must be given to any new proposal for fortification; for example, too enthusiastic fortification with vitamin D might be harmful for young children consuming excess amounts of this nutrient.

The 1973 Policy Statement of the Food and Nutrition Board in regard to Improvement of Nutritive Quality of Foods

. . . endorses the addition of nutrients to foods in order to achieve enrichment or fortification when all of the following conditions are met:

1. The intake of the nutrients is below the desirable level in the diets of a significant number of people;
2. The food used to supply the nutrients is likely to be consumed in quantities that will make a significant contribution to the diet of the population in need;
3. The addition of the nutrients is not likely to create a dietary imbalance;
4. The nutrient added is stable under customary conditions of storage and use;
5. The nutrient is physiologically available from the food;
6. The enhanced levels attained in the total diet will not be harmfully excessive for those who may employ the foods in varying patterns of use; and
7. The additional cost is reasonable for the intended consumer.

Thus the enrichment of flour, bread, degerminated corn meal, corn grits, whole grain corn meal, white rice, and certain other cereal grain products with thiamin, riboflavin, niacin, and iron; the addition of vitamin D to milk, fluid skim milk, and nonfat dry milk; the addition of vitamin A to margarine, fluid skim milk, and nonfat dry milk; and the addition of iodine to table salt [are endorsed]. The protective action of fluoride against dental caries is recognized and the standardized addition of fluoride to water in areas in which the water supply has a low fluoride content is endorsed.[26]

**Table 11-13. Nutrient Composition of Homemade and Homebaked Sugar Cookies**

| Food | Weight (g) | Household Measure | Energy (kcal) | Protein (g) | Fat (g) | Carbohydrate (g) | Calcium (mg) | Iron (mg) | Vitamin A (IU) | Thiamin (mg) | Riboflavin (mg) | Niacin (mg) |
|---|---|---|---|---|---|---|---|---|---|---|---|---|
| Homemade sugar cookies* | 20 | 2″ diam | 89 | 1.2 | 3.3 | 16 | 15 | 0.3 | 22 | 0.03 | 0.03 | 0.2 |
| Homebaked sugar cookies† | 20 | 2″ diam | 90 | 0.7 | 4.5 | 12 | 6 | 0.06 | 14 | 0.004 | 0.006 | 0.04 |

*Values (Handbook No. 8, USDA, 1963) calculated from a recipe using enriched flour.

†Dough, chilled unbaked, commercial, unenriched.

(Figures courtesy Preschool Nutrition Survey; Owen GM et al: Preschool Nutrition Survey. Pediatrics (Suppl) 53: Apr, 1974)

## Study questions and activities

1. The Food and Nutrition Board of the National Research Council has recommended dietary allowances for certain specific nutrients. Which ones are listed in Tables 11-1 to 11-3? What are the differences in rationale for the figures in each table?

2. These allowances are listed for different age and sex categories. For which of these are the allowances as great for young children as for a grown man? Why?

3. How were the single-valued nutrient allowances per 1000 kcal established?

4. Choose any dietary pattern with which you are familiar and plan a day's menu according to the Daily Food Guide (Fig. 11-1), using foods well liked by the people for whom it is intended.

5. Which nutrients are most difficult to obtain in sufficient quantities in low-cost meals in your locality at the season of the year when you are studying this chapter?

6. List the foods you ate yesterday and check to see whether all four food groups were adequately represented.

7. For what reason were the US-RDA established?

8. What are food composition tables? How are protein values calculated? What does "total carbohydrate by difference" mean? List two commonly used food composition tables and show how they differ.

9. How may preparation affect the amount of fat in a serving of pork chops? A serving of eggs? Of gravy?

10. What is meant by fortified milk? By enriched bread?

## References

1. Food and Nutrition Board: Recommended Dietary Allowances, 9th rev ed. Washington, DC, NAS-NRC, 1980
2. Canadian Council on Nutrition: Dietary standards for Canada. Can Bull Nutr 6:1, 1964 (Suppl, 1974)
3. FAO/WHO Expert Group: Calcium requirements. WHO Tech Rep Ser, no. 230. Geneva, World Health Organization, 1962
4. Joint FAO/WHO Expert Group: Requirements of vitamin A, thiamine, riboflavin and niacin. WHO Tech Rep Ser, no. 362. Geneva, World Health Organization, 1967
5. Joint FAO/WHO Expert Group: Requirements of ascorbic acid, vitamin D, vitamin $B_{12}$, folate and iron. WHO Tech Rep Ser, no. 452. Geneva, World Health Organization, 1970
6. Joint FAO/WHO Ad Hoc Expert Committee: Energy and protein requirements. WHO Tech Rep Ser, no. 522. Geneva, World Health Organization, 1973
7. WHO Expert Committee: Trace elements in human nutrition. WHO Tech Rep Ser, no. 532. Geneva, World Health Organization, 1973
8. Campbell JA: J Am Diet Assoc 64:175, 1974
9. Hansen RG, Wyse BW: J Am Diet Assoc 76:223, 1980
10. Hansen RG: Nutr Rev 31:1, 1973
11. Sorenson AW et al: J Am Diet Assoc 68:236, 1976
12. Guthrie HA: J Am Diet Assoc 71:14, 1977
13. Wyse BW, Hansen RG: J Am Diet Assoc 75:242, 1979
14. Essentials of an Adequate Diet, rev ed. Washington, DC, USDA, Consumer and Food Economics Research Division, 1964
15. Pennington JAT, Church HN: Food Values of Portions Commonly Used, 13th ed. Philadelphia, JB Lippincott, 1980
16. Sweeney JP, Marsh AC: J Am Diet Assoc 59:238, 1971
17. Farrow RP et al: J Food Sci 38:595, 1973
18. Watt BK, Murphy EW: Food Tech 24:675, 1970
19. Murphy EW, Willis BW, Watt BK: Abstract of paper presented at the 57th annual meeting of the American Dietetic Association, Philadelphia, Oct 8, 1974
20. Fabietti LG: J Am Diet Assoc 60:135, 1972
21. Hertzler AA, Hoover LW: J Am Diet Assoc 70:20, 1977
22. Witschi J et al: J Am Diet Assoc 78:609, 1981
23. Marston RM, Peterkin BB: Nutrient Content of the National Food Supply, pp 21–25. National Food Review, Washington, DC, USDA, Winter, 1980
24. Standal BR et al: J Am Diet Assoc 56:392, 1970
25. Nutritive Value of Foods. Home and Garden Bulletin No. 72. Washington, DC, USDA, United States Government Printing Office, 1981
26. Food and Nutrition Board: General Policies in Regard to Improvement of Nutritive Quality of Foods. Washington, DC, National Academy of Sciences, 1973

## Supplementary readings

Campbell JA: Approaches in revising dietary standards—Canadian, U.S. and international standards compared. J Am Diet Assoc 64:175, 1974

Food, Home and Garden Bulletin No. 228. Washington, DC, USDA, United States Government Printing Office, 1979

Food and Nutrition Board: Recommended Dietary Allowances, 9th rev ed. Washington, DC, NAS-NRC, 1980

Guthrie HA: Concept of a nutritious food. J Am Diet Assoc 71:14, 1977

Guthrie HA, Scheer JC: Validity of a dietary score for assessing nutrient adequacy. J Am Diet Assoc 78:240, 1981

Hansen RG, Wyse BW: Expression of nutrient allowances per 1000 kilocalories. J Am Diet Assoc 76:223, 1980

Hertzler AA, Anderson HL: An historical review: Food guides in the United States. J Am Diet Assoc 64:19, 1974

Leverton RM: The RDAs are not for amateurs. J Am Diet Assoc 66:9, 1975

Mertz W: The new RDAs: Estimated adequate and safe intake of trace elements and calculation of intake of iron. J Am Diet Assoc 76:128, 1980

Munro HN: How well recommended are the Recommended Dietary Allowances? J Am Diet Assoc 71:490, 1977

Munro HN: The status of the elderly—Major gaps in nutrient allowances. J Am Diet Assoc 76:137, 1980

Peterkin BB, Patterson PC et al: Changes in dietary patterns. J Am Diet Assoc 78:453, 1981

Sorenson AW et al: An Index of Nutritional Quality for a balanced diet. J Am Diet Assoc 68:236, 1976

Windham CT, Wyse BW, et al: Consistency of nutrient consumption patterns in the United States. J Am Diet Assoc 78:587, 1981

*For further references see Bibliography in Part 4.*

# Meal Management

## 12

Planning
Purchasing
Storage
Preparation
Meal Service

If mealtimes are to fulfill the nutritional needs of the various family members, as well as the many other purposes associated with such occasions in our culture, the manager, particularly when inexperienced, may need assistance from the nutrition educator in meal management. This chapter outlines the steps that have proven helpful in achieving successful family meals. As skill in this area is developed, some of the steps may be combined.

## Planning

Successful meal management implies efficient use of the manager's resources—knowledge, skill, time, money, and equipment—to accomplish predetermined goals. Goals for family or group meals may differ widely depending on individual life-styles, but most managers would agree on the following three goals, although perhaps not in the order specified. Family or group meals should meet the nutritional norms established for each individual member, fit within the available food budget, and be acceptable to each member.

Planning is the key to each step of the process, which includes the preparation of menus and shopping lists, the purchasing and storing of food, and the preparation and service of meals. Because the amount of time spent in planning is most directly related to the knowledge, skill, and experience that the manager brings to the task, it decreases as these are gained. Taking time at the beginning to plan the various steps often pays dividends later by saving time as well as money and energy when one is shopping or preparing meals.

### Menu planning

Using a guide, such as the Daily Food Guide (see Fig. 11-1), the manager may plan a week's menus, which take into consideration the group's preference as well as the time, energy, and money available. Because there are many food patterns that meet the RDA (see Chap. 11), menu plans that do not conform to the Daily Food Guide should be evaluated in terms of amounts of specific nutrients and not merely food groups. Suggested changes in family menus should also be made with due consideration for the family's food pattern, rather than for stereotyped food guides. Any pattern that suits the group is a good one if it provides for regular meals and allows for a variety of foods that meet nutritional requirements.

Meal patterns in many areas of the United States have come to vary widely from the traditional three meals a day. For many Americans one or two meals plus additional "minimeals" appear to have become the accepted norm. This phenomenon, perhaps, offers the greatest challenge to the nutrition planner, who must provide foods adequate in essential nutrients while recognizing the need to count calories. Because many of the foods included in these minimeals are so-called snack foods, the nutrient composition of these should be of great concern to the meal manager. It is expected that increased and improved nutritional labeling will assist the planner in evaluating the contribution to the diet of these foods as well as many others. Nutrition labeling when appropriately used by the planner provides helpful information for relating serving size to calories and to amounts of essential nutrients (see Chap. 15).

Cultural preferences also determine the esthetic qualities that require consideration in menu planning. Variation in flavor, color, texture, shape, and temperature are factors that the manager should recognize in creating meals that will be acceptable to the group. Although no set rules can be applied to these elements, the manager's sensitivity to them and her creativity in dealing with them cannot be overlooked by the nutrition educator. Magazines, newspapers, and cookbooks are often helpful in these respects, especially to the inexperienced planner. Menu planning help is also available from government publications, especially from the Home and Garden Bulletins of the USDA (see the *Supplementary Readings* at the end of this chapter) and the State Cooperative Extension Services, and from food trade associations, such as the Cereal Institute and the National Dairy Council.

### Food plans

For more than 40 years, the USDA has published food plans as guides for determining food needs and estimating food costs of families and other population groups. Four food plans at different cost levels are shown in Tables 12-1–12-4. They include the thrifty, low, moderate, and liberal cost food plans. The homemaker can choose the appropriate food plan according to the amount of money the family has budgeted for food costs.

As shown in the tables, there are 15 food groups in each of the food plans, and the amounts suggested in each food group vary according to age and sex of family members and the cost level of the plan selected. When properly used, the food plans provide the recommended dietary

allowances for energy, protein, calcium, vitamin A, thiamin, riboflavin, niacin, and ascorbic acid. The RDA for iodine can be met if iodized salt is used. Iron intake may be low, especially for women of childbearing age; iron supplements for this group may be required. Iron-fortified cereal is recommended for infants and children 1 to 2 years of age. It is estimated that at least 80% of the RDA for vitamin $B_6$ and magnesium is provided and that further adjustments in the food groups may be appropriate when additional food composition data is available. Similarly, insufficient information about the amounts of folacin, zinc, vitamin D, and vitamin E in foods makes impossible reliable estimates of the levels of these nutrients provided by the plans.

Homemakers may find it more beneficial to start with the appropriate food plan rather than the Daily Food Guide, estimate the amount needed in each food group, and then prepare menus and shopping lists based on the food plan.

Table 12-5 shows the weekly quantities of food suggested according to the low-cost food plan for a family of four—mother, age 30; father, age 32; girl, age 6; and boy, age 12. The specific foods selected within each of the food groups will then depend on the availability and cost of the individual foods as well as the preferences of the family. Menus and shopping lists based on the suggested amounts of food from each of the food groups for a family of four are shown in Tables 12-6 and 12-7.

### Shopping lists

Until some experience has been gained in knowing the types and amounts of food required for various menu items, the homemaker may save time, money, and heartache by making a shopping list based on the week's menus. Most local markets usually advertise in the newspaper; these ads are most helpful in indicating the foods available and their prices. The homemaker should substitute for foods that may not be in the market or that may be priced too high for the consumer's food budget. Shopping lists are good deterrents to impulse buying in the supermarket, especially if the spouse and children accompany the shopper.

### Purchasing

Most communities offer a variety of different markets, and the wise shopper soon learns where to buy certain items. The newspaper advertisements also tell where to find specials on various foods. Usually one or two markets in close proximity to the shopper are the most appropriate choices when transportation costs are included.

If adequate refrigeration and freezer storage are available, most consumers find weekly grocery shopping most convenient. Although many stores are open 7 days a

**Table 12-1. Thrifty Food Plan—Amounts of Food for a Week**

| Family Member | Milk, Cheese, Ice Cream* | Meat, Poultry, Fish† | Eggs | Dry Beans and Peas, Nuts‡ | Dark-Green, Deep-Yellow Vegetables | Citrus Fruit, Tomatoes | Potatoes | Other Vegetables, Fruit | Cereal | Flour | Bread | Other Bakery Products | Fats, Oils | Sugar, Sweets | Accessories§ |
|---|---|---|---|---|---|---|---|---|---|---|---|---|---|---|---|
| | qt | lb | no | lb | lb | lb | lb | lb | lb | lb | lb | lb | lb | lb | lb |
| *Child:* | | | | | | | | | | | | | | | |
| 7 months to 1 year | 4.95 | 0.39 | 1.2 | 0.15 | 0.41 | 0.55 | 0.09 | 2.49 | 1.02// | 0.02 | 0.08 | 0.04 | 0.04 | 0.19 | 0.05 |
| 1–2 years | 3.30 | 0.83 | 3.3 | 0.17 | 0.22 | 0.89 | 0.65 | 2.26 | 1.02// | 0.31 | 0.78 | 0.24 | 0.11 | 0.30 | 0.37 |
| 3–5 years | 3.54 | 0.95 | 2.5 | 0.28 | 0.20 | 0.92 | 0.88 | 2.28 | 1.03 | 0.37 | 0.94 | 0.53 | 0.38 | 0.74 | 0.59 |
| 6–8 years | 4.22 | 1.27 | 2.4 | 0.49 | 0.22 | 1.10 | 1.23 | 2.50 | 1.12 | 0.62 | 1.42 | 0.79 | 0.51 | 0.94 | 0.84 |
| 9–11 years | 4.92 | 1.61 | 3.4 | 0.53 | 0.28 | 1.52 | 1.48 | 3.38 | 1.34 | 0.81 | 1.82 | 1.10 | 0.60 | 1.20 | 1.10 |
| *Man:* | | | | | | | | | | | | | | | |
| 12–14 years | 5.18 | 1.79 | 3.6 | 0.67 | 0.33 | 1.45 | 1.59 | 3.30 | 1.22 | 0.81 | 2.07 | 1.13 | 0.77 | 1.21 | 1.45 |
| 15–19 years | 5.08 | 2.35 | 4.0 | 0.43 | 0.32 | 1.70 | 2.10 | 3.43 | 0.98 | 0.99 | 2.36 | 1.46 | 1.00 | 1.05 | 1.73 |
| 20–54 years | 2.57 | 3.03 | 4.0 | 0.44 | 0.39 | 1.80 | 2.02 | 3.69 | 0.89 | 0.92 | 2.29 | 1.33 | 0.95 | 0.86 | 1.24 |
| 55 years and over | 2.37 | 2.45 | 4.0 | 0.25 | 0.51 | 1.85 | 1.75 | 3.77 | 1.09 | 0.80 | 1.90 | 1.12 | 0.79 | 0.94 | 0.73 |
| *Woman:* | | | | | | | | | | | | | | | |
| 12–19 years | 5.35 | 1.80 | 3.8 | 0.28 | 0.42 | 1.74 | 1.22 | 3.61 | 0.72 | 0.76 | 1.49 | 0.84 | 0.51 | 0.74 | 1.36 |
| 20–54 years | 2.81 | 2.41 | 4.0 | 0.27 | 0.52 | 1.86 | 1.51 | 3.39 | 0.90 | 0.67 | 1.41 | 0.67 | 0.57 | 0.57 | 1.18 |
| 55 years and over | 2.85 | 1.84 | 4.0 | 0.19 | 0.60 | 2.02 | 1.26 | 3.73 | 1.12 | 0.68 | 1.30 | 0.58 | 0.37 | 0.45 | 0.66 |
| Pregnant | 5.25# | 2.69 | 4.0 | 0.42 | 0.56 | 2.17 | 1.89 | 4.03 | 1.13 | 0.58 | 1.41 | 0.66 | 0.59 | 0.58 | 1.48 |
| Nursing | 5.25# | 3.00 | 4.0 | 0.38 | 0.57 | 2.36 | 1.92 | 4.27 | 0.98 | 0.63 | 1.56 | 0.82 | 0.80 | 0.75 | 1.54 |

* Fluid milk and beverage made from dry or evaporated milk. Cheese and ice cream may replace some milk. Count as equivalent to a quart of fluid milk: Natural or processed cheddar-type cheese, 6 oz; cottage cheese, 2½ lb; ice cream or ice milk, 1½ qt; unflavored yoghurt, 4 cups.

† Bacon and salt pork should not exceed ⅓ lb for each 5 lb of this group.

‡ Weight in terms of dry beans and peas, shelled nuts, and peanut butter. Count 1 lb of canned dry beans—pork and beans, kidney beans, and so on—as 0.33 pound.

§ Includes coffee, tea, cocoa, soft drinks, punches, ades, leavenings, and seasonings.

// Cereal fortified with iron is recommended.

# For pregnant and nursing teenagers, 7 qt are recommended.

(Amounts are for food as purchased or brought into the kitchen from garden or farm to prepare *all* meals and snacks for the week. Amounts allow for a discard of about 5% of the *edible* food as plate waste, spoilage, and so forth.)

## Table 12-2. Low-Cost Food Plan—Amounts of Food for a Week

| Family Member | Milk, Cheese, Ice Cream* (qt) | Meat, Poultry, Fish† (lb) | Eggs (no) | Dry Beans and Peas, Nuts‡ (lb) | Dark-Green, Deep-Yellow Vegetables (lb) | Citrus Fruit, Tomatoes (lb) | Potatoes (lb) | Other Vegetables, Fruit (lb) | Cereal (lb) | Flour (lb) | Bread (lb) | Other Bakery Products (lb) | Fats, Oils (lb) | Sugar, Sweets (lb) | Accessories§ (lb) |
|---|---|---|---|---|---|---|---|---|---|---|---|---|---|---|---|
| **Child:** | | | | | | | | | | | | | | | |
| 7 months to 1 year | 5.70 | 0.56 | 2.1 | 0.15 | 0.35 | 0.42 | 0.06 | 3.43 | 0.71// | 0.02 | 0.06 | 0.05 | 0.05 | 0.18 | 0.06 |
| 1–2 years | 3.57 | 1.26 | 3.6 | 0.16 | 0.23 | 1.01 | 0.60 | 2.88 | 0.99// | 0.27 | 0.76 | 0.33 | 0.12 | 0.36 | 0.68 |
| 3–5 years | 3.91 | 1.52 | 2.7 | 0.25 | 0.25 | 1.20 | 0.85 | 2.95 | 0.90 | 0.30 | 0.91 | 0.57 | 0.38 | 0.71 | 1.02 |
| 6–8 years | 4.74 | 2.03 | 2.9 | 0.39 | 0.31 | 1.58 | 1.10 | 3.67 | 1.11 | 0.45 | 1.27 | 0.84 | 0.52 | 0.90 | 1.43 |
| 9–11 years | 5.46 | 2.57 | 3.9 | 0.44 | 0.38 | 2.13 | 1.41 | 4.81 | 1.24 | 0.62 | 1.65 | 1.20 | 0.61 | 1.15 | 1.89 |
| **Man:** | | | | | | | | | | | | | | | |
| 12–14 years | 5.74 | 2.98 | 4.0 | 0.56 | 0.40 | 1.99 | 1.50 | 3.90 | 1.15 | 0.67 | 1.88 | 1.25 | 0.77 | 1.15 | 2.61 |
| 15–19 years | 5.49 | 3.74 | 4.0 | 0.34 | 0.39 | 2.20 | 1.87 | 4.50 | 0.90 | 0.75 | 2.10 | 1.55 | 1.05 | 1.04 | 3.09 |
| 20–54 years | 2.74 | 4.56 | 4.0 | 0.33 | 0.48 | 2.32 | 1.87 | 4.81 | 0.93 | 0.71 | 2.10 | 1.47 | 0.91 | 0.81 | 2.11 |
| 55 years and over | 2.61 | 3.63 | 4.0 | 0.21 | 0.61 | 2.38 | 1.72 | 4.92 | 1.02 | 0.62 | 1.73 | 1.23 | 0.77 | 0.90 | 1.16 |
| **Woman:** | | | | | | | | | | | | | | | |
| 12–19 years | 5.63 | 2.55 | 4.0 | 0.24 | 0.46 | 2.17 | 1.17 | 4.57 | 0.75 | 0.63 | 1.44 | 1.05 | 0.53 | 0.88 | 2.44 |
| 20–54 years | 3.02 | 3.21 | 4.0 | 0.19 | 0.55 | 2.34 | 1.40 | 4.17 | 0.71 | 0.55 | 1.31 | 0.94 | 0.59 | 0.72 | 2.13 |
| 55 years and over | 3.01 | 2.45 | 4.0 | 0.15 | 0.62 | 2.54 | 1.22 | 4.57 | 0.97 | 0.58 | 1.24 | 0.86 | 0.38 | 0.64 | 1.11 |
| Pregnant | 5.25 | 3.68 | 4.0 | 0.29 | 0.67 | 2.80 | 1.65 | 4.99 | 0.95 | 0.66 | 1.52 | 1.06 | 0.55 | 0.78 | 2.56 |
| Nursing | 5.25 | 4.16 | 4.0 | 0.26 | 0.66 | 2.99 | 1.67 | 5.33 | 0.78 | 0.61 | 1.55 | 1.16 | 0.76 | 0.91 | 2.70 |

* Fluid milk and beverage made from dry or evaporated milk. Cheese and ice cream may replace some milk. Count as equivalent to a quart of fluid milk: natural or processed cheddar-type cheese, 6 oz; cottage cheese, 2½ lb; ice cream, 1½ qt.

† Bacon and salt pork should not exceed ⅓ pound for each 5 pounds of this group.

‡ Weight in terms of dry beans and peas, shelled nuts, and peanut butter. Count 1 pound of canned dry beans—pork and beans, kidney beans, and so on—as 0.33 pound.

§ Includes coffee, tea, cocoa, punches, ades, soft drinks, leavenings, and seasonings. The use of iodized salt is recommended.

// Cereal fortified with iron is recommended.

(Amounts are for food as purchased or brought into the kitchen from garden or farm. Amounts allow for a discard of about one-tenth of the *edible* food as plate waste, spoilage, and so forth. Amounts of foods shown to two decimal places to allow for greater accuracy, especially in estimating rations for large groups of people and for long periods of time. For general use, amounts of food groups for a family may be rounded to the nearest tenth or quarter of a pound.)

# Table 12-3. Moderate-Cost Food Plan—Amounts of Food for a Week

| Family Member | Milk, Cheese, Ice Cream* | Meat, Poultry, Fish† | Eggs | Dry Beans and Peas, Nuts‡ | Dark-Green, Deep-Yellow Vegetables | Citrus Fruit, Tomatoes | Potatoes | Other Vegetables, Fruit | Cereal | Flour | Bread | Other Bakery Products | Fats, Oils | Sugar, Sweets | Accessories§ |
|---|---|---|---|---|---|---|---|---|---|---|---|---|---|---|---|
| | qt | lb | no | lb | lb | lb | lb | lb | lb | lb | lb | lb | lb | lb | lb |
| *Child:* | | | | | | | | | | | | | | | |
| 7 months to 1 year | 6.46 | 0.80 | 2.2 | 0.13 | 0.41 | 0.49 | 0.06 | 3.98 | 0.64// | 0.02 | 0.06 | 0.05 | 0.05 | 0.19 | 0.08 |
| 1–2 years | 4.04 | 1.69 | 4.0 | 0.15 | 0.29 | 1.24 | 0.59 | 3.44 | 1.03// | 0.26 | 0.81 | 0.33 | 0.12 | 0.28 | 0.79 |
| 3–5 years | 4.74 | 1.88 | 3.0 | 0.22 | 0.30 | 1.46 | 0.85 | 3.51 | 0.74 | 0.27 | 0.82 | 0.73 | 0.41 | 0.81 | 1.42 |
| 6–8 years | 5.79 | 2.60 | 3.3 | 0.34 | 0.37 | 1.94 | 1.17 | 4.39 | 0.84 | 0.39 | 1.14 | 1.11 | 0.56 | 1.03 | 1.97 |
| 9–11 years | 6.68 | 3.31 | 4.0 | 0.38 | 0.45 | 2.61 | 1.40 | 5.76 | 1.03 | 0.51 | 1.47 | 1.51 | 0.66 | 1.31 | 2.63 |
| *Man:* | | | | | | | | | | | | | | | |
| 12–14 years | 7.02 | 3.77 | 4.0 | 0.48 | 0.48 | 2.44 | 1.52 | 4.66 | 0.94 | 0.56 | 1.69 | 1.54 | 0.85 | 1.34 | 3.65 |
| 15–19 years | 6.65 | 4.65 | 4.0 | 0.29 | 0.47 | 2.73 | 2.00 | 5.45 | 0.80 | 0.67 | 1.98 | 1.82 | 1.05 | 1.15 | 4.41 |
| 20–54 years | 3.38 | 5.73 | 4.0 | 0.29 | 0.59 | 2.92 | 1.94 | 5.93 | 0.76 | 0.65 | 1.97 | 1.65 | 0.95 | 0.96 | 2.95 |
| 55 years and over | 2.97 | 4.64 | 4.0 | 0.19 | 0.70 | 2.91 | 1.69 | 5.88 | 0.89 | 0.53 | 1.58 | 1.45 | 0.87 | 1.05 | 1.50 |
| *Woman:* | | | | | | | | | | | | | | | |
| 12–19 years | 6.22 | 3.32 | 4.0 | 0.24 | 0.53 | 2.62 | 1.21 | 5.38 | 0.68 | 0.56 | 1.34 | 1.22 | 0.56 | 0.97 | 3.36 |
| 20–54 years | 3.35 | 4.12 | 4.0 | 0.19 | 0.62 | 2.84 | 1.35 | 4.94 | 0.54 | 0.49 | 1.28 | 1.08 | 0.65 | 0.81 | 2.89 |
| 55 years and over | 3.35 | 3.21 | 4.0 | 0.14 | 0.72 | 3.09 | 1.17 | 5.50 | 0.81 | 0.52 | 1.20 | 0.98 | 0.45 | 0.73 | 1.39 |
| Pregnant | 5.44 | 4.57 | 4.0 | 0.25 | 0.91 | 3.52 | 1.60 | 6.13 | 0.73 | 0.83 | 1.77 | 1.28 | 0.46 | 0.85 | 3.50 |
| Nursing | 5.31 | 5.01 | 4.0 | 0.26 | 0.91 | 3.76 | 1.73 | 6.52 | 0.74 | 0.81 | 1.84 | 1.42 | 0.69 | 1.00 | 3.79 |

* Fluid milk and beverage made from dry or evaporated milk. Cheese and ice cream may replace some milk. Count as equivalent to a quart of fluid milk: natural or processed cheddar-type cheese, 6 oz; cottage cheese, 2½ lb; ice cream, 1½ qts.

† Bacon and salt pork should not exceed ⅓ pound for each 5 pounds of this group.

‡ Weight in terms of dry beans and peas, shelled nuts, and peanut butter. Count 1 pound of canned dry beans—pork and beans, kidney beans, and so on—as 0.33 pound.

§ Includes coffee, tea, cocoa, punches, ades, soft drinks, leavenings, and seasonings. The use of iodized salt is recommended.

// Cereal fortified with iron is recommended.

(Amounts are for food as purchased or brought into the kitchen from garden or farm. Amounts allow for a discard of about one-sixth of the *edible* food as plate waste, spoilage, and so forth. Amounts of foods are shown to two decimal places to allow for greater accuracy, especially in estimating rations for large groups of people and for long periods of time. For general use, amounts of food groups for a family may be rounded to the nearest tenth or quarter of a pound.)

**Table 12-4.  Liberal Food Plan—Amounts of Food for a Week**

| Family Member | Milk, Cheese, Ice Cream* (qt) | Meat, Poultry, Fish† (lb) | Eggs (no) | Dry Beans and Peas, Nuts‡ (lb) | Dark-Green, Deep-Yellow Vegetables (lb) | Citrus Fruit, Tomatoes (lb) | Potatoes (lb) | Other Vegetables, Fruit (lb) | Cereal (lb) | Flour (lb) | Bread (lb) | Other Bakery Products (lb) | Fats, Oils (lb) | Sugar, Sweets (lb) | Accessories§ (lb) |
|---|---|---|---|---|---|---|---|---|---|---|---|---|---|---|---|
| *Child:* | | | | | | | | | | | | | | | |
| 7 months to 1 year | 6.94 | 0.97 | 2.3 | 0.14 | 0.43 | 0.60 | 0.06 | 4.71 | 0.64// | 0.02 | 0.05 | 0.06 | 0.05 | 0.20 | 0.09 |
| 1–2 years | 4.26 | 2.07 | 4.0 | 0.17 | 0.31 | 1.50 | 0.59 | 4.10 | 1.07// | 0.28 | 0.82 | 0.35 | 0.13 | 0.27 | 0.95 |
| 3–5 years | 5.08 | 2.35 | 3.1 | 0.23 | 0.32 | 1.77 | 0.85 | 4.18 | 0.76 | 0.27 | 0.79 | 0.78 | 0.45 | 0.85 | 1.74 |
| 6–8 years | 6.25 | 3.18 | 3.4 | 0.36 | 0.40 | 2.35 | 1.18 | 5.21 | 0.85 | 0.39 | 1.08 | 1.23 | 0.60 | 1.08 | 2.41 |
| 9–11 years | 7.21 | 4.04 | 4.0 | 0.39 | 0.48 | 3.15 | 1.41 | 6.83 | 1.04 | 0.51 | 1.39 | 1.67 | 0.71 | 1.38 | 3.21 |
| *Man:* | | | | | | | | | | | | | | | |
| 12–14 years | 7.57 | 4.57 | 4.0 | 0.50 | 0.51 | 2.94 | 1.52 | 5.52 | 0.95 | 0.56 | 1.60 | 1.71 | 0.92 | 1.40 | 4.47 |
| 15–19 years | 7.18 | 5.59 | 4.0 | 0.31 | 0.50 | 3.29 | 2.01 | 6.45 | 0.84 | 0.69 | 1.92 | 2.05 | 1.07 | 1.20 | 5.36 |
| 20–54 years | 3.64 | 6.83 | 4.0 | 0.32 | 0.62 | 3.51 | 1.95 | 6.99 | 0.79 | 0.66 | 1.91 | 1.86 | 0.95 | 1.00 | 3.54 |
| 55 years and over | 3.24 | 5.54 | 4.0 | 0.19 | 0.76 | 3.52 | 1.68 | 6.97 | 0.89 | 0.54 | 1.49 | 1.57 | 0.94 | 1.09 | 1.82 |
| *Woman:* | | | | | | | | | | | | | | | |
| 12–19 years | 6.72 | 3.97 | 4.0 | 0.25 | 0.56 | 3.15 | 1.21 | 6.34 | 0.71 | 0.59 | 1.31 | 1.35 | 0.54 | 0.98 | 4.09 |
| 20–54 years | 3.62 | 4.86 | 4.0 | 0.20 | 0.66 | 3.41 | 1.35 | 5.81 | 0.56 | 0.51 | 1.24 | 1.22 | 0.66 | 0.84 | 3.47 |
| 55 years and over | 3.65 | 3.79 | 4.0 | 0.15 | 0.76 | 3.71 | 1.14 | 6.42 | 0.74 | 0.54 | 1.17 | 1.12 | 0.48 | 0.77 | 1.66 |
| Pregnant | 5.91 | 5.43 | 4.0 | 0.26 | 0.96 | 4.22 | 1.57 | 7.17 | 0.70 | 0.87 | 1.70 | 1.45 | 0.46 | 0.87 | 4.20 |
| Nursing | 5.76 | 5.97 | 4.0 | 0.28 | 0.97 | 4.51 | 1.72 | 7.66 | 0.75 | 0.84 | 1.76 | 1.58 | 0.68 | 1.02 | 4.52 |

\* Fluid milk and beverage made from dry or evaporated milk. Cheese and ice cream may replace some milk. Count as equivalent to a quart of fluid milk: natural or processed cheddar-type cheese, 6 oz; cottage cheese, 2½ lb; ice cream, 1½ qts.

† Bacon and salt pork should not exceed ⅓ pound for each 5 pounds of this group.

‡ Weight in terms of dry beans and peas, shelled nuts, and peanut butter. Count 1 pound of canned dry beans—pork and beans, kidney beans, and so on—as 0.33 pound.

§ Includes coffee, tea, cocoa, punches, ades, soft drinks, leavenings, and seasonings. The use of iodized salt is recommended.

// Cereal fortified with iron is recommended.

(Amounts are for food as purchased or brought into the kitchen from garden or farm. Amounts allow for a discard of about one-fourth of the *edible* food as plate waste, spoilage, and so forth. Amounts of foods are shown to two decimal places to allow for greater accuracy, especially in estimating rations for large groups of people and for long periods of time. For general use, amounts of food groups for a family may be rounded to the nearest tenth or quarter of a pound.)

**Table 12-5.  Weekly Quantities of Food for a Family of Four According to the Low-Cost Food Plan**

| | Milk, Cheese, Ice Cream (qt) | Meat, Poultry, Fish (lb) | Eggs (no) | Dry Beans and Peas, Nuts (lb) | Dark-Green, Deep-Yellow Vegetables (lb) | Citrus Fruit, Tomatoes (lb) | Potatoes (lb) | Other Vegetables, Fruit (lb) | Cereal (lb) | Flour (lb) | Bread (lb) | Other Bakery Products (lb) | Fats, Oils (lb) | Sugar, Sweets (lb) | Accessories (lb) |
|---|---|---|---|---|---|---|---|---|---|---|---|---|---|---|---|
| Mother (30 yrs) | 3.02 | 3.21 | 4.0 | 0.19 | 0.55 | 2.34 | 1.40 | 4.17 | 0.71 | 0.55 | 1.31 | 0.94 | 0.59 | 0.72 | 2.13 |
| Father (32 yrs) | 2.74 | 4.56 | 4.0 | 0.33 | 0.48 | 2.32 | 1.87 | 4.81 | 0.93 | 0.71 | 2.10 | 1.47 | 0.91 | 0.81 | 2.11 |
| Girl (6 yrs) | 4.74 | 2.03 | 2.9 | 0.39 | 0.31 | 1.58 | 1.10 | 3.67 | 1.11 | 0.45 | 1.27 | 0.84 | 0.52 | 0.90 | 1.43 |
| Boy (12 yrs) | 5.74 | 2.98 | 4.0 | 0.56 | 0.40 | 1.99 | 1.50 | 3.90 | 1.15 | 0.67 | 1.88 | 1.25 | 0.77 | 1.15 | 2.61 |
| Total | 16.24 | 12.78 | 14.9 | 1.47 | 1.74 | 8.23 | 5.87 | 16.55 | 3.90 | 2.38 | 6.56 | 4.50 | 2.79 | 3.58 | 8.28 |

## Table 12-6. Shopping Lists for a Low-Cost Food Plan

| *Food and Quantity Required* (See Table 12-5) | *Quantity Purchased* | *Food and Quantity Required* (See Table 12-5) | *Quantity Purchased* |
|---|---|---|---|
| *Milk, Cheese, Ice Cream (16.24 qt)* | | *Cereal (3.90 lb)* | |
| Nonfat dry milk (2 lb) | 10 qt | Cornflakes (1 box) | ½ lb |
| Homogenized milk | 4 qt | Oatmeal (1 box) | 1 lb |
| Swiss cheese (6 oz) | 1 qt | Cornmeal (1 box) | 1 lb |
| Processed cheese (12 oz) | 2 qt | Macaroni (1 box) | ½ lb |
| Total | 17 qt | Rice | 1 lb |
| | | Total | 4 lb |
| *Meat, Poultry, Fish (12.78 lb)* | | | |
| Ground Beef (regular) | 1 lb | *Flour (2.38 lb)* | |
| Frozen perch | 1 lb | White flour, all purpose | 2 lb |
| Stewing chicken | 3–3½ lb | | |
| Pork liver | 1 lb | *Bread (6.56 lb)* | |
| Canned clams (one 8-oz can) | ½ lb | White, enriched (4 loaves) | 4 lb |
| Frankfurters | 1 lb | Whole wheat rolls (two 12-oz packages) | 1½ lb |
| Tuna (one 7-oz can) | ½ lb | French bread, enriched (1 loaf) | 1 lb |
| Turkey roll | 2–3 lb | Total | 6½ lb |
| Sausage | 1 lb | | |
| Total | 12–12½ lb | *Other Bakery Products (4.50 lb)* | |
| | | Graham crackers (1 box) | 1 lb |
| *Eggs (14.9 eggs)* | | Saltines, enriched (1 box) | 1 lb |
| Eggs (large) | 1½ doz | Chocolate chip cookies | 1 lb |
| | | Waffles, frozen (one 10-oz package) | 10 oz |
| *Dry Beans and Peas, Nuts (1.47 lb)* | | Total | 3⅝ lb |
| Peanut butter (1 large jar) | 1 lb | | |
| Dry beans | ½ lb | *Fats, Oils (2.79 lb)* | |
| Total | 1½ lb | Margarine | 1 lb |
| | | Cooking oil (1 pt) | 1 lb |
| *Dark-Green, Deep-Yellow Vegetables (1.74 lb)* | | Salad dressing (½ pt) | ½ lb |
| Carrots | 1 lb | Suet | ¼ lb |
| Squash, winter | 1 lb | Total | 2¾ lb |
| Spinach, fresh | 10 oz | | |
| Total | 2⅝ lb | *Sugars, Sweets (3.58 lb)* | |
| | | Sugar | 2 lb |
| *Citrus Fruit, Tomatoes (8.23 lb)* | | Jelly (1 jar) | ½ lb |
| Grapefruit (2) | 2 lb | Syrup, maple-flavored (½ pt) | ½ lb |
| Orange (1) | ½ lb | Molasses (½ pt) | ½ lb |
| Tomato juice (one 46-oz can) | 3 lb | Strawberry gelatin (one 4-oz package) | ¼ lb |
| Frozen orange juice (two 6-oz cans) | 12 oz | Total | 3¾ lb |
| Stewed tomatoes (one no. 2½ can) | 1½ lb | | |
| Lemon juice (one 1-pt bottle) | ½ lb | *Accessories (8.28 lb)* | |
| Total | 8¼ lb | Coffee | 1 lb |
| | | Cinnamon | 1 can |
| *Potatoes (5.87 lb)* | | Salt (1 box) | 1 lb |
| White potatoes | 5 lb | Vinegar | 1 pt |
| | | Vanilla | 1 bottle |
| *Other Vegetables, Fruits (16.55 lb)* | | Baking powder | 1 can |
| Lettuce | 1 lb | Pepper | 1 can |
| Celery | 1 lb | Fruit-flavored juice, enriched (one 46-oz can) | 3 lb |
| Cabbage | 2 lb | | |
| Raisins | 1 lb | | |
| Apples | 4 lb | | |
| Pineapple | 2 lb | | |
| Bananas | 2 lb | | |
| Onions | ½ lb | | |
| Cranberries | 1 lb | | |
| Yellow beans (one no. 303 can) | 1 lb | | |
| Green beans (one no. 303 can) | 1 lb | | |
| Peas (frozen) | 10 oz | | |
| Total | 17⅛ lb | | |

week and more than 12 hours a day, frequently there are certain times and days when choices on various items may be limited. There may be no butcher in the meat department after 6 P.M. on weekdays or on Sunday. Many supermarkets have only leftover fresh produce on Monday. Modifications in the family menus may be made when necessary to reduce food costs. Intelligent adjustments can ensure that meals are still nutritionally adequate and acceptable to the family. Unit pricing, which allows the purchaser to compare the cost per unit of different brands and different size containers, is available in supermarkets. Open dating of perishable products, such as

### Table 12-7. Menus for 1 Week of Low-Cost Meals

| | *Breakfast* | *Lunch* | *Dinner* |
|---|---|---|---|
| *Monday* | Half Grapefruit<br>Cornflakes with Skim Milk<br>Coffee   Milk | Peanut Butter and Jelly Sandwich<br>Carrot and Celery Sticks<br>Apple<br>Skim Milk | Meat Loaf<br>Baked Potato<br>Spinach<br>Bread   Margarine<br>Strawberry Fluff<br>Coffee   Milk |
| *Tuesday* | Applesauce<br>Waffles with Syrup<br>Coffee   Milk | Tomato Soup<br>Egg Salad Sandwich<br>Banana<br>Skim Milk | Broiled Perch with Lemon<br>Baked Squash<br>Cole Slaw<br>Cornbread   Margarine<br>Baked Custard<br>Coffee   Milk |
| *Wednesday* | Oatmeal with Raisins<br>Coffee   Milk | Macaroni and Cheese<br>Tomato Aspic<br>Chocolate Chip Cookies<br>Skim Milk | Chicken with Dumplings<br>Peas<br>Fruit Salad<br>Bread   Margarine<br>Rice Pudding<br>Coffee   Milk |
| *Thursday* | Orange Juice<br>Cornmeal Mush<br>Coffee   Milk | Chicken Sandwich<br>Cole Slaw<br>Oatmeal Cookies<br>Skim Milk | Broiled Liver with Onions<br>Boiled Potato<br>Yellow Beans<br>Whole Wheat Rolls<br>Margarine<br>Baked Apple<br>Coffee   Milk |
| *Friday* | Pineapple Slices<br>Poached Egg on Toast<br>Coffee   Milk | Manhattan Clam Chowder<br>Whole Wheat Rolls<br>Indian Pudding<br>Skim Milk | Tuna Rice Casserole<br>Carrots<br>Apple-Celery Salad<br>Cheese Biscuits<br>Margarine<br>Lemon Pudding Cake<br>Coffee   Milk |
| *Saturday* | Tomato Juice<br>Cornflakes with Skim Milk<br>Coffee   Milk | Potato Pancakes with Sausages<br>Applesauce<br>Coffee   Milk | Baked Beans with Frankfurters<br>Green Salad<br>Bread   Margarine<br>Fruit Cup<br>Coffee   Milk |
| *Sunday* | Orange Juice<br>French Toast with Syrup<br>Coffee   Milk | Tomato Cheese Fondue<br>Tossed Salad<br>Coffee   Milk | Roast Turkey<br>Mashed Potatoes<br>Green Beans<br>Cranberry-orange Salad<br>Whole Wheat Rolls<br>Mince Pie<br>Coffee   Milk |

(Foods for snacks are included in the shopping list, for example, crackers, juice, peanut butter, jelly, cheese, and so on.)

bread, milk and other dairy products, and eggs, also assists the consumer by indicating how fresh a food is at the time of purchase. The date itself usually refers to the last day the product should be offered for sale in the market.

## Milk and dairy products

Either evaporated or nonfat dry milk (fortified with vitamins A and D) is cheaper than fresh milk and is entirely satisfactory for cooking. Each product can also be used as a beverage, especially when reconstituted dry milk is mixed with equal amounts of fresh milk. It is also economical to buy dry milk in as large a package as can be stored and used without waste. Premeasured units of the nonfat dry milk cost more than the bulk form. Fresh fluid milk sold at retail food and dairy stores usually costs less than home-delivered milk or that sold at small special service stores. The $\frac{1}{2}$- or 1-gal containers, if they can be stored properly and used efficiently, usually provide some savings per quart when compared with the 1-qt container. Inexpensive cheeses are as good a source of protein as more expensive types. Processed cheeses may be cheaper than natural cheeses, especially those natural cheeses that have been aged and are labeled *sharp*. Cheese foods and cheese spreads may, according to their standards of identity, contain more moisture than processed cheeses.

## Meat, poultry, fish, and eggs

One-third or more of the food dollar in the United States is spent for meat, poultry, and fish. Less expensive cuts of meat may be used when it is necessary to cut food costs. The consumer should buy meat according to grade when possible. It is important to learn to identify cuts; bones are an excellent guide for identification. A rough estimate of the cost of the edible portion of some of the apparently cheapest cuts may disclose that the cheapest cut is not always the one that has the lowest price per pound. Variety meats, such as liver, are often good buys. Fish may be cheaper than meat. Poultry today is less expensive per pound than most cuts of meat. An average 3-oz serving of cooked meat, fish, or poultry requires 4 to $4\frac{1}{2}$ oz of fat-free and bone-free uncooked lean meat. The amount of meat that must be purchased to yield this depends on the amount of inedible fat and bone in a cut and on the amount of skin on poultry and fish. Table 12-8 indicates the cost of 3 oz of cooked lean from specified meat, poultry, and fish at June, 1980 prices. Current prices may be substituted for the "retail price per pound" in column 1, and current costs (column 3) may easily be calculated by multiplying each retail price per pound by the factor in column 2, the "part of pound for 3 oz of cooked lean."

The price wise consumer often substitutes other kinds of main dishes for meat. Macaroni products, rice, or

## Table 12-8. Cost of 3 Ounces of Cooked Lean from Specified Meat, Poultry, and Fish at June, 1980 Prices

| Food | Retail Price Per Pound* | Part of Pound for 3 Ounces of Cooked Lean | Cost of 3 Ounces of Cooked Lean |
|---|---|---|---|
| Beef liver | $1.03 | 0.27 | $0.28 |
| Chicken, whole, ready to cook | .67 | 0.49 | .33 |
| Turkey, ready to cook | .86 | 0.44 | .38 |
| Ham, whole, bone in | 1.15 | 0.35 | .40 |
| Pork, shoulder, smoked, bone in | .89 | 0.46 | .41 |
| Ground beef, regular | 1.50 | 0.28 | .42 |
| Chicken breasts | 1.31 | 0.36 | .47 |
| Ground beef, lean | 1.89 | 0.26 | .49 |
| Ocean perch, fillet, frozen | 2.21 | 0.25 | .55 |
| Ham, canned | 2.20 | 0.25 | .55 |
| Haddock, fillet, frozen | 2.43 | 0.25 | .61 |
| Chuck roast of beef, bone in | 1.50 | 0.45 | .68 |
| Pork loin roast, bone in | 1.33 | 0.51 | .68 |
| Pork chops, center cut | 1.87 | 0.45 | .84 |
| Rump roast of beef, bone out | 2.53 | 0.34 | .86 |
| Round beefsteak, bone in | 2.70 | 0.34 | .92 |
| Veal cutlets | 4.48 | 0.25 | 1.12 |
| Rib roast of beef, bone in | 2.54 | 0.45 | 1.14 |
| Sirloin beefsteak, bone in | 3.06 | 0.43 | 1.31 |
| Porterhouse beefsteak, bone in | 3.59 | 0.52 | 1.87 |
| Lamp chops, loin | 4.08 | 0.46 | 1.88 |

*U.S. average retail price of food item estimated using information provided by the Bureau of Labor Statistics (United States Department of Labor) and United States Department of Agriculture.

(From USDA, Science and Education Administration, Human Nutrition, Consumer Nutrition Center, Hyattsville, MD 20782)

corn, when combined with eggs, milk, cheese, or small amounts of fish, poultry, or meat, make good substitutes for the more expensive cuts of meat. When their prices are right, dried beans, peas, or nuts may also add variety to economically planned meals. A comparison of the costs of the amounts of various foods that supply 20 g of protein is given in Table 12-9. In many instances, a meal will include protein from more than one of these sources; for example, 2 tbsp (1 oz) peanut butter (8 g of protein); 2 slices (2 oz) enriched bread (4 g of protein); 1 cup (8 oz) milk (8.5 g of protein). Based on the prices given in the table the 20 g of protein in this meal would cost approximately 26 cents.

Eggs of graded size show considerable variation in price—sometimes small ones are the best buy, sometimes large ones. If large eggs are 95 cents per dozen, medium eggs are a good buy if they cost less than 83 cents per dozen. Extra large eggs would be a good buy if they cost less than 12 cents more than large eggs per dozen. Grade B eggs, suitable for cakes, casseroles, and scrambling, are less expensive than Grade A.

**Table 12-9. Cost of 20 Grams of Protein from Specified Meats and Meat Alternates at June, 1980 Prices**

| *Food* | *Market Unit* | *Price Per Market Unit** | *Part of Market Unit To Give 20 Grams of Protein†* | *Cost of 20 Grams of Protein* |
|---|---|---|---|---|
| Dry beans | lb | $0.59 | 0.24 | $0.14 |
| Eggs, large | doz | .77 | 0.25 | .19 |
| Peanut butter | 12 oz | .91 | 0.23 | .21 |
| Bread, white enriched‡ | lb | .47 | 0.51 | .24 |
| Chicken, whole, ready to cook | lb | .67 | 0.37 | .25 |
| Beef liver | lb | 1.03 | 0.24 | .25 |
| Turkey, ready to cook | lb | .86 | 0.33 | .28 |
| Pork, shoulder, smoked, bone in | lb | .89 | 0.32 | .29 |
| Milk, whole fluid§ | ½ gal | 1.07 | 0.29 | .31 |
| Ham, whole, bone in | lb | 1.15 | 0.30 | .34 |
| Bean soup, canned | 11.25 oz | .37 | 0.96 | .36 |
| Chicken breasts | lb | 1.31 | 0.29 | .38 |
| Tuna, canned | 6.5 oz | .98 | 0.44 | .43 |
| American processed cheese | 8 oz | 1.16 | 0.38 | .44 |
| Pork loin roast, bone in | lb | 1.33 | 0.33 | .44 |
| Ground beef, lean | lb | 1.89 | 0.25 | .48 |
| Chuck roast of beef, bone in | lb | 1.50 | 0.35 | .52 |
| Ham, canned | lb | 2.20 | 0.24 | .53 |
| Liverwurst | 8 oz | .94 | 0.60 | .56 |
| Frankfurters | lb | 1.63 | 0.36 | .59 |
| Pork sausage | lb | 1.13 | 0.52 | .59 |
| Salami | 8 oz | 1.21 | 0.50 | .61 |
| Round beefsteak, bone in | lb | 2.70 | 0.23 | .62 |
| Ocean perch, fillet, frozen | lb | 2.21 | 0.29 | .63 |
| Bacon, sliced | lb | 1.22 | 0.52 | .63 |
| Pork chops, center cut | lb | 1.87 | 0.35 | .65 |
| Rump roast of beef, bone out | lb | 2.53 | 0.26 | .66 |
| Sardines, canned | 4 oz | .73 | 0.94 | .69 |
| Haddock, fillet, frozen | lb | 2.43 | 0.29 | .71 |
| Bologna | 8 oz | 1.09 | 0.73 | .79 |
| Rib roast of beef, bone in | lb | 2.54 | 0.33 | .84 |
| Sirloin beefsteak, bone in | lb | 3.06 | 0.28 | .86 |
| Veal cutlets | lb | 4.48 | 0.23 | 1.05 |
| Porterhouse beefsteak, bone in | lb | 3.59 | 0.34 | 1.22 |
| Lamb chops, loin | lb | 4.08 | 0.32 | 1.31 |

*U.S. average retail price of food item estimated using information provided by the Bureau of Labor Statistics (United States Department of Labor) and United States Department of Agriculture.

†One-third of the daily amount recommended for a 20-year-old man, assuming that all meat is eaten.

‡Bread and other grain products, such as pasta and rice, are frequently used with a small amount of meat, poultry, fish, or cheese as main dishes in economy meals. In this way the high-quality protein in meat and cheese enhances the lower quality of protein in cereal products.

§Although milk is not used to replace meat in meals, it is an economical source of good-quality protein.

(From USDA, Science and Education Administration, Human Nutrition, Consumer Nutrition Center, Hyattsville, MD 20782)

## Fruits and vegetables

To determine the best buy in fruits and vegetables, comparisons must be made among fresh, frozen, canned, and dehydrated products in the cost per serving. Table 12-10 shows the number of servings obtained from the usual purchasing unit. Count as a serving one medium-size apple, orange, banana, peach, or pear; 2 or 3 apricots, figs, or plums; $\frac{1}{2}$ cup canned fruit with liquid.

Fresh fruits and vegetables in season and when plentiful are usually cheaper than canned or frozen ones. Home frozen and canned foods are economical when the food is homegrown or purchased at the peak of the season.

Help from the agents and publications of the Cooperative Extension Service is available in most communities to assist the inexperienced person with home preservation of food. Bruised or overripe soft fruits and vegetables usually involve excessive waste and for this reason are rarely economical to purchase. Blemishes on fruits and vegetables which may be discarded with the skin or rind, however, may influence grade and be good buys.

Prices of frozen, canned, and dehydrated fruits and vegetables vary according to brand, grade, type of process and other added ingredients. The nutritive value of cheaper standard grades of canned fruits and vegetables is

### Table 12-10. Number of Servings of Fruits and Vegetables from Usual Purchasing Unit

| Fresh Vegetables | Servings Per Pound as Purchased |
|---|---|
| Asparagus | 3 or 4 |
| Beans, lima (in pods) | 2 |
| Beans, snap | 5 or 6 |
| Beets, diced (without tops) | 3 or 4 |
| Broccoli | 3 or 4 |
| Brussels sprouts | 4 or 5 |
| Cabbage: | |
| Raw, shredded | 9 or 10 |
| Cooked | 4 or 5 |
| Carrots: | |
| Raw, diced or shredded (without tops) | 5 or 6 |
| Cooked | 4 |
| Cauliflower | 3 |
| Celery: | |
| Raw, chopped or diced | 5 or 6 |
| Cooked | 4 |
| Kale (untrimmed) | 5 or 6 |
| Okra | 4 or 5 |
| Onions, cooked | 3 or 4 |
| Parsnips (without tops) | 4 |
| Peas (in pods) | 2 |
| Potatoes | 4 |
| Spinach, (prepackaged) | 4 |
| Squash, summer | 3 or 4 |
| Squash, winter | 2 or 3 |
| Sweet potatoes | 3 or 4 |
| Tomatoes, raw, diced, or sliced | 5 |

| Frozen Vegetables | Servings Per Package (9 or 10 oz) |
|---|---|
| Asparagus | 2 or 3 |
| Beans, lima | 3 or 4 |
| Beans, snap | 3 or 4 |
| Broccoli | 3 |
| Brussels sprouts | 3 |
| Cauliflower | 3 |
| Corn, whole kernel | 3 |
| Kale | 2 or 3 |
| Peas | 3 |
| Spinach | 2 or 3 |

| Canned Vegetables | Servings Per Can (16 oz) |
|---|---|
| Most vegetables | 3 or 4 |
| Greens, such as kale or spinach | 2 or 3 |

| Dry Vegetables | Servings Per Pound |
|---|---|
| Dry beans | 11 |
| Dry peas, lentils | 10 or 11 |

| Fresh Fruit | Servings Per Market Unit as Purchased |
|---|---|
| Apples | |
| Bananas | |
| Peaches | 3 or 4 per pound |
| Pears | |
| Plums | |
| Apricots | |
| Cherries, sweet | 5 or 6 per pound |
| Grapes, seedless | |
| Blueberries | |
| Raspberries | 4 or 5 per pint |
| Strawberries | 8 or 9 per quart |

| Frozen Fruit | Servings Per Package (10 or 12 oz) |
|---|---|
| Blueberries | 3 or 4 |
| Peaches | 2 or 3 |
| Raspberries | 2 or 3 |
| Strawberries | 2 or 3 |

| Canned Fruit | Servings Per Can (16 oz) |
|---|---|
| Served with liquid | 4 |
| Drained | 2 or 3 |

| Dried Fruit | Servings Per Package (8 oz) |
|---|---|
| Apples | 8 |
| Apricots | 6 |
| Mixed fruits | 6 |
| Peaches | 7 |
| Pears | 4 |
| Prunes | 4 or 5 |

(From Your Money's Worth in Foods, Home and Garden Bulletin No. 183. Washington, DC, USDA, revised 1979)

essentially the same as that of the more expensive fancy grades, and they are equally wholesome. Compare unit prices and the nutrition labeling on the can or package. The USDA publication HERR 42, *Buying Food—A Guide for Calculating Amounts to Buy and Comparing Costs in Household Quantities,*\* is helpful in determining the most economical buys.

### Breads and cereal products

In general, foods prepared at home are less expensive than foods purchased ready to eat. Products made from whole or enriched grains are more nutritious than unenriched products, so it is worthwhile to check the label or ask the baker for nutrition information. Breakfast cereals cooked at home are almost always cheaper than "instant" ones. Ready-to-eat cereals in individual boxes may cost twice as much per ounce as the same cereal in a larger box. Large packages are economical for big families but not for small ones, as the contents may become stale and have to be discarded. Unsweetened cereals usually cost less per ounce than presweetened ready-to-serve cereals. Day-old bakery products may represent savings to large families who consume many loaves of bread each week. Sweet rolls, buns, and coffee cakes are expensive types of bread.

In most instances, the cost of service adds to the price of commercially prepared mixes. The convenience value of a prepared mix differs according to the experience, skill, and interest of the individual cook and must be evaluated accordingly.

### Storage

Because many staple foods have a long storage life, large economical packages can be purchased if storage facilities are adequate. In general, these storage spaces should be away from water, drain, or heating pipes and should be kept clean, dry, reasonably cool, and free from insects and rodents. Household chemicals and cleaning supplies should *never* be stored with food.

Special attention should be paid to the storage of perishable items. Refrigerators should maintain a temperature of 45°F or below. Fresh meat should be stored in the refrigerator loosely wrapped; all containers should be closed or covered. Many food dollars are wasted on food that spoils before it can be consumed and must be discarded. This is particularly true of frozen foods when there is not adequate freezer space in the home. A temperature of 0° F or below is required if frozen foods are to be stored for long periods of time. Frozen concentrated orange juice can be stored for a year without losing more than 5% of its ascorbic acid if it is kept frozen throughout the period. Fresh meats and, especially, poultry and fish

require freezing if they are not cooked and consumed within a day or two of purchase.

The manner in which fresh produce is stored may alter nutritive values. Table 1 in Part 4 gives the average values for nutrients in foods. Averages, however, do not reveal that half the vitamin C in leafy dark green vegetables and broccoli is lost if they are stored in the refrigerator for 5 days or more. Raw cabbage stores well even at room temperature and storage may even increase the vitamin A value of sweet potatoes. Berries lose their ascorbic acid rapidly if they are capped or bruised.

### Preparation

A reliable cookbook is a necessity for an inexperienced cook. Careful attention should be given to recipe amounts and instructions until the cook has developed sufficient skill to make adjustments. (See Table 12-11 for general directions for following a recipe.) It is important to realize that those ingredients that determine the shape, texture, consistency, and tenderness of a mixture are proportional; these proportions cannot be altered without changing the basic characteristics of the product. However, flavoring agents may be varied according to the preference of the family or individual. Knowledge of the terms used in recipes (Table 12-12) is important for following directions accurately.

The successful cook also selects carefully the essential equipment for food preparation.

For accurate measuring the following utensils are essential: an 8-oz measuring cup divided into fourths and thirds or a set of measuring cups of these volumes; tablespoons and teaspoons of regulation sizes or, preferably, a set of measuring spoons.

To measure dry material by the cup, fill lightly with a spoon to brim or to indicated cup level. Do not shake the cup to level the material. This is particularly important in the case of flour sifted before measurement. Granulated sugar may be measured easily, but brown sugar should be packed firmly into the cup. Before measuring honey or syrup, rinse the cup with cold water.

Measurement of butter and margarine, when in $\frac{1}{4}$-lb sticks, may be made by accurate division. One stick corresponds to the measurement of $\frac{1}{2}$ cup. To measure bulk fat, pack firmly into cup to the desired mark of measurement. Except for that used in pastry, fat should be at room temperature. (An easy way of measuring $\frac{1}{2}$ cup of shortening is to fill the cup to the one-half mark with cold water and add shortening enough to cause water to rise to the 1-cup mark. To measure $\frac{1}{4}$ cup, fill with cold water to the three-quarter mark.)

To measure dry ingredients by the tablespoon or the teaspoon, fill until heaping and, with the back edge of the knife, level off all that extends above the edge of the spoon. If one-half spoonful is desired, divide the contents of the spoon lengthwise and push off one half. If one-fourth is wanted, divide the remaining half crosswise and push off the portion not desired. If one-eighth is desired, divide the remaining one-fourth crosswise and push off the portion not needed. If one-third of a spoonful is desired, divide the contents of the spoonful crosswise into thirds, pushing off the undesired portion.

To measure spoonfuls of liquid, dip the spoon into the liquid.

To measure butter or other solid fats, pack solidly into the spoon and level with a knife.

So that all the foods to be served for a meal are ready at the appointed time, the cook plans the work according to the amount of preparation and cooking time each item requires. The ability to organize a meal is one of the true tests of the cook-manager. Many beginners actually write down their work plan before they begin so that they can perform each task at the appropriate time without wasting time or energy.

## Milk and dairy products

Because at high temperatures some of the protein in milk coagulates into a film on top and a coating on the sides of the pan, milk should be heated or cooked slowly at a low temperature and not allowed to boil. It can be heated in a double boiler or, with care, over direct heat. Overcooking may cause off-flavors or scorching. Similarly, when baking casseroles containing a large proportion of milk it is necessary to use low oven temperatures. Cream sauces or gravies thickened with flour or cornstarch require constant stirring while cooking to prevent lumping. Care must also be taken in adding any acid foods, such as tomato or lemon juice, to milk because they often cause it to curdle. Add small amounts of the acid ingredient to the milk or sauce just before serving.

Evaporated milk may be substituted for fresh milk by diluting it with an equal amount of water before use. Nonfat dry milk may be sifted with the dry ingredients or reconstituted and used as a liquid.

When cheese is used in cooking, it is usually grated or finely flaked or cut into small pieces. For cooking on top of the stove, it is generally best to use a double boiler and to cook the cheese over hot water. For baked cheese dishes, a low temperature is suggested; sometimes directions call for placing the dish containing the cheese mixture in a pan of hot water. When a high temperature is used, as in toasting an open cheese sandwich under the broiler, the cooking period should be short. The texture of cheese will toughen and become stringy when it is overcooked by any method.

## Meat, poultry, fish, and eggs

As previously indicated, protein foods are coagulated by heat. Low-temperature cooking produces a tender product, whereas high temperatures tend to cause toughening. This is best illustrated in egg cookery; an egg cooked below the boiling point is more tender than a boiled egg. For baking or roasting meat, cookery experts recommend temperatures between 300° and 325° F to achieve more tender meat as well as to lessen shrinkage.

### Meat

All cuts of meat, including the inexpensive ones, provide acceptable main dishes when they are properly prepared. The use of moderate temperatures and the

## Table 12-11. General Directions for Following a Recipe

1. Select tested recipes from reliable sources, and read them carefully.
2. Turn on the oven to the correct temperature if the product is to be baked or roasted, so that the oven will be at the desired heat when the mixture is ready for cooking.
3. Check supplies and collect the necessary ingredients in one work area.
4. Collect the needed mixing, measuring, and cooking equipment in one work area.
5. If baking or roasting, prepare the pan for the product, using the size indicated in the recipe for best results.
6. Check to see if there is anything that should be done to ingredients before adding them to the mixture, such as melting fat or chocolate, beating egg whites, or sifting dry ingredients together.
7. Use level measurements; measure exactly—dry ingredients first, then liquids, if possible, to save washing of extra utensils.
8. Combine the ingredients, following the procedure given in the recipe.
9. Bake or cook exactly as directed. Follow cooking times and temperatures given, testing for doneness as directed. Thermometers for roasting, deep-fat frying, and candymaking will be found helpful.
10. Handle finished product as directed, such as removing from pans, molding, chilling; cooling or chilling before serving; or serving at once.

## Table 12-12. Terms Used in Recipes

**Baste:** to pour liquid over the surface of food that is being baked or roasted.

**Blanch:** to let food stand in hot water 3 to 5 minutes to loosen skin, remove strong flavors, or set color.

**Cream:** to soften shortening and to blend with sugar by rubbing with a wooden spoon or in an electric mixer.

**Cut in:** to blend shortening with flour with pastry blender or two knives.

**Dice:** to cut in small square pieces.

**Fold:** to add whipped cream or beaten egg whites with a careful folding motion.

**Mince:** to cut or to chop fine.

**Pan-broil:** to cook in a heated pan or on a griddle with little or no added fat.

**Pan-fry:** to cook in a shallow pan with just enough added fat to prevent sticking and aid browning.

**Parboil:** to boil in water until it is partially cooked.

**Purée:** to press through a sieve.

**Sauté:** to cook in a small amount of fat.

**Scald:** to heat milk until bubbles appear around the edge.

**Sear:** to brown quickly over direct heat or in an oven.

**Shred:** to cut or to tear in thin strips.

**Simmer** or **stew:** to cook in liquid just below boiling point.

**Steep:** to let stand in hot liquid below boiling point.

selection of the correct method of cooking for each cut of meat are essential. Dry heat (oven roasting, oven broiling, pan broiling, and pan frying) should be used only with the tender and, therefore, usually more expensive cuts of meat. Moist heat (braising, pot roasting, stewing) and the use of meat tenderizers make the less tender and less expensive cuts almost equally acceptable.

No additional moisture or fat is required for oven roasting and oven broiling. The use of low oven temperatures, checked by an oven thermometer, for roasting prevents overcooking, shrinkage in size, and the loss of vitamins and palatability that occur with high-temperature cooking. When the more tender cuts are pan-fried or pan-broiled, a small amount of fat is needed to prevent adherence to the frying pan. Some types of utensils are now made to be used without added fat. A nonfat spray preparation may also be used with regular utensils by the cook who is restricting fat in his diet.

In moist heat cookery, such as braising, pot roasting, or stewing, the addition of an acid—either vinegar or lemon or tomato juice—to the liquid used in cooking increases the tenderizing effect of this method.

Fresh pork should be cooked until every vestige of the pink coloring of the flesh has disappeared, to prevent infection with *Trichina spiralis*. Of all food animals, only pigs or hogs are susceptible to trichinosis infection, which may be passed on to humans if sufficient heat is not applied to kill any parasites present. Present methods of slaughtering and handling do not ensure against infection. For this reason, thorough cooking of all pork products in the home kitchen is essential.

The *Meat Cookery Guide* presented in Fig. 12-1 suggests the most desirable cooking methods for a variety of cuts and types of meat.

### Poultry

Chickens, the most commonly used type of poultry, are known by various terms, which indicate size and, to some extent, tenderness. This is shown in the following chart:

| | |
|---|---|
| Squab | $3/4$–$1\frac{1}{4}$ lb |
| Broiler | $1\frac{1}{4}$–$2\frac{1}{2}$ lb |
| Fryer | $2\frac{1}{2}$–$3\frac{1}{2}$ lb |
| Roaster | 3 lb or over |
| Fowl | 4 lb or over |

Proper cooking, which develops and holds the delicate flavor of the meat, is important in preparing chicken. Young chicken may be broiled or pan fried in a small amount of fat. Older birds should be roasted or simmered, and serve sliced, hot or cold; boiled chicken may be used for fricassee or creamed chicken. A very palatable broth can be made from the bones of roast chicken or turkey.

### Fish

The general rule for cooking fish may be summed up in one sentence—short cooking just before serving is most important. This rule is particularly applicable in the case of broiled and pan-broiled fish, which after cooking dries out quickly. The test for doneness is simple. When tried with a fork, the flesh should flake. Sliced or quartered lemon is the chosen garnish for both appearance and flavor. Suggestions for cooking fresh fish are given in Table 12-13.

### Eggs

Low temperature and short cooking are also desirable for most egg dishes, as the texture is more delicate and tender under these conditions. For this reason, soft-cooked eggs generally are coddled by being allowed to stand covered in water that has been brought to the boiling point. Hard-cooked eggs, prepared by boiling, have a firmer texture and are easier to slice or to stuff.

When they are part of a meal, eggs should be prepared just before they are to be served. Coddled eggs in their shells should be opened just before they are to be eaten.

## Fruits and vegetables
### Fruits

Most fresh fruits may be eaten raw. Fruits such as apples, pears, peaches, plums, grapes, and cherries should be washed thoroughly to remove any traces of insecticide spray residue. Berries should be washed just before serving. Strawberries should be washed before being hulled. Peaches, pears, and apples may be served whole or peeled and sliced or sectioned. They, and bananas, should be peeled or sliced just before serving or they will discolor due to oxidation. Sprinkling or dipping them in lemon juice or ascorbic acid solution or adding sugar at the time of slicing prevents discoloration.

A melon should be tested for ripeness by feeling the "softness" of the stem end, or by the sound it makes—rather dull and thick—when slapped. Melons should be washed and chilled in the refrigerator before serving. Cantaloupe and medium-sized melons are served in halves or wedges after the seeds are carefully removed. Watermelon is served in 1-in or $1\frac{1}{2}$-in slices or, if small, in half of a lengthwise wedge. Cut portions of leftover melon should be wrapped tightly in plastic wrap so that their aroma will not permeate other foods in the refrigerator.

Pineapple may be kept at room temperature unless it is very ripe. The easiest method of preparation is to cut the fruit in thick slices or wedges, pare each piece and remove the "eyes," then cut it into bitesize pieces.

Fresh pineapple should not be used with gelatin, as it contains a proteolytic enzyme, which "digests" the gelatin and keeps it from setting. The enzyme is destroyed in canned fruit or juice.

When large oranges or grapefruit are cut in half for serving, the segments should be loosened with a curved knife made for the purpose. It should be run between the pulp and the fiber membranes, although the fiber partitions should never be cut. Oranges and grapefruit may also be served in sections by themselves or in combination with other fruits in a fruit plate or salad. They should be peeled with a sharp or serrated knife, round and round, directly into the flesh, and the sections between the membranes removed with a sharp knife.

Dried fruits should be prepared according to the directions on the package, or they may be purchased already prepared. Canned fruits, prepared with heavy or medium syrup or without added sugar, are available, and may be served in the syrup or drained for use in salads. Cooked fruits are usually stewed or baked. One should make sure that frozen fruits are thoroughly thawed before they are served.

### Vegetables

Vegetables should be washed thoroughly to remove soil and traces of spray. Root vegetables should be

| Cooking Methods | Beef Cuts | Veal Cuts | Pork Cuts | Lamb Cuts | Variety Meats |
|---|---|---|---|---|---|
| **Roasting** | Standing Rib<br>Rolled Rib<br>Sirloin<br>Chuck Ribs<br>  (high quality)<br>Rump<br>  (high quality)<br>Loaf | Rolled Shoulder<br>Cushion Shoulder<br>Arm Roast<br>Blade Roast<br>Rib<br>Loin<br>Rump<br>Leg | Loin<br>Rolled Shoulder<br>Cushion Shoulder<br>Fresh Ham (pork leg)<br>Smoked Picnic<br>Smoked Shoulder Butt<br>Smoked Ham<br>Sausages<br>Sliced Salt Pork | Cushion Shoulder<br>Rolled Shoulder<br>Breast with<br>  Pocket<br>Rolled Breast<br>Rack<br>Leg | Liver (beef-veal-<br>pork-lamb) |
| **Broiling and Pan Broiling** | Rib Steaks<br>Club Steaks<br>T-Bone Steaks<br>Porterhouse<br>  Steaks<br>Sirloin Steaks<br>Chuck Steaks<br>  (high quality)<br>Rump Steaks<br>  (high quality)<br>Patties | Veal is not<br>  broiled or<br>  pan-broiled | Fresh pork is not<br>  broiled or pan-<br>  broiled<br>Smoked Ham Slices<br>Sliced Bacon<br>Sliced Canadian-<br>  style Bacon<br>Smoked Shoulder<br>  Butt Slices | Rib Chops<br>Loin Chops<br>Shoulder<br>  (arms or blade)<br>Leg Steaks<br>Patties<br>Choplets<br>  (from breast<br>  stuffed with<br>  ground lamb) | Liver (veal-lamb)<br>Kidney (lamb)<br>Sweetbreads<br>  (beef-veal-<br>  lamb) |
| **Frying** | Thin Steaks (tender<br>  or pounded)<br>Patties | Chops<br>Cutlets<br>Steaks<br>Patties | Sausage<br>Sliced Salt Pork | Thin Chops<br>  or<br>Thin Steaks | Liver (all kinds<br>  if cut thin)<br>Tripe (after pre-<br>  cooking in water)<br>Sweetbreads<br>Brains |
| **Braising** | Chuck<br>  (arm or blade)<br>Rump<br>Round<br>Heel of Round<br>Brisket<br>Plate<br>Short Ribs<br>Flank<br>Shanks<br>Ox-joints | Breast<br>Rib Chops<br>Loin Chops<br>Shoulder Chops<br>Cutlets<br>Patties | Rib Chops<br>Loin Chops<br>Shoulder Chops<br>  or Steaks<br>Fresh Ham<br>  Slices | Breast<br>Neck Slices<br>Shanks<br>Riblets<br>Shoulder<br>  (arm or blade) | Liver (beef-pork)<br>Kidney (beef-veal-<br>  pork)<br>Heart (beef-veal-<br>  pork-lamb)<br>Tripe (beef)<br>Sweetbreads<br>  (beef-veal-lamb) |
| **Cooking In Liquid** (Stews and Large Cuts) | Neck<br>Shank<br>Plate<br>Brisket<br>Flank<br>Heel of Round<br>Ox-joints<br>Corned Beef | Neck<br>Shoulder<br>Shanks<br>Flank | Hocks<br>Shanks<br>Feet<br>Backbones<br>Neck Bones<br>Spareribs<br>Smoked Picnic<br>Smoked Shoulder<br>  Butt<br>Smoked Ham Shanks<br>Smoked Spareribs<br>Smoked Hocks | Neck<br>Steaks<br>Shoulder<br>Breast | Kidney (beef-<br>  veal-pork-lamb)<br>Heart (beef-veal-<br>  pork-lamb)<br>Tongue (beef-<br>  veal-pork-lamb)<br>Tripe (beef)<br>Sweetbreads (for<br>  precooking)<br>Brains (for pre-<br>  cooking) |

**Fig. 12-1.** Meat cookery guide. A pressure cooker may be used for "cooking in liquid." Follow directions as given in the pressure cooker guidebook.

scrubbed; asparagus, spinach, and other greens should be washed under running water to remove sand. Vegetables, such as potatoes and carrots, should not be pared or scraped until just before they are to be used. Peas and beans should not be shelled or corn husked until just before they are to be cooked. Outer leaves of cauliflower and cabbage should not be removed until just before they are to be used. A larger loss of vitamins occurs when vegetables are cut in small pieces. Grated carrots, for instance, lose vitamins more quickly than the sliced vegetable.

Salad greens should be separated and thoroughly washed under cold running water and allowed to drain or to be dried with a clean towel. Placing them in a plastic bag in the refrigerator will help to keep them crisp. Salads should be prepared for serving just before the meal and the dressing added at the last moment. They should be cold and crisp and attractive to the eye. They should be simple rather than elaborate, and they should have a dressing that is well but moderately seasoned.

Vegetables should be cooked as short a time as possible, as long cooking destroys vitamins and changes flavor,

## Table 12-13. Suggestions for Cooking Fresh Fish

| Kind of Fish | Preparation at Market | Methods of Cooking | Sauce or Garnish |
|---|---|---|---|
| Bass, black | Split | Broil | Lemon |
| Bass, sea | Split* | Broil | Lemon |
| | Whole | Stuff and bake | Tomato sauce |
| Bluefish | Split | Broil, bake, plank | Sliced tomatoes |
| | Whole | Stuff and bake | Sliced pickles |
| | | | Parsley sauce |
| Cod, small | Whole | Stuff and bake | Anchovy sauce |
| large | Steaks* | Broil, bake | Melted butter |
| | | | Lemon sprinkled with paprika |
| Flounder | Fillets* | Bake | Lemon, parsley |
| Haddock, small | Whole | Stuff and bake | Mock Hollandaise sauce |
| large | Fillets* | Bake | Grilled tomatoes |
| large | Steaks* | Bake, broil | Tartar sauce |
| Halibut | Steaks* | Broil, bake, pan-fry | Cucumber sauce |
| | Thick slice* | Steam | Hollandaise sauce |
| Mackerel | Split* | Broil, bake | Sliced cucumbers |
| Pompano | Split | Broil, plank | Melted butter |
| | Fillets* | Bake | Minced parsley |
| | | | Lemon, parsley |
| Salmon | Steaks* | Broil | Sliced cucumbers |
| | Thick slice* | Steam | Egg sauce |
| Scrod | Split* | Broil | Melted butter |
| | | | Pepper relish |
| Shad | Split | Bake, plank | Lemon |
| | | | Radishes |
| Shad roe | | Parboil, then bake | Bacon |
| | | | Lemon |
| Smelts | Whole* | Broil, bake, pan-fry | Tartar sauce |
| Sole | Fillets* | Broil, bake | Melted butter |
| | | | Grilled tomatoes |
| Snapper, red | Split | Bake, broil, plank | Sliced cucumbers |
| Swordfish | Steaks* | Broil, pan-fry | Cucumber sauce |
| Trout, lake and sea | Split | Broil, bake | Melted butter |
| | | | Minced parsley |
| Tuna, fresh | Steak* | Bake, broil | Lemon sprinkled with paprika |
| | Thick piece* | Steam | Hollandaise sauce |
| Weakfish | Split* | Broil, bake | Sliced tomatoes |
| Whitefish | Split | Broil, bake, plank | Lemon |
| | Whole | Stuff and bake | Parsley sauce |

*Especially adapted to service in small family.

(From Heseltine M, Dow UM: The Basic Cookbook, 5th ed. Boston, Houghton Mifflin, 1967)

color, and texture. The use of baking soda in the cooking of green vegetables is not recommended because an alkali, such as soda, hastens the destruction of the B vitamins and ascorbic acid.

Only a small amount of water should be used for boiling most vegetables. There is little evaporation if the utensil is tightly covered and if the cooking is done over low heat. (See Table 12-14.)

Although boiling is the most common method of preparing vegetables, other methods can be used to add interest and palatability to everyday meals. Potatoes, winter squash, onions, and tomatoes are especially attractive and flavorful when baked in the oven. Sautéeing or frying such vegetables as eggplant, summer squash, parsnips, mushrooms, or peppers may add special appeal to a meal. Steaming spinach and cabbage helps to retain the natural flavor and texture as well as the nutritive value of these products. There are numerous popular vegetable combinations: two or more vegetables cooked together, or vegetables combined with protein foods, such as eggs, cheese, meat, or fish, with sauces or garnishes. Imagination on the part of the homemaker can often bring about enthusiastic acceptance of vegetables where only mere tolerance existed before.

For maximum retention of nutrients in canned vegetables, the liquid should be poured out and heated and the vegetables added to the liquid and heated just before serving. Directions for preparation of frozen vegetables are given on each package.

### Breads and cereal products

Most of the bread used in the home is purchased ready-made from the supermarket. Many kinds of commercially baked breads are available to the consumer. Some are of the "brown and serve" variety, which require a short baking time before serving. Other hot breads, such as biscuits and muffins leavened with baking powder rather than yeast, are frequently prepared in the home. Enriched all-purpose flour, which forms gluten when it is mixed with liquid, gives the structure to these products. Fat and sugar tenderize and help produce the characteristic texture. Baking powder or soda is used for leavening, and some salt is added for flavor. Depending on the characteristics of the product, eggs may or may not be added.

Ready-to-eat cereals require no additional preparation in the home. A wide assortment is found on most grocery shelves. Milk and sugar as well as fruit may be added, depending on individual choice.

When cooking porridge-type cereals, such as oatmeal, farina, or cornmeal, use the proportions of ingredients shown on the package and follow the directions for cooking times.

Regular rice should not be washed before cooking. Use only the amount of water that the rice absorbs during cooking, and do not rinse after cooking. Directions for cooking converted rice and instant rice are found on the package.

To make a smooth cornmeal mush, blend the cornmeal with cold water before stirring it into hot boiling water. It may be served as mush or chilled, sliced, and fried.

Macaroni products and pasta should be cooked until tender but firm. To achieve this consistency, add the pasta to rapidly boiling, salted water, and cook only until tender. The less water that is used in cooking pasta, the

### Table 12-14. General Rules for Boiling Vegetables

1. Use only enough water barely to cover the vegetables. (Exceptions to this rule are noted by an asterisk.) Spinach and other tender greens need no water.
2. Bring water to boiling point and add salt before vegetable is added.
3. Cover tightly and cook over low heat only until vegetables are tender.
4. Use any remaining liquid of mild-flavored vegetables for soup or sauce.
5. Vegetables may be baked in tightly covered casseroles when the oven is being used for some other purpose. The time of cooking will be about one and a half times again as long as for boiling.
6. Variations from the general rules:
   Whole artichokes, beets, the cabbage family, onions, parsnips, turnips, potatoes, and corn on the cob should be cooked in water to cover, and the water discarded. Keeping the pot tightly covered will prevent spreading the strong cooking odors of some of these vegetables through the house.
   Stalks of asparagus and broccoli may be laid side by side in a skillet with one inch of water, or tied and placed upright in the top of a tall double boiler with 1 to 2 inches of water. The skillet or pot should be tightly covered.
7. When a pressure saucepan is to be used, the time chart provided with the utensils should be followed exactly for best results.

### Timetable for Boiling

As vegetables differ in texture according to maturity, directions for cooking time can only be approximate.

| Vegetable | Minutes | Vegetable | Minutes |
|---|---|---|---|
| Artichokes | | | |
|   American or Jerusalem | 15–20 | Dandelion greens | 10–20 |
|   French or Globe* | 20–30 | Eggplant | 10–15 |
| Asparagus* | 15–20 | Kohlrabi | 20–30 |
| Beans | | Mushrooms | 7–10 |
|   String | 15–30 | Okra | 20–25 |
|   Lima | 20–30 | Onions* | 20–40 |
| Beets* | 20–60 | Parsnips* | 30–50 |
| Beet greens | 10–20 | Peas | 8–15 |
| Broccoli* | 15–25 | Potatoes* | |
| Brussels sprouts* | 10–20 |   White | 20–30 |
| Cabbage* | 5–10 |   Sweet | 20–30 |
| Carrots | 15–30 | Spinach | 6–10 |
| Cauliflower* | 10–30 | Squash | |
| Celery | 10–15 |   Summer | 10–20 |
| Corn* | 5–10 |   Winter | 20–30 |
| Cucumbers | 10–15 | Turnips* | 15–60 |

*See General Rules for Cooking, No. 6, above.

more vitamins that are retained. Thick pasta, such as lasagna noodles, require more water for cooking; follow directions on the package.

### Variations in food values

Food values for prepared dishes are based on standard recipes, but people do not always use standard recipes. Obviously, cream of tomato soup made with heavy cream has a higher calorie and fat value, and a lower calcium and protein value, than cream of tomato soup made with skim milk. Cooking methods also affect the nutritive value of food. Broiling in place of frying may greatly reduce the amount of fat and, accordingly, the calorie value of a serving of hamburger. Broiling it to the welldone stage rather than rare further reduces the amount of fat in a serving. Water-soluble vitamins and minerals may be lost in the cooking water when vegetables or meats are cooked in liquid and the liquid is, discarded.

## Meal service

The temperature and the appearance of food as it is placed before the family can be determining factors whether or not the meal will be consumed and enjoyed or wasted. The cook who wishes to please the group will take special pleasure in presenting the meal attractively. Children and people who are ill are especially sensitive to the appearance of the plate.

The type of meal service is usually determined by the life-style of the family and may vary drastically from one meal to another. Breakfast may be an individual effort, with each member preparing and serving his own food, whereas dinner may be served more formally to the group as a whole. In any case, responsibility for serving the meal as well as for its preparation and cleanup is frequently a shared one in today's American family. Men and women alike appear to find enjoyment in the creative aspects of meal management and also in sharing the other work involved in providing food for the family.

## Study questions and activities

1. List your goals for family meal management.
2. What are the steps involved in providing successful family meals?
3. Using the Moderate-cost Food Plan (Table 12-3), plan a week's menus and shopping lists for a family of four consisting of mother, age 28; father, 30; girl, 8; boy, 6. Calculate the cost of the week's food at current market prices.
4. Calculate the costs per quart of milk purchased as follows: 1 qt homogenized milk; $\frac{1}{2}$ gal homogenized milk; 1 gal homogenized milk; 13-oz can evaporated milk; nonfat dry milk (bulk), one 1-lb box; nonfat dry milk (premeasured), 1 lb.

5. Calculate the vitamin C content and the cost per serving of $\frac{1}{2}$ grapefruit; $\frac{1}{2}$ cup frozen orange juice reconstituted according to directions; 1 orange; $\frac{1}{2}$ cup canned tomato juice; $\frac{1}{2}$ cup canned grapefruit; $\frac{1}{2}$ cup canned grapefruit juice.
6. What is the recommended procedure for storing fresh meats, potatoes, and bread in the home?
7. Describe the most appropriate methods for cooking tender cuts of meat and less tender cuts of meat.
8. What effect does heat have on protein foods? What precautions must be taken in cooking cheese mixtures?
9. How may cooking methods change the nutritive value of food?

## Supplementary readings

Bennion M, Hughes O: Introductory Foods, 6th ed. New York, Macmillan, 1975

Kinder F, Green N: Meal Management, 5th ed. New York, Macmillan, 1978

Lane S, Vermeersch J: Evaluation of the thrifty food plan. J Nutr Educ 11:96, 1979

McWilliams M: Food Fundamentals, 2nd ed. New York, John Wiley & Sons, 1970

Medved E: Food in Theory and Practice. Fullerton, CA, Plycon, 1978

Vail GE, Phillips JA, Rust LO et al: Foods—An Introductory College Course, 6th ed. Boston, Houghton Mifflin, 1973

### Cookbooks

General Mills: Betty Crocker's New Good and Easy Cookbook. New York, Golden, 1962

General Mills: Betty Crocker's New Picture Cookbook. New York, McGraw-Hill, 1961

Heseltine M, Dow V: The Basic Cookbook, 5th ed. Boston, Houghton Mifflin, 1967

Rombauer IS, Becker MR: Joy of Cooking. New York, Bobbs-Merrill, 1962

### USDA Home and Garden Bulletins

Single copies of the following publications can be obtained free from the Office of Communication, U.S. Department of Agriculture, Washington, D.C. 20250.

Family Fare—A Guide to Good Nutrition (HG 1)
Home Canning of Fruits and Vegetables (HG 8)
Home Freezing of Fruits and Vegetables (HG 10)
Freezing Combination Main Dishes (HG 40)
Money Saving Main Dishes (HG 43)
How to Make Jellies, Jams and Preserves at Home (HG 56)
Home Care of Purchased Frozen Foods (HG 69)
Food and Your Weight (HG 74)
Storing Perishable Foods in the Home (HG 78)
Conserving the Nutritive Value in Foods (HG 90)
Making Pickles and Relishes at Home (HG 92)
Freezing Meat and Fish in the Home (HG 93)
Family Food Budgeting—For Good Meals and Good Nutrition (HG 94)
Eggs in Family Meals: A Guide for Consumers (HG 103)

Vegetables in Family Meals: A Guide for Consumers (HG 105)

Home Canning of Meat and Poultry (HG 106)

Poultry in Family Meals: A Guide for Consumers (HG 110)

Cheese in Family Meals: A Guide for Consumers (HG 112)

Beef and Veal in Family Meals: A Guide for Consumers (HG 118)

Lamb in Family Meals: A Guide for Consumers (HG 124)

Fruits in Family Meals: A Guide for Consumers (HG 125)

Milk in Family Meals: A Guide for Consumers (HG 127)

How to Buy Nonfat Dry Milk (HG 140)

How to Buy Fresh Fruits (HG 141)

How to Buy Fresh Vegetables (HG 143)

How to Buy Eggs (HG 144)

How to Buy Beef Steaks (HG 145)

How to Buy Beef Roasts (HG 146)

Baking for People with Food Allergies (HG 147)

Cereals and Pasta in Family Meals: A Guide for Consumers (HG 150)

How to Buy Poultry (HG 157)

Pork in Family Meals: A Guide for Consumers (HG 160)

Keeping Food Safe to Eat (HG 162)

How to Buy Meat for Your Freezer (HG 166)

How to Buy Beans, Peas and Lentils (HG 177)

Your Money's Worth in Foods (HG 183)

Breads, Cakes and Pies in Family Meals: A Guide for Consumers (HG 186)

How to Buy Canned and Frozen Fruits (HG 191)

How to Buy Cheese (HG 193)

How to Buy Lamb (HG 195)

How to Use USDA Grades in Buying Foods (HG 196)

How to Buy Potatoes (HG 198)

How to Buy Dairy Products (HG 201)

Food for the Family—A Cost Saving Plan (HG 209)

Aunt Sammy's Radio Recipes (HG 215)

Food is More than Just Something to Eat (HG 216)

Drying Foods at Home (HG 217)

Food (HG 228)

Como Comprar Los Comestibles/How to Buy Food—A Bilingual Consumers Aid (HG 976N)

Food Makes the Difference: Ideas for Economy-Minded Families (HG 934)

Cooking for Two (PA 1043)

Fun with Good Foods (PA 1204)

Food for Thrifty Families (unnumbered)

*For further references see Bibliography in Part 4.*

# The Helping Process in Nutrition Services

*13*

**Clair Agriesti Johnson**

## Responsibility of the nutrition counselor

The chief responsibility of the health-care team is to maintain or to reestablish a positive state of wellbeing in the population it serves. The nutrition counselor (see Chap. 1), as a member of this team, must focus on the reinforcement or modification of food habits that promote good health. Because nutritional requirements change throughout the life span from infancy to old age, most people need to monitor their food practices throughout their lives. Because knowledge about nutrition is constantly increasing, most people also need help to modify their food practices at one time or another.

The public receives nutrition information from a variety of sources other than health practitioners. Chief among these are the public communications media, which bring broad health issues to public attention and attempt through advertising to persuade consumers to change food choices. Few would argue that during the 1960s the media were chiefly responsible for changing the type of fat consumed by an entire nation. Nutrition counselors might well look to this experience as a model for implementing change. In this case, the mission of the advertising industry was to persuade the public to use one type of fat rather than another while the food industry provided an acceptable alternative.

The mission of the nutrition counselor, however, is not only to encourage the client to select among options, but to discontinue one type of behavior in favor of another and to sustain this change over a lifetime. Discontinuance of smoking and curtailment of eating are examples of changes that health practitioners have historically found difficult to implement because most people find these changes difficult to accept. Therefore, the chief responsibility of the nutrition counselor is to translate nutrition knowledge into information the client can accept and subsequently adopt.

## Determining the role of the nutrition counselor

Nutrition counseling is a multidisciplinary effort, and, as such, counseling roles will change in relation to the context of clinical practice. Nutrition counselors can practice in a variety of settings. Some of these are: *the primary health-care setting,* such as neighborhood health clinics, prenatal and child health clinics, and health maintenance organizations where the type of care delivered is essentially *preventive* in nature; *the secondary health-care setting,* such as community hospitals and extended-care facilities where the type of care delivered is essentially crisis and *rehabilitative* in nature; and *the tertiary health-care setting,* such as major medical teaching centers, where the type of care delivered is essentially complex and *crisis* in nature. This is not to say that preventive care cannot be delivered in a tertiary setting nor crisis care in a primary setting. The point is that before the role of the nutrition counselor can be defined it is important to know the needs of the clients served. Specifically, does the client need *preventive, rehabilitative,* or *crisis* care?

Another related consideration in role definition is the power invested in the counselor and that invested in the client. Here it becomes necessary to define power. Power is not a negative concept but rather a reality of the situation in which both the counselor and client find themselves. In other words, who is most in control? In a crisis, it is the practitioner who is most in control and has the most power to change the situation. In a rehabilitative situation, there is almost equal control and, therefore, equal

power. In a preventive situation, it is the client who is in control and who has the power to accept or reject what the counselor advocates. The counselor's role then is a dynamic one and will change as the client's needs change.

## Practitioner-managed vs. client-managed care

Clients enter the health-care system at many points. Figure 13-1 demonstrates how a client can enter at one point in the system and progress or be referred to another. If, for example, a person with diabetes mellitus enters the crisis-care setting in a state of ketoacidosis, all efforts of the team are focused on the immediate treatment and care. In this situation, the care given can be said to be *practitioner-managed;* the primary goal at this point is to reestablish, as quickly as possible, physiological homeostasis. Once this is achieved, the health goal is the reestablishment of psychological equilibrium so that the client can begin to assume the responsibility for the continued implementaton of the primary goal—a sustained positive state of wellbeing.

It is good to remember that during a medical crisis the client often progresses from the passive phase to the collaborative phase of his treatment and care. The nutrition counselor working in a crisis-care setting needs to be aware of these phases so that she can help the client pass through them at his own pace and with dignity. During the period of passivity the care needed can be described as essentially practitioner-managed, but as soon as the client shows an interest in the rationale of his treatment, it is time for the nutrition counselor to encourage him to accept responsibility for his own management. In doing this the nutrition counselor moves from the caring role to the helping role. As this shift occurs, the client begins to move from a passive role to an active one, and true counseling begins. The counselor's objective at this time changes again and becomes one of helping the client determine his own goals and participate completely in his own care. In other words, the care delivered is client-managed.

When one compares the number of persons in crisis care or institutional settings to those in preventive care or noninstitutional settings, it is obvious that there is a greater need for clients to know how to care for themselves than for the practitioner to care for them. Yet the present health-care system is better organized to deliver crisis care than to deliver preventive care. The reason for this is understandable. In a developing nation the chief mission of health personnel is the eradication of infectious disease. As this becomes a reality, life expectancy increases, and health professions are faced with the growing problem of chronic diseases which, by their very nature, require the client to manage his own care to prevent,

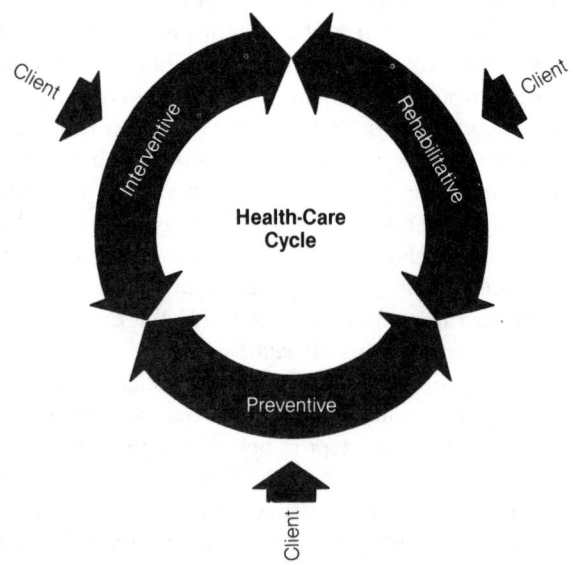

**Fig. 13-1.**   Continuity of care. This health-care cycle was developed to demonstrate how a client, having entered at one point within the cycle, can proceed or be referred to another, thus establishing continuity of care.

delay, or treat them. This type of care implies competence on the part of the client; and, if the delivery of this care is to become a reality, the counselor must see to it that the client becomes competent at caring for himself. Nutrition counselors who hope to become effective in helping the client to manage his care need to be as competent in the preventive setting as they have historically been in the crisis setting. This requires the nutrition counselor to assume the predominant role of change-agent.

As a change-agent, the counselor must understand and use the helping process. In nutrition counseling the helping process can be defined as a process of intervention in which the counselor makes available to an individual the means for establishing or modifying his food practices. And, to carry out the process, the counselor must enter into a helping relationship with the client.

## Nature of the helping relationship

A relationship refers to a connection between people, ideas, or things. A helping relationship demands a regularized pattern of interaction between counselor and client and is built up over time. A single exchange of information does not meet these criteria. By the same token, a system involving multiple exchanges of information between the client and a variety of counselors does not lend itself to the firm establishment of the helping relationship. This has been demonstrated in research studies that suggest that patient compliance is better in private practice than in clinics because the continuing relationship of client and practitioner is well established.[1]

In 1960 Feinstein reviewed the literature of the treatment of obesity published in professional journals from 1940 to 1959.[2] From his analysis of various approaches to the treatment of obese patients, he concluded that the most significant factors in successful weight reduction were the patient himself and the therapeutic relationship. Feinstein pointed out that an external source of motivation may be the decisive factor in assisting the majority of obese patients to lose weight. The external source of motivation for many of these individuals is a continuing therapeutic relationship with a clinician. He identified the clinician as the health professional with an adequate knowledge of the energy value of foods and the ability to establish a positive relationship with the client. Feinstein emphasized that the clinician must see the patient frequently, or as it is described today, there must be "continuity of care" and that the clinician must be accepting of the patient's needs and problems.

More recently the disciplines of psychiatry and psychology have been studying behavior modification as an approach to the treatment of obesity. An underlying premise of this approach is that major changes in eating and exercise behaviors are necessary to ensure long-term weight control. The success of these programs have been documented for short-term weight loss but has yet to be demonstrated for long-term control.[3] Yet, one can assume that the success that has been documented can be attributed to the frequency and duration of client–clinician interaction as described by Feinstein.

What Feinstein calls the *therapeutic relationship*, others call the *helping relationship*. The work of Rogers[4] and others has shown that the helping person must first establish a climate of trust between herself and the client. To achieve this the helping person must believe that all people can change and be able to communicate this to the client. It is important to accept *unconditionally* the client's feelings and personal meanings as the client sees them. The counselor must be warm, caring, and genuinely interested in the client. Finally, the counselor must help the client make decisions rather than have the client become dependent on her. The reason that the development of the helping relationship is so crucial to the delivery of nutritional care is that most nutritional care is implemented outside the institutional setting by the client in the context of his social environment. Therefore, the nutrition counselor is advocating a process, not a solution.

## Elements of the helping process

The remainder of this chapter delineates the process of delivering client-managed nutritional care. This process is made up of several critical components (Chap. 1): *establishing and maintaining the relationship; collecting and assessing information; planning change; implementing change; and evaluating effectiveness.* It must be remembered that these components are not discrete steps toward a solution but a series of highly interrelated functions systematically planned to implement a process that has evaluation criteria built in. Simply stated, a person who needs to lose weight must be helped to implement and evaluate a weight reduction program. A critical step in helping the client is to determine how much weight is to be lost and at what rate. This then becomes the ultimate criterion by which both client and counselor evaluate the effectiveness of their collaboration.

### Establishing the helping relationship

Collaboration implies that the client and counselor are working together. An important first component of the helping process is the generation of a climate conducive to the achievement of this end. That this function is a continuous process is shown by the fact that the counselor does not simply establish the relationship and then move on to the next step. The helping relationship is one that requires constant building, and it permeates the entire process.

The first interaction with the client, however, is most critical because at this time the direction of the helping process is established. Before the nutrition counselor can do anything, she must find the answers to two important questions: what does the client expect from her and what does she expect from the client? Although one of these questions is directed to the counselor and the other to the client, it is the responsibility of the counselor to determine these answers as well as reconcile any existing differences.

If the client seeks out the counselor's help, then the counselor's task is greatly simplified. In the case of the nutrition counselor, however, the client often enters the health-care system expecting a solution to a problem and is referred to the nutrition counselor because of a complicating factor. A classic example of this is the client who seeks medical attention due to fatigue and shortness of breath with the expectation that the health-care team will "get him well." In order to meet the client's expectations, the physician refers him to the nutrition counselor for a weight-reduction program. The nutrition counselor then finds herself in a situation where she is face-to-face with a client who has come for a solution, not a process.

Here, the nutritional counselor has three major tools which can be used to help the client: force, knowledge, and client values. These can be translated into three kinds of health arguments that the counselor can use: an argument based on fear, one based on reason, and one based on trust. Health personnel have been, and continue to be, criticized for relying heavily on fear and reason, while ignoring client values. This may well be the case, but those who would advocate the third to the exclusion of the first and second are ignoring the variability of human nature as well as the reality of the clinical setting.

It is the client's need that should dictate the health argument used. Often, it is fear that brings the client into the health-care setting. In the preventive setting it is usually fear of losing his health; in the crisis setting, it is fear of losing his life. Both of these fears are motivating forces because they are rooted in basic values. Accordingly, in the preventive setting, the nutrition counselor might well focus on the fear motive, whereas, in the crisis setting this is impossible. It is not, however, a question of which argument is best to employ, but which best meets the needs of a client at a particular point of time. Often, the client's self-generated fear is motive enough to establish a collaborative relationship with the counselor. When fear is not sufficient, then the counselor may try reason and, in turn, trust. It is imperative in establishing the relationship that the nutrition counselor start where the client is, not where she would like him to be.

No matter where the client is, he will eventually be outside the health-care setting managing his own care; and for sustained change to occur, the client's value system must be made known to the counselor. Hence, it is important to develop a climate of trust so that this kind of information can be analyzed for its significance to the problem.

## Collecting and assessing information

Collecting and assessing information provides the basis for the development of the counseling plan and, as in the establishment of the relationship, is a continuing process. Here the nutrition counselor has two major sources—secondary and primary.

### Secondary sources

Information that can be obtained from sources other than the client or his family is described as secondary. Such sources include the client's records in any health-care setting; continuity of care or referral reports; or the information shared in health team conferences. The nutrition counselor not only uses this information but also contributes to it. She uses it to develop a nutritional care plan and contributes to it to ensure continuity of care.

Analysis of the secondary information about a client and his family reveals the health problem, the objectives of care, and the resources available for the solution of the problem. *Health problems* are conditions or situations that obstruct the maintenance or reestablishment of a positive state of wellbeing. They are usually stated in a problem list and can include such conditions as poor dental hygiene or obesity. *Health objectives* are those goals that the health-care team wants accomplished. For example, the objectives for an obese person who has habitually practiced poor dental hygiene might be "full-mouth extraction" and "25% reduction in weight." The health-care team then looks to resource persons who can help meet these objectives. *Health resources* are those persons, departments, or agencies within or outside the health-care setting that can either solve the client's problems or help him deal with them. It is through the analysis of secondary information that the nutritional counselor can determine the health problems that will be encountered, the objectives to be achieved, and the resources to be identified for the client.

### Primary sources

Relevant nutritional care information that is not recorded must be obtained from primary sources. These are the client himself and those persons who will help him implement his care. The nutrition counselor gathers this information in any health-care setting and must be a skilled interviewer. The counselor uses this information to develop a counseling plan as well as to keep the team informed of client progress. Analysis of primary information reveals the client's *nutritional needs*, *problems*, and *resources*.

*Nutritional needs* can be defined as that nutrient intake that best promotes or reestablishes physiological homeostasis. They can be stated as a dietary prescription or implied in the problem list. For example, the problem of obesity implies the need for a deficit in energy intake; the problem of less than adequate weight gain in an infant without organic disease implies underfeeding; a potential nutritional need may be dictated by a socioeconomic problem. In addition, nutrient monitoring may be warranted if the client is from a high-risk population, such as the pregnant teenaged girl.

*Nutritional problems,* on the other hand, are reasons why the nutritional needs exist. Obesity may be the health problem but not the nutritional problem. For example, one client may be obese because he is a compulsive eater, while another may be too old to move about, have inadequate kitchen facilities, or be living on a limited budget. These clients obviously have similar nutritional needs but quite different nutritional problems related to these needs. Therefore, they will likely need different resources.

*Client resources* are those persons or attitudes that can assist the client in dealing with the nutritional problem, hence, in meeting the nutritional need. The person who is a compulsive eater may have strong support at home, and the person with inadequate kitchen facilities may be an active member of a church or fraternal organization. Persons too old to move about or living on inadequate funds who also have limited personal resources may need to be referred to agencies outside their primary social environment. It is through the analysis of primary and secondary information that the nutrition counselor can reconcile the differences between objectives which are defined by the health-care team and objectives which are defined by the client. Such mutually defined objectives then become the basis for the counseling plan.

## Planning change

A critical component of the helping process is the development of a plan of action. The concept of planned change implies that the change-agent knows, in advance, where she is going (*objectives*), how she will get there (*action*), and how she will know she has arrived (*evaluation*). In client-managed nutritional care it is important that the user of change becomes the agent of change. In other words, it is not enough to produce an attitude change in the client. To move from attitude to action, a meaningful plan is necessary. This point is extremely important. There is experimental evidence from studies of antismoking communications that both a message of threat and instructions for action are necessary to reduce or stop smoking.[5]

### Objectives

Health-care objectives are directly related to the client's health problem and should reflect the common objectives of the health-care team. However, if the client is to manage his own care, then the team's objectives must be congruent, whenever possible, with the client's. For example, the health-care team in a prenatal clinic may have breast-feeding as an objective whereas a mother who plans to return to work 4 weeks after the birth of her baby

may reject this objective. Equally important is the need for the nutrition counselor and the client to work together on the nutritional aspects of the health-care objectives.

Objectives are written in the client's record and vary from client to client. There is one health-care objective, however, that is so universal that it is rarely specified. That objective is to preserve the *psychological equilibrium* of the client and his family. Viewed in this way, the importance of involving clients in the formulation of their own goals is more than an effective change strategy; it is the foundation upon which their health maintenance or recovery from disease rests.

### Action

Once the client has developed his objectives, he must be shown how to achieve them. It is important that the nutrition counselor help the client find a way that is least disruptive to his life-style, yet conducive to health maintenance or the reestablishment of physiological homeostasis. Just as health objectives are related to health problems and client objectives to client problems, the action to be taken is related to both health and client objectives. It is at this point that the counselor must identify the specific information the client needs in order to manage his care, determine the sequence in which this will be shared with the client, and offer a variety of alternatives to the client for achieving his goals.

### Evaluation

Critical components of any plan are the evaluation criteria by which progress toward the objectives is measured. As such, evaluation criteria are directly related to the objectives. How much and what foods will the teenaged girl eat for breakfast before going to school each morning? Is the business executive to lose 1 lb per week? In addition, how long should the client sustain these changes? Both client and counselor need this information. The client needs it to guide him toward his goal, and the counselor needs it to assess the client's progress. Although evaluation criteria are usually the *last* of the components mentioned in any health-care plan, they should comprise the *first* components. Objectives and evaluation criteria should be developed simultaneously so that both the health-care team and the client know the ultimate goal, and so that the team and client can reconcile any differences.

## Implementing change

Once the change has been planned, the next step in the helping process is counseling the client in how to implement the needed change. This process is not unlike teaching children to form new ideas. But, whether teaching adults or children, the nutrition counselor is involved in a process that is commonly referred to as "adult education." Adults are free to retreat from a learning environment that they do not find satisfying. New concepts, therefore, cannot be taught in the health setting as they have traditionally been taught in the classroom. In order for the nutrition counselor to meet commonly defined objectives, she must be aware of some fundamental principles of adult education that are applicable to any learner in an open environment.

## Perception

This is the process by which humans become aware of their environment. It is mediated through the five senses to the sensory area of the brain where an impression is formed on the mind. These impressions are called *percepts*, which are the basic components of *concepts*. Hearing is the most critical to concept formation, followed by seeing. The other modalities are less critical to learning but still play a role. Generally, the more sense organs stimulated, the more effective the learning.[6] The use of visuals is a practical application of this theory. These need not be elaborate. In fact, very few professionally developed materials can be used with all clients without some modification. Therefore, a blackboard in a formal counseling area or a flip chart in the clinical area as well as food models, labels, and scales are indispensable aids for the nutrition counselor.

People with a perceptual loss are particularly challenging to the nutrition counselor. Hearing loss has a more profound effect on cognitive development than loss of any other modality. When interacting with persons with absolute deafness, the counselor needs either special training or a resource person who can help with the teaching process. When working with people with only impaired hearing, several simple rules can help.

- Raise volume but not pitch of voice.
- Exaggerate the formation of words with the lips.
- Give nonverbal cues.
- Stand facing the light.
- Focus on one concept at a time.
- Use a variety of visual aids.

## Memory

This is an important factor in learning. The fact that we learn implies that we remember. Yet, we tend to forget things over a period of time. This is a continuous process and seems to be selective.[6] For example, we remember what we value. There are several theories related to memory. The theory of disuse suggests that something learned that is not used will disappear. Thus, learned behavior that is not practiced will be forgotten. Interference theory, which is opposed to the theory of disuse, refers to the phenomenon that what is learned will remain intact unless some new event occurs to interfere with it. Therefore, the recall of a previous learning can be obliterated by new learning. The reverse can also occur, especially if previously learned information is highly valued. Therefore, the nutrition counselor must be assured that the client has

and remembers necessary facts. Although persons may not act on knowledge they possess, they certainly cannot act on knowledge they do not have. Some rules to follow are:

- Encourage clients to do something that forces them to use what you have taught.
- Provide for distributed practice. Four 15-minute periods are likely to yield better recall than one 60-minute period.
- Assess the degree and validity of previously learned knowledge.

## Readiness

Physical and mental readiness is necessary for learning.[7] It must be remembered that humans do not have easily identifiable characteristics to suggest intellectual readiness. The nutrition counselor needs to distinguish between lack of readiness and lack of motivation. Some people will appear unmotivated when, in actuality, they cannot cope with the abstractness of a concept that is entirely new to them. A good rule is to use concrete illustrations in teaching abstract concepts. Giving an example, such as: "Sodium is like a sponge in the body," enables the learner to translate the abstraction into meaningful, everyday, terms.

Another impediment to readiness is the client's physical condition. Biochemical changes profoundly affect mental ability. For example, persons who are in impending hepatic coma, a state of diabetic acidosis, or renal failure have biochemical changes affecting the brain. In such cases the underlying biochemical problem must be dealt with before intellectual function, hence teaching, can be resumed.

## Conditioning

In the pavlovian sense this refers to the process through which a response aroused by a specific stimulus can be aroused by an entirely different stimulus if the two stimuli are presented simultaneously over a given period of time. Behavioristic theory was developed in light of Pavlov's experiments. The use of behavior modification techniques is an application of this theory. These techniques have been used primarily in the treatment of obesity, but they also have been successful in the treatment of hypertension.[8] A distinction between behavioral therapy and the use of behavioral modification techniques needs to be made. *Behavior therapy* is defined here as a systematic method of changing maladaptive behavior, usually conducted by or in conjunction with a psychiatrist or psychologist, whereas the term *behavior modification techniques* is defined as a method by which clients motivate themselves through self-monitoring and other means of behavioral control. The essence of behavior modification is that clients monitor their own behavior. In nutrition counseling this is translated into certain activities that provide a positive stimulus for a desired response.

The hope is that these activities will lead to changes in the behaviors being monitored.

Keeping records of food intake, physical activity, body weight, and conditions that influence eating are examples of self-monitoring behavior. But these techniques alone are not usually sufficient to modify behavior. Clients also need to be taught to control various stimuli that they have found to promote excessive food intake. These include the sight and smell of food, the time of day, and the eating location. Hypertensive clients, for example, would be counseled not to keep salted snack foods and preserved meats and fish in the house. Obese persons would be counseled to keep low-calorie snack foods readily available and to eliminate high-calorie foods entirely from their shopping lists. If watching television, or reading, for example, is associated with excessive eating, obese clients would be counseled to eat in a prescribed place at a prescribed time of day. Another type of behavior modification technique for obese persons is eating more slowly so that they can become more aware of the eating process. Clients can develop their own methods for accomplishing this, such as pausing between bites, counting bites, and pausing between courses.

Positive reinforcement is the cornerstone of any type of nutrition counseling. Many clients, however, are in a double bind. The positive consequences of eating a hot fudge sundae or a bag of potato chips, for example, is immediate, whereas, the negative consequence of such foods for the obese or hypertensive person is more remote. The nutrition counselor's role in such cases is much like that of a clergyman trying to convince people that suffering in this life will lead to a rich reward at a later date. Two methods for dealing with such conflicting goals are the use of social rewards in the form of approval from self-help organizations (see Chap. 28) and the use of strong family support. Therefore, involving the family or significant others in planning, implementing, and evaluating nutritional objectives is one of the most potent counseling techniques the nutrition counselor can use.

Whether dealing with obesity, hypertension, or preventive nutrition, the nutrition counselor needs to consider cognitive restructuring of the client's attitudes. How clients feel about themselves and their ability to change has profound implications for success or failure. If persons feel that they are not in control of a situation, are weak-willed, or are bound to fail, they can use these feelings to justify a given condition. Such feelings lead to self-defeating behavior, which the nutrition counselor must help the client to deal with through positive reinforcment. On the other hand, if the nutrition counselor suspects that the client's self-defeating behavior is so maladaptive that it is out of her therapeutic range, she needs to refer the client elsewhere. Weight loss has more than cosmetic overtones. Persons who have such feelings often are the ones who fail to maintain weight loss once achieved; they go on and off diets, and their weight fluctu-

ates widely. Stunkard maintains that if people cannot maintain weight loss, they would be better off not trying to lose weight. Stunkard's rationale for this position is based on human research suggesting that the deleterious effects of obesity are exerted primarily during periods of weight gain and that research on animals has shown the danger to the cardiovascular system of the kind of weight loss-weight gain cycle that characterizes many obese people.[3]

Implementing change, then, requires the client to participate actively in the therapeutic process. It is recognized that this is time-consuming, for it involves more than handing the client a list of instructions, commonly referred to as "giving diet instructions." Giving does not imply accepting.

## Evaluating effectiveness

The effectiveness of the collaboration is tested during subsequent client-counselor encounters. At this point the nutrition counselor needs to determine whether or not the client is progressing toward his goals. If this is not being achieved, it is important for them to determine together where the relationship became ineffective.

Many nutritional care plans fail because the client's needs, problems, and resources have not been accurately identified. Some questions are so basic that they are often not asked. "Does a need exist?" is such a question. If there is evidence that the client is adequately managing his own nutritional care, it is pointless and can be disruptive to initiate a new plan of action. Some clients seen by nutrition counselors have often been counseled before. Others sustain a positive state of wellbeing through their own resources. Therefore, before a counseling plan is developed, it must be determined whether change is needed, as well as the nature of that change.

Weed defines a health problem as a situation that requires the health-care team to do one of three things—obtain more information, treat, or educate.[9] Many nutritional care plans are not effective because there is insufficient data to identify the client's problem. In these cases there is clearly a need for more information. On the other hand, some plans fail because the client cannot care for himself and needs to be treated or cared for by someone else. When it is determined that the client's problem is lack of information, then there is a need to educate. Also, the client's resources may not have been assessed correctly.

The client has two types of resources available to him—those within his primary social environment, or the family, and those within his extended social environment, or the community. When the client is an infant, it is obvious that the persons counseled are the parents or other caretakers. When the client is an adult, the persons to be counseled will vary depending on certain factors. For example, when a self-directed adult lives alone, he is the person who should be counseled. Yet, when the client is a dependent adult living with a parent, an offspring, or a spouse, counseling efforts need to be directed at both the client and his primary resource person. When the client is not in control and is being referred to an extended-care facility or a community agency, the nutritional care plan should be communicated to those persons who will care for him.

When the proper relationship has not been established, an otherwise effective care plan is doomed to failure. There are times when, despite efforts on the part of the nutrition counselor, a helping relationship cannot be established with the client. When this is the case, many nutritional counselors might make a sincere attempt to proceed with the plan as best they can. Effective professional counselors, however, recognize that in these circumstances it is wiser, when possible, to refer the client to another practitioner who can better help him. Before this decision is made, the nutrition counselor should be certain that the client wants to be referred to another practitioner. She must also reassure the client that she will be available at any time the client needs her. Often this open gesture of concern is enough to identify the problem obstructing the development of the helping relationship, and effective counseling can proceed.

## Interviewing

Interviewing is a component of counseling, and the two cannot be separated. For our purposes here, however, interviewing is defined as the information-gathering portion of the counseling process. Interviewing is the method used to gather primary information from the client about usual food choices and the environmental factors that directly affect them. Interviewing is a form of interpersonal communication that differs from social conversation in that it is guided by goals defined either by the counselor or the client and agreed upon by both. The interviewer is responsible for *guiding*, rather than *controlling*, the interview. The goal of the interview should control the process.

### Direct interviewing

If one needs to gather precise information, if the client starts to ramble, or if clarification is needed, one can use a direct line of inquiry. In this technique the chief problem to avoid is interviewer bias.[10] Rules to keep in mind are:

- *Do not* suggest a response, such as "Do you use butter on your toast?"
- *Do* seek qualifying information by using terms like: "How do you eat it? Cook it? Anything on it? In it? With it?"
- *Do not* suggest a judgment, such as "You *always* eat watching television?"
- *Do* use such questions as "Where? In what circumstances? With whom?"

- *Do not* suggest intensified interest, such as: "You mean you ate a *whole* watermelon?"
- *Do* respond with: "How many? How often? How big? Show me."

During the history-taking process the interviewer may need to intervene to obtain precise information, and this may require asking direct questions. Direct questions need not be closed, however. The interviewer is cautioned about using a direct line of inquiry too early in the interview or using this technique too often. By intervening too early the interviewer can destroy the client's initiative in telling his own story. Keep in mind that a great deal of specific history information can be gleaned through indirect interviewing techniques.

### Indirect interviewing

The clinical interview has a double goal—to obtain valid, reliable, and precise information relevant to the client, and to promote a helping relationship. A direct line of inquiry can lead to precise information and possibly valid and reliable information. Yet, skill in indirect interviewing is the *sine qua non* of an effective counselor, for it leads to both valid and reliable information while, at the same time, promoting a helping relationship.

When the interviewer needs to seek specific information, it is logical to assume that the most efficient way to go about this is to ask direct questions. Interviewers skilled in indirect interviewing can develop a line of inquiry leading to specific information that is not only precise but valid and reliable as well. This is done by starting with a general exploratory question, like: "How do you start your day?" and gradually restricting the open-endedness of a series of questions until the client gives the specific information needed. This can happen at any point in the sequence. For example, suppose that the specific information needed is related to the relationship between an 85-year-old farm wife and her husband. Starting at the periphery and working toward the center may yield the following information:

Interviewer: "How do you and your husband manage such a large farm?"

Client: "Oh, my son and his wife manage it now. Dad and I just take it easy."

Interviewer: "Easy?"

Client: "Yes, I tend the chickens, and Dad runs the dairy, and when I'm finished I go into the house and fix breakfast and spend most of the rest of the day preparing for lunch and supper . . . canning, you know."

As can be seen, the client, in her own words, not only gave the interviewer the information she was seeking, but also added a whole set of new and important data as well as opening up another area of questioning that the interviewer needs to pursue.

## Summary

For more specific interviewing techniques the reader is referred to the supplementary readings listed at the end of this chapter. The following summary statements relate to developing a helping relationship with clients within the interviewing and counseling role.

- The role of the nutrition counselor is to help the client become self-sufficient or to help significant others help the client do so.
- Counseling is no special prerogative of any one discipline; it is simply a method of interaction that occurs in every helping situation.
- The nutrition counselor is concerned mainly with affecting long-range eating behavior, not in affecting alterations in maladaptive reactions.
- When the nutrition counselor suspects that a client's behavior is maladaptive, the client must be referred to the appropriate clinician.
- A helping relationship is a collaborative one, and for such a relationship to occur, the client needs to have contact with the same clinician long enough for the client to understand, accept, and adopt the necessary changes.
- For collaboration to occur, the clinician needs to be a warm, caring person, have a genuine interest in the client, and permit the client to plan, implement, and evaluate his own behavior.
- In order for clients to plan their own care, they must be given the information needed, helped to determine their own objectives, shown how to meet them, and given precise criteria by which to evaluate their own effectiveness.
- In order to help clients in this way, the nutrition counselor needs to operate from a valid and reliable data base, which is best accomplished through indirect interviewing.
- Direct interviewing may be used to elicit precise information, but this should be done in a way so that client's responses are not biased by the interviewer.
- Indirect interviewing skills are essential to the nutrition counselor. This assumes that the counselor develops a line of inquiry that proceeds from the general to the specific, permitting the clients to tell their own story.
- Interviewing skills are critical to the success of the nutrition counselor, and refining them is a lifelong challenge.

## Study questions and activities

1. In a prenatal clinic or a family health clinic, interview a client to obtain information about his or her usual food practices. With your instructor, formulate nutritional care objectives and observe your instructor interacting with the client to validate whether or not your objectives are congruent with the client's.
2. Review a client's record and identify the nutritional component of his health-care needs. Does the information in the record indicate that the client is aware of his needs?
3. Without counseling other members, plan and implement a change in your family's usual food practices. Did your family accept or reject this change?
4. Visit a congregate meals program for the elderly and *listen* to the participants discuss the food served. Analyze the discussion with your instructor.
5. Record your own food practices for a 3-day period. Analyze your record and plan and carry out *one* minor change for 2 weeks. Were you successful? Why or why not?

## References

1. Blackwell D: N Engl J Med 289:249, 1973
2. Feinstein A: J Chronic Dis 11:349, 1960
3. Stunkard AJ, Penick SB: Arch Gen Psychiatry 36:801, 1979
4. Rogers C: Personnel and Guidance J 37:6, 1958
5. Leventhal H et al: J Pers Soc Psychol 6:313, 1971
6. Mouly GJ: Psychology for Effective Teaching. New York, Holt, Rinehart & Winston, 1973
7. Gagne RM: The Conditions of Learning. New York, Holt, Rinehart & Winston, 1977
8. Alderman MH, Schoenbaum EE: N Engl J Med 293:65, 1975
9. Weed LL: Arch Intern Med 127:101, 1971
10. Enelow AJ, Swisher SN: Interviewing and Patient Care. New York, Oxford University Press, 1972

## Supplementary readings

Bernstein L, Dana RH: Interviewing and the Health Professions. New York, Appleton-Century-Crofts, 1970

Biltz PA, Derelian DV: Changing dietitians' attitudes toward client counseling. J Am Diet Assoc 73:239, 1978

Brill NI: Working with People: The Helping Process. New York, JB Lippincott, 1973

Collins M: Communication in Health Care. St Louis, CV Mosby, 1977

Danish SJ et al: The anatomy of a dietetic counseling interview. J Am Diet Assoc 75:626, 1979

Evans RJ, Hall Y: Social-psychologic perspective in motivating changes in eating behavior. J Am Diet Assoc 72:378, 1978

Ferguson J: Dietitians as behavior-change agents. J Am Diet Assoc 73:231, 1978

Glanz K: Dietitians' effectiveness and patient compliance with dietary regimens. J Am Diet Assoc 75:631, 1979

Mason M, Wenberg BG, Welsch PK: The Dynamics of Clinical Dietetics. New York, John Wiley & Sons, 1977

Pohl M: Teaching Function of the Nursing Practitioner. Dubuque, C Brown, 1968

Skipper JK, Leonard RC: Social Interaction and Patient Care. Philadelphia, JB Lippincott, 1965

*For further references see Bibliography in Part 4.*

# Regional, Cultural, and Religious Food Patterns

## 14

## Factors influencing food habits

The factors that determine individual food habits are varied and complex. The nutrition counselor must develop an understanding of them if she is to fulfill her function successfully. The following brief discussion indicates some of the influences that help to establish food habits.

### Cultural factors

Culture may be defined as the way of life of a group of people—usually of one nationality or from a particular locality. Food habits are a deeply rooted aspect of many cultures. One culture may consider food only as a means of satisfying hunger; another may consider eating a duty, a virtue, or a form of pleasure; still another may feel eating is a means of family or social sharing.

Culture is transmitted from one generation to another by institutions such as family, school, and church. Over periods of time various degrees of change occur within any given culture. The preservation of individual cultures is an important goal of many minority groups today. The revival of interest in the American Indian culture, the "Black is Beautiful" concept, and the activities of Italian-American groups represent attempts to identify and to transmit to future generations certain aspects of a cultural identity. It is important to understand that culturally determined food practices, which vary from group to group, may nevertheless meet the basic biologic needs that are similar for all peoples.

### Economic factors

Rising food costs and food shortages have had their impact on the food patterns of many American families. As agricultural surpluses disappeared and the world food crisis became apparent, consumers began to reexamine their buying practices and to look for substitutes for scarce and expensive foods. Although there is still a tremendous variety of foods available in supermarkets, increased prices make the selection of food for the family a real challenge.

**ADI:** Acceptable Daily Intake

The homemaker who has little or no concept of nutritional value bases choices on cost and on cultural and family preferences. If the food budget is unlimited so are the choices; but the homemaker who must stay within a limited budget especially needs information about nutritive values as they relate to the cost per serving of individual food items. Consumerism is rapidly developing in the United States, and consumer groups are active in demanding greater honesty in the marketplace. Nutrition labeling and unit pricing are examples of programs introduced to assist the consumer. The nutrition counselor should help the homemaker take advantage of this information provided in the marketplace to make wise food selections.

### Social factors

If one recognizes that individuals belong to various social groups, the effect of group behavior cannot be overlooked when considering factors that influence food habits. The organization of society, with its many structures and accompanying value systems, plays an important part in the acceptance or rejection of food patterns.

The social groups to which one belongs—club, church, union, or fraternal organization—often have meals together, and the menus are apt to reflect the tastes of the group. For instance, union members, such as those who work in heavy industry, may be used to hearty but simple meals, either at home or in groups. On the other hand, an upper middle class club may be used to exotic foods and delicacies quite unfamiliar to the first group.

If people accept obesity or overweight as natural—in women as the accompaniment of maturity and in men as a sign of strength—it will be difficult for the nutrition counselor to persuade them to change their eating habits to lose weight. By contrast, a business executive or professional person, warned of the health hazard of excess weight and too little exercise, will often seek advice and be motivated to follow it. Although socially people in such occupations may be exposed to too much or too rich food on occasion, they are able to exert self-control and to avoid overeating.

### Psychological factors

Food habits are an important part of human behavior. Individuals are motivated to act in terms of what they perceive as being relevant to meet their needs. Maslow[1] has defined a hierarchy of five levels of human need: basic physiologic survival, security, belongingness, self-esteem, and self-actualization. Because minimum satisfaction of each level of need must be met before a person seeks satisfaction at the next level, a thorough understanding of the person is necessary to determine effective motivation. Weight reduction for the purpose of improving self-esteem will probably not motivate the unemployed father of a large family when he is primarily concerned with his and his family's survival. Self-esteem, however, may be the motivating force for the mature woman returning to a career.

Assuming that the person has been motivated, his ability to change behavior, that is, food habits, will be affected by knowledge or cognition. In this case, he must have the information to select appropriate kinds and amounts of food. Thus, although a knowledge of nutrition is indispensable in affecting the desired change, information itself is useless unless a person has accepted the need for change and is motivated to act accordingly (see Chap. 13).

## Food patterns in America

Before discussing specific food patterns, it is important to consider some factors that have influenced American eating habits in general. The large number of people of different national backgrounds living together in urban areas have made tamales, frankfurters, pizza, chow mein, sukiyaki, and many other dishes of foreign origin as American as apple pie. Just as it is difficult to define the typical American in terms of national origin, color, religion, or local region, it is equally difficult to define the "typical" American food pattern. As each national group brought its native food habits to this country and adapted them to available foods, it also dispersed them to its neighbors.

Also, because this country stretches across an entire continent, it has a variety of geographic conditions that have resulted in relatively varied regional food patterns. Fish, an important source of protein in coastal regions, is less widely used as one moves away from the sea. Soft wheat, indigenous to the South, which makes good "hot breads" but poor yeast breads, has determined regional food preferences that cannot be changed easily.

When large numbers of people of similar national origins or ethnic backgrounds settle in their own communities, they tend to be less influenced by the food habits of indigenous groups or of other cultural groups. Because of the demand for foods they are used to, their own retail stores evolve, such as the German delicatessen, the Italian fruit and vegetable market, the Chinese restaurant, and the kosher meat market.

It may also be noted that transplanted people usually arrive poor and that it may take several generations before opportunities are available for them to achieve "middle class status." In the meantime, the frugality necessary to stretch the food dollar may develop food habits that are retained even after economic reasons for them have disappeared. French and Chinese cuisines were evolved not from unlimited food resources but rather from a set of restrictions growing out of geographic, economic, and social factors; as someone once noted, these two great national cuisines were indeed based on poverty. The evolution of "soul food" from the black culture has some of the same characteristics today.

No story of American food practices, however, is complete without mentioning the highly developed food technology that makes all foods, in a variety of forms, available in all parts of the country during all seasons of the year. Hence, the choice available to the American public is nearly unlimited, even though each person's selection may normally derive from cultural practices.

Also, mention must be made of the effect of mass media advertising on the changing food habits of the American family. Young children, especially, are besieged by television commercials that advertise not only a food item but also "prizes" included in the package. Certain display techniques are used in retail stores to entice the shopper to buy an item or select a brand on the spur of the moment. Such impulse buying can increase the cost of the family's food and may at the same time reduce its nutritive value.

Mention must also be made of the increased use of alcoholic beverages and drugs among certain groups of Americans today. The high cost of such items and the physiological consequences to the people who use them excessively are well known. In cases of true alcoholism and drug addiction the appetite is reduced or perverted, and cases of frank malnutrition often result.

## Regional food patterns in the United States

Anyone who has traveled in different parts of the United States and has eaten meals typical of various regions is aware of differences in menus, food preparation, and local terms for foods or special dishes. Part of the joy of travel is eating the traditional foods of each locality. However, national advertising in magazines and on TV has tended to popularize certain foods so that diets are not as regional in character as they once were.

People who are ill are much more likely to want familiar foods cooked in a traditional manner with familiar seasoning. Therefore, the nutrition counselor should recognize the existence of regional differences and make some adjustments in the diet so as to provide essential nutrients from familiar foods.

### The South

In the South, hot breads are served at nearly every meal, and baker's yeast breads are not popular. Corn and rice are common sources of carbohydrates. There is a preference for vegetables that have been cooked a long time and often with fatback. Undoubtedly, some vitamins are destroyed by this process, but the common use of pot liquor conserves the nutrients, which are in solution. The wide variety of greens used contributes significantly to the intake of calcium and vitamins. Pork is the most popular

meat, although chicken and fish are frequently served. Less cheese is consumed in the south than in other regions of the country. Twelve times more margarine than butter was purchased by Southern households.[2] Buttermilk is liked and used when available. Southern black families recently reported purchasing significantly less fluid and nonfat dry milk than white families in the same region.[3]

Because many black Americans now living elsewhere came from the South, their food customs reflect some of the practices of this region, as discussed later in the chapter.

### The Southwest

The Mexican influence here is shown in the use of beans and highly seasoned dishes. Again, milk production is limited, and, although drinking fresh milk was not the custom originally, it is being introduced gradually. Mexican foods, such as tortillas, tamales, enchiladas, and a wide variety of beans, are popular in American homes of the southwest as well as in Mexican families. More details of Mexican foods are given later in this chapter.

### The Far West

The infiltration of Oriental cultures in the Far West has influenced food habits. The use of a wide variety of garden produce and locally grown citrus fruits, the short-time cooking of vegetables typical of Oriental cooking, and the serving of generous salads as the first course are features to be commended.

### The North Central States

There is a mixed cultural background here with a strong northern European and Scandinavian heritage in many localities. Homes still maintain characteristic native dishes, perhaps modified by the choice of regional ingredients. Many of these states produce and use large quantities of dairy products, especially cheeses of several varieties closely resembling European types. The so-called typical American diet is really an adaptation of much of the northern European food pattern. This is only natural because climatic conditions and crops are similar. Locally grown fruits and vegetables are used in season and preserved for winter use. This is a good custom and should be encouraged.

### The East Coast and New England

Many traditional dishes that have come down from the Pilgrim settlers are still enjoyed in this part of the country. The practice of using cornmeal in Indian pudding and johnnycake was acquired from the Indians by their new neighbors. Baked beans, codfish cakes, clam or fish chowder, and turkey for festive occasions are all old New England traditions, some of which have been adopted nationally. A smaller variety of green, leafy vegetables is used in New England than in many other areas, but yellow vegetables, such as squash, turnips, and carrots, are popular. Apples were the chief fruit in the area and were used to make cider. In New York the Dutch added doughnuts and crullers, and the Germans contributed coleslaw, knockwurst, hamburgers, and frankfurters. The custom of the Pennsylvania Dutch of "hiding the tablecloth" was an expression of providing quantities of a wide variety of food.[4]

### Isolated communities

In any part of the country, unusual food habits may be encountered. Malnutrition may result from a limited variety of foods grown locally, especially if the economic status prohibits extensive use of foods from other producing areas. Sporadic outbreaks of actual deficiency diseases have been reported occasionally. National attention has been called to such problems in Appalachia, on Indian Reservations, and among the Eskimos in Alaska. State and federal agencies are recognizing their responsibilities for these conditions quite as much as for the control of communicable disease.

### Metropolitan areas

A great variety of food patterns may be found in large cities. There may be whole sections in which the inhabitants follow as closely as possible the food customs of the country of their origin. This influence is retained to some extent by the second generation. People who come to the city from regions of the United States where there are definite preferences for certain types of foods attempt to continue following the diet to which they have been accustomed. Usually they can be persuaded to supplement their meals with foods that are more generally available in the city than in the part of the country where their food habits were established.

## Cultural food patterns
### American Indian food

Over 50% of our present food plants originated with the Indians of South, Central, and North America. These include corn, potatoes, tomatoes, peppers, squash, pumpkins, beans, cranberries, wild rice, groundnuts, and cocoa. The Indians also consumed a variety of wild fruits, acorns, lily bulbs, nuts, herbs, maple sugar, small and large game, sheep and goats, wild fowl, fish, and other seafood. Jerky and pemmican were also used by the Indians and introduced to the frontiersmen. The food patterns and feeding practices of various tribes differed according to their geographic location, their occupations (whether they were hunters, shepherds, fishermen, or settled agricultural groups), and their particular historical experience. "Feast or famine" is an expression that can be used to describe the quality of their early experience because they depended primarily on what was immediately avail-

able and had little provision for storing food. There are accounts of Indians fasting and gorging; however, on the whole the traditional Indian diet was probably more nutritionally adequate than many of their diets are today. Just as the trading posts introduced new items, such as tea, coffee, sugar, lard, flour, and tinned milk and meat to the Indians, so did the European settlers adopt many of the Indian foods. Corn is an outstanding example of a crop developed by the American Indians and adopted and transplanted around the world by European adventurers.[5]

The Indians used open-fire cooking for their game and fish, and the clambake, an Indian invention, is still popular in New England. Because of extensive food acculturation, it is difficult today to identify a typical Indian food pattern; however, dietary customs have persisted so that not only are traditional foods prepared, but they are also preferred. Many of the traditional foods retain their religious and ceremonial significance and are featured on feast days. There is great interest in reviving the traditional foods and methods of preparation as part of a cultural reawakening and a desire to understand and appreciate the Indian heritage.

Because the native Indian foods are, for the most part, higher in nutritive value than those adopted from the European culture, it is to the nutritional advantage of the Indians to encourage the use of their traditional foods. The increased buying of expensive foods, such as soft drinks, sweets, cakes, potato chips, and crackers uses a great portion of the limited food budget of the Indians and contributes little but calories to their diets.

Soups and stews made with game or other meat and vegetables are usually well liked by Indians. They may be served with bread, especially the Indian "fry bread" (biscuit dough fried in deep fat) or cornbread. Wasna, a native dish, consists of dry berries, powdered dried meat, fat, and sugar. Fruits and vegetables that provide a source of vitamins A and C should also be encouraged rather than highly processed expensive snack foods. Wajupi is a traditional fruit pudding made from berries, sugar, and cornstarch. The practice of breast feeding infants is a good one and should receive support from the nutrition counselor. The use of milk in children's diets after weaning rather than the carbonated beverages so popular with Indian children would be a good food habit to encourage. Recent studies[6-8] of traditional Hopi foods and their nutrient content indicate the nutritional advantages of the traditional foods.

Nutrition surveys of various tribes indicate mild to marked deficiencies in a number of specific nutrients. Intake of calories, calcium, riboflavin, and vitamins A and C were frequently below recommended amounts. The growth of children in all the surveys was below the norms for North American children.[9] Infant mortality rates are three times that of the general population. The incidence of disease, especially tuberculosis, still is high.[10]

## The black experience

The food habits of the black American reflect the region of the country from which he comes. Southern blacks have the same distinctive food habits that are typical of the rest of the population in the same geographic locale. The northern black may evidence little identification with the regional patterns of the South, or he may have adapted many of these in his present environment. This fact was made exceptionally clear to one of the authors when planning menus with a group of paraprofessionals in a preschool center in the North. In developing a feeding program that would be supportive of the cultural backgrounds of black children, many of the "soul food" items planned and prepared by staff were new and strange to many northern blacks and whites alike, although completely familiar to blacks and whites with considerable experience of the South.

With many exceptions, the following represents what, in general, might be considered the black experience in food customs. Breakfast patterns are similar to the breakfasts of many other groups except for the very frequent use of grits in some form. If eggs and bacon, or another form of pork, are available, they are served with the grits. Hot breads, biscuits, muffins, and cornbread take the place of yeast bread at most meals.

The family usually has one main meal at a time that is determined by the activities of the family members. Greens—mustard, turnip, collard, and kale—cooked in a pot liquor with some form of pork, such as fatback, salt pork, or "streak of lean," are popular. Although fresh greens are used in the South, a wide variety of frozen greens are available in northern markets. Cornbread is traditionally served with greens. Sweet potatoes, squash, lima beans, snap beans, fresh corn, and cabbage are also popular vegetables. Sweet potatoes and squash are often used in pies as the New Englander uses pumpkins. Fruits, such as oranges, watermelon, and peaches are enjoyed when available.

Grits, rice, or potatoes provide the chief source of carbohydrate, whereas black-eyed peas and other dried beans may be used and contribute both carbohydrate and protein. Fried fish of all kinds, particularly that caught by members of the family in streams and lakes, are considered most acceptable. Poultry, cured and fresh pork, and some wild game, such as rabbit, woodchuck, and pheasant, are served when available. Use of meats high in bone or connective tissue with little lean tissue, such as pig's ears, tails, feet, and chin bone, oxtails, neckbones, spareribs, hog maws (stomach), and chitterlings (intestines) is frequent. Frying, barbecuing, and stewing are the most popular methods of preparation even when an oven is available. Milk, milk products, and cheese are not used extensively; buttermilk, evaporated milk, and ice cream are the preferred forms. Sweets—particularly molasses, other syrups, cakes, pastries, and candy—are consumed in large quantity. Sweetened, flavored drinks often take the place of fruit juice and milk as a beverage.

"Soul food," a descriptive term for many of these dishes, connotes special feelings and emotions. It suggests the spirit of the provider or cook, which creates an atmosphere of love and wellbeing for those who are to be fed. There is also the implication that from limited food resources, much happiness and enjoyment can be achieved by giving special care to the preparation of food.

Because large amounts of fat and carbohydrate are consumed, adequate or more than adequate calories are, as a rule, provided. Because relatively small amounts of meat, milk, and fish may be available, the protein content of the diet of a poor southern black family is often limited. Minerals, iron, and calcium have been found inadequate in many southern black dietaries, as have vitamins A and C.[11]

## Dietary habits of Mexicans and other Latin Americans

The Mexicans freely use many varities of beans, especially the pinto, as well as rice, potatoes, peas, and some vegetables. Chili, a variety of pepper, is also popular. The chili plant is sacred to the Mexican, who is supposed to be blessed in health if he uses it plentifully. The tomato is always prominent in Mexican cookery. Mexicans use little meat and practically always cook it with vegetables. They have a strong aversion to meat that is not perfectly fresh and slaughtered in the approved Mexican style. Chili con carne is a favorite meat dish. It consists of beef seasoned with garlic and chili peppers and cooked several hours. Tamales are also popular. They are made of corn meal and ground pork, highly seasoned, and are rolled in corn husks and steamed. Tortillas, made with ground whole corn, which has been soaked in lime water and baked on a griddle, serve as bread. Enchiladas, another favorite, are made by filling tortillas with cheese, onion and shredded lettuce. Tacos, a similar dish, is prepared by adding meat and a sauce to the tortilla. Thus, some calcium is provided in tortillas and in beans in a diet that includes very little milk or cheese. The use of milk for the children should be encouraged when and if a change to the American-type of bread is made. Vitamin A deficiency has been reported as the most prevalent nutritional problem among Mexican-American children.[12]

The influx of Cuban refugees into our southern states creates a need for the nutrition counselor to recognize and adjust nutrition advice and special diets to Cuban preferences. Their food pattern is similar to that of other West Indian groups where the Spanish influence predominates.

It should be noted, however, that many of the more prosperous eastern South American peoples have a meat and milk consumption as high or higher than the United States. Spanish and Portuguese influences are evident in the liberal use of peppers and spices.

On the west coast of South America the situation is

quite different. A few cities are prosperous, but agriculture is handicapped by desert, mountains, and jungles. The native Indian populations of the Andes in Ecuador, Peru, and Chile are short of food and especially of adequate sources of protein.

## Puerto Rican dietary habits

The dietary pattern in Puerto Rico is similar to that of other Caribbean Islands and some Latin American countries. From the extensive work of Dr. Lydia Roberts in Puerto Rico, information is available on a typical moderate cost food supply for an adult for 1 day (Table 14-1). The nutrient value comes close to meeting the United States recommended allowances.

When Puerto Ricans migrate to the United States, as they have in great numbers, they may modify this pattern considerably according to what is available and what they can afford.

Rice, beans, and viandas (starchy root vegetables and plantains) are the staple foods used daily. Salt codfish is used more often than fresh fish and is served with viandas, oil, and vinegar. Chicken, pork, and beef are favorite meats and are used when there is money to purchase them. Tomatoes, peppers, onions, garlic, salt pork, and seasonings (sofrito), cooked with different varieties of dried peas and beans, is a common dish. Bananas, oranges, and pineapple are popular and relatively inexpensive in Puerto Rico. Even more important are some of the native fruits, which are not as familiar in the North, such as mango, papaya, and the West Indian cherry, or acerola, which is now recognized as the richest known natural source of ascorbic acid.

Milk is not popular as a beverage except perhaps, when income permits, as *café con leche*, a combination of coffee and hot milk. Sweetened cocoa and chocolate made with milk are also consumed occasionally.

Puerto Ricans living in northern United States may have to adjust to different fruits in season and to canned fruits. They may well be encouraged to use more milk and cheese, and cheaper cuts of meat, to supplement the protein at meals when rice and beans are served. Acceptance of canned tomatoes in place of more expensive fresh ones out of season, margarine in place of butter, and cheaper cuts of meat would provide better nutrition for less cost.

Puerto Ricans in New York City and other urban areas are often among the lower economic groups because, having come from a more rural culture, many of them are unskilled laborers. Their poor and crowded housing may provide inadequate cooking and refrigeration facilities. As a result, they may be unable to provide their families with food as good as they had at home. Malnutrition, rickets, and tuberculosis are not uncommon among Puerto Rican children living under such conditions. The nutrition counselor can suggest how they can improve nutrition within their budgets.

## Italian dietary habits

Italian-Americans, few of them today born in Italy, have adopted many food customs of the United States. Similarly, the popularity of Italian spaghetti and pizza in this country testifies to the influence that Italian food customs have had on Americans. Italians here continue to use pastas in a great variety of shapes and with many different sauces and cheeses. Similarly, bread is still an essential part of an Italian meal, although crusty white bread is now more popular than the dark breads that were a former standby.

Southern Italians may use more fish and highly seasoned foods, whereas northern Italians use more root vegetables and more meat. The liberal use of eggs, cheese, tomatoes, green vegetables, and fruits in the Italian cuisine is to be commended. More milk and meat might be used, both of which are popular. In general, northern Italians have better food habits than those from the south.

Italians have a strong sense of individuality. We may think of spaghetti as a typically Italian food, but not all Italians like spaghetti. They dislike foods that are not prepared to their particular tastes. They are particularly sensitive to the lack of close family ties in a hospital and therefore dread hospitalization more than one may suspect. Most Italians eat a very light breakfast: black coffee

## Table 14-1. Moderate Cost Diet for a Day for a Puerto Rican Adult

| Food | Amount of Edible Portion | Weight (g) |
|---|---|---|
| Rice | 3 cups cooked | 668 |
| Plantain or root vegetable | 1 serving | 200 |
| Bean, broad, kidney, or other type | 1 cup | 256 |
| Onion | 1 medium | 110 |
| Eggplant | 1 small | 100 |
| Green pepper | 2 small | 100 |
| Tomato | 1 medium | 100 |
| Mango | 1 medium | 200 |
| Banana | 2 medium | 300 |
| Salt codfish | 1 oz dry | 30 |
| Goat's milk | 1 cup | 224 |
| Lard | ½ cup | 50 |
| Olive oil | 2 tbsp | 28 |

The value of this diet is approximately:

| | | | |
|---|---|---|---|
| Energy | 2506 kcal | Vitamin A | 33,500 IU |
| Protein | 69 g | Thiamin | 1.0 mg |
| Fat | 77 g | Riboflavin | 1.0 mg |
| Calcium | 0.6 g | Niacin | 13.3 mg |
| Iron | 12.5 mg | Vitamin C | 195 mg |

(Adapted from information provided by Dr. Lydia Roberts, formerly of University of Puerto Rico, and Miss Ethel Robinson, formerly a teacher in rural Puerto Rico)

for adults and milk for children, with perhaps bread without butter. Some like the main meal at noon, others at night, but bread and cheese with coffee or wine is an acceptable light meal.

## Western European and Scandinavian dietary habits

Most western European peoples, including Scandinavians, have food patterns not unlike those of northeastern and central North America, where immigrants from these areas have settled during the past two centuries. Many American food customs of today have been derived from these countries. The lists of meats, vegetables, fruits, and grain products used by them would be a mere recital of those in our markets. To be sure, they make more frequent use of dark breads, potatoes, fish, and cheese than native Americans do. For western Europeans the differences in culinary methods, seasonings, and attitudes toward food are never serious hurdles in adjusting to American food patterns.

## Central European dietary habits

In many of the central European countries grains and potatoes provide 60% to 70% of the total calories for the rural and the lower income groups. Rye and buckwheat are used, as well as wheat, for their breads. Pork and pork products, including highly seasoned sausages, are popular. Cabbage may be used raw, cooked, or as sauerkraut, and other vegetables—onions, turnips, peppers, carrots, beans, squash, and greens—are often cooked with small amounts of meat. Eggs, fresh milk, sour cream, and yogurt (known by a different name in each country), cottage cheese, and other cheeses are widely used. Central Europeans bring with them many good food habits that are to be encouraged.

## Dietary habits of the Middle East

The inhabitants of the Middle East—the Lebanese, Armenians, Turks, Greeks, Iranians, and Arabs—are outdoor people. Many of them are farmers; they raise their own sheep, goats, cattle, chickens, ducks, and geese; they produce their own grains and grow fruits and vegetables in abundance, wherever water is plentiful. In some Arab countries meals are served on the floor and eaten with the fingers. Grains, rice, or wheat products furnish the major source of energy. The whole wheat is parboiled and cracked for use as a staple starchy food at the main meal. Chickpeas in the form of homous are popular. Eggs, butter, and cheese are also produced on the farm. Lamb is the favorite meat. Olive and sesame oil are used extensively in cooking. Matsoon, leben, or yogurt, a sour milk preparation, is used almost universally by these people; sweet milk is seldom used. Milk from goats and camels is available in certain rural areas. Eggplant, tomatoes, okra, beets, and spinach are all popular vegetables. Cabbage or grape leaves stuffed with rice and meat are served with the main meal in some areas. Dates, olives, and figs are well known in this part of the world. Black coffee, heavily sweetened, in which the pulverized bean is retained—often called Turkish coffee—is the preferred beverage in many countries of the Middle East. Rose water is often used in sweets. Each country has its own distinctive flavorings in the form of spices, herbs, and extracts.

## Chinese dietary habits

The Chinese diet is varied, consisting of eggs, meat, fish, cereals, and a large variety of vegetables. Many plants and weeds, such as radish leaves and shepherd's purse, are used, as well as various sprouts (*e.g.* bean, bamboo). None of these vegetables is ever overcooked, and no cooking water is discarded; as a result, nutrients are well retained. The soybean is abundant, and some 30 or more products are manufactured from it. The protein content is high and of good quality for a vegetable protein.

Rice is used freely and takes the place of American bread, particularly in southern China. In northern China, wheat, corn, and millet seed are used in abundance. The millet seed (ground or whole) is made into cakes or a thin mush, the latter being the form in which it is given to children. Noodles are widely used. Grains and, in some areas, sweet potatoes constitute the chief source of calories in the Chinese diet; grain and potato together provide from 70% to 90% of the total calories.

The quantity of meat eaten is small, and usually it is served with vegetables. All ingredients are cut into small pieces in conformity with an ancient law laid down by Confucius, the philosopher, specifying that food should not be eaten unless first chopped or cut into small pieces. Pork is the chief meat of the poorer classes. Lamb and goat meat and other animal foods are used when available, but beef is uncommon. Small amounts of meat and vegetables are often enclosed in wonton wrappers and fried in a wok.

In certain parts of China, a child rarely tastes cow's milk, but water buffalo milk is used to some extent. Soybean milk and cheese are more common. In this country, the Chinese readily accept the use of dairy products for children and adults.

The Chinese use practically every part of the animal as food (with the exception of the hair and the bones); the brain, the spinal cord, and the various internal organs, as well as the skin and the blood, are used. Coagulated blood is sold in the market in pieces similar to liver, and because this is one of the inexpensive foods, it is used frequently. Fish and shellfish are also in common use. They are sold alive, for the Chinese have a strong aversion to dead fish and consider them unfit for food.

Eggs, including hen, duck, and pigeon eggs, are used in abundance, when they can be afforded. The Chinese prepare what are known as "fermented" eggs, much relished by them, as well as other types of preserved eggs, which are eaten much as we in this country eat sweets.

Soy sauce, highly flavored and salted, is a frequent accompaniment to meals. It may present problems to the Chinese patient who must omit salt from his diet. This is true also of the Japanese diet.

### Japanese dietary habits

During the past 30 years there have been spectacular changes in Japanese food habits, influenced by Western culture. Typical diets formerly included rice, bean paste soup, bean curd, vegetables and fruit, raw or cooked fish, and pickles. Now the trend is to bread as well as rice, milk, cheese, meat, and eggs. Instant foods and frozen items are available. Seafoods are served raw, smoked, fried, and, recently, as fish sausage. Japanese make a whole meal of wheat or buckwheat noodles cooked in broth and garnished with a few bits of vegetables and fish sausage and served with salty pickles. Sushi—vinegared, sweetened cold rice—is a popular food for both meals and snacks. Sukiyaki—sautéed meat and vegetables—has become a familar dish in the United States. Japanese are fond of steamed egg custards that include small pieces of meat or fish. Meat, fish, and vegetables are often cooked tempura style by dipping in batter and frying. The very extensive use of shoyu (soy sauce) results in high intakes of sodium. Although they are traditional tea drinkers, many Japanese now prefer coffee, and they like to drink milk when it is available. Many kinds of crisp salty snack foods made from rice or wheat flour, seaweed, and other delicacies are popular. A Japanese or Chinese meal is complete without dessert, but at New Year's and other holidays the Japanese relish their "decoration cakes." Even the simplest one-dish meal is attractively served, and an elaborate party meal, served in 10 or 12 separate and colorful dishes of different shapes, it truly a work of art.

### South and Southeast Asian habits

Indian food habits vary from region to region. Many Indians are vegetarians and do not consume meat, fish, or poultry, although milk, milk products, and eggs are included in their diets. Indian meals are not served in courses, but many different dishes are put out at the same time. Indians pick up food with their fingers or small pieces of bread. A great many combinations of spices, *masalas*, are used in Indian cookery. Rice, beans, peas, and lentils are used extensively in Indian meals. Breads, chapati, made from wheat are often deep fried in vegetable oil or on a hot griddle. Curries of meat, fish, or vegetables are ubiquitous in this region. *Ghee*, clarified butter, and yogurt are included in many Indian recipes. The fruits and vegetables vary from region to region. Chutneys, made from mangoes or other fruits and vegetables, accompany the meal.

The food habits of the peoples from Southeast Asia have been influenced by both the Chinese and the Indians. The Vietnamese, Thais, Cambodians, and Laotians, for example, have many common food practices. Rice is their staple food; curries are popular main dishes, although the various spices used are distinctive to the different countries. The wok is used to deep fry or sauté many foods. Meat, primarily pork and chicken, and fish are used in small amounts. Fruits and vegetables abound in these tropical countries. Coconut is used in many different forms in a wide variety of dishes. *Nuac nam*, fermented salted fish sauce, is used by the Vietnamese as soy sauce is used by the Chinese. Soy bean curd is also frequently eaten in this area. Many of the foods familiar to Vietnamese families are now found on the shelves of supermarkets in the United States or, in many cities, in the now popular Oriental food stores. The nutrition counselor working with a Vietnamese family should become knowledgeable about their food practices and assist them in the economical selection of appropriate foods. Purchasing rice in large quantities may be a good practice for an Asian family who consumes it two or three times a day compared to a typical American family by whom it is only used occasionally. As much as a pound of rice per person per day may be consumed by an Asian family.

## Religious food patterns
### Jewish dietary habits and laws

In the United States today Jewish families differ in food habits according to whether they belong to Orthodox, Conservative, or Reform groups. Food habits may also be influenced by the country from which they or their forefathers came, as well as by Biblical and rabbinical regulations, known as the Jewish dietary laws.

According to Kaufman:

> Variations in observance are due largely to differences in interpretation and importance placed on dietary laws by the three schools of thought among American Jews today. Orthodox Jews still place great value on traditional and ceremonial practices of their religion, and observe the dietary laws under all conditions. Reform Jews place much less emphasis on rules which they consider to be purely ceremonial and tend to minimize the significance of the dietary laws. Conservative Jews stand between these two groups and, while nominally adhering to dietary laws, sometimes draw the distinction between the observance of the rules in the home and outside.

> Regulations include selection, preparation and service of the foods involved. The Bible gives no reason for these rules, but observant Jews feel that the rules known as Kashruth and hallowed since the time of Moses, are a positive means of self-purification and of service to their God. Although many hygienic and ethical bases have been alleged for these rules, the spiritual factors of sanctification and self-discipline are the primary motivations for those who adhere to them.[13]

Miss Kaufman also gives some definitions of Jewish terms and special foods. A brief outline of some of the specific rules to which the Orthodox Jews conform follows.

Certain meats, poultry, and fish are allowed or prohibited. Quadrupeds with the cloven hoof that chew a cud are allowed. These include cows, sheep, goats, and deer. Pork in all forms including lard and bacon is prohibited. The poultry allowed includes chicken, turkey, goose, pheasant, and duck. All meats and poultry must be freshly slaughtered according to prescribed ritual and soaked in salted water to remove all trace of blood. This process is known as koshering (meaning clean), and many Jewish markets sell koshered meat and poultry. Prescribed methods of preparing meats and other foods are given in most Jewish cookbooks. The fish prescribed in the Bible are those with fins and scales. Thus, all shellfish and eels are excluded.

Certain food combinations are allowed or prohibited. The command, "Thou shalt not seethe a kid in its mother's milk," repeated several times in Exodus and Deuteronomy, is the basis for never combining meat and milk in the same meal or even cooking them in the same utensils. Eggs, fruits, vegetables, cereals, and all other foods may be used without restrictions.

A striking characteristic of the Jewish diet is the richness of the food, including pastries and cakes, foods rich in fats, and preserves and conserves, as well as stewed and canned fruits. Butter, a product of milk, must not be served with meat. Most vegetables, therefore, are cooked with the meat. Cooked vegetables are most often served in soup. Borscht, a soup made with "sour salt" (tartaric acid) and vegetables to which sour cream is added, is a favorite dish but is not served with the meat meal. Cereals, especially barley and millet, are frequently served as a vegetable with meat or in soup.

Noodles and other egg and flour mixtures are used extensively, as are crusty rolls.

Dried fruits, as well as fresh fruits, are popular.

Fish is served frequently, especially cod, haddock, carp, salmon, and whitefish, smoked and salted fishes—herring, salmon, and sturgeon. Gefilte fish is a delicacy prepared in almost all Jewish homes. Chicken is considered almost an essential for the Sabbath evening meal.

Because milk in any form cannot be served with meat at the same meal, the diet of children in Jewish families that rigidly observe the dietary laws may lack the proper amount of milk. The use of more green vegetables and more milk for the children should be stressed. The continued use of rye bread, legumes, coarse cereals, dried fruits, and a variety of fish, which are characteristic of the Jewish diet, is advantageous.

Dietary laws for the Jewish Sabbath and religious holidays are often observed by even the less orthodox groups and, therefore, merit comment. No food may be cooked on the Sabbath. This means that all cooking for both Friday and Saturday is done on Friday. This need has led to the development of foods such as Sabbath Kugel or Sholend, Petshai, and many others. During Passover week no leavened bread or its product or anything that may have touched leavened bread, may be eaten. A complete new set of dishes is used during the week. Cutlery, silver, or metal pots may be used during this holiday if properly koshered or sterilized. In actual practice, this means that in every orthodox Jewish household there are four sets of dishes—the usual sets for meat and for milk foods, in addition to duplicate Passover sets.

Fast Days include Yom Kippur (the Day of Atonement) on which no food or drink may be taken for 24 hours. The Fast of Esther precedes the Feast of Purim and is now observed only by the very pious. The Feast of Purim is universally observed.

## Roman Catholic

Because the Church liberalized the dietary restrictions and fast days, customs may vary in different localities. Catholics in the United States are required to abstain from eating meat on Ash Wednesday and the Fridays of Lent. It is well to conform to local custom with regard to foods allowed on other fast days and days of abstinence.

## Eastern Orthodox

The Christians who originated in the Middle East, Greece, Russia, and the Balkans are often followers of this religion. The Orthodox laws have not been changed in recent years but are interpreted somewhat more liberally. The use of meat, fish, poultry, eggs, and dairy products is still restricted on Fridays and Wednesdays and during Lent and Advent.

## Seventh Day Adventists

Adventists in general are ovo-lacto-vegetarians; that is, they allow the use of eggs, milk, and cheese as good sources of animal protein, but they eat no meat, fish, or poultry. They also use nuts and legumes as sources of protein. Tea, coffee, and alcoholic beverages are also considered harmful. Meat analogs made from soybean are frequently used by this group.

## Latter-Day Saints

The Mormons make no food restrictions but prohibit the use of alcohol, tobacco, tea, and coffee.

## Islam

Although the youngest major religion in the world, Islam is the second largest religion in number of members. It is the major religion of Saudi Arabia, its birthplace, Iraq, Jordan, Syria, Kuwait, Iran, Egypt, Algeria, Morocco, Libya, Pakistan, Indonesia, and Malaya.

Moslems practice several dietary restrictions. Pork and all pork products are prohibited. Other meats and poultry should be slaughtered according to specified rules. The consumption of alcoholic beverages is forbidden. Fasting is observed for 1 month, Ramadan, every year. The religious Moslem abstains from any food or drink from dawn until after dark during Ramadan.

### Hindu

Although most pious Hindus are vegetarians and consume no meat, fish, or poultry, beef is the especially forbidden food. This is because of the sacredness of the cow in the Hindu religion. All life is considered sacred because any animal might contain the soul of an ancestor who has been reborn in that form. Even eggs are not consumed by some devout Hindus because to eat an egg would represent taking a life. The vast majority of Hindus live in the Indian subcontinent.

## Understanding and using food patterns

Characteristic food habits of every regional, cultural, or religious group should be respected; there are good nutritional practices in each of them and nutritional needs may be met by many different patterns of eating. Emphasis should be placed on the desirable features of the established food pattern and on methods of preparation that preserve maximum food values. Although choice of foods and methods of preparation may differ from those to which we are accustomed, it often happens that the foods used fall into the Four Food Groups and provide nutrients that meet recommended allowances.

Unfamiliar foods and methods of preparation need to be studied and possible values recognized before changes are suggested. A family may be encouraged to continue its own methods of preparation and seasoning when these are not incompatible with health; later it may gradually be helped to institute necessary changes to correct any poor practices, if these exist.

Therapeutic diets should be interpreted for the patient or the homemaker in terms of the regional, cultural, or religious food pattern. A woman of foreign birth or one from a different part of the country may have little contact outside her home and little opportunity to learn how to use foods that are new to her. The marked improvements in homes where the mother has had the opportunity to learn to adjust to local foods and customs show that instruction, as well as understanding, is an important phase of nutrition work.

In this chapter special attention is given to regional, cultural, and religious food patterns that are distinctive. A knowledge of these food preferences and attention to them may help to build the bridge of understanding between the nutrition counselor and the family in need of assistance.

### Vegetarian diets

Vegetarian diets are not new, nor are they unusual in the United States today. They have been followed throughout history by various groups. The Seventh Day Adventists and the Trappist monks subscribe to vegetarianism on the basis of religion. In the 19th century the Utopian groups advocated this dietary pattern. Among their followers were the breakfast cereal manufacturers, W.K. Kellogg and C.W. Post. Today many young people are adopting, for health, ecological, or philosophical reasons, one type of vegetarian diet or another. The practice in some instances is a belief or regulation of quasi-religious or cultist groups. Some of these groups are also natural or organic food followers or adherents of the Zen-Macrobiotic diet (see below).[14]

Vegetarian diets usually include vegetables, fruits, cereals and breads (often whole grain), yeast, dry beans, peas and lentils, nuts and peanut butter, seeds, vegetable oils, and sugars and syrups. They may also include more unusual types of food, such as seaweed and bean curd, and some may permit certain animal products.

*Vegans,* or the strict vegetarians, avoid all food of animal origin including meat, poultry, fish, eggs, and dairy products, such as milk, ice cream, and cheese.

*Lacto-vegetarians* eat dairy products but not meat, poultry, fish, or eggs.

*Ovo-lacto-vegetarians* include eggs and dairy products in their diets while excluding meat, poultry, and fish.

Because vitamin $B_{12}$ is known to occur naturally only in foods of animal origin, a person following strict vegetarianism should use cereals fortified with vitamin $B_{12}$ or a vitamin preparation that includes it. Because the chief source of calcium in our diet is milk, vegans who exclude milk products need to include daily relatively large amounts of certain dark green, leafy vegetables, such as kale, collards, mustard, turnip, or dandelion greens. Soybeans, almonds, broccoli, okra, and rutabaga are also moderately good sources of calcium. Pregnant women and children, especially, need adequate calcium and should have milk in their diet. Similarly, pregnant women, infants, and young children need to include a source of vitamin D, such as homogenized milk or margarine fortified with vitamins A and D. Yeast that has been heated or cooked to inactivate it can help supply some of the riboflavin usually supplied by milk and meat. Green leafy vegetables, asparagus, broccoli, Brussels sprouts, okra, and winter squash are also good sources of riboflavin if consumed frequently in large quantity. Whole grain and enriched cereal also contribute riboflavin.[15] The availability of certain minerals, such as zinc, may be marginal in vegetarian diets due to the large amount of phytate in these diets.

If milk and eggs are included in the vegetarian diet, obtaining adequate quality and quantity of protein is not difficult. However, vegans must exercise great care in selecting and combining vegetable proteins to achieve adequate quality protein. Soybeans and chickpeas provide good quality protein, almost comparable to animal sources. Combining several kinds of vegetable sources, such as beans with corn or rice, and peanuts or peanut butter with wheat contributes a better mixture of amino acids than either cereals or legumes alone. Meat analogs made from textured vegetable proteins (see Chap. 4) may also be used to improve the quality of proteins.[15]

The more restricted the vegetarian diet is, the greater the commitment to it usually is, and the greater the challenge to achieve nutritional adequacy. If the nutrition counselor is to be helpful, the restrictions on food choices imposed by these dietary patterns must be accepted and the person guided to make the best choices within the limitations. In other words, the counselor must work within the client's value system.

## Unusual dietary practices

More and more young American adults have adopted unusual dietary practices that are of particular concern to the nutrition counselor. Some of the more popular of these patterns will be discussed in this section.

### "Natural" foods

So-called natural foods have become especially popular in recent years. Natural food enthusiasts use raw sugar or honey in place or refined sugar or sea salt in place of table salt, without realizing that the trace minerals that may be present in the impurities of such natural products are widely available in most foods. The use of olive oil in place of other fats or stone ground wheat instead of whole wheat may taste better but have little nutritional significance. The question of the safety of raw milk has increased the demand for certified unpasteurized milk. This is costly, and there is no absolute assurance as to its safety.

Certain vegetable juices have been credited with virtues they do not possess, such as celery juice as a treatment for rheumatism and garlic juice for high blood pressure. Juices, extracted from vegetables or fruits, have essentially similar nutritive values as the original product except for the cellulose. There is no evidence that certain vegetables or their juices have special curative properties other than as sources of nutrients.

Although it must be admitted that the number and variety of processed foods now available is often confusing, the prejudice expressed against processed foods is quite unwarranted. In general, processing aims at improving preservation, flavor, texture, nutritive value, or convenience in preparation. Seldom does such processing significantly reduce nutritive value. Moreover, as recently reported, many of the so-called natural vitamin preparations do have synthetic chemicals added. Rose hip vitamin C tablets are made from natural rose hips plus the same

chemical ascorbic acid used in standard vitamin preparations; synthetic B vitamins are added to the yeast and other natural bases; and chemical solvents are used for the extraction and separation of the vegetable oils used for vitamin E preparations.[16] There is no legal definition for these natural products because the vitamins themselves are identical, but the product may cost the consumer more. For these reasons, labels should be carefully read.

### "Organic" foods

The craze for so-called organic foods has reached such a point that even wayside markets are advertising food grown "organically." This means that crops are grown without chemical fertilizers or pesticides and processed without the use of food chemicals or additives. People seldom realize that all organic material—compost, manure—used in growing foods organically must be broken down to inorganic elements before plants can absorb nutrients from the soil. Scientific tests have shown that such foods show no significant difference in nutritive value from those grown with commercial fertilizers. Salmonella contamination can result from the use of organic farming techniques.

Pesticides aid in the production of good quality foods and of increased yields, thus making larger quantities of products even more widely available to our growing population. The use of pesticides to prevent destruction of crops by infestations of fungi, microorganisms, or insects is carefully monitored, and pesticide levels well below international standards for acceptable daily intake (ADI) are reported.

Meat is considered organically grown when produced from animals raised without antibiotics or hormones and dressed without the use of chemicals. People should be aware that our regular market meats are inspected regularly; also, the constant vigilance of law-enforcing agencies regulates the use of all additives and medical agents to be sure that they are within safe limits.

The whole cult of natural and organic foods has puzzled scientific nutritionists for years because all the evidence points to the fact that fertilizers and pesticides increase yield and that plant genetics determine the color, flavor, and nutritive value of the crop.

According to an article that appeared in the *New York Times*, the FDA takes the following position concerning organic foods:

> Organic or natural foods are not considered to be significantly different from other foods, in terms of their nutritional qualities. The FDA feels that if you want them and can afford them, they're there in the marketplace for you to buy. But they must be labeled in a manner that's neither false or misleading, and no attempt can be made in promoting these foods to suggest that they offer special health benefits. There's just no evidence to show that people living on organic or natural foods will be protected from chronic

disease problems, or that they can expect better health. Nevertheless, the interested and alert consumer can get good and nutritious food either from the so-called organic food store or the modern supermarket. The choice is and should remain open to the individual. But the main point is that we cannot hope to feed today's population with yesterday's production methods. We must use the technical advances that science and chemistry have given us if we hope to produce and preserve enough food to meet today's requirements.

The cost of organically grown groceries may be 30% to 100% more than for their nonorganic counterparts.[17]

## Macrobiotic diet

This diet is an outgrowth of an interpretation of Zen Buddhism introduced into the United States and Europe from Japan by Ohsawa. According to the macrobiotic system there are 10 diet plans (Diet No. −3—10% cereal, 30% vegetables, 10% soup, 30% animal products, 15% salads and fruits, and 5% desserts, to Diet No. 7—100% cereal), which may be followed to establish a healthy and happy life. In progressing from Diet No. −3 to Diet No. 7, one gradually gives up in the following order: desserts, salads and fruits, animal foods, soups, and, finally, vegetables, at the same time increasing the amount of cereal grains to be consumed. There is no scientific basis for the restrictions or recommendations of the macrobiotic system. Part of the plan for all the diets is the consumption of as little beverage as possible. Only organically produced fresh vegetables, fruits, or animal products are used. Foods are classified into Yang (the male principle) or Yin (the female principle), and a 5:1 balance between these is considered to be important. Because sweets and many fruits are Yin foods, the amount of these in the macrobiotic diet is small.

Most of the diet plans are low in ascorbic acid. Diet No. 7 (in which whole grain cereal, usually brown rice, is the only food consumed) is grossly inadequate in many of the essential minerals and vitamins, as well as in good quality protein. Fortunately, not too many follow No. 7 diet plan for very long. Another danger in the macrobiotic concept is that, because the various diet plans promise to cure the body of disease and purge it of all poisons, adequate medical care may be postponed when it is needed. The American Medical Association has warned of the hazards of following this regimen.[18]

Because it is possible to have an adequate intake of nutrients on certain macrobiotic diet plans, emphasis should be placed on essential nutrients in maintaining health and wellbeing, and followers of this system should be counselled to select their macrobiotic foods in keeping with this principle of good nutrition. One must work within the value system or philosophy of these groups if change is to be expected. The *Hip Health Handbook* is a resource for workers in this field.[19]

## Food fads

In this scientific age quackery still flourishes in the field of nutrition as well as in the area of drugs and medical devices. Quacks thrive by misinterpreting scientific authorities in order to sell their ideas and their products. It is estimated that some 10 million Americans spend $1 billion a year on worthless and sometimes dangerous drugs, treatments, dietary fads, and other quackery. This section focuses attention on those nutrition fads that are most widespread.

### Vitamin concentrates and food supplements

The promotion of vitamin and mineral supplements and special diet foods is misleading millions of people who have little need for such products. This type of deceptive advertising, which until recently appealed mainly to the "golden-agers," is now deceiving people of all ages, even teenagers. Many people are attempting self-medication for imaginary or real illness with a multitude of irrational products. They are apt to spend much more for such products than they would for beneficial nutrients provided in an adequate diet.

### Fact and fancy

There is no magic in any specific food item. It makes little difference whether one obtains his nutrients from fluid milk or milk powder, from milk products, such as cheese, yogurt, or ice cream, or whether he gets them from meat, fish or fowl, wheat germ, whole grains, or blackstrap molasses. The essential point is to get an adequate supply of each nutrient from food that tastes good.

Complicating and encouraging food fads today is the growing number of false nutritional ideas, or folklore, built up by pseudoscientific books, pamphlets, and periodicals on diets of various sorts. Some tell us that calories don't count or that arthritis can be cured by oils to lubricate joints; others tempt the unwary with a drinking man's diet or with martinis and whipped cream. In some unreliable books there is enough of the true mixed with the false about food values and human needs to make it difficult for the average person to judge what is valid.

Many dietary fads may be relatively harmless but senseless. Too often they detract from the pleasure of eating, an important element of good nutrition. Variety is in itself a safeguard, and, when variety is severely limited, as it is by some fads and self-imposed restrictions, certain nutritive factors are apt to be low or absent. When fads lead to delay in seeking necessary medical advice, they can be dangerous indeed. In any event, food fads may increase food costs unduly and result in the omission of foods really needed. The consequences are the same whether one is led to food faddism by the enthusiasms of the uninformed neighbor or the profit seekers.

Hence, attention is again called to the Recommended Dietary Allowances as the nutritional norms against which any dietary pattern may be measured. If a given food plan compares favorably with the RDA, the basic nutrients for health and wellbeing will be supplied, and one need not be concerned with a person's specific dietary pattern.

## Study questions and activities

1. Why is it essential that the nutrition counselor be able to adjust her advice on nutrition to various regional and cultural food patterns?
2. After noting the regional dietary habits in the United States, which ones in the South and in the Southwest would you recommend and encourage, and what changes would you recommend?
3. How has the transplanting of various cultures influenced the food habits of those in various regions of the United States?
4. Why is the Jewish diet one of the most difficult problems for the health worker? What are some of the dietary laws which must be respected?
5. How does the use of grains, potatoes, and animal protein vary among the different regions of Europe and Asia?
6. How can you help others to gain respect for the food habits and favorite dishes of cultural groups other than their own?
7. Which one of the unusual dietary practices mentioned in this chapter is most restrictive? Why? Is there a danger that nutritional deficiencies will result from following this regimen? Explain.
8. What are the types of vegetarian diets practiced by many young people today? What nutritional problems may be found among these adherents?

## References

1. Maslow AH: Motivation and Personality. New York, Harper & Row, 1954
2. Kreidler PL et al: J Am Diet Assoc 77:46, 1980
3. Kreidler PL et al: J Am Diet Assoc 77:41, 1980
4. Lowenberg ME, Lucas BL: J Am Diet Assoc 68:207, 1976
5. Farr T: Food Management 9:45, 1974
6. Kuhnlein HV et al: J Am Diet Assoc 75:37, 1979
7. Kuhnlein HV, Calloway DH: Ecol Food Nutr 6:159, 1977
8. Calloway DH et al: Ecol Food Nutr 3:203, 1974
9. Moore WM, Silverberg MM, Read MS: Nutrition, Growth and Development of North American Indian Children. DHEW Publ. No. (NIH) 72-26, Washington, DC, 1972
10. Bass MA, Wakefield LM: J Am Diet Assoc 64:36, 1974
11. Mayer J: Nutr Rev 23:161, 1965
12. Larson LB et al: J Am Diet Assoc 64:29, 1974
13. Kaufman M: Am J Clin Nutr 5:676, 1957
14. Dwyer JT et al: J Am Diet Assoc 65:529, 1974
15. Raper NR, Hill MM: Nutr Rev (Suppl) 32:29, July, 1974
16. Kamil A: Nutr Rev (Suppl) 32:34, July, 1974
17. Review: Nutr Rev (Suppl) 32:53, July, 1974
18. Statement: JAMA 218 #3, 1971. Reprinted in Nutr Rev 32:27, 1974
19. J Am Diet Assoc 61:126, 1972

## Supplementary readings

American Dietetic Association position paper on food and nutrition misinformation on selected topics. J Am Diet Assoc 66:277, 1975

Bass MA, Wakefield LM: Food and nutrient intake of reservation Indians. J Am Diet Assoc 64:36, 1974

Brittin HC, Zinn DW: Meat-buying practices of Caucasians, Mexican-Americans and Negroes. J Am Diet Assoc 71:623, 1977

Cantoni M: Adapting therapeutic diets to the eating patterns of Italian Americans. Am J Clin Nutr 6:548, 1958

Chang B: Some dietary beliefs in Chinese folkculture. J Am Diet Assoc 65:436, 1974

Committee on Nutrition, American Academy of Pediatrics: Nutritional Aspects of vegetarianism, health foods and fad diets. Pediatrics 59:460, 1977

Day ML et al: Food acceptance patterns of Spanish-speaking New Mexicans. J Nutr Educ 10:121, 1978

Dwyer JT et al: Mental age and I.Q. of predominantly vegetarian children. J Am Diet Assoc 76:142, 1980

Dwyer JT et al: The new vegetarians: The natural high? J Am Diet Assoc 65:529, 1974

Fathauer GH: Food habits—An anthropologist's view. J Am Diet Assoc 37:335, 1960

Foley C et al: Attitudes and food habits—A review. J Am Diet Assoc 75:13, 1979

Frankle RT, Owen AY: Nutrition in the Community. St Louis, CV Mosby, 1978

Grivetti LE, Paquette MB: Nontraditional ethnic food choices among first generation Chinese in California. J Nutr Educ 10:109, 1978

Harland BF, Peterson M: Nutritional status of lacto-ovo-vegetarian Trappist monks. J Am Diet Assoc 72:259, 1978

Helmick SA: Family living patterns—Projections for the future. J Nutr Educ 10:155, 1978

Kuhnlein HV, Calloway DH: Composition of traditional Hopi foods. J Am Diet Assoc 75:37, 1979

Larson LB et al: Nutritional status of Mexican-American children. 64:29, 1974

Lowenberg ME: The development of food patterns. J Am Diet Assoc 65:263, 1974

Lowenberg ME, Lucas BL: Feeding families and children 1776–1976. A bicentennial study. J Am Diet Assoc 207, 1976

Lowenberg ME et al: Food and People, 3rd ed. New York, John Wiley & Sons, 1979

Macgregor FC: Uncooperative patients: Some cultural interpretations. Am J Nurs 67:88, 1967

Mills ER: Psychosocial aspects of food habits. J Nutr Educ 9:67, 1977

Natow AB et al: Integrating the Jewish laws into a dietetics program. Kashruth in a dietetics curriculum. J Am Diet Assoc 67:13, 1975

Reaburn JA et al: Social determinants in food selection. J Am Diet Assoc 74:637, 1979

Sakr AH: Fasting in Islam. J Am Diet Assoc 67:17, 1975

Schafer R, Yetley EA: Social psychology of food faddism. Speculations on health food behavior. J Am Diet Assoc 66:129, 1975

Schafer RB, Keith PM: Influences on food decisions across the family life cycle. J Am Diet Assoc 78:144, 1981

Tabor LAH, Cook R: Dietary and anthropometric assessment of adult omnivores, fish-eaters and lacto-ovo-vegetarians. J Am Diet Assoc 76:21, 1980

Torres RM: Dietary patterns of the Puerto Rican people. Am J Clin Nutr 7:349, 1959

Wheeler M, Harder SQ: Buying and food preparation patterns of ghetto blacks and Hispanics in Brooklyn. J Am Diet Assoc 75:560, 1979

White PL (ed): Nutrition misinformation and food faddism—A special supplement. Nutr Rev (Suppl 1) 32:1, July, 1974

Wilson C: Food-custom and nurture—An annotated bibliography on sociocultural and biocultural aspects of nutrition. J Nutr Educ (Suppl 1) 11:211, 1979

Valassi KV: Food habits of Greek-Americans. Am J Clin Nutr 11:240, 1962

Yang G I-P, Fox HM: Food habit changes in Chinese persons living in Lincoln, Nebraska. J Am Diet Assoc 75:420, 1979

*For further references see Bibliography in Part 4.*

# Ecology of Food

## 15

Food Spoilage and Deterioration
Care and Preservation of Foods
Effects of Food Processing on Nutrient
   Composition
Foodborne Diseases and Toxins
Safeguarding the Food Supply

**BAI:** Bureau of Animal Industry
**BHA:** Butylated hydroxyanisole
**GMP:** Good Manufacturing Practices
**GRAS:** Generally Recognized as Safe
**PCB's:** Polychlorinated biphenyls
**BHT:** Butylated hydroxytoluene
**EPA:** Environmental Protection Agency
**FDA:** Food and Drug Administration
**FTC:** Federal Trade Commission

The production and processing of food in the United States today is a highly developed scientific business. The 296 billion pounds of food produced each year to feed the 210 million people in this country is accomplished almost entirely by scientific farming methods using chemical fertilizers and pesticides. It would be impossible to achieve these production levels using so-called organic farming methods (the growing of food without the use of chemical aids) alone. In the first place, the gigantic quantities of manures and composts that would be required for our vast farm system do not exist; as a result, the crop yield would be drastically reduced. Without the insecticides and herbicides, the amount of crop loss from insect and fungi infestation would increase, and food shortages such as exist in the underdeveloped countries would occur.

Selective breeding of plants, another aspect of scientific farming, has developed strains of cereals, fruits, and vegetables appropriate for varying climatic and soil conditions. Other specific characteristics, such as increased resistance to certain diseases, increased amino acid content, and decreased perishability, also result from selective breeding. The nutritive value of individual foods is determined chiefly by their genetic character and not by the soil or type of fertilizer used.

Animals, too, have been bred for certain desired characteristics, for example, the lean, meat-type hog and steer, and the more tender, meatier chicken and turkey. In the United States the per capita consumption of beef has increased by approximately 70% and that of chicken by 100% in the last 20 years.

Most of the food consumed in American homes today has undergone some form of commerical processing—canning, freezing, or drying (Fig. 15-1). The TV dinner is perhaps the ultimate in commercial processing, but even the fresh fruits purchased in the supermarket may have had a heat or chill treatment before shipping to preserve their quality. In the processing of foods to produce specific properties there may be significant changes in the characteristics and composition of the original food, such as in the milling of the whole wheat kernel to make white flour

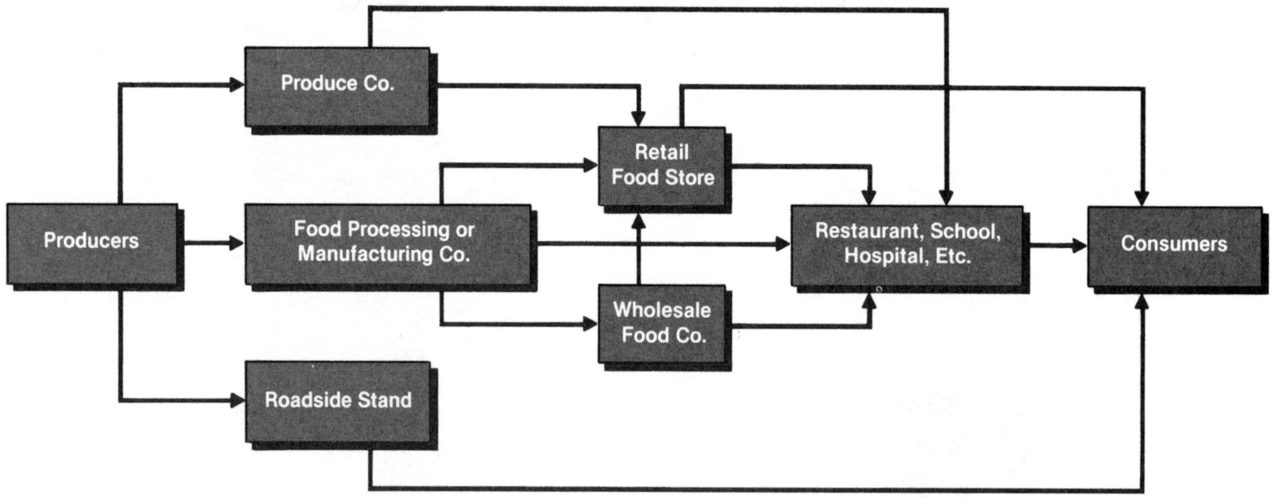

**Fig. 15-1.** How foods get to the consumer—the principal supply routes. (Protecting Our Food, Yearbook of Agriculture, U.S. Department of Agriculture, 1966, p 239)

with good bread-making properties. Food additives may also be used as preservatives, antioxidants, stabilizers, emulsifiers, and coloring and flavoring agents.

All of these factors involved in the production and processing of food provide the American consumer with an almost limitless choice of food items throughout the year, but they also make laws and regulations essential in order to protect the safety of this food supply.

This chapter reviews the factors that cause food spoilage and deterioration, the methods used for the care and preservation of food, foodborne diseases, and finally government laws and regulations that control food production and marketing.

## Food spoilage and deterioration

Any change that renders a food undesirable or unfit for human use may be called *food spoilage.* Although one usually thinks of spoilage as being caused by microorganisms, it can also be caused by chemical or physical changes, by enzymes, and by contamination with any foreign matter. A distinction should be made between foods *unfit* for consumption by anyone and foods which may be considered *distasteful* or *undesirable* by most Americans. For instance, snails, squid, fried grasshoppers, and fermented eggs may be delicacies in certain cultures but undesirable in others.

### Microbial food spoilage

Food spoilage may be caused by three different groups of microorganisms—bacteria, yeasts, and molds. The stale odor of spoiled meat, the foul odor of a spoiled egg, and the souring of milk are familiar examples of bacterial spoilage. The spoilage of canned foods also is usually traced to bacterial causes.

Yeasts and molds are most familiar as causes of spoilage of fresh foods, dried foods, and foods of high sugar content. The fermentation of catsup and cider is due to yeast growth. The fuzzy growths on bread and cheese and on the surface of jams and jellies indicate mold spoilage. The spoilage of citrus fruits and other fruits and vegetables is often due to the growth of molds.

### Enzymic food spoilage

Spoilage due to enzymic action is much more widespread than most people realize. Enzymic spoilage appears most often in loss of quality rather than as frank spoilage. The hay-like flavor of frozen vegetables after long or improper storage is due to enzymic activity. The softening or ripening of fruits and vegetables during storage may be the result of either enzymic action or mold growth. Because high temperatures destroy enzyme activity, the blanching of vegetables before freezing helps to prevent spoilage.

### Chemical food spoilage

Chemical causes of spoilage include flavor changes due to oxidation; swelling of cans due to production of hydrogen by the action of food acids on the metal of the container; discoloration from the reaction of metal ions from the container with the products, such as crabmeat or corn to produce discoloration; and oxidative rancidity of fats.

Most of these situations can be prevented by using a lining in the can to protect the can and the contents; "fruit" enamel prevents the bleaching of highly colored fruits; "corn" enamel prevents corn from discoloring. Antioxidants are added to foods subject to rancidity to prevent oxidation of unsaturated fatty acids.

## Physical causes of food spoilage

The spoilage of foods by physical changes usually involves a change of state from a solution to a precipitate, such as "sandy" ice cream caused by the formation of large lactose crystals during storage at fluctuating temperatures.

Exposure to light can cause spoilage in beer bottled in clear glass, resulting in an off odor described by the industry as "skunky." Sunlight can cause a tallowly off flavor in milk left too long on the doorstep and, at the same time, can destroy a high percentage of its riboflavin content.

## Spoilage by animals and insects

One means by which the Federal Food and Drug Administration (FDA) checks the sanitary conditions under which a product has been packed is to examine the product for rat hairs and droppings, insects and insect fragments, and mold hyphae. If these are present, the FDA can confiscate an entire shipment of food and prohibit future shipments until the unsanitary conditions are corrected to the satisfaction of the Food and Drug inspector.

A food may not be condemned due to the presence of foreign matter in amounts below the irreducible minimum if all precautions have been taken. The *food defect action levels* are established on the basis of a product's presenting *no hazard to health* and are modified as industry performance improves. The FDA proceeds with regulatory action whether or not the product exceeds the defect action level if poor manufacturing processes are evident.

## Care and preservation of foods

The methods of food preservation may be divided into two general classes—bactericidal and bacteriostatic. Bactericidal methods are those that destroy the organisms. These include cooking, canning, making jams and jellies, smoking, and the addition of chemical preservatives. Bacteriostatic methods make conditions unsuitable for microbial growth by reducing the temperature (refrigeration and freezing), removing water (dehydration), addition of acid (pickling), or adding substances to inhibit growth (salt or sugar).

### Refrigeration

All perishable food products and especially those potentially hazardous foods that consist in whole or in part of milk or milk products, eggs, meat, poultry, fish, and shellfish require refrigeration. To prevent the growth of microorganisms, refrigeration temperatures should be maintained at 7° C (45° F) or below if food is to be stored up to 3 or 4 days and at 4° C (40° F) if food is to be kept longer. At temperatures between 7° C (45° F) and 60° C

(140° F) (Fig. 15-2) both infectious bacteria and toxin-producing microorganisms grow rapidly. Within this range, for every 10° C (18° F) increase in temperature, a tenfold increase in the rate of growth of microorganisms may occur. Food may also undergo a doubling of the bacterial growth every 15 to 30 minutes.

Almost all fresh foods sold in the United States have been refrigerated during part of their journey from the producer to the consumer. If high-quality foods are to reach the consumer, the enzyme action of the fruits and the vegetables must be reduced (for these products are made up of living cells), growth of microorganisms must be inhibited, and chemical and physical changes must be prevented or slowed down.

Usually, fresh foods are stored at the lowest temperature possible at which no adverse physiological changes take place. Bananas, for example, are stored at higher temperatures during ripening, 17° C–21° C (62° F–70° F), then are held at 13° C (56° F) to 16° C (60° F) for storage after ripening. If they are chilled below 13° C (56° F) before ripening, they develop a smoky, dull color, and if chilled after ripening, the skin turns brown rapidly.

Apples and some other fruits are usually stored at

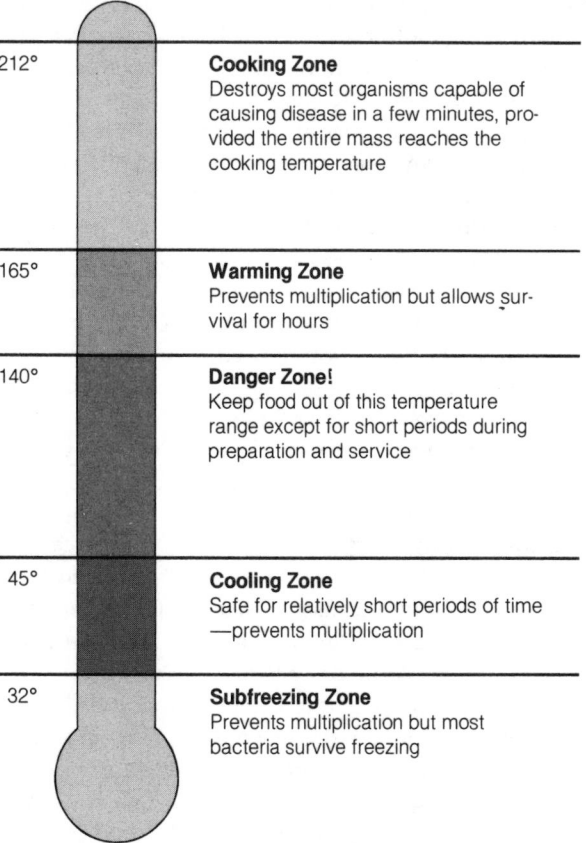

**Fig. 15-2.** Thermometer for control of bacteria. (Protecting Our Food, Yearbook of Agriculture, U.S. Department of Agriculture, 1966, p 189)

−1° C (30° F) to 0° C (32° F) in a nitrogen atmosphere for best results. In order to maintain crispness or an attractive appearance, the humidity is usually maintained as high as possible to prevent loss of moisture, but it must also be low enough to discourage mold growth. Most fruits and vegetables are maintained at 85% to 90% relative humidity.

### Freezing

Because certain varieties of fruits and vegetables have characteristics that make them better able to withstand freezing and thawing and because freezing does not improve a product that was of poor quality to start with, foods for the freezer should be carefully selected for appropriate variety and quality. Vegetables are blanched before freezing to inactivate the enzymes, and fruits are either placed in a sugar syrup or treated with an antioxidant, such as ascorbic acid, to keep them from darkening. Some foods, such as peas, beans, or shrimp, may be frozen before they are packaged, but most foods are placed in cartons and then frozen rapidly at temperatures of −40° C (−40° F) or below. Frozen foods should be stored at 0° F or below.

Cooked prepared foods require special care in preparation and sanitary handling because frequently they contain potentially hazardous mixtures (see *Refrigeration*) and may not be thoroughly cooked before serving Most bacteria survive freezing, but their growth is inhibited at such low temperatures. However, *Trichinella*, a parasite that may infect pork, is destroyed by freezing.

When foods are allowed to thaw and are kept at room temperature, spoilage actually occurs more rapidly than one might expect because, due to a partial breakdown of cell walls and tissues, the thawed food is an excellent medium for the growth of bacteria. Most foods should not be refrozen once they have thawed.

*Dehydrofreezing* is a process that removes about 50% of the water from fruits and vegetables before they are frozen. The reduction in weight and volume allows them to be shipped and stored more economically.

### Cooking and baking

Nearly all the microorganisms in a food are destroyed by proper cooking. Because this lengthens the time that a food will keep, cooking may be regarded as a method of preservation. In some cases it is a mixed blessing, as a study of food poisoning quickly shows that most cases of food poisoning are caused by consumption of a cooked food that has not been properly refrigerated. Cooking destroys the organisms that would ordinarily compete with, and hold in check, the growth of food-poisoning organisms. If cooking is inadequate, for example, in roasting a prestuffed turkey, or if the cooked food is contaminated after cooking, from the hands or nasal discharge of a food handler, the toxin-producing organisms can then grow without hindrance.

### Pasteurization

The time–temperature relationship of pasteurization is based on the time at a given temperature during which all the organisms that will produce disease are destroyed. Milk as it comes from the pasteurizer is not sterile. The total bacterial count has been reduced, and all the disease-causing organisms are destroyed.

Two methods are used for milk pasteurization—the *holding* method consists of heating milk to 63° C (145° F) and holding that temperature for 30 minutes; the *high-temperature short-time* method consists of heating milk to 71.1° C (160° F) and holding for 17 seconds.

The reduction in bacterial count plus refrigeration increases the shelf life of many foods other than milk, such as beer and wines. Mild heat treatment of concentrated citrus juices before freezing is practiced by many packers to control the enzymes that may cause clarification or gelation of the concentrate if it is mishandled (allowed to remain above freezing) during storage and marketing.

### Canning

Canning has probably done more than any other discovery to help mankind maintain an adequate food supply throughout the year.

The canning industry has continually improved the quality and the retention of nutrients in food by increasing the rate of heating and cooling. Canned foods are sterilized by heating with steam under pressure [5 lb, 108° C (227° F); 10 lb, 116° C (240° F); 15 lb, 121° C (250° F)]. Agitation of the can during heating also permits faster heat penetration of the cans' contents, shortening processing time.

Originally food was preserved by boiling jars of food for hours. Now food can be sterilized in less than a second at temperatues up to 135° C (275° F) in a specially designed heat exchanger, cooled immediately, and then sealed into sterile containers aseptically. This method, known as *aseptic canning*, is now used on a small scale to process purees and baby foods, but its use is limited because of the high cost of the equipment required and the short packing periods of most canneries.

Since 1973 all commercial processors of *low-acid foods* (*p*H value greater than 4.6) in airtight containers are required to register their plants and products with the Food and Drug Administration. They must also file process information (*e.g.*, cooking time and temperatures) for each low-acid product.

### Dehydration

In the past, dehydration was looked upon as one of the least desirable methods of preservation. Technological advances during and after World War II have made possible much improved products with the attributes of low cost, reduced weight, convenience, and keeping quality. The absence of water prevents the growth of microorganisms in dehydrated products.

The use of dehydrated foods has increased rapidly. Certain dehydrated products are used by some consumers to the exclusion of their counterparts preserved by other methods. An example of this is instant coffee, which now constitutes at least 50% of coffee used.

Of particular interest to the nutritionist is the availability of nonfat dried milk, an excellent food, which is brought to the consumer at a low price in an easily soluble form with good flavor and keeping qualities.

Certain fruits, such as prunes, peaches, apricots, apples, raisins, figs, and dates are also popular consumer items. Dried legumes, onions, and parsley are available. Fish and meat may also be preserved by drying.

Other items in this multimillion dollar business include cake, muffin, cornbread, pancake, and roll mixes (which are mixtures of dehydrated ingredients); instant potato, fruit-flavored juices and dessert mixes; precooked dehydrated cereals, rice, and tapioca; soups; and dried active yeast. Dried stabilized eggs (whole eggs, egg yolk, or egg white) are used widely in bakery products but have not yet reached wide distribution on a retail scale.

### Freeze drying

This process consists of first freezing the food and then removing the water with a vacuum. The food is packaged in the presence of an inert gas, such as nitrogen. Freeze-dried foods rehydrate very readily and retain their original shape and volume. The most widely used freeze-dried product today is coffee, although seafoods, meats, poultry, fruits, and vegetables have been tested and found acceptable.

### Chemicals as preservatives

Chemical preservatives are among the oldest forms of food preservation, with salt, sugar, and vinegar as the most familiar ones. Other types of chemical preservatives are also used. Some are effective for a particular type of food or against a particular spoilage organism. They are called *antioxidants*, *inhibitors*, *fungicides*, and *sequestrants*. Ascorbic acid is frequently used an an antioxidant in commercial canning and freezing to prevent the enzymatic browning of fruits and vegetables. Sorbic acid is used to prevent mold growth on cheese, and sodium benzoate is used to preserve cider from yeast fermentation and margarine from spoilage by mold. Sodium propionate, calcium propionate, or sodium diacetate are used in bread to prevent mold growth. In general, however, chemical preservatives have faced stiff opposition to their retention in foods due to adverse public opinion about their use and strict regulation by the Food and Drug Administration. When a food can be preserved satisfactorily without chemicals, chemical preservatives are not allowed. For example, catsup will keep because of the preservative effects of acids, sugars, and spices; for this reason sodium benzoate, which for years had been added to catsup, may no longer be used.

The present dilemma about the use of nitrites, which may be carcinogenic, in bacon and other meat products is the result of not having available an equally effective substitite for inhibiting the growth of deadly *Cl. botulinum* spores in these products. The FDA has had to move very slowly in banning nitrites while at the same time encouraging industry to develop equally safe means of preserving these products.

### Radiation

The newest method of food preservation is still in the experimental stage. The Armed Forces Food and Container Institute at Natick, Massachusetts, has been doing extensive research on food irradiation in one of the best equipped laboratories in the world for this purpose. They are testing various types of foods in different designs of containers to determine levels of irradiation that will safeguard the food without changing its flavor. Obviously, food does not become radioactive in the process. F. P. Mehrlich, Technical Director, explains,

> The radiation preservation process involves exposing food to electrons so the food itself is not cooked in the process. Raw foods remain raw. Different effects are obtained, depending on the level of irradiation provided.
>
> At the lowest levels, in the order of 7500 rads, sprouting of potatoes and onions is inhibited, extending their postharvest storage life well into the next harvest. At slightly higher levels, human pathogens like trichinosis-causing worms and liver flukes are destroyed, making infested pork and fish safe for human consumption. At still higher levels, insect larvae and eggs are destroyed, eliminating insect damage in packaged cereal and permitting previously infested fruits across quarantine barriers.
>
> At even higher levels, pathogenic bacteria like Salmonella are inactivated. At the same time so are most of the bacteria present, thereby extending the refrigerated shelf life and marketing radius of fresh foods.
>
> Finally, at the highest levels, in the order of 4.5 million rads, all bacteria are killed and prepackaged food can be kept without bacterial spoilage, in the absence of refrigeration. The military and civilian advantages of such a process are readily apparent.[1]

A *rad* is a unit of absorbed ionizing radiation. It corresponds to an energy absorption of 100 ergs per gram of material. A lethal dose for man is between 500 and 600 rads.

Since many foods become unacceptable at radiation levels above 500,000 rads due to off flavor and odor, it is probable that research will develop a combination of heat, radiation, and refrigeration to retain the highest quality of certain foods. Heat destroys enzymes that are resistant to destruction by radiation.

The use of radiation has been defined as "addition of chemicals to food;" accordingly, this method of food preservation is subject to the rules that regulate food additives (see *Food Additives*). Extensive studies must be conducted to prove the safety and wholesomeness of food preserved in this manner.

## Microwaves

Heat energy in foods exposed to microwaves is produced by the intermolecular friction created when molecules in food oscillate as they attempt to align themselves with the rapidly alternating current field. Temperature increase alone cannot explain the detrimental effect that microwaves have on microorganisms; further studies of this phenomenon are currently underway. In addition to its use in homes and institutions, the food industry employes microwave energy for such processes as cooking, blanching, puffing.

# Effects of food processing on nutrient composition

## Canning

Properly canned fruits and vegetables have approximately the same nutrient composition as fresh ones. It is possible that the canned products might be better than the fresh if the latter are not protected in shipment from farm to market or are stored incorrectly and cooked by the homemaker. Some nutritive loss, especially of the heat-labile water-soluble vitamins, ascorbic acid, thiamin, vitamin $B_6$, and pantothenic acid, occurs during the canning process. Additional losses occur during storage depending on the temperature at which canned goods are stored. Canned fruits and vegetables stored for a year at 18° C (65° F) or below lose much less ascorbic acid and thiamin than if stored at 27° C (80° F). The use of the liquid from canned fruits and vegetables also reduces the loss of water-soluble nutrients.

The caloric value of most canned fruits is greater than fresh due to the addition of sugar during processing. The majority of canned vegetables differ in sodium composition when compared with fresh ones because salt (NaCl) is added during processing.

Losses of heat-labile water-soluble vitamins, such as thiamin and vitamin $B_6$, also occur in the canning and storage of meat, poultry, and fish products. However, because the cooking of fresh meat, fish, and poultry in the home also results in similar losses, these products have approximately the same nutritive composition. NaCl is usually added to these foods in processing.

## Freezing

Frozen vegetables and fruits may also lose small amounts of the water-soluble vitamins during the blanching and freezing process; however, this loss is similar to the loss from fresh foods prepared in the home. The temperature at which frozen foods are stored also affects nutrient losses. Freezers should be maintained at −18° C (0° F) or below if food is to be stored for more than a few days.

Frozen fruits, vegetables, meat, fish, and poultry are comparable in nutrient composition to the fresh products if other food items are not added. Plain frozen vegetables, without the addition of butter or sauces for seasoning, are equal to fresh or canned ones. Salt, and in some instances monosodium glutamate, may be added to plain frozen vegetables. When salt is added, it is listed on the label. Frozen fruits may or may not have sugar added during processing. Frozen orange juice concentrate does not have sugar added, but most of the orange-flavored breakfast drinks do have sugar added. The caloric value of frozen meat, fish, or poultry can be greater than fresh if a gravy or sauce has been added or if the product is breaded and fried before freezing, such as frozen fish sticks.

## Dehydration

Drying and storing of protein foods, such as milk, fish, meat, and legumes, may result in some reduction of biologic value or a reduction in the protein efficiency ratio (PER).

Ascorbic acid losses in dehydrated fruits and vegetables are considerable. Thiamin levels may also be decreased in dehydrated products. Some loss of fat-soluble vitamins A and E have been reported in dehydrated foods.[2]

# Foodborne diseases and toxins

Foods may be contaminated by a variety of pathogenic organisms. These contaminants may be various worms, molds, bacteria, viruses, and other organisms or the toxins produced by them. The appearance, taste, and smell of the food so infected may show no change and, for this reason, give no warning to the consumer.

These infections may be present in the food at its source, such as animals infected with tuberculosis, brucellosis, salmonellosis, tularemia, tapeworms, or trichinae, and may be carried to the consumer if the food is undercooked.

Food may also be infected by food handlers who are convalescent from infectious diseases. They may be in apparent good health but still carry infectious organisms. The organisms may be distributed on food by hands soiled with urine or feces or by spray of oral and nasal secretions by coughing and sneezing over the food being prepared. Contamination may also come from the butcher block or from the handling of an infected animal before working with the food in question.

Dust falling on uncovered foods and the feces and the bodies of insects may also convey pathogenic organisms to a food supply. Covering of cooked foods and refrigeration can do much to cut down on the number of pathogenic organisms in foods. Cooked foods should be cooled as quickly as possible by pouring or sorting into flat pans and prompt refrigeration rather than by allowing them to cool at room temperature. Often the period required for cooling in a warm kitchen is sufficient for bacteria to grow rapidly.

## Contamination of food and water by nonsporeforming bacteria

### Salmonella

Salmonella infection is a term used to cover a large group of infections caused by several species of the salmonella organism common to humans and several animals and birds. Salmonellosis is an infection of the intestinal tract, and symptoms begin to appear from 8 to 48 hours after contaminated food has been eaten. Symptoms typically are headache, vomiting, diarrhea, fever, and cramps. An attack may last a few hours or several days. Infants and debilitated older people may be most seriously affected, and death may result. Antibiotics do little to relieve an attack; fluids and a bland diet are the usual treatment.

The Center for Disease Control in Atlanta, Georgia, reported that salmonellosis has become a major national problem, whereas a generation ago it was seldom recognized as such. Even today cases go unreported because they are mistaken for "24-hour flu" or "stomach upset." They state that some 20,000 cases of salmonella infection are reported each year but that the actual incidence is probably 2 million cases per year. In this decade salmonellae have been traced to well water, frozen turkey, fresh chicken, eggs, smoked fish, ground beef, and a contaminated batch of powdered milk.

Many varieties of salmonella may be carried by contaminated foods. Because these bacteria grow easily in moist foods of low acidity and may continue to be viable even in some dry foods, strict control of food sanitation and cooking procedures at home and in institutions, especially, is essential. The usual path of infection is from animals or animal products to humans. Precautions for utensils, dishwashing, and food handling are outlined by Werrin and Kronick.[3] Salmonellae are readily destroyed by usual cooking procedures and by pasteurization but not by freezing. Note the incident of turkeyborne multiple infection below.

### The typhoid bacillus

This is a strain of salmonella that may be carried by contaminated water or shellfish. In the United States, however, an outbreak of typhoid fever can usually be traced to a food handler who is a "carrier" of the organism. Fortunately, the disease responds to an antibiotic, and the course is not as serious as it once was.

### Shigellosis

Closely related to salmonellosis, shigellae also are enteric bacteria and are the etiologic agents of bacillary dysentery in man. Young children and newborn animals are most seriously affected. Symptoms include diarrhea, abdominal pain, fever, and vomiting and usually appear within 36 hours after ingestion of the contaminated food. Shigellae are transmitted by personal contact, flies, and water as well as by food. In the United States, potato salad has been an important vehicle for shigellae. The following sequence takes place—an infected food handler with poor personal hygiene touches the food, which is not subsequently cooked and is held for several hours at a temperature range in which shigellae can grow.

### Escherichia coli

Certain strains of *E. coli* can cause illness in man, either by producing a cholera-like enterotoxin or by penetrating the epithelium similar to shigellae.[4]

### Staphylococcus food poisoning

Staphylococcus bacteria are responsible for many cases of food poisoning. Most people are sensitive to the exotoxins produced by these bacteria, and serious illness can result if enough of the toxin is present in the food. The toxin affects only the gastrointestinal tract, and the onset of symptoms occurs within 1 to 8 hours after infected food is eaten. The symptoms are severe nausea, vomiting, and abdominal cramps. This kind of food poisoning is rarely fatal.

Most outbreaks of this type of food poisoning have been caused by the bacteria in prepared or unheated foods, such as custard-filled pastries, cream pies, salads, precooked meats like ham, sandwiches, and creamed dishes. The bacteria get into food from boils, infected cuts, coughing, and sneezing by food handlers followed by improper storage and inadequate reheating of foods before service. The flavor and appearance of the food may not change. Control of this type of food poisoning is largely a matter of educating food handlers.

### Vibrio infections

*Vibrio parahaemolyticus*, which inhabits the marine environment especially in warm coastal waters, can be the cause of food poisoning. Gastroenteritis can occur 2 to 48 hours after consumption of the contaminated seafood. Raw fish are particularly subject to contamination, and the number of viable organisms multiply rapidly if the fish is not kept continually refrigerated or frozen. Because cooking destroys the microorganism, this form of food poisoning is more common in countries like Japan, where raw seafood is regularly consumed.[4]

*Vibrio cholerae* is the microorganism responsible for cholera. Water is the most important vehicle for the spread of cholera. It is contaminated by human feces containing *V. cholerae.* Very early diagnosis and treatment with antibiotics, fluid, electrolyte, and carbohydrate replacement reduces the high mortality rate from cholera. Cholera is said to occur in pandemics, spreading especially to the warmer countries of the world. The last pandemic (7th) spread from the Southwest Pacific (1961) to the Middle East (1965) to North and West Africa and Eastern Europe (1970). It is endemic in countries, such as India, where it has a seasonal pattern. It is a disease that strikes primarily the lower socioeconomic groups because of poor sanitary standards. The provision of a safe water supply is the most essential measure to prevent cholera epidemics.[4]

### Streptococcal infections

Hemolytic streptococcus is the type most commonly carried by food. Food and utensils may be contaminated by a carrier, from nasal discharge or skin infection. Strep sore throat, strep ear infections, and scarlet fever are all caused by strains of hemolytic streptococci.

### Tularemia

Sometimes called rabbit fever, Tularemia is caused by infection with *Pasteurella tularensis.* It is transmitted from rodents by flies, fleas, and ticks and may be acquired by humans from the handling of infected animals. It is characterized by an ulcer at the site of inoculation, followed by inflammation of the lymph glands and by headache, chills, and fever. It is recommended that hunters use rubber gloves when dressing wild game.

## Contamination of food and water by sporeforming bacteria

### Botulism

Botulism is a rare form of food poisoning. It occurs when nonacid foods have been underprocessed. Botulin (the toxin) may also be found in some meat products, such as sausage (the Latin word for sausage is botulus). Because *Cl. botulinum* is a strict anaerobe, it can grow only under conditions in which air is excluded, such as in a can or deep inside a product.

Spores of *Cl. botulinum* are widely distributed in nature, and one must assume that any raw food is contaminated with the spores. The survival of a single spore in a processed nonacid food cannot be tolerated because the spore is capable of producing a lethal toxin if stored for a period of time in the absence of oxygen. Unfortunately, the botulinogenic food may show no sign of spoilage. Absolute sterilization at high temperatures is necessary in canning nonacid foods. Sodium nitrate has been used to prevent botulism in bacon and other meat products.

In recent years commercially processed foods have been relatively free of any poisoning caused by *Cl. bot-*

*ulinum.* However, in 1963 two cases were caused by canned tuna fish and one by smoked fish frozen in polyethylene bags.

In 1971 two cases were reported as the result of the use of canned soup and resulted in a massive recall of all soups and sauces processed by that particular company.

In 1973 to 1974 30 cans of mushrooms were found to contain *Cl. botulinum* toxin.

The toxin produced is one of the most deadly biologic poisons known. On average, mortality is about 25% for the diagnosed and reported cases. Occasionally, entire families are killed by botulism. A quadrivalent antitoxin containing types A, B, E, and F antitoxins should be administered to anyone known to have eaten botulinogenic foods even if symptoms have not developed. Administration of antitoxin has reduced the mortality rate from botulism.

Home-canned foods account for the vast majority of the 10 to 20 botulism outbreaks that occur each year. Lowacid foods should be preserved only by a pressure cooker process. Boiling canned foods for 10 minutes also destroys the toxin.

The toxin is absorbed directly from the stomach and the intestinal tract. In about 8 to 72 hours it affects the nervous system, causing double vision, difficulty in swallowing, loss of speech and, when lethal, respiratory failure in from 3 to 6 days.

*Infant botulism* was diagnosed as a distinct clinical entity in the United States in 1976. From 1976 to 1978 58 cases were reported in 15 states, more than half in California. Only one case was fatal. All the infants were less than 6 months old. The toxin is produced after *Cl. botulinum* multiplied in the gastrointestinal tract. The clinical symptoms include constipation, refusal to eat, lethargy, weakness, weak or altered cry and loss of head control. The factors that predispose the infant to this disease are unknown.[4] Although no definite association with any specific food item has been established, honey was suspected in a number of cases. Because some *Cl. botulinum* spores were found in honey, the recommendation was made not to feed honey to infants less than a year old.

### Clostridium perfringens

Perfringens poisoning, which results in gastrointestinal disturbances, is caused by certain strains of *Clostridium perfringens*, a spore-forming bacterium that grows in the absence of oxygen. The spores are resistant to heat, ordinary cooking, drying, freezing, curing of meats, and irradiation. To prevent their growth, meats should be cooked rapidly and refrigerated promptly below 4° C (40° F).

The symptoms of *Cl. perfringens* food infection are mild gastroenteritis, abdominal cramps, and diarrhea 8 to 16 hours after eating infected food, and are rarely accompanied by nausea and headache. The illness is usually mild and of short duration, with recovery within 24 hours.

A report of three consecutive outbreaks of foodborne disease in 1 week was recently investigated and traced to turkey infected with both salmonella and *Cl. perfringens.* The turkey, which was prepared ahead and served at three banquets in 1 week, caused food poisoning in 23% of the persons present at the first, in 35% of those at the second, and in 69% of those at the third banquet. The 20-lb to 22-lb turkeys had been purchased frozen, thawed at room temperature, boiled for 4 hours and allowed to cool in water overnight. They were stored in a refrigerator but were probably at room temperature for some time during preparation and prior to reheating before service at each banquet. This is an example of poor food handling, if not poor sanitation.[5]

## Bacillus cereus

This organism is commonly found in soil and on vegetation and has been isolated in several countries from a wide variety of samples of food, including uncooked rice. Ingestion of small numbers of the microorganism is not harmful. Immediate consumption of freshly cooked food produces no problems from *B. cereus.* However, because cooking at temperatures not exceeding 100° C (212° F) (boiling) does not destroy all of the spores of *B. cereus*, there is potential danger in slow cooling without refrigerated storage of large batches of rice and other cereal or starch-containing foods if contaminated with surviving spores. Both vomiting and diarrheal types of gastroenteritis have been linked to *B. cereus* food poisoning. The incubation period for the diarrheal type is 10 to 12 hours after ingestion of the contaminated food, whereas, for the vomiting type it is 1 to 5 hours after consumption of contaminated food. The importance of proper food handling, especially in institutions and restaurants, is emphasized in preventing outbreaks of food poisoning from *B. cereus.* It is speculated that many cases of food poisoning would be removed from the "causal agent unknown" category if investigators examined food remnants and specimens of feces and vomitus for *B. cereus* as well as for salmonellae, staphylococci, clostridia, and vibrios.[4]

## Toxins from molds (Mycotoxins)

Aflatoxin, a toxin produced by *Aspergillus flavus*, a fungus found on nuts, corn, and other grains has been found to be carcinogenic in rats. Several possible cases of acute aflatoxicosis have been reported in the Philippines, Taiwan, and Thailand. Recent epidemiological studies in Asia and Africa show a positive relationship between the aflatoxin intake and the incidence of human liver cancer.[4]

Because mycotoxins have been recognized as important food contaminants, greater efforts to control or eliminate the growth of molds on food crops have been made.

The FDA has proposed new stricter regulations for monitoring aflatoxin levels in human and animal foods. Commercial peanut products designed for human consumption in the United States are toxin-free, even if produced from contaminated nuts, because any trace of aflatoxin is removed in the refining process.

## Naturally occurring toxins

It is well known that many varieties of mushrooms are poisonous and have been mistaken for edible types with disastrous results. There is no simple test that will identify edible types other than botanical characteristics.

A few plants used as foods are safe at one time and not at another. The young white shoots of pokeweed frequently are eaten with safety as greens in the early spring, but the later green shoots may cause severe illness. The green leaves of rhubarb may contain enough oxalic acid to cause illness, but the succulent leaf stems are eaten without any untoward effects. Clams and mussels on the Pacific coast may build up toxins during the summer due to an infection from certain plankton (red tide).

## Viral infections

Infectious hepatitis, or hepatitis A, is the most common of viral infections spread by contaminated food. It may be spread by the consumption of contaminated water, milk, or other food. Contaminated shellfish has been identified as the vehicle for the virus in a number of outbreaks. These shellfish came from contaminated waters and in most cases were consumed with little or no cooking. A food handler who is a carrier may contaminate food; this may not be discovered for some time. The incubation period is from 10 to 50 days, and the virus may be in the blood 2 to 3 weeks before the onset of the disease.

## Parasitic infections

Parasitic infections are not confined to the tropics as is sometimes thought. They may be transmitted by food or drink, often by infected meat, fish, shellfish, or crustacea.

## Trichinosis

Trichinosis is the parasitic disease most likely to be encountered in the United States and is caused by improperly cooked pork from pigs that were infected with *Trichinella spiralis.* Symptoms of the infection in humans include fever, muscle pain, sweating, chills, vomiting, and swollen eyelids. Outbreaks have been reported from homemade sausage and other pork products improperly cured. Trichinosis can be avoided if pork is well cooked [internal temperature of at least 58° C (137°F)] or properly cured or frozen.

## Anisakiasis

Anisakiasis caused by the anisakis larvae has been recognized in Holland. These parasites may be present in raw, pickled, or smoked herring or other marine fish.

## Protozoan infections

### Amebic dysentery

Amebic dysentery, caused by *Entamoeba histolytica*, is another infection that may be carried by food and food handlers. It is common in the tropics. Once it is acquired, the organism remains in the tissues of the intestinal tract and causes intermittent attacks until the person is treated. Abscesses of the liver may be a complication.

## Safeguarding the food supply

The food industry is the nation's largest industry and depends upon the work of thousands of scientists and experts to predict needs and regulate food production and processing in the United States. Most people do not have the means or the skills to examine how meats are handled, or to check fruits and vegetables for residues of pesticides or processed foods for harmful preservatives or accidental contaminants or packaged goods for insect infestation. Through Congress, however, laws have been passed making certain federal agencies responsible for protecting the safety of our food supplies. Such agencies as the Food and

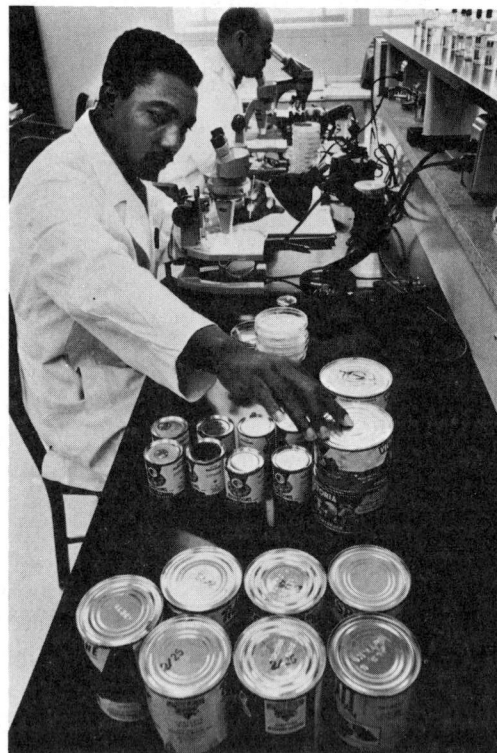

**Fig. 15-3.** FDA's enforcement effort for foods is mainly concerned with food plant sanitation and the wholesomeness of ingredients and finished products. The Federal Food, Drug, and Cosmetic Act (1938) makes it illegal to ship in interstate commerce a food that comes from unsanitary premises. To enforce this section of the Act, FDA inspects food processors to ensure that the factories are sanitary. FDA is responsible for establishing safety standards for additives in foods. (FDA Publ. No. 1. U.S. Department HEW, Washington, D.C.)

Drug Administration, the Federal Trade Commission, and the Department of Agriculture have extensive programs for safeguarding our foods.

## U.S. Department of Health and Human Services— Food and Drug Administration

### Federal Food, Drug, and Cosmetic Act

Under the Food, Drug, and Cosmetic Act, the Food and Drug Administration (FDA) of the Department of Health and Human Services (HHS) has jurisdiction over the safety of foods shipped interstate or manufactured in a territory of the United States or the District of Columbia. Federal regulations also control imported and exported foods. The act prohibits distribution in the United States or importation of articles that are adulterated or mislabeled. Foods manufactured and sold within a state's boundaries are not subject to federal regulation but are controlled by the food regulations of the state in which they are produced (Fig. 15-3).

***Adulteration of Foods.*** A food is considered to be adulterated if it is filthy, putrid, or decomposed, if noncertified colors are used, if the container is made of a substance injurious to health (*e.g.*, lead), if there is dilution or substitution, or if there is omission of a valuable ingredient. Food is also considered to be adulterated if it contains meat from a diseased animal or one that died by means other than slaughter.

### Good Manufacturing Practice

Regulations issued by the FDA are an important part of the Food and Drug Law. The Good Manufacturing Practice (GMP) regulations, which set requirements for sanitation, inspection of materials and finished products, and other quality controls are examples of especially important regulations. Detailed GMPs are available for low-acid foods, smoked fish and frozen raw breaded shrimp. Processing of these foods is always critical because of the menace of foodborne pathogens.

***Standards*** of identity, quality, and fill have been established under federal regulations. A *standard of identity* defines what a food product is. It determines what ingredients must be included, the minimum and maximum amounts of each, and additional ingredients that are optional. Standards of identity have been set for such products as milk and cream; cheese and cheese products; eggs and egg products; margarine; mayonnaise, French dressing and salad dressing; frozen desserts; flours; macaroni and noodle products; jellies and preserves; canned fruit and fruit juices; vegetables and vegetable products. Only the optional ingredients used in these products must appear on the label. Hence, the nutrition educator needs to know that even though salt may not appear in the list of ingredients on the label of the catsup bottle, it is included in the standard of identity; therefore, catsup is a food to be avoided on a sodium-restricted diet. The FDA is planning to request legislation to require that mandatory ingredients in standardized foods be declared on product labels.[6]

**Standards of quality** have been established chiefly for canned fruits, vegetables, and meats. Foods that do not meet the minimum standards for quality must be labeled substandard. These foods are not usually sold in the retail market.

**Standards of fill** are specifications for the amount of food that must be in a container. They were established to prevent the use of deceptive containers and to provide guidelines for foods, such as cereals and crackers that tend to "shake down" after being packaged.

**Pesticide control.**  An amendment to the Food, Drug, and Cosmetic Act of 1938 was passed in 1954 to establish safe limits of pesticide chemical residues on fresh fruits and vegetables. The chemical pesticide sprays range in their toxicity to humans from virtually harmless to extremely toxic and dangerous. To control their use the FDA has published a list of more than 2000 tolerance levels for pesticide chemicals and has established a zero tolerance for certain pesticides, such as cyanides, mercury-containing compounds, and selenium-containing compounds, which are extremely dangerous.

To protect the consumer, foods that are shipped in violation of FDA regulations are subject to recall or seizure. The manufacturers may be fined or imprisoned or both, depending on the circumstances. The FDA works with the Environmental Protection Agency (EPA), USDA, and the individual states in residue monitoring and enforcement.

**Food Additives.**  The Food Additives Amendment of 1958 and the Color Additive Amendment of 1960 govern the use of intentional and incidental food additives. These amendments are designed to protect the public from the presence in foods of any substance not demonstrated to be safe under the recommended conditions of use as judged by competent experts.

Food additives are prohibited specifically by the Food, Drug, and Cosmetic Act where they are used to mask faulty processing and handling techniques, to deceive the consumer, and to aid processing at the expense of a substantial reduction of the nutritional value of the product, and, where good manufacturing practices do not require the use of an additive, to produce a food item economically.

**Intentional food additives** include nutrients, preservatives, antioxidants, stabilizers, emulsifiers, leavening agents, humectants, maturing and bleaching agents, anticaking agents, and coloring and flavoring agents. Over 2800 such additives are being used in food processing today, and these are continually being investigated by the Food and Drug Administration. An additive is intentionally used in food for one or more of the following four purposes; to maintain or improve nutritive value; to main-

tain freshness; to help in processing or preparation; and to make food more appealing.

The *GRAS list*, published by the FDA, is a list of approximately 675 substances used in food which are *generally recognized as safe*. Other approved food additives not on the GRAS list are known as regulated food additives. All GRAS list items are currently under review to determine their usage rates in the American food supply and the relative safety of the amounts consumed. Most of the substances reviewed so far present no hazards to health from current or future uses. However, several substances originally on the GRAS list have been removed by the FDA, and an additional number have been identified by the Select Committee on GRAS substances of the Federation of American Sciences for Experimental Biology as of concern because of adverse effects on test animals or because there is a lack of significant scientific data on their safety.

Cyclamates, which originally appeared on the GRAS list, were banned from food as a result of finding that they produced bladder cancer in rats. Saccharin was removed from the GRAS list to an "interim regulated additives" list in the early 1970s. When additional information regarding the carcinogenicity of saccharin became available, the FDA proposed a ban that would have eliminated the use of saccharin in foods, beverages, and cosmetics likely to be ingested and in drugs as a nonmedical ingredient to improve taste. The proposal would have permitted continued marketing of saccharin as a single-ingredient drug, available without prescription, provided that manufacturers prove it is medically effective for such uses as controlling diabetes and obesity. Due to public outcry opposing the ban, Congress in November, 1977, passed an 18-month moratorium known as the *Saccharin Study and Labeling Act*. The moratorium should have ended in May, 1979, but was extended until June, 1981, after the FDA announced its intention to re-propose the ban—a regulation-making process that could take 15 to 18 months. The saccharin story has been a long and controversial one but probably did more to make the public aware of the federal government's role in food safety than any other recent issue.

The use of nitrates and nitrites in bacon and other cured meat is another serious problem. Since the 1960s evidence has been available that nitrite, when combined with certain chemicals, can form nitrosamines, a family of chemicals known to produce cancer in test animals. Nitrites, however, prevent the spore formation from *Cl. botulinum* in these meat products. The FDA must continue to evaluate nitrites, but at the same time it must ensure that the industry develop equally safe ways of processing these products or remove them from the market.

Additional additives, such as brominated vegetable oil, BHT (butylated hydroxytoluene), BHA (butylated hydroxyanisole), and mannitol have been given interim status while FDA requires additional studies to determine their safety. FDA has affirmed a number of GRAS substances including sorbitol, a sweetener, and dill and garlic, two familiar flavoring agents, and has proposed to affirm an additional number including mustard, a flavoring agent, and gelatin, a thickener.

The manufacturer has the burden of proof for the usefulness and safety of a proposed additive. The proposed new additive must first be subjected to a battery of chemical tests to determine whether it does what is intended and to make sure it can be analyzed and measured in the finished food product. Then the additive must be fed in large doses over an extended period to at least two kinds of animals, usually rodents and dogs. These feeding studies are designed to determine whether the substance causes cancer, birth defects, or other injury to the animals. After a manufacturer submits the results of all these tests to FDA and if they indicate the additive is safe, the FDA establishes regulations for its use in food. A basic rule is a 100-fold margin of safety for any food additive. This means that the manufacturer may use only one-hundreth the maximum amount of an additive that has been found not to produce any harmful effects in test animals. The Delaney Clause states that a substance shown to cause cancer in humans or animals may not be added to food in any amount. The banning of cyclamates as a food additive was based on this regulation.

Although safety of food additives is a problem of extreme importance, it is practically impossible to demonstrate absolute proof of safety of an additive for all people in a population that may include a few very sensitive people and others in poor physiological condition, as well as those suffering from a disease of one sort or another.

**The incidental additives,** usually undesirable, which may appear in food products, include:

1. Pesticides (used for plant and animal pest control)
2. Fertilizers (used by plants)
3. Feed adjuvants and drugs (antibiotics, hormones, tranquilizers, and enzymes)
4. Chemicals used in packaging materials (may migrate into the food)

These regulations are monitored by FDA, EPA, and USDA officials, and the public is protected when foods that do not conform to them are found.

## Pollution

The hazards of environmental pollution to our food supply have become a national concern. The rapid increase in the contamination of air, water, and soil as a result of increased population and technological advances requires diligent monitoring by those persons responsible for safeguarding the nation's health.

Of special concern is the possible presence of *radioactive materials* in food. For example, the milk supply requires constant radiation surveillance because of the possible presence of strontium-90 or iodine-131, two potentially harmful substances, especially in infants and children. Although most of the Sr-90 is excreted from the body, small amounts may be deposited in bones. Larger amounts of I-131 are absorbed and have a carcinogenic effect on the thyroid gland. Currently, the amounts of radioactive fallout in our food supply are well below danger levels. The EPA monitors levels of radioactivity accidentally released from nuclear facilities.

Another problem of environmental contaminants involves the toxic metals (see Chap. 6), including mercury, lead, and cadmium. The FDA has alerted the public to the excessive amounts of *mercury* in certain types of fish. Swordfish, in particular, had been identified as containing potentially harmful levels and had been temporarily removed from the market. Although the presence of mercury has been detected in tuna fish, these amounts are not as alarming, and tuna fish has remained available. In fact, most of the fresh tuna fish is now examined before it is canned, and only that fish that is below guideline levels, is canned for the consumer market.

The pollution of inland lakes and streams and coastal waters from industrial wastes and sewage has not only reduced the available supply of fish from these sources but has also increased the health hazard from the consumption of that supply which remains. The FDA monitors for levels of Mirex and PCBs (polychlorinated biphenyls) in fish, and if they discover amounts above the "action or tolerance levels," they remove them from the market.

**Drinking water.** FDA and EPA share responsibility for drinking water. EPA has complete authority over drinking water supplied to the public. This authority covers all additives contained in the water. Some additives are chemicals, such as chlorine, lime and alum, used to treat water. Other additives enter water indirectly by leaching from paints and coatings, from pipes, tanks, and other equipment. Under law, EPA has the authority to set and enforce maximum contamination levels and treatment techniques for drinking water. The use of pesticides and other toxic chemicals is also regulated by EPA. FDA will continue to regulate the purity of bottled water. For this purpose bottled water is considered a "food," the purity of which is controlled under the Food, Drug, and Cosmetic Act. FDA will also retain its responsibility for water used in food and food processing.

## Fair Packaging and Labeling Act

The Fair Packaging and Labeling Act of 1966, known as the "truth in packaging" law, provides for more informative and more prominent labeling of packaged foods. The regulations concerning labeling include the following requirements: the common name of the food with appropriate descriptions, such as "whole," "sliced," "diced," or "chopped," must appear in bold type on the principal display panel; the name and address of the manufacturer, packer, and distributor must be conspicuous on the package; the net contents of the package must be stated in terms of standard measure and the number and size of servings (no misleading statements such as "giant quart" or "jumbo pound" may be used); the common names of ingredients must be listed in legible type in decreasing order of their prominence in the food.

### Nutrition labeling

All prepared and packaged foods shipped in interstate commerce after July, 1975, on which label or advertising claims are made must carry nutrition labeling. The objectives of this labeling program are to provide consumers with nutrition information about packaged foods; to assist in the nutrition education of the consumer; to encourage improvement of the nutritional content of foods; and to safeguard the nutritional value of the food supply.

Although nutritional labeling for most foods is voluntary, it must be used for all fortified and enriched foods, such as fortified milk and enriched flour. If, however, enriched flour is one of the many ingredients in a product, nutrition labeling is not mandatory. The sodium content of a food may appear on the label without full nutrient disclosure.

Formats for the nutrition label, exemplified in Table 15-1, have been standardized and must include the following:

Serving size
Servings per container
Calorie content per serving
Protein content per serving—grams
Carbohydrate content per serving—grams
Fat content per serving—grams
Percentages per serving of the US-RDA of protein, vitamin A, vitamin C, thiamin, riboflavin, niacin, calcium, and iron

Other optional nutrients may be included—vitamin D, vitamin E, vitamin $B_6$, folic acid, vitamin $B_{12}$, phosphorus, iodine, magnesium, zinc, copper, biotin, and pantothenic acid. The fatty acid composition or cholesterol content of a food or both may also appear on the label.

Several types of foods may be presented with two sets of figures. Foods, such as bread, that reliable data has established are consumed more that once a day, may carry an additional set of figures, which show the nutrients in a day's intake. A product that requires preparation in the home may carry a second column of figures showing the nutrient value of the finished product, provided that the directions for its preparation are given on the package. Table 15-2 shows the current status of food labeling and the proposed changes.

The US-RDA (see Chap. 11) was adopted as the standard reference for all nutrition labeling. As shown in Table 15-3, these standards recognize differences in protein quality by establishing two levels of recommended intakes. One recommended intake level is for protein with a protein-efficiency ratio (PER—a biological index of protein quality) less than casein; a lower recommended intake level is given for food protein sources with a PER value equal to or greater than casein. For products whose protein quality is less than 20% that of casein, the statement, "not a significant source of protein," must be inserted in place of grams per serving.

Nutritional labeling is a most valuable consumer program; however, it must be recognized that the costs of implementing, sustaining, and regulating the program are in the millions of dollars. An estimate of one cent per case of product has been suggested, and this cost has to be shared by the consumer. Thus, for the consumer to get his

### Table 15-1. Example of Nutrition Information on Cereal Package

| | *Nutrition Information per Serving** | |
| | *Corn Flakes* | |
| | *1 oz* | *with $\frac{1}{2}$ cup whole milk* |
| --- | --- | --- |
| CALORIES | 110 | 190 |
| PROTEIN | 2 g | 6 g |
| CARBOHYDRATES | 24 g | 30 g |
| FAT | 0 g | 4 g |

| | *Percentage of U.S. Recommended Daily Allowance (US-RDA)* | |
| | *Corn Flakes* | |
| | *1 oz* | *with $\frac{1}{2}$ cup whole milk* |
| --- | --- | --- |
| PROTEIN | 2 | 10 |
| VITAMIN A | 25 | 25 |
| VITAMIN C | 25 | 25 |
| THIAMIN | 25 | 25 |
| RIBOFLAVIN | 25 | 35 |
| NIACIN | 25 | 25 |
| CALCIUM | † | 15 |
| IRON | 10 | 10 |
| VITAMIN D | 10 | 25 |
| VITAMIN $B_6$ | 25 | 25 |
| FOLIC ACID | 25 | 25 |
| PHOSPHORUS | † | 10 |
| MAGNESIUM | † | 4 |

*SERVING SIZE: One ounce ($1\frac{1}{3}$ cups) corn flakes alone and in combination with $\frac{1}{2}$ cup vitamin D fortified whole milk.
SERVINGS PER CONTAINER: 12

†Contains less than 2% of the US-RDA of these nutrients.

(Cereal Institute, Inc.)

## Table 15-2. The Food Labeling Picture at a Glance

| | *Current Status* | *Proposed Change* |
|---|---|---|
| *Ingredient List* | Not all ingredients are required to be listed on standardized foods, *i.e.*, foods for which a basic "recipe" has been established. If "optional" ingredients are used, FDA can require that they be listed. | Request legislation to require that mandatory ingredients in standardized foods be declared on product labels. |
| *Colors, Spices, Flavors* | Colors, spices, and flavors do not have to be listed on labels by specific name. Artificial color may be used in butter, cheese, or ice cream without listing it on the label. | Require food labels to carry specific names of all colors and spices and of flavors that are known to cause health problems, such as allergies. |
| *Quantity of Ingredients* | All ingredients in a food must be listed on labels in descending order of predominance by weight, but are not required to be stated as percentages. However, labels can be required to list the percentage of some "characterizing" ingredients, such as shrimp in shrimp cocktail. | Expand use of percentage labeling of characterizing ingredients. Also seek explicit authority to require quantitative ingredient labeling and authority to examine a company's formulas and records to ensure that labeling is truthful and accurate. |
| *Order of Predominance* | FDA and USDA require the ingredients be listed on food labels in descending order of predominance, but many consumers are unaware of this fact. | Require a label statement that ingredients are listed in descending order of predominance. (Some manufacturers have voluntarily done this.) |
| *Fats and Oils* | A processor is sometimes allowed to use the term "and/or" when one or more fat or oil ingredient is used in a food product. This means that the name of any fat or oil present must be used, but a fat or oil not actually present in a food can also be named in the ingredient list. For foods in which fats or oils constitute the predominant ingredient, the specific fat or oil ingredient used in the food must be declared in descending order of predominance. | Permit foods containing less than 10% total fat (dry weight basis) to continue to use the flexible "and/or" labeling. For foods containing more than 10% total fat, the specific source of fat or oil used in the food must be declared. |
| *Fresh Fruits and Vegetables* | Colors, preservatives, and waxes used on fresh fruits and vegetables must be declared on placards and leaflets at the point of sale. | FDA will continue to encourage compliance with this law, but will not seek authority to impose similar requirements for pesticides and fertilizers as was suggested. |
| *Nutrition Labeling* | Nutrition labeling is required when nutrients are added to a food or nutrition claims are made. Otherwise nutrition labeling is voluntary. | FDA and USDA will seek legislation to expand their authority to require nutrition labeling on more foods. |
| *Nutrition Format* | Nutrition information on the label must be accurate and conform to a prescribed format, which includes listing the serving size, the number of servings in the container, the amount of calories, protein, carbohydrates, and fat per serving, the "U.S. Recommended Daily Allowances" and protein and seven specific vitamins and minerals. | Determine what changes, if any, consumers want, and encourage the industry to experiment, in collaboration with FDA and USDA, with graphic and other formats. |
| *Serving Sizes* | Nutrition information is expressed on a per serving basis. The label specifies size of serving (cups, ounces, spoonfuls)—but these sizes are not uniform within a product class. | FDA will publish serving size regulations for some beverage products, cereals, and meal replacements. Regulations will also be proposed for classes and types of foods. FDA will publish uniform serving sizes for additional foods for the purpose of nutrition labeling. |
| *Sugars* | FDA has jurisdiction over most sugar-sweetened products, but lacks authority to require quantitative labeling of sugars on all foods. | Require disclosure of total sugars content of a product as part of nutrition labeling when contained above a specified level. Seek authority to require sugars content labeling on the basis of public health considerations. |

## Table 15-2.  The Food Labeling Picture at a Glance (Continued)

| | *Current Status* | *Proposed Change* |
|---|---|---|
| *Sodium (Salt) and Potassium* | Sodium content labeling is optional unless a claim is made about sodium content, in which case the label must list sodium content per 100 g and per serving. | Require quantitative labeling of sodium and potassium as part of the nutrition label. Seek authority to require declaration of sodium and potassium on the basis of public health significance. |
| *Fatty Acid and Cholesterol* | Fatty acid and cholesterol content is optional in nutrition labeling. If any claims are made concerning these substances the information becomes mandatory. | Require fatty acid labeling whenever cholesterol is declared or vice versa. Seek authority to require cholesterol/fatty acid content labeling on the basis of public health significance. |
| *Open Date Labeling* | Open dating (date when food was packaged or should be sold or used) is voluntary under Federal law, but required by some State and local governments. | Seek legislation to require open dating on classes of foods as is found necessary. Study various kinds of open dating and formats and legislative approaches. |
| *Imitation and Substitute Foods* | A new food that is similar to and substitutes for an existing food does not have to be called "imitation" if it is not nutritionally inferior to the original product. This policy permits manufacturers flexibility in developing foods that may be substituted for a traditional or standardized food while maintaining the food's nutritional quality. | This policy, though basically sound, is recognized to have some drawbacks. Public comment is sought on other approaches. |
| *Food Fortification* | FDA has limited control over food fortification, namely, the addition of nutrients to foods. | Seek legislation for explicit discretionary authority to control the fortification of food when deemed necessary. |
| *"Natural" and "Organic" Claims* | FDA does not attempt to control claims that foods are "natural" or "organic" because it believes such terms are too variously defined. USDA does not permit use of "natural" and "organic" claims on the labels of meat, poultry, and egg products. FTC is developing rules designed to set standards for using these terms in advertising. | FDA and USDA agree with FTC that claims that foods described as "natural" and "organic" are inherently superior in their nutrient content or safety should be prohibited because they are false and misleading. The agencies are evaluating FTC rulemaking efforts in this field. |

(FDA CONSUMER February, 1980)

money's worth from nutrition labeling, a large-scale educational program was introduced. All nutrition educators share responsibility for assisting the consumer in understanding and using the information provided. At the present time many fresh foods do not contain nutrition labeling so that an equal amount of emphasis by the nutrition educator must be placed on the nutritive values of these foods if the homemaker is to select an adequate diet for the family.

### Foods for special dietary uses

Any food intended to be used for special dietary needs must be labeled with all the information concerning its nutrient content and other dietary properties that FDA regulations require; in this way, the label must inform consumers of the food's value for such purposes, or it will be classed as mislabeled. Food for special dietary use may be classed as follows: supplying a special dietary need that exists because of a physical, physiological, pathologic or other condition, such as disease, convalescence, pregnancy, lactation, infancy, allergic hypersensitivity to food,

underweight, or the need to control intake of sodium; supplying a vitamin, mineral, or other ingredient to supplement the diet by increasing the total dietary intake; or supplying a special dietary need due to its use as the sole item of the diet. Regulations under this section prescribe the nutrients for infant formulas. Food labeled *low-calorie* and *reduced calorie* must meet precise standards. Low-calorie foods must contain no more than 40 calories per serving. To be labeled reduced calorie a food must be at least one-third lower in calories than a similar food in which the calories have not been reduced. Reduced calorie foods must not be nutritionally inferior to their full-calorie equivalent foods.

### Other laws administered by the Food and Drug Administration

The Radiation Control for Health and Safety Act

The Radiation Control for Health and Safety Act protects the public from unnecessary exposure to radiation from medical x-ray and electronic products, such as microwave ovens.

### The Public Health Service Act

The Public Health Service Act regulates the sanitary practices of interstate carriers and provides for a sanitation program to control public health problems associated with the production, processing, and distribution of products by the food service, milk, and shellfish industry.

### The Tea Importation Act

The Tea Importation Act regulates the quality of imported tea.

### The Milk Import Act

The Milk Import Act demands certification that imported milk products meet United States' requirements.

## Federal Trade Commission

False advertising of foods, drugs, and cosmetics through media, such as television and radio, is under the jurisdiction not of the FDA but the Federal Trade Commission (FTC). The FTC has been investigating and attempting to set regulations for the advertising of certain foods on children's television programs.

## U.S. Department of Agriculture

### Federal Meat Inspection Act

Through the Bureau of Animal Industry (BAI), the Secretary of Agriculture administers regulations concerning the meat industry. Formerly, laws provided for the inspection of all cattle, sheep, swine, and goats slaughtered for transportation or sale as articles of interstate or foreign commerce. A law passed in late 1967 provides for similar inspection and regulation of all meats sold for human consumption anywhere in the United States. The carcasses and parts of all such animals found to be sound, healthful, wholesome, and fit for human food are stamped "Inspected and Passed." Animals found to be unfit for human food are separated and stamped "Inspected and Condemned." Carcasses that have been condemned for food purposes must be destroyed under the supervision of a federal inspector.

The Secretary of Agriculture also enforces the regulations concerning imported and exported meat and meat products, as well as those concerning the labeling of horsemeat. Horsemeat may be used for human food, but strict labeling is required to prevent its use as a substitute for beef.

## Table 15-3. U.S. Recommended Daily Allowances (US-RDAs) for Essential Nutrients

|  | Infants Birth to 12 Months (Tentative) | Children Under 4 Years of Age | Adults and Children 4 or More Years of Age | Pregnant or Lactating Women |
|---|---|---|---|---|
| *Nutrients that MUST be declared on the label\** | | | | |
| Protein, "low quality protein" (g) | 28 | 65 | 65 | 65 |
| Protein, "high quality protein" (g) | 20 | 45 | 45 | 45 |
| Protein, "proteins in general" (g) | 28 | 65 | 65 | 65 |
| Vitamin A (IU) | 1500 | 2500 | 5000 | 8000 |
| Vitamin C (ascorbic acid) (mg) | 35 | 40 | 60 | 60 |
| Thiamin (vitamin $B_1$) (mg) | 0.5 | 0.7 | 1.5 | 1.7 |
| Riboflavin (vitamin $B_2$) (mg) | 0.6 | 0.8 | 1.7 | 2.0 |
| Niacin (mg) | 8 | 9 | 20 | 20 |
| Calcium (g) | 0.6 | 0.8 | 1.0 | 1.3 |
| Iron (mg) | 15 | 10 | 18 | 18 |
| *Nutrients that MAY be declared on the label* | | | | |
| Vitamin D (IU) | 400 | 400 | 400 | 400 |
| Vitamin E (IU) | 5 | 10 | 30 | 30 |
| Vitamin $B_6$ (mg) | 0.4 | 0.7 | 2.0 | 2.5 |
| Folic acid (Folacin) (mg) | 0.1 | 0.2 | 0.4 | 0.8 |
| Vitamin $B_{12}$ (mcg) | 2 | 3 | 6 | 8 |
| Phosphorus (g) | 0.5 | 0.8 | 1.0 | 1.3 |
| Iodine (mcg) | 45 | 70 | 150 | 150 |
| Magnesium (mg) | 70 | 200 | 400 | 450 |
| Zinc (mg) | 5 | 8 | 15 | 15 |
| Copper (mg) | 0.6 | 1 | 2 | 2 |
| Biotin (mg) | 0.05 | 0.15 | 0.3 | 0.3 |
| Pantothenic acid (mg) | 3 | 5 | 10 | 10 |

\*Whenever nutrition labeling is required.

A law passed in 1957 provides for compulsory inspection of poultry and poultry products and is similar in nature to the Meat Inspection Act.

## USDA grade standards and inspection service for processed foods

The Fruit and Vegetable Division of the Agricultural Marketing Service, United States Department of Agriculture, develops grade standards for processed foods and supplies an inspection service for processed fruits, vegetables, and related foods.

The federal grading of foods aids in informing processors, sellers, brokers, distributors, and buyers about the class, the quality, and the condition of the product. The grades serve as a basis for arriving at the value of a product for securing a loan, payment of damages, or sale of the product.

## State regulations

It is the responsibility of the states to regulate food production and processing of certain products that do not leave the state. The state also controls such aspects as pasteurization of milk, inspection of cattle and goats for brucellosis and tuberculosis, and regulations concerning the sale of margarine. Many state food regulations are similar to the federal regulations, but others may prohibit some things which are allowed by federal law. Food processors must satisfy the regulations of the state in which they operate and the states in which the food is sold, as well as the federal regulations. Oregon was the first state to adopt regulations defining organic foods. In New York, mandatory unit pricing of most food items sold in large-volume retail stores began in 1975.

Local municipal sanitary codes may also regulate food production and processing to the extent that they may be more restrictive than state or federal codes, but not less so.

## Study questions and activities

1. List three techniques that are used in scientific farming to increase food production. How is the safety of these methods regulated to protect the consumer?
2. Which foodborne bacteria, carried most often in eggs or poultry, have been responsible for recent outbreaks of gastrointestinal disease?
3. What disease carried by water, milk, or food is due to a virus? How long after exposure may it take to develop?
4. Name some of the activities of the FDA stemming from the Federal Food, Drug and Cosmetic Act.
5. What is meant by standards of identity? What implications are there for the nutrition counselor in relation to labeling and standards of identity?
6. What types of food additives may be considered "intentional"? Why are they used and how are they controlled?
7. How would you answer someone who questioned the safety of the many additives foods contain today? Of the use of pesticides and the danger of traces of these being present in food?
8. What labeling procedures must be followed as a result of the "truth in packaging" law?
9. What is nutrition labeling? What is the standard reference for nutrition labeling?

## References

1. Mehrlich FP: Protecting Our Food. In Yearbook of Agriculture, p 204. Washington, DC, USDA, 1966
2. Labuza TP: Food Tech 27:20, 1973
3. Werrin M, Kronick DA: Am J Nurs 65:528, 1965
4. Reimann H, Bryan FL (eds): Food-borne Infections and Intoxications. New York, Academic Press, 1979
5. Note: Nutr Rev 25:94, 1967
6. Corwin E: FDA Consumer 14:4, Feb, 1980
7. Wright CV: Public Health Rep 77:628, 1962

## Supplementary readings

Coon JM: Natural food toxicants—A perspective. Nutr Rev 32:321, 1974

Eyl TB: Alkyl mercury contamination of foods. JAMA 215:287, 1971

Food and Drug Administration: Fact Sheets (available from FDA consumer representative). Washington, DC, DHHS

Hodges RE: The toxicity of pesticides and their residues in food. Nutr Rev 23:225, 1965

Lehmann P: More than you ever thought you would know about food additives. Part I. FDA Consumer 13:10, Apr, 1979; Part II, FDA Consumer 13:18, May, 1979; Part III, FDA Consumer 13:12, June, 1979

Moore JL, Wendt PF: Nutrition labeling—A summary and evaluation. J Nutr Educ 5:121, 1973

Public Health Service, DHEW: You Can Prevent Foodborne Illness. Folder, 1967, Hot Tips on Food Protection. Folder, 1966. United States Government Printing Office, Washington, DC 20201

Pyke M: Food technology and society. Nutr Rev 28:31, 1970

Requirements of Laws and Regulations Enforced by the U.S. Food and Drug Administration. DHEW PHS-FDA Publ. No. (FDA) 79-1042. Washington, DC, Superintendent of Documents, United States Government Printing Office, 1979

Scientific Status Summary by the Institute of Food Technologists' Expert Panel on Food Safety and Nutrition. Chicago. Botulism, 1972; Mercury in food, 1973; Nitrites, nitrates, and nitrosamines in food—a dilemma, 1972; Nutrition labeling, 1973

Stephenson, M: Making food labels more informative. FDA Consumer 9:13, October 1975

*For further references see Bibliography in Part 4.*

# Application of Nutrition to Critical Periods Throughout the Life Span

# Part 2

# Growth and Development

## 16

## Relationship of nutrition to the growth process

The terms, *growth* and *development*, imply all the complex physiological changes that take place during conception (when a single-celled ovum is fertilized by a single sperm), during embryogenesis (as cells divide and differentiate to form the structures of the fetus), and during fetal life (as growth and maturation of the fetus occur). These terms also apply to the complex physiological, psychological, and sociological changes that take place during infancy, throughout childhood and adolescence, and into young adulthood.

Growth and development depend on both the genetic or hereditary background of the individual and the physical and cultural environment into which he is born. The food that provides the nutrients required for physical growth is one environmental factor essential for growth and development, whereas the feeding process itself, at least during infancy and childhood, is an integral part of psychosocial development. A poor environment—for example, one providing inadequate nutrition—can prevent a child from reaching his full genetic potential, not only in physical size and strength but also, according to all indications of contemporary research, in mental development as well.

### Growth

Growth occurs continuously from conception to full maturity, but it is not a uniform process. It consists of two periods of rapid growth separated by a period of more or less uniform but slower increase in size. The first period of rapid growth occurs in fetal life and early infancy and the second during adolescence.

Physical growth may be defined as an increase in the size of a person as measured by changes in weight or height or both. It is an exceedingly complicated process brought about by an increase in the number of cells as a result of cell division and by the enlarging of the size of cells from increases in their protein content. Winick discusses four phases of normal growth.

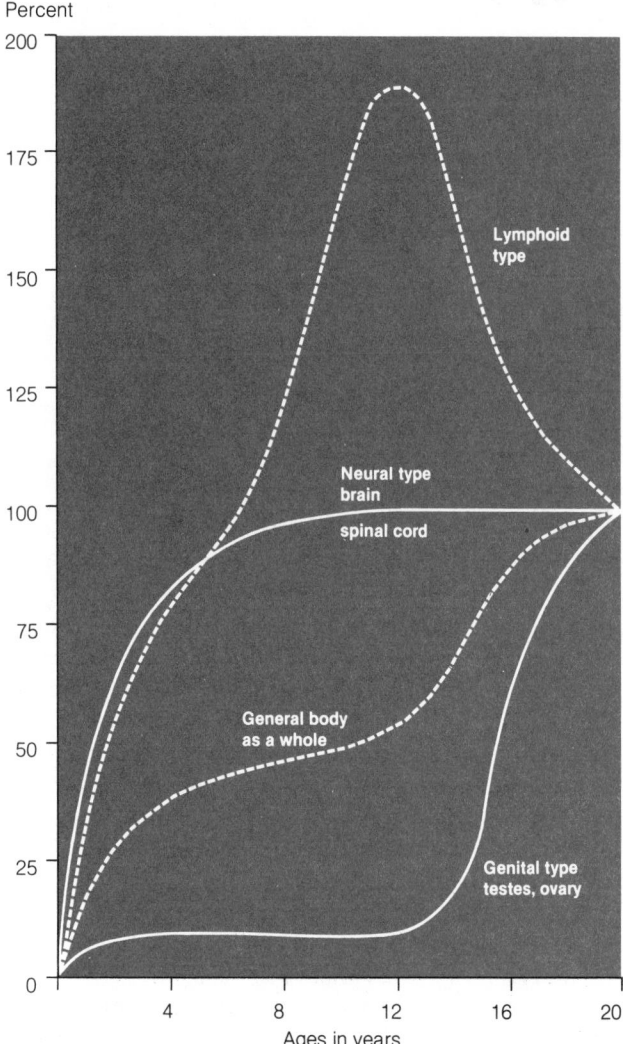

**Fig. 16-1.**   Growth of various body tissues. (Scammon RE: The Measurement of Man. Minneapolis, University of Minnesota Press)

1. Hyperplasia—rapid cell division with cell size remaining constant. The cell number is determined by measuring the total amount of DNA in an organ and dividing it by the DNA content per diploid cell for the particular species (6.0 picograms (pg) in the human).
2. Hypertrophy—an increase in cell size accompanied by a slowing down of cell division. Cell size increases due to an increase in protein content. The average weight per cell or protein content per cell is determined by weighing the organ or by determining its total protein content and then dividing by the number of cells.
3. Cessation of cell division while individual cells continue to grow from increased protein content.
4. Cessation of growth (maturity) as protein synthesis and degradation come into equilibrium.[1]

Both animal research and limited studies of humans have shown that different organs are at various phases of growth at different times. However, during prenatal life

and for variable periods into postnatal life, all organs are undergoing cell division. Growth by cell division in the human brain begins to slow down at birth but continues until about 10 months of age. Hypertrophy, increase in size of cells, continues after hyperplasia ceases, and in humans the brain growth spurt continues until at least the second birthday. (The relationship of nutrition to mental development is discussed later in this chapter.) Nerve and lymphoid tissue grow most rapidly in the early years, the body as a whole more slowly; genital tissues remain almost dormant until puberty. Figure 16-1 shows the different rates of growth for various body tissues.

Due to the differential growth of various body parts, there are changes in body proportions during growth. Figure 16-2 shows the increases in size of the different portions of the body from birth to maturity.

Obesity in adults may well be related to these phases of growth. There is evidence that infants who are overnourished at the stage when adipose tissue cells are rapidly increasing accumulate more fat cells in their bodies than infants whose weight gain is more carefully controlled. It is believed that this excess of adipose tissue cells persists throughout life with, of course, persistent problems of overweight.[2,3] Infant feeding is discussed in Chapter 18.

For this reason, the nutrition counselor should recognize, when working with mothers, that undernutrition or overnutrition during the critical phases of growth for an organ can affect the ultimate number of cells in that organ, and this, in turn, may have permanent effects on its function. If undernutrition or overnutrition occurs at a later phase of growth, the size of the organ may be temporarily smaller or larger but returns to normal when the nutritional needs of the individual are met.

### Development

Development or maturation refers to the progressive increase in the capacity to function both physically and mentally and is closely associated with growth. Changes in body composition and biochemical function occur in the process of development. The body's nitrogen, calcium, and phosphorus content increases proportionately more than total body size. The concentration of iron in the newborn is higher than that in the adult. Water concentration decreases throughout gestation and after birth, whereas the concentration of fat increases in the latter part of pregnancy and after birth. Changes in enzyme activity also occur as part of biochemical maturation. The growth process or growth cycle as it is used in this chapter refers also to development.

### The growth cycle
#### Fetal growth during pregnancy

During the first 2 months of pregnancy when the cells for the various organs and for the arms, legs, eyes, and ears are differentiating, the growth rate is relatively slow, and the quantitative nutritional demands are small.

*Qualitatively*, however, they are extremely important. Animal research indicates that severe malnutrition during embryonic development can produce spontaneous abortions or congenital abnormalities in the newborn. Although these findings have not been proven in humans, there remains the implication that, because this critical period occurs at an earlier stage in pregnancy than when most women seek medical advice, it is most desirable for young women to acquire good dietary habits before pregnancy.

The next 7 months of pregnancy are often referred to as the growth period because the weight of the fetus increases 500-fold, from about 6 g at 9 weeks to approximately 3500 g at birth. Skeletal development begins during the second month of intrauterine life and continues after birth until the end of puberty. Fatty tissue begins to build up by the sixth month. A maternal weight gain of about $1/2$ to 1 lb per week is normal during the last two trimesters of gestation. Inadequate nutrition of the fetus during this time may result in stillbirths, prematurity, or small-for-date babies. This period of growth, due to its greater nutritional demands, is more sensitive to *quantitative* nutritional inadequacies than the earlier period of differentiation.[4]

Throughout the course of pregnancy there is also growth of the maternal tissue. About half of the weight gained during a normal pregnancy represents increases in the mother's tissues—growth of tissues in the uterus, the breasts, and maternal stores. Nutritional needs during pregnancy are discussed in Chapter 17.

## Infancy—growth and development during the first year

Rapid cell division continues into the postnatal period for varying amounts of time for different organs. During the early months of life growth is more rapid than at any other time. Infants double their birth weight in about 5 to 6 months. After that their weekly gain is slower—4 to 5 oz—for the rest of the year, and they will usually triple the birth weight by the end of the first year.

The infant grows in length, from 20 in to 22 in at birth to 30 in to 32 in by the end of a year. At birth the head is large in proportion to the rest of the body and continues to grow. This is the time when the brain and nervous system are developing rapidly, and during this period a supply of essential nutrients is crucial for normal mental development.

The gastrointestinal system of a fullterm infant can digest protein, emulsified fats, and simple carbohydrates.

The body of the newborn infant contains a higher proportion of water than that of older children. The muscles are poorly developed, and although the amount of subcutaneous fat is limited, it increases during the first year. The skeleton is not fully calcified, and there is a high percentage of cartilage. Girls have a greater skeletal maturity at birth than boys by about 1 month. A fullterm infant has a store of iron and a high hemoglobin level—nature's

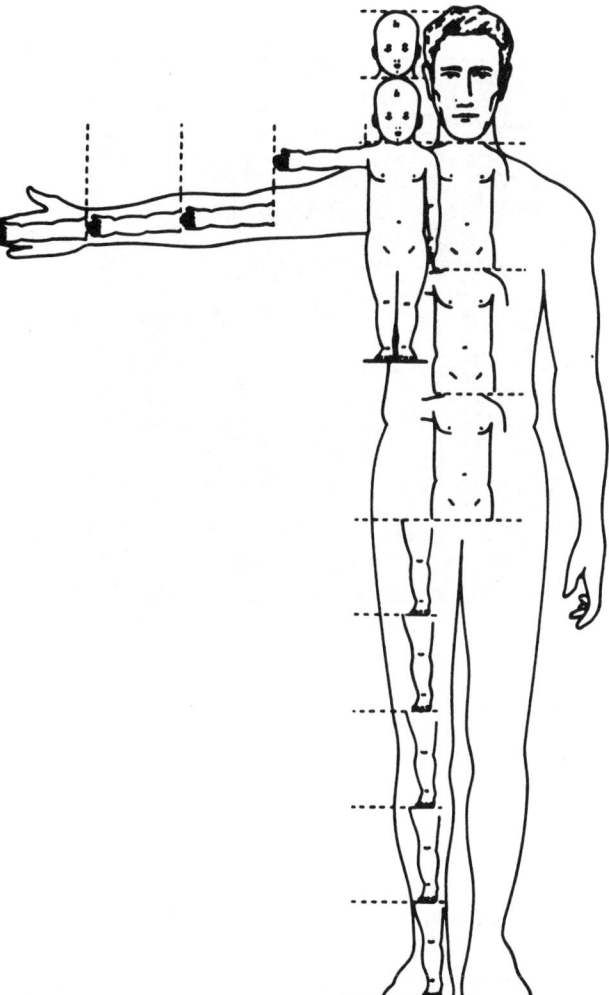

**Fig. 16-2.** Differential growth of different portions of the body. (Valadian I, Porter D: Physical Growth and Development. Boston, Little, Brown and Co.)

way of providing for the early months on milk, which is low in iron. The iron stores are gradually depleted, however, unless either the milk is supplemented with iron in some form or iron-rich foods are added 4 to 6 months after birth (see Chap. 18).

## Preschool and school age growth (one to nine years)

Growth during the second year of life slows down, and a weight gain of 8 lb to 10 lb is considered average. For example, infants who triple their weight during the first year will be approximately four times their birth weight at the end of 2 years. From about 2 to 9 years the average annual weight gain is approximately 5 lb.

Annual increments in height gradually decrease from birth to maturity except during the period of the adolescent growth spurt. Birth length is usually doubled by 4 years. The average gain is about $2\frac{1}{2}$ in per year until adolescence.

Body composition changes during childhood; baby fat disappears at the same time that muscles increase in

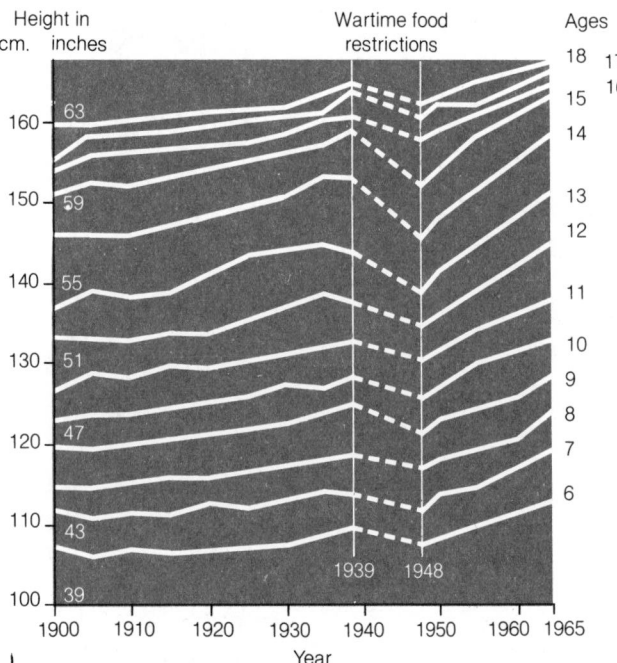

**Fig. 16-3.** Secular changes in the height of Japanese boys of school age, 1900–1965. (Japanese Ministry of Education Report for 1965. Tokyo, 1965)

size and bones harden. Body proportions also become more like the adult form as legs lengthen at a rapid rate while head growth decelerates (Fig. 16-2). Motor coordination progresses at a fast rate, as does intellectual development.

### The adolescent growth spurt

It is during adolescence that the second very rapid growth period occurs. This is usually between the ages of 10½ and 13 for girls and 13 and 16 for boys, although it may be sooner for early-maturing children and somewhat later for late-maturing children. Girls grow approximately 3 in per year, whereas boys may grow as much as 4 in per year during the growth spurt. From ages 13 to 16 years girls continue to grow but at a much slower rate. In contrast, boys' growth rate declines less rapidly and they continue to grow until the late teens.

The growth spurts occur in all directions—in length and weight of bones, in muscle mass, in the laying down of body fat in the soft tissues, in the widening of the shoulders in boys and the broadening of the hips in girls, and in the accelerated growth of genital tissue. Hands and feet are usually the first to grow, followed by hips, chest, and shoulders. By age 10 girls will have undergone a fivefold increase in muscle cell number; further increase in either number or size will be small. Boys, in contrast, at age 18 will have 14 times as many muscle cells as at birth, and they may continue to increase in size for another 5

years.[5] Girls will have increasingly greater proportions of fat. Increases in height due to lengthening of the long bones, particularly the femur and tibia, occur until the epiphyses of the bones close at the end of puberty.

When the nutrients supplied by the bloodstream are inadequate to permit optimum growth of these long bones, merely shorter stature may be found without obvious signs of malnutrition. Protein is essential for the formation of the new cartilage cells in the epiphysis of the long bones, which later become calcified to form bone. Evidence that the adolescent growth spurt may be slowed down by nutrient and especially protein limitation has been reported by Mitchell.[6] The changes in stature over 65 years of Japanese youth show a remarkable parallelism with the food limitations during the war years and subsequent increase in consumption of animal protein, which has more than doubled during prosperous years. Fig. 16-3, showing the changes in stature in Japanese boys over a period of 65 years (including World War II and later), suggests that teenagers are more susceptible than younger children to limitations and more responsive to postwar improvements in food. The response of girls was similar but not quite as striking. The commonly accepted association of calcium with bone growth needs to be supplemented by the need for good quality protein for the lengthening of bone before calcification occurs.

Biologic age at this period is a much better guide to growth and development than chronologic age. The total period of rapid adolescent growth seldom lasts more than 2 or 3 years, when adult build and stature are reached. However, growth in skeletal muscle mass continues. A further "lengthening out" may occur in both men and women up to age 30. Garn and Wagner point out that, "In a growth sense, adolescence does not terminate with college entrance but continues well beyond, to age 25 to 30 for muscle mass, to age 30 for stature, to age 30 to 40 for skeletal mass, and life long for skeletal volume."[7]

Physical growth is usually measured by changes in height and weight with age. Stature is the more significant criterion because variations in build and the amount of adipose tissue may cause wide variations in weight. However, Cheek and co-workers report that the growth of adipose tissue in normal children is so predictable and uniform that weight can be a good measure of "metabolic size" in boys and girls from 5 to 17 years.[8] Development other than physical growth is more difficult to measure: it deals with muscle strength and coordination, with mental health, and with adaptations and attitudes.

## Nutrition in brain development and behavior

One of the most interesting and dramatic aspects of nutrition today is its relationship to central nervous system development. Evidence indicates a close relationship between energy-protein malnutrition and impaired brain growth and development, but the role of nutrition *per se* in behavior and cognitive development has not been clearly defined.

The brain and central nervous system grow rapidly from the end of the second trimester of pregnancy into the second year of postnatal life. During the growth spurt the brain weight is increasing at its highest rate, and other developmental processes are rapidly occurring. At birth the infant's brain has approximately 75% of the adult number of brain cells. Different regions of the brain, each made up of their characteristic cell types and each controlling different functions, show their own specific cell division growth patterns. Nerve cells (neurons) and glial cells are the chief cellular constituents of the brain. Multiplication of the neurons occurs first. This is followed by the elaboration of synaptic connections between nerve cells, glial cell multiplication, and nerve myelination.[9] In addition, for normal brain function the neurons must also be able to synthesize and release neurotransmitter molecules (Fig. 16-4). *Neurotransmitters*, such as serotonin and acetylcholine, relay impulses among neurons that have no direct contact with one another. They are the chemical links by which nerve cells communicate with each other. As a result, along with increase in size there is a continuous complex evolution of the anatomy, biochemistry, and physiology of the brain. By the time a child is 4 years old, some 90% of the brain has been formed. The formation and functioning of the brain and nerve fibers and the laying down of the myelin sheath demand that adequate nutrients be available at this critical period.[10]

During the early formative years as the brain acquires each new specific function it integrates the process into its total pattern of performance and experience. Experimental evidence suggests that the timing of this overall procedure is of utmost importance. Each new function seems to make its appearance chronologically at a critical period of development. Therefore, any disruption of the normal sequence may result in limitation of the capacity of the brain in some specific ability. This damage may not be evident immediately but may show up at a later age.

Studies of the brains of young children who have died of malnutrition and others who died accidentally indicate that severe malnutrition during early life can result in reduced numbers of brain cells in malnourished infants compared with normal children.[11]

Winick suggests three different effects of malnutrition on brain growth depending on when it occurs.

1. Marked reduction in brain cell number when fetal malnutrition (low-birth-weight infants) and severe malnutrition during the first year of life occur
2. Moderate reduction in brain cell numbers as a result of severe malnutrition during the first year in normal-birth-weight infants
3. No reduction in brain cell numbers when malnutrition occurs after the first year, but possible reduction in cell size[12]

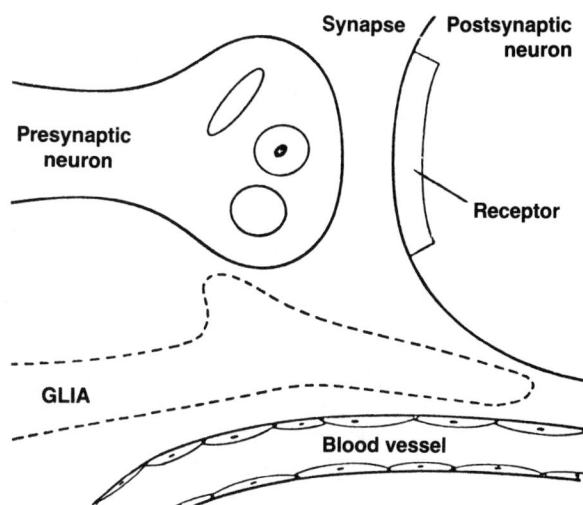

**Fig. 16-4.** Schematic diagram illustrating a typical synapse in the mammalian central nervous system. Choline circulating in the blood vessel is transported into or out of the brain by a low-affinity uptake system located within the blood-brain barrier (in the endothelia of the central nervous system capillaries). Choline then enters the extracellular space of the brain, where it can be taken up probably by all cells (for use in synthesizing membrane lecithins). A portion diffuses into the synaptic cleft and is taken up by high- and low-affinity systems in terminals of presynaptic neurons, where it is converted to acetylcholine through the catalytic action of the enzyme choline acetyltransferase (CAT). The acetylcholine may be stored in synaptic vesicles or, perhaps, in association with a cytoplasmic macromolecule. When the presynaptic neuron becomes depolarized, it releases acetylcholine into the synaptic cleft; a portion of these molecules reaches receptor sites on post-synaptic neurons, whereas other portions are inactivated by hydrolysis, catalyzed by the enzyme acetylcholinesterase. (From Nutrition Reviews 37:130, 1979)

Early malnutrition has also been found to reduce the total number of synapses and the number of synapses per neuron. It should also be pointed out that environmental factors, such as sensory stimulation, can also influence synaptic numbers.[13] Similarly, the rate of myelin formation and numerous biochemical features of the nervous system are altered by early malnutrition.

Recent research has demonstrated that the ability of the brain neurons to make and release certain neurotransmitters is dependent on the concentration of certain nutrients in the blood and, therefore, on the composition of the diet. The rate at which neurons synthesize the neurotransmitter, serotonin, is dependent on the level in the brain of the essential amino acid, tryptophan, its precursor.[14] Similarly, the synthesis of acetylcholine is accelerated by increasing the level in the brain of its precursor, choline.[15] More recent studies show that the production and release of other neurotransmitters, dopamine and norepinephrine, can also be influenced by the level of their dietary precursor, the amino acid tyrosine.[16] Clinical application of these findings are being tested in the treatment of brain diseases.[17]

The significance of the various brain abnormalities and their effects on brain function are not clearly understood. A report of the National Research Council summarizes the "possible modes of interference with learning and behavior by malnutrition" as follows:

First, abnormalities of morphologic, biochemical, and/or physiological characteristics may so alter normal brain function as to reduce learning abilities. Secondly, the developmental process may be impaired by decreased exposure and responsiveness to environmental stimuli during critical periods when essential sequences of experience must be acquired to provide for continued orderly development. Third, the learning process may be disrupted by adverse changes in personality, emotionality, and behavior of the child. These changes may interfere with the interpersonal relationships that are necessary for learning experience. Furthermore, malnutrition among the persons in social contact with the child may militate against their providing adequate learning experience.[18]

Thus, the relationship between malnutrition and mental development in humans is extremely complicated because the environment of poverty in which we find severe malnutrition is almost always lacking in those other characteristics that are also important for a child to reach full mental potential. The disadvantaged child is therefore at high risk not only for limited physical growth but also for psychosocial and cognitive development.

Ricciuti summarizes the current understanding of the relationship between malnutrition and cognitive development as follows:

When the concern about malnutrition as a possible major cause of mental retardation reached a peak in the late 1960s and early 1970s, it was assumed by many that the brain changes produced by malnutrition led directly to an impairment of learning ability and thus to retarded intellectual development. However, on the basis of results obtained in human as well as animal research since that time most investigators tend to discard this view in favor of the hypothesis that malnutrition may exert its major influence on behavioral competencies through dysfunctional changes in attention, responsiveness, motivation, and emotionality rather than through a more direct impairment of the basic ability to learn. In short, the malnourished child's interaction with its environment may be altered in ways that make him less likely to seek out, utilize, and respond to opportunities for learning and social interaction available in his environment. This state of events would imply hopeful prospects for reversibility or remediation, since it should be possible to manipulate the environment so as to make the child's interaction with it more intellectually facilitative. . . .[19]

As more and more types of intervention programs for the young child are initiated, particularly in infant and child care centers, it is important that the total growth process of the child be considered by those responsible for program planning.[20] Equal emphasis and attention must be given to the physical, emotional, social, and intellectual development of the infant and child. All who are involved in the physical care of infants should understand the intimate relationship between the various components of the developmental process. Cuddling, smiling, and talking to the baby while he is being fed a nutritionally adequate diet all contribute to his total development.

## Study questions and activities

1. What is meant by physical growth? How is it accomplished?
2. What are the phases of growth? How do these relate to brain size? to obesity?
3. When do the two periods of most rapid growth occur? At what age does muscle mass growth cease?
4. What are the differences in nutritional demands during the two stages of pregnancy—differentiation and growth? What are the effects if these demands are not met?
5. What effect does severe malnutrition during infancy have on brain growth?
6. What are neurotransmitters? How are they influenced by dietary components?
7. What kinds of growth occur during adolescence?

## References

1. Winick M: Malnutrition and Brain Development. New York, Oxford University Press, 1976
2. Hirsch J, Knittle JL: Fed Proc 29:1516, 1970
3. Eid EE: Br Med J 2:74, 1970
4. Giroud A: The Nutrition of the Embryo. Springfield, IL, Charles C Thomas, 1970
5. How Children Grow. NIH-PHS DHEW Publ. No. (NIH) 73-166. Washington, DC, 1973
6. Mitchell HS: J Am Diet Assoc 44:165, 1964
7. Garn SM, Wagner B: The adolescent growth of the skeletal mass and its implications to mineral requirements. In Heald F (ed): Adolescent Nutrition and Growth, pp 139–161. New York, Appleton-Century-Crofts, 1969
8. Cheek DB et al: Body composition: anthropometric growth and heat production. In Heald F (ed): Adolescent Nutrition and Growth, pp 163–176. New York, Appleton-Century-Crofts, 1969
9. Nutr Rev 33:6, 1975
10. Coursin DB: Undernutrition and brain function. Borden's Rev Nutr Res 26:1, 1965
11. Rosso P, Hormazabal J, Winick M: Am J Clin Nutr 23:1275, 1970
12. Winick M: Med Clin North Am 17:69, 1970
13. Dyson SE, Jones DG: Prog Neurobiol 7:171, 1976
14. Wurtman RJ, Fernstrom JD: Nutr Rev 32:193, 1974
15. Growdon JH, Wurtman RJ: Nutr Rev 37:129, 1979
16. Carlsson A, Lindguist M: Arch Pharm 303:157, 1978
17. Growdon JH: In Wurtman RJ, Wurtman JJ (eds): Nutrition and the Brain, Vol 3, pp 117–170. New York, Raven Press, 1979

18. Food and Nutrition Board: The Relationship of Nutrition to Brain Development and Behavior. Washington, DC, NAS-NRC, 1973

19. Ricciuti HN: In Brozek J (ed): Behavioral Effects of Energy and Protein Deficits. DHEW Publ. No. (NIH) 79-1906, Washington, DC, 1979

20. Dibble MV, Lally JR: J Nutr Educ 5:200, 1973

## Supplementary readings

Beal V: Nutrition in the Life Span. New York, John Wiley & Sons, 1980

Brozek J (ed): Behavioral Effects of Energy and Protein Deficits. DHEW Publ. No. (NIH) 79-1906, Washington, DC, 1979

Brozek J: Nutrition, malnutrition and behavior. Annu Rev Psychol 29:157, 1978

Growden JH, Wurtman RJ: Nutrients and neurotransmitters. Contemp Nutr 4, No. 12:1, Dec, 1979

Hurley L: Developmental Nutrition. Englewood Cliffs, NJ, Prentice-Hall, 1980

Lowrey GH: Growth and Development of Children, 7th ed. Chicago, Yearbook, 1978

Nutrition and behavior. Dairy Council Digest 50, No. 5:25, Sept-Oct, 1979

Ricciuti HN: Adverse environmental and nutritional influences on mental development. J Am Diet Assoc 79:115, 1981

Valadian I, Porter D: Physical Growth and Development from Conception to Maturity. Boston, Little, Brown, 1977

Winick M: Malnutrition and Brain Development. New York, Oxford University Press, 1976

*For further references see Bibliography in Part 4.*

# Nutrition in Pregnancy and Lactation

# 17

## Nutritional demands of pregnancy

Pregnancy makes many demands on the prospective mother, not the least of which are her nutritional needs and those of the unborn infant. Although an undernourished mother may produce a healthy child, studies of nutrition of women during pregnancy have shown a definite relationship between the diet of the mother and the condition of the baby at birth. These studies have also shown that some of the complications of pregnancy, such as anemia, toxemia, and premature delivery, may result from a diet inadequate for the nutritional needs of the mother and the baby. Moreover, if the mother has always eaten a diet adequate in all essentials and is in good health, she has a much better chance of bearing a healthy baby than does the mother who has consistently had a poor food intake.

Epidemiologic studies show that maternal height, prepregnancy weight, and weight gain during pregnancy all influence the infant's birth weight. Tall, normal-weight women who gain an appropriate amount of weight during pregnancy give birth to heavier infants and have fewer low-birth-weight infants than short, underweight women who fail to gain enough weight during pregnancy. Thus, the mother's nutritional status before and during pregnancy is important to the outcome of pregnancy.

### The teenaged mother

In the United States there are approximately 200,000 babies born each year to teenaged mothers 17 years of age and younger. These young mothers represent a high-risk population because there are more cases of toxemia and an increased number of premature deliveries and low-birth-weight infants in this age group. It has been found that preeclampsia and essential hypertension occur more often in the white teenaged patients than in patients between 21 and 25 years of age. Weight gain over 25 lb is more common in young black girls, and anemia and essential hypertension are frequent complications in this group.

**ICEA:** International Childhood Education
  Association

The percentage of low-birth-weight babies (under 2500 g) born to young teenaged mothers is considerably higher than those born to more mature mothers. The highest percentage of low-birth-weight infants were born to nonwhite mothers under 15 years of age. Infant mortality rates are also higher for infants born to young mothers, particularly to young girls who have had repeated pregnancies.

Many of these teenage pregnancies occur out of wedlock. Society has imposed certain stigmas upon them and has developed punitive attitudes toward them. The pregnant teenager often has to drop out of school; she may be rejected by her family and may find medical care difficult to obtain. Hence, many young people do not have the guidance of a physician or a prenatal clinic early in their pregnancy, and adequate counseling often comes too late for the prevention of complications. To help solve these problems many communities have introduced health and education programs to meet the particular needs of the pregnant adolescent.

Nutritional requirements for the adolescent during pregnancy vary widely, depending on the rate of growth and stage of maturation of the expectant mother. Early-maturing girls who reach menarche at the peak of their growth spurt may conceive before their skeletal, including pelvic, maturation has been completed. Because calorie requirements parallel the growth curve (see Figs. 19-3 and 19-4), these girls have high caloric needs. Protein and calcium requirements are also high. Calorie restrictions imposed on these teenagers may not only affect the birth weight of their infants but their own adult stature. Approximately 10% to 12% of pregnant teenagers are overweight, and an equal number are underweight. Even for the obese teenager, who must meet her own nutritional demands as well as those of the fetus, normal weight gain should be allowed during pregnancy.[1] The special care that should be given to the diet plans for these young girls is discussed later in this chapter.

## Nutrition studies in pregnancy

The effect of food intake on the condition of the newborn is best illustrated by the now classic studies of Burke and her co-workers at the Harvard School of Public Health and the Boston Lying-In Hospital.[2] In a study of 284 women, it was found that those on good or excellent diets (42 mothers) had babies in good or excellent condition at birth, with only two exceptions. The mothers on fair diets (202 patients) had babies rated largely as good or fair. Those mothers on poor to very poor diets (40 patients) had babies rated as fair or poorest, with only three exceptions. The poorest infants were those who were stillborn or born prematurely, who died within 3 days of birth, who had congenital defects, or who were functionally immature.

The question sometimes is asked, "What is meant by a *poor* diet?" Such a diet is usually low in most necessary food nutrients; there may even be one food group, such as milk, entirely missing. An example is that of a young, pregnant woman, living in a housing development, whose husband leaves for work early. Usually she gets up and joins him in a cup of coffee and a piece of Danish pastry for breakfast. In the morning and again in the afternoon she visits her neighbors, at which time more pastry and coffee are consumed. Often she is not hungry at lunch, nor does she enjoy preparing food only for herself, so that frequently lunch either is skipped or takes the form of a piece of fruit. Fortunately, she may have a good dinner when her husband returns in the evening, but this is not sufficient to meet her nutritional needs, except perhaps for calories. Another woman may drink up to 15 cups of tea daily, each with 2 teaspoonfuls of sugar and, consequently, is seldom hungry for other food.

It can be seen from the foregoing that the importance of nutrition in pregnancy is poorly recognized by a large section of the population and that nutrition counselors, as well as many others in the medical field, must assume more responsibility for teaching this group better nutrition.

## Nutritional requirements

Table 17-1 shows the Recommended Dietary Allowances for girls and women at various ages with added allowances for pregnancy. The RDA varies with the weight, the age, and the activity of the woman and should be used only as a guide. See Chap. 11.

### Calories

If the physical activity of the woman remains the same during the second and third trimesters of pregnancy, an additional 300 calories daily is suggested to meet the gross energy cost of 80,000 kcal for a 9-month pregnancy. The building of new tissue in the woman, the placenta, and the fetus, an increased work load associated with the activity of the woman, and an increased basal metabolic rate contribute to increased energy needs. Nutrition intervention in the form of food supplements providing additional calories resulted in an increase of the average birth weights of infants born to malnourished mothers.[3] However, among well nourished women decreased physical activity, particularly during the third trimester, may more than compensate, to the point that no additional calories may be needed. Blackburn and Calloway state:

> If a pregnant woman's occupation involves externally paced work, such as on an assembly line or with a production quota, her energy expenditure will increase according to the increment in body weight. Left to her own inclination a pregnant woman will slow her pace so that she works at a comfortable rate; her daily energy expenditure will be greater, equal to, or less than her nonpregnant level according to the use to which she puts the excess time left after performing a fixed number of tasks.[4]

Although the pregnant adolescents in this study were extremely sedentary, many pregnant women today are employed in strenuous occupations, in addition to their household work. Many are also actively involved in the care of small children. The physician, by carefully observing weight changes, is best able to recommend necessary calorie modifications. For adequate protein utilization, energy intake should not go below 36 kcal per kilogram of pregnant body weight. In any case, the calorie increase is small, and food must be carefully chosen if the other nutrient increases are to be met while keeping the total calories within the recommended allowance.

### Protein requirement

The protein intake must be increased in pregnancy due to its specific contributions to growth and because, as a rule, a diet low in protein is lacking in other nutrients.

Studies indicate that approximately 925 g of protein are deposited in the fetus and accessory tissues of the woman. The amount increases throughout successive quarters of pregnancy as follows: 0.6 g, 1.8 g, 4.8 g, and 6.1 g per day.[5] There is also evidence that during early pregnancy protein may be stored in maternal tissue and used later when the needs for growth of the fetus are greatest. An additional allowance of 30 g of protein is therefore recommended to provide the protein that is accumulated by the fetus and accessory tissues during pregnancy.

Extra protein in the diet is supplied by additional milk, meat, poultry, fish, and eggs (Table 17-2). Skim milk, liquid or dried, can be used to increase protein without adding considerably to the total calorie intake. Inexpensive dried skim milk can be used in creamed soups and casserole dishes; 1 or 2 tablespoonfuls can also be added to regular milk to increase the protein content.

### Calcium and phosphorus requirements

The pregnant woman must be supplied with calcium and phosphorus in quantities large enough for her own needs and those of the bony framework of the growing fetus' body and for the formation of its teeth. Approximately 30 g of calcium are found in the fullterm infant, most of which (300 mg daily) is deposited during the last trimester. In addition, the mother may store calcium in

## Table 17-1. Recommended Daily Dietary Allowances for Girls and Women at Various Ages, with Added Allowances for Pregnancy

| | Recommended Daily Allowances for Nonpregnant Women | | | | Recommended Daily Allowances Added for Pregnancy |
|---|---|---|---|---|---|
| | *11–14\* Years Old* | *15–18† Years Old* | *19–22‡ Years Old* | *23–50§ Years Old* | |
| Energy (kcal) | 2200 | 2100 | 2100 | 2000 | 300 |
| Protein (g) | 46 | 46 | 44 | 44 | 30 |
| Vitamin A (mcg RE)// | 800 | 800 | 800 | 800 | 200 |
| Vitamin D (mcg)# | 10 | 10 | 7.5 | 5 | 5 |
| Vitamin E (mg $\alpha$-TE)** | 8 | 8 | 8 | 8 | 2 |
| Ascorbic acid (mg) | 50 | 60 | 60 | 60 | 20 |
| Folacin (mcg) | 400 | 400 | 400 | 400 | 400 |
| Niacin (mg NE)†† | 15 | 14 | 14 | 13 | 2 |
| Riboflavin (mg) | 1.3 | 1.3 | 1.3 | 1.2 | 0.3 |
| Thiamin (mg) | 1.1 | 1.1 | 1.1 | 1.0 | 0.4 |
| Vitamin $B_6$ (mg) | 1.8 | 2.0 | 2.0 | 2.0 | 0.6 |
| Vitamin $B_{12}$ (mcg) | 3 | 3 | 3 | 3 | 1 |
| Calcium (mg) | 1200 | 1200 | 800 | 800 | 400 |
| Phosphorus (mg) | 1200 | 1200 | 800 | 800 | 400 |
| Iodine (mcg) | 150 | 150 | 150 | 150 | 25 |
| Iron (mg) | 18 | 18 | 18 | 18 | ‡‡ |
| Magnesium (mg) | 300 | 300 | 300 | 300 | 150 |
| Zinc (mg) | 15 | 15 | 15 | 15 | 5 |

\*Weight, 46 kg; height, 157 cm.

†Weight, 55 kg; height, 163 cm.

‡Weight, 55 kg; height, 163 cm.

§Weight, 55 kg; height, 163 cm.

//Retinol equivalents. 1 retinol equivalent = 1 mcg retinol or 6 mcg beta-carotene.

#As cholecalciferol. 10 mcg = 400 IU of vitamin D.

**Alpha-tocopherol equivalents. 1 mg d-alpha-tocopherol = 1 $\alpha$-TE.

††1 NE (niacin equivalent) is equal to 1 mg niacin or 60 mg of dietary tryptophan.

‡‡It is recommended that the diet supplemented with 30 mg to 60 mg of iron per day.

(Adapted from Food and Nutrition Board: Recommended Dietary Allowances. Washington, DC, National Academy of Sciences/National Research Council, 1980)

her own body as a reserve for the high demands of lactation. An additional allowance of 0.4 g of calcium and phosphorus per day is recommended at this time. Again, a quart of milk a day will supply a large proportion of the needed calcium and phosphorus, as well as a good proportion of the necessary protein.

## Magnesium requirement

The NRC-RDA recommends an additional 150 mg of magnesium per day during pregnancy. The additional milk, meat, whole grain cereals, vegetables, and fruit can supply the extra amount.

## Iron requirement

An adequate iron supply during pregnancy is no less important than that of calcium. Besides the woman's need for iron, the developing fetus is building its own blood supply. When the baby is born its blood has a hemoglobin content of from 20 g to 22 g per 100 ml. This high level is needed in fetal life for oxygen uptake at the placenta, where oxygen is at lower pressures than it is in the lungs. Soon after birth some of the hemoglobin begins to break down until a normal level of 13 g to 14 g per 100 ml of blood is reached. The iron from the hemoglobin breakdown is stored in the infant's liver to serve as a

## Table 17-2. Suggested Pattern Dietary During Pregnancy

*Whole or skimmed milk:* 1 qt (1 oz of cheddar cheese is equivalent to 8 oz milk.)

*Lean meat, fish, poultry, eggs, dried peas, beans, and nuts:* One liberal or two small servings (4 oz) of meat, fish, or poultry; liver is desirable at least once each week. One egg equals approximately one-half of a small serving. Dried peas, beans, or nuts may be used as meat substitutes.

*Fruit:* Two or more servings (1–1½ cups, 200 g–300 g) each day. One large serving should be citrus fruit or other good source of ascorbic acid.

*Vegetables:* Two or more servings of cooked or raw vegetables (1–1½ cups, 200 g–300 g) each day; these should include dark-green leafy or deep-yellow vegetables; in addition, a medium potato (150 g) should be eaten daily.

*Bread and cereal:* Whole grain or enriched bread, at least four slices daily (½ cup of cereal is equivalent to one slice of bread).

*Butter or margarine:* 1 to 2 tablespoons.

*Additional foods:* Consisting of either more of the foods already listed or other foods of one's own choice adjusted to individual energy needs and in relation to desired weight gain.

*Vitamin D:* Some form of vitamin D to supply 400 IU such as 1 qt of milk would supply.

supply during the first few months of life when the diet of milk provides little iron. If the woman's intake of iron is low, this is reflected in the level of her own hemoglobin.

Menu planning should take into consideration the various factors that determine the availability of iron in individual meals. Heme iron, estimated to be approximately 40% of the iron in meat, poultry, and fish, is more readily absorbed than nonheme iron, the remaining iron in meat, poultry, and fish and all the iron in other foods. In addition to providing more available iron, the amount of meat, fish, and poultry in a meal also influences the availability of the nonheme iron in the meal. Similarly, increasing the amount of ascorbic acid also increases the absorption of iron in an individual meal (see Chap. 6). For this reason, including 1 to 3 oz of meat, fish, or poultry and 25 mg to 75 mg of ascorbic acid in each meal may result in greater availability of iron than providing the same foods in different meals. Because it is difficult to obtain sufficient iron from food alone, even with very careful planning, the Food and Nutrition Board recommends a supplement in the range of 30 mg to 60 mg per day, the actual amount to be determined by the physician responsible for prenatal care.

## Iodine requirement

Iodine is also an important element in the diet of the pregnant woman. An additional 25 mcg of iodine per day is recommended during pregnancy. A deficiency of this element during pregnancy may cause goiter in the pregnant woman. The use of iodized salt is suggested for those who live in areas where the soil and the drinking water are known to be deficient in iodine.

## Zinc requirement

An additional 5 mg of zinc per day is recommended during pregnancy. It is based on the calculated additional 0.75 mg required daily for growth of the fetus and placenta. The allowance includes a large safety factor for diets with poor availability of zinc, assuming only 15% absorption of dietary zinc. Meat, poultry, dry beans, eggs, and milk are good sources of zinc.

## Vitamin requirements

All vitamins are essential for the metabolism of living tissue and doubly so in growth.

Nutritional assessment studies indicate increased need during pregnancy for thiamin, riboflavin, and niacin. The increased requirement for protein necessitates an increase in vitamin $B_6$ of 0.6 mg per day for the pregnant woman. Because the added burden of pregnancy is known to increase the risk and incidence of folacin deficiency among populations with low or marginal intakes, an added allowance of 400 mcg per day is recommended. An oral supplement of folacin is suggested to meet the RDA of 800 mcg. The added allowance of 1 mcg per day of vitamin $B_{12}$ for the pregnant woman is based on fetal demands and the increased metabolic needs of the mother. Pregnant women should also receive at least the amounts of biotin and pantothenic acid that are estimated as safe and adequate daily dietary intakes; 100 mcg to 200 mcg and 4 mg to 7 mg, respectively.

During pregnancy the placenta transfers ascorbic acid from the mother to the fetus at a rate that results in 50% higher plasma vitamin C levels in the fetal blood than the maternal. An additional allowance of 20 mg of ascorbic acid is recommended to provide for fetal need. This enhancement of ascorbic acid intake may also prevent the fall in maternal plasma vitamin C levels, which often accompanies pregnancy.

The vitamin A allowance is increased 200 RE during pregnancy to compensate for the storage of vitamin A in the fetus. Similarly, the added amount of vitamin E, 2 mg alpha-TE per day, provides for the amount deposited in the fetus. The estimated safe and adequate intake of vitamin K for the adult, 70 mcg to 140 mcg, is also important for the pregnant woman.

Foods rich in vitamins are those that have been discussed as essential for other nutrients: milk and milk products, eggs, meat, fish and poultry, and especially liver, whole grain and enriched breads, green and yellow vegetables, citrus fruits, tomatoes, cabbage, and potatoes. All these must be supplied liberally in the diet of the pregnant woman if she is to meet her own nutritional needs as well as those of the growing fetus.

The proper utilization of calcium and phosphorus depends on the inclusion of a certain amount of vitamin D in the diet. Most areas today offer both whole and skim fluid milk to which 400 IU (10 mcg) of vitamin D per quart has been added. Due to evidence indicating a relationship between abnormal calcium deposition in infants and excessive vitamin D intakes during pregnancy, the pregnant woman should be cautioned against overdosage with supplements.

Mineral oil in any form interferes with the absorption of the fat-soluble vitamins and should be avoided.

The use of vitamin supplements (except for folic acid and possibly vitamin D) is not necessary unless, because of illness or other problems, the woman is unable to eat an adequate diet. The physician is best able to determine whether or not supplements are needed.

## Food selection in pregnancy

Table 17-2 lists the foods and the quantities of each that, if consumed daily by the pregnant woman, meets the Recommended Dietary Allowances except for iron and folic acid. Such a food intake represents the so-called excellent diet found by investigators to be most likely to produce a healthy infant and to maintain the woman's health at an optimum. Salt restriction or rigid weight control should not be necessary if the pregnancy is proceeding normally.

Two menus based on the foregoing table, one for adult pregnant women and one for pregnant adolescent girls, are presented in Table 17-3. It is assumed that both groups are of normal weight. Note that calories and calcium have been increased in the menu for pregnant adolescent girls to provide for their own growth needs and those of the fetus.

### Nutrition counseling

The needs of pregnant girls or women for nutrition counseling varies. The mother having her second or third baby, who feeds her family with good judgment will probably do the same for herself. All she may need is a review of dietary essentials with perhaps some suggestions for adapting her diet during pregnancy.

The most urgent nutritional problem is that of the very young pregnant woman. It has been said that "nutrition for pregnancy begins before conception," and, above all, this is true of the mother under 18. The diet of many teenaged girls is low in calcium and vitamin C. There is also a tendency to an inadequate iron intake. The young girl needs help in understanding her body's new needs, and possibly the help of the social worker or community agency in providing a good diet.

The first step in nutrition counseling of the pregnant woman is to determine her usual dietary practices, including her consumption of snacks and beverages. Such information as who shops for food, who prepares the meals and eats together, and when and where may need to be considered in assisting the woman adapt her diet to the needs of pregnancy. If someone other than the pregnant woman is responsible for meal planning, such as the mother of the pregnant teenager or the husband of the working woman, the nutrition counselor may wish to include them in counseling.

A woman with culturally different food habits, limited financial resources, or strong likes or dislikes may find it difficult to follow the suggested dietary pattern. The nutrition counselor can help make adaptations that will not impair the nutritive value of the diet. Cheese, buttermilk, and plain yogurt are good replacements for milk at mealtimes or for snacks.

The woman who asks for calcium pills because she does not like milk needs to be taught that milk and milk products are rich sources of other needed nutrients besides calcium and to be encouraged to use a variety of methods for including them in her diet. On the other hand she may be allergic to milk or may be lactase insufficient and may require calcium pills.

Dried peas and beans used by many groups in the United States as well as in other countries serve as a partial substitute at lower cost for meat, poultry, and fish. However, small amounts of those animal proteins do enhance both the protein quality and the availability of iron in the diet. Whole grain or enriched cereal products, including rice and cornmeal, also may be used combined with small amounts of meat, poultry, fish, egg, milk, or cheese as the main dish in a meal.

Fresh, frozen or canned vegetables and fruits may be used interchangeably in the diet. In the Southeastern section of the United States, the frequent use of greens and their accompanying pot liquor provides a good source of calcium and vitamin C. Raw fruits and vegetables can replace snack foods of higher caloric density and be used frequently throughout the day to satisfy the craving for nibbling and to meet the suggested dietary pattern for fruits and vegetables.

Desserts made from milk, eggs, and fruit may give a psychological lift to the pregnant woman.

The nutrition counselor should be aware of community resources available for assisting the pregnant woman with limited income. A referral to the local Social Services or Welfare Department to determine her eligibility for financial assistance should be made if the family income is inadequate to purchase the necessary foods. Her eligibility to participate in the Food Stamp Program and the Special Supplementary Program for Women, Infants and Children (WIC) may also be evaluated. The purpose of the WIC Program is to improve the nutrient intake of women, prenatally and postnatally, lactating mothers, infants, and children under 5 years who are at risk. Nutri-

tional risk may apply to women and children who have poor food habits, a previous history of miscarriage or preterm birth, nutritional anemia, or an abnormal growth pattern, such as obesity or underweight. It would also include those who are eligible for low cost medical care. Participants receive a WIC Food Package or vouchers, which can be used in a grocery store to purchase the designated foods. Food supplements for women include milk and cheese, eggs, vitamin C rich fruit or vegetable juice, and iron-fortified cereals. WIC is administered by the Health Department at the local level, although the USDA Food and Nutrition Service is the responsible Federal agency.

## Alcohol

The consumption of alcohol during pregnancy has been shown to be associated with a pattern of altered growth and development in the infants of drinking mothers and has been referred to as the "fetal alcohol syndrome." Clinical symptoms have ranged from severe abnormalities in ocular and facial structures, limb and heart malformations, renal anomalies, and permanent physical and mental retardation to milder degrees of mental and growth deficiencies. Alcohol crosses the placenta and enters the fetal bloodstream in the same concentration as it exists in the mother. The fetus, however, lacks the enzyme, alcohol dehydrogenase, that metabolizes alcohol in the body. Thus, the damaging effects of

### Table 17-3. Sample Menus for Pregnancy

| *For Pregnant Women of Normal Weight* | *For Pregnant Adolescent Girls of Normal Weight* |
|---|---|
| Breakfast | Breakfast |
| Orange juice—4 oz | Orange juice—4 oz |
| Sausage | Cornflakes or grits |
| Toast—1 slice | Scrambled egg |
| Butter or margarine | Toast—1 slice |
| Coffee (decaffeinated) | Milk—$\frac{1}{2}$ pint |
| Midmorning | Midmorning |
| Milk—$\frac{1}{2}$ pint | Milk—$\frac{1}{2}$ pint |
| Lunch | Lunch |
| Meat, cheese, or peanut butter sandwich | Hamburger on a bun |
| Carrot sticks | Cole slaw |
| Oatmeal cookies | Oatmeal cookies |
| Milk—$\frac{1}{2}$ pint | Milk—$\frac{1}{2}$ pint |
| Midafternoon | Midafternoon |
| Milk—$\frac{1}{2}$ pint | Frankfurter on a bun |
| | Milkshake or fruit juice—$\frac{1}{2}$ pint |
| Dinner | Dinner |
| Roasted or broiled beef, pork, liver, or fish | Roasted or broiled beef, pork, liver, or fish |
| Broccoli or greens | Broccoli or greens |
| Baked potato | Baked or french-fried potatoes |
| Butter or margarine | Butter or margarine |
| Green salad with French dressing | Green salad with French dressing |
| Fresh or canned fruit | Fruit |
| Coffee (decaffeinated) or milk | Milk—$\frac{1}{2}$ pint |
| Bedtime | Bedtime |
| Milk—$\frac{1}{2}$ pint | Fruit juice—$\frac{1}{2}$ pint |

alcohol have a much longer period of activity within the fetus than in the adult. Although evidence indicates that the greater the alcohol consumption, the greater the chance of severe multiple symptoms, the amount of alcohol needed to produce defects in the fetus has not been determined. Because no safe level of alcohol ingestion has been established, women should be urged to abstain throughout their pregnancy.

### Caffeine

Birth defects have been observed in pregnant rats fed a diet containing caffeine. Although caffeine has yet to be established as toxic to the human fetus, it is known to cross the placenta and for this reason may be harmful to the developing fetus. The FDA has advised pregnant women to avoid caffeine or use it sparingly pending further studies. Coffee, tea, cocoa, and cola beverages contain caffeine. The March of Dimes Foundation urged pregnant women and those who might become pregnant to limit caffeine intake to no more than 444 mg per day. They estimated the amount of caffeine per cup of beverage as follows: coffee 74 mg, tea 32 mg, cocoa 13 mg, and cola beverages 32 mg. Meanwhile, the FDA has urged the industries involved to support research for birth defect studies.

### Cigarette smoking

Cigarette smoking has been shown to limit fetal development and reduce birth weight. Although the mechanism for this action has not been established, a direct relationship appears to exist between the number of cigarettes smoked and the effect on the newborn.

### Pica

An abnormal craving for nonfood substances (pica), such as laundry starch and clay, has been reported by certain women during pregnancy. This practice appears to be most prevalent among black women, particularly in the South, where it is often a traditional practice accepted within the immediate community. A study by Edwards and associates in Alabama showed that the caloric intake of pregnant women who consumed starch and clay was reduced when these substances were omitted from the diet, indicating that they were either appetite stimulators or that deprivation of them was so emotionally upsetting as to reduce appetite.[6] In general, the diets of these women tended to be low in protein, iron, and calcium. Although the birth weight and length of the infants born to these mothers were similar to those of the control groups' infants, fewer babies born to the starch- and clay-eating mothers were rated in good condition at birth. Ice eating is another form of pica found among pregnant women. Pica is often associated with iron-deficiency anemia. However, whether it is cause or effect or simply coincidental has not been established.

### Weight control during pregnancy

Pregnancy usually is a time of wellbeing and often is accompanied by an excellent appetite. The average weight gain during pregnancy of 24 (20–25) lb includes the following:

| | |
|---|---|
| Fullterm baby | 7.7 lb |
| Placenta | 1.4 lb |
| Amniotic and body fluids | 1.8 lb |
| Enlarged uterus | 2.0 lb |
| Enlarged breasts | 0.9 lb |
| Blood volume increase | 4.0 lb |
| Interstitial body fluids | 2.7 lb |
| Maternal storage—fat | 3.5 lb |

Figure 17-1 shows a pattern of normal prenatal gain in weight. Although a maternal weight gain of 20 lb to 25 lb is normal and desirable, especially if the mother is to nurse her infant, certain factors contribute to some variability in weight gain. Teenaged mothers tend to slightly higher gains than more mature women; thin women gain more than obese women. Women having their first pregnancy gain more than women having second, third, or fourth babies.

The Committee on Maternal Nutrition has stated the following in relation to nutrition and weight gain during pregnancy:

> An average weight gain during pregnancy of 24 lb (range 20–25 lb) is commensurate with a better than average course of pregnancy. This would be a gain of 1.5 lb to 3.0 lb during the first trimester and a gain of 0.8 lb per week during the remainder of pregnancy. There is no scientific justification for routine limitation of weight gain to lesser amounts. . . .
>
> The pattern of weight gain is of greater importance than the total amount—a sudden sharp increase after about the 20th week of pregnancy may indicate water retention and the possible onset of preeclampsia. There is no evidence that the total amount of gain during pregnancy has, per se, any causal relationship to preeclampsia.
>
> Severe caloric restriction, which has been very commonly recommended, is potentially harmful to the developing fetus and to the mother and almost inevitably restricts other nutrients essential for growth processes. Weight-reduction regimes, if needed, should be instituted only after pregnancy has terminated.[7]

Care must be taken that any calorie restriction in pregnancy is not so severe that the protein in the diet is used partly for energy instead of for growth. Oldham has shown that this occurs when the diet is below 1500 calories, even when the protein of the diet is adequate.[8] Probably no diet in pregnancy should fall below 1800 calories.

If there is a tendency to gain too much weight, such foods as sugar, candy, jelly and other sweets, salad dress-

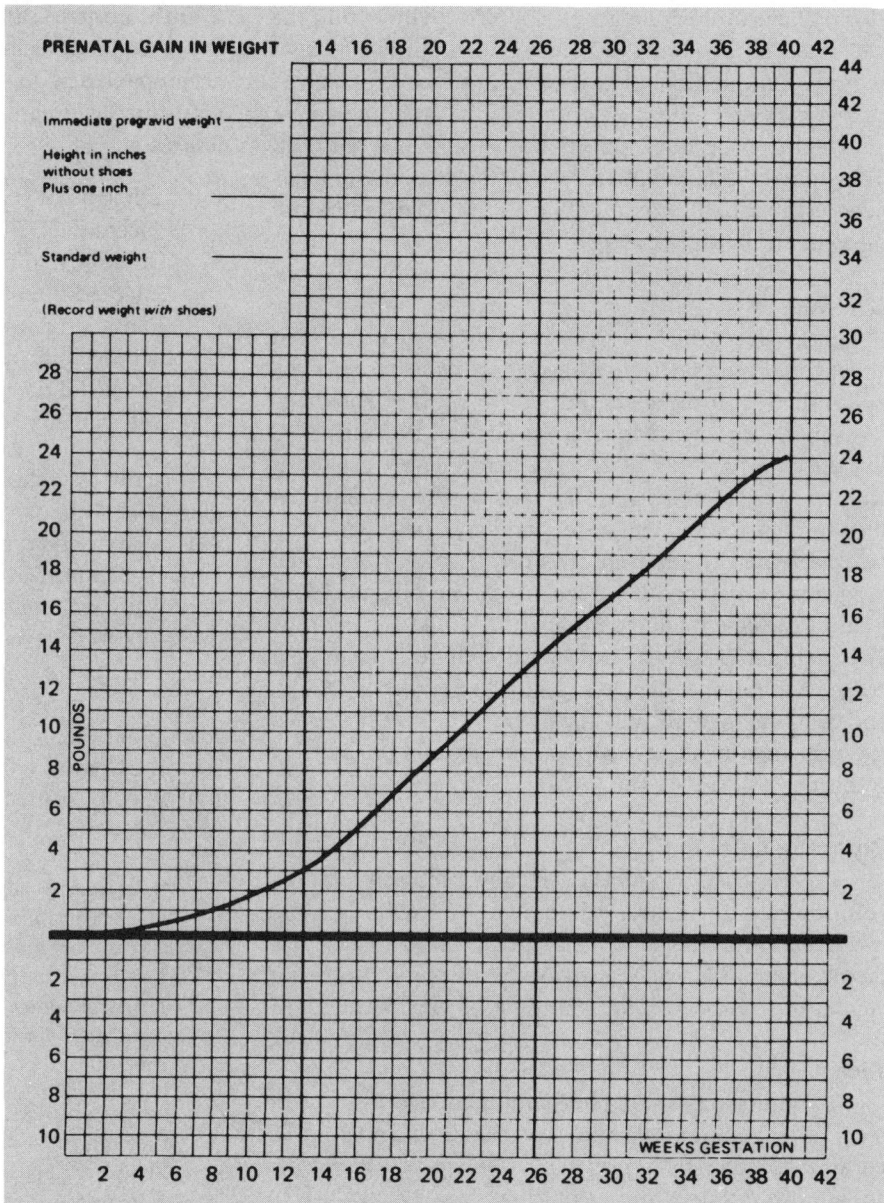

PRENATAL GAIN IN WEIGHT

Immediate pregravid weight ———

Height in inches
without shoes
Plus one inch          ———

Standard weight       ———

(Record weight *with* shoes)

POUNDS

WEEKS GESTATION

**Fig. 17-1.**   Weight-gain grid. Pattern of normal prenatal gain in weight. (U.S. Department HEW, Social and Rehabilitation Service, Children's Bureau)

ings, fried foods, fatty meats, cake, pie, and desserts, and carbonated beverages should be limited or omitted entirely.

A problem arises with the woman who believes that milk is "fattening" and reduces or omits it in her diet. As explained earlier, the substitution of calcium pills for milk markedly lowers the protein and the vitamin content of the diet and should be discouraged.

### Underweight in pregnancy

The severely underweight woman and the woman who does not gain normally during her pregnancy are of great concern. The reason for the underweight may be economic; this may often be discovered by the nutrition worker, who can direct the client to a community agency

for help (see p. 303, *Nutrition Counseling*). If the cause is psychological—such as a severe depression—or physical, the physician should take the appropriate measures.

### Nutrition education

Hospitals or community health centers frequently provide group education for expectant parents. Nutrition education should be an integral part of such a program. In addition to focusing on nutritional needs and the selection of an adequate diet during pregnancy, the nutrition education component may also include consideration of breast feeding. A number of teaching aids are available for parents' classes. Providing information about other community groups of interest to expectant parents may also assist individuals in meeting special needs.

## The International Childbirth Education Association (ICEA)

A volunteer, nonprofit organization, ICEA is devoted to promoting family-centered maternity care. Local affiliates offer a series of classes on prepared childbirth that cover the anatomy and physiology of pregnancy, labor and delivery, and other birth-related topics. Publications and lending libraries are also available. The organization works actively with local medical professionals in an attempt to create an environment that will meet the needs of prospective parents.

## The La Leche League International, Inc.

A nonprofit, nonsectarian organization that encourages mothers to breast-feed their babies, La Leche League sponsors a series of monthly meetings. They present the advantages of breast-feeding to mothers and babies, the art of breast-feeding, the family and the breast-fed baby, and nutrition and weaning. Some groups have a special meeting for fathers only. Nursing babies are welcome to come with their mothers. A telephone service is available that offers breast-feeding help. Most groups have a lending library of appropriate material. La Leche League publications are approved by a board of medical consultants. *The Womanly Art of Breast-feeding* is one of the League's best known publications.

# Complications of pregnancy involving diet
## Vomiting

During the first trimester of pregnancy the prospective mother may be troubled with nausea. Certain foods that previously have been eaten without difficulty now may cause distress. Fats are a common cause of upset. Fluids taken with meals may also precipitate vomiting. Dry toast or a few unsalted crackers eaten before arising may be of help. Fluids should be drunk between meals, not with the meal. Skim milk may be tolerated better than whole milk. Often the nausea disappears by the middle of the day, and the woman can make up her dietary needs by increasing her food intake in the late afternoon, at dinner, and before bedtime.

Vomiting, if it persists and becomes pernicious, should be treated by a physician.

## Anemias of pregnancy

During pregnancy there is a slight lowering of the hemoglobin content of the woman's blood due to physiological adjustments. Her total blood volume increases considerably to provide for the placental circulation. This is accompanied by a smaller increase in red blood cells; consequently, a degree of hemodilution occurs. Normal hemoglobin values for the pregnant woman are lower than for the nonpregnant woman.

True anemia occurring during pregnancy is due most often to an iron deficiency. Even healthy American women usually do not have iron stores large enough to meet the demands of pregnancy. Iron supplementation can aid greatly in maintaining the hemoglobin at normal levels in these patients. During the second and third trimester of pregnancy, an oral iron supplement of 30 mg to 60 mg of ferrous salts is recommended. It is also essential, however, that the woman be urged to include foods rich in iron and protein in her diet, or other deficiencies may appear.

Megaloblastic anemia of pregnancy may be due to poor food intake, vomiting, or the fetal demands for folacin. It is characterized by an extremely low red blood cell count and an equally low hemoglobin and has some other findings associated with pernicious anemia, with which it may be confused. The administration of folic acid causes an immediate and dramatic rise in red blood cells and hemoglobin, and in appetite. Studies indicate that the folic acid requirement during pregnancy is greatly increased compared with the minimum adult requirement.[9] The Committee on Maternal Nutrition suggests a supplement of 400 mcg of folacin per day. If the woman does not receive treatment before the birth of the infant, the infant also will show some of the symptoms of megaloblastic anemia. The infant may be treated with folic acid, or, if the mother is being treated while nursing, the infant will receive enough folic acid from its mother's milk to restore its blood components to normal.

## Toxemia of pregnancy

The cause of toxemia of pregnancy is not known. It occurs during the third trimester of pregnancy and is characterized by an elevation in blood pressure, proteinuria, and rapid weight gain due to edema. Because of these symptoms it has recently been termed edema-proteinuria- and hypertension-gestosis (EPHG). In the eclamptic stage there may be convulsions and coma. A marked decrease in the incidence of eclampsia has occurred in the last 30 years in the Western world. The Collaborative Prenatal Study reported only 26 cases among the black (23 cases) and white (3 cases) women in the group who numbered over 51,000.[10] There is considerable controversy over the influence of nutrition on the development of toxemia. Toxemia occurs more frequently in pregnant women on poor diets, and particularly in those on low protein intakes, than in corresponding groups on good diets. Epidemiologic studies show a direct relationship between the incidence of toxemia and an individual state's per capita income. The poorer the state the greater the number of cases of toxemia reported.[11]

Findings of Burke and Kirkwood show that 44% of the women on poor or very poor diets, 8% on fair diets, and none on good or excellent diets developed symptoms of toxemia.[12] Tompkins and Wiehl have shown that supplementation of the diet with protein and vitamins greatly reduced the incidence of toxemia in their patients.[13] Although McGanity and his group in Nashville, Tennessee, were not able to relate nutritional status to health during pregnancy as clearly as other investigators, they do report an increased incidence of toxemia in mothers who ate less than 1500 calories and 50 g of protein per day during the last trimester.[14]

Recent epidemiological observations and new clinical and experimental studies have revived the hypothesis that calcium intake is related to the pathogenesis of toxemia of pregnancy.[15]

In the past few years a question has arisen about the relation of salt intake to toxemia. Robinson,[16] studying over 2000 pregnant women, advised half to increase their salt intake and half to lower it. He found a lower incidence of toxemia in those having the higher salt intake. Mengert placed 48 patients with proven toxemia either on a high salt intake or on a very low one. No difference in the progress of the disease was noted between the two groups of women in this study.[17] It is now recognized that pregnancy increases sodium requirements and that attempts to restrict sodium stress the normal renin-angiotensin-aldosterone adjustments. The Committee on Maternal Nutrition discourages the routine use of salt restriction and diuretics during pregnancy.

### Cardiac disease and pregnancy

It should be remembered that the nutritional requirements of the pregnant woman with cardiac disease are the same as those of the noncardiac pregnant woman. See Chapter 31 for diet modifications in Cardiovascular Diseases.

### Table 17-4. Recommended Dietary Allowances for the Lactating Woman 23 to 50 Years, 55 kg, 163 cm

| Nutrient | Amount |
| --- | --- |
| Energy (kcal) | 2500 |
| Protein | 64 g |
| Vitamin A | 6000 IU (1200 RE) |
| Vitamin D | 10 mcg (400 IU) |
| Vitamin E | 11 mg $\alpha$-TE |
| Ascorbic acid | 100 mg |
| Folacin | 500 mcg |
| Niacin | 18 mg |
| Riboflavin | 1.7 mg |
| Thiamin | 1.5 mg |
| Vitamin $B_6$ | 2.5 mg |
| Vitamin $B_{12}$ | 4 mcg |
| Calcium | 1.2 g |
| Phosphorus | 1.2 g |
| Iodine | 200 mcg |
| Iron | 18 mg |
| Magnesium | 450 mg |
| Zinc | 25 mg |

### Diabetes and pregnancy

The diabetic woman's diet must be increased to meet her larger needs and those of the growing fetus. The insulin dosage must be augmented accordingly. For further discussion of pregnancy and diabetes see Chapter 29.

### Diet during labor

During the early part of labor, if feeding by mouth is permitted by the physician, the diet should consist mainly of carbohydrates, as they leave the stomach quickly. Protein and fat tend to remain in the stomach considerably longer, which may result in aspiration if anesthesia is given. The diet may be soft or liquid and may include white bread toast with jelly, soda crackers, canned or cooked fruits, gelatin, fruit juices, ginger ale, broth, and tea or coffee with sugar but no milk or cream. By the time the patient is in active labor, most obstetricians prefer that no food be given by mouth in order to prevent the possibility of vomiting and of aspiration of food into the trachea. Intravenous fluids are given to maintain water balance if labor is prolonged.

### Diet following delivery

A liquid diet usually is given for the first meal after delivery. After that, there is a return to the normal diet. If the mother nurses the infant, there must be an even greater allowance of food than there was during pregnancy.

### Diet in lactation

Lactation makes even greater demands in some respects on the maternal organism than does pregnancy. After birth the child still may be fed from the mother's body, the food now being produced by the mammary glands instead of being supplied through the bloodstream, as before birth. As the infant gains in weight and becomes increasingly active, the food supply from the mother must increase.

### Supply of mother's milk

A normal infant consumes daily $2\frac{1}{2}$ oz of mother's milk for each pound of its weight. An 8-lb infant consumes approximately 20 oz, whereas a 15-lb one consumes about 35 oz. Because human milk has a caloric value of 20 calories per ounce, it is readily seen that a nursing mother must have several hundred additional calories per day to supply food for the infant.

### Dietary requirements

The recommended dietary allowance for energy for the nursing mother producing 850 ml of milk daily is 500 additional calories above her normal needs for the first 3 months of lactation. This recommendation is based on the 80% efficiency with which maternal dietary energy is

## Table 17-5. Sample Menu for a Day for a Lactating Mother

| *Breakfast* | *Lunch* | *Dinner* |
|---|---|---|
| Orange juice | Vegetable beef soup | Green salad |
| Oatmeal or grits with milk | Cottage cheese with fruit salad | Baked ham |
| Poached egg or chicken livers on toast | Biscuit with butter or margarine | Scalloped potatoes |
| Milk, Coffee if desired | Gingerbread with topping | Green beans |
| | Milk, Coffee if desired | Bread with butter or margarine |
| | | Sliced peaches |
| | | Milk, Coffee if desired |
| Midmorning | Midafternoon | Bedtime |
| Milk | Fruit juice | Milk |

converted into energy in milk. The production of 100 ml of milk requires approximately 90 kcal. It also takes into account the calories available (200–300 per day for 100 days) from the 3.5 lb of fat stored by the mother who gained 24 lb during pregnancy. Thus the allowance provides for the production of milk as well as for the readjustment of maternal body fat stores following pregnancy. If lactation continues beyond 3 months or if the mother's weight falls below ideal weight for height, the mother's energy allowance should be increased.[18]

Besides the increase in energy requirements, there are also increases in the requirements for protein, minerals, and vitamins. To cover the needs of milk production and to allow for 70% efficiency of protein utilization, an additional 20 g of protein is recommended. Increasing maternal protein intake in very poorly nourished mothers has been shown to increase the volume of breast milk produced, whereas the proximate amount of protein in human milk remains relatively constant.[19] Similarly, vitamins and minerals which are to be used in milk production must be supplied in adequate amounts or the mother's own tissues may become depleted. Supplements of vitamin A, vitamin C, thiamin, and riboflavin given to malnourished mothers have resulted in increased amounts of these nutrients in the milk.[20] Low levels of vitamin $B_{12}$ have been found in the breast milk of Indian women who were lacto-vegetarians.[21] Table 17-4 shows the recommended dietary allowances for the lactating woman.

Feedings between meals often are advisable during lactation. Plenty of fluids should be taken to replace the water secreted in the milk. A typical sample menu for a day is shown in Table 17-5.

It should be remembered that the mother must return to a normal food intake when she weans the infant or she will gain excess weight.

## Study questions and activities

1. Even the normal healthy woman who has been eating an adequate diet will require more dietary essentials during pregnancy. Review the Recommended Dietary Allowances for women in various conditions. Which allowances increase in ratio to the energy allowance? What other essentials should be increased during pregnancy?
2. Discuss the importance of providing an adequate calorie allowance during pregnancy.
3. Give several reasons why the adolescent may have serious nutrition problems in pregnancy. Name some of the ways in which these can be met.
4. List maternal characteristics that influence the birth weight of the infant.
5. Discuss the increased protein needs during pregnancy. How can the normal diet be modified to meet the protein allowance for pregnant women?
6. The mineral requirement is naturally larger during pregnancy. How may the calcium and the phosphorus requirements be fulfilled? What are the food sources of iron? How may the iodine requirements be met?
7. Describe the pregnant women who may need the most nutrition counseling.
8. List the foods and the quantity of each that must be included daily in the diet of the pregnant woman.
9. Plan a menu for a day for a healthy pregnant woman of average weight with a limited income.
10. Using Chapter 14 as a guide, write a menu for a day for a pregnant woman with a food pattern not typically American. Be sure that it is adequate for the needs of pregnancy.
11. During the first trimester there may be trouble with nausea. How may the menu be modified to relieve this?
12. Write what you would tell the pregnant women about the consumption of alcoholic beverages and caffeine-containing beverages.
13. During the third trimester toxemia may appear. Is there anything to indicate that diet may act as a preventive? If so, state the evidence.
14. Lactation makes greater demands upon the mother than does pregnancy. What food increases should be made to provide for the supply of milk? Plan a menu differing in content from the sample menu in Table 17-5, but equivalent to it in other respects.

## References

1. Committee on Maternal Nutrition, Food and Nutrition Board: Maternal Nutrition and the Course of Pregnancy. Washington, DC, NAS-NRC, Summary Report, 1970
2. Burke BS et al: J Nutr 38:453, 1949
3. Lechtig A et al: Am J Clin Nutr 28:1223, 1975
4. Blackburn ML, Calloway DH: J Am Diet Assoc 65:24, 1974
5. Hytten FE, Leitch I: The Physiology of Human Pregnancy, 2nd ed. Philadelphia, FA Davis, 1971
6. Edwards CH et al: J Am Diet Assoc 44:109, 1964
7. Committee on Maternal Nutrition, Maternal Nutrition and the Course of Pregnancy, p 13
8. Oldham H: Bull Matern Welf 4:10, 1957
9. Alperin JB et al: Arch Intern Med 117:681, 1966; Willoughby MLN, Jewell FJ: Br Med J 5529:1568, 1966
10. Niswander K, Gordon M: The Women and Their Pregnancies. The Collaborative Perinatal Study of the National Institute of Neurological Diseases and Stroke. Philadelphia, WB Saunders, 1972
11. Committee on Maternal Nutrition, Maternal Nutrition and the Course of Pregnancy, p 163
12. Burke BS, Kirkwood BB: Am J Public Health 40:960, 1950
13. Tompkins WT, Wiehl DG: Am J Obstet Gynecol 62:898, 1951
14. McGanity WJ et al: Am J Obstet Gynecol 67:501, 1954
15. Review: Nutr Rev 39:124, 1981
16. Robinson M: Am J Obstet Gynecol 76:1, 1958
17. Mengert WF: Am J Obstet Gynecol 81:601, 1961
18. Food and Nutrition Board: Recommended Dietary Allowances. Washington, DC, NAS-NRC, 1974
19. Jelliffe DB, Gurney M, Jelliffe EFP: Cajanus 6:156, 1973
20. Belavady B: Indian J Med Res 57:63, 1969
21. Jathar VS et al: Arch Dis Child 45:236, 1970

## Supplementary readings

American Academy of Pediatrics, Committee on Adolescence: Statement on teenage pregnancy. Pediatrics 63:795, 1979

Beal VA: Nutrition in the Life Span. New York, John Wiley & Sons, 1980

Endres JM, Sawicki M, Casper JA: Dietary assessment of pregnant women in a supplemental food program. J Am Diet Assoc 79:121, 1981

Grant JA, Heald FP: Complications of adolescent pregnancy— Survey of the literature on fetal outcome in adolescence. Clin Pediatr 11:567, 1972

Kaminetzky HA, Baker H: Micronutrients in pregnancy. Clin Obstet Gynecol 20:363, 1977

Moghissi KS, Evans TN (eds): Nutritional Impacts on Women Throughout Life with Emphasis on Reproduction. Hagerstown, MD, Harper & Row, 1977

Pitkin RM: Calcium metabolism in pregnancy: A review. Am J Obstet Gynecol 121:724, 1975

Pitkin RM: Nutritional support in obstetrics and gynecology. Clin Obstet Gynecol 19:489, 1976

Rosso P: Maternal nutrition, nutrient exchange and fetal growth. In Winick M (ed): Nutritional Disorders of American Women. New York, John Wiley & Sons, 1977

Rush D, Stern Z, Susser M: A randomized controlled trial of prenatal supplementation in New York City. Pediatrics 65:683, 1980

Snowman MK, Dibble MV: Nutrition component in a comprehensive child development program. I. The home visitor's role in the prenatal intervention phase. J Am Diet Assoc 74:119, 1979

Widdowson EM: Prenatal nutrition. Ann NY Acad Sci 300:188, 1977

Worthington BS, Vermeersch J, Williams SR: Nutrition in Pregnancy and Lactation, 2nd ed. St Louis, CV Mosby, 1981

*For further references see Bibliography in Part 4.*

# Nutrition During Infancy and Early Childhood— from Birth to 3 Years

# 18

Because of the rapid rate of growth during the first year, infancy is one of the most critical periods in the life cycle as far as food is concerned. Nutrient needs in relationship to size are high, and optimum nutrition at this time is very important to health and vigor throughout life. Many mothers feel insecure with their first babies and are concerned about what and how to feed the infant. The nutrition counselor should be able to advise and help the mother develop skills in this area.

## Nutritional requirements of infants

### The energy requirement

Infants require much greater energy per unit of body weight than older children or adults. During the first year energy allowances range from 120 kcal per kilogram at birth to 100 kcal per kilogram at the end of the year. The RDA for energy is, therefore, stated as 115 kcal per kilogram for the first 6 months and 105 kcal per kilogram for the second half of the first year (Table 18-1). This is from $3\frac{1}{2}$ to $2\frac{1}{2}$ times the adult requirement per unit of weight.

There are several reasons for this difference in requirements. The infant is growing rapidly, but is doing so at a decreasing rate, which is reflected by the reduction in kcal per kilogram during the first year.

He has a greater surface area in proportion to his weight than the adult and, for this reason, a greater heat loss. Additional energy is also needed for increased activity. The accompanying table (Table 18-2) shows the approximate distribution of the energy needs of the infant at the 120 kcal per kilogram level.

The caretaker should recognize that these recommendations are averages and approximate allowances for feeding groups of infants. Longitudinal growth studies indicate wide ranges of intakes among healthy infants. The intake for an individual infant is best determined by observing his appetite, activity, growth, and weight gain.

Both breast milk and infant formulas (normal dilution) supply approximately 20 calories per ounce (67 kcal per 100 ml); thus 24 oz of human milk or formula supply about 480 calories or 120 calories per kilogram for the 4-kg infant (120 kcal × 4 kg = 480 kcal).

### The fluid requirement

Normal healthy infants require about 1.5 ml per kilogram of fluid in 24 hours. Most of this amount is usually consumed in the formula or from the breast. If extra water is lost from the skin, lungs, or gastrointestinal tract, such as in hot weather, fever, or diarrhea, additional water should be given. When solid foods replace formula or breast milk in the infant's diet, some extra fluids may also be necessary. This is especially true if the solid food is high in protein, sodium chloride, or potassium[1] (see Chap. 5 and 35 for a discussion of fluid and electrolyte balance in the normal and in the sick child).

### Table 18-1. Recommended Dietary Allowances for Infants During the First Year

|  | 0–6 Months 6 kg–60 cm | 6–12 Months 9 kg –71 cm |
|---|---|---|
| Energy (kcal) | 115 kcal/kg (690) | 105 kcal/kg (945) |
| Protein (g) | 2.2 g/kg (13.2) | 2.0 g/kg (18) |
| Vitamin A (RE) | 420* (1400 IU) | 400 (2000 IU) |
| Vitamin D (mcg) | 10 (400 IU) | 10 (400 IU) |
| Vitamin E (mg α-TE) | 3 | 4 |
| Ascorbic Acid (mg) | 35 | 35 |
| Folacin (mcg) | 30 | 45 |
| Niacin (mg NE) | 6 | 8 |
| Riboflavin (mg) | 0.4 | 0.6 |
| Thiamin (mg) | 0.3 | 0.5 |
| Vitamin $B_6$ (mg) | 0.3 | 0.6 |
| Vitamin $B_{12}$ (mcg) | 0.5 | 1.5 |
| Calcium (mg) | 360 | 540 |
| Phosphorus (mg) | 240 | 360 |
| Iodine (mcg) | 40 | 50 |
| Iron (mg) | 10 | 15 |
| Magnesium (mg) | 50 | 70 |
| Zinc (mg) | 3 | 5 |

*Assumed to be all as retinol in milk during the first 6 months of life. All subsequent intakes are assumed to be half as retinol and half as beta-carotene when calculated from international units. As retinol equivalents, three-fourths are as retinol and one-fourth as beta-carotene.

(Adapted from Food and Nutrition Board: Recommended Dietary Allowances. Washington, DC, National Academy of Sciences/National Research Council, 1980)

### Table 18-2. Distribution of the Energy Needs of the Infant

|  | Calories/kg of Body Weight/24 hr |
|---|---|
| Basal metabolism | 60 |
| Activity | 25 |
| Growth | 30 |
| Loss in stools | 5 |
| Total | 120 |

### The protein requirement

In the first year of life the infant's protein requirement is greater per unit of body weight than at any other time of life. It gradually decreases from 2.2 g per kilogram during the first 6 months to 2.0 g per kilogram for the second half of the first year. The RDA for protein during infancy (Table 18-1) is based on the "amount of protein provided by the quantity of milk required to ensure a satisfactory rate of growth."[2] The protein content of the body increases during the first year from 11% to 14.6% while there is a 7-kg increase in body weight.

Most of the infants in the United States today who are not breast-fed receive a modified cow's milk formula, which closely simulates human milk. Because protein provides from 9% to 11% of the total calories in the usual infant formulas, 1 oz of formula supplies approximately 0.5 g of protein. As a result, the 4-kg infant receiving 24 oz of formula (20 kcal per ounce) gets approximately 12 g of protein per day (RDA = 8.8 g).

### Fat requirement

No specific requirement for fat can be stated, but the energy value of fat is essential during the early months of life when energy requirements per unit of body weight are high. Human milk provides 48% to 54% of its energy as fat, cow's milk—46% to 50%. Most commercial formulas provide 35% to 50% of the energy as fat. In order for infants to acquire adequate energy from the limited amount of formula they are able to consume, at least 15% of the energy provided must come from fat. The fat must be in an easily digestible form, preferably emulsified. Fomon[3] points out that loss of fat in the stools may be excessive if whole or evaporated milk without added carbohydrate is fed to the infant and suggests that the change from formula to whole milk be delayed until the infant is taking two jars of carbohydrate-rich commercially prepared strained food or the equivalent in table food.

Fat is also a carrier of fat-soluble vitamins. As described in Chapter 3, the infant requires small amounts of the essential fatty acid (EFA)—linoleic acid. Human milk is an excellent source of EFA, providing 6% to 9% of total energy as linoleate, whereas cow's milk provides 1% to 2%. The American Academy of Pediatrics recommends 3% of energy as the minimum amount of essential fatty acid in infant formulas.[4]

### Carbohydrates in infant feeding

In human milk 37% of the energy is from carbohydrate, whereas 29% in cow's milk and approximately 42% in commercially prepared infant formula are from carbohydrate.

Lactose, the natural carbohydrate of mammalian milks, has many advantages. It provides calories in nonirritating and easily available form. Its slow breakdown and absorption probably have a beneficial effect on calcium absorption in the intestinal tract. Most commercial formulas use lactose as the preferred carbohydrate, although a variety of other carbohydrates that modify the flavor (sucrose, corn syrup solids, dextrose, dextrins, maltose) or consistency (arrowroot starch, cornstarch, modified cornstarch and tapioca starch, banana powder, carrageenan) may be added to commercially prepared formulas. For economy and for the convenience of the mother preparing a formula at home, cane sugar (sucrose), or corn syrup can be used, the amount calculated according to the caloric need.

## Minerals

### Calcium—Phosphorus—Magnesium

The recommended dietary allowances for calcium, phosphorus, and magnesium during the first year of life apply to bottle-fed infants. These recommendations are given in Table 18-1. To prevent hypocalcemic tetany during the first week of life, a calcium to phosphorus ratio similar to that of human milk (2:1) is more desirable for the newborn than the Ca to P ratio (1.2:1) found in cow's milk. The NRC's recommendation for a Ca to P ratio of at least 1.5:1 for the first weeks of life is found in several commercial formulas. For later infancy, the cow's milk Ca to P ratio is suggested. The approximate amounts of these minerals supplied by human milk and by cow's milk are shown in Table 18-3.

### Iron

The fullterm infant is born with approximately 75 mg per kilogram of total body iron; about 25% of this amount is in iron stores. The high concentration of hemoglobin found in the newborn declines during the first 6 to 8 weeks of life to the lowest levels observed during any period of development, approximately 11.0 g per deciliter. The rate of decrease in hemoglobin level is closely related to the lifespan of the red blood cells that were synthesized before birth. Due to the very limited amount of erythropoiesis (production of red blood cells) occurring during this period, the iron from senescent (old) red blood cells temporarily goes into storage iron. Because large iron stores decrease the intestinal absorption of iron, the amount of dietary iron absorbed during this stage (Stage I) is less than in later infancy. From about 2 to 4 months the decrease in hemoglobin concentration is reversed. The production of red blood cells increases, and hemoglobin concentration rises to about 12.5 g per deciliter, where it remains for the rest of the first year. Iron stores in the fullterm infant are available to meet a large part of the iron needs during this stage (Stage II). After 4 months there is a much greater dependence on dietary iron. By this stage (Stage III) iron stores have been used up due to the

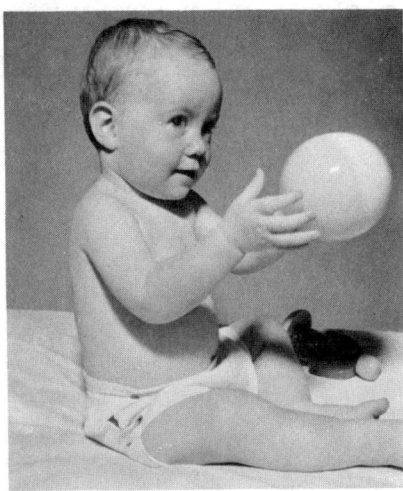

**Fig. 18-1.** Signs of good nutrition. Note the straight back, well-developed body, alertness, and good coordination of this child. (The New York Hospital)

infant's rapid growth rate and the low iron content of milk. The increase in hemoglobin level seen in Stage II will be reversed if dietary iron is inadequate after 4 months. Iron deficiency anemia is most prevalent between 6 months and 2 to 3 years of age.[5]

In the low-birth-weight infant the iron stores are less at birth. Because these infants also experience a greater growth rate after birth, their iron stores are depleted at an earlier age, and they become more dependent on dietary iron by about 3 months of age.[5]

The RDA for infants is based on an average need of 1.5 mg/kg per day during the first year of life. However, the Food and Nutrition Board has recognized that "the normal term infant can maintain optimal hemoglobin levels with an iron intake of 1 mg per kilogram per day, starting about the third month of life."[2] The American Academy of Pediatrics[4] recommends an intake of 1 mg per kilogram body weight per day to a maximum of 15 mg per day, beginning no later than 4 months of age and continuing until 3 years.

Both human and cow's milk contain small amounts of iron (Table 18-3), however, differences in the percentage absorbed by the infant are great and have an important impact on infant feeding. Approximately 50% of the iron in breast milk is absorbed compared to 10% to 12% from cow's milk. As a result, infants receiving a cow's milk formula need the introduction of a good source of iron in their diets by 3 to 4 months, whereas recent evidence[6] supports the observation that breast-feeding can provide adequate iron for fullterm infants through the first 6 months of life (see *Breast-Feeding*). Commercial infant formulas fortified with 11 mg to 12 mg of iron per liter are available. They are recommended by many physi-

**Table 18-3. Comparative Nutritive Value of Human Milk and Cow's Milk**

| Constituent (g/l Except Where Stated) | Mature Human Milk | | | Cow's Milk | | |
|---|---|---|---|---|---|---|
| | Mean | Range | s.d. | Mean | Range | s.d. |
| *Energy* (kcal/l) | 747 | 446–1192 | 93 | 701 | 587–876 | |
| (MJ/l) | 3.127 | 1.867–4.989 | 0.389 | 2.934 | 2.457–3.666 | |
| *Protein* | | | | | | |
| Total | 10.6 | 7.3–20 | 4.6 | 32.46 | 28.16–36.76 | |
| *Casein* | 3.7 | 1.6–6.8 | 0.8 | 24.9 | 21.90–28.0 | |
| Lactalbumin | 3.6 | 1.4–6.0 | 1.0 | 2.4 | 1.40–3.3 | |
| Lactoglobulin | 2.0* | | | 1.70 | 0.7–3.7 | |
| *Amino acids* | | | | | | |
| Total | 12.8 | 9.0–16.0 | | 33.0 | 27.0–41.0 | |
| *Essential total* | 5.39† | | | 19.59† | | |
| Histidine | 0.24 | 0.12–0.30 | 0.041 | 1.2 | 1.1–1.3 | |
| Isoleucine | 0.61 | 0.41–0.92 | 0.121 | 2.5 | 2.1–2.9 | |
| Leucine | 0.97 | 0.65–1.47 | 0.174 | 3.6 | 3.2–3.9 | |
| Lysine | 0.70 | 0.36–0.93 | 0.127 | 2.6 | 2.3–3.1 | |
| Methionine | 0.12 | 0.07–0.16 | 0.023 | 0.8 | 0.6–0.9 | |
| Cystine | 0.29* | 0.23–0.25 | | 0.29* | | |
| Phenylalanine | 0.40 | 0.24–0.58 | 0.069 | 1.8 | 1.5–2.2 | |
| Tyrosine | 0.62* | 0.46–0.52 | | 1.9* | | |
| Threonine | 0.52 | 0.30–0.66 | 0.085 | 1.7 | 1.3–2.2 | |
| Tryptophan | 0.19 | 0.14–0.26 | 0.030 | 0.6 | 0.4–0.8 | |
| Valine | 0.73 | 0.45–1.14 | 0.155 | 2.6 | 2.4–2.8 | |
| *Fats* | | | | | | |
| Total (g) | 45.4 | 13.4–82.9 | 10.0 | 38.0 | 34.0–61.0 | |
| *Essential total* (% weight of total fatty acids) | 12.02† | | | 4.2† | | |
| Linoleic (18:2) | 10.6 | | 2.9 | 2.1 | | 0.7 |
| Linolenic (18:3) | 0.85 | | | 1.7 | | 0.7 |
| Arachidonic (20:4) | 0.57 | | | 0.4 | | |
| *Saturated total* | 50.3† | | | 70.9† | | |
| C4:0–C10:0 | 1.4 | | | 9.1 | | 1.1 |
| Luric (12:0) | 4.7 | | 2.2 | 3.6 | | 1.5 |
| Myristic (14:0) | 7.9 | | 1.5 | 11.8 | | 4.7 |
| Palmitic (16:0) | 26.7 | | 2.7 | 36.6 | | 3.2 |
| Stearic (18:0) | 8.3 | | 1.7 | 8.1 | | |
| Arachidic (20:0) | 1.3 | | | 1.7 | | |
| *Unsaturated* | | | | | | |
| C10:1–C16:1 | 3.8 | | | 5.2 | | |
| Oleic (18:1) | 37.4 | | 3.7 | 17.7 | | 4.2 |
| Eicosenoic (20:1) | 0.9 | | | 1.0 | | |
| Cholesterol | 0.139 | 0.088–0.202 | 0.025 | 0.110 | 0.070–0.170 | |
| *Carbohydrates* | | | | | | |
| Lactose | 71 | 49–95 | | 47 | 45–50 | |
| Citric acid | | 0.35–1.25 | | 2.45 | 2.15–2.90 | |
| *Minerals* | | | | | | |
| *Electropositive* (mEq/l) | 41 | | | 149 | | |
| Sodium (g/l) | 0.189 | 0.080–0.350 | 0.006 | 0.768 | 0.392–1.390 | |
| Potassium (g/l) | 0.553 | 0.425–0.735 | 0.070 | 1.430 | 0.380–2.870 | |
| Calcium (g/l) | 0.271 | 0.207–0.372 | 0.030 | 1.370 | 0.560–3.810 | |
| Magnesium (g/l) | 0.035 | 0.018–0.057 | 0.007 | 0.130 | 0.070–0.220 | |
| *Electronegative* (mEq/l) | 28 | | | 108 | | |
| Phosphorus (g/l) | 0.141 | 0.068–0.268 | 0.025 | 0.910 | 0.560–1.120 | |
| Sulphur (g/l) | 0.140 | 0.050–0.300 | 0.030 | 0.300 | 0.240–0.360 | |
| Chlorine (g/l) | 0.375 | 0.088–0.734 | 0.090 | 1.080 | 0.930–1.410 | |

## Table 18-3.  Comparative Nutritive Value of Human Milk and Cow's Milk (Continued)

| Constituent (g/l Except Where Stated) | Mature Human Milk | | | Cow's Milk | | |
|---|---|---|---|---|---|---|
| | Mean | Range | s.d. | Mean | Range | s.d. |
| *Excess electropositive* | | | | | | |
| Elements (mEq/l) | 13 | | | 41 | | |
| pH | 7.01 | 6.4–7.6 | | 6.6 | | |
| | | | | | | |
| *Trace elements* | | | | | | |
| Cobalt ($\mu$g/l) | trace | | | 0.6 | | |
| Iron (mg/l) | 0.50 | 0.20–0.80 | | 0.45 | 0.25–0.75 | |
| Copper (mg/l) | 0.51 | | 0.046 | 0.102 | | |
| Manganese (mg/l) | trace | | | 0.02 | 0.005–0.067 | |
| Zinc (mg/l) | 1.18 | 0.17–3.02 | | 3.9 | 1.7–6.6 | |
| Fluorine (mg/l) | 0.107 | 0.0–0.24 | | | 0.10–0.28 | |
| Iodine (mg–l) | 0.061 | 0.044–0.093 | | 0.116 | 0.036–1.05 | |
| Selenium (mg/l) | 0.021 | | | 0.04 | 0.005–0.067 | |
| | | | | | | |
| *Vitamins* | | | | | | |
| Vitamin A (mg/l) | 0.610 | 0.150–2.260 | 0.230 | 0.270 | 0.170–0.380 | |
| Carotenes (mg/l) | 0.250 | 0.020–0.770 | 0.110 | 0.370 | 0.120–0.790 | |
| Vitamin D ($\mu$g/l) | | 0.1–2.5 | | | 0.1–1.0 | |
| Tocopherol (mg/l) | 2.4 | 1.0–4.8 | | 0.6 | 0.2–1.0 | |
| Thiamin (mg/l) | 0.142 | 0.081–0.227 | 0.024 | 0.430 | 0.280–0.900 | |
| Riboflavin (mg/l) | 0.373 | 0.198–0.790 | 0.087 | 1.560 | 1.160–2.020 | |
| Vitamin $B_6$ (mg/l) | 0.180 | 0.100–0.220 | | 0.510 | 0.400–0.630 | |
| Nicotinic acid (mg/l) | 1.83 | 0.66–3.30 | 0.48 | 0.74 | 0.50–0.86 | |
| Vitamin $B_{12}$ ($\mu$g/l) | trace | | | 6.6 | 3.2–12.4 | |
| Folic acid ($\mu$g/l) | 24.0 | 7.4–61.0 | | 37.7 | 16.8–63.2 | |
| Biotin ($\mu$g/l) | 2 | 1–3 | | 22 | 14–29 | |
| Pantothenic acid (mg/l) | 2.46 | 0.86–5.84 | 0.63 | 3.4 | 2.2–5.5 | |
| Ascorbic acid (mg/l) | 52 | 0–112 | 19 | 11 | 3–23 | |

*From Macy IG, Kelly HJ: Human milk and cows' milk in infant nutrition. In Kon SK, Cowie AT (eds): Milk: The Mammary Gland and Its Secretion, p 265. London, Academic Press, 1961.

†Calculated by D. Burman in McLaren DS, Burman D (eds): Textbook of Paediatric Nutrition. Edinburgh, Churchill Livingstone, 1976

(Adapted from Documenta Geigy Scientific Tables, 7th ed. Basle, Switzerland, Ciba-Geigy Ltd, 1970)

cians as the chief source of iron during the first 6 months of infancy when the RDA is 10 mg per day.

Infant (dry) cereals, also fortified with iron, may be introduced by 4 to 6 (the second or third month for low-birth-weight infants) months. Because many of these supply approximately 1 mg of iron per tablespoon, they provide the additional iron recommended for the 6 to 12 month infant (15 mg of iron for a 9-kg infant), assuming the iron-fortified formula is continued.

If the 6- to 12-month infant is to get 15 mg of iron as specified in the RDA, both the iron-fortified formula and infant cereal must be continued throughout the first 12 months rather than making a change at 4 to 6 months to whole cow's milk and using other forms of cereal, as is the current practice. Approximately 5 mg to 6 mg of iron is supplied by the fortified formula, 5 mg to 6 mg by the fortified cereal, and 4 mg to 5 mg by the addition of meat, vegetables, and fruits carefully selected for their iron content. The inclusion of some meat and a good source of ascorbic acid improves the availability of the iron in the diet.

### Iodine

Table 18-1 gives the recommended dietary allowance for iodine during the first year. Although the amount of iodine in human milk and cow's milk varies depending on the quantity that has been consumed in food and water, the breast-fed infant of an adequately nourished mother is assumed to receive at least the recommended amounts. In regions of the United States where the soil is low in iodine, feeding practices in dairies may increase the amount of iodine in cow's milk. The introduction of strained foods to the infant's diet may also be a source of iodine depending on the nature of the soil in which they were grown.

### Zinc

Human and cow's milk contains approximately the same amount of zinc. Low zinc concentrations in hair have been found in infants with a history of poor appetite and growth retardation.[7] Breast-fed infants receive 2 mg or more per day of zinc in a highly available form; for this reason, the allowance for infants during the first 6 months of life was set at 3 mg per day. Acrodermatitis enteropathica is a rare disease caused by an inherited recessive gene defect in zinc metabolism, which results in a serious zinc deficiency state. Treatment involves zinc supplementation.

## Fluorine

In technically advanced countries the magnitude of the dental caries problem exceeds that of all other nutritional diseases. It has been dramatically demonstrated that children 6 years old born after fluoridation started in one community had significantly fewer cavities than children 10 or 11 years old using the same water supply but born before fluoridation started.[8] These differences suggest that fluoride prophylaxis during infancy is desirable. The advisable intake proposed by Fomon,[9] 0.5 mg per day, is approximately the amount that would be ingested by infants fed formulas diluted with equal parts of water fluoridated at the usual level of 1 ppm. Ranges of 0.1 mg to 1.0 mg during the first year of life are suggested as adequate and safe.[2]

Other trace elements—copper, chromium, manganese, molybdenum, and selenium—are assumed to be essential for the infant in extremely small amounts, which are supplied by the usual diet. See Table 11-3 for Estimated Safe and Adequate Allowances for these trace minerals.

## Electrolytes

Both the Food and Nutrition Board[2] and the American Academy of Pediatrics[4] have set minimum and maximum levels for sodium, potassium, and chloride intakes for infants. Table 11-3 shows the Estimated Safe and Adequate Dietary Allowances for these electrolytes. Recently a number of cases of hypochloremic metabolic alkalosis occurred in infants receiving formulas low in chloride.[10]

## Vitamins

The recommended dietary allowances for the vitamins (Table 18-1) may be met by human milk or cow's milk formulas consumed at a rate of approximately 850 ml per day, with the following exceptions.

*Vitamin D.* The breast-fed infant should receive a supplement of 10 mcg or 400 IU of vitamin D per day after about 5 days of age. If the infant is bottle-fed with a commercial formula already fortified providing this amount of vitamin D, no further supplement is necessary.

*Vitamin E.* Human milk is higher in vitamin E content (2 IU to 5 IU of $\alpha$-tocopherol per liter) and meets the infant's requirement, whereas cow's milk is relatively low (only about $\frac{1}{10}$ to $\frac{1}{2}$ of the amount in human milk) in vitamin E content and does not meet the RDA. Most of the commercial infant formulas have had vitamin E added to them and supply approximately 1.3 mg per 100 ml. Some vitamin preparations for infants also include vitamin E.

Low-birth-weight infants require additional amounts of vitamin E.[2]

*Vitamin K.* The Committee on Nutrition of the American Academy of Pediatrics[11] recommends that every newborn infant receive a single oral dose of 1.0-2.0 mg of vitamin K or a intramuscular dose of 0.5 mg to 1.0 mg of phytylmenaquinone (vitamin K) soon after birth. This is especially important for breast-fed infants because human milk (15 mcg per liter) provides much less vitamin K than cow's milk (60 mcg per liter); as a result, vitamin K deficiency in the newborn period is more common in breast-fed infants.[12] It is recommended that all infant formulas contain a minimum of 4 mcg per 100 kcal.[4]

Precautions are necessary in the use of the fat-soluble vitamins, which should be given in the amounts recommended but not in excess of them, because an excess of these factors can be toxic (see Chap. 7).

*Ascorbic Acid.* Ascorbic acid is a limiting factor for bottle-fed infants whose homemade formulas are subjected to high-heat processing. Infants should receive a supplementary source of ascorbic acid by the tenth day of life. A synthetic source of this vitamin rather than orange juice is frequently recommended for small infants because it minimizes any sensitizing reaction. Most commercially prepared infant formulas have had ascorbic acid added to them, and because these require no further heat processing, the vitamin C is available. When used according to the directions on the label, 1 quart of prepared formula supplies approximately 50 mg of ascorbic acid.

*Folacin.* The recommended dietary allowance for folacin during the first year is supplied by either human milk or cow's milk, both of which are relatively good sources of this nutrient. Because folic acid is heat-labile, infants receiving boiled homemade formulas should receive a supplement. Folic acid has been added to the prepared commercial formulas in amounts to supply 100 mcg of folacin per liter of formula. Estimated Safe and Adequate Daily Dietary Intakes of biotin and pantothenic acid are given in Table 11-3.

## Breast-feeding

Among American mothers the downward trend in breast-feeding, which had been in progress since the 1950s, was reversed in the 1970s. Breast-feeding is reported more common among white women and among women with 12 or more years of education. Although breast-feeding has become more popular, it continues to be of relatively short duration, with fewer than 5% of the mothers reporting that they breast-fed for 3 months or more.[13]

## Psychological factors

There is much evidence that the earliest experiences of the newborn infant are of great importance to his total growth and development. This is particularly true of the way he obtains his food. Even at this early stage, he reacts to the emotions of the mother, and this is of more importance than whether he is breast- or formula-fed. If the mother is relaxed and confident, the infant will respond to her and, through her, to the world about him with trust and confidence. On the other hand, if the mother is tense and overanxious, or if the feeding is hurried, the infant becomes aware of discomfort. In response, he may become fretful or cry, which could prevent his taking the food he needs.

Certain psychological advantages have been attributed to breast-feeding. Many mothers derive satisfaction from feeling they are the source of their infant's nutriment. Also, breast-feeding permits early establishment of an intimacy with the child that bodes well for the mother–child relationship.

A mother should be encouraged to breast-feed her infant, but she should not be made to feel guilty if she prefers to bottle-feed him. If he is cuddled and made comfortable when he is being fed, whether by breast or by bottle, he will feel warm and comforted.

### Nutritional factors

Human milk from a well nourished mother, when consumed in amounts sufficient to fulfill caloric needs, meets the recommended intakes for all nutrients, and there is no need for supplementation except for vitamin D and possibly fluoride during the first 4 to 6 months of life.

The nutritive composition and the interaction of nutrients in human milk may result in certain advantages of breast feeding compared to formula feeding. Human milk contains about one-third the amount of protein in cow's milk. It has a much higher proportion of whey proteins to casein than cow's milk—60:40 compared to 18:82. The essential amino acids constitute 45% of the total amino acids in human milk. The protein content is highest in colostrum (secretions first 3–5 days after delivery) and decreases during the rest of lactation. Similarly, the growth rate of the infant decreases as the amount of milk he ingests increases.

The amount of carbohydrate, lactose, in human milk (42% of calories) is greater than in cow's milk (32% of calories). Mature milk contains more lactose than colostrum. Lactose is responsible for enhancing the growth of fermentative rather than putrefactive bacteria in the intestinal tract. It also lowers the $pH$ and thereby improves absorption of minerals, such as calcium and magnesium.

Although the total fat content of human and cow's milk is similar, the amount of fat absorbed from human milk is greater. Several factors appear to be responsible for the decreased fecal loss of fat from human milk. Human milk contains a lipase which is active even at 4°C. There is a greater degree of unsaturation in human milk fat, 12% compared to 4% in cow's milk. There is also a difference in the position of palmitic acid on the glycerol base. Pancre-

atic lipase hydrolyzes fatty acids in the 1 and 3 positions, resulting in free fatty acids and 2-monoglycerides. Palmitic acid is better absorbed as 2-monopalmitin because the free fatty acid combines with calcium to form an insoluble soap, which is lost in the stools. Of the palmitic acid in human milk 74% is on the 2 position, in contrast with only 39% in cow's milk. Human milk contains 5% more essential fatty acids than cow's milk, which contains 1%. Colostrum supplies much less fat than mature milk. There is also considerable variation in the fat content of human milk during a feeding with the fat content being higher at the end of a feeding compared to the first milk from a breast. This may make it easier for the breast-fed infant to regulate his calorie intake and reduce the incidence of excessive weight gain in early infancy. The fatty acid composition of human milk is affected by the maternal diet. If calories are restricted, the fatty acid composition reflects maternal fat stores.

The mineral content of cow's milk is about three times greater than that of human milk, but there are considerable differences in the relative amounts of the various elements, Table 18-3. There is almost seven times more phosphorus, three times more calcium, sodium, and magnesium and twice as much potassium, sulfur, chloride, manganese, zinc, iodine, and selenium in cow's milk than in human milk. Copper is higher in human milk, and iron is approximately the same in cow's milk and human milk. Equally significant are the differences in the absorption of minerals from the two milks. Approximately 50% of the iron in human milk is absorbed compared to 10% in cow's milk; 50% to 70% of the calcium in breast milk is absorbed in contrast to 10% to 55% in cow's milk. The calcium to phosphorus ratio of 2:1 in human milk compared to 1.2:1 in cow's milk accounts for the fact that infantile tetany occurs almost exclusively in formula-fed infants.

The B-complex vitamins are higher in cow's milk, whereas vitamins A, C, and E are higher in human milk. Human milk, however, meets the needs for all these vitamins. Levels of vitamins D and K in human milk are low and, for this reason, requirements for these nutrients must be met in other ways for the breast-fed infant.

### Immunological factors

In poor areas or where medical aid is not available, breast milk may be safer than a poor formula or one unhygienically prepared. Breast milk also has the advantage of freedom from contamination and of requiring no preparation. The bifidus factor in human milk is often referred to as the "intestinal guardian" because it appears to inhibit growth of certain pathogenic organisms by creating an acid environment in the gastrointestinal tract. The lysozyme content of human milk, which is much higher than cow's milk, may also have a bactericidal effect. Lactoferrin, an iron-binding protein in milk, has been shown to inhibit the growth of bacteria by denying them iron. Human milk also contains antibodies important in immunizing the infant against certain infectious diseases. Moreover, human milk is less likely to cause allergic reactions.

## Other factors

The lactating woman will find that she needs more food than a nonlactating woman of her age and size, and it may cost her more per week to feed herself during the time that she is sharing her nutriment with her infant. The cost of feeding the mother extra nutrients may be less than the cost of purchasing commercial infant formula for the infant.

Because certain drugs may pass from the mother's blood to her milk, it is recommended that nursing mothers not receive certain medications. The Food and Drug Administration is requiring that information for nursing mothers be provided in the "Precautions" section of prescription drug labeling. All drugs that are absorbed through the gastrointestinal tract have labeling for the physicians that includes all that is known about excretion of the drug in human milk and the effects on the nursing mother.

Drugs that are known to affect the breast-fed infant are chloral hydrate, diazepam (Valium), phenobarbital, bromide, chlorpromazine (Thorazine), primidone (Mysoline), caffeine, penicillin, propoxyphene (Darvon), and most laxatives.

Nursing is contraindicated in women taking such drugs as chloramphenicol, metronidazole, lithium, reserpine, and antithyroid drugs.

An infant can become addicted to heroin if the mother is taking large doses of the drug while nursing. Similarly, nursing can help break the infant's addiction to heroin if the mother is using methadone.[14]

## The process of lactation

The decision of whether to breast-feed or bottle-feed the infant should be made during pregnancy. If the mother decides to breast-feed, instructions for the preparation of her breasts prior to delivery should be given by the nurse. Some young mothers will breast-feed their infants if careful teaching and psychological as well as physical preparation is instigated early in pregnancy. Moreover, the nursing mother must be sure to have the proper diet (see Chap. 17) and get sufficient sleep and relaxation; otherwise she will not produce enough milk.

Table 18-4 shows the approximate quantity of milk consumed by an average infant under normal conditions, proving that the mother must eat properly if she is to produce this quantity of milk.

Lactation is under the control of hormonal and psychological factors. Prolactin is the major hormone involved in milk production, and it rises after delivery when there is a fall in maternal blood levels of estrogen and progesterone. Oxytocin is the hormone responsible for milk ejection; it causes the transfer of milk from the epithelial cells of the alveoli into the ducts and sinuses, thereby making it available to the infant. The infant's sucking causes the let-down reflex, and milk in the sinuses and ducts can be withdrawn easily. Psychological factors, such as hearing the infant cry, or thoughts of the infant, may also elicit the let-down reflex and cause milk to be ejected.

The thick, yellowish fluid that appears the first few days of nursing (colostrum) nourishes the baby until the milk comes a few days later. The infant should be laid beside the mother with his cheek close to her breast. He will turn his head toward the breast trying to find the nipple (*rooting reflex*), and the mother can help him by holding the breast so that he can get the nipple into his mouth. To express the milk and prevent nipple irritation, most of the areola should be in the infant's mouth, not just the tip of the nipple.

Nursing the baby will in itself increase the milk supply of the mother, and she will be able to satisfy his needs with an ever increasing supply as he keeps growing. At first the infant may be satisfied after he has emptied only one breast, but if he does not give signs that he is full, he should be given the other breast. He should be started on this breast at his next feeding to be sure it is emptied.

## Formulas—types and sources

The physician usually determines the type of formula for the newborn infant. Various factors, such as availability, ease of preparation, cost, and (most important) the infant's needs, should be considered in recommending the type and amount of feeding to be given.

### Fresh cow's milk

Although there is a tendency toward the earlier introduction of undiluted fresh, whole homogenized, or skim milk, this is rarely the form prescribed for the newborn (see Chap. 35).

Because whole cow's milk contains more protein and mineral salts and less milk sugar than human milk, it is usually modified for the newborn by dilution with water and the addition of some form of sugar. Most homogenized milk is fortified with 400 IU of vitamin D per quart.

### Evaporated whole milk

Although it has much to recommend it for use in infants' formulas, evaporated whole milk is less used than it formerly was. Because evaporated milk is already sterilized, it is easy to prepare. The heat processing and homogenizing it undergoes results in both a soft, easily digested curd and well distributed digestible fat. Evaporated milk contains 400 IU of vitamin D per reconstituted quart and is less expensive than commercial formula.

Evaporated milk formula, however, is deficient in folic acid, and infants on this type of formula should receive supplementation. It is available in two different size cans—$5\frac{1}{2}$-oz and 13-oz.

### Condensed cow's milk

With its high sugar content, condensed cow's milk is considered undesirable for infant feeding.

### Skim milk

Deficient in calories as well as in essential fatty acids, skim milk is not recommended for infant feeding.

### Prepared commercial formulas

These are by far the most popular type of infant feeding for the newborn. They are available in a variety of forms: powdered, concentrated-liquid, ready-to-feed, and in feeding bottles, ready-to-feed. Their cost is related to their ease of use. Currently, the two most popular forms are the concentrated-liquid, and the ready-to-feed. Several brands are marketed, with and without added iron. The American Academy of Pediatrics[4] has recommended standards for the Food and Drug Administration's regulations on nutrient levels of infant formulas.

Commercial formulas may also be modified in one or more of the following ways. Butterfat may be removed, and a vegetable oil or oils added to increase the amount of unsaturated fatty acid, particularly the essential fatty acid, linoleic acid. This makes the cow's milk formula more like breast milk in essential fatty acid content, and fat in this form is better tolerated by the infant. The protein may be treated to produce a softer, more flocculent curd, which is more easily digested by the infant. The milk may be diluted to reduce the calcium and, to make up for this dilution of calories, sugar—usually lactose—is added. Both of these modifications make the formula more like breast milk. Dialysis may be used to reduce the sodium content of cow's milk. Examples of commercially prepared formulas are given in Table 18-5.

Only by carefully reading the labels on the individual brands can one be sure of the exact nutritive content of the formula. The nutrition counselor should urge the mothers to follow the specific directions for the form she is using. Dilution of a ready-to-feed can of formula may reduce the infant's nutritive intake, whereas failure to dilute the concentrated liquid form may result in too strong a formula, which the infant may vomit. Care should also be taken to sterilize the bottles, nipples, and can opener. Water, if it is to be added, should be sterilized if there is any question about its safety.

If facilities for sterilizing bottles or refrigeration are unavailable, as, for instance, in a home emergency or when traveling, the individual 4-oz, 6-oz, or 8-oz bottles called nursettes may be an excellent way to ensure a safe supply of milk for the infant.

### Goat milk

Seldom used today in the United States for infant feeding, goat milk is still used in many parts of the world. Experience shows that it is nutritionally adequate in most respects, except for folacin. Infants receiving goat milk as their major source of calories should receive folacin supplements. Goat milk was formerly used to feed infants who had an allergy to cow's milk; it is still used occasionally today and is available in drug and grocery stores. Goat milk fat differs from fat in cow's milk in that it contains more essential fatty acids and has a greater percentage of medium- and short-chain fatty acids. These differences suggest that the fat of goat milk may be more readily digested than that of cow's milk.

### Milk substitutes

Certain infants are born with a sensitivity to the proteins of all milks. This may be mild enough to cause irritability only, or it may be severe enough to cause violent illness and even death. Several preparations have been devised as formulas to approximate human milk in carbohydrate, protein, fat, mineral, and vitamin content. These contain no milk at all. Soybean preparations are used most commonly. Usually, the protein in the soybean can be taken by infants allergic to the proteins of milk. A milk substitute having meat protein as a base, with added vitamins and minerals, has also proved to be adequate nutritionally for such infants (see Table 35-4, Chap. 35).

If these milk substitutes are properly supplemented, infants do as well on them as on other formula feedings.

Galactosemia and lactose intolerance in infants and children are discussed in Chapters 26 and 35.

### Temperature for feeding

The formula may be given at room temperature or warmed to body temperature if desired. If the formula has been stored in the refrigerator, it should be allowed to stand long enough to reach room temperature, or the

**Table 18-4. Approximate Quantities of Milk Consumed by an Average Infant During the First 6 Months of Life**

|  | g | oz |
|---|---|---|
| 1st day | 10 | $\frac{1}{3}$ |
| 2d day | 90 | 3 |
| 3d day | 190 | $6\frac{1}{3}$ |
| 4th day | 300 | 10 |
| 5th day | 350 | $11\frac{1}{2}$ |
| 6th day | 390 | 13 |
| 7th day | 470 | $15\frac{2}{3}$ |
| 3d week | 500 | 16 |
| 4th week | 600 | 20 |
| 8th week | 800 | $26\frac{1}{2}$ |
| 12th week | 900 | 30 |
| 24th week | 1000 | 33 |

bottle may be placed in warm water until it reaches the desired temperature.

The temperature of milk should be tested by shaking a few drops on the inside of the wrist. The older infant may tolerate his formula straight from the refrigerator.

### How often to feed

Much has been said in recent years about so-called self-demand schedules of feeding. For many years infants were fed by the clock, no matter whether they were hungry earlier or later than the scheduled time. Today we recognize that the time to feed an infant is when he is hungry, whether the interval is 2, 3, 4, or even 5 hours. The inexperienced mother may need help in recognizing the difference between a hunger cry and a cry for something else.

A newborn infant may wake up to be fed eight to ten times in 24 hours. By the time he is a month old, there may be 3 hours between feedings. Most infants establish themselves on a schedule of 4-hour feedings by the time they are between 2 and 3 months old. During this time, too, the infant begins to sleep through the night after a late evening feeding. The nutrition counselor should also recognize that the frequency of feeding is influenced by the attitude of the mother as well as by other demands on her time.

### Burping the infant

Once or twice during a feeding, the infant should be given a chance to bring up any swallowed air. Holding him up so that his stomach is against the mother's shoulder and gently patting him on the back helps to eliminate

### Table 18-5. Average Nutrient Content of Commercially Prepared Milk-Based Formulas (Per 100 ml)

|  | Enfamil† | Similac‡ | SMA§ |
|---|---|---|---|
| Energy, kcal | 67 | 68 | 67 |
| Protein, g | 1.5 | 1.55 | 1.5 |
| Type of protein | nonfat cow milk | nonfat cow milk | demineralized whey and nonfat cow milk |
| Fat, total, g | 3.7 | 3.6 | 3.6 |
| Saturated, g | 1.2 | 1.4 | 1.6 |
| Unsaturated, g | 2.5 | 2.2 | 2.0 |
| Type of Fat | soy, coconut | coconut, soy | oleo, coconut, soy, safflower |
| Cholesterol, mg | 1.4 | 1.6 | 3.3 |
| Carbohydrate, g | 7.0 | 7.2 | 7.2 |
| Type of carbohydrate | lactose | lactose | lactose |
| Ash, g | 0.4 | 0.4 | 0.3 |
| Calcium, mg | 55 | 51 | 44 |
| Phosphorus, mg | 46 | 39 | 33 |
| Iron, mg | 0.15 | 0.15 |  |
|  | (1.27)* | (1.2)* | (1.3)* |
| Iodine, mcg | 46 | 10 | 7 |
| Copper, mcg | 63 | 60 | 48 |
| Magnesium, mg | 4.7 | 4.1 | 5.3 |
| Zinc, mg | 0.42 | 0.50 | 0.37 |
| Sodium, mg | 28 | 22 | 15 |
| Potassium, mg | 70 | 78 | 56 |
| Vitamin A, IU | 251 | 250 | 264 |
| Vitamin D, IU | 42 | 40 | 42 |
| Vitamin E, mg | 1.3 | 1.5 | 1.0 |
| Vitamin K, mcg | 7 | 9 | 6 |
| Ascorbic acid, mg | 5.5 | 5.5 | 5.5 |
| Thiamin, mcg | 53 | 65 | 71 |
| Riboflavin, mcg | 63 | 100 | 106 |
| Niacin equiv., mg | 0.8 | 0.7 | 1.0 |
| Pyridoxine, mcg | 42 | 40 | 42 |
| Pantothenic acid, mg | 0.32 | 0.30 | 0.21 |
| Vitamin $B_{12}$, mcg | 0.21 | 0.15 | 0.11 |
| Folacin, mcg | 10.6 | 10.0 | 5.3 |

*Sold as "Iron Fortified."

†Producer, Mead-Johnson Laboratories, Evansville, IN 47721.

‡Producer, Ross Laboratories, Columbus, OH 43216.

§Producer, Wyeth Laboratories, Philadelphia, PA 19101.

the air. An even better method is for the mother to hold the infant in a sitting position on her knee, with his chin held in the palm of her hand. By leaning the infant forward and gently stroking or patting his back, swallowed air is released.

### Psychosocial aspects of infant feeding

If the mother is feeding her infant by bottle, she should hold him as though she were breast-feeding him, cradled in her arm, in order to give him the same sense of nearness and companionship. It is important that she feel relaxed and unhurried and that she enjoys this time with her infant. It is particularly important that the bottle-fed infant not be overfed. Because the mother cannot tell how much the breast-fed infant has consumed, she is inclined to assume that the infant is satisfied when he stops sucking, whereas the mother who is feeding her infant by bottle may urge him to completely finish the bottle. This early training may be the beginning of overfeeding and one of the causes of obesity in later life.

Moreover, the infant should not be allowed to eat by himself from a bottle propped up beside him. His nutritional needs may be met this way but not his need for love and contact.

By feeding "on demand," the mother also eliminates the infant's frustration caused by hunger and helps him develop trust and security in the feeder. Talking and repeating sounds to the infant while he is being fed is a valuable learning experience and may be an important aspect of his later intellectual development.

## Feeding difficulties in infants

### Vomiting and regurgitation

Vomiting may result from a number of causes and may or may not be a serious symptom. In regurgitation only small amounts of food are lost, whereas in vomiting the contractions are sufficiently strong to empty the stomach. Regurgitation may be avoided by burping the infant once or twice during a feeding. Occasional vomiting is usually caused by overdistention of the stomach due to the ingestion of too large or too frequent feedings or to the swallowing of air. It may also be caused by an imbalance of the food constituents, especially an oversupply of fat, which delays emptying of the stomach. Persistent vomiting may be a symptom of infection, obstruction, or other serious ailment and should be referred promptly to the physician. The cause should be determined and the feedings adjusted accordingly.

### Colic

An infant who has hard crying spells shortly after eating is said to be "colicky." The colic, or severe abdominal cramping pain, may be caused by distention due to the

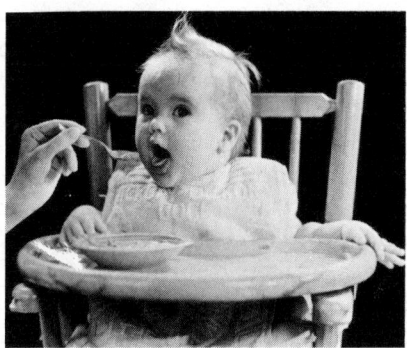

**Fig. 18-2.**  The right start for the baby. Liking comes through learning to like. Teach the flavor of a variety of foods early. (Gesell A, Ilg, FL: Behavior of Infants. Philadelphia, JB Lippincott)

swallowing of air; to gas formed by bacterial fermentation of undigested food; to overfeeding or underfeeding; to cold, excitement, or fatigue. The infant may have to be burped again. Making sure he is warm may help. Mothers are apt to think that his feeding is wrong, but changing the feeding usually does not help. Spock[15] says that these babies seem to grow and gain weight better than most, and that generally, the condition disappears at the age of 3 to 4 months.

### Diarrhea

Loose stools may be serious, and the doctor should be consulted at once. See Chapter 35 for diseases in which diarrhea is a symptom.

### Constipation

Constipation in infancy is not infrequent. Many mothers are concerned when the infant has only one bowel movement per day or on alternate days. The number of movements per day is not of so much importance as the consistency of the stools. If the feces are hard and expelled with difficulty, then the child may be said to be constipated and should be treated accordingly. Increasing the amount of fruit in the diet and giving additional water usually relieves constipation. If it persists, the doctor should be consulted.

## Introduction of solid foods

Fomon[16] has introduced the German word *Beikost*— other than milk or formula—to describe the semisolid or transitional foods used in infant feeding. Because these terms may be unfamiliar to the readers of this text, the authors will continue to refer to such foods as *solids* or *semisolids*.

Opinions about the time for the addition of supplementary foods to the diet of the breast- or formula-fed infant have undergone marked changes in the past 60 years. Whereas prior to the 1920s, no solid foods were introduced until the end of the first year, the pendulum swung all the way to the opposite extreme of offering the infant semisolids during the first month of life. The availability of commercially prepared infant foods introduced in the 1920s no doubt contributed to this practice. In the 1950s Beal[17] found that the early introduction of solid foods tended to meet resistance from the infant. The average infant's willing acceptance of cereal and fruit occurred at $2\frac{1}{2}$ to 3 months, of vegetables at 4 to $4\frac{1}{2}$ months and of meat and meat soups at $5\frac{1}{2}$ to 6 months.

Later studies, however, indicated that most infants were fed some solid foods before they were 2 months old and that they began to eat foods from the family table before the end of the first year.

Recently, there are indications that pediatricians and nutrition counselors are advising that the introduction of semisolid foods be delayed until 4 to 6 months of age for the formula-fed infant and until 6 months of age for the breast-fed infant. By 4 months of age the extrusion reflex disappears and the infant is able to move food from the front of the mouth to the pharynx efficiently, which makes feeding easier. By waiting for this neuromuscular readiness other problems associated with the early introduction of semisolid food may be avoided. Food intolerances and allergies may be reduced if semisolid foods and fresh milk are withheld until the intestinal permeability of the neonate has decreased and there is an increased production of IgA antibody. Early feeding of semisolid food may also create problems of overnutrition and result in excessive weight gain in early infancy. There is no scientific evidence that the early introduction of semisolid food causes the infant to sleep through the night. In fact, there is no known nutritional reason for starting solid food before 3 months of age or later if the infant's nutritional needs are being met with breast milk or a quart or less of formula per day.[18] It is usually not necessary to start semisolid foods until the infant is at least 6 kg to 7 kg. Because the introduction of semisolid food to the breast-fed infant appears to interfere with the absorption of iron from human milk,[19] some pediatricians are suggesting a delay in these foods until about 6 months; at this time additional iron is needed for hemoglobin synthesis, and the quantity of breast milk alone is not sufficient to meet the energy needs in the larger, growing infant.

In any case, semisolid foods should be introduced slowly. Each new food should be introduced separately, and 4 to 5 days should elapse before starting another new food so that any intolerance to an individual food may be easily identified. Although there is no set order for introducing new foods, it is common practice to start with infant rice cereal, then fruits, then vegetables, and finally meats. Due to the infant's ability to chew and swallow, texture should be an important consideration. Excessive sugar and salt should be avoided. All mealtimes should be pleasant experiences.

## Cereals

Cereals are usually added to the infant's diet between 4 and 6 months of age. Dry, precooked cereal preparations are fortified with iron, whereas the "wet-packed" jars of cereal may or may not be iron-fortified.

Dry, precooked cereals must be mixed with warm formula or whole milk, whereas others may need only to be warmed. Only a small amount of cereal should be used at first, and this is generally given with the midmorning feeding. The original small amount may be increased gradually to $\frac{1}{4}$ to $\frac{1}{2}$ cup, and in a few weeks it may be of a thicker consistency.

## Fruits

Cooked, strained fruits, and ripe banana may be added to the infant's diet when he is between 4 and 6 months old. Like cereals, these may be purchased in cans or jars, all ready for infant use, or they may be prepared at home without the addition of excessive amounts of sugar. Cooked fruits should be put through a sieve or strainer to puree them. Strained apple sauce, prunes, peaches, pears, and apricots are suitable. Ripe mashed banana may also be given. Starting with a teaspoonful once or twice a day, the infant will soon take 2 to 3 tablespoonfuls. Most infants like fruit and take it readily. This helps them to accept the taste of other solid foods, which may not appeal to them quite as much.

## Vegetables

By the fifth or sixth month, strained vegetables are usually introduced. Those added first are peas, string beans, spinach, carrots, and squash. Fresh, frozen, or canned vegetables are suitable. If prepared at home, they should be cooked in a small amount of water, as would be done for the family meal, and the infant's portion put through a sieve or a strainer before the addition of salt. Again, these and other varieties of vegetables are available in cans or jars in most grocery stores, prepared and ready for serving after they are warmed. Starting with a teaspoonful at one feeding, the infant will soon be taking 2 to 3 rounded tablespoonfuls. Potatoes, both sweet and white, may be added a little later, but potatoes in any form are one of the last vegetables to be accepted by most infants.

## Meats

Meats are usually the last food group introduced. The most convenient way of serving meat to the infant is in cans; strained beef, beef heart, liver, lamb, chicken, veal, and pork preparations are available in cans and jars at most grocery stores. To prepare meat for the infant at home, the mother should buy a lean cut of beef, pork, lamb, veal, or poultry. It may be simmered or pan broiled and then put in a blender with sufficient water to achieve the desired consistency. Liver may be prepared in the same way. If a blender is not available, a fork or dull knife may be used to scrape meat off fibers from the surface of a cooked or cleaned raw piece of meat. If raw meat is used, the resulting meat pulp may be heated until it is brown in a custard cup set in a small pan of water over heat.

Meats add protein, iron, and some of the B complex vitamins to the infant's diet. Again, it is best to begin slowly with a teaspoonful or less, increasing the quantity as the infant grows older.

### Handling and storage of home-prepared baby foods

Particular care must be taken in preparing and storing home-prepared baby food. The food should be sufficiently cooked (boiled) to destroy any microorganisms that might be present in the raw food. Only utensils that have been thoroughly washed and scalded with boiling water should be used to process the food. Individual portions of the food may be frozen in ice cube trays. When frozen solid they may be transferred to plastic bags and sealed.

### Widening variety in the infant diet

By the time they are 6 months old, most babies are introduced to some semisolid foods. They may also be starting to take some milk or fruit juice from a cup. In addition to milk, a good meal plan for an infant of this age is to give him cereal and fruit at breakfast, vegetable and meat for lunch, and cereal and fruit for supper. The quantities depend on his appetite.

#### Additional foods, 6 to 12 months

The infant welcomes a piece of dried bread, toast, or an infant teething biscuit to hold in his hands and chew on, particularly if his teeth are beginning to appear. If potato has not already been given, it can be added at this time, mashed fine. Puddings made mainly with milk, such as junket, cornstarch, tapioca, and rice pudding, may also be added occasionally for variety. A small piece of fish, such as flounder, haddock, or halibut, may be substituted for meat now and then. It should be poached gently in water to cover until it flakes, and *all bones carefully removed.*

By the time he is 9 months old, it is time to try serving some of the junior foods, or foods mashed with a fork, instead of strained foods. The change should be made gradually and should not be forced. Vegetables and fruits may be tried this way first. Meat is better served strained until after the first year, because it is so much more difficult to swallow.

Babies often enjoy a piece of crisp bacon or a bit of raw, *peeled* apple when they are allowed to hold it in their hands and suck on it.

Mixed dishes, either junior foods or appropriate ones from the family table, may also be added. These include spaghetti with meat sauce, macaroni and cheese, and tuna fish and noodles.

As the infant becomes acquainted with a variety of things, including his food, he will want to explore it with the tools that he has at his command. To quote Rabinovitch:[20] "In the second half of the first year, the baby will begin to mess with food, to feel its texture and consistency, to finger-feed himself as he recognizes his growing dexterity. Such experimentation, often difficult for the cleanliness-and-germ-conscious mother, is essential for the child as he learns to relate to food by messing, smelling and pouring. That a high degree of parental fortitude is necessary to allow for these developmental realities goes without saying."

#### Weaning

The weaning of an infant from sucking from a nipple to taking milk from a cup is not an abrupt transition as infants are fed today. As soon as the infant is introduced to the supplementary foods discussed earlier, he is on the way to being weaned. Although he may have learned to drink from a cup by the time he is 7 to 9 months old, he may still be fed from a bottle or the breast until he is a year old. Milk should be restricted to no more than 3 cups (750 ml) per day.

## Other considerations in infant feeding

### Commercial baby foods

The widespread use of commercial baby foods by mothers in the U.S. today makes knowledge of these foods especially important. Anderson and Fomon[21,22] have discussed the many factors that must be considered in using them, such as the differences and similarities between various groups of infant foods. Table 18-6 compares the proximate composition of the commercially prepared infant foods and similar foods prepared at home. Note the much lower calorie, protein, and fat content of the commercially prepared foods, due to the higher water content, compared with the same items prepared at home.

### Salt and sugar in commercial baby foods

Most of the commercially prepared single-ingredient baby foods do not have salt or sugar added to them. Mothers should read the labels on all baby foods in order to determine the ingredients. Excess salt and sugar should be avoided.

### Satiety

This mechanism, by which the infant is made aware that he has had enough, varies widely in infants. In some, the reaction is sharp, and they actively resist further feeding attempts. In others, satiety is less sharply defined, and interest in eating wanes gradually after a period of playfulness. Still others do not seem to know when they have had enough and vomit what they cannot handle. Remember, overfeeding in infancy may establish an undesirable food pattern for later life.

**Table 18-6. Proximate Composition of Selected Commercially Prepared Baby Foods and Home-Prepared Foods of the Same Name**

| Product | Energy kcal/100 g | Proximate Analysis (g/100 g) | | | |
|---|---|---|---|---|---|
| | | *Water* | *Protein* | *Fat* | *Carbohydrate* |
| Chicken and noodles, cooked from home recipe* | 152 | 71.0 | 9.2 | 7.5 | 10.8 |
| Strained chicken noodle dinner† | 57 | 87.0 | 2.4 | 1.5 | 8.5 |
| Spaghetti with meatballs in tomato sauce cooked from home recipe* | 133 | 70.0 | 7.7 | 4.8 | 15.7 |
| Junior spaghetti, tomato sauce, and meat† | 63 | 84.7 | 2.8 | 1.1 | 10.9 |

*From Adams CF, Richardson M: Nutritive Value of Foods. Home and Garden Bulletin No. 72. Washington, DC, USDA, 1981 (items 215 and 497).

†From Gerber Products Co, Fremont, MI 49412.

## Criteria for judging nutritional adequacy

The criteria for judging adequate nutrition in an infant are a steady gain in weight; a moderate increase in subcutaneous fat; the development of firm muscles; good elimination; and an infant who is happy, sleeps well, and shows normal curiosity about his surroundings.

## Overnutrition

The nutrition counselor should be particularly aware of the hazards of overnutrition. She must be able to relate these to the mother, who may look upon a fat baby as a healthy, happy baby and sees no cause for alarm.

Infants who show an excessive weight gain from overfeeding even as early as 6 weeks of age are reported to have a greater tendency toward overweight and obesity later in childhood.[23] As previously discussed in Chapter 16, there may also be an increase in the total number of fat cells in the body of an infant who is overnourished during the phase of rapid fat cell division, and this condition may persist throughout his life. Although the reasons are not clear, there is evidence that obese infants also have a higher incidence of respiratory infections than those of normal weight.[24]

# The toddler

## Nutritional requirements of early childhood

The recommended dietary allowances for infants 1 to 3 years old are shown in Table 18-7.

### Calories

The calorie needs from 1 to 3 years are relatively low (Table 18-7), and in order to ensure a diet adequate in other nutrients, careful selection of the toddler's food is essential.

### Protein

Protein needs for growth of muscles and other tissue are relatively high during this period. They are easily met, however, if the toddler consumes a pint of milk and 1 oz to 2 oz of meat each day.

### Minerals

*Calcium, phosphorus,* and *magnesium* recommendations also depend on the inclusion each day of 1 pint of milk and 1 oz to 2 oz of meat.

The recommended dietary allowance for *iron*, 15 mg, is not easily met with the usual diet at this age, and a supplement may be necessary.

Meat and seafood are important sources of available *zinc.*

In areas where iodine in the soil is limited, a small amount of iodized salt in cooking and seasoning adequately provides for the recommended amounts of *iodine.*

**Table 18-7. Recommended Dietary Allowances for the 1- to 3-Year-Old**

| | 1–3 Years (13 kg) |
|---|---|
| Energy (kcal) | 1300 |
| Protein (g) | 23 |
| Vitamin A (RE) | 400 |
| Vitamin D (mcg) | 10 |
| Vitamin E (mg $\alpha$-TE) | 5 |
| Ascorbic acid (mg) | 45 |
| Folacin (mcg) | 100 |
| Niacin (mg) | 9 |
| Riboflavin (mg) | 0.8 |
| Thiamin (mg) | 0.7 |
| Vitamin $B_6$ (mg) | 0.9 |
| Vitamin $B_{12}$ (mcg) | 2.0 |
| Calcium (mg) | 800 |
| Phosphorus (mg) | 800 |
| Iodine (mcg) | 70 |
| Iron (mg) | 15 |
| Magnesium (mg) | 150 |
| Zinc (mg) | 10 |

(From Food and Nutrition Board: Recommended Dietary Allowances. Washington, DC, National Academy of Sciences/National Research Council, 1980)

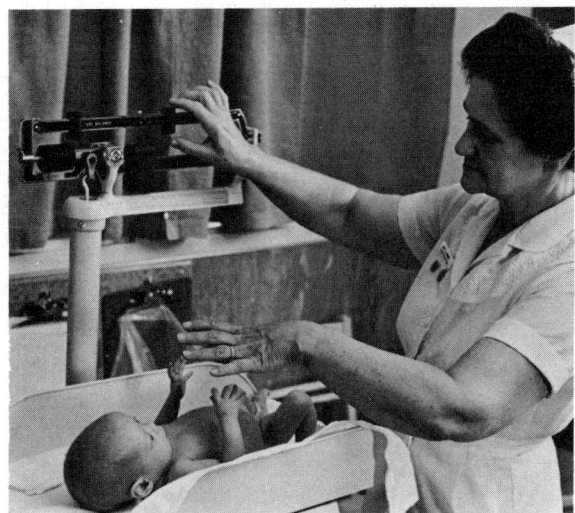

**Fig. 18-3.** The rate at which a child gains weight is dependent on many factors. As long as he gains weight and length steadily and exhibits the other signs of good nutrition, there is no cause for worry. (Broadribb V: Foundations of Pediatric Nursing, 2nd ed. Philadelphia, JB Lippincott, 1972)

### Vitamins

A varied menu such as that shown in Table 18-8 provides an adequate intake of vitamins if the toddler's appetite permits its consumption. Foods high in ascorbic acid and vitamin A should be served each day. If fortified milk is not used, a vitamin D supplement is necessary.

### Feeding the toddler

The 1 year old begins to show a decided change in appetite and interest in food. Beal[25] has shown that, on the average, girls at 6 months and boys at 9 months decrease their milk intake markedly. For girls this persists until 2 to 3 years of age and then slowly milk intake begins to rise. In contrast, boys have a somewhat steeper decrease in milk intake than girls but recover more rapidly and by 2½ years have reached a higher level than girls. Other foods, too, are not taken as eagerly as formerly, and some may be refused altogether. This should not be interpreted as a poor appetite but rather, the normal appetite for that age.

All this is due in large measure to a decrease in growth rate and, therefore, to the quantitative need for food. Also, at this age, the young child is becoming increasingly intrigued by his surroundings—parents, sisters, and brothers, and the paraphernalia of the home, all of which vie for his attention. He wants to play with his food to feel its texture, and he tries to feed himself with his hands, refusing the same food when it is offered on a spoon.

This can become an anxious time for the inexperienced mother, accustomed to the voracious appetite of infancy. Unless the mother is guided correctly, food and eating may become a battleground between the child and

her and may lay the groundwork for the anorexia and emotional upsets related to food and eating that so often occur in the preschool years. It is important for her to understand that changes in food acceptance and the need for exploration are a part of the normal growth pattern and that all children go through this process.

Physically, the child is learning a motor mastery of his body—eye, hand, and mouth coordination, chewing, swallowing, the use of mouth and throat muscles. He "puts everything into his mouth." From his earliest days his mouth has served him as a sensory organ. He now uses it to explore whatever is within reach. Moreover, from the very beginning his feedings establish his primary relationships with other people. If the mother is helped to understand and is able to enjoy her baby's developing skills and interests even when she is frustrated by the spilled milk, the dropped spoons, and the gleeful contrariness, she is less likely to worry about the food that he does or does not eat.

### Table 18-8. Suggested Meal Plan for the 1- to 3-Year-Old

*Breakfast*
Fruit or juice
Cereal with milk
Toast
Butter or margarine
Milk

*Lunch or Supper*
Main dish—mainly meat, eggs, fish, poultry, dried beans
   or peas, cheese, peanut butter
Vegetable or salad
Bread
Butter or margarine
Dessert or fruit
Milk

*Dinner*
Meat, poultry or fish
Vegetable
Relish or salad
Bread
Butter or margarine
Fruit or pudding
Milk

*Snacks Between Meals*
Dry cereal, with milk or out of the box
Simple cookie or cracker
Raw vegetables
Canned, fresh or dried fruit
Cheese wedge
Fruit sherbet or ice cream
Toast, plain or cinnamon
Fruit juice
Fruit drinks made with milk and juice

(From Your Child from 1 to 3. Children's Bureau, DHEW, Washington, DC, 1966. Revised 1967; reprinted 1969)

## The diet of the 1 year old

This differs only slightly from that described. It includes not much more than a pint of milk a day plus foods from each of the other four food groups. His vegetables and fruits are mashed or chopped instead of strained, and he has started on "finger foods." He is introduced to the family meal schedule with a midmorning and a midafternoon snack of fruit juice or milk. The cup largely supplants the bottle, and he may start to try feeding himself with a spoon.

## The second year

More solid foods are added during the second year, such as chopped or sliced fruits and vegetables; ready to eat cereals as well as hot cereals; chopped liver, lean meat, fish, and poultry instead of the strained variety. Eggs, cottage cheese, and other mild cheeses may be used. Butter or fortified margarine is used with toast. The 2 year old child also enjoys custard, puddings, and ice cream.

## Food from the family table

By the time the infant reaches his first birthday his usual food is often from the family table. It is important that the family food fed to the toddler is appropriate both in nutritive value and in consistency. Because caloric intake is limited, the 1 year old child cannot afford calories that do not contribute equal amounts of other nutrients. Soft drinks, candy, many types of cookies, pastries and cakes supply too many calories and not enough protein, vitamins, or minerals for the toddler. The nutrition counselor should discourage mothers from feeding the toddler these foods except, perhaps, on special occasions.

When the toddler's meat comes from the family table it should be tender and cut into small pieces. Rich gravies and sauces are not appropriate for this age. Except for finger items, other foods should be cut into bite-size pieces.

Very small portions (1 to 2 tablespoonfuls) seem to encourage the toddler to eat. He should have the option of refusing certain foods as well as having additional servings of those he likes.

## Making foods easy to eat

Beginners appreciate food that helps them to develop independence in feeding themselves and prevents accidents. Small plastic cups or tumblers are easier to handle than glass or china. If they are not filled too full, there will be less spilling.

## Overuse of milk

Earlier in this chapter it is stated that most children decrease their milk intake in favor of other foods sometime during the first year. Because milk is the center of the diet in infancy, there is a tendency to think that it must continue to be so. When milk continues to provide the largest part of the 1 to 2 year old diet, nutritional anemia may result. The 1 to 2 year old may cut his milk intake down to a pint or even less a day and, instead, eat a variety of other foods, many of which help supply his need for iron. He slowly resumes milk drinking, but it will be some years before he is able to consume a full quart and still eat a variety of other foods.

## Abnormal cravings—pica

Pica is a craving for unnatural foods or for nonfood substances, such as clay or chalk. It is most apt to occur in children between the ages of 18 and 24 months of age. Lourie and co-workers[26] found no correlation between the occurrence of pica and nutritional deficiencies. Gutelius and co-workers[27] supplemented the diet of some pica children with vitamins and minerals but failed to reduce the incidence of this craving among their subjects. These workers agree that pica is a complicated environmental, cultural, and psychological problem most apt to occur among children of mothers who also practice pica themselves.

## Study questions and activities

1. Why is breast-feeding considered to be highly desirable for both mother and infant?
2. What should the mother's attitude be if she bottle-feeds the infant?
3. What foods in what quantity should be included in the mother's diet if she is nursing her infant? (See Chap. 17.)
4. How much iron should a 9 month old infant get per day? How can this be supplied by food?
5. Is there evidence that fluoride in an infant's diet has any prophylactic effect during later childhood?
6. Which nutrients are most apt to be the limiting factor in breast-fed infants?
7. Discuss iron needs in the breast-fed infants during the first 6 months of life.
8. Prepared commercial formulas are used generally in artificial feeding. How do they compare in composition with human milk?
9. Supplementary foods are introduced into the infant's diet gradually. What is the first supplement generally advised and in what amount? In what order are other foods introduced?
10. Why are we concerned today about overnutrition in infants?
11. What changes take place in the small child's food habits at about one year of age? Why does this occur?
12. Why do later emotional problems with food and appetite often have their origin at this period?

13. How can the nutrition counselor help to allay the mother's anxiety and sense of frustration about her child's food habits at ages one to three years?

14. How much milk is the 1 to 2 year old likely to be willing to drink? What may happen if he is forced to drink a quart of milk daily?

## References

1. Fomon SJ: Infant Nutrition, p 261. Philadelphia, WB Saunders, 1974
2. Food and Nutrition Board: Recommended Dietary Allowances. Washington, DC, NAS-NRC, 1980
3. Fomon, Infant Nutrition, p 166
4. Committee on Nutrition, American Academy of Pediatrics: Pediatrics 57:278, 1976
5. Dallman PR et al: Am J Clin Nutr 33:86, 1980
6. McMillan JA et al: Pediatrics 58:686, 1976
7. Hambridge M et al: Pediatr Res 6:868, 1972
8. Dunning JM: N Engl J Med 272:30, 1965
9. Fomon, Infant Nutrition, p 350
10. Simopoulos AP, Barter FC: Nutr Rev 38:201, 1980
11. Committee on Nutrition, American Academy of Pediatrics: Pediatrics 66:1015, 1980
12. Keenan WJ et al: Am J Dis Child 121:271, 1971
13. Advance Data—Vital and Health Statistics of the National Center for Health Statistics, No. 59, Mar 28, 1980. Hyattsville, MD, Department of Health and Human Services, 1980
14. Hecht A: FDA Consumer 13, No. 9:21, 1979
15. Spock B: Baby and Child Care, rev ed. New York, Hawthorn Books, 1968
16. Fomon, Infant Nutrition, p 408
17. Beal VA: Pediatrics 20:448, 1957
18. American Academy of Pediatrics: Pediatric Nutrition Handbook. Evanston, American Academy of Pediatrics, 1979
19. Oski F, Landaw SA: Am J Dis Child 134:459, 1980
20. Rabinovitch RD, Fischoff J: J Am Diet Assoc 28:614, 1952
21. Anderson TA, Fomon SJ: J Am Diet Assoc 58:520, 1971
22. Anderson TA, Fomon SJ: J Pediatr 78:788, 1971
23. Nutr Rev 28:184, 1970
24. Tracey VV et al: Br Med J 1:16, 1971
25. Beal VA: J Nutr 53:499, 1954
26. Lourie RS et al: Children 10:143, 1963
27. Gutelius MF et al: Am J Clin Nutr 12:388, 1963

## Supplementary readings

American Academy of Pediatrics, Committee on Nutrition: Pediatric Nutrition Handbook, Evanston, American Academy of Pediatrics, 1979

Andrew EM, Clancy KL, Katz MG: Sources of kilocalories and macronutrients in the infant diet. J Am Diet Assoc 79:131, 1981

Beal VA: Nutrition in the Life Span. New York, John Wiley & Sons, 1980

Burman D: Nutrition in early childhood. In McLaren DS, Burman D (eds): Textbook of Pediatric Nutrition. Edinburgh, Churchill Livingstone, 1976

Dallman PR, Siimes MA, Stekel A: Iron deficiency in infancy and childhood. Am J Clin Nutr 33:86, 1980

Ernst JA, Wynn RJ, Schreiner RL: Starvation with hypernatremic dehydration in two breast-fed infants. J Am Diet Assoc 79:126, 1981

Fomon SJ: Infant Nutrition, 2nd ed. Philadelphia, WB Saunders, 1974

Hall B: Changing composition of human milk and early development of an appetite control. Lancet 1:779, 1975

Jelliffe DB: World trends in infant feeding. Am J Clin Nutr 29:1227, 1976

Lawrence RA: Breast-Feeding—A Guide for the Medical Profession. St. Louis, CV Mosby Co, 1980

McMillan JA, Landaw SA, Oski F: Iron sufficiency in breast-fed infants and availability of iron from human milk. Pediatrics 58:686, 1976

Oski F, Landaw SA: Inhibition of iron absorption from human milk by baby food. Am J Dis Child 134:459, 1980

Pipes PL: Nutrition in Infancy and Childhood, 2nd ed. St Louis, CV Mosby, 1981

Pollitt E, Wirtz S: Mother–infant feeding interaction and weight gain in the first month of life. J Am Diet Assoc 78:596, 1981

Review: Nutritional composition of breast milk produced by mothers of preterm infants. Nutr Rev 38:312, 1980

Review: Zinc therapy of depressed cellular immunity in acrodermatitis enteropathica. Nutr Rev 79:168, 1981

Widdowson EM: Nutrition and lactation. In Winick M (ed): Nutritional Disorders of American Women. New York, John Wiley & Sons, 1977

*For further references see Bibliography in Part 4.*

# Nutrition for Children and Youth

**19**

Nutritional Requirements of Children
   and Youth
Food Habits and Eating Practices
Child Nutrition Programs

Children and youth constitute approximately 35% of the total population of the United States today. The youth-oriented society of the 1970s and 1980s has increasingly focused attention on the needs of young people. New and innovative programs dealing with all aspects of childhood and adolescence, from comprehensive medical care projects for children and youth to coordinated health and educational centers for teenaged mothers and their infants, have been developed in many communities. Of particular concern to all of these programs are the needs of the disadvantaged child and the opportunities available to him. Nutritional assessments, dietary counseling, and nutrition education should be an integral part of all programs for children and youth.

This chapter examines nutritional requirements of various age groups through adolescence and food habits and eating practices as they are related to nutritional requirements and developmental levels. The role and influence of child nutrition programs is also discussed.

## Nutritional requirements of children and youth

The Recommended Dietary Allowances, Table 19-1, for children from 4 through 10 years are the same for boys and girls. There is a gradual increase in growth, accordingly, in the recommended amounts for most nutrients throughout childhood. However, because the adolescent growth spurt is markedly different for boys than it is for girls, separate recommendations are given for each, starting at age 11.

If the Daily Guide to Foods Needed by Children and Their Families (Table 19-2) is followed, using appropriate servings for different age groups, as well as other foods suggested in the guide, the recommended dietary allowances for children and youth will be met.

### Calories

The RDA for calories during childhood, 4 through 10 years, is based on an allowance of 80 calories per kilogram of body weight. After age 10 there is a decrease in the calories per kilogram for both boys (45 calories per kilogram) and girls (38 calories per kilogram).

It is important to understand, however, that these recommendations represent average amounts for groups of children. An individual child may require more or less calories than the RDA, depending on his size, activity, and rate of growth.

Adequate calories must be supplied if growth is to proceed normally. When caloric intake is below the requirement, protein foods are used for energy instead of for tissue building. Macy and Hunscher[1] have shown that "a difference in intake of as few as 10 calories per kilogram of body weight per day (or approximately 4 calories per pound) may make the difference between progress and failure in satisfactory growth."

Figs. 19-1 and 19-2, which compare differences in increments of height and calorie intake between early- and late-maturing boys and girls, illustrate well why food intake of individual children must be adjusted to specific needs.

If a *growth chart*, such as Fig. 19-3, is used for recording height and weight, deviations from normal patterns can readily be seen. The chart shown is for boys from age 2 to 13. Similar charts have been constructed for girls of this age, for infants, for both boys and girls, and for adolescent boys and girls. They are based on careful measurements of a selected group of children followed for the years specified and, as can be seen, show a wide range of variation.

The 50th percentile in both height and weight curves represents the median of all children measured. A child of stocky build is below the median for height and may be slightly above the median for weight. On the other hand, the tall, rangy child is well above the median for height and may or may not be below the median for weight.

The height and the weight recorded on such a chart at 6-month or yearly intervals show graphically how a child is progressing within his particular growth pattern. For example, a drop to a lower percentile in weight from one measuring period to the next may indicate inadequate energy intake, particularly if the height trend is in the same direction. The nutrition counselor should determine the reason for this deviation. Similarly, a shift in weight to a higher percentile, if not accompanied by a similar height increase, may signal overnutrition.

The basic foods listed in Table 19-2 need to be supplemented by varying amounts of butter or margarine, salad dressings, jams, jellies, desserts, and, occasionally, other sweets to meet the energy needs of different age groups.

## Protein

The RDA for protein decreases from 1.5 g/kg of body weight for 4 to 6 year olds to 0.8 g/kg of body weight at 18 years. Total protein needs, however, increase with growth, and protein intake should rise as calories are increased if there is a variety of foods in the diet. The milk and meat groups, including fish, eggs, cheese and peanut butter, meet protein needs adequately. However, if calories are obtained largely from carbohydrates, including candy and soft drinks in excess, both the quantity and the quality of the protein intake suffers.

## Minerals

Calcium and phosphorus allowances are set at 800 mg for children 1 to 10 years and are increased to 1200 mg for the preadolescent and adolescent 11 to 18 years. Milk in the amounts recommended is the main source of *calcium* and *phosphorus* and, together with meat, contributes significant amounts of magnesium and zinc. *Iron* needs for children can be met by an adequate intake of

## Table 19-1. Recommended Dietary Allowances for Children and Youth

| Age (Years) | *Males and Females* | | *Males* | | *Females* | |
|---|---|---|---|---|---|---|
| | *4–6* | *7–10* | *11–14* | *15–18* | *11–14* | *15–18* |
| Energy (kcal) | 1700 | 2400 | 2700 | 2800 | 2200 | 2100 |
| Protein (g) | 30 | 34 | 45 | 56 | 46 | 46 |
| Vitamin A (mcg—RE) | 500 | 700 | 1000 | 1000 | 800 | 800 |
| Vitamin D (mcg) | 10 | 10 | 10 | 10 | 10 | 10 |
| Vitamin E (mg—$\alpha$TE) | 6 | 7 | 8 | 10 | 8 | 8 |
| Ascorbic acid (mg) | 45 | 45 | 50 | 60 | 50 | 60 |
| Folacin (mcg) | 200 | 300 | 400 | 400 | 400 | 400 |
| Niacin (mg—NE) | 11 | 16 | 18 | 18 | 15 | 14 |
| Riboflavin (mg) | 1.0 | 1.4 | 1.6 | 1.7 | 1.3 | 1.3 |
| Thiamin (mg) | 0.9 | 1.2 | 1.4 | 1.4 | 1.1 | 1.1 |
| Vitamin $B_6$ (mg) | 1.3 | 1.6 | 1.8 | 2.0 | 1.8 | 2.0 |
| Vitamin $B_{12}$ (mcg) | 2.5 | 3.0 | 3.0 | 3.0 | 3.0 | 3.0 |
| Calcium (mg) | 800 | 800 | 1200 | 1200 | 1200 | 1200 |
| Phosphorus (mg) | 800 | 800 | 1200 | 1200 | 1200 | 1200 |
| Iodine (mcg) | 90 | 120 | 150 | 150 | 150 | 150 |
| Iron (mg) | 10 | 10 | 18 | 18 | 18 | 18 |
| Magnesium (mg) | 200 | 250 | 350 | 400 | 300 | 300 |
| Zinc (mg) | 10 | 10 | 15 | 15 | 15 | 15 |

(From Food and Nutrition Board: Recommended Dietary Allowances. Washington, DC, National Academy of Sciences/National Research Council, 1980)

meat, green leafy vegetables, whole grain and enriched breads, and cereals and potatoes. Dried beans, peas, and peanut butter contribute a share of iron if these products are a staple of the diet. Adolescent boys may be able to meet the RDA for iron if they consume large quantities of foods to meet energy needs. Due to the positive effect that ascorbic acid, meat, fish, and poultry have on the availability of iron in the diet, attention should be given to including these items in the meals of children and adolescents. The adolescent girl, however, probably needs an iron supplement, particularly after menstruation begins, and iron is lost from the body. The necessary *iodine* is supplied by the use of iodized salt in cooking or as seasoning.

## Vitamins

Vitamin needs are more likely to be met when a variety of foods is included in the diet. Milk, butter, fortified margarine, and green and yellow vegetables and fruits provide vitamin A. Milk fortified with vitamin D ensures a sufficient intake of this vitamin. The B-complex vitamins are included if good quality protein foods, as well as enriched bread and cereals, appear frequently in the diet. Children and adolescents who consume strictly vegetarian diets (vegans) may not receive adequate amounts of vitamin $B_{12}$. In Southern states, where cornmeal rather than wheat flour is frequently used, it is important to obtain enriched cornmeal when possible. In at least one Southern state, rice must be enriched by law.

Citrus fruits and tomatoes may be expensive sources of vitamin C when not in season. Many of the fruit-flavored juices, which are popular drinks with children, do supply significant amounts of ascorbic acid in the amounts consumed. If these are used to replace citrus juices, their vitamin C content should be investigated. Raw potatoes are a good source of this vitamin but lose a large percentage of it in commercial processing, and the processed form of potato is the one most frequently found in

## Table 19-2.  A Daily Guide to Foods Needed by Children and Their Families

| Type of Food | | Each Day |
|---|---|---|
| *Milk Group* | | |
| Milk, whole or skim | Children under 11 | 2 to 3 cups |
| | Children 11–18 | 3 or more cups |
| Dairy products such as: | | |
| Cheddar cheese, cottage cheese, and ice cream | | May be used sometimes in place of milk |
| *Vegetable–Fruit Group* | | 4 or more servings |
| Include: | | |
| A fruit or vegetable that contains a high amount of vitamin C: Grapefruit, oranges, and tomatoes (whole or in juice), raw cabbage, green or sweet red pepper, broccoli, and fresh strawberries | | |
| A dark-green or deep-yellow vegetable or fruit for vitamin A: You can judge fairly well by color—dark green and deep yellow: broccoli, spinach, greens, cantaloupe, apricots, carrots, pumpkin, sweet potatoes, winter squash | | |
| Other vegetables and fruits, including potatoes | | |
| *Meat and Meat Substitutes* | | 2 or more servings |
| Include: | | |
| Meat, poultry, fish, or eggs | | |
| Dried beans or peas, peanut butter, and nuts can be used as meat substitutes | | |
| *Breads and Cereals* | | 4 or more servings |
| Whole grain, enriched, or restored bread and cereals or other grain products such as cornmeal, grits, macaroni, spaghetti, and rice | | |
| *Plus Other Foods* | | |
| To round out meals and to satisfy the appetite, many children will eat more of these foods, and other foods not specified will be used, such as butter, margarine, other fats, oils, sugars, and unenriched refined grain products. These "other" foods are frequently combined with the suggested foods in mixed dishes, baked goods, desserts, and other recipe dishes. They are a part of daily meals, even though they are not stressed in the food plan. | | |

(Adapted from Your Child from 6 to 12. Children's Bureau, DHEW, Publ. No. 324. Washington, DC, 1966)

the diets of children and adolescents. Cabbage and other leafy vegetables, raw especially, contribute some of this vitamin to the diet.

## Food habits and eating practices
### The preschool child—3 to 5 years

The daily food guide (Table 19-2) serves as the basis of the diet for the child 3 to 5 years old, although size of servings is about half the average size used for older children and adults. A good estimate for size of a serving at meals is approximately 3 tablespoons for the 3 year old and 4 tablespoons for the 4 year old. The child 3 to 5 years old should be encouraged to drink 1 to $1\frac{1}{2}$ pints of milk (regular or skim) a day. Some of this milk requirement may be provided in creamed soups and custards or other desserts included in his meals. Helping to prepare and serve "instant puddings" is fun for the preschooler and is also an excellent way to increase milk consumption in this age group.

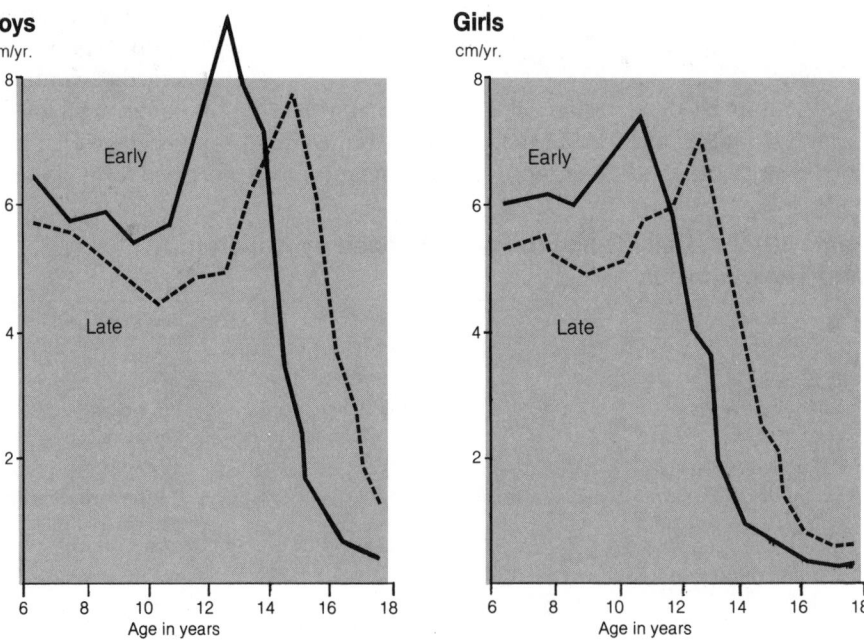

**Fig. 19-1.**   Increments in the height of early- and late-maturing boys and girls (means of 20 in each group). (Mitchell HS et al: the adolescent growth spurt and nutrient intake. Presented at the International Congress of Nutrition, Hamburg, Germany, August 8, 1966)

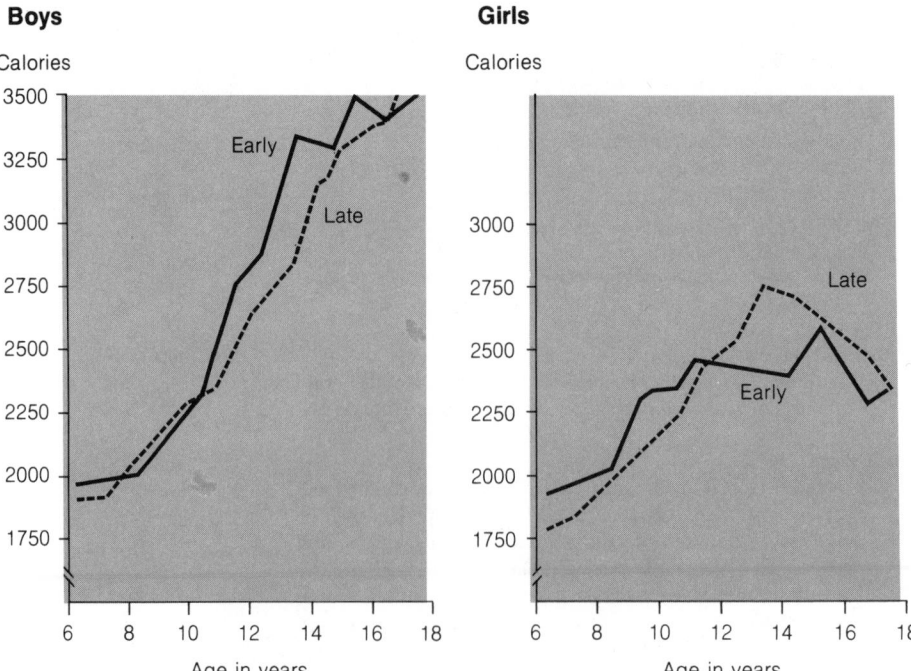

**Fig. 19-2.**   Total caloric intakes of early- and late-maturing boys and girls (means of 20 in each group). (Mitchell HS et al: The adolescent growth spurt and nutrient intake. Presented at the International Congress of Nutrition, Hamburg, Germany, August 8, 1966)

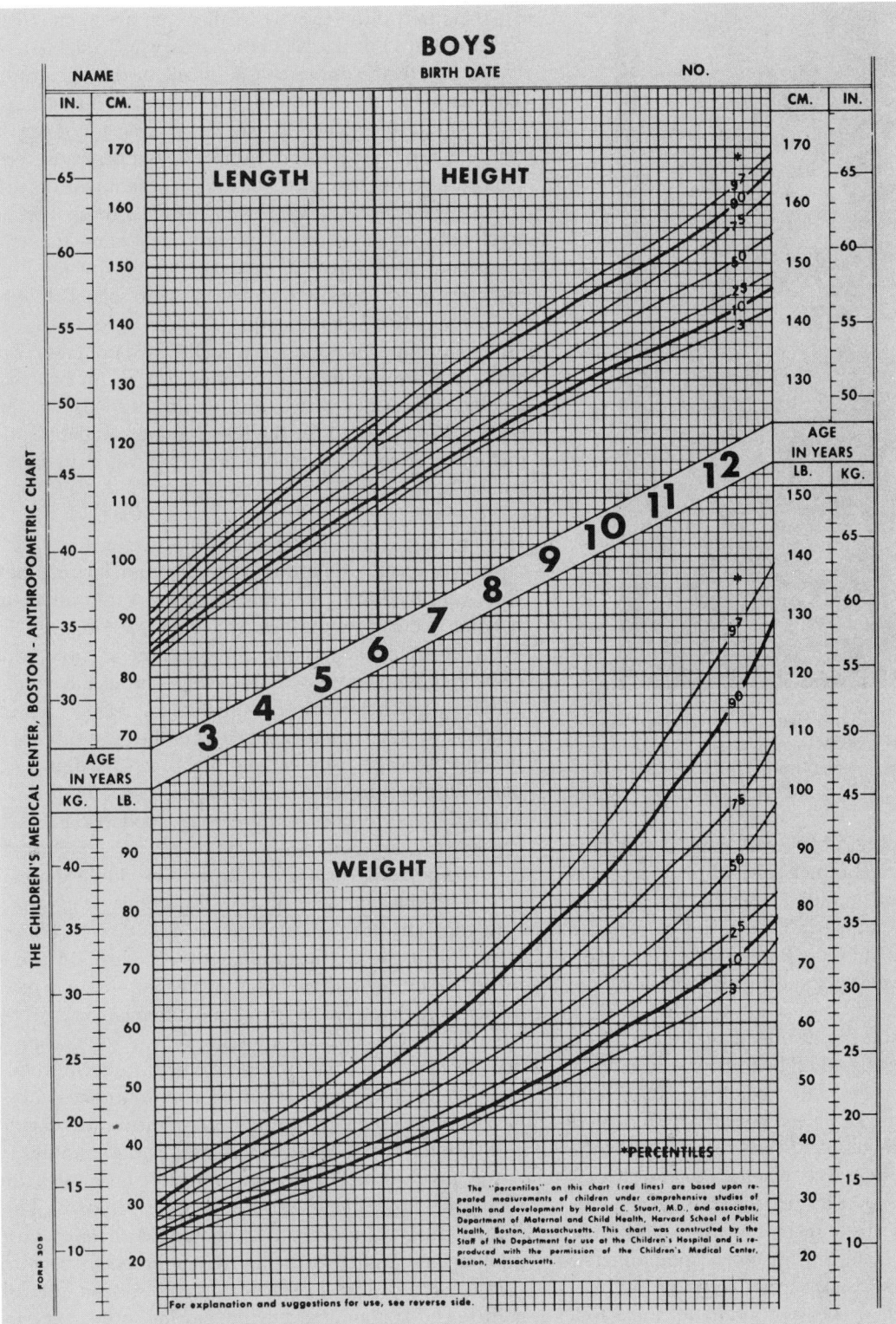

**Fig. 19-3.** Anthropometric height–weight chart for boys. For explanation of use, see text. The break in height at the 6-yr level occurs because up to that time the length of the child is measured as he lies recumbent, whereas after this age the standing height is measured. The 50th percentile is the median range. Most children fall somewhere between the 10th and 90th percentiles. (Children's Medical Center, Boston, Mass.)

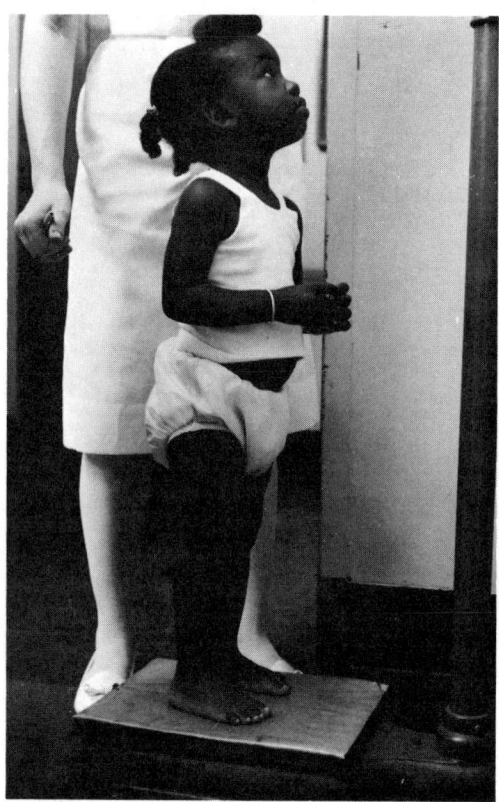

**Fig. 19-4.** A healthy child at the Pediatric Clinic, The New York Hospital. Note sturdy build, straight back, and alert interest in being weighed. (Children's Bureau photograph)

Whole fruits and vegetables, both cooked and raw, should begin to appear in his menu. Meat should be cut in small pieces rather than ground. Remember that often at this age, a child gladly eats such foods as raw carrots and lettuce with his fingers but refuses them if he has to use a fork or a spoon because it is too difficult to manage the food with them.

It is usually desirable for the preschool child to have a midmorning, midafternoon, and bedtime snack in addition to his regular meals. Some pediatricians feel that there is room for further study and research on the question of the number of meals best suited to the needs of the preschool child. Stitt[2] wonders "whether good nutrients distributed fairly evenly over the waking hours may not be what many children seem to reach toward." Milk, if not consumed at a regular meal, or fruit juice accompanied by bread, crackers, or plain cookies, may form a good light meal or snack. Desserts, to be appropriate for the 3 to 5 year old child, should furnish essential protein, minerals, and vitamins as well as calories. They should not be given as rewards for finishing a meal or withheld as punishment for not doing so, but perhaps even offered with the meal if the child prefers. Birch and co-workers have recently shown that presenting food as a reward to children in preschool enhanced the children's preference for that food.[3]

Children differ greatly in their natural preferences for food, but some patterns emerge clearly. "Finicky" food habits and food jags are characteristic of this age group. They may want to eat nothing except peanut butter sandwiches and fruit juice, or two to three hard cooked eggs at a sitting, but these patterns usually do not persist for very long, and soon they will settle down again to normal meals. The overall pattern of food intake from week to week and month to month is more important than the occasional food binge or refusal. Fig. 19-4 shows the monitoring of the growth of a healthy preschool child.

Project Head Start, serving children aged 3 to 5, has offered an opportunity of studying the food preferences of children from low income families. These children usually lack experience with a wide variety of foods. For this reason, any program for the disadvantaged child should include a variety of new foods as well as culturally familiar foods.

### Preschool day care centers

As a result of the intensive demand for adequate child-care facilities, more and more day care centers are opening in our communities. The *Child Development Center*, a term currently being used for some of these, indicates their focus on the total development of the child— physical, psychosocial, and intellectual. Many of these centers not only serve meals as part of the physical care of the child but also use food and mealtimes as an integral part of the learning and socializing processes. They afford excellent opportunities for developing good food habits in children.

The breakfast or lunch or both served in the day care center provides an opportunity to introduce children to fruit juices, fruits in season, and raw vegetables. Children are pretty sure to like the familiar and simple main dishes, bread and butter, and milk. Eating in company with other children, perhaps for the first time, often encourages the less venturesome to try something new. A story about a new food and a small sample served attractively may make the difference between rejection and acceptance. Parent involvement in the programs of the center provides a chance for nutrition education of the entire family.

A professionally qualified nutrition consultant should be available to group day-care programs on a regular basis. The consultant should participate in developing and implementing written policies for the nutritional care of the children. These should include guidelines for planning, buying, storing, preparing, and serving food to meet nutritional needs, training of food service workers, and nutrition education programs for staff, children, and parents. A nutritional assessment, including dietary practices, should be made at the time each child enters the program and, if necessary, an individualized nutritional care plan should be established. The child's growth progress, food pattern, and mealtime behavior should be recorded and included in regular staff and parent conferences. Opportunities should be provided for parents to visit the center and to participate in mealtime activities. Menus should be posted in appropriate places in the center and made available to parents to facilitate planning of meals served in the home[4] (see *Special Food Service Program for Children*, p. 343).

## The school age child—5 to 10 years

The basic food plan (Table 19-2) is the same for the school age child and the preschooler, except that serving sizes increase until they are equal to or greater than the average adult serving.

The meal patterns for the school age child may vary depending on what the school provides and to what extent these services are used by the family. In any case, the mother needs to plan the family's meals around the school situation.

Breakfast for the child going off to school is an important meal. Because many mothers today have a variety of responsibilities, the preparation of this meal is often shared with the whole family. The school age child with a minimum of help can prepare a simple breakfast. Many schools in low income areas have introduced a breakfast program to provide disadvantaged children with a good start for the school day.

Under certain circumstances, especially if the school does not have a school lunch program, a bag lunch has to be carried from home. Incorporating foods selected from the food guide, the bag lunch should be planned to supplement breakfast and dinner. Many children still need and enjoy snacks during this period. The after-school snack, particularly, is important and should be planned so that it does not interfere with the evening meal.

Children's food habits develop along with other aspects of their growth. The 5 to 7 year olds prefer plain foods, such as meat, potatoes, raw vegetables, milk, and fruits. Although most casserole dishes, mixtures of all kinds, fat meats, and gravies are not liked, spaghetti and meat sauce, pizza, tacos, and macaroni and cheese are notable exceptions. By 6 or 7 years, they are willing to try new foods and to accept foods previously disliked. By 8 years, there is a ravenous appetite with few refusals but strong preferences. Food may be judged by odor or color, and food served attractively makes an impression. By 9 years, the child usually has a keen interest in food, likes to help prepare it, and is positive in his likes and dislikes. Some eat everything at this age, but plain foods are still preferred.

One of the best methods for developing good food habits in children is for the whole family to eat wisely. If the mother and father, knowing that they can expect variations in acceptance of foods by their children, maintain a reasonably firm stand about overall behavior, mealtime can and should be one of the pleasant times of day for the whole family.

Children are great imitators. Although they may object to being asked to conform, they may, on the other hand, be heard to say proudly to some friend, "My mother won't let me eat that." The absence of variety in choices of food offered in the fast-food restaurants, especially fruits and vegetables, would suggest that visits to them be limited for the child who is still developing his food habits.

### Role of the elementary school

For many children, elementary school is an introduction to group feeding. This can be difficult if the school does not make special provisions for the first and, perhaps, second graders. The hurry and confusion of most school cafeterias does not provide a conducive atmosphere for the average 6 year old child to eat and enjoy his lunch. A smaller group in a quieter place, such as the classroom, is a more satisfactory arrangement for this age. This arrangement also affords an opportunity to use the luncheon meal as an educational tool to develop the child's interest in food.

The nutritional contributions of the school lunch are particularly important to those children who do not receive adequate food at home. However, all children can share the social aspects of group feeding, and this in itself may be enough incentive for a child to try an unfamiliar food or to drink his milk because the other children do. The National School Lunch Program is discussed on page 341. Hyperactivity in the school age child is discussed in Chapter 35.

## The challenges of youth—10 to 18 years

Because the growth spurts of girls and boys usually occur at different ages (11–13 or 14 years for girls and 12–15 years for boys), their nutritional requirements during adolescence also vary. Before the spurt, the recommendations are only slighly higher than for 7 to 10 year olds and after the growth spurt taper off to the adult level.

All the foods included in the Daily Guide to Foods Needed by Children and Their Families (Table 19-2) are essential in the diet of the adolescent but in markedly increased quantities. A rapidly growing boy needs a quart of milk or its equivalent each day to meet his calcium requirement, and girls during their period of rapid growth also need a quart of milk daily. Skim milk may be substituted for whole milk if excess weight, real or imaginary, is a factor. The increased milk intake provides good-quality protein for growth as well as calcium. All the other foods listed, eaten in sufficient quantity, provide for the greatly increased physiologic needs during this period of growth and stabilization.

In addition to adequate calcium, protein, and calories, girls need an iron supplement when menses begin. An adequate amount of foods high in iron, such as lean meats, liver, eggs, green leafy vegetables, enriched breads, and cereals and potatoes, should also be included in the daily food intake. This is a period when the young girl, who may be looking forward to marriage and motherhood, should be helped to realize that good nutrition is an important factor in the bearing of healthy babies.

During the period of rapid physical growth and sexual development, there is a concurrent maturing of the whole personality, with its attendant strains and stresses. The identity crisis of the teenager results in a drive for independence from parental restriction, coupled with an increased need for guidance and reassurance. There is a tremendous need for peer group approval, and fads in food habits are prevalent. The adolescent must be given the opportunity to make his own decisions, and parents should be understanding of this urge for independence, yet they should also be willing to help when needed.

Because boys and girls differ in their response to this growth period, they are discussed separately.

### Boys

As shown in Fig. 19-5, the diets of adolescent boys at all ages were generally found to be adequate for protein, calcium, vitamin A, riboflavin, thiamin, and ascorbic acid; however, calories and iron were low in the diets of certain age groups.

The adolescent spurt stimulates appetite, as is well recognized. The energy and nutrient requirement for this spurt in any one boy is not known. If the increments of height gained as shown in Fig. 19-1 are compared with the caloric intake for the same boys (Fig. 19-2), it is not surprising that the early maturers experienced an earlier increase in food intake than the late maturers.[5]

### Girls

With many girls the story is different. Despite the abundance of food in the United States and the inclusion of nutrition education in most elementary and high schools, the HANES Survey (Fig. 19-5) shows that teenaged girls, at all ages, constitute one of the most poorly fed groups in our population. The most serious deficits are in iron and calories, with smaller numbers deficient in protein. This finding is particularly critical in pregnant teenagers (see Chap. 17), because of the additional nutritional demands being made on the young mother's body.

The caloric intake of adolescent girls shows quite a different picture from that of boys (see Figs. 19-1 and 19-2). One can almost read into these graphs the psychology of the early-maturing girls who are concerned about their rapid growth and increase in height ahead of boys their age. As a result, they curtail their total food intake and often choose foods unwisely with respect to essential nutrients. The late-maturing girls do not make so drastic a reduction in caloric intake until much later.

The concern of teenage girls often centers on weight reduction, whether necessary or not. There is probably no great harm in this, if the essential foods to meet nutritional needs are included in the diet. However, if soft drinks, candy and other sweets are substituted for milk, fruits, and vegetables, as is often the case, there may be a reduction in essential minerals and vitamins though not in calories.

### Adolescent obesity

A word of warning concerning adolescent obesity is necessary in any discussion of nutritional needs of this age group. Although the basic cause of juvenile-onset obesity is not well-understood, the fact that most fat children remain fat adults indicates an urgent need to prevent the development of obesity when possible and to treat it promptly when it occurs.

A minority of boys and girls have the habit of consuming more calories than they can use for energy and growth, becoming overweight for their height and age. Whether this is due to underactivity, to overeating, or to a combination of the two, adolescent obesity presents a real problem to the teenager's social and emotional adjustment as well as to future health. Obese adolescents are discriminated against in many ways. They are rejected by their peer group, harassed by their parents, set apart from the average by the fashion industry, laughed at in movies and on television, and generally excluded from the mainstream of teenage life.[6]

Improving the poor self-image that the obese adolescent frequently has is usually the first step in his treatment. As his self-confidence is developed, his determination to effect change can often be depended on to motivate him through the long and difficult struggle with weight control. Although adolescent weight control is more successful with parental understanding and cooperation, the teenager must be the one responsible for his food intake. Weight control is discussed in Chapter 28, as is anorexia nervosa, a serious psychological problem of adolescents, which results in self-starvation. Adolescent pregnancy is discussed in Chapter 17.

### Oral contraceptives

Because many adolescent girls use oral contraceptive agents at some time, it is important for the nutrition counselor to recognize the drug's influence on the nutritional status and health of young women. Oral contraceptives include combinations of different estrogens and progestogens. The lack of agreement in the reported effects of oral contraceptives is no doubt related to the differences in dosage, frequency of use and duration of administration as well as to the type of progestogen. The nutritional status of the individual previous to administration of the drug also appears to have an effect on the results. The metabolism of practically all the nutrients is influenced by these agents. Increased levels of cholesterol, triglycerides, phospholipids, and free fatty acids have been reported in users of oral contraceptives. The relationship between higher lipid levels and increased risk of thromboembolic disease in users of the "pill" is not well

| Sex and age | Calories | | | Protein (gm) | | | Calcium (mg) | | | Iron (mg) | | |
|---|---|---|---|---|---|---|---|---|---|---|---|---|
| | All income | Below poverty level[1] | Above poverty level[1] | All income | Below poverty level[1] | Above poverty level[1] | All income | Below poverty level[1] | Above poverty level[1] | All income | Below poverty level[1] | Above poverty level[1] |

**Male**

1 year
2-3 years
4-5 years

6-7 years
8-9 years
10-11 years

12-14 years
15-17 years
18-19 years

20-24 years
25-34 years
35-44 years

45-54 years
55-64 years
65 years and over

**Female**

1 year
2-3 years
4-5 years

6-7 years
8-9 years
10-11 years

12-14 years
15-17 years
18-19 years

20-24 years
25-34 years
35-44 years

45-54 years
55-64 years
65 years and over

**KEY**
- Below by 1-10%   •• Below by 21-29%
- • Below by 11-20%   ••• Below by 30% or more

[1]Excludes persons with unknown income.

**Fig. 19-5.**  Mean intake of calories and selected nutrients as a percent below the standard for persons aged 1 to 74 years, by income level, sex, and age, United States, 1971 to 1974. (Caloric and Selected Nutrient Values for Persons 1 to 74 Years of Age: First Health and Nutrition Examination Survey, United States, 1971 to 1974. U.S. Department of Health, Education and Welfare, Public Health Service, 1979)

defined because higher concentrations of blood coagulation factors also occur in women taking these drugs.[7,8] However, as the dosage of estrogen is reduced, the risk of thrombosis is lowered.

Some women on the pill have demonstrated an abnormal glucose tolerance test (GTT). This finding may be related to alteration in tryptophan metabolism, which precipitates a relative or absolute vitamin $B_6$ deficiency. Supplements of two to three times the RDA of vitamin $B_6$ have been found to improve glucose tolerance in these cases.[9]

Changes in protein metabolism observed in users of oral contraceptives appear to be similar to the alterations seen in pregnancy. The blood levels of certain amino acids (proline, glycine, lysine, histidine, alanine, valine, tyrosine, and ornithine) are decreased; serum albumin levels are generally lowered. Concentrations of carrier proteins are increased, and this influences the results of laboratory tests for iron, copper, zinc, and vitamin A. For example, the rise in serum levels of retinol-binding protein may account for the higher serum vitamin A levels in pill users. Moreover, this effect may result in further tissue depletion of vitamin A in women deficient in vitamin A.[10] Plasma-carotene levels have also been found to decrease in women administered oral contraceptives, perhaps due to greater conversion to vitamin A.

In users of oral contraceptives, plasma-zinc levels have been shown to decrease at the same time the level of erythrocyte zinc increases. Investigators suggest a redistribution of zinc in the body rather than a change in total body zinc.[10] The decreased menstrual loss of iron together with the estrogenic effect of oral contraceptives result in higher serum iron levels and increased total iron binding capacity. Estrogens increase serum levels of copper and ceruloplasmin, the copper transport protein. The latter may be responsible for catalyzing the oxidation of ascorbic acid, thereby lowering the level of vitamin C in the plasma and tissues.[10]

Oral contraceptives have also been found to reduce the urinary excretion of riboflavin and thiamin.[10] Estrogen may also increase the requirement for vitamin $B_6$, probably by raising the level of circulating cortisol, which, in turn, stimulates the conversion of tryptophan to niacin. This reaction requires a vitamin $B_6$ coenzyme. Caution, however, is advised in routine supplementation of vitamin $B_6$ for pill users because vitamin $B_6$ supplementation may further complicate the nutritional status of women with protein malnutrition.[11] The metabolism of folic acid is altered when oral contraceptives are taken. Severe megaloblastic anemia has been identified in some cases. Malabsorption of polyglutamic form of folic acid has been implicated by some investigators. Other research workers have suggested an increased rate of metabolism of folic acid by the intestine. More recently, a folate-binding protein in serum and leukocytes that sequesters the folate has been identified in women taking oral contraceptives. The latter would explain why women who are marginally deficient in folic acid develop megaloblastic anemia when using these drugs. Women who become pregnant soon after discontinuing the pill probably are at greater risk of folic acid deficiency.[10]

Although few investigations have studied adolescents who take oral contraceptives, the evidence that marginal nutritional status probably increases the risk of harmful nutritional effects from oral contraceptives implies close, individualized nutritional supervision of adolescents for whom oral contraceptives are prescribed. Although there is not general agreement on supplementation, many investigators have emphasized the importance of providing a diet adequate in all nutrients for all users of oral contraceptives.

### Alcohol and drugs

Alcohol consumption among teenagers has increased during the 1970s. A national study indicated that approximately 39% of the teenagers in school were moderate drinkers, and 28% appeared to be problem drinkers.[12] The nutritional status of the teenager can be seriously affected by the continual consumption of alcohol. Alcohol, which contributes 7 kcal per gram (Chap. 2), may replace food that contains the essential nutrients. For this reason, the chronic teenaged drinker's dietary intake may be low in the protein, vitamins, and minerals that the adolescent needs for growth and development. Appetite may also be decreased, as well as the absorption and utilization of certain nutrients. The alteration in the chronic alcoholic of the metabolism of nutrients, such as zinc (see Chap. 6) may lead to specific deficiencies. Alcoholics also run the risk of eventual liver disease. Programs for rehabilitation of the teenaged alcoholic should provide for nutrition counseling, because malnutrition is frequently a problem among this group.[13]

Teenagers who abuse alcohol may also be using drugs, and the combination can be synergistic in its effects. Drug abusers have been found to have a craving for high-carbohydrate, low-nutrient-density snack foods including candy, cookies, cakes, potato chips, and pretzels. Addicts report that these foods enhance the drug effect. Because the addict must have money for drugs, he may not have it for food. So-called fast foods, hot dogs and hamburgers, available on the street are the types of food consumed when money is available. Users of drugs and alcohol are at high risk for liver disease and nutritional deficiencies. Drug rehabilitation programs should emphasize nutrition by providing for a highly nutritious diet and nutrition counseling.

### Athletics

Currently there is great interest in the relation between nutrition and sports and physical fitness; nutritionists, physicians, and trainers are exchanging ideas and studying the nutritional implications of various types of physical activity associated with different sports. One area of common interest has been muscle physiology and the metabolic processes within muscle cells. Muscles are made up of many filamentous cells or fibers. Each cell contains many nuclei lying between the cell membranes (sarcolemma) and the cytoplasm (sarcoplasm). Embedded in the sarcoplasm and running the entire length of the cell are many fine fibers called myofibrils. Within each myofibril are long parallel rows of contractile proteins, actin, and myosin. The smallest contractile unit in a myofibril is called a *sarcomere*. During muscle contraction, brought about by the release of acetylcholine at the synapse of the neuromuscular junction, actin filaments slide into spaces between myosin filaments, pulling in the ends of the sarcomere. Cell membrane permeability to sodium and calcium is increased, and potassium leaks out of the cell. Immediately after this contraction acetylcholinesterase breaks down the acetylcholine, readying the muscle for reactivation.

ATP (adenosine triphosphate) is the source of energy for the actin-myosin contractile process. Both glucose and fatty acids are metabolized in the muscle cell to produce the ATP (see Chap. 9, *Metabolism*). The proportion of each depends on the metabolic state and nutrient supply to the muscle, the type of physical exercise, and the type of muscle cell. After a meal when plenty of glucose is available, it is taken up by the muscle cell in quantity, both converted to glycogen and, along with fatty acids, used to produce ATP. In the postabsorptive state when blood glucose levels drop, more fatty acid is taken into the cell and oxidized at the same time glucose uptake and utilization decrease.

During light to moderate exercise the muscle cell readily takes up and oxidizes fatty acids for ATP. As the work load increases, however, there is a relatively greater metabolism of glucose (from glycogen stores) than fatty acids. This is because glucose is the most efficient fuel in using oxygen.

Two types of muscle cells have been identified, according to the speed at which they contract—fast-twitch and slow-twitch fibers. Fast-twitch fibers, which contract and relax quickly, are said to have more contractile fibers and fewer mitochondria. They tend to be used for tasks that require short bursts of intense energy under conditions where relatively little oxygen is available. Glucose from glycogen stores is the chief fuel used in these cells. Slow-twitch cells contract at a slower rate and have a greater proportion of mitochondria to contractile fibers. Fatty acids are their choice as a source of fuel for ATP. When sufficient oxygen is available during endurance activities, more of these cells are used. Both types of cells exist in muscles, such as biceps and calf muscles. However, it appears that different amounts of each type of cell are found in different individuals. It may be that certain athletes were born to run the marathon by their greater percentage of slow-twitch muscle cells, whereas others have a natural adaptation for the sprint due to their number of fast-twitch cells.

Training can increase the cross-sectional dimension of the muscle cell, the size of the mitochondria, the number of capillaries bringing oxygen, glucose and fatty acids to the cells, the activity of the enzyme systems for metabolizing fatty acids and glucose, and the amount of glycogen stored per unit of muscle weight. This is the reason that a high degree of efficiency in procuring and using energy sources can be achieved by training.

In reviewing muscle physiology as it pertains to physical performance, one should not lose sight of the other parts of the body equally important to a satisfying performance. The heart must be healthy and strong to pump blood containing nutrients to all the organs; the lungs supply oxygen to the blood and remove carbon dioxide; the liver regulates the supply of glucose and fatty acids; and the brain transmits the messages, defining which muscles will do what.

There are *general rules in nutrition* that should be applied for maintaining health in the adolescent athlete.

**Adequate fluids** are essential (Chap. 5). Water is used by the body to rid itself of excess heat through evaporation of sweat. The energy expended during exercise produces a great amount of heat and causes the athlete to sweat large quantities of water. If this water is not replaced, dehydration, increased body temperature, and eventually heat stroke may occur. Performance usually suffers after about 3% of total body water is lost. Frequent, intermittent fluid replacement should be practiced.

Plain water is preferred, but if sugar solutions are used, the American College of Sports Medicine recommends they provide less than 2 g to 5 g glucose per 100 ml water, less than 10 mEq sodium and less than 5 mEq potassium per liter of solution. Most commercial electrolyte drinks exceed these values and, for this reason should be diluted with an equal amount of plain water. Salt tablets are not recommended, because in most instances electrolyte depletion does not occur. In addition, if fluid intake is not sufficient, they can increase risk of dehydration.

Wrestlers attempting to "make weight" are often in a state of dehydration. Many techniques, for example, induced sweating, vomiting, spitting, and diuretics, are used to lose pounds quickly by creating a negative fluid balance. Because the water is frequently not replaced between the time of weight certification and the match, the wrestler enters competition in a negative fluid balance. The immediate and long term effect of this practice on the adolescent has not been adequately investigated, but the nutrition counselor should be aware of the risks.

**Nutrient needs** of the adolescent athlete are next in importance. A diet that supplies adequate amounts of all the nutrients required for growth and development (see Table 19-1) of the adolescent is essential if the teenaged athlete is to reach optimum performance levels. Additional *kilocalories* are needed by the athlete to provide the energy required for training and performance. *Weight control* can be an important aspect of many sports. Because the sprinter is more efficient when he carries a minimum of weight, he strives to achieve a very low percentage of body fat. Wrestlers have to make a certain weight and are very conscious of weight control. Football players, particularly defensive linebackers, are more effective if they carry extra weight—muscle, not fat.

As previously stated, ATP is the source of energy for muscular activity. This is supplied from glucose and fatty acid metabolism in muscle cells (see Chap. 9). In strenuous physical exercise when the heart and lungs cannot supply adequate oxygen to the cells, glucose from glycogen stores is used anaerobically (without oxygen) to product ATP. Intensive training by athletes for endurance events improves their utilization of oxygen and increases their efficiency in using fatty acids as a source of ATP. Thus the well conditioned athlete is able to spare some glycogen by metabolizing more fat. Protein is not used as a source of energy during exercise.

The amount of additional kilocalories required by the athlete depends on the type, intensity, and duration of the exercise as well as on the skill of the athlete. During periods of intense training and competition in football, soccer, cross-country skiing, and distance running, an athlete may expend up to twice the number of calories required by the nonathlete. Reported caloric intakes of over 6000 kcal have not been unusual from college football players. These additional calories are provided by increased amounts of the basic food groups plus use of high-calorie snacks. The usual distribution of calories from carbohydrate (45%–55%), fat (35%–40%) and protein (10%–15%) is suggested for the athletes' regular food pattern.

The *pregame meal* for events of moderate and long duration may be more beneficial if it is relatively high in carbohydrate and eaten about 3 hours before the event. In this case the stomach will be empty by the start of the event, and energy intake should be sufficient to prevent hunger and weakness during competition. In short events the body is not dependent on substances synthesized from this meal, and there is no evidence that the content of the pregame meal has any effect on performance. Concentrated sugars and sugar solutions should be avoided, because they may cause extra water to enter the gut and result in discomfort and diarrhea.

*Glycogen loading* has been tried by some athletes competing in moderate to long duration events. Stores of glycogen in the muscle can be greatly increased by following a glycogen-loading regimen for a week before an event. For the first 3 days of the regimen a diet low in

carbohydrate (10%) and high in protein and fat is consumed, while moderate to heavy exercise (using the same muscles required for the event) is performed to deplete muscle glycogen stores. The last 3 days before the event a high carbohydrate (70%) diet is consumed, and exercise is tapered off to very light in order to load fully the muscles with glycogen. This practice is not without hazard and should be attempted only under medical supervision, and then very infrequently, perhaps for the one or two major events of a year. Remember that the heart is a muscle, and the long term effects of glycogen loading are not known.

*Protein* needs are not increased as a result of physical activity. However, during training and competition when the muscle mass is increasing and the blood volume is expanding, there is some additional retention of amino acids. Increased losses of nitrogen in sweat as well as in athletes who temporarily exhibit proteinuria and hemoglobinuria may also indicate slightly increased protein needs. How very small these demands are on the actual amounts of protein can be seen in Table 19-3.[14] The athlete consuming 3000 kcal per day and receiving 10% of these from protein consumes 75 g of protein, more than adequate to meet the needs of an athlete. This amount of protein is found in 1 quart of milk (32 g), 4 oz of meat (28 g), 6 slices of bread (12 g), and 1 potato (3 g). The majority of athletes consume far more protein than they actually need. Where there is concern about dehydration, excess protein consumption causing increased urinary excretion could provide a problem.

The only *vitamin* needs that appear to increase in the athlete are those for B vitamins related to energy metabolism. The suggested allowances per 1000 kilocalories are shown in Table 11-4 and can be used to estimate the need for athletes requiring energy in excess of 3000 kcal.

The *minerals* that require some consideration for athletes are the electrolytes, sodium and potassium, and the trace mineral, iron. The loss of sodium and potassium due to sweating requires replacement of these electrolytes to maintain fluid and electrolyte balance (see Chap. 5). Salt (NaCl) can usually be replaced by salting foods to taste. Electrolyte drinks may be diluted and consumed during or immediately following an event. Salt tablets are not recommended because frequently fluids are not consumed in amounts adequate to maintain homeostasis. During vigorous exercise in high temperature and humidity, potassium depletion can occur from profuse sweating, if potassium is not replaced by foods and beverages containing liberal amounts of this mineral (see Table 1, Part 4).

Due to the role that iron metabolism appears to play in physical performance and endurance, good iron status in the athlete is important. Because the female athlete loses greater amounts of iron due to menstruation, a diet providing good sources of iron, including some meat and fruits and vegetables high in ascorbic acid (to increase the

**Table 19-3. Estimated Daily Protein Need of the Large, Rapidly Growing Male Athlete with a Developing Muscle Mass**

| *Basis for Need* | *Protein (g)* |
|---|---|
| Replacement of nitrogen lost through urine, feces, skin, and other sites (for 70-kg man) | 24.5 |
| Provision of 30% extra protein for individual variation (for 70-kg man) | 7.5 |
| Replacement of nitrogen lost through sweat during 4 hours of strenuous exercise (for 70-kg man) | 7.5 |
| Coverage of increased protein need of growing muscle mass (for 70-kg man) | 7.5 |
| Coverage for extra protein associated with rapid growth in adolescence (liberal estimate) | 10.0 |
| Extra protein allotment for the exceptionally large male (liberal estimate) | 10.0 |
| TOTAL | 67.0 |

(From Worthington-Roberts B: Nutritional considerations for children in sports. In Pipes P: Nutrition in Infancy and Childhood, pp 205–223. St Louis, CV Mosby, 1981; Data obtained in part from Durnin JVGA: Protein requirements and physical activity. In Parizkova J, Rogozkin VA (ed): Nutrition, Physical Fitness, and Health. Baltimore, University Park Press, 1978)

availability of iron), is especially important for her. Reports indicate that menstruation may be delayed in the young female competitive athlete[15] and that amenorrhea may occur in cases of severe weight loss.[16] Continued suppression of menstruation by inadequate dietary intake may seriously affect the future health and reproductive performance of these young women and should be viewed with caution.

## Child nutrition programs

The Food and Nutrition Service of the U.S. Department of Agriculture (USDA) is responsible for the Child Nutrition Programs, which were authorized either by the National School Lunch Act of 1946 or the Child Nutrition Act of 1966. The purpose of these programs is to safeguard the health and wellbeing of the nation's children. The Child Nutrition Programs include the National School Lunch Program, the School Breakfast Program, the Special Milk Program, and the Special Food Service Program for Children.

In order to participate in Child Nutrition Programs, schools and child-care institutions must agree to the following regulations:

1. To operate the food service on a nonprofit basis for all children without regard to race, color or national origin
2. To provide free or reduced-price meals to children unable to pay the full price. These children must not be identified nor discriminated against in any way; and
3. To serve meals that meet the minimum nutritional requirements established by the Secretary of Agriculture (This does not apply to schools and institutions that participate only in the special milk program.)

Generally, these programs are administered through the State Education Departments; however, in those states where the law and other restrictions prohibit agencies from administering programs in private schools and child-care institutions, the Food and Nutrition Service, USDA, directly administers the program.

The *National School Lunch Program* assists schools in providing nutritionally adequate lunches to children by making available direct financial aid, donated foods, nonfood assistance, and technical guidance. The lunches served must meet the requirements for the "Type A lunch pattern." This pattern has been designed to provide approximately one-third of the RDA for children and includes as a minimum:

1. One-half pint of fluid milk as a beverage. Recent regulations define this to mean "fluid types of unflavored whole milk or lowfat milk or skim milk or cultured buttermilk, which meet State and local standards for such types of milk and flavored milk made from such types of milk which meet such standards."
2. Two ounces (edible portions as served) of lean meat, poultry, or fish; 2 oz of cheese; one egg; one-half cup of cooked dry beans or peas; 4 tablespoons of peanut butter; or an equivalent combination of these foods. To be counted in meeting these requirements these foods must be served in a main dish or in a main dish and one other menu item. When an egg or one-half cup of cooked dry peas or beans is served, it is nutritionally desirable to have an additional source or protein, such as meat, cheese, or peanut butter
3. A three-fourths cup serving that consists of two or more vegetables or fruits or both. Full strength vegetable or fruit juice may be counted to meet not more than one-fourth cup of this requirement
4. One slice of whole grain or enriched bread; a serving of cornbread, biscuits, rolls, or muffins made of whole grain or enriched meal or flour

Since 1977 different size portions may be served to children in different grade levels, Table 19-4. High school students may also select three of the five items from the Type A lunch. It is anticipated that these changes will

## Table 19-4. School Lunch Pattern Requirements—Minimum Amounts of Foods to Serve Children of Various Ages and Grades

| Food Components | Preschool Children | | Elementary School Students | | Secondary School Students |
| | Group I | Group II | Group III Grades K-3 | Group IV Grades 4-6 | Group V Grades 7-12 |
| | Age 1-2 | Age 3-4 | Age 5-8 | Age 9-11 | Age 12 and up |
|---|---|---|---|---|---|
| Meat and meat alternate | 1 oz | $1^1/_2$ oz | $1^1/_2$ oz | 2 oz | 3 oz |
| Vegetables and fruits | $^1/_2$ c | $^1/_2$ c | $^1/_2$ c | $^3/_4$ c | $^3/_4$ c |
| Bread and bread alternates | 5 slices/wk | 8 slices/wk | 8 slices/wk | 8 slices/wk | 10 slices/wk |
| Milk, fluid | $^1/_2$ c | $^3/_4$ c | $^3/_4$ c | $^1/_2$ pt | $^1/_2$ pt |

(From Rules and regulations, school lunch pattern requirements. Federal Register 43:163, Aug 22, 1978)

reduce the amount of food wasted in the School Lunch Program.

The number of children participating in the school lunch program has steadily risen, although recently the need to increase the price of lunches has resulted in decreased pupil participation. Future changes in the program will probably aim at increasing the participation of children from low-income families and of teenagers. There is also a movement underway—although not likely to be implemented in the near future—for a universal school lunch program that would guarantee each child at least one nutritionally adequate, free meal each day. Bettelheim,[17] in support of such a concept, discusses the ways in which food and the manner of its delivery may influence present and future behavior of children.

> . . . in order to make going to school attractive and learning feasible, I would suggest that we first concentrate on feeding all children there. And by this I do not mean something akin to existing food programs, which provide food as food, and not as an essential part of the educational enterprise. Instead I suggest centering the school experience around satiation of the children's needs, building the school day around meals, beginning with breakfast in the morning, a snack at midmorning, lunch at noon, and another snack at the end of the school day. Money spent on such programs would pay off much better than that spent on practically any other expense, be it textbooks, teaching machines, etc. I would give it priority even over school buildings. But this program would have to be entirely different from the mass feeding that is characteristic of most of our food programs. The meals I have in mind are not just filling of the stomach, but an enrichment of the total personality around a common meal—which requires that only a small group should eat together, and eat with those who are supposed to educate not only their minds, but nurture their total personalities.

Many innovative changes have already occurred in school feeding programs and these as well as future ones will require careful evaluation in terms of the goals of the program. Satellite feeding systems have been used whereby those schools which do not have adequate kitchens are served from other schools where kitchen facilities are available. Similarly, some school systems have established central kitchens not located in school buildings, which provide food for the entire school system. Commercially prepared convenience foods both canned and frozen in individual-sized containers have been introduced to meet the needs of schools where facilities are inadequate. Food service management companies and caterers also provide the food for some schools under the National School Lunch Program. To increase flexibility without reducing standards, menu planning techniques designed to meet predetermined nutrient requirements are being developed and tested as an option to the Type A pattern. Alternate or engineered foods have also been introduced. These include enriched macaroni with fortified protein and textured vegetable protein products (Chap 4).

The USDA's proposed rule for foods sold in competition with the School Lunch (snack bars and vending machines) is that the food must provide at least 5% of the US-RDA for any one or more of the eight nutrients—protein, vitamins A and C, niacin, riboflavin, thiamin, calcium, and iron. There has been much concern expressed by nutritionists about this rule due to the low nutrient density and high fat and sugar content of some of the foods permitted, such as potato chips, chocolate bars, and pastry.

### The school breakfast program

Established in 1966 to assist schools in providing breakfasts to pupils from low-income families or to children who had to travel long distances to school, the program is available today to all schools.

According to the regulations, the breakfast pattern must include as a minimum each of the following:
1. One-half pint of fluid milk served as a beverage, or on cereal, or used in part for each purpose
2. A one-half cup serving of fruit or full-strength fruit or vegetable juice
3. One slice of whole grain or enriched bread or an equivalent serving of foods such as cornbread, biscuits, rolls, muffins made of whole grain or enriched meal or flour; three-fourths cup serving of whole grain or enriched or fortified cereal; or an equivalent quantity of any combination of these foods

To improve the nutrition of participating children, school breakfasts should also include as often as practicable: one egg; or a 1-oz serving (edible portion as served) of meat, fish, or poultry; or 1 oz of cheese; or 2 tablespoons of peanut butter; or an equivalent quantity of any combination of any of these foods. Additional foods may be served with breakfast as desired.

An "alternate breakfast" consisting of a formulated grain-fruit product called *fortified breakfast cake* has been approved for use in breakfast programs, especially in those schools without kitchen facilities. These products when served with one-half pint of milk provide, with the exception of calories, approximately one-fourth the US-RDA for children. Critics of this program have been concerned not only about encouraging the use of cake for breakfast but also about giving credence to the idea that all cakes are equally nutritious.

All pupils in participating schools can buy breakfast at a reasonable price. Children from low-income families are eligible for free or reduced-price breakfasts under the same guidelines established for the school lunch program.

### The special milk program

In order to encourage the consumption of milk by children, all public and private schools and child-care institutions are eligible to participate in this program. Schools and other institutions are reimbursed in part for all the milk sold to children at reduced cost.

### The special food service program for children

This program assists all public and nonprofit child care institutions in providing nutritionally adequate meals—breakfast, lunch, dinner, and between meal supplements. Guidelines for participation are similar to those of the school lunch program and must include specific types of foods in minimum amounts according to the ages of the children.

- Breakfast: milk, fruit or juice, and bread or cereal
- Lunch or Supper: milk, meat or alternate, two or more vegetables or fruits, bread and butter or margarine
- Between Meals: milk or fruit or vegetable or juice, and bread or cereal

Institutions may receive assistance in the form of donated commodities, cash reimbursements, or financial help to buy food service equipment and technical guidance to establish and operate the food service program.

In 1977 Nutrition Education and Training, Section 19, became a part of the National School Lunch Act. The purpose of this amendment is to encourage effective dissemination of scientifically valid information to children participating in the school lunch or related child nutrition programs. In order to receive funds each state was required to develop a state plan, including a needs assessment. Nutrition educators have been employed in many school districts to train teachers in the preparation and use of nutrition education materials. Future funding of this program is in jeopardy due to Federal budget cuts, especially in Child Nutrition Programs. However, there has been real progress in the training of teachers and in the amount and quality of nutrition education materials available to them.

### Study questions and activities

1. What are some food preferences and prejudices of children at various ages?
2. What is the probable effect of a poor breakfast on the total food intake? Why do American families so often eat an inadequate breakfast?
3. Why do you think adolescent girls eat so much more poorly than boys in the same age group? Have you had experience with this problem yourself?
4. What are the food needs of the teenager? Do girls have additional nutritional needs as compared with boys? What are these, why do they occur, and how may they be met?
5. How is the Daily Guide to Foods Needed by Children and Their Families adapted to meet the nutritional needs of the various age groups?
6. Why is adolescent obesity of particular concern to the nutrition counselor?
7. Observe a preschool child during mealtime either in the hospital or at a day-care center. What was the menu served to the child? What were the portion sizes? Approximately how much of the various items did the child eat? Describe his eating skills. Were there any opportunities for socializing during the meal?
8. Describe four programs included in the Child Nutrition Programs. What is the Type A pattern lunch? Plan a week's menus for lunch which meets the Type A pattern for elementary school children.
9. What forms of assistance are available to day-care centers through the Special Food Service Program for Children? Discuss the role of the nutrition consultant to group day-care programs.
10. Why is nutrition counseling an important part of teenage drug and alcohol rehabilitation programs?
11. Discuss the fluid and nutrient needs of the adolescent athlete.

### References

1. Macy IG, Hunscher HA: J Nutr 45:189, 1951
2. Stitt PG: Nutrition Education Conference, Washington, DC, Jan 29, 1962
3. Birch LL et al: Child Dev 51:856, 1980
4. Dibble MV, Lally JR: J Nutr Educ 5:200, 1973
5. Mitchell HS et al: Proceedings VII, International Congress of Nutrition, 1967
6. Peckos PS: Food Nutr News 42:1, Dec–Jan, 1970–1971
7. Mann JI, Inman WHW: Br Med J 2:245, 1975
8. Mann JI et al: Br Med J 2:241, 1975
9. Spellacy WN et al: Contraception 6:265, 1972
10. Prasad AS et al: Effect of oral contraceptives on micronutrients and changes in trace elements due to pregnancy. In Moghissi KS, Evans TN (eds): Nutritional Impacts on Women Throughout Life with Emphasis on Reproduction, pp 160–188. Hagerstown, MD, Harper & Row, 1977
11. Belsey MA: Hormonal contraception and nutrition. In Moghissi and Evans, Nutritional Impacts on Women Throughout Life, pp 189–200.
12. Harford TC: Postgrad Med 60:73, 1976
13. Frankle R, Christakis G: Some nutritional aspects of "hard" drug addiction. Dietetic Currents 2, No. 3:1, July–Aug, 1975
14. Worthington-Roberts B: Nutritional considerations for children in sports. In Pipes P: Nutrition in Infancy and Childhood, pp 205–223. St. Louis, CV Mosby, 1981
15. Malina RM et al: Med Sci Sports 10:218, 1978
16. Feicht CB et al: Lancet 2:1145, 1978
17. Bettelheim B: Food to Nurture the Mind. Washington, DC, The Children's Foundation, 1026 17th Street, NW, 1970

### Supplementary readings

American Academy of Pediatrics, Committee on Nutrition: Calcium requirements in infancy and childhood. Pediatrics 62:826, 1978

American Academy of Pediatrics, Committee on Nutrition: Nutritional aspects of vegetarianism, health foods and fad diets. Pediatrics 59:460, 1977

Beal VA: Nutrition in the Life Span. New York, John Wiley & Sons, 1980

Birch LL, Zimmerman SI, Hind H: The influence of social-affective context on the formation of children's food preferences. Child Dev 51:856, 1980

Clancy-Hepburn K, Hickey AA, Nevill G: Children's behavior responses to TV food advertisements. J Nutr Educ 6:93, 1974

Consolazio CF et al: Protein metabolism of intensive physical training in the young adult. Am J Clin Nutr 29:29, 1975

Crawford PB et al: Serum cholesterol of 6-year-olds in relation to environmental factors. J Am Diet Assoc 78:41, 1981

Dibble MV, Lally JR: Nutrition in a family-oriented child development program. J Nutr Educ 5:200, 1973

DuRant RH, Linder CW: An evaluation of five indexes of relative body weight for use with children. J Am Diet Assoc 78:35, 1981

Dwyer JT el al: Risk of nutritional rickets among vegetarian children. Am J Dis Child 133:134, 1979

Greger JL et al: Nutritional status of adolescent girls in regard to zinc, copper and iron. Am J Clin Nutr 31:269, 1978

Hanley DF: Athletic training—And how diet affects it. Nutr Today 14, No. 6:5, Nov-Dec, 1979

Kirksey A et al: Vitamin $B_6$ nutritional status of a group of female adolescents. Am J Clin Nutr 31:946, 1978

Lane HW, Cerda JJ: Potassium requirements and exercise. J Am Diet Assoc 73:64, 1978

Leibel RL: Behavioral and biochemical correlates of iron deficiency. J Am Diet Assoc 71:398, 1977

Marino DD, King JC: Nutritional concerns during adolescence. Pediatr Clin North Am 27:125, 1980

McKigney JI, Munro HN (eds): Nutrient Requirements in Adolescence. Cambridge, MIT Press, 1976

Parizkova J, Rogozkin VA (eds): Nutrition, Physical Fitness and Health. Baltimore, University Park Press, 1978

Pipes P: Nutrition in Infancy and Childhood, 2nd ed. St Louis, CV Mosby, 1981

Smith NJ: Gaining and losing weight in athletes. JAMA 236:149, 1976

*For further references see Bibliography in Part 4.*

# Nutrition for Older Persons

## 20

**Margaret Knight Snowman**

As they age, people realize that they are going to lose independence, that they are going to get older and have disabilities, that they are going to have to accept the loss of their image of themselves (Fig. 20-1). Health professionals can help the aging to recognize their ability to adjust, to change, to accept. Nonetheless, these adjustments are difficult.

> People say that our adapting power ... has gone down a bit, that we have adjusted to many changes. Probably they think we are all cozy and content. . . . But the door is closed! The door is closed. Opportunities are narrowing, constantly. When I was 40, the world was my oyster. I could do anything! When I was 50—well, I began to realize that maybe I'd gone as far as I could go, with my capacities. When I was 60, I thought, Oh dear God, I am so tired. When I was 70, I was ready for a retirement community. And it's that ability to accept and know what's going on that is important. But you don't like it, believe me.[1]

Older Americans are the most rapidly growing segment of our population. The absolute number of people over age 65 and the proportion of the total population that they represent have increased dramatically in recent decades and will continue to increase in the near future. In 1970, there were 20 million people in the United States over the age of 65, representing 10% of our population. The estimate for 1980 is over 25 million or 11% of the population. By the year 2000, we expect to have almost 32 million people over 65, representing 12% of that population.

Medical science, which is largely responsible for the increase in the number of older persons alive today, is also challenged to learn more about the degenerative and chronic diseases common in this group. The social sciences also have a responsibility to help make the later years of life worthwhile.

Unfortunately, the elderly are often the target of *agism*—stereotypes and discrimination against people

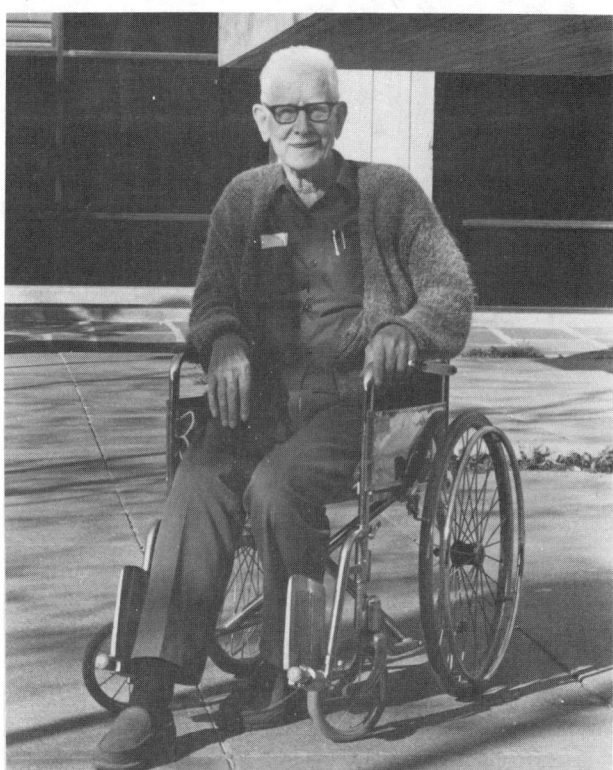

**Fig. 20-1.** The ability to adjust has helped this man to accept the disabilities of older age. (Photo Syracuse University, Gerontology Center)

because they are old. Dr. Robert Butler has sensitively discussed these prejudices in *Why Survive? Being Old in America.*[2] The elderly are often thought of as sick, living alone, housebound and lonely, or confined to nursing homes, dependent, and perhaps senile. In reality, about 5% of the elderly live in nursing homes and other institutions. Most noninstitutionalized elderly people live with relatives. The most common marital status for men is married and living with their wives. Because women live longer and tend to marry older men, most older women are widows. Most elderly people report that their health is good to excellent.

Although the nutritional requirements for older adults are not fundamentally different from those of the young adult, several aspects of nutrition deserve consideration. First, can dietary alterations delay aging? Second, what is the relationship of diet to some of the chronic diseases associated with aging? Third, what special dietary considerations are needed for elderly persons?

## Nutrition and aging
### Search for the fountain of youth

A modern search for the fountain of youth is occurring in the laboratories of biochemists around the world. Life expectancy in laboratory animals can be increased significantly by caloric restriction. Ross,[3] for example, was able nearly to double the life expectancy of rats by imposing a regimen of severe underfeeding throughout the animals' post-weaning life. Some rats survived more than 1800 days, which corresponds to about 180 years for humans. His experiments suggested that it is possible to extend the period of life prior to the onset of some diseases commonly associated with aging. However, the adverse effects of severe underfeeding were serious enough so that this practice has little applicability for humans. Infant mortality was high, growth was stunted and impairments of behavior developed. There was also greater susceptibility to bacterial and parasitic diseases. Whereas the limited diet reduced the incidence of some types of tumors, a higher proportion of the tumors that did occur were malignant.

The composition of the diet also affected the length of life and susceptibility to diseases associated with aging. The timing of dietary changes was important too. Diets that were compatible with long life when started at the time of weaning became progressively less so when begun at later ages. Dietary restriction started in old age actually shortened life.[3,4] Thus there may be a critical period early in life when diet most affects longevity.

Although nutritional changes in diet can affect longevity in animals, the causal relationships remain to be identified. Some researchers feel that dietary changes may produce neuroendocrine and immunologic changes, which affect the aging process.[5] Studies in rats have shown that tryptophan-deficient diets lowered mortality rates. (Tryptophan, an essential amino acid, is a precursor of the neurotransmitter serotonin.) However, the tryptophan-deficient animals aged more rapidly than controls once they were restored to a normal diet.

Animal studies have shown that changes in the quality, composition and timing of the diet can modify aging. However, these findings are far from practical application in humans. Many years of carefully controlled testing on various species are needed first. In addition, dietary modifications represent only one area of environmental research on aging. For example, temperature modifications also affect life expectancy.

### Theories of biologic aging

What causes aging? No one really knows. A number of theories have been developed in an attempt to explain the process of aging—some environmental, others genetic. To date, however, there is no generally accepted theory, partly due to the difficulty of separating external causes from internal ones.

In the laboratory, cells are able to replicate themselves only a certain number of times before they lose this ability. Genetically induced aging may be due to the failure of genetic material to function normally, with resulting errors in replication. Some believe that the body has a pacemaker or "biological death clock," possibly located in the cell membranes or in the hypothalamus. Others believe that aging is caused by cellular mutations resulting from external causes, such as ionizing radiation, heat, chemicals, or perhaps viruses, such as RNA virus.[6-8] A detailed discussion of theories of biologic aging is beyond the scope of this chapter. However, two theories with nutritional implications are discussed briefly.

### Free-radical theory

According to the free-radical theory, radiation entering the body can strike polyunsaturated fatty acids within the cell, knocking loose hydrogen atoms and initiating peroxidation, which results in formation of free radicals. A free radical is very reactive and flies around within the cell until it strikes another molecule, damaging it. Cross-linkages may form between molecules, forming dense aggregates, which no longer function normally. Cell membranes may be disrupted, the cell nucleus may be distorted, or mitochondria may be destroyed. Free radicals may also damage the lysosomes, which then attack the cell and destroy it. After the cell is burned out by peroxidation, all that remains may be a "clinker" or ash of the lysosome, which holds colored pigments. According to this theory, such antioxidants as vitamin E, ascorbic acid, or, perhaps, selenium or the food additive, BHT, may be able to protect the polyunsaturated lipids, thus delaying the aging of the cell.[8,9]

### Immune system and neuroendocrine changes

Changes in the immune system may result in autoimmune reactions, which cause the body to attack itself. These changes might be slowed by manipulating the immune system by diet, heat, or other methods. Another promising area of research is that of neuroendocrine changes. Diet may affect the synthesis of neurotransmitters (such as serotonin, norepinephrine, and dopamine), which may affect mechanisms that regulate the aging process. Understanding these changes may make it possible to devise drug therapies to control aging.[5]

## The aging process

### Aging continues throughout the life span

The changes associated with aging generally begin as soon as the growth and development of a particular body subsystem are completed. In other words, there is no plateau of optimal functioning during the middle years. People do not stay "in their prime" for 20 or 30 years and then suddenly age. Instead, loss of function is uniform into the eighth and ninth decades. Elderly people are losing function at the same rate as younger people—an 80 year old person is aging at the same rate as a 30 year old; he has simply aged longer.[10]

### People tend to differ more as they grow older

Babies resemble each other more in behavior and physical growth than do adolescents. The elderly show still more individual variations, as Dr. Swanson[11] has pointed out:

> A person at 70 is an historical record of all that has happened to him—his injuries, infections, nutritional imbalances, fatigues, and emotional upsets. Old people, therefore, differ from each other much more than do younger folk. All this needs to be considered in food planning for any older person. Each one is an individual, quite unlike anyone else.

### Individuals age at different rates

Chronological age is a poor predictor of functional ability. Some 80 year olds function as well as the average 40 year old, and some 40 year olds perform like the average 80 year old.[10]

### Age-related changes occur in practically every part of the body[6,10,12-14]

The following illustrate a few of the body parts that are affected. The bones decrease in density. Lean body mass tends to be lost, whereas adipose tissue and connective tissue generally increase. The heart may pump blood less efficiently. Blood flow may be reduced because of atherosclerotic deposits in the blood vessels and less elastic walls. The rate of renal blood flow is often reduced, and the kidneys are less efficient in removing waste products from the blood. Nerve signals are transmitted at slower speed. The lenses of the eyes lose the ability to focus at near distances, and elderly people usually need brighter light to see without glasses than do young adults. Hearing loss is common, especially for high tones. Smell and taste may become less acute,[15-17] and loss of teeth may make chewing difficult. Digestion may become slightly impaired as a result of decreased hydrochloric acid secretion by the parietal cells and decreased bile secretion. Loss of tone in the gastrointestinal tract may result in constipation. Some systems, however, show little change with age. For example, liver function tests do not change with age, and there is no decline in hematocrit with advancing age up until the ninth or tenth decade.

### Various parts of the body age at different rates

Recent studies suggest that learning, memory, reaction time, and problem-solving ability decline very late in life. The rate of change in function varies not only from one person to another, but within a person, from one individual organ to another. For this reason, knowing the condition of a person's kidneys tells little about the state of his heart.

### Loss of function is more apparent during stress

In spite of the large number of changes that occur during aging, most activities in normal resting people are affected to only a modest degree by aging. However, the young have a strikingly more effective response to physiologic challenges. Such challenges justify the impression that marked physiologic deterioration occurs during aging.[13]

### It is difficult to distinguish normal changes due to aging from changes caused by disease

Because many studies of aging people have not excluded diseased persons, there has been a confusion between changes related to age and disease. For example, declines in the functioning of the central nervous system, which are generally believed to be part of aging, may instead be due to Parkinson's disease or Alzheimer's disease, which are more common in the aged than in the young. Alternatively, some changes related to age mimic disease states. Glucose tolerance is frequently impaired in the elderly. Failure to use criteria adjusted for age can result in the over-diagnosis of diabetes mellitus in elderly people, causing concern and unnecessarily limiting the person's dietary choices.[10]

## Nutrition and chronic disease

Many elderly people suffer from chronic disease. Approximately 80% of people over 65 have one or more chronic diseases, in contrast to 40% of those under 65. In addition, illnesses in older people are likely to involve a larger number of organ systems than in younger people.[18] However, age is not synonymous with illness. Only 21% of those over 65 identified poor health as a very serious problem.[6] Two-thirds of noninstitutionalized elderly people reported that their health was good to excellent.[19]

A variety of diseases are more common among elderly Americans, for example, atherosclerosis and heart disease, hypertension and stroke, diabetes mellitus, cancer, diverticular disease, arthritis, osteoporosis, periodontal disease, and cataracts and other visual disturbances. Nutritional components have been implicated in the etiology of many of these diseases, although controversy exists about the relative importance of nutrition in the prevention of disease.

In spite of a number of studies on the use of cholesterol and saturated fat, their relationship to the development of atherosclerotic disease is still very controversial. Other factors, such as exercise, fiber, and various minerals, are also being investigated. Although high-sodium diets and, more recently, high-fat diets and obesity have been suggested as possible contributing factors in hypertension in genetically susceptible people, the role of diet in the prevention of hypertension is still uncertain. Weight control is generally considered important in the prevention and treatment of diabetes mellitus. The possible role of chromium in the prevention of adult-onset diabetes is currently being explored. Recent attention has focused on the possible effects of high-fat and low-fiber diets on some types of cancer. Recent theories have linked low-fiber diets with diverticular disease and other diseases of Western civilization. These topics are discussed in more detail elsewhere in this text.

Even if further research demonstrates that nutritional factors play specific causative roles in these diseases, it is unlikely that dietary modifications late in life are able to halt or reverse these diseases; they may, however, stabilize them. Instead, nutrition is likely to play its most significant role during youth and middle age. Although these diseases are regarded as geriatric problems, their prevention may well be a pediatric concern.

### Arthritis

Although diet plays a part in gout, there is no evidence that nutrition can cause or cure osteoarthritis. In spite of this, many elderly people spend large sums of money on special foods and vitamins, hoping that their arthritis will be helped. Because obesity can cause increased stress on arthritic joints, weight reduction diets may benefit overweight people with arthritis.

Arthritis pain and deformities may limit mobility, making food preparation and shopping difficult. Hands crippled with arthritis may require specially adapted utensils to facilitate eating. Habitual aspirin use for arthritis may cause gastrointestinal bleeding, increasing the risk of anemia.

### Osteoporosis

Osteoporosis is a common problem among the elderly, especially women. Estimates of the prevalence of osteoporosis range from 15% to 50%. At least 10% of the population over 50 has osteoporosis severe enough to cause vertebral, hip or long bone fractures.[20] Bone loss occurs gradually and is asymptomatic in the early stages. Advanced osteoporosis may not be noticed until spontaneous fractures occur. In postmenopausal women, the first symptoms are progressive loss of height (Fig. 20-2).

Bone loss is affected by activity levels, hormonal levels (especially estrogen and parathyroid hormone), high intakes of phosphorus and low intakes of protein, vitamins A, C, and D, fluoride, and calcium. Researchers disagree about whether osteoporosis is a normal consequence of advancing age or can be prevented by dietary modifications. The Committee on Dietary Allowances, Food and Nutrition Board NAS-NRC[21] has stated that the role of long-term nutrient intake in the cause of osteoporosis remains uncertain, and it has continued to recommend intakes of 800 mg per day of calcium for adult and elderly men and women. Other researchers support the view that liberal intakes of calcium may be important, especially for elderly women, and recommend

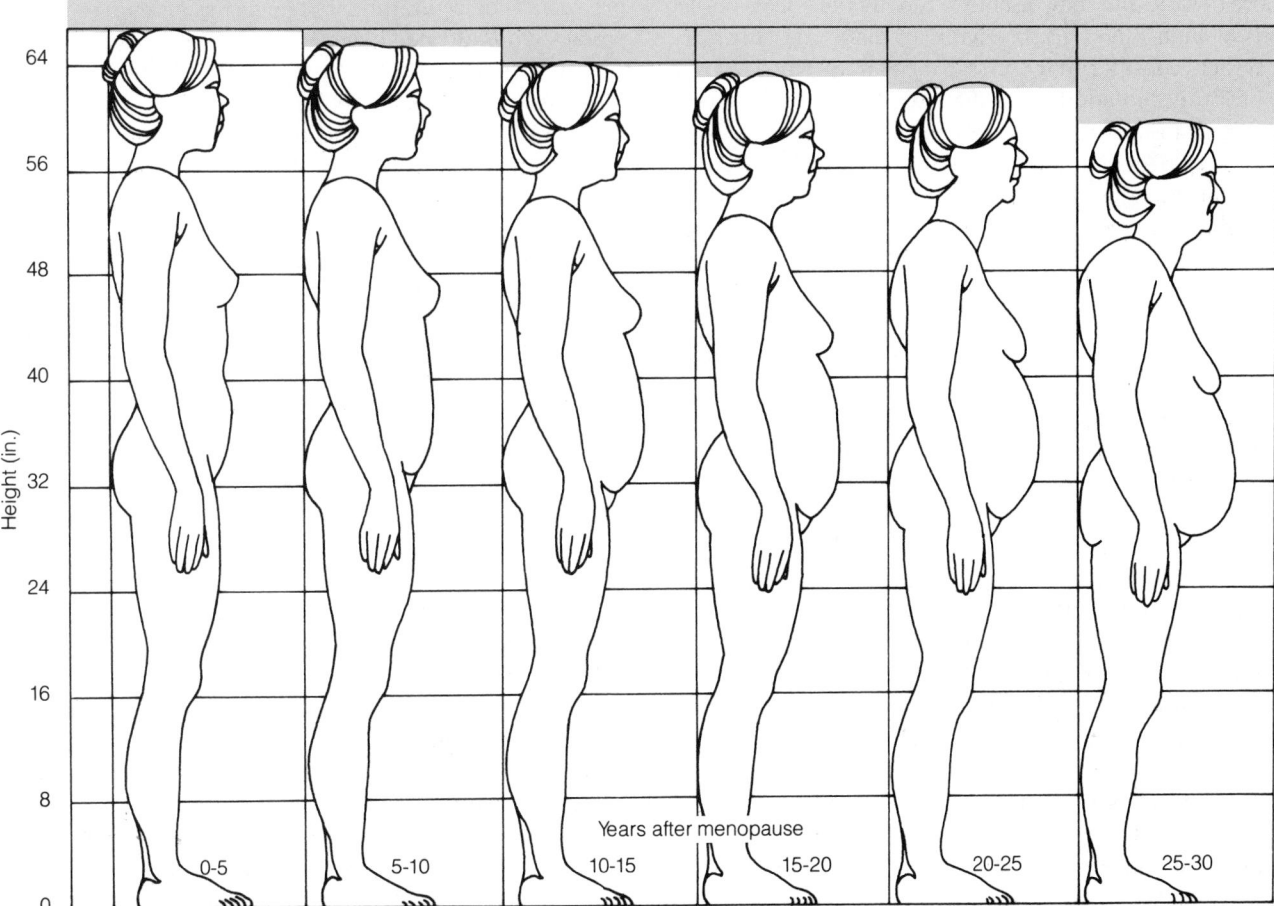

**Fig. 20-2.** The osteoporotic process causes progressive loss of height and kyphosis in women in the years following menopause. (Albanese AA, Lorenze EJ, Wein EH, Reprinted from the October 1978 issue of *American Family Physician,* published by the American Academy of Physicians)

levels as high as 1000 mg for the average person[20] and 1400 mg per day for the postmenopausal woman.[22] To achieve these levels, a person would have to consume a quart or more of whole or skim milk or an equivalent amount of cheese. An alternative is daily administration of a calcium supplement.

Prevention of osteoporosis, starting in youth, has been advocated because treatment after diagnosis has generally shown little effect in slowing or reversing bone loss, due in part, perhaps, to decreased calcium absorption in the elderly. Recent studies by Albanese and associates,[20] however, have indicated that daily supplements of 750 mg calcium and 375 IU of vitamin D administered over a 3-year period to women aged 79 to 89 resulted in increases in bone density that have been verified by x-ray.

Some researchers feel that calcium-to-phosphorus ratio may be the critical factor because excess phosphorus accelerates bone loss. Although milk intake is decreasing, dietary intakes of phosphorus are increasing in the American diet due to high consumption of meat, carbonated beverages, and the addition of phosphates to processed foods and snack foods. As it is difficult to ingest foods with a calcium-to-phosphorus ratio higher than one, dietary calcium supplements may be necessary.[23]

### Periodontal disease

Periodontal disease causes the loss of teeth in approximately 35 million Americans, most of them elderly. Recent data suggest that periodontal disease may be an early form of generalized nutritional osteoporosis. Bone loss in the jaw may lead to loosening of the teeth with later infection of the gums. These changes have been demonstrated in dogs fed high-phosphorus, low-calcium diets. If this research proves applicable to humans, periodontal disease may provide an early warning of osteoporosis, so that appropriate dietary treatment could be instituted to prevent further changes.[24]

### Cataracts

Researchers have hypothesized that dietary factors may play a role in the development of cataracts. Gunby[25] has suggested that vitamin E may make lens membranes more flexible and may be able to modify the effects on the lens of high blood glucose levels in diabetics. Other researchers consider that excess calories may play a part by contributing to adult-onset diabetes. Some consider that excess lactose, galactose, arabinose, or xylose may have harmful effects. Tryptophan may modify the effect of sugar on the lens. The roles of tryptophan, calcium, selenium, zinc, and vitamin deficiencies, especially tryptophan, are also being investigated.[26]

### Senility

Senility is often mistakenly considered an inevitable consequence of growing old. *Senility* is not an accurate medical diagnosis, but a lay term used to describe a large number of conditions ranging from simple confusion through irreversible organic dementia or chronic organic brain syndrome.

Elderly people with reversible conditions are frequently labeled senile and sent to institutions for the rest of their lives.[2] If confusion is noted, a complete physical workup should be done to rule out temporary problems. Drug reactions, for example, frequently cause confusion. Functional illnesses like depression may be mistaken for senility. A variety of physical disorders can trigger seemingly senile behavior. Eldery patients may show confusion and disorientation as early signs of a variety of conditions such as infection, heart failure, electrolyte imbalance, dehydration, diabetic acidosis, hypothyroidism, or anemia.

#### Nutritional deficiencies can cause mental confusion

Classic niacin deficiency, pellagra, is characterized by poor memory, hallucinations, irritability, delusions of persecution, and finally dementia. Irritability and forgetfulness are seen in folic acid deficiency. Severe thiamin deficiency is a well documented cause of dementia. Mental depression may be caused by pernicious anemia (failure to absorb vitamin $B_{12}$), deficiencies of pantothenic acid and vitamin $B_6$. Iodine deficiency can result in apathy and slow mental performance. Protein undernutrition can also impair psychological performance. Misdiagnosis of senility is tragic because it delays or prevents treatment, which could restore the elderly to normal functioning.

Howell and Loeb[27] have suggested that awareness on the part of the elderly and their families that behavior, emotions, and intellectual functions could be related to diet might prove a powerful incentive to improving and maintaining good dietary habits in aging adults.

#### Organic dementia

About 10%* of the population over 65 have organic dementia. Half of the cases are severe. One-fifth require hospitalization. Senile dementia of the Alzheimer's type accounts for at least half of all dementia in old age. The prevalence of senile and other forms of dementia increases with advancing age.[28]

In recent years, there have been radical changes in ideas about dementia. Dementia is no longer seen as a degeneration or exaggerated aging of the brain. Instead it is viewed as a disease process. Active searches for causes of dementia hasten the possibility that effective treatments will be developed.

A variety of hypotheses are now being explored, among them one that dementia may be caused by an infection (perhaps a slow-acting virus) or by alterations in the body's immune system. Several hypotheses have dietary implications, for example, that dementia may be caused by toxic agents, such as aluminum. Raised aluminum concentrations have been noted in some brain regions of victims of Alzheimer's disease. High serum levels of aluminum in elderly humans are associated with poor long-term memory and impaired visual–motor coordination. Levick[29] has raised the question whether aluminum can be absorbed from corrosive pitting of aluminum cookware. Studies testing this hypothesis are not yet available. However, aluminum has been implicated as a causative agent in dementia of patients on dialysis who are receiving aluminum-containing phosphate-binding gels. Normally functioning kidneys have been assumed to be efficient in ridding the body of aluminum, but this assumption is currently being reexamined.[30]

Another hypothesis with dietary implications is that senile dementia may be due to a specific neurotransmitter defect. Recent studies have shown that the composition of meals can cause daily fluctuations in the synthesis of brain neurotransmitters. There is some evidence for a cholinergic deficiency in dementia. (Choline is a key part of lecithin and is a precursor of the neurotransmitter acetylcholine. It is widespread in our food supply. It is found in muscle meats and grains; legumes are good sources, and egg yolks and organ meats are particularly high.) Choline and lecithin are currently being tested in patients with Alzheimer's type dementia and in people with mild to moderate memory defects. Preliminary data suggest that large doses of lecithin or choline slightly improve memory and social behavior in some subjects.[31]

Because dietary tyrosine can enhance the formation of the neurotransmitters dopamine and norepinephrine, it may play a role in motor coordination and in the perception of reality. Although these studies are stimulating considerable interest, it will be years before we know whether dietary changes can help to combat the fogetfulness seen in some elderly people.

## Dietary intakes and requirements of older people

The nutritional state of people at 70 or 80 years reflects not only their current food practices, but all of their previous dietary history as well. This can be observed

---

*Other estimates range from 5% to 25%.

by anyone with a long close association with older persons. As Dr. Swanson[11] comments,

> The older a person grows, the longer and more complex is his dietary history. The variations in nutritional status and dietary needs of a group of adults thus are bound to be greater than corresponding variations in a group of young people. Recommendations for the food needs of this age group must be pointed especially to the needs of individuals.

> The same nutritional principles that describe adequate diets for earlier periods of life apply to the diets of adults. Even though the adult has grown up—matured—his basic food supply still must provide all the nutrients necessary for maintaining body structure and for operating its machinery.

Good nutrition is only one of the habits which help to maintain strength and vigor, and it can be practiced three times a day—but it is abused more frequently than any other.

It has been demonstrated repeatedly that older people can adjust to different circumstances, learn new skills, and adopt new food habits. We cite a few examples: the 80 year old man who learned to eat salads when a thoughtful housekeeper chopped them to make them easier to eat yet kept them colorful and attractive; the elderly homemaker still trying new gadgets and ready-prepared foods to make work easier and also to add interest and variety to meals for two. "Never too old to learn" is a far truer adage than "You can't teach an old dog new tricks."

None of us is too young to begin thinking about improving our health prospects for later years. People invest money to protect their future; why shouldn't they consider other steps which may give even greater security and comfort?

## Dietary intakes of older persons

It is not unusual for elderly Americans to consume less than the RDA for energy, calcium, iron, ascorbic acid, thiamin, and vitamin A. In general, however, there is less information available on the dietary intakes of the elderly than for younger groups. Most studies have been done on noninstitutionalized people; some have reported on the intakes of nursing home residents.[32-35] The studies vary in methodology, although most use 24-hour dietary recalls, a method that relies on ability to recall accurately and, for this reason, tends to underestimate caloric consumption. O'Hanlon and Kohrs[36] have summarized dietary surveys that assess the nutrient intakes of older Americans and have discussed the results of different methodologies and standards used. Food energy and calcium were the nutrients most often found to be below standards. Mean caloric intake was below the standards in all large national surveys and a number of smaller studies. Calcium was low in many of the studies, with more women than men having inadequate intakes. Niacin and protein were most often found to be sufficient. The mean intake of

protein was adequate in the studies reviewed, with the exception of the Ten-State Survey.[37] However, several studies reported that at least one-third of their subjects had low protein intakes.

Other studies have suggested that the zinc nutriture of older Americans may be less than ideal.[16,17,38] This is of particular interest because several changes associated with aging resemble the symptoms of zinc deficiency, namely decreased taste acuity and delayed wound healing. Preliminary studies, however, have failed to reveal significant correlations between taste acuity and dietary zinc levels.[16,17]

### Susceptibility to fads

Unfortunately, many adults in late middle age, or older, are misled in their search for "eternal youth" or relief from their aches and pains. They hear and believe the television and radio promotions of various panaceas—elixirs or multivitamin and mineral mixtures claimed to be remedies for all sorts of ills. They read and believe the fad health books, especially those that have been flooding the book market during the past decade. It is well known that food and nutrition quackery thrives in areas where middle income retired people congregate. So-called health food stores may carry many desirable food items, but they also stock a variety of items promoted by the faddists. The cost of fad foods may divert money from other food items or from other needs. Indiscriminate use of vitamin and mineral supplements may also cost the older person money that could more appropriately be used to purchase a better quality diet, one more generally beneficial to health.

### Food requirements change with age

The dietary requirements of later life are influenced by a number of factors, such as general health; degree of physical activity; changes in ability to chew, digest, and absorb food; efficiency in the use of nutrients by the tissues; alteration in the endocrine system; emotional state; and mental health. The nutrient and calorie allowances that maintain one person in optimum health may be inadequate or more than adequate to meet the needs of another, apparently similar, person.

## Calorie needs

The major physiologic change occurring with age is a decrease in the number of functioning cells, which results in a slowing down of metabolic processes. This, together with a decrease in physical activity, may reduce the energy needs of the older adult. For example, a woman over 76 years of age weighing 120 lb may need only 1600 kcal, whereas she needed about 1800 kcal at age 60 and 2000 kcal at age 23. If she does not reduce her caloric intake to conform to her needs, she will store the excess as fat.

## When calories need to be reduced

The food sources of reduced calories must be chosen with care to include all essential factors, in higher proportion than those needed in former years because the total food consumed is less. There is an obvious need for foods that carry a full quota of proteins, minerals, and vitamins. It is essential to reduce consumption of empty calories—sugar, rich desserts, sweet rolls, candies, fats, and alcohol.

Reduction in total calories involves a most difficult task of alteration of food habits. For the majority of persons, habit is perhaps one of the greatest obstacles in the path to an optimal diet. The longer the habits are continued, the more fixed they become. The food habits of older people are apt to be so fixed that it is difficult to change them unless the way is made easy.

Whoever is planning or preparing the meals for overweight persons—the homemaker herself, a health aide or housekeeper—can eliminate some calories behind the scenes (if necessary) while still keeping meals attractive and in the familiar pattern. If people do not see the high calorie foods, one psychological barrier has been overcome. By substituting for rich cakes and pastries such items as puddings and custards made with skim milk, angel food cake and more fruit desserts, gelatins, whips, calories are saved without sacrificing flavor. Also, low-calorie salad dressings, less butter or margarine on vegetables, and gravies made with a minimum of fat are devices for the cook to use before the food reaches the table.

When appropriate, the nutrition counselor concerned with the continuing education of the patient may make specific suggestions along this line in keeping with the socioeconomic status of the patient and his cultural pattern of eating.

## When calories need to be increased

Quite another problem exists for the disabled and shut-in, who may not get enough food to meet energy or other nutritional requirements. If they live alone or have poor cooking facilities, they may have little incentive or opportunity to shop and cook for themselves.

Sometimes appetite fails to tempt the elderly to eat enough food or the right kind of food. The reduced calories in such cases seldom carry enough of the essential nutrients.

The undernutrition that may occur can be relieved by attention to foods with low bulk and concentrated calories that are high in protein, vitamins, and minerals and are prepared in a tasty way. This may not be easy for the person living alone to achieve; even for someone living with a large family, attention to the younger members of the family may seem more important to the homemaker than tempting the appetite of an elderly grandmother. For others the same problem may stem from the necessity of eating in hotels or restaurants where food does not appeal to the appetite or may be too expensive.

## Protein requirements

Apparently, protein needs are not reduced appreciably with age; in spite of this, many older people eat less protein than they did when younger. This is most likely to happen where marketing is difficult, cooking facilities are poor, or the money for food is limited. It can also happen among those with a better economic status when denture troubles, lack of appetite, or too little energy prevent the preparing or the eating of meats or other protein foods.

Some good-quality protein is essential at each meal no matter what the age. The Recommended Dietary Allowances (0.8 g per kilogram body weight) suggest no reduction in protein with age, in contrast to calories. As a result, the proportion of protein making up the total calories is increased.

Cheng and associates[39] found no significant differences in protein requirement, efficiency of protein use, or the ability to adapt to changes of protein intake in the elderly. Others believe that the requirement for certain amino acids may even be increased to meet changes in body function with age. Bigwood[40] found the methionine and lysine requirements of six male subjects 50 to 70 years of age to be substantially greater than that of younger males. For a more detailed discussion of protein needs, see Young.[41]

Special attention may be needed in meeting the protein requirements of the older person if he is sharing family meals planned to meet the higher caloric food habits of younger members of the family. An extra glass of skim milk at meals or between meals may be consumed to supplement smaller servings of meat, fish, or other high protein main dishes. If the person lives alone, milk, yogurt, cheese, and eggs are often used as substitutes for meat, fish, or poultry due to ease of preparation. Because adequate calories tend to spare protein, the total food intake should always be taken into account.

## Mineral requirements

Postmenopausal women need less iron than younger women; for this reason, the RDA for iron is 10 mg for women over 51 years, compared to 18 mg for younger women. The recommendations for remaining minerals are the same for elderly and younger adults. Due to inadequate studies of nutrient requirements among the elderly, these allowances are extrapolations from the nutrient needs of younger adults. The NAS-NRC Food and Nutrition Board has not made any recomendations for dietary changes to prevent diseases, such as osteoporosis, because it feels that the role of long-term nutrient intake remains uncertain.

## Vitamin requirements

Unfortunately, little is known about the vitamin requirements of older people and whether there is a change associated with age or with chronic disease. However, there is no evidence that vitamin requirements are reduced with advancing years, and it is safe to assume that older people need all the vitamins they did in earlier years.

If there has been merely a marginal supply of any vitamin in the diet for many years, a reduction in total food eaten may be sufficient to precipitate minor nutritional deficiencies. The time factor of advancing age may permit cumulative effects to show up.

### Fluid and fiber requirements

Adequate fluid and fiber are necessary to prevent constipation, a common complaint among the elderly. The NAS-NRC Food and Nutrition Board recommends 1 ml of water for each kilocalorie of food consumed for people of all ages. More fluid is needed for comatose patients, people with fevers, vomiting, diarrhea, or polyuria, and for those using diuretics or high-protein diets. Additional fluid is needed in hot environments.

Much recent attention has been focused on fiber intakes in relation to diseases, but it is not yet possible to recommend a specific intake of fiber. Johnson and associates[42] have studied the dietary fiber content of the diets of older women and found that most had adequate intakes to maintain normal laxation. Women who used laxatives regularly, however, generally had lower fiber intakes. They concluded that a normal diet containing fruits, vegetables, nuts and whole grains should provide adequate dietary fiber for most people.

## Planning meals for older people

The planning of menus to meet the needs of the older age group presents problems that are as varied as the circumstances in which elderly people live. They may be living alone, with one or two other older people, marketing and preparing meals for themselves; they may be the older member in a younger family; they may be cared for by a practical nurse or a housekeeper. Whoever is responsible for planning and preparing their food should be aware of individual likes and dislikes, and special needs and limitations. There are multiple factors, such as ignorance of nutritional facts, food prejudices, fear of new foods, lack of money, limited cooking facilities, poor dentition, and poor appetite, which should be considered. The Daily Food Guide described in Chapter 11 is as important for meeting the nutritional needs of older people as for younger ones. The nutrition counselor may be able to advise or help with the planning where such problems seem to interfere with adequate nutrition.

The elderly person may require some special foods or food preparation, but so far as possible he or she should be a member of the family at mealtime and eat foods prepared for the family. If digestive ability is limited, the family meals should be planned so that the older person may avoid foods that disagree with him. When lack of appetite at mealtime makes an adequate food intake difficult, a midmorning and a midafternoon snack, such as hot chocolate or orange juice, may be offered. A hot drink at bedtime may be welcomed by an older person and may help to induce sleep.

Making simple food attractive and appropriate to the specific needs of an elderly person may be appreciated far out of proportion to the effort involved. This is particularly important when an event in his honor is celebrated, such as a birthday, anniversary, or other special occasion. By considering the texture and consistency of various menu items as well as their relationship to any diet modification, appropriate meals that will be enjoyed by all can be planned.

### Frequent use of therapeutic diets

Special diets are commonly used by the elderly. For example, diabetic or weight-control diets are frequently prescribed. Levels of dietary fiber or fat may also be modified. Sodium-restricted diets are often prescribed for hypertension and heart or kidney problems. Use of diuretics for these conditions may necessitate monitoring of dietary potassium levels. Loss of teeth or poorly fitting dentures may necessitate modifications in consistency.

Multiple dietary restrictions are not uncommon. Several diets may have been prescribed over the years, often by different physicians, who did not coordinate their advice. Food choices may be unnecessarily limited by attempts to follow past diets prescribed for conditions that no longer require dietary modifications. In addition, some people may have placed themselves on modified diets in an effort to cure or prevent a variety of problems. Financial considerations and personal likes and dislikes may further restrict the diet until the limited variety of foods consumed makes it difficult to secure an adequate intake of nutrients.

Combining dietary restrictions prescribed for a variety of conditions requires considerable skill since some aspects of the diets may conflict. Priorities need to be established, and the diet may need to be simplified to prevent confusion or unnecessary hardships. Diets prescribed in the past may need updating to take advantage of recent advances in diet therapy. For example, ulcer diets are usually much more liberal now than they were in the past. High-fiber diets rather than low-fiber diets may now be prescribed for several intestinal disorders.

Individualization of diets is important to ensure compliance and avoid unnecessary restrictions. A clinical dietitian can help to set priorities and individualize the diet, adjusting modifications to likes and dislikes, personal resources, and life-styles. A dietitian can also assist in budgeting and in advising how to stretch food dollars.

### Use of drugs

The elderly use more drugs than any other age group. People over 65 years spend about four times more money for drugs than do younger people. Drugs represent a significant expense for people on fixed incomes and may limit the amount of money available for food. The elderly also are more likely to suffer adverse side effects from drugs, including food–drug interactions. Not only do they take more medications, but their less efficient liver function may cause the drugs to accumulate. Nonprescription drugs are commonly used and may contribute to serious adverse side-effects.[18,43]

## Use of alcohol

Alcohol is the most commonly used nonprescription drug, with the possible exception of aspirin. Although overall reported alcohol use decreases with age, problem drinking and alcoholism are still found in over one million elderly in the United States. Treatment is difficult for older alcoholics. They are difficult to spot because they are more likely to drink alone, to drink at home, and to be binge drinkers. In addition, treatment centers are not geared to the needs of the elderly. Malnutrition is more common among heavy drinkers. Heavy alcohol use can alter the therapeutic effects of many drugs and may adversely affect many disease processes. The older brain appears to be more susceptible to alcohol than the younger one. The same dose of alcohol results in higher peak blood alcohol. The older drinker's thought processes may be more susceptible to the effects of alcohol.[18]

The consequences of alcohol consumption in old age vary with how much a person drinks. An occasional drink is not usually considered harmful to older people in good health. Some studies have attributed beneficial effects to moderate alcohol consumption in a social setting.[44-47]

## Elderly hospital patients

The elderly use hospitals more than three times the rate of the rest of the American population. More than one-third of all days of care provided by hospitals is devoted to the elderly, even though this age group represents only about 11% of the total population. During hospitalization, the elderly require more assistance, particularly nursing care.

During hospitalization, individualization of diets is important. Likes and dislikes should be considered, and the diet should be adjusted to the elderly person's physical limitations and cultural and religious patterns. A careful nutritional assessment should be made, beginning with a dietary history that considers the potential problems of elderly clients. Food intakes should be monitored.

Nutritional counseling about normal or modified diets should be practical and should take into account the elderly person's food habits, dental status, and possible limitations in finances, transportation, shopping, cooking skills, and appetite. Written instructions should summarize all verbal directions to aid failing memories. The writing should be sufficiently large to be seen easily, preferably in black lettering on white paper.

The high cost of hospital care necessitates that hospital stays be kept to a minimum. Patients are discharged as soon as feasible. Continuity of care should be ensured by using transfer or discharge forms that summarize the patient's nutritional status, diet prescription, diet instructions, food preferences, and degree of dietary compliance. Suggestions should be made to appropriate community agencies. Elderly people living alone may need temporary assistance from public health nurses or visiting nurses, home health aides, or home-delivered meals, as well as assistance in obtaining groceries.

## Elderly clients in nursing homes

Most elderly people will never live in a nursing home. Only 5% of the elderly reside in institutions; nontheless this represents over a million people. Elderly residents of extended care facilities have different needs from patients in acute care facilities. The less acute nature of their problems often makes it appropriate to liberalize therapeutic diets for elderly clients. Occasional meals without dietary restrictions may increase overall dietary compliance.

Due to their longer stays, more careful attention needs to be given to individual food preferences and religious and cultural customs. The food should be attractive and palatable. More variety and flexibility are needed in the menu, for example, longer menu cycles, selective menus, and more choices of menu items. Seasonal changes of menu items are welcome. Variety in color, texture, and flavor are also appreciated.

Portion sizes should vary according to the needs of the clients, and appropriate substitutions should be offered when menu items are refused. Supplements between meals make important contributions to overall daily intakes. Timing of meals is important. Meals should not be served too close together so that too much time is left between dinner and breakfast. Some nursing homes offer four or five meals a day instead of the traditional three.

Nursing homes should be as home-like and pleasant as possible. Because food is important to basic feelings of security, mealtime should be treated as a recreational activity. Celebrations of birthdays, holidays, and special events create a more home-like atmosphere. Occupational therapy and activities programs can sometimes be joined with dietary services for the planning of outdoor barbecues, picnics, Hawaiian luaus, and other ethnic festivals.

Food is an important medium of socialization. It is not only important *what* the older person eats, but *with whom* he eats. Whenever possible, clients should eat with others in the dining room or in small groups near their rooms rather than alone. Residents often focus their activities around the meal, sometimes waiting in the hall near the dining room for an hour or more before mealtime.

Seating arrangements and dining room decorations are important. Krasa[48] observed that behavior in the dining room improved and complaints about food and service were reduced by the presence of an observer during the serving of meals. As a result, supervisory staff in the dietary department decided to spend time in the dining room during mealtime conversing with the residents. The style of serving was also changed so that residents chose individual portions from specially designed food carts wheeled around the dining room. This created a more pleasant mealtime and won the enthusiasm of the residents.

Moderate amounts of alcoholic beverages have been found to increase social interactions among institutionalized geriatric patients, especially if they are offered in a pleasant atmosphere. As a result, some nursing homes have instituted a cocktail hour.

Foods should be seasoned to meet the tastes of residents. In an effort to reduce the number of extra food items that must be prepared for special diets, some nursing homes prepare all dishes with a minimum of added salt and seasoning. For practical purposes, all residents are served bland diets with no added salt. In view of the decreased taste sensitivity noted in studies of the elderly, increased attention given to seasoning food to make it more palatable might well spark appetites and result in more adequate food intakes. Client surveys can help to ascertain preferred levels of seasonings. Elderly residents should be invited to participate on taste panels and menu planning committees.

Nursing home menus are planned to meet the NAS-NRC RDA. However, adequately planned menus do not ensure that all residents have adequate intakes. Clarke and Wakefield[32] found that some nursing home residents ate good diets, whereas others ate poor diets. More than half had intakes below 67% of the RDA for at least one nutrient.

Several additional studies have evaluated the dietary intakes of nursing home residents.[33-35,49] Caloric intakes tended to be considerably lower than the RDA for energy. Because menus are planned on the assumption that all foods will be eaten, refusal of part of the menu may result in inadequate intakes of some nutrients. The tendency to eat fewer calories than the RDA should be kept in mind, and foods of high nutrient density should form the basis of the menu.

Individual food intakes should be monitored to detect poor intakes, not only for people on special diets but for those on regular diets as well. Weights should be monitored regularly to detect changes, which means the home should have a chair scale and a bed scale in addition to the usual models.

State and federal standards have considerable influence on the nutritional care of the elderly in nursing homes. Nutrition consultants have been hired to meet Medicare and Medicaid requirements in many nursing homes. Smith[50] summarized the historical development of nutritional care services and pointed out that one deterrent to effective consultation seems to be that many facilities have no one with sufficient training in foodservice supervision to carry out the consultant dietitian's recommendations. Few consultant dietitians spend significant time on nutritional care activities because most of their visit in the facility is focused on writing regular and therapeutic diet menus. Supervisors who had no sense of participation in writing the menus frequently changed them or sometimes ignored them completely. A recent trend has been toward larger, more modern extended-care facilities, which emphasize team effort. Professional dietitians and nutritionists have an important part in this comprehensive picture.

## Special problems
### Mentally disturbed residents

Surveys have shown that between 15% to 35% of those over 65 suffer from some form of mental disorder. Up to 60% of the elderly residents of nursing homes and hospitals may have mental impairments.[51] Some with long-standing psychiatric problems have recently been released from state mental hospitals, which are cutting back on the number of inpatients and attempting to reintegrate many patients into the mainstream of society. Others have developed mental problems for the first time late in life. Many have chronic organic brain syndromes, but a surprising number have reversible brain disorders and functional illnesses like depression. Accurate diagnosis is essential to ensure appropriate treatment.

Feeding large numbers of confused and disturbed clients presents complex management problems. Some clients are collectors and hoarders, compulsively taking food, napkins, and paper goods. They may steal food from others' plates. Psychiatric patients may fear that food is being poisoned or may attribute symbolic meanings to foods. Medications used may stimulate or depress appetites so that clients eat excessive amounts of food or refuse to eat at all.

Noise levels in dining areas may be high, with clients yelling at each other and mimicking one another's behavior. Some wander from their seats. Seating arrangements are important because some residents may eat only when seated in a particular area. Some clients irritate others. Confused and disturbed residents may be happier when they can select their friends and choose where to sit. Pleasant dining environments are important in bolstering self-esteem and raising morale. Background music may be soothing and may decrease yelling.[51]

Some disturbed residents can feed themselves, often preferring to do this with spoons and fingers. Others may need to be fed. Some residents eat only when fed by particular staff members. Staff members need sensitivity in helping to decode nonverbal behavior and in learning the wishes and idiosyncrasies of clients. This is important in motivating residents to eat and helping them to reach their maximum potential.

### Self-feeding skills for handicapped persons

Self-feeding skills may need to be retaught to persons recovering from strokes, to blind or mentally confused clients, and to those with Parkinson's disease, severe arthritis, or limited cardiac or respiratory reserves. Manning and Means[52] described a self-feeding program for geriatric patients. Occupational and physical therapists can provide valuable assistance in helping disabled clients to achieve as much independence as possible. Clients can be trained to use self-help devices such as plate guards, spoons and forks with enlarged or jointed handles, and weighted mugs that resist tipping. It may be necessary to modify the texture and consistency of food to make it easier to eat. Finger foods are welcome. Because eating may be a slow process, it is important to allow sufficient time for the meals.

Difficulties in swallowing and the threat of choking may make modifications in consistency necessary. Some foods may need to be chopped, ground, or blended. In general, however, these substitutions should be kept to a minimum to ensure palatability. Regular menu items that are chopped or blended are usually tastier than commercial pureed foods.

### Incontinence

Incontinence is a common problem of elderly clients, although it is often concealed due to embarrassment and fear of social consequences. Fecal incontinence usually results in admission to an institution. However, it can often be prevented or controlled. Gross constipation is a common cause of fecal incontinence. A large, solid mass of stool may form in the rectum or sigmoid colon and act like a ball valve, allowing drainage of a mucous-type diarrhea caused by irritation from the fecal mass. Thus, one cause of diarrhea can be fecal impaction. Increased fluid and fiber may prevent constipation and, accordingly, incontinence. When incontinence is due to loss of nervous control, it is sometimes possible to retrain the person's bowel habits. Medications as well as enemas may allow more predictable and manageable bowel function.

Some nursing homes use cranberry juice in an effort to reduce the odor of urinary incontinence. Incontinence necessitates strict hygiene procedures. Retraining programs may be able to control some forms of urinary incontinence.

### Decubitus ulcers

Decubitus ulcers or bedsores, which are caused by tissue anoxia, are a potential problem in paralyzed, chronically ill and bedridden patients, particularly when nursing care is less than optimal. Poor nutrition may increase the risk of developing decubitis ulcers due to the development of anemia, the increased likelihood of edema, and muscular weakness and lack of mobility. Once formed, decubitus ulcers can produce a significant drain on the body's resources, particularly if they are neglected or badly infected. Increased levels of protein and vitamins may be needed for the healing of wounds.

### Refusal to eat

Aggressive feeding measures, such as gastrostomy, are sometimes advocated to provide nourishment for elderly patients who cannot or will not eat.[53] However, these measures may not be acceptable to some clients or their families. A patient's right to refuse treatment and the ethical and legal implications of self-starvation need to be considered by health professionals working with the elderly. *Gramp*[54] sensitively explores the issue of self-starvation by an elderly man from the viewpoint of his family.

### Care of the terminally ill

The hospice movement for care of the dying began in England in the late 1950s and the early 1960s and is now growing in this country. Hospices provide palliative and supportive care for terminally ill people of all ages and their families. They focus on the family unit, recognizing differences in life-style, and include the family in the client's care. Support is given to the grieving family as well as to the client. The atmosphere is friendly and home-like. Children and even pets are welcome. Emphasis is placed on increasing the quality of life.[55]

High-quality food is offered to stimulate the client's appetite. Clients are asked what they like to eat and favorite meals are offered. Selective menus are often used, as this is one of the few opportunities for choice still available to the client. Alcoholic beverages may be permitted. Families are encouraged to eat together. Special kitchen facilities may be available where family-prepared meals may be warmed and served.

Clients are kept as symptom-free as possible. Careful attention is given to the relief of pain. Diet modifications may help to control such distressing symptoms as nausea, vomiting, dry or sore mouths, peptic ulcers, flatus, diarrhea, constipation, and impactions.

Hospices offer continuity of care in a variety of settings—inpatient and outpatient care, discharge planning, and home visits. Whenever possible, the dying person is allowed to finish his life at home. A multidisciplinary team may be available 24 hours a day, 7 days a week to assist families in home care. Families may need counseling on diet modifications, food preparation, and feeding of the terminally ill person. Some require assistance with transportation, shopping, and food preparation.

New models that emphasize continuing health care are being explored, not only for terminally ill clients but for chronically ill patients. Day-care centers and day hospitals are also being developed to support family efforts to provide home care and to prevent institutionalization.[56]

## Preventing institutionalization

Institutionalization of the elderly is tremendously costly, not only to society in terms of dollars and manpower, but to the individual person's loss of independence, dignity, and feelings of self-worth. The trend is to prevent institutionalization by supporting the strengths of the elderly person and his family. Todhunter[57] pointed out that the ability to obtain or prepare meals that are adequate to maintain nutritional health is a major factor in enabling the elderly to continue independent living.

### Day-care

Day-care centers for senior citizens are a relatively new approach to avoiding institutionalization. Day-care programs are designed for older persons who need some help in a protected environment but who do not require the services of a nursing home. The person returns home to his family at night. Some programs offer occasional overnight or weekend services if the family must be away.

### Congregate living

Group living is becoming more common for elderly people. By the year 2000, half of elderly Americans may be living in some form of congregate housing. In addition to the 5% now living in nursing homes, many older Americans live in retirement communities, retirement homes, residence hotels, boarding houses, adult homes, and domiciliaries. Meal service and nutritional support services in these facilities vary widely in form and quality.

Retirement communities are rapidly growing in number and offer a variety of services for independent living to those with adequate financial resources to afford these facilities. Elderly residents may own their own apartments, often with small kitchens provided for those who want to fix meals. Finding convenient places to buy groceries can be a problem, however, especially for those without cars. Meal service is usually available in dining rooms and coffee shops, but adjusting to group eating arrangements can be bothersome. Some find it difficult to go into the dining room alone.

Although these communities offer advantages, such as financial and health-care security, safety, group activities, and a variety of social supports, the decision to enter a retirement community is difficult, as is pointed out in an article by Rynbergen.[1] Living in an age-segregated retirement community, she longs for a community of people of all ages and kinds. "The trouble, though, living only with people of your own age is that they get sick, and you're surrounded by the breakdown not only of bodily function but of mental function." Being with young people is what she misses most.

## Community food and nutrition programs for older people

Many communities have programs that provide services especially appropriate for the older adult. The following discussion indicates the variety of opportunities that may be available to the senior citizen in his community. The nutrition counselor should become knowledgeable about the resources in the local area.

### Food stamps

Low-income people of all ages can use food stamps to stretch their food dollars. Many older adults, living on very limited incomes, are eligible for this program. Local welfare departments determine eligibility and the amount of stamps received, depending on the size and income of the family unit. The stamps or coupons may be used to buy food in any cooperating retail store. Although food stamps represent a real saving in food dollars, many older citizens hesitate to participate in the program. This aspect of food budgeting is one in which the nutrition counselor may be able to help the older client understand the long-term advantages of such a program.

### Home health aides

For the person capable of remaining in his own home where assistance in meal management can be furnished, home health or neighborhood aides have been made available by certain community agencies. These aides are trained to go into homes to assist with such matters as marketing, food preparation, handling and storage, uses of equipment, and budgeting. Nurses together with other members of the home care team, such as dietitians, nutritionists, or home economists, help to train and supervise home health aides. The provision of these services enables elderly persons to continue to maintain themselves for longer periods of time in their own homes than could be possible otherwise.

### Transportation services

Because transportation is a problem for many older Americans, many cities are providing special transportation to the elderly. A survey of the elderly in Philadelphia, for example, revealed that 30% needed transportation, 40% were handicapped, and 6% were wheelchair-bound.[58] Many cities offer public transportation at reduced rates for senior citizens. Special transportation may be available for the handicapped. In some cities, local supermarkets charter buses to help groups of senior citizens shop for groceries. In Boston, a bookmobile was made into a mobile market and serves some 500 older Bostonians who find shopping at local supermarkets difficult. The prices at the "foodmobile" are the same as those at the supermarket as the costs of the vehicle and staff are covered by grants and city subsidies.[59]

### Congregate meal programs

A variety of community group feeding projects provide older adults with good nutrition in a social atmosphere. For the older person who is able to go to the center and is interested in meeting people, these programs offer recreational as well as nutritional benefits. Many of these centers also include nutrition or consumer education programs and health services, such as blood pressure screening.

Federal grants have helped to sponsor congregate feeding programs in different locations throughout the country. In 1968, research and demonstration nutrition programs were initiated under Title IV of the Older Americans Act of 1965.[60,61] As a result of these projects, the Title VII Nutrition Program for the Elderly (P.L. 92-258) was established in 1972. The goal of this program was to provide older Americans with low-cost, nutritionally sound meals served in strategically located centers, such as schools, churches, community centers, senior citizen centers, and other public and private facilities where the elderly could obtain other social and rehabilitative services. Besides promoting better health among the older segment of the population through improved nutrition, this program was designed to reduce the social isolation of old age by offering older Americans an opportunity to live with dignity and companionship.

The 1978 amendments to the Older Americans Act (P.L. 95-478) repealed Title VII and incorporated its contents into various parts of Title III. Title III provides for home-delivered meals as well as for meals in congregate settings. Hot (or other appropriate) meals supplying at least one-third of the RDA are served at least 5 days a week. Special menus may be provided as needed to accommodate special diets or ethnic preferences. Up to 20% of the project's funds may be used for supportive services, such as transportation and nutrition education. People aged 60 or over or their spouses can participate, no matter what their income level. Charges for meals are permitted because many elderly people are reluctant to participate in meals labeled "free." Money collected is used to increase the number of meals that are served by the project. Advisory committees, consisting of older participants, professionals, gerontologists and others, are mandated.

An important feature of the nutrition programs is the outreach service. Outreach tries to seek out and identify the maximum number of hard-to-reach, isolated, and withdrawn eligible individuals and to provide them with the opportunity to participate in the program.[62,63] Congregate meal programs have been shown to improve nutrient intakes. Kohrs and associates[64] found that nutrient intakes were greater for those who ate at the meal site on the day of the study than for those who did not. Dietary ratings on food records indicated that participants had better overall diets than nonparticipants. Another important effect of eating at the meal program was the reduction of differences in nutrient intakes related to various socioeconomic factors, such as education, occupation, age and sex.[65]

Experience with congregate meals has pointed out the importance of socialization. Some programs have had success with welcoming committees and "introductions tables," where newcomers sit for the first few days or weeks until they become familiar with the program. Participants' committees can serve a variety of functions and foster identification with the project. Seating arrangements are important. Small tables of four to six people contribute to an atmosphere of sociability. The site of the program affects participation. The safety of the neighborhood is an important consideration because many elderly persons are reluctant to go out alone. An efficient transportation system can improve attendance at meals. If possible, sites should be within walking distance. A familiar site is an important asset. Church sites may have more limited participation than more neutral community locations.

Schneider[62] has recommended that less emphasis should be placed on regular attendance. Not all elderly people will participate on a regular basis. Some prefer to drop by for a meal from time to time.

### Home-delivered meal programs

Approximately 3 to 4 million elderly people who are eligible for congregate feeding programs are unable to participate because they are ill, handicapped, homebound, or otherwise prevented from doing so. Home-delivered meals can play an important role in improving the nutrition of these people.[66]

Many cities have a long tradition of "meals-on-wheels" programs, which provide home-delivered meals for homebound people of all ages who cannot prepare their own meals. They are usually a community service and make extensive use of volunteers. Some are funded by grants. Fees for meals may be based on ability to pay. Home-delivered meal programs are eligible for Title III funding, and additional programs are being developed in many areas. Two meals a day (one hot and one cold) are usually provided 5 days a week, although some programs offer frozen dinners for weekends. Modified diets may be available for people on therapeutic diets. Because breakfasts and weekend meals are not usually included, participants in these programs should have some additional resource for providing meals in the home.

Food technology that grew out of the manned space program of the National Aeronautics and Space Administration (NASA) has been used to develop pleasant tasting, easily transportable, shelf-stable meals designed to complement existing group feeding and meals-on-wheels programs. Packages of seven single-meal units can be mailed or personally delivered to the elderly. Each meal includes an entree, two side dishes, dessert, and a beverage to supply one-third of the RDA. The food items are freeze-dried, dehydrated, canned or in foil-polyethylene layered pouches and require few utensils and minimal skills to prepare. Results of a pilot project using NASA meals revealed that participant reaction was very favorable. Meals were considered convenient, easy to prepare and tasty. Most found the hot meals equal to or superior to meals received in meal programs or prepared by themselves. The cost was competitive with congregate and meals-on-wheels programs.[66]

Home-delivered meals are particularly useful as crisis intervention, for example, during periods of convalescence. These meals may prevent or postpone institutionalization. However, many elderly clients are socially isolated and home-delivered meals do not solve their problems of loneliness. In addition, when clients have severe enough problems to warrant home-delivered meals, they often need a variety of social services that are not met by nutritional programs alone. Active systems of referral to other agencies may be required to address these needs.

## Study questions and activities

1. Summarize current thinking about possible relationships between nutrition and aging.
2. How are aging and chronic disease related? What is the role of diet in chronic diseases which are common among older people?
3. Why is the caloric requirement of older people reduced? How much reduction in caloric intake is recommended between ages 23 and 51?
4. What advice would you give an older person who should reduce his calorie intake? How may calories be increased for the underweight older person?
5. If an older person shares the family meals but eats less of everything than younger members, which nutrients may be lower than recommended? How can this be remedied?
6. In what circumstances may the use of vitamin or mineral supplements be justified?
7. If an older person with whom you are associated is a food faddist, how would you attempt to correct his or her false ideas? What reliable sources of information would you recommend?
8. What special dietary considerations are appropriate for elderly residents in nursing homes?
9. What are some of the dietary problems of mentally disturbed elderly people?
10. What does it feel like to be aged and handicapped? Play the role of a handicapped person. Try using a blindfold to simulate blindness, gloves to simulate impaired touch sensation, and weights on your arms to simulate weakness. Use adaptive eating devices or let someone else feed you.
11. What nutrition services for older people are available in your community?

## References

1. Klein M, Overholser MO, Rynbergen H: Geriatric Nurs 1:114, 1980
2. Butler RN: Why Survive? Being Old in America. New York, Harper & Row, 1975
3. Ross MH: In Behnke JA, Finch CE, Moment GB (eds): The Biology of Aging, p 173. New York, Plenum Press, 1978
4. Moment GB: In Behnke, Finch, and Moment, Biology of Aging, p 1
5. Kent S: Geriatrics 76:141, 1976
6. Rowe D: J Am Diet Assoc 72:478, 1978
7. Shock NW: In Birren JE, Schaie KW (eds): Handbook of the Psychology of Aging, p 103. New York, Van Nostrand Reinhold, 1979
8. Harman D: Age 1:143, 1978
9. Tappel A: Nutr Today 2:2, 1967
10. Rowe JW: Professional Nurse 1:3, May, 1980
11. Swanson P: In Food, The Yearbook of Agriculture, p 311. Washington, DC, USDA, 1959
12. Finch CE, Hayflick L: Handbook of the Biology of Aging. New York, Van Nostrand Reinhold, 1977
13. Masoro E: In Winick M (ed): Nutrition and Aging, p 61. New York, John Wiley & Sons, 1976
14. Cape R: Aging: Its Complex Management, p 13. Hagerstown, MD, Harper & Row, 1978
15. Schiffman SS, Hornack K, Reilly D: Am J Clin Nutr 32:1622, 1979
16. Gregor JL, Sciscoe BS: J Am Diet Assoc 70:37, 1977
17. Gregor JL, Geissler AH: Am J Clin Nutr 31:633, 1978
18. Eckardt MJ: In Behnke, Finch, and Moment, Biology of Aging, p 191
19. Kovar MG: Public Health Rep 92:9, 1977
20. Albanese AA, Lorenze EJ, Wein EH: Am Fam Pract 18:160, 1978
21. Food and Nutrition Board: Recommended Dietary Allowances, 9th rev ed. Washington, DC, National Academy of Sciences, 1980
22. Jowsey J: Geriatrics 33:43, Aug, 1978
23. Jowsey J: In Winick, Nutrition and Aging, p 131
24. Lutwak L: In Winick, Nutrition and Aging, p 145
25. Gunby P: Med News JAMA 243:1025, 1980
26. Bunce GE: Nutr Rev 37:337, 1979
27. Howell SC, Loeb MB: Nutrition and aging—A monograph for practitioners. Gerontologist 9:77, 1969
28. Amaducci L, Davidson AN, Antuono P (eds): Aging of the Brain and Dementia. New York, Raven Press, 1980
29. Levick SE: Letter to the Editor. N Engl J Med 303:164, 1980
30. Bowdler NC et al: Pharmacol Biochem Behav 10:505, 1979
31. Growdon JH, Wurtman RJ: Nutr Rev 37:129, 1979
32. Clarke M, Wakefield LM: J Am Diet Assoc 66:600, 1975
33. Stiedmann M, Jansen C, Harrill I: J Am Diet Assoc 73:132, 1978
34. Justice CL, Howe JM, Clark HE: J Am Diet Assoc 65:639, 1974
35. Brown PT et al: J Am Diet Assoc 71:41, 1977
36. O'Hanlon P, Kohrs MB: Am J Clin Nutr 31:1257, 1978
37. Ten-State Nutrition Survey, 1968–1970: V. Dietary. DHEW Publ. No. (HSM) 72-8134, 1972
38. Wagner PA et al: Am J Clin Nutr 33:1771, 1980
39. Cheng AHR et al: Am J Clin Nutr 31:12, 1978
40. Bigwood EJ: Nutritio et Dieta 8:226, 1966
41. Young VR et al: In Winick, Nutrition and Aging, p 77
42. Johnson CK et al: J Am Diet Assoc 77:551, 1980
43. Cape R: Aging: Its Complex Management. Hagerstown, MD, Harper & Row, 1978
44. Volpe A, Kastenbaum R: Am J Nurs 67:100, 1967

45. Turner TB: JAMA 226:779, 1973
46. Black AL: Northwest Med 68:453, 1969
47. Chien CP, Cole JO: Am J Psychiatry 127:1070, 1971
48. Krasa EJ: J Geriatr Psychiatry 9:81, 1976
49. Ford MG, Neville JN: J Am Diet Assoc 61:292, 1972
50. Smith CE: J Am Diet Assoc 73:115, 1978
51. Lissitz S: Gerontologist 9:114, 1969
52. Manning AM, Means JG: J Am Diet Assoc 66:275, 1975
53. Pomerantz MA, Salomon J, Dunn R: J Am Geriatr Soc 28:104, Mar, 1980
54. Jury M, Jury D: Gramp. New York, Penguin Books, 1978
55. Krant MJ: N Engl J Med 299:546, 1978
56. McNamara EM: Hospitals 52:79, Apr 1, 1978
57. Todhunter EN: In Winick, Nutrition and Aging, p 119
58. Stirner FW: Gerontologist 18:207, 1978
59. "Foodmobile" serves the elderly. J Am Diet Assoc 70:487, 1977
60. Pelcovits J: J Am Diet Assoc 58:17, 1971
61. Pelcovits J: J Am Diet Assoc 60:297, 1972
62. Schneider RL: Gerontologist 19:163, 1979
63. Kohrs MB: J Am Diet Assoc 75:534, 1979
64. Kohrs MB, O'Hanlon P, Eklund D: J Am Diet Assoc 72:487, 1978
65. Kohrs MB et al: J Am Diet Assoc 75:537, 1979
66. Rhodes L: Gerontologist 17:333, 1977

## Supplementary readings

Behnke JA, Finch CE, Moment GB: The Biology of Aging. New York, Plenum Press, 1978

Butler RN: Why Survive? Being Old in America. New York, Harper & Row, 1975

Howell SC, Loeb MB: Nutrition and aging—A monograph for practitioners. Gerontologist 9:77, 1969

Kent S: Is diabetes a form of accelerated aging? Geriatrics 31:140, 1979

Munro HN: Major gaps in nutrient allowances. J Am Diet Assoc 76:137, 1980

O'Hanlon P, Kohrs MB: Dietary studies of older Americans. Am J Clin Nutr 31:1257, 1978

Rockstein M, Sussman M: Biology of Aging. Belmont, CA, Wadsworth, 1979

Rowe D: Aging—A jewel in the mosaic of life. J Am Diet Assoc 72:478, 1978

Shock NW: Biological theories of aging. In Birren JE, Schaie KW (eds): Handbook of the Psychology of Aging, p 103. New York, Van Nostrand Reinhold, 1979

Weinberg J: Psychologic implications of the nutritional needs of the elderly. J Am Diet Assoc 60:293, 1972

Winick M (ed): Nutrition and Aging. New York, John Wiley & Sons, 1976

*For further references see Bibliography in Part 4.*

# Malnutrition—A World Problem

# 21

**CSM:** Corn Soy Milk
**DSM:** Dry Skim Milk
**EPM:** Energy-protein Malnutrition
**PEM:** Protein-energy Malnutrition
**WSB:** Wheat-soy Blend

## Nutrition planning: A priority in national development

Estimates indicate that there are a billion and a half women, men, and children in the world today suffering from severe, moderate, or mild malnutrition.[1] Most of these people live in developing countries. The capacity for work of malnourished adults may be significantly reduced and their potential as family providers and as bearers of children equally affected. Some children die from malnutrition; larger numbers suffer physical and, possibly, mental retardation and are more susceptible to infectious diseases.[2] Due to the synergistic effect of malnutrition and infection, malnourished children are not only more apt to contract infectious diseases, such as diarrhea, upper respiratory infections, bronchitis, and measles, but are also less able to withstand the effects of such diseases than children who are adequately nourished. The high mortality rate among children from infectious disease in developing countries is a reflection of the nutritional status of these children.

Findings of a 5-year study, The Inter-American Investigation of Mortality in Children, identified nutritional deficiency as the most important factor contributing to the very high childhood mortality in Latin America. Low birth weight or malnutrition was either a primary or secondary cause of death in more than half of the 35,000 deaths of children under the age of 5 years.[3] Due to improved medical care in the last 30 years, more children may survive severe episodes of illness during early life, but at school age these survivors show signs of physical underdevelopment and appear to be withdrawn and uninterested in their environment.[4]

Consequently, the degree to which long-term effects of malnutrition may relate to the socioeconomic development of a nation is becoming a matter of increasing concern to government planners in developing countries. Low productivity, poor quality of life, increased expenditures for health and medical care, and low returns from educational investments are some costs paid by a nation that is not concerned with improving the nutritional status of its poor. For economic as well as for humanitarian reasons, then, nutrition should have a high priority in national development plans. Nutrition intervention programs can be planned to be cost effective—an important consideration as they compete for the limited resources available for development in poorer countries. Moreover, government decision makers must realize that expanding employment opportunities and larger incomes would increase consumption among low income groups. Forecasts to 1985 of the growth rate of the food supply compared to the projected demand indicate that, although there are adequate levels of food supplies available for human consumption, the major problem remains one of distribution[5]—among nations, among rich and poor within a nation, and even among individual family members. Government decisions about food policies will largely determine whether individual nations and the world as a whole will have a surplus or a deficit of food in the future. These complex issues must be examined by nutritionists, agricultural specialist, food technologists, economists, bankers, and development planners before political decisions on policy can be made and implemented by individual nations.

Latham[6] states that a national food and nutrition policy should have the following goals:

1. To improve food production so that there is an adequate supply of the right kind of food to satisfy all the nutritional requirements of its population
2. To increase the purchasing power of low-income families and enable them to improve their nutrition
3. To control infections and parasitic diseases that are significant in malnutrition.

Lack of protein no longer looms as the most important nutrition problem. Malnutrition in most developing countries is due primarily to inadequate food intake. At least 400 million people do not receive a sufficient quantity of foods to meet their energy needs.[5] If calorie needs are met by modest increases in cereal grains, legumes, and vegetables, the prevalence of malnutrition in the developing countries can be greatly reduced. Labor-intensive projects, which employ large numbers of people and thereby increase the amount of money the poor have to spend for food, are more beneficial in most developing countries than capital-intensive ones, which often benefit those who are already economically advantaged.

## Identification of nutrition problems

The extent of malnutrition in the world today is difficult to determine because specific deficiency diseases with obvious clinical signs are not encountered as frequently as they were a half century ago. Instead, the presence of more moderate and less clearly identified forms of malnutrition is the foremost threat to public health. Health workers are challenged not only to identify and treat nutritional deficiencies but also to understand and prevent the causes of malnutrition before children and adults are handicapped by its effects.

Surveys of the daily consumption of nutrients at the family and individual levels, combined with a physical examination and appropriate laboratory tests, remain the most important tools in diagnosing individual nutritional problems. Morbidity and mortality statistics can give helpful information regarding the prevalence of malnutrition. Physical growth data may also be used as indicators of the status of a community's nutrition. Because few countries have these sophisticated data available to them, planners frequently must rely on "food disappearance" data from food balance sheets. This information reveals little about the distribution of food in a country The causes of malnutrition are multiple and frequently overlap in a given situation. They include problems related to the physical environment, social structure, family development and child rearing patterns, agricultural practices, or natural disasters. An understanding of how these various factors interrelate in specific communities is important for all health personnel. The encouragement of breast feeding at the same time that more emphasis is placed on immunization programs could, in many instances, improve the nutritional status of large numbers of young children.

Nutritional problems may be classified into three main groups according to their geographical range and prevalence. First, there are those that are common to most of the developing countries: protein-energy malnutrition (PEM), nutritional anemia, endemic goiter, ariboflavinosis, and dental problems. Second, there are those found in certain areas of developing countries: xerophthalmia and rickets. Finally, there are those limited to very specific areas: pellagra, beriberi, and scurvy.[4]

According to Bengoa[4] there are four conditions that, due to their prevalence, social significance, and feasible prevention (Fig. 21-1), should have the highest priority from an international point of view:

1. Protein-energy malnutrition has a high prevalence, a high mortality rate, and can produce irreversible physical and mental damage in those who survive. Although the feasibility of eradicating PEM at the present time is recognizably low, the consequences of this problem, if ignored, are so extreme that it must be given priority.
2. Xerophthalmia is less prevalent but more easily prevented than PEM. This disease not only contributes to childhood mortality but also causes irreversible blindness in its victims.
3. Nutritional anemias, which, like PEM, have a high prevalence and contribute to mortality primarily caused by many other conditions, also have nega-

tive effects on a person's working capacity. The feasibility of prevention is similar to that of xerophthalmia.

4. Endemic goiter has less social significance than the first three conditions. It is as prevalent as PEM and the nutritional anemias, but its prevention is more feasible.

## Protein-energy malnutrition (PEM)

The term, *protein-energy malnutrition* (PEM), is used to identify a complex group of related nutritional problems, as shown in Table 21-1. Because energy intake is regarded by many authorities as the more important problem in childhood malnutrition today, the term, *energy-protein malnutrition* (EPM) is also used to describe these conditions.[7] According to Kimm,

> The controversy goes beyond the semantic one. It is now felt that the previous rather simplified view of PCM (PEM) as a protein deficiency disease has led to the formulation of strategies which are almost identical to those which have been successful in controlling other nutritional diseases. It is becoming evident, however, that the programs to increase the protein supply in the diet or to enrich the diet with protein or amino acid supplementation have not significantly altered the global prevalence of protein-calorie malnutrition. The word *malnutrition* implies that the problem is caused by an insufficient food supply, either in quantity (calories) or quality (proteins in this particular situation) and also that food alone will be effective in its cure or prevention. This narrow interpretation has misled politicians, economists, and national planners into believing that children will not suffer from PCM (PEM) if they get enough food to eat without alteration of the other environment conditions detrimental to health.
>
> Protein-calorie malnutrition is now generally viewed as a broader ecological problem which is in part due to the inadequate availability of food or specific nutrients but which is also a function of generalized poverty, deficient social organization, poor environmental sanitation, and ignorance of proper feeding and care of the child.[8]

The ecology of PEM in the urban and rural settings is described in Table 21-2. Children with PEM are always retarded in their growth and development, but other clinical symptoms vary with age and condition of the child and the intensity of the causal factors. A severe deficiency of both energy and protein results in nutritional marasmus, whereas a severe protein deficiency with more adequate energy intake may result in kwashiorkor. Both of these are severe; the latter, however, is an acute disease from which the child either dies quickly or, with suitable medical care, recovers quickly. Nutritional marasmus may also terminate in death if not treated. Some children present symptoms of an intermediate or mixed form of PEM, showing clinical signs of both marasmus and kwashiorkor. Most of the children suffering from PEM

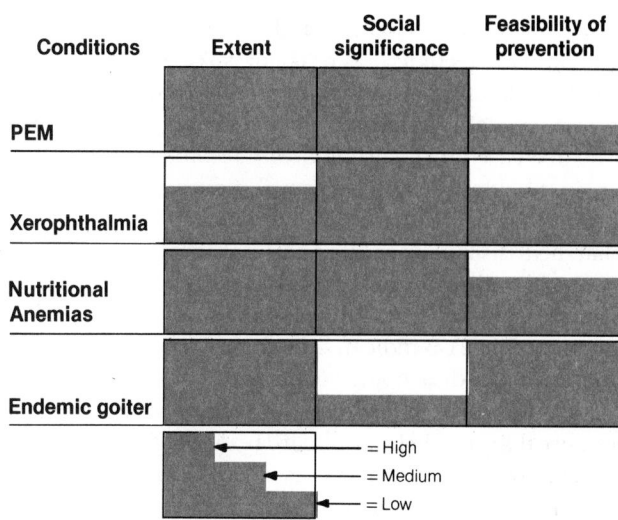

**Fig. 21-1.** Priorities among nutritional conditions. (Bengoa JM: Berg A, Scrimshaw NS, Call DL (eds): In Nutrition, National Development and Planning. Cambridge, MIT Press, 1973)

present a moderate form of the disease, and many cases may go unrecognized unless an infectious disease, famine, or some other factor precipitates a more severe form. In community studies made between 1963 and 1972 in Latin America, Africa, and Asia, it was estimated that 100 million children between birth and 4 years of age were suffering from severe or moderate protein-energy malnutrition. In addition, the number of children in these areas who show signs of nutritional dwarfing is unknown.[4]

### Nutritional marasmus

The age of a child is an important factor in determining whether severe protein-energy malnutrition appears as nutritional marasmus or kwashiorkor. Marasmus is

### Table 21-1. Simplified Classification of PEM

| Categories | Body Weight % of Standard | Body Height | Edema | Deficit of Weight for Height |
|---|---|---|---|---|
| Kwashiorkor | 80-60 | Affected | + | ++ |
| Marasmus | <60 | Affected | 0 | ++ |
| Mixed forms (marasmic kwashiorkor) | <60 | Affected | + | ++ |
| Underweight child (moderate PEM) | 80-60 | Affected | 0 | Minimal |
| Nutritional dwarfing | <60 | Pronounced deficit | 0 | Minimal |

(Reprinted from Benjoa JM: In Berg A, Scrimshaw NS, Call DL (eds): Nutrition, National Development and Planning, pp 103–125. Cambridge, MIT Press, 1973, by permission of the MIT Press, Cambridge, MA)

more likely to develop in children under 1 year of age when breast-feeding fails or is not carried on for a sufficient length of time, and suitable foods for weaning either are not available or feeding practices discourage their use. The decreased incidence of breast-feeding among mothers in developing countries contributes greatly to the high proportion of deaths due to nutritional deficiency and diarrheal disease. Records of hospital admissions in many countries indicate that the number of cases of marasmus is increasing, whereas kwashiorkor is becoming less frequent. Table 21-3 indicates the factors that contribute to marasmus in developing countries.

As indicated in Table 21-1, the infant with marasmus is more than 40% below standard body weight. There is an absence of subcutaneous fat, evidence of muscle wasting, and diminution of height or length (see *Undernutrition*, Chap. 35). Edema is not noticeable and appetite is often good.[4] The marasmic infant looks like a little old man, with a big head and huge eyes, wrinkled face, and tiny body. Such infants are particularly susceptible to infectious disease, and their mortality rate is high.

## Kwashiorkor

In 1933, Dr. Cicely Williams, a British pediatrician working in West Africa, first described this disease in children from 1 to 4 years of age. She called it by its local name, "kwashiorkor." and found that milk could cure it. The name means "the disease the deposed baby gets when the next one is born."[9] The picture of a mother from Uganda (Fig. 21-2) is a striking example—the healthy infant in arms and the "deposed" one by her side.

Although kwashiorkor was first described and named in Africa, it has also been recognized in Latin America and Asia. Severe protein-energy malnutrition tends to appear as kwashiorkor rather than marasmus when the child is over 1 year old. The presence of edema is its most distinguishing characteristic, Table 21-1. Invariably, growth is retarded, although the presence of edema may conceal the degree of emaciation. Kwashiorkor is caused by severe protein deficiency relative to energy intake; however, it may be superimposed on any degree of marasmus and is frequently precipitated by the occurrence of an infectious disease. Kwashiorkor is an acute

## Table 21-2. Ecology of PEM (Urban and Rural Differences)

| | Urban Setting | Rural Setting |
|---|---|---|
| Culture | Rapid acculturization, with loss of traditional patterns of life | Traditional pattern of life, with less rapid change |
| | Alienation from the existing social structure | Participation in an established social structure |
| | More working mothers | Mothers working at home or in the field nearby |
| | Pregnancies in more rapid succession | Longer interval between pregnancies |
| Economic structure | Market money economy ("No job means no food for the family") | Subsistence agrarian economy |
| Role of environmental sanitation | Very critical | Less critical |
| | Adverse role of crowded living quarters | Crowding not as prevalent, thus less critical |
| | Repeated infections, especially gastroenteritis | Predominantly, acute infections rather then weanling diarrhea |
| Feeding practices | Breast-feeding declining with early weaning; bottle feeding increasing; diluted, dirty formula | Breast-feeding more prevalent; adequate nutrition for the first 4 to 6 months of life |
| Major dietary inadequacy | Limited calories | Predominantly protein when the family staple diet consists of starchy foods |
| Age of onset of PEM | Second 6 months of life or earlier | After 1 year of age and usually before 2 years |
| Common clinical type | Marasmus or marasmic kwashiorkor | Kwashiorkor |

(From Kimm S: Control of protein–calorie malnutrition. In Mayer J, Dwyer J (eds): Food and Nutrition Policy in a Changing World, pp 155–177. New York, Oxford University Press, 1979)

condition of short duration in which recovery or death occurs relatively rapidly. The mortality rate even among hospitalized children is high. The child is apathetic and miserable. There may also be disorders of pigmentation of the skin and hair and some liver enlargement. Diarrhea and anorexia may accompany the disease. Anemia and other deficiencies are frequently found in children with kwashiorkor.

Kwashiorkor is found in areas where starchy roots or tubers are the staple food, or less commonly, where cereals are the staple food. Although cereal grains are better sources of protein than starchy roots or tubers, many cereal grains do not have sufficient good quality protein relative to their bulk and energy value to serve as appropriate weaning foods for young children when milk is not available.[10]

## Mixed forms of severe protein-energy malnutrition

As shown in Table 21-1, some children show clinical signs of both marasmus and kwashiorkor. They present a weight deficit of more than 40% of standard weight, which is indicative of nutritional marasmus; in addition, they have edema and other symptoms of kwashiorkor. It has been recognized that an infant with marasmus may develop kwashiorkor as a result of protein losses incurred during acute infection. Similarly, an infant in whom kwashiorkor has been diagnosed may, when edema disappears during treatment, appear marasmic.[4]

## Moderate form of protein-energy malnutrition

More children suffer from the moderate form of PEM than the severe form. Although there is not total uniformity in the diagnosis of this form, a weight deficit of 25% to 40% below standard is the general criterion used to determine it. Children with moderate PEM may become severely malnourished as a result of diarrhea or other infectious diseases. The practice of feeding the sick child a very limited diet consisting primarily of carbohydrate can precipitate acute malnutrition in the preschool age group.

## Nutritional dwarfing

Children who have survived PEM and a series of infectious diseases during infancy and the toddler and preschool periods often show signs of nutritional dwarfing when they reach school age. It is difficult to distinguish between the child who has suffered permanent growth retardation and the one who could catch up if his marginal subsistence diet were improved. The distinguishing characteristic of nutritional dwarfing is the pronounced deficit in body height as compared to standard heights. Children with this condition are often thought to be years younger than their actual chronological age, although their facial expressions may be more mature.

Diets that are inadequate, particularly in protein, among teenagers may also result in retarded growth during the adolescent spurt. This situation seems to have occurred in Japan from 1939 to 1948, resulting in shorter stature, especially of teenagers, at the end of World War II than before.[11]

## Prevention and treatment of protein-energy malnutrition

Because PEM has been found to occur in early infancy in developing countries where breast-feeding is no longer common, mothers should be encouraged to breast-feed

### Table 21-3. The Marasmus Cycle—Factors that will Precipitate Malnutrition in Young Infants in Developing Countries

*Factors That Make Correct Bottle Feeding Impossible*

Poverty

Poor environmental sanitation

Poor cooking facilities

Lack of clean water supply

Lack of education oriented to use of manufactured products

Lack of familiarity with standardized measurements

Lack of equipment

*Factors That Interfere With Normal Breast-Feeding Pattern*

*Industry*
Advertising in hospitals and via all mass media; distribution of funds, free milk samples, baby books, pamphlets, calendars, diaries; employment of "milk nurses," who advise on bottle feeding in hospitals and homes

*Community*
Lack of funds; pressure by peers; imitation of "socioeconomic superiors"; availability of other options; multiplicity of products on market; advice from grocers, pharmacists, and others; visits from "milk nurses"; lack of nutritional knowledge on the part of local midwives

*Medical Services*
Indifferent teaching due to a lack of nutritional knowledge generally and especially of the physiology of lactation; introduction of prelacteal feeds and formulas in nurseries; separation of mother/child dyad; no psychological support to newly delivered mothers

*Individual Problems*
Lack of information; welcome availability of other options if there is a need to work, or to engage in social intercourse; pressure by husband or lover; desire to remain sexually attractive; anxiety, poor "letdown" reflex, discouragement

*Government*
Ineffective legislation regarding pregnancy and lactation benefits; inappropriate advertising permitted; lack of creches in government plants and in industry; inappropriate distribution of milk

(From Jelliffe EFP: The impact of the food industry on the nutritional status of young children in developing countries. In Mayer J, Dwyer J (eds): Food and Nutrition Policy in a Changing World, pp 197–222. New York, Oxford University Press, 1979)

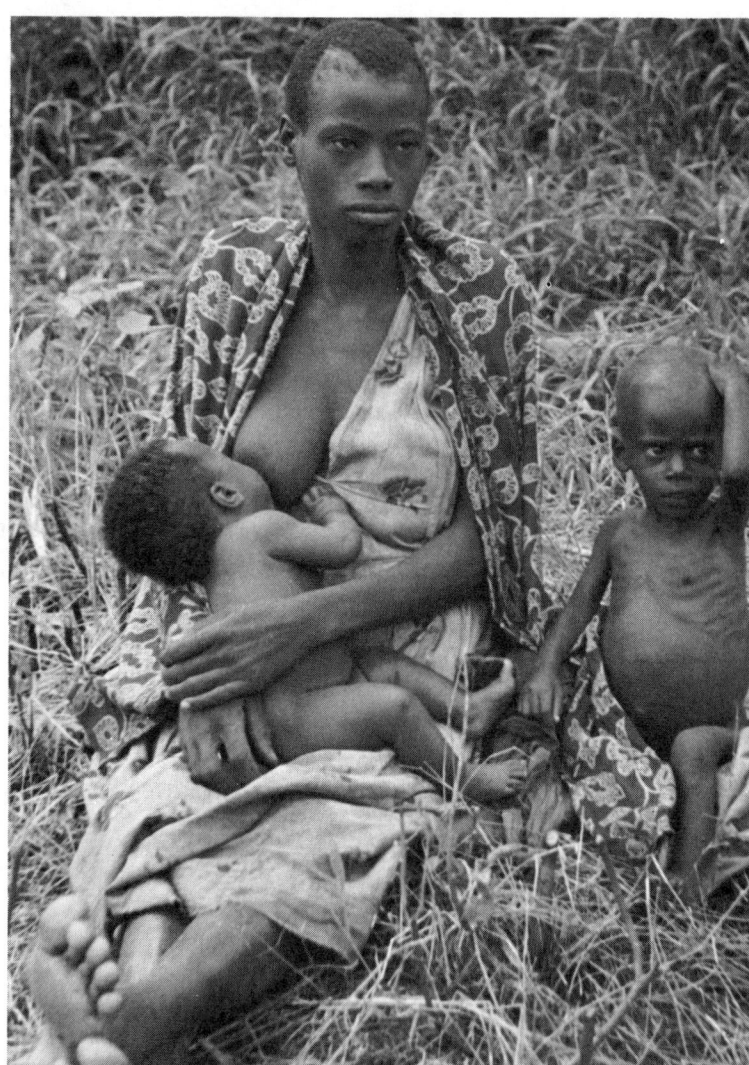

**Fig. 21-2.**   The older child in this picture shows the protein calorie deprivation and the malnutrition that occurred when he was "deposed" or replaced at the mother's breast by the new baby. He is subsisting on starchy foods and a few vegetables. (Dr. John Bennett, Nutrition Unit, Ministry of Health, Kampala, Uganda)

their infants as long as they can.[12] They should also be encouraged to add other appropriate foods to the infant's diet at about four or five months of age. These foods should be of a consistency suitable for the infant and should be free of contamination with harmful pathogens. Mixtures of cereals and legumes, such as rice and red peas, made into a porridge and rubbed through a strainer, may be used in combination with fruits and vegetables, such as mashed bananas and sweet potatoes. By the time the infant is six months old, he may be fed many of the same foods the rest of the family consumes provided that they are soft or tender, not too highly seasoned, and provided that he continues to be breast-fed.[13] Table 21-4 shows the FAO/WHO recommended daily intakes for calories and protein.

The feeding of the sick child is also an important factor in the prevention of PEM. It is the cultural practice in many areas to feed the child with diarrhea or other infectious disease a very limited diet, often consisting of a thin gruel, such as rice or barley water. Because these illnesses tend to be frequent and severe among children living in poverty with poor housing and unsanitary conditions, the dietary treatment is extremely important, and mothers need to be made aware of the increased nutritional needs during these periods. If possible, the infant should be fed his usual diet of breast milk and other soft bland foods. Because loss of body fluids during diarrhea may be the most critical factor, he should be given additional water that has been boiled, with perhaps barley or rice to make a very thin gruel.

In the absence of adequate amounts of animal milk, the availabilty of appropriate "weaning food" (those foods that will replace breast milk) is critical to the prevention of malnutrition in the toddler and the preschool child. Cereal and legume mixtures are relatively bulky foods for their amount of calories and proteins, and young children may not be able to consume large enough quantities of them to meet their needs if other sources of calories and proteins are not also included in the diet. Due to the bulk of these foods and the small capacity of the child's stomach, frequent feeding is an important aspect of nutritional care. Four or five meals per day for the child rather than one or two, which may be the common adult practice, is advisable.[4] Moreover, additional, more concentrated sources of both energy and proteins should be added. Starches, tubers and roots, other vegetables, and fruits can contribute additional calories as well as essential vitamins and minerals. Small amounts of eggs, meat, fish (including fish protein concentrate), unfortunately considered inappropriate foods for children by some cultures, would add good-quality protein to the child's diet. Peanuts (ground nuts) and soy bean products can also provide good sources of high-quality protein. Of course, if milk is

available and tolerated, the young child should receive generous amounts of it. Because fresh milk is easily contaminated with harmful bacteria which grow readily in it, it should be pasteurized or boiled for the young child. Dry skim milk (DSM) has been widely distributed by various international agencies, such as UNICEF, Catholic Relief Services, and Church World Service, and can be added to other foods to increase their protein content.

In some developing countries, especially in urban areas, a processed, protein-rich mixture is available as a substitute for milk as a weaning food. The problem, however, is that although this food may cost less than milk or meat, it does usually cost more than the cereals it replaces and, as a result, it is often more expensive than the lowest income groups can afford to purchase in suffi-

## Table 21-4. Recommended Intakes of Nutrients (FAO/WHO)

| Age | Body Weight | Energy (1) | | Pro-tein (1, 2) | Vitamin A (3, 4) | Vitamin D (5, 6) | Thia-min (3) | Ribo-flavin (3) | Niacin (3) | Folic Acid (5) | Vitamin B₁₂ (5) | Ascor-bic Acid (5) | Calcium (7) | Iron (5, 8) |
|---|---|---|---|---|---|---|---|---|---|---|---|---|---|---|
| | kilo-grams | kilo-calories | mega-joules | grams | micro-grams | micro-grams | milli-grams | milli-grams | milli-grams | micro-grams | micro-grams | milli-grams | grams | milli-grams |
| *Children* | | | | | | | | | | | | | | |
| <1 | 7.3 | 820 | 3.4 | 14 | 300 | 10.0 | 0.3 | 0.5 | 5.4 | 60 | 0.3 | 20 | 0.5–0.6 | 5–10 |
| 1–3 | 13.4 | 1360 | 5.7 | 16 | 250 | 10.0 | 0.5 | 0.8 | 9.0 | 100 | 0.9 | 20 | 0.4–0.5 | 5–10 |
| 4–6 | 20.2 | 1830 | 7.6 | 20 | 300 | 10.0 | 0.7 | 1.1 | 12.1 | 100 | 1.5 | 20 | 0.4–0.5 | 5–10 |
| 7–9 | 28.1 | 2190 | 9.2 | 25 | 400 | 2.5 | 0.9 | 1.3 | 14.5 | 100 | 1.5 | 20 | 0.4–0.5 | 5–10 |
| *Male adolescents* | | | | | | | | | | | | | | |
| 10–12 | 36.9 | 2600 | 10.9 | 30 | 575 | 2.5 | 1.0 | 1.6 | 17.2 | 100 | 2.0 | 20 | 0.6–0.7 | 5–10 |
| 13–15 | 51.3 | 2900 | 12.1 | 37 | 725 | 2.5 | 1.2 | 1.7 | 19.1 | 200 | 2.0 | 30 | 0.6–0.7 | 9–18 |
| 16–19 | 62.9 | 3070 | 12.8 | 38 | 750 | 2.5 | 1.2 | 1.8 | 20.3 | 200 | 2.0 | 30 | 0.5–0.6 | 5–9 |
| *Female adolescents* | | | | | | | | | | | | | | |
| 10–12 | 38.0 | 2350 | 9.8 | 29 | 575 | 2.5 | 0.9 | 1.4 | 15.5 | 100 | 2.0 | 20 | 0.6–0.7 | 5–10 |
| 13–15 | 49.9 | 2490 | 10.4 | 31 | 725 | 2.5 | 1.0 | 1.5 | 16.4 | 200 | 2.0 | 30 | 0.6–0.7 | 12–24 |
| 16–19 | 54.4 | 2310 | 9.7 | 30 | 750 | 2.5 | 0.9 | 1.4 | 15.2 | 200 | 2.0 | 30 | 0.5–0.6 | 14–28 |
| *Adult man* (moderately active) | 65.0 | 3000 | 12.6 | 37 | 750 | 2.5 | 1.2 | 1.8 | 19.8 | 200 | 2.0 | 30 | 0.4–0.5 | 5–9 |
| *Adult woman* (moderately active) | 55.0 | 2200 | 9.2 | 29 | 750 | 2.5 | 0.9 | 1.3 | 14.5 | 200 | 2.0 | 30 | 0.4–0.5 | 14–28 |
| *Pregnancy* (later half) | | +350 | +1.5 | 38 | 750 | 10.0 | +0.1 | +0.2 | +2.3 | 400 | 3.0 | 30 | 1.0–1.2 | (9) |
| *Lactation* (first 6 months) | | +550 | +2.3 | 46 | 1200 | 10.0 | +0.2 | +0.4 | +3.7 | 300 | 2.5 | 30 | 1.0–1.2 | (9) |

[1]Energy and Protein Requirements. Report of a Joint FAO/WHO Expert Group, FAO, Rome, 1972.—[2]As egg or milk protein.—[3]Requirements of Vitamin A, Thiamine, Riboflavin and Niacin. Report of a Joint FAO/WHO Expert Group, FAO, Rome, 1965.—[4]As retinol.—[5]Requirements of Ascorbic Acid, Vitamin D, Vitamin B₁₂, Folate and Iron. Report of a Joint FAO/WHO Expert Group, FAO, Rome, 1970.—[6]As cholecalciferol.—[7]Calcium Requirements. Report of a FAO/WHO Expert Group, FAO, Rome, 1961.—[8]On each line the lower value applies when over 25 percent of calories in the diet come from animal foods, and the higher value when animal foods represent less than 10 percent of calories.—[9]For women whose iron intake throughout life has been at the level recommended in this table, the daily intake of iron during pregnancy and lactation should be the same as that recommended for nonpregnant, nonlactating women of childbearing age. For women whose iron status is not satisfactory at the beginning of pregnancy, the requirement is increased, and in the extreme situation of women with no iron stores, the requirement can probably not be met without supplementation.

cient quantities for child feeding. One of the first of these was prepared at the Institute of Nutrition of Central America and Panama (INCAP) in Guatemala City. This mixture, called *Incaparina*, consists of cornmeal and defatted cottonseed or soy flour with added vitamins and minerals and is available in several Central American countries.

Other mixtures of vegetable proteins that have been developed include *Pronutro* in South Africa, *Faffa* in Ethiopia, *Superamine* in Algeria, *Columbiharina* in Columbia, and *Bal Ahar* in India. A corn-soy milk (CSM) and a wheat-soy blend (WSB) have been commercially produced in the United States for distribution throughout the world. *Vitasoy* is a protein-rich beverage bottled and marketed in Hong Kong accounting for 25% of the soft drink sales.

Because generous amounts of good-quality protein are required for the treatment of kwashiorkor, milk or a protein-rich milk substitute is essential. Specific dietary treatment depends on the severity of the disease and other deficiency symptoms that may be present. The child may be too sick in the beginning to consume more than small, frequent feedings of relatively dilute mixtures of milk or other formula. As his condition improves, he will be able to take larger quantities of more concentrated mixtures.

## Vitamin deficiencies
### Vitamin A deficiency—xerophthalmia

The prevention of xerophthalmia has been given the second highest priority by J. M. Bengoa, Chief Medical Officer of the Nutrition Division of the World Health Organization.[4] It is not unusual for protein-energy malnutrition and vitamin A deficiency to occur together, with severe consequences. When xerophthalmia accompanies PEM, the mortality may be as high as 80%, whereas it is about 15% in a group equally malnourished but not deficient in vitamin A.

The signs of vitamin A deficiency are predominantly ocular, and the preschool child (30–36 months is the age of peak incidence) is especially vulnerable to the severe forms that cause blindness. Xerophthalmia due to vitamin A deficiency is the most important single cause of blindness in many developing countries. It has been widely reported in various parts of the world, especially Southeast Asia, India, the Middle East, parts of Africa, and Latin America. One must recognize that in human suffering and economic loss, the cost of blindness is incalculable. In comparison, the cost of prevention is almost negligible.

### Classification of stages of xerophthalmia

The ocular signs of vitamin A deficiency include night blindness, conjunctival xerosis, Bitot's spots, corneal xerosis, and keratomalacia. The classification proposed for general use is as follows:[15]

| *Classification* | *Signs —primary* |
| --- | --- |
| X1A | Conjunctival xerosis—dryness or lack of luster, loss of ability to retain moisture no matter whether tears are present or absent, loss of transparency, thickening, wrinkling, pigmentation, accumulation of debris |
| X1B | Bitot's spot with conjunctival xerosis—a small plaque with a silvery gray hue and a foamy surface; it is quite superficial and is raised above the general level of the conjunctiva |
| X2 | Corneal xerosis—follows conjunctival xerosis. The corneal surface has a rough, fine pebbly appearance and lacks luster. Later, cellular infiltration of the corneal stroma contributes to the intense haziness of the cornea, which frequently has a bluish, milky appearance |
| X3A | Corneal ulceration with xerosis—involving loss of substance of a part or of the whole of the corneal thickness |
| X3B | Keratomalacia—consists of a characteristic softening of the entire thickness of a part or, more often, the whole of the cornea, leading to deformation or destruction of the eyeball. The process is a rapid one, the corneal structure melting into a cloudy gelatinous mass which may be dead white or dirty yellow in color |
| | *Signs —secondary* |
| XN | Night blindness—impairment of the ability to adapt to the dark |
| XF | Xerophthalmia fundus—multiple lesions, sometimes glaring white, scattered profusely along the course of the vessels |
| XS | Corneal scars—resulting from the healing of irreversible corneal changes |
| XB | Bitot's spot—(see X1B) |

Stage XN, or *night blindness*, indicates a functional impairment of the retina and is difficult to diagnose in the young child (1–4 yr) unless the mother is aware that the child cannot see well at night. As a method of screening, the child may be asked to walk into a darkened room.

The first sign of xerophthalmia is xerosis of the conjunctiva (stage X1A). This dryness and dullness associated with the stability of the precorneal film is considered complete alteration of the reflection of light from the conjunctiva. Night blindness (XN) and Bitot's spots (accumulation of debris and fatty material near the edge of the eye) are frequently present at stage X1B. At stage X2, when there is xerosis of the cornea itself, the precorneal film fails to cover the cornea, which now appears dry and opaque. Small erosions or perforations begin to occur if treatment with massive doses of vitamin A (100,000 IU/day, orally or intramuscularly) is not provided within 1 to 3 days of inception, and irreversible damage will soon result. However, if treated, the corneal xerosis will clear up within a short period of time.

Irreversible damage occurs once deeper layers of the cornea are involved, as in stage X3A. The cornea may liquefy and melt away, resulting in large perforations and extrusion of the iris, the lens, and the vitreous (X3B). The permanent scarring effects (stage X5) may differ depending on whether or not intraocular pressure was restored at stage X3B. It is essential that medical and paramedical personnel be alert to the signs of xerophthalmia and that treatment be instituted immediately when symptoms are recognized in order to prevent blindness.

## Etiology of xerophthalmia

The development of xerophthalmia is complex and often involves dietary as well as nondietary factors. It frequently results from deficiencies of protein and energy as well as vitamin A; its onset is often precipitated by infectious disease. Young children are the most vulnerable group, and males are more susceptible than females.

The reduction in serum proteins found in kwashiorkor includes a reduction in the amount of retinol-binding protein and, for this reason, also a decrease in the amount of vitamin A or retinol in the blood. When increased levels of protein are fed without additional vitamin A, the concentration of vitamin A in the blood increases, apparently due to the utilization of previously unavailable stores. In marasmus, however, xerophthalmia is not associated with low levels of serum protein but rather with a lack of vitamin A. Consequently, in xerophthalmia and marasmus, only administration of vitamin A at the proper time will cure the xerophthalmia.[16,17]

Because breast-feeding protects the infant from xerophthalmia, the greatest incidence occurs in children over 1 year old. There is also a seasonal variation in the incidence which appears to relate both to seasonal availability of the food sources of carotene and vitamin A and to the occurrence of infectious diseases.

## Treatment and prevention of xerophthalmia

Due to the extremely serious consequences of vitamin A deficiency and the high cost of identifying specific cases, four methods of prevention have been suggested; one as a short-term measure and the others as long-range goals.[18] Presently, the most practical and immediate method of controlling vitamin A deficiency in high risk children appears to be the periodic (usually at 6-month intervals) oral administration of large doses (200,000 IU) of retinol to preschool children 1 to 5 years of age. This may be done as part of routine procedures in child health programs. India, Indonesia, Bangladesh, and certain other areas have mass campaigns employing special mobile units participating in the project. Because vitamin A can be stored in the liver, children treated by this method maintain enhanced serum levels of vitamin A for 4 to 6 months. In areas where large doses of vitamin A have been given to children, the incidence of xerophthalmia has been greatly reduced. It is important, however, that all health personnel working in the programs are aware of the risks of overdosage and are supervised by medically qualified personnel.[14]

Fortification of a staple foodstuff is also a possibility, provided there is a food regularly consumed by children in sufficient quantity. The enrichment of sugar with vitamin A, as is currently being done in Guatemala, should be carefully evaluated for its overall nutritional effect on children. Fortifying tea with vitamin A has been suggested in several Indian states. In Cebu, Philippines, vitamin A has been added to monosodium glutamate (MSG). All skim milk products shipped from the United States must be fortified with vitamin A. Wheat flour produced in the United States for overseas shipment is also fortified with vitamin A. A new "premix" method of fortifying white rice with vitamin A has been developed.

Horticultural approaches to the eradication of vitamin A deficiency include developing agricultural policies that will ensure that crop production and distribution is related to the nutritional needs of the population as well as encouraging the establishment of small family gardens. There is a need to identify and promote the cultivation of those vegetables and fruits that are acceptable to the people in an area and that are high in available provitamin A.[18]

The long-term goal should be to improve the child's diet to ensure adequate intake of vitamin A. The success of this method will depend on the effectiveness of nutrition education. Dietary sources of vitamin A should be emphasized in programs directed toward pregnant and lactating women and infants and preschool children. Instruction in nutrition should also become a part of the formal educational system. Other instructional media that may be used are posters, demonstrations, radio, and television programs. Green leafy vegetables and yellow fruits and vegetables are all good sources of vitamin A and may be used to satisfy the vitamin A requirements of children (see Table 21-4). Another good source of carotene is the red palm oil available in certain parts of Africa. Ultimately, in order to increase the amount of vitamin A in young children's diets, the nutrition educators will have to face the difficult task of modifying culturally determined child feeding practices.

## Night blindness and day blindness
### Incidence

Mild deficiencies of vitamin A with a variety of manifestations still occur in more prosperous areas of the world. One of the early signs long associated with this deficiency is night blindness (*Nyctalopia*). In Labrador and Newfoundland, where the condition has been recognized for generations, the popular remedy is fish liver, which the people rarely eat as a food but will take as medicine. Varying degrees of night blindness are discovered among children and adults in the United States when instruments for detecting and measuring adjustment to dull light are used for routine examinations of large groups. In general, it tends to be more prevalent among low-income groups, but some cases are found in almost any group.

Day blindness (*hemeralopia*), closely related and essentially similar to night blindness, was recognized when automobile drivers complained of being unable to drive at night because of the glare of headlights (Fig. 21-3). During World War II pilots were examined especially for this condition, and a liberal intake of vitamin A was recommended as a preventive.

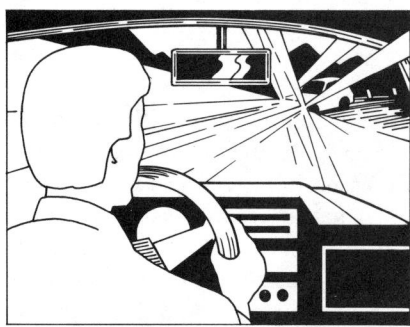

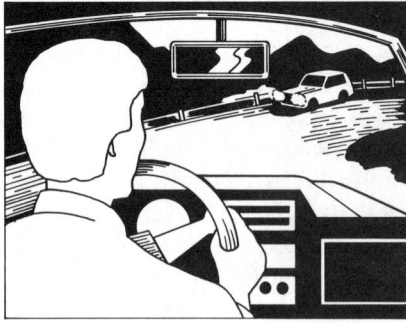

**Fig. 21-3.** (*Top*) "Glare blindness" often is a symptom of vitamin A deficiency. Headlights dazzle the eyes and cause discomfort. The driver is blinded temporarily by oncoming headlights, and the edge of the road is seen with difficulty. (*Bottom*) An adequate intake of vitamin A protects against "glare blindness" or remedies it. Properly focused headlights no longer dazzle so blindingly, and the road edge can be seen almost immediately after the headlight glare has passed.

### Etiology and pathology

Both nyctalopia and hemeralopia are functional disorders resulting from the slowed regeneration of visual purple in the retina of the eye. The difficulty is usually due to an insufficient supply of vitamin A to function with the protein of the retina for the regeneration of visual purple, which is bleached to visual yellow under the influence of bright light. Regeneration of visual purple takes place in the dark, but replenishment of vitamin A from the bloodstream is essential to continue the reaction, that is, to permit adaptation in the shortest possible time (see Chap. 7).

### Symptoms and diagnosis

A person may have a mild degree of either night or day blindness and not be aware of it unless his attention is drawn to it by some circumstance or special test. One person may be slower than another in adjusting to the dull light of a movie theater, but neither is aware of a difference. This is not a condition that causes discomfort severe enough to prompt one to seek medical advice unless it reaches an advanced stage.

### Treatment

A daily intake of 5000 IU of vitamin A is more than enough to prevent night blindness or any related condition.

## Other conditions due to vitamin A deficiency
### Cutaneous lesions

These may appear early in adults and have a characteristic appearance. Papules tend to form around hair follicles on outer surfaces of arms, legs, shoulders, and lower abdomen, and are described as having a "gooseflesh" appearance. They usually disappear when an adequate food source of vitamin A is provided.

### Epithelial tissue changes

Possibly as a result of vitamin A deficiency, normal secretory epithelium is replaced by dry, keratinized epithelium, which is more susceptible to invasion by infectious organisms.

### Genitourinary tract changes

In the female, the epithelial cells in the vagina may undergo changes that interfere with the normal estrus cycle, and in the male atrophic changes in the testes may occur, resulting in permanent damage. These changes have also been connected to vitamin A deficiency.

For food sources of vitamin A and further discussion of the subject, see Chapter 7 and Table 1, Part 4.

## Thiamin deficiency
### Incidence

Mild or chronic thiamin deficiency is more often part of a depletion of the whole group of B complex vitamins. Such a chronic multiple deficiency may be a contributing factor in malnutrition in children. It also should be recalled that the thiamin allowance is related to total calorie intake (see Chap. 8).

## Beriberi

The frank deficiency disease known as *beriberi* is of special significance among the rice eaters of the Orient, where it still occurs, although less frequently than formerly.

Beriberi is described in Chinese history, and some of the earliest attempts to treat it are reported from Japan and the Philippines. The recognition of its cause and of its possible cure by better diet is one of the landmarks in the history of nutrition. The story is well told by Dr. R. R. Williams in his book, *Toward the Conquest of Beriberi.*[19] This account of Dr. Williams's own 26-year search for what proved to be a vitamin, its identification and eventual synthesis, is a classic in nutrition research. Prior to his death in 1965 Dr. Williams had been the moving spirit behind the practical use of thiamin and other factors of the B complex for the enrichment of rice in the Philippines and some other oriental countries. This has resulted in a marked reduction in the incidence of beriberi. In fact, beriberi has almost disappeared from Japan, where the prophylactic use of thiamin and enrichment of rice are common.

> "In Thailand, Malaysia, and Vietnam, however, beriberi has increased in recent years as more efficient small mechanical mills replace hand pounding, which left some of the germ and hull. Moreover, most of the increase has been in infantile beriberi, with its recognized high mortality."[20]

According to Scrimshaw:

> . . . infantile beriberi is one of the most dramatic deficiencies, for a child may be apparently well and die from this condition in a few hours. It is due to low thiamin levels in breast milk. Recovery is equally dramatic when the mother is given thiamin. [The initial stage is characterized by] vomiting, restlessness, pallor, anorexia and insomnia. . . . In the subacute form further vomiting, puffiness of the face and extremities, oliguria, abdominal pain, dysphasia, aphonia and convulsions may appear. This type may go on to a fatal episode or may become chronic.

> There need be no signs of beriberi in the mothers of infants affected.

### Symptoms and pathology

Three main types of beriberi occur in adults and older children: the chronic dry, atrophic type generally found only in older adults, often associated with pro-longed consumption of alcohol; the acute fulminating wet type, which is more serious and dramatic but occurs rarely; and the mild subacute form, which is most common. This third type

> has characteristic nervous manifestations, including alterations in tendon reflexes. Paresthesia is common. . . . Sensations of fullness and tightening of the muscles and muscle cramps are common at night. Cardiovascular signs and symptoms range from breathlessness on exertion and palpitation to tachycardia, cardiac dilation and some degree of congestive heart failure. Coexisting deficiencies of ascorbic acid, riboflavin, niacin and vitamin A are common.[20]

### Treatment

Adequate food sources of thiamin are sufficient to prevent any of the deficiency conditions described, but, when the pathologic symptoms appear, more concentrated sources of thiamin usually are necessary for prompt recovery. Anorexia and nausea are often so severe that they preclude an adequate food intake until symptoms have been relieved by the administration of concentrates.

Because most of the cases diagnosed as beriberi in regions where it is prevalent are suffering from multiple deficiencies, it is customary for the physician to prescribe B complex concentrates rather than pure thiamin and to seek improvement in the diet. The dosage for therapeutic purposes is often several times the recommended allowance of thiamin, with other factors in proportion (see Table 21-4 for recommended allowances of vitamins for different age and sex categories; see Chap. 8 for rich food sources of thiamin and other fractions of the B complex).

### Beriberi heart disease

Beriberi heart disease is described as a distinct clinical entity by Gubbay.[21] The pathology includes right heart failure, edema, and peripheral vasodilation. Beriberi heart disease is due to a deficiency and is curable if the deficiency is corrected in time.

## Nutritional disorders of the central nervous system

Several acute disorders of the central nervous system have been associated with alcoholism. Similar disturbances may also occur in the absence of alcoholism when there is a prolonged deficiency of food intake, as in gastric carcinoma or when anorexia is a complication of other conditions, such as pregnancy.

Experimental work in pigeons in 1938 first demonstrated that a severe thiamin deficiency could produce brain lesions. In 1942 British prisoners of war developed nervous disorders that disappeared with small doses of thiamin.

Subsequent clinical research has identified the lesion

in man as polioencephalitis, an inflammatory disease of the gray substance of the brain. This is due in most, if not all, cases to a thiamin deficiency.

### Polyneuropathy

A disease that involves many nerves and affects the peripheral nerves, the symptoms of polyneuropathy are remarkably similar to those of classical beriberi and are frequently relieved by thiamin or vitamin B complex therapy. Under some circumstances a deficiency of pyridoxine or pantothenic acid may give rise to similar symptoms. The chief ones are weakness, numbness, partial paralysis, and pain in the legs. The legs are affected earlier than the arms. Motor, reflex, and sensory reactions are lost in most cases. Recovery is a slow process involving weeks or months, and a year may pass before a patient is able to walk unaided. Recently multiple causes have been suggested for peripheral neuropathy, including genetic predisposition, nutritional deficiency and direct neuropathic effect of alcohol.[22]

### Wernicke's disease

Wernicke's disease is closely associated with Korsakoff's psychosis, and the combination is often referred to as the Wernicke-Korsakoff syndrome. The specific nutritional factor primarily involved is thiamin. This syndrome may occur apart from alcoholism but is most frequently encountered in chronic alcoholics (see Chap. 33). The chief symptoms are ophthalmoplegia (paralysis of the eye muscles), nystagmus (involuntary rapid movement of the eyeballs), and ataxia (failure of muscular coordination). The ophthalmoplegia is relieved promptly after a few adequate meals; the other symptoms respond more slowly to thiamin therapy, indicating, perhaps, some structural damage to the nerve tissue. Wernicke's disease is a medical emergency, and massive doses of thiamin (as much as 250 mg per day) may be prescribed. Mental symptoms, such as apathy, drowsiness, inattentiveness, and inability to concentrate or sustain a conversation seem to clear up upon thiamin administration.

### The Korsakoff syndrome

This is characterized by memory defect and confabulation (a form of mental confusion consisting of giving answers and reciting experiences without regard to truth). These symptoms may not respond to thiamin therapy as do the other mental symptoms mentioned in the preceding paragraph. There is evidence that the damage to the nervous system in the Korsakoff syndrome may be structural rather than biochemical, and that thiamin deficiency of long standing may be responsible.

### Amblyopia (dim vision)

The amblyopia accompanying alcoholism and formerly attributed to the toxic effects of alcohol and tobacco is probably of nutritional origin.[23] Clinical experiments

have demonstrated recovery following improved nutrition, and have identified vitamin B complex—and, more specifically, thiamin—as the important factor.

## Riboflavin deficiency

### Incidence

No well defined deficiency syndrome or disease with a long history, such as scurvy or beriberi, is associated with a lack of riboflavin. However, dietary and clinical evidence of riboflavin deficiency or borderline intake has been reported from Taiwan, Korea, the Philippines, East Pakistan, and Turkey.[24] Riboflavin deficiency was the deficiency most commonly reported from these countries, which are predominantly rice-eating. Ariboflavinosis as it exists today is seldom fatal, but it is a serious handicap. It must be remembered that a person with a riboflavin deficiency is likely to have associated deficiencies of thiamin and niacin.

### Symptoms and pathology

Before any true clinical symptoms appear, a mild riboflavin deficiency may be responsible for a type of light sensitivity and dimness of vision, followed later by itching, burning, and eyestrain. Other eye symptoms include proliferation and engorgement of the limbic plexus, followed by superficial vascularization of the cornea and the production of interstitial keratitis. Later clinical manifestations are angular stomatitis, cheilosis, seborrheic dermatitis, scrotal dermatitis, and erythema of buccal and palatal mucosa and tongue.

### Treatment and prevention

Common food sources of riboflavin are listed in Chapter 8. Milk and organ meats are the richest natural sources. Enriched bread is also a good economical source.

## Niacin and tryptophan deficiency—pellagra

### Incidence

Pellagra is still found in India, South Africa, and Egypt where there are large numbers of poor peasants living on maize or, sometimes, on millet. It has become rare in recent years in Yugoslavia and Romania where wheat has replaced some of the maize in the diets of these Eastern Europeans. The enrichment of bread and other cereal grains resulted in the disappearance of pellagra in the United States and Western Europe.[25] There is also a low incidence of pellagra in those areas of the world, for example, Mexico and Central America, where maize is treated with lime, which apparently makes the niacin content more available.[26]

Isolated cases of pellagra may occur in any area in persons restricted to a diet low in protein and niacin. This can happen in older people with self-imposed restrictions or in someone with allergies to a number of protein foods. Alcoholic pellagra is essentially identical with endemic pellagra. It is caused by the substitution of alcohol for food.

## Symptoms and pathology

On exposure to sun, persons whose diets supply inadequate tryptophan and are deficient in niacin acquire a scaly, pigmented dermatitis over the exposed areas. Depending on the type of clothing and extent of exposed skin, the areas most affected are the face, neck, back of hands, elbows, knees, and ankles. The classic "three D's," *dermatitis*, *diarrhea*, and *dementia*, may still describe the symptoms, although dementia is rare. Anemias are frequent, probably due to associated deficiencies. Glossitis (sore tongue) suggests a relationship to the disease, *blacktongue*, in dogs.

## Treatment and prevention

Large doses of niacin, usually in the form of niacinamide, are used in the treatment of pellagra. The addition of milk, eggs, meat, nuts, and certain vegetables (see Chap. 8) can supply the factors missing in the typical pellagra-producing diet.

The best method of preventing pellagra has been the improvement of the socioeconomic status of people living chiefly on maize diets. When a more varied diet is introduced, perhaps where individuals have gained some land of their own to raise additional foods or money with which to purchase more expensive items in the diet, endemic pellagra disappears. Roe summarizes the situation as follows:

> It is not, however, the opportunity for social, economic, and agricultural progress that determines the decline of pellagra but rather the extension of the benefits of progress to all members of society. The current situation in India, South Africa, and Egypt points up the fact that pellagra will be with us until the dispossessed achieve their right to freedom from want and can choose to eat the foods that prevent the disease.[25]

## Ascorbic acid deficiency and scurvy

### History and incidence

Scurvy is probably the oldest recognized deficiency disease. Although its specific relationship to ascorbic acid was not recognized until the 20th century, its prevention by the use of fresh foods was practiced much earlier. Prevalent in Europe during the 19th century and earlier, scurvy was attributed for centuries to a limited food supply. On the long voyages that followed the discovery of America, sailors were often forced to subsist for long periods on salt fish and meats and hardtack or other breadstuffs, entirely deprived of any fresh food. The outbreaks of scurvy on such voyages were frequently so severe that there were scarcely enough of the crew left to man the vessel. In 1772, however, Captain Cook commanded a voyage, which lasted three years, during which not one man was lost due to scurvy. This fact he attributed to the use of a "sweet wort" made from barley and sauerkraut. Subsequently, limes or lemons were included in the supplies, after they had been found to be antiscorbutic, that is, preventing scurvy.

Scurvy probably was responsible for most of the deaths among the pilgrims in the Massachusetts Bay Colony during that first hard winter. There was an outbreak of mild scurvy in northern Maine during the depression years, the early 1930s. Outbreaks of the disease have also been associated with famine or war areas, when the food supply was limited. Historically, its occurrence was reported during polar expeditions or other circumstances in which supplies of fresh food were unavailable. Expert dietetic advice was sought in planning the food supplies for the more recent polar expeditions in order to avoid the possibility of a vitamin C shortage because scurvy is greatly dreaded by explorers.

Eskimos on their native diets seldom have scurvy but are susceptible to it when they adopt the "white man's diet." On their native diets they may include organ meats and mosses that supply ascorbic acid. It is also reported that some groups eat meat raw or undercooked, thereby retaining the slight amount of ascorbic acid that may be present.

The only cases of scurvy in adults reported in this country are in men living alone and preparing inadequate meals or in psychoneurotic individuals on bizarre diets. During the 1960s an increased number of cases of infantile scurvy was reported in the medical literature from such areas as Canada, Newfoundland, and Australia. A survey in Canada during 1961 to 1963 found 87 cases of infantile scurvy.[27] These cases occurred mostly in small communities where there was ignorance, poverty, and poor health supervision. As a result of these findings, Canada has enacted a regulation permitting the addition of ascorbic acid to evaporated milk, commonly used in infant feeding.

Scurvy is relatively rare in the underdeveloped areas of the world. Many of these countries are in the tropical and subtropical zones where fruits and vegetables are plentiful and widely consumed.

Frank scurvy is so rare in the United States today that medical students seldom have a chance to observe the disease. Yet the history of this disease and its prevention are worthy of note.

## Symptoms and pathology

The principal symptoms of scurvy in order of occurrence are weakness, fatigue, listlessness, neurotic behavior; aching in bones, joints and muscles; dry rough skin; petechiae and ecchymoses of the arms, legs, and conjunctivae; hemorrhages in muscles; swollen, blue red friable gums where teeth are present; loosening of the teeth; neuritis due to nerve hemorrhages; failure of wounds to heal; peripheral stasis of blood and cyanosis of extremities; convulsions, shock, and death. Anemia may occur as a result of blood loss.

Marginal symptoms of this disease are sallow skin, muddy complexion, lack of energy, and fleeting pains in limbs and joints. Irritability, retarded growth, and tooth defects may also accompany this dietary deficiency.

Mild manifestations of ascorbic acid deficiency in adults may easily be overlooked or ignored. Tendency to bruise easily, slow healing of minor wounds, and pinpoint hemorrhages may be indications that tissues are depleted of this factor.

### Treatment

An adequate supply of ascorbic acid is the obvious treatment for all these conditions, but what is an adequate supply? This problem is reflected in the differences between the Recommended Dietary Allowances of the National Research Council, Table 11-2, and the FAO/WHO Recommended Intake of Nutrients, Table 21-4. For rich food sources of ascorbic acid and for a discussion of its properties and losses in cooking, see Chapter 8. Ascorbic acid in tablet form is stable and relatively inexpensive. It is useful when fresh foods are not available or must be omitted from the diet for any reason. This synthetic form has been used to promote wound healing and to act as a food supplement in emergency rations.

### Vitamin D deficiency—rickets

"The disappearance of rickets" is the title of an article[28] reviewing the history and prevention of vitamin D-deficient rickets as a triumph of medicine and nutrition. As late as 1940 rickets was still a common disease of early childhood in northern climates.

One cannot be complacent, however, about the overall decrease in rickets, because in the 1960s a survey by the committee on Nutrition of the American Academy of Pediatrics[29] reported 843 cases of rickets in 5 years among hospital pediatric admissions. The general use of antirachitic supplements in infant feeding was expected to preclude this deficiency from still being a public health problem. Of course, the widespread use of vitamin D supplements in infant feeding has reduced the incidence in northern climates. Although it is generally rare in tropical countries, where children spend more time out of doors and expose more of their skin to the sun, a 1967 survey in North Africa reported that 45% to 60% of the children examined showed some signs of rickets.[30] Children of dark-skinned races living in northern climates are even more susceptible to rickets than light-skinned children. In Ethiopia local child rearing practices contribute to a high incidence of rickets. Children are deliberately not exposed to sunlight, and dietary intake of vitamin D is low.[8]

### Symptoms and pathology

Rickets is a disease of infancy and early childhood in which the bones do not calcify properly as they grow. They become pliable, malformed, and distorted, which results in such evident deformities as pigeon chest, enlarged wrists and ankles, and bowed legs or knock knees when the leg bones are not strong enough to support the child learning to walk. All these symptoms are shown in the schematic drawing of a child with rickets (Fig. 21-4). The enlargement or beading of the ribs, frequently called *the rachitic rosary*, may be less evident in a plump infant than in an emaciated one, but is characteristic. Profuse sweating and restlessness are early symptoms of rickets in infants. Growth may not be retarded at first, because nature seems to allow the bones to increase in length to keep up the growth in soft tissues if other nutrients are adequate. Prolonged and severe cases usually show stunted growth.

### Treatment and prevention

The major factors involved in the prevention of rickets—calcium, phosphorus, and vitamin D—have been discussed in Chapters 6 and 7. Because the geographic incidence of rickets and practical experience indicate that more often a deficiency of vitamin D causes rickets in children, attention must be directed to adequate and reliable sources of this factor in regions where sunshine cannot act as the natural preventive agent. Obviously, when children can be exposed to an adequate source of ultraviolet light (sunshine or ultraviolet lamp), sufficient vitamin D may be synthesized to regulate the utilization of minerals for bone building. Vitamin preparations containing vitamins A and C in addition to vitamin D are readily available for infants in the United States.

Vitamin D milk is a convenient and reliable antirachitic agent. Because milk contains the minerals calcium and phosphorus and is a natural food for children, it seems to be the most suitable carrier for added vitamin D. Fortified evaporated milk is especially convenient for use in areas where fresh vitamin D milk is not available. Dry skim milk may also be fortified with vitamin D.

### Precautions

It is wise to caution mothers against the simultaneous use of several supplementary sources of vitamin D because it is possible to give too much (see Chap. 7).

### Osteomalacia

***Incidence and pathology.*** Prolonged deficiency of dietary calcium and vitamin D or sunlight may result in osteomalacia, sometimes called *adult rickets*. This condition is characterized by poor calcification of the bones with increasing softness, so that they become flexible, leading to deformities of limbs, spine, thorax, or pelvis. These bone changes may be accompanied by rheumatic pains and exhaustion.

Osteomalacia is rare in Western countries but still occurs in the Middle East and the Orient, especially among women after several pregnancies and when they nurse their infants for extended periods of time. The high incidence of osteomalacia among women in certain parts of India where the rite of purdah is still practiced and among Bedouin Arab women who wear long black garments and live in dark tents testifies indirectly to the protective action of sunshine on exposed skin. In many of these same areas the diet consists largely of cereals and root vegetables low in calcium.

Osteomalacia is often confused with osteoporosis, which may occur in older women in any country, even the most prosperous. The etiology of osteoporosis is not well understood but is more likely due to a metabolic or endocrine disturbance than to a deficiency (see Chap. 20).

***Prevention and treatment.*** Preventon of osteomalacia, like rickets, is entirely possible by means of a diet adequate in calcium and phosphorus and with a supply of vitamin D or exposure to sunlight. The diet of patients suffering from osteomalacia should be adequate in all respects but especially in calcium and vitamin D. In countries where milk is not readily available other food sources of calcium and the protective vitamin should be supplied.

## Mineral deficiencies
### Nutritional anemia

As a world problem nutritional anemias, particularly iron deficiency anemia, are widespread and are generally more serious than has previously been recognized. They are responsible for considerable ill health and some mortality in most areas of the world, including the more developed countries. The groups most at risk for iron deficiency anemia are pregnant women, infants, and young children. It is estimated that 20% of the United States' population, and between 10% to 25% of European women, are affected by iron deficiency anemia. In Africa, 6% to 17% of the adult men, 15% to 50% of the adult women, and 30% to 60% of the children under 15 years of age suffer from iron deficiency anemia. Similar figures are also reported for Asia, where it is estimated that as high as 92% of the children under 2 years of age are affected. Reports from the Middle East indicate that 20% to 25% of pregnant women and 25% to 70% of the children are anemic. Mortality as high as 10, 20 and 40 per 100,000 population is reported in some South American countries.[2]

Chapters 6 and 35 include discussion of the etiology and dietary treatment of anemias. See Chapter 6 for information on iron requirements, dietary sources, and methods of assessments.

To increase the amounts of iron in the diets of children and women during childbearing years the enrichment of wheat and other grains with iron has been adopted in many developed countries. More information on the availability of iron in various foods and in supplements used for fortification is important. Although the general practice of enriching staple foods should be rec-

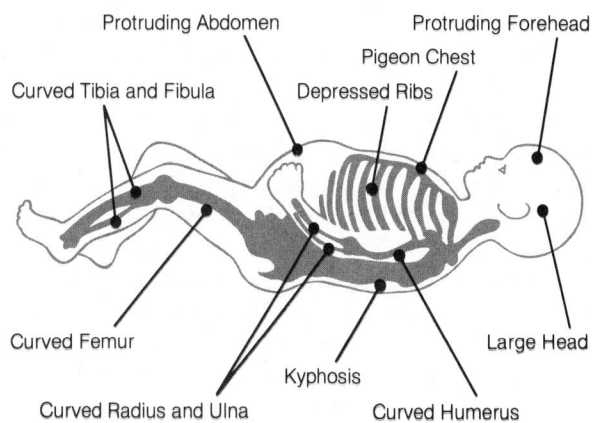

**Fig. 21-4.** The symptoms of rickets. (Abbott Laboratories)

ommended in countries where the food iron content of the diet is less than 6 mg per 1000 calories, the extent and level should be determined by the individual countries, depending on the general composition of the national diet.

Additional suggestions for preventing iron deficiency in the high-risk groups include encouraging prolonged breast-feeding; avoiding excessive amounts of fresh cow's milk in the diet of infants and children; including enhancers of iron absorption in the diet; and avoiding excessive weight gain in pregnancy.[31]

### Endemic goiter and cretinism—iodine deficiency—incidence

The cause of simple goiter is failure of the thyroid gland to obtain a supply of iodine sufficient to maintain its normal structure and function. The lack of iodine is usually a result of environmental deficiency of iodine.

Because iodine in surface soil shows a very uneven distribution and plants absorb iodine from the soil, the iodine content of foodstuffs varies with the locality in which they are grown. For this reason, we find simple goiter most common in those parts of the world where the surface soil is low in iodine and where salt water fish are not commonly eaten. Due to increased facilities for food distribution in the United States today, city people are less confined to food grown in one locality, and the incidence of simple goiter seems to be decreasing.

Iodized salt, which is on the market in most areas of the United States, has proved beneficial in reducing the incidence of goiter, as shown by examination of schoolchildren. In one state where goiter was almost eliminated, it again became prevalent when the emphasis on the use of iodized salt was relaxed. If the spectacular decrease in the incidence of goiter that resulted from the use of iodized salt in the United States is to continue, effective nutrition education must support its use.

Similar programs using iodized salt have been successful in reducing sharply the incidence of endemic goiter in Argentina, Czechoslovakia, France, Guatemala, New Zealand, Switzerland, and Yugoslavia. Injection of iodized oil has also been used successfully as a prophylactic agent in such areas as New Guinea and Zaire. There are, however, many parts of the world where endemic goiter continues to be an important medical problem. They include the Middle East, Southeast Asia, the Himalaya region, most of Central Africa, and many of the Latin American countries (Fig. 21-5). It should be recognized that where the incidence of moderately severe and severe endemic goiter is high, endemic cretinism and deaf mutism are also found among the population. Stanbury and co-workers[32] suggest that in certain areas of Zaire, the Andes, New Guinea, and Southeast Asia 5% of all surviving persons are significantly retarded. The implications of this finding are serious for the economic and social development in these countries.

### Symptoms and pathology

Many criteria have been suggested for identifying the prevalance of simple goiter. Enlargement of the thyroid may exist in 5% to 10% of the adolescent or preadolescent population, even when ample iodine is available in their diets. For this reason, guidelines are essential to determine the scope of the problem. The following scheme of classifying thyroid conditions has been suggested.[33]

Grade Oa: Thyroid not palpable or, if palpable, not larger than normal

Grade Ob: Thyroid distinctly palpable but usually not visible with the head in a normal or raised position; considered to be definitely larger than normal, that is, at least as large as the distal phalanx of the subject's thumb

Grade I: Thyroid easily palpable and visible with the head in a normal or a raised position. The presence of a discrete nodule qualifies a patient for inclusion in this grade

Grade II: Thyroid easily visible with the head in a normal position

Grade III: Goiter visible at a distance

Grade IV: Monstrous goiter

The thyroid, as a result of iodine deficiency, becomes enlarged and, with chronic stimulation over time, becomes nodular. Hypothyroidism may also result if the deficiency is sufficiently severe. In the female, endemic goiter appears to persist throughout the life span, whereas it decreases in the male following adolescence. In addition to iodine deficiency, dietary goitrogens and perhaps genetic factors may influence the severity of the disease.

Endemic goiter may be said to exist in a community when more than 5% of the adolescents or preadolescents have Grade I goiter or when more than 30% are assigned to Grade Ob or above. Urinary excretion of iodine may be used to confirm this finding. If large numbers of the sample population excrete less than 50 mcg of iodine every 24 hours (or per gram of creatinine) the conclusion that endemic goiter due to iodine deficiency exists would be reinforced.[32]

Where the incidence of endemic goiter, as defined by Grade I or above thyroid enlargement, is greater than 20% of the population, endemic cretinism can also be diagnosed. The symptoms of endemic cretinism may include all or a combination of the following: mental retardation, deafness, deaf mutism, retarded growth, neurological abnormalities, and hypothyroidism. Cretins are usually deaf-mute, but it is not certain whether deaf mutism without mental retardation can be the result of endemic cretinism. As a result, it is difficult in field surveys to trace and identify cretins. It is believed that cretinism results when the fetus receives insufficient iodine. Although proof is still lacking, cretinism may also be the result of low levels of thyroid hormone in the maternal blood.[32]

### Prevention

Both endemic goiter and cretinism can be prevented by supplying adequate amounts of iodine. The most successful programs have been those where sodium or potassium iodide have been added to table salt. Various countries have found different concentrations to be beneficial. In the United States one part of iodide is added to 10,000 parts of salt; in Finland, one part of iodide is added to 25,000 parts of salt; and in India, the concentration used is one part iodide to every 40,000 parts salt. Iodide may be lost during storage of salt that is high in moisture or other impurities.

In remote areas of the world where the distribution of iodized salt is not practicable, intramuscular injection of iodized oil has proved effective. It has been administered to women up to the age of 45 and to men up to 20 years of age. Amounts currently used in this program require new injections approximately every 3 years.

Iodine prophylactic programs should be carefully monitored by health personnel. Surveillance of the target population is particularly important after administration of iodized oil due to the large initial dose. Persons over the age of 40, especially, should be examined after 3 to 6 months so that any cases of thyrotoxicosis can be diagnosed and treated. Surveys by trained personnel every 2 or 3 years should be carried out to evaluate the effectiveness of the iodized salt or oil program in reducing the incidence of endemic goiter and cretinism. Reports from Tasmania, Australia, point out that improved iodine nutriture can reduce the rate of stillbirths in a population before similar change is seen in the rate of infant deaths from congenital anomalies. The delay in lowering infant death rates from birth defects is explained as due to long-standing iodine deficiencies in childhood and adolescence, which increase the body's tendency to store iodine in the thyroid gland. In the pregnant woman, therefore, the availability of iodine is reduced to the fetus, even when the woman's present intake is adequate; increased excretion of iodine during pregnancy also contributes to the problem.[34]

### Goitrogens

The availability of dietary iodine may be affected by goitrogenic substances that interfere with iodine utilization. These are found in a number of plant species, including cabbage, Brussels sprouts, soy beans, and peanuts. They are of significance only when the intake of iodine is borderline, and their effect can be compensated for by an adequate intake of iodine.

In central Africa, studies indicate that iodine deficiency and a goitrogenic agent (thiocyanate) from underprocessed cassava are responsible for endemic goiter and related cretinism. Public health measures for treatment and prevention call for not only the use of iodized salt but also for the administration of iodized oil where salt intake is low and for improvement in the processing of cassava.[35]

## Dental caries

### Incidence

Dental caries is probably the most common disease that affects human beings. Authorities estimate that only about 2% of the people of the United States have escaped having at least one dental cavity. Contrary to the regional and the endemic incidence of some other deficiencies, dental caries is so common that nearly everyone has experienced it. Few adults in western civilization have absolutely perfect teeth. Figures on incidence of caries among population groups vary according to locality and race. The prevalence among blacks is lower than among whites of comparable age in the same locality. In the underdeveloped countries, primitive peoples as a rule show a lower incidence than do civilized populations. However, as soon as primitive populations are touched by civilization, and native foods are replaced by processed foods, an increase in dental caries follows.

### Etiology

Dental caries has been variously attributed to inheritance, metabolic disturbances, specific or multiple food deficiencies, conditions in the mouth, including composition of saliva, and lack of fluorine in the water supply. None of these entirely explains the high incidence or varying degree of susceptibility to caries encountered among children of the same family with similar dietary and mouth hygiene habits.

Extensive research has been conducted in an attempt to understand carious changes in teeth and thereby to be able to prevent or inhibit them better. It is now generally agreed that dental caries is of bacterial origin with certain other contributing factors. Bacterial metabolism and

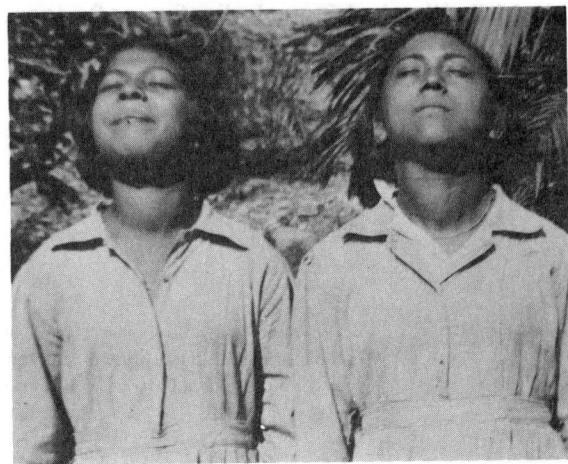

**Fig. 21-5.** Goiter is so common among youth of mountainous regions of South America that a child without goiter is ridiculed as a "bottleneck." (Photo FAO, Rome)

growth in the mouth lead to destruction of both tooth enamel and dentin. Carbohydrates must be present in the crevices of the teeth for caries-producing organisms to grow. Heredity and nutrition during the period of tooth development will affect the resistance to decay at a later date. Saliva is protective, but much is yet to be learned about hereditary, nutritional, endocrine, and other variables that determine the physical consistency, the chemical composition, and the rate of flow of saliva. It is now also recognized that teeth are more resistant to caries when the fluoride ion is incorporated in the crystal lattice of the enamel and the dentin.

The inverse relationship between incidence of dental caries and the fluorine content of drinking water has given impetus to the use of fluorine as a prophylactic agent. A review of caries control in the United States[36] indicated that controlled fluoridation had reduced the incidence of caries by 50% to 70% among young people whose teeth had been formed during the period of fluoridation.

### Prevention

It is generally agreed that fluorine is the only known agent ordinarily included in food and water that is capable of exercising mass control of dental caries. It is effective during the period of calcification of the crown of the tooth and through the period of eruption.

Among the authorities who have studied the problem, it is agreed that the simplest, cheapest, and most far-reaching method of ensuring adequate fluoride is through the fluoridation of drinking water. This procedure will supplement, but not supplant, other dental health measures.

The level of fluorine that seems to be protective without being harmful is 1.0 part per million (ppm) of drinking water. Mottled enamel (dental fluorosis) is apt to occur when fluorine in the water supply exceeds 2 ppm, as

## Table 21-5.  Physical Signs Indicative or Suggestive of Malnutrition

| *Body Area* | *Normal Appearance* | *Signs Associated with Malnutrition* |
| --- | --- | --- |
| *Hair* | Shiny; firm; not easily plucked | Lack of natural shine; hair dull and dry, thin and sparse; hair fine, silky, and straight; color changes (flag sign); can be easily plucked |
| *Face* | Skin color uniform; smooth, pink, healthy appearance; not swollen | Skin color loss (depigmentation); skin dark over cheeks and under eyes (malar and supra-orbital pigmentation); lumpiness or flakiness of skin of nose and mouth; swollen face; enlarged parotid glands; scaling of skin around nostrils (nasolabial seborrhea) |
| *Eyes* | Bright, clear, shiny; no sores at corners of eyelids; membranes a healthy pink and are moist. No prominent blood vessels or mound of tissue or sclera | Eye membranes are pale (pale conjunctivae); redness of membranes (conjunctival injection); Bitot's spots; redness and fissuring of eyelid corners (angular palpebritis); dryness of eye membranes (conjunctival xerosis); cornea has dull appearance (corneal xerosis); cornea is soft (keratomalacia); scar on cornea; ring of fine blood vessels around corner (circumcorneal injection) |
| *Lips* | Smooth, not chapped or swollen | Redness and swelling of mouth or lips (cheilosis); especially at corners or mouth (angular fissures and scars) |
| *Tongue* | Deep red in appearance; not swollen or smooth | Swelling; scarlet and raw tongue; magenta (purplish color) of tongue; smooth tongue; swollen sores; hyperemic and hypertrophic papillae; and atrophic papillae |
| *Teeth* | No cavities, no pain; bright | May be missing or erupting abnormally; gray or black spots (fluorosis); cavities (caries) |
| *Gums* | Healthy; red; do not bleed; not swollen | "Spongy" and bleed easily; recession of gums |
| *Glands* | Face not swollen | Thyroid enlargement (front of neck); parotid enlargement (cheeks become swollen) |
| *Skin* | No signs of rashes, swellings, dark or light spots | Dryness of skin (xerosis); sandpaper feel of skin (follicular hyperkeratosis); flakiness of skin; skin swollen and dark; red swollen pigmentation of exposed areas (pellagrous dermatosis); excessive lightness or darkness of skin (dyspigmentation); black and blue marks due to skin bleeding (petechiae); lack of fat under skin |
| *Nails* | Firm, pink | Nails are spoon-shape (koilonychia); brittle, ridged nails |
| *Muscular and skeletal systems* | Good muscle tone; some fat under skin; can walk or run without pain | Muscles have "wasted" appearance; baby's skull bones are thin and soft (craniotabes); round swelling of front and side of head (frontal and parietal bossing); swelling of ends of bones (epiphyseal enlargement); small bumps on both sides of chest wall (on ribs)—beading of ribs; baby's soft spot on head does not harden at proper time (persistently open anterior fontanelle); knock-knees or bow-legs; bleeding into muscle (musculoskeletal hemorrhages); person cannot get up or walk properly |
| *Internal Systems:*<br>Cardiovascular | Normal heart rate and rhythm; no murmurs or abnormal rhythms; normal blood pressure for age | Rapid heart rate (above 100 tachycardia); enlarged heart; abnormal rhythm; elevated blood pressure |
| Gastrointestinal | No palpable organs or masses (in children, however, liver edge may be palpable) | Liver enlargement; enlargement of spleen (usually indicates other associated diseases) |
| Nervous | Psychological stability; normal reflexes | Mental irritability and confusion; burning and tingling of hands and feet (paresthesia); loss of position and vibratory sense; weakness and tenderness of muscles (may result in inability to walk); decrease and loss of ankle and knee reflexes |

(From Christakis G (ed): Nutritional assessment in health programs. Am J Public Health (Suppl)63:Nov, 1973)

it does naturally in communities in several Western states. Indeed, it was the absence of caries in persons with mottled enamel that first called attention to the protective action of fluorine (see Chap. 6).

Consideration has been given to media other than water as possible means of administering fluorides to children where the community water supply is not fluoridated. Rusoff and co-workers[37] tried milk as a vehicle for administering fluoride in the school lunch program. The amount added was 1 mg of fluoride per $1/_2$ pint of milk. This was tried on 171 children over a period of $3^1/_2$ years and resulted in a 70% reduction in caries incidence in teeth erupting after the initiation of the experiment.

Calcium, phosphorus, or vitamin D deficiencies during and preceding the eruption of teeth undoubtedly account for some faults in structure.

## Early diagnosis and treatment of nutritional failure

The insidious development and delayed clinical evidence of malnutrition make the problem particularly serious. This subject is of great concern to nutritionists, public health nurses, physicians, and others who are frequently in close contact with children and with families living on low incomes and an inadequate food supply. There is ample room for further study and observation of these marginal deficiencies among all groups of the population, but especially among lower income groups, in which the vicious circle of malnutrition, lack of strength and possibilities for self-improvement, and continued low income offers little opportunity for real positive change.

Before clinical signs of nutritional deficiencies appear, there must be biochemical abnormality. Although specific biochemical lesions are difficult to detect, low levels of certain nutrients in blood or urine or both can be determined by laboratory tests and indicate probable deficiency states (Table 11, Part 4, gives current guidelines for criteria of nutritional status for laboratory evaluation). These low levels may persist for varying periods of time before clinical symptoms (Table 21-5) of a deficiency manifest themselves. The pattern for the development of nutritional deficiencies is shown in Fig. 21-6.

## Study questions and activities

1. What are the relationships between malnutrition and infectious diseases? Explain nutritional dwarfing.
2. List three goals for a national food and nutrition policy.
3. What are the most prevalent nutritional deficiencies in the world today?
4. What age group is most susceptible to marasmus? Why? Discuss the marasmus cycle.

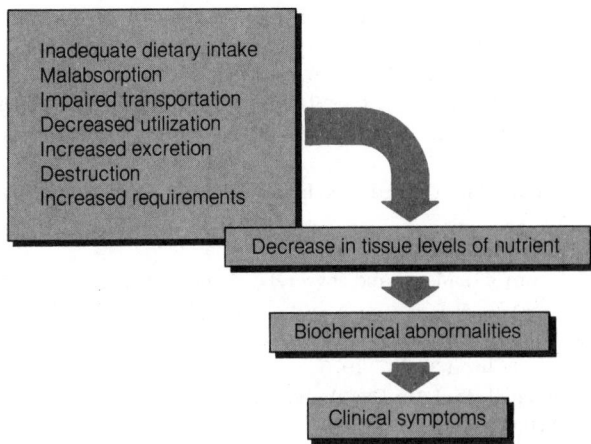

**Fig. 21-6.** Pattern for development of nutritional deficiencies.

5. What are the most likely symptoms of kwashiorkor? What is the meaning of the word kwashiorkor and where did it come from?
6. What contributions has INCAP made in the control and treatment of PEM or kwashiorkor? What is the chief problem in the use of weaning foods in developing countries?
7. What other deficiency may complicate the picture in PEM?
8. Which vitamin deficiency is most widespread and most serious in the world today? What are the consequences?
9. What diseases other than beriberi may result from a thiamin deficiency? What is a common complication?
10. Why is pellagra not as serious a problem in the United States today as it was formerly? Is it found elsewhere in the world? What food pattern is most apt to be found associated with pellagra?
11. Which deficiency disease is widespread in the developed countries? What means have been used to combat its incidence in the United States?
12. What progress is being made in the control of dental caries? What stands in the way of greater success in this area?
13. What is the world distribution of common goiter? Is there a proved method of control and how successful has it been?
14. What steps might be or are being taken toward earlier diagnosis or detection of mild forms of nutritional failure?

## References

1. Berg A: The Nutrition Factor: Its Role in National Development. Washington, DC, Brookings Institute, 1973
2. Bengoa JM: WHO Chron 28:3, 1974
3. Pan American Health Organization: Patterns of Mortality in Childhood. Scientific Publ. No. 262. Washington, DC, 1973

4. Bengoa JM: In Berg A, Scrimshaw NS, Call DL (eds): Nutrition, National Development and Planning, pp 103–125. Cambridge, MIT Press, 1973

5. Toro J: In Mayer J, Dwyer JT (eds): Food and Nutrition Policy in a Changing World, pp 33–66. New York, Oxford Press, 1979

6. Latham M: In World Food Issues. Ithaca, Cornell University, 1979

7. McLaren DS: Lancet 2:93, 1974

8. Kimm S: In Mayer and Dwyer, Food and Nutrition Policy, pp 155–177

9. Williams CD: Lancet 2:1151, 1935

10. WHO Chron 27:487, 1973

11. Mitchell HS: J Am Diet Assoc 44:165, 1964

12. WHO Chron 27:276, 1974

13. Williams C: Cajanus 7:37, Feb, 1974

14. WHO Chron 27:28, 1973

15. WHO/USAID: Vitamin A deficiency and xerophthalmia. WHO Tech Rep Ser, no. 590. Geneva, World Health Organization, 1976

16. Zaklama MS et al: Am J Clin Nutr 26:1202, 1973

17. Oomen HAPC: Nutr Rev 32:161, 1974

18. International Vitamin A Consultative Group: Guidelines for the Eradication of Vitamin A Deficiency and Xerophthalmia. New York, Nutrition Foundation, 1980

19. Williams RR: Toward the Conquest of Beriberi. Cambridge, Harvard University Press, 1961

20. Scrimshaw NS: N Engl J Med 272:137, 1965

21. Gubbay ER: Can Med Assoc J 95:21, 1966

22. Review: Nutr Rev 39:237, 1981

23. Victor M, Adams RD: Am J Clin Nutr 9:379, 1961

24. Williams RR: J Am Diet Assoc 36:31, 1960

25. Roe DA: A Plague of Corn: The Social History of Pellagra. Ithaca, Cornell University Press, 1973

26. Joint FAO/WHO Expert Committee: Requirements of vitamin A, thaimine, riboflavin and niacin. WHO Tech Rep Ser, no. 362. Geneva, World Health Organization, 1967

27. Demers P et al: Can Med Assoc J 93:573, 1965

28. Harrison HE: Am J Public Health 56:734, 1966

29. Report: Pediatrics 29:646, 1962

30. Joint FAO/WHO Expert Committee: Nutrition—Seventh report. WHO Tech Rep Ser, no. 377. Geneva, World Health Organization, 1967

31. Dallman PR: Iron Deficiency in Infancy and Childhood. Washington, DC, USAID, 1979

32. Stanbury JB et al: WHO Chron 28:220, 1974

33. Perez C et al: Technique of endemic goitre surveys. In Endemic Goitre, pp 369–383. WHO Monogr Ser, no. 44. Geneva, World Health Organization, 1960

34. Potter JD et al: Int J Epidemiol 8:137, 1979

35. Ermans AM et al: Role of Cassava in the Etiology of Endemic Goitre and Cretinism. Ottawa, International Development Center, 1980

36. Dunning JM: N Engl J Med 272:30, 84, 1965

37. Rusoff LL et al: Am J Clin Nutr 11:94, 1962

*For further references see Bibliography in Part 4.*

## Supplementary readings

Berg A: The Nutrition Factor: Its Role in National Development. Washington, DC, Brookings Institute, 1973

Berg A, Scrimshaw NS, Call DL (eds): Nutrition, National Development and Planning. Cambridge, MIT Press, 1973

Chandra RK: Immunodeficiency in undernutrition and overnutrition. Nutr Rev 39:225, 1981

FAO/WHO: Handbook on human nutritional requirements. FAO Nutritional Studies no. 28. WHO Monogr Ser, no. 61. Rome, FAO, 1974

Food Composition Tables: Updated Annotated Bibliography. Rome, FAO of the U.N., 1975

Mayer J, Dwyer JT (eds): Food and Nutrition Policy in a Changing World. New York, Oxford University Press, 1979

McClure FJ: Water Fluoridation. Bethesda, DHEW, National Institutes of Health, National Institute of Dental Research, 1970

Olson RE (ed): Protein-Calorie Malnutrition. New York, Academic Press, 1975

Oomen HAPC: Vitamin A deficiency, xerophthalmia and blindness. Nutr Rev 33:161, 1974

Raphael D (ed): Breastfeeding and Food Policy in a Hungry World. New York, Academic Press, 1979

Review: Depression of serum levels of retinol and retinol binding protein during infection. Nutr Rev 39:165, 1981

Roe, DA: A Plague of Corn: The Social History of Pellagra. Ithaca, Cornell University Press, 1973

Solomons NW, Keusch GT: Nutritional implications of parasitic infections. Nutr Rev 39:149, 1981

Stansbury JB et al: Endemic goiter and cretinism: Public health significance and prevention. WHO Chron 28:220, 1974

WHO/USAID: Vitamin A deficiency and xerophthalmia. WHO Tech Rep Ser, no. 590. Geneva, World Health Organization, 1976

Winikoff B: Nutrition and National Policy. Cambridge, MIT Press, 1978

*For further references see Bibliography in Part 4.*

# Diet in Disease

# Part 3

# Nutritional Care and Diet Therapy for the Hospitalized Patient

# 22

The Registered Dietitian
Hospital Organization for Nutritional Care
Classification of Dietary Modifications
Quality Assurance
Professional Standards of Practice

The community general hospital is viewed today not only as a medical care facility but also as a community center for health education. Therefore, the food served to patients in the hospital should exemplify proper meal planning for the community as well as provide for the nutritional needs of each patient. At the same time, well prepared and attractively served food acceptable to the majority of patients enhances the hospital's image in the community.

## The registered dietitian

The registered dietitian (RD) has been educated in the science and art of human nutrition to assume responsibility for the nutritional care of individuals and groups; she has successfully completed the registration examination and maintains registration through participating in approved continuing education activities.

As defined by the American Dietetic Association[1] the:

*Administrative dietitian* is a member of the management team (of a hospital or other health care facility) and affects the nutritional care of groups through the management of food service systems that provide optimum nutrition and quality food; the *clinical dietitian* is a member of the health care team and affects the nutritional care of individuals and groups for health maintenance. The clinical dietitian assesses nutritional care plans, and evaluates these results appropriately. When functioning in an organization that provides food service, the clinical dietitian cooperates and coordinates activities with those of the department's management team.

In large hospitals in the United States menu planning, food purchasing and preparation, and the delivery of meals to the clinical units are directed by a qualified administrative dietitian, whereas the clinical dietitian is the primary nutrition counselor in the health-care team. She is prepared to enter into the helping relationship (see

**JCAH:** Joint Commission on Accreditation of Hospitals
**PSRO:** Professional Standards Review Organization
**RD:** Registered Dietitian

Chap. 13) with a patient to assist him in modifying his usual food choices as part of the treatment of his medical problem. The clinical dietitian may interact with patients in the in-patient or out-patient facilities of a hospital, in a health maintenance organization, in a neighborhood health center, or in any other medical care setting. She may share her *functions* with, or delegate them to, another member of the health-care team, such as the physician, nurse, nurse practitioner, social worker, dietetic technician or aide, or the home health aide. However, the therapeutic dietitian is never privileged to delegate her *responsibility* for the quality of nutritional care of any patient to another member of the team.

With the knowledge explosion in both management science and in food, nutrition, and related biomedical sciences, the nutritional care of patients in large hospitals today requires the expertise of both the administrator of dietetic services and the clinical dietitian. Together these two members of the dietetics profession plan and implement the nutritional care of patients. At the same time all the members of the health-care team, including dietitians, must coordinate their services for the comfort and satisfaction of the patient. For example, interrupting a 4-year-old child's lunch to draw blood can be as hazardous to his nutritional care as serving an inadequate diet; or serving breakfast trays a half hour later than scheduled can disrupt a variety of treatment schedules for many of the patients in a clinical unit. Communication and cooperation among patient-care services are achieved most effectively by a patient nutritional care committee that is responsible for establishing routines that best serve the patient.

## Hospital organization for nutritional care
### The diet order

A patient's diet prescription is ordered by his physician and can be found in the orders written by him at the time the patient is admitted to the hospital. The order that the physician writes depends on the patient's condition and may vary from nothing by mouth (NPO, *nil per oris*) to a normal or regular diet. The diet order is changed as the patient's condition changes. If he is known to have a disease that requires the modification of his diet as a part of his treatment, or if diagnostic procedures during hospitalization indicate a disease that can be treated by diet therapy, a therapeutic diet will be ordered.

In most but not all instances, the patient with a prescription for a therapeutic diet requires counseling prior to discharge from the hospital so that he can manage this aspect of his treatment at home. To avoid inadequate initial counseling, those who are working with the patient must anticipate his discharge and consult the physician about his plans for the patient. Some physicians anticipate discharge when they write the therapeutic diet prescrip-

tion, for example, "diabetic diet and instruct for discharge." In any situation, counseling begins with the interpretation of the diet prescription to the patient when the physician writes the order.

The physician is legally responsible for the patient's medical care plan, including the diet order. He may delegate the formulation of the diet order to the clinical dietitian or he may formulate the prescription in consultation with the dietitian. However, he cannot delegate his ultimate responsibility for the order to the dietitian or to any other member of the team. If the clinical dietitian is to participate in the formulation of the diet order, she is responsible for familiarizing herself with the patient's medical problem before making any decisions or recommendations about the order. At the same time the dietitian is responsible for keeping up with current theory and practice of therapeutic dietetics.

### The diet manual

The diet manual is a compilation of routine and therapeutic diet plans and includes an explanation of the rationale for each plan. It is used to facilitate communication by the members of the health-care team. The manual serves as a guide to the kinds and amounts of foods and beverages the dietary department provides to fulfill the patient's diet order. A copy of the manual used by a hospital is usually available in each clinical unit for the convenience of doctors and nurses. Under Medicare, in the Conditions of Participation for Hospitals, the dietary department is required to have an up-to-date manual, which has been approved jointly by the medical and dietary staffs.

In teaching hospitals and in many large hospitals, physicians, dietitians, and other members of the health-care team working together in committee frequently compile a diet manual for use in their institutions. In some communities a committee of physicians and dietitians representing all the hospitals compile a manual for community-wide use. Many of these diet manuals are available for purchase. Diet manuals have also been compiled by state or district dietetic associations or by state health or welfare agencies for use by small hospitals, extended-care facilities, and nursing homes (see partial list of diet manuals at the end of this chapter).

As a general rule, the first section of a manual describes routine diet plans for infants, children, and adults, including soft and liquid diet plans. Subsequent sections describe a variety of therapeutic diets used in the treatment of disease, test diets required by certain diagnostic procedures, and food composition tables. Diet manuals often differ in terms used to describe diets and in the recommendations for the foods used in a diet plan. These differences reflect variations in interpretation of theory relating to therapeutic dietetics or regional or cultural variations in food acceptance.

## The patient's medical record

A record or chart for each hospitalized patient is available in the clinical unit. These charts have been standardized by the American Hospital Association and include demographic data obtained on admission—the patient's name, address, sex, age, physician, admitting or provisional diagnosis, and so on; graphic data—temperature, pulse, respiration, and fluid intake and output; nursing notes—reports of treatment procedures, food acceptance, and any expression of psychosocial problems, either observed by the nurse or verbally communicated to her by the patient or his relatives and friends; the medical history elicited by the physician, the diagnosis, and the physician's daily progress notes; laboratory data and x-ray reports; reports of any operative procedures; and consultants' comments and progress notes. The patient's orders may be a part of his chart during hospitalization, or the orders for all patients in a clinical unit may be kept in one folder or notebook in the unit office. The patient's record is available to all qualified professional personnel working with the patient; all personnel are equally responsible for sharing information and *protecting the confidentiality* of this information.

The dietitian's notes are recorded on a page identified by the hospital Records Committee. Because the medical record is a legal document, any note should be *legible*, in the *third* person, *concise*, and *factual*, with no expression of opinion or judgment of the patient's behavior. For example, noting that the patient "cheats on his diet" reflects a judgment. A more appropriate recording is: "The patient is unable to manage his diet because . . .," followed by an identification of the reason for his behavior, such as "he cannot afford to purchase food required" or "he does not understand reason for therapeutic diet." The notes should include the patient's diet history, acceptance or rejection of food, food intolerances, diet order and any therapeutic diet plan, progress, and counseling notes. If the physician is using the problem-oriented medical record system in his daily progress notes, it is advisable for the dietitian to use the same problem identification in labeling her notes, and use the SOAP format (Subjective, Objective, Assessment, and Plan).[3,4]

## Food service

### Food service management systems

Two management systems are used in hospitals today. Under one system the hospital administers all aspects of the dietary department, including both the nutritional care of patients and employee food service. All the members of the dietary department staff are employees of the hospital, and the director of the department is directly responsible to the hospital administrator or one of his assistants.

Under a second system the hospital contracts with a food service or catering company to manage all aspects of the dietary department. In many situations all employees of the dietary department including the dietitians are employees of the food service company. However, it would seem advisable for the clinical dietitian to be an employee of the hospital because her counseling services to patients are not in all instances directly related to daily food service; for example, the dietitian giving service in the ambulatory care clinics of the hospital, or the one who is a member of the team in a clinical research center. Either system, properly managed, can provide quality food service to patients and employees and expert dietary counseling to both inpatients and outpatients.

### Food service delivery systems

Two types of food delivery systems, centralized and decentralized, are used to deliver food to the patient area. In centralized service, a patient's tray is completely assembled in or near the food production area and delivered to the patient area in a specially designed cart or by a conveyor system or dumbwaiter. The tray is delivered to the patient directly from the cart or from a service pantry.

Decentralized service refers to the method by which bulk food is transported from the production area to a service kitchen in the patient area. The patient's tray is assembled in the service kitchen and delivered to the bedside. Either system requires that nursing and dietary departments carefully coordinate their schedules so that patients receive palatable, attractive food.

In some hospitals the patient's tray is delivered to the bedside by a dietary department employee, in others by an employee of the nursing service. In either situation the individual who delivers the tray needs to know of any recent change in the patient's status, and must be informed if meals are to be delayed or omitted for tests and treatments. Errors of this type in the delivery of trays can add to the discomfort of the patient and the cost of medical care by increasing the time the patient is required to stay in the hospital. At the same time any personnel responsible for the delivery of the tray to the patient must be trained to help the patient and to protect both himself and the patient from infection.

### Selective menus

The hospital patient is offered a daily menu from which he can select his meals. Two or more items in each section of the menu are usually offered; for example, at dinner there may be choice of roast beef or fried chicken, mashed or baked potato. The printed menus are marked by the patient each day, usually for service the next day. In some hospitals menu items for soft and liquid diets may also be included on the regular diet menu (see the following section, *"Progressive Hospital Diets"*).

Selective menus, even when selections are limited, have improved patient food acceptance. Patients with poor vision or who cannot read need assistance. All selective menus need to be evaluated daily to ensure adequate nutrient intake by the patient. The patient who consistently selects a less-than-adequate diet needs professional guidance.

In some but not all hospitals, the patient requiring a therapeutic diet is also offered a selective menu. This patient must be guided by the dietitian so that his menu selections fulfill his diet plan. This system provides the dietitian with the opportunity to guide the patient early in his hospital stay to become familiar with his therapeutic diet and to counsel the patient appropriately. The selective menu can serve as a "paper and pencil test" of a patient's knowledge of his therapeutic diet and identify for the dietitian, as counseling progresses, areas where reinforcement is needed.

## Progressive hospital diets
### Regular, standard, general diet

Various terms are in current use to describe the normal hospital diet, which provides a patient with the energy and nutrients he needs. This diet is intended for the patient whose condition does not require a therapeutic diet. The pattern dietary, Table 22-1, reproduced here for the convenience of the reader (see Chap. 11), illustrates the basic pattern used to plan the regular hospital diet. This pattern furnishes the nutrients needed to meet the NAS-NRC Recommended Dietary Allowances for an adult, with the exception of calories and iron.

It is expected that additional items will be chosen from the selective menu to meet a patient's needs for calories. A limited number of items, such as milk and sugar for coffee and a cookie served with canned fruit for dessert, need to be added to this 1400-calorie diet plan for an older patient, who requires 1600 to 1700 calories per day. On the other hand, a patient requiring 2400 calories per day may select more bread or rolls and butter, a simple dessert, and a larger serving of meat to meet his energy needs. In any situation it is well to remember that some patients may require fewer calories than usual because even ambulatory patients are less active during hospitalization than they are at home or at work.

The nutritional adequacy of a regular diet depends not only on the patient's selection of foods and the amount served but also on the protection of the nutrients in food during preparation and cooking, including the time and temperature of these processes (see Chap. 12). The foods chosen for the regular diet reflect the preferences characteristic of the cultural background and the economic status of the majority of those served by the institution. For example, two hospitals may serve the same cut of beef, one as pot roast and the other as sauerbraten. The choice of food is further determined by its suitability for quality and quantity of preparation, its availability, and current market costs and conditions.

The regular diet may be modified with regard to selection, methods of preparation, and consistency for patients who cannot tolerate a regular diet but do not require a therapeutic diet. These modifications of the regular diet are the *light or convalescent diet*; the *soft diet*, including the surgical soft, medical soft, and dental soft diets; and the *full liquid* and *clear liquid diets*. Table 22-2, *Foods Used in Progressive Hospital Diets*, illustrates the types of food included in regular, light, soft, and full liquid diets; and Table 22-3, *Typical Menus for Progressive Hospital Diets*, illustrates how these foods are used in menu plans.

### The light, or convalescent, diet

A light, or convalescent, diet is intended for convalescent patients not yet able to tolerate the regular diet and for those with minor illnesses. It must be appetizing and readily digested. The chief difference between this diet and the regular diet is the method of preparation. The foods are cooked simply, and fried foods and rich pastries are omitted. Other fatty foods, such as nuts, avocado, and salad dressing, are avoided. Bran and strong or gas-forming vegetables are to be avoided, as well as most raw vegetables and fruits. All foods included in the soft and the liquid diets may be served on the light diet. In some hospitals this classification is omitted.

### The soft diet

The soft diet is soft in texture and consists of liquids and semisolid foods. It is an intermediate step between the liquid and the light or regular diets. It is indicated in certain postoperative cases, in acute infections, and in some gastrointestinal conditions; also, it may be ordered for the debilitated patient because it is easy to eat.

The soft diet is low in residue and is readily digested. Few or no spices or condiments are used in the preparation. It is somewhat more restricted than the light diet in fruit, meat, and vegetables.

The foods included in the medical soft diet are generally the same as those in the soft diet in Table 22-2. In the surgical soft diet tougher meats and certain vegetables and fruits may be puréed or blenderized.

### The dental or mechanical soft diet

The regular diet may need modification for patients with poor teeth or none, or with dentures which they are unable or unwilling to wear. Additional cooked vegetables or juices should be substituted for salads, and no whole meats should be served, unless the physician approves of the patient's eating whole tender meats. Otherwise the diet should follow the foods used in the light diet.

### The full liquid diet

The liquid diet is usually prescribed for the postoperative patient, or the patient acutely ill with an infection, a gastrointestinal tract disturbance, or a myocardial infarction. See Table 22-2 for the kinds of fluids used and Table 22-3 for a suggested menu.

## The clear liquid diet

If the patient's condition requires it, only clear fluids may be offered him. In addition to water, clear broth, fruit juices, thin gruels made with water, plain gelatin, and tea and coffee are generally used. Carbonated beverages may or may not be included, depending on the policy set by the physicians and dietitians. In some hospitals simple solids, such as plain crackers or dry toast, are served with the clear liquid diet.

***Special problems with liquid diet.*** Both the clear and the full liquid diets are low in nutritive value. The clear liquid diet is used for only limited periods of time, usually no longer than 24 to 36 hours. When the full liquid diet must be given for a period of time, special attention must be provided to improve its nutritive value. Skim milk powder, protein supplements, cream, and sugars may be used to increase its protein and calorie content.

Patients receiving liquid diets will require a feeding every 2 to 3 hours during the day and evening. When it is not possible for the dietary department personnel to serve these patients other than at regularly scheduled mealtimes, nurses have found it helpful to remind themselves of a patient's need for an interval feeding by noting this at the proper time interval in the nursing care plan. Also, when the dietitian or nurse observes that a patient is ready for more than a liquid diet, either one can tactfully suggest this to the physician so that he will revise the patient's diet order.

## Fluid intake

Fluids are essential to all body functions and must be provided by foods and beverages each day (see Chap. 5). Unless the physician prescribes otherwise, adult patients should drink 1000 ml to 1500 ml of fluid per day as beverages served with meals and as water available in the patient's unit. Some patients need to be reminded to drink

## Table 22-1. Evaluation of a Pattern Dietary for Its Nutritive Content

| Food Group | Amount in g | Household Measure | Energy (kcal) | Pro-tein (g) | Fat (g) | Carbo-hydrate (g) | Cal-cium (mg) | Phos-phorus (mg) | Magne-sium (mg) | Iron (mg) | A (IU) | Thia-min (mg) | Ribo-flavin (mg) | Niacin (mg NE) | Ascorbic Acid (mg) |
|---|---|---|---|---|---|---|---|---|---|---|---|---|---|---|---|
| Milk or equivalent* | 488 | 2 c (1 pint) | 320 | 17 | 17 | 24 | 576 | 452 | 63 | 0.2 | 700 | 0.16 | 0.84 | 0.3 | 5 |
| Meat, fish, poultry, or egg† | 120 | 4 oz, cooked | 376 | 30 | 31 | | 13 | 212 | 104 | 3.3 | 280 | 0.14 | 0.23 | 6.1 | |
| Vegetables: | | | | | | | | | | | | | | | |
| Potato, cooked | 100 | 1 medium | 65 | 2 | | 15 | 6 | 48 | 22 | 0.5 | | 0.09 | 0.03 | 1.2 | 16 |
| Deep green or yellow, cooked‡ | 75 | ½ c | 21 | 2 | | 6 | 44 | 28 | 29 | 0.9 | 4700 | 0.05 | 0.10 | 0.5 | 25 |
| Other, raw or cooked§ | 75 | ½ c | 45 | 2 | | 10 | 16 | 41 | 18 | 0.9 | 300 | 0.08 | 0.06 | 0.6 | 12 |
| Fruits: | | | | | | | | | | | | | | | |
| Citrus‖ | 100 | 1 serving | 44 | 1 | | 10 | 18 | 16 | 12 | 0.3 | 140 | 0.06 | 0.02 | 0.3 | 43 |
| Other# | 100 | 1 serving | 85 | | | 22 | 10 | 21 | 16 | 0.8 | 365 | 0.03 | 0.04 | 0.5 | 4 |
| Bread, white, enriched | 100 | 4 slices | 270 | 9 | 3 | 50 | 84 | 97 | 20 | 2.5 | | 0.25 | 0.21 | 2.4 | |
| Cereal, whole grain or enriched** | 130 / 30 | ⅔ c cooked or 1 oz dry | 89 | 3 | 1 | 18 | 12 | 95 | 34 | 0.9 | | 0.08 | 0.03 | 0.7 | |
| Butter or margarine | 14 | 1 tbsp | 100 | | 11 | | 3 | 2 | 2 | | 460 | | | | |
| Totals | | | 1415 | 66 | 63 | 155 | 782 | 1012 | 335 | 10.3 | 6945 | 0.94 | 1.56 | 12.6†† | 105 |
| Compare with recommended allowances‡‡ | | | | | | | | | | | | | | | |
| Men (70 kg, 23–50 yrs old) | | | 2700 | 56 | | | 800 | 800 | 350 | 10.0 | 5000§§ | 1.40 | 1.60 | 18 | 60 |
| Women (55 kg, 23–50 yrs old) | | | 2000 | 44 | | | 800 | 800 | 300 | 18.0 | 4000‖‖ | 1.00 | 1.20 | 13 | 60 |

*Milk equivalents mean evaporated milk and dried milk in amounts equivalent to fluid milk in nutritive content; cheese, if water-soluble minerals and vitamins have not been lost in whey; and food items made with milk.

†Evaluation based on the use of 700 g of beef (chuck, cooked), 200 g of pork (medium fat, roasted), 200 g of chicken (roaster, cooked, roasted), and 100 g of fish (halibut, cooked, broiled) per 10-day period, and egg occasionally.

‡Evaluation based on figures for cooked broccoli, carrots, spinach, and squash (all varieties).

§Evaluation based on figures for raw tomatoes and lettuce, and cooked peas, beets, lima beans, and fresh corn.

‖Evaluation based on figures for whole orange and grapefruit, and orange and grapefruit juices.

#Evaluation based on figures for banana, apple, unsweetened cooked prunes, and sweetened canned peaches.

**Evaluation based on figures for shredded wheat biscuit and oatmeal.

††The average diet in the United States, which contains a generous amount of protein, provides enough tryptophan to increase the niacin value by about one-third.

‡‡From the National Research Council Recommended Dietary Allowances, revised 1980.

§§5000 IU equals 100 RE.

‖‖4000 IU equals 800 RE.

(From Composition of Foods. Handbook No. 8. USDA, revised 1963)

this quantity because their usual routines—coffee breaks, stopping for a drink each time they pass a water fountain, having a glass of beer or carbonated beverage at bedtime—have been interrupted by hospitalization.

In situations where fluid intake is critical and the daily amount of oral fluid intake is defined in the physician's orders for a patient, close communication between dietary and nursing services is required to carry out the

**Table 22-2. Foods Used in Progressive Hospital Diets**

| Type of Food | Regular Diet | Light Diet | Soft Diet | Full Liquid Diet |
|---|---|---|---|---|
| Fruits | All | All cooked and canned fruits, citrus fruits, bananas | Fruit juices, cooked and canned fruits (without seeds, coarse skins or fiber), bananas | Fruit juices, strained |
| Cereals and cereal products | All | Cereals: dry or well-cooked, spaghetti and macaroni, not highly seasoned | Same as light diet | Gruels, strained or blended |
| Breads | All | Enriched and whole-wheat bread, crackers | Same as light diet | |
| Soups and broths | All | All | Broth, strained cream soups | Same as soft diet, or blended |
| Meat, fish, and poultry | All | Tender steaks and chops, lamb, veal, ground or tender beef, pork, chicken, sweetbreads, liver, fish | Tender chicken, fish and sweetbreads, beef, lamb, and pork | |
| Eggs | Eggs cooked all ways | Soft-cooked eggs | Same as light diet | Eggnog* |
| Dairy products | Milk or buttermilk; cream; butter; cheese, all kinds | Milk or buttermilk; cream, butter, cottage and cream cheese, cheddar cheese used in cooking | Same as light diet | Milk or buttermilk, cream |
| Vegetables | All, including salads | Cooked vegetables: asparagus, peas, string beans, spinach, carrots, beets, squash | Cooked vegetables: same as light diet | Vegetable juices |
| | | Salads: tomato and lettuce | Salads: none | |
| | | Potatoes: boiled, mashed, creamed, scalloped, baked | Potatoes: same as light diet | |
| Desserts | All | Ices, ice cream, junket, cereal puddings, custard, gelatin, simple cakes, plain cookies | Same as light diet | Ices, ice cream, gelatin, junket and custard |
| Beverages | All | Tea, coffee, cocoa; coffee substitutes; milk and milk beverages; carbonated beverages | Same as light diet | Same as light diet |

*Because of the danger of salmonella infection when raw egg is used, a pasteurized commercial eggnog preparation is recommended.

order for fluids and, at the same time, satisfy the patient. Water is not a popular beverage in our society today, and the order to force fluids to 3000 ml per day may be difficult to achieve without the use of coffee, tea, fruit juices, or carbonated beverages between meals, in addition to fluids served with meals. The problem is even more critical for the patient in chronic renal failure when fluid intake is limited to 500 ml or 800 ml per day. This patient usually wants as much fluid with his meals as possible within the limitations of any concurrent sodium and potassium restrictions, whereas the nursing service needs some water for administering medications. In this situation the dietitian and the nurse must work together with the patient to carry out the order for fluids and to satisfy the patient. Where applicable, critical problems of fluid intake, other than infection, are discussed in succeeding chapters.

### Infection

In patients with acute infection, excessive fluid loss may occur through the skin and lungs and the gastrointestinal tract (diarrhea), which can result in dehydration if the fluid is not replaced. Electrolyte depletion or retention can also occur. Severe dehydration with electrolyte imbalance can lead to death. Asiatic cholera is a dramatic example; this infection produces a sudden, massive diarrhea, which within a few hours leads to shock (hypovolemia) and death.

### Table 22-3.  Typical Menus for Progressive Hospital Diets

| Regular Diet | Light Diet | Soft Diet | Full Liquid Diet |
|---|---|---|---|
| | | Breakfast | |
| Fresh pear | Orange | Orange juice | Orange juice, strained |
| Oatmeal with milk or cream | Oatmeal with milk or cream | Oatmeal with milk or cream | Strained oatmeal gruel with milk or cream |
| Scrambled eggs | Soft scrambled eggs | Soft scrambled eggs | Coffee with cream and sugar |
| Buttered whole-wheat toast | Buttered whole wheat toast | Buttered whole-wheat toast | 10 A.M. |
| Coffee with cream and sugar  . | Coffee with cream and sugar | Coffee with cream and sugar | Eggnog* |
| | | Dinner | |
| Vegetable soup | Vegetable soup | Strained vegetable soup | Broth |
| Roast veal | Roast veal | Ground veal | Ginger ale with ice cream |
| Mashed potato | Mashed potato | Mashed potato | Coffee with cream and sugar |
| Buttered carrots | Buttered carrots | Buttered carrots | 3 P.M. |
| Tomato salad with French dressing | Tomato salad with French dressing | Bread: whole-wheat or white | Malted milk or buttermilk |
| Bread: whole-wheat, rye, or white | Bread: whole-wheat, rye, or white | Butter | |
| Butter | Butter | Vanilla ice cream with chocolate sauce | |
| Peppermint stick ice cream | Peppermint stick ice cream | Milk | |
| Milk | Milk | | |
| | | Supper | |
| Cream of pea soup with crackers | Cream of pea soup with crackers | Cream of pea soup with crackers | Strained cream of pea soup |
| Macaroni au gratin | Macaroni au gratin | Macaroni au gratin | Plain gelatin with whipped topping |
| Head lettuce salad with Russian dressing | Head lettuce salad with French dressing | Buttered beets | Tea with cream and sugar |
| Bread | Bread | Bread | 9 P.M. |
| Butter | Butter | Butter | Hot cocoa |
| Fruit gelatin | Fruit gelatin | Plain gelatin with whipped topping | |
| Tea with cream and sugar | Tea with cream and sugar | Tea with cream and sugar | |

*See note, Table 22-2.

Severe dehydration due to infection is usually treated by intravenous fluids (dextrose and water or electrolyte solutions or both). At this stage many patients cannot tolerate fluids by mouth. When oral fluids are tolerated, not only water but broth, tea, coffee, carbonated beverages, fruit and vegetable juices, and milk should be offered. These beverages, in addition to adding variety, also contribute to the patient's electrolyte intake (100 g canned tomato juice contains approximately 200 mg sodium and 227 mg potassium; see Tables 1 and 4, Part 4). Most of these fluids also contribute to the patient's carbohydrate intake.

In addition to fluid and electrolyte loss, an elevation in body temperature is always accompanied by an increase in metabolism. In most febrile conditions (acute or chronic) the basal metabolic rate is increased 7% for each degree Fahrenheit rise in temperature (12% for each degree Centigrade). As a result, the carbohydrate stores are quickly exhausted, and body protein and fat are used for energy if insufficient food is eaten. As soon as the patient with an infection can tolerate food as well as fluids, he should be assisted in selecting food that will meet his energy and other nutrient needs.

## Classification of dietary modifications

Diet therapy is the component of the treatment of a patient with an acute or chronic disease that involves the modification of food intake. It may be the primary mode of therapy, such as the energy-restricted diet for uncomplicated obesity. It may be used in conjunction with therapeutic agents, such as diet combined with insulin to treat diabetes. Or, diet therapy may support other modes of treatment, such as the progression from a liquid to a regular diet following surgery.

Traditionally, therapeutic diets have been classified according to the disease being treated—for example, diabetic diet, cardiac diet, ulcer diet, renal diet. These labels indicate a patient's diagnosis but do not indicate the nutritional problem associated with the disease process or the modification in food or nutrient intake required in the treatment of the disease. Moreover, these labels do not indicate the nutritional problems which may be common to a number of diseases. The patient with the renal complications that may occur in long-standing diabetes, the patient with the renal complications of severe cardiac failure, and the patient with primary renal disease all have similar problems with the excretion of the end products of protein metabolism and with fluid and electrolyte balance. All of these patients require some modification of their protein, fluid, sodium, and, in many situations, potassium intake.

The patient's diagnosis continues to be the primary focus of the physician's medical plan of care, although those physicians who are using the problem-oriented patient record may also identify the nutritional problem.[2] For example, hyperglycemia is often one of the problems listed in the physician's progress notes for the patient with diabetes. As this trend of physicians identifying the nutritional problem continues, the labeling of therapeutic diets today and in the future should reflect the modifications of food and nutrient intake required to treat the problem, not the disease *per se.* Although the chapter headings in this section appear to contradict this statement, the food and nutrient modifications required to treat the nutritional problems associated with diseases are presented at the beginning of each chapter.

Therapeutic diets may be modified in consistency or bulk, in energy content, or in the kinds and amounts of nutrients, such as protein, fat, carbohydrate, minerals, vitamins, and fluids and electrolytes.

### Consistency or bulk

Foods are modified in consistency or bulk for patients with difficulty in chewing and swallowing and with diseases of the gastrointestinal tract, such as peptic ulcer, diarrhea, or constipation. Modification in consistency may vary from a liquid diet administered by nasogastric tube to a diet of well cooked food. Modification in bulk may vary from a diet totally devoid of fiber to a diet high in fiber (nondigestible residue). See the discussion of fiber in foods in Chapter 2, *Carbohydrates.*

### Energy

The energy content of a diet is modified for overweight (overfat) and underweight patients. The obese patient requires a diet restricted in energy but adequate in all nutrients. The underweight patient requires an increase in energy intake with a reasonable distribution of protein, fat, and carbohydrate and adequate amounts of minerals and vitamins. In many complex situations the energy content of the diet pattern must be given the same consideration as other nutrients. For example, in chronic renal failure the basal energy needs must be met. Otherwise amino acids will be deaminized to provide carbon units for the citric acid cycle and the nitrogen from such amino acids will contribute to the amount of urea the kidney has to excrete (see Chap. 9).

The chronically ill older person living alone or the disturbed person admitted to the psychiatric unit often requires total nutritional rehabilitation, including an increased energy intake. These patients may also be dehydrated as well as underfed and require rehydration as well as a diet adequate in calories and all nutrients.

Modification in energy intake is also used as a preventive measure. Any adult who reduces his energy expenditure for any reason requires a decrease in energy intake. For most adult patients hospitalization reduces energy expenditure.

## Kinds and amounts of nutrients

The kinds and amounts of nutrients are modified when problems of nutrient utilization occur. Problems involving the digestive-absorptive process occur frequently. Interference with the flow of bile into the duodenum usually requires a modification in the amount and, in some situations, the kind of fat intake. Total fat intake may be reduced, or medium chain triglycerides may be substituted for long chain ones. Patients who have an insufficient amount, or a total lack, of the digestive enzyme, lactase, require a diet reduced in the amount, or totally devoid, of the disaccharide, lactose.

Problems of nutrient utilization in intermediary metabolism require a variety of modifications. In the diet of the patient with diabetes mellitus the amount of protein and the amount and kinds of fat and carbohydrate are modified to achieve a reasonable level of blood glucose and lipids. For the infant with phenylketonuria, the amount of the essential amino acid phenylalanine is restricted to meet the minimum need for this essential nutrient. Such an infant is unable to metabolize excessive amounts of phenylalanine through the tyrosine pathway due to a lack of the enzyme phenylalanine hydroxylase.

Problems in the utilization of lipids also occur. The polyunsaturated fatty acid composition of a diet may be increased and saturated fatty acid decreased either to prevent or to treat patients with atherosclerosis; the amount of cholesterol in a diet is reduced in the treatment of a patient with familial hypercholesterolemia.

Problems also occur in fluid and electrolyte balance and in the excretion of the end products of metabolism. The patient in chronic renal failure faces both problems. He requires a diet restricted in fluid, electrolytes, and protein. However, the food selected to supply the limited amount of protein must contain protein of high biological value to provide the essential amino acids needed by the patient; it must also limit the nonessential amino acids to reduce the amount of nitrogen to be excreted by the kidneys.

Whatever the modification, care must be taken to ensure the nutritional adequacy of the therapeutic diet. When such a diet cannot for any reason provide an adequate intake of vitamins and minerals, the physician should be informed so that he can supplement the diet with vitamin and mineral preparations.

## Quality assurance

### Rosita Schiller

*Quality assurance* is a relatively new term in the vocabulary of health professionals that can be attributed to dynamic and potentially opposing forces at work in the United States during the 1970s. Many new health specialties emerged, each responsible for a smaller but increasingly complex segment of health care, resulting in a sharp rise in the cost of care and the fragmentation of services. At the same time, consumer advocates fought to protect the rights of the consumers of health-care services. Quality assurance programs have been established as a universal remedy for these and many other problems in the health-care delivery system. We can address the complexities of these programs by posing several questions.

*What is quality care?* Generally, the term *quality care* implies that appropriate patient care will be provided by competent and qualified health-care personnel using acceptable procedures and up-to-date technology to achieve the desired outcome. Standards for quality care, such as diagnosis, treatment, and length of hospitalization, have been established for each disease category as listed in the International Classification of Disease, Clinical Modification[5] with contingency sets of standards to be used when complications occur. Although quality care may be an inclusive term, its application differs from one patient to another depending on each one's needs.

*Who determines quality?* Only those familiar with the complex nature of diseases, diagnostic tests, and professional services can set standards of quality. Physicians must agree on the specifications of quality medical care; nurses set standards for quality nursing care; registered dietitians are responsible for determining what is quality nutritional care.

In some hospitals "interdisciplinary" committees, including representatives from several disciplines, set the standards of quality care. Usually physicians chair these committees, and input may be requested from other health-care professionals not represented. Generally, only minimum standards of quality are set by these committees, and only the fundamental aspects of care are included. As a result, the nutrition standards for quality care of a diabetic may simply require that a diet be prescribed and instruction given. It is the common practice among health-care professionals, including dietitians, to define in greater detail what they consider to be the elements of quality practice for their own profession. These standards are known as "monodisciplinary" because they are established and monitored by members of a single professional group.

*How is quality measured?* It is assumed that the components of acceptable care can be defined—that is, that requirements can be set for what should be done, who should do it, in what manner, and for what purpose. We also assume that it is possible to determine whether or not requirements are being met. Physicians, nurses, dietitians, and other health-care professionals have made great progress in determining how the quality of their services should be measured. There are two major types of evaluation: assessment of outcomes and assessment of professional practice.

One way to evaluate the quality of care is to measure

its outcomes, that is, effect of care on the patient. For example, if the medical problem is identified and treated with achievement of anticipated results, it is concluded that quality care was provided. If a cachectic patient achieves the desired weight gain in a given period, it is assumed that this occurred as a result of high-quality nutritional care. There are, however, some problems with this approach. When the goal is for a hospitalized patient to return to a normal state of health within a given length of time, but the goal is not achieved, can we say the patient has not been given quality care? Again, if a patient develops an unexplained symptom during the course of hospitalization, does it mean that proper care was lacking? If an obese patient fails to achieve anticipated weight loss, is the dietitian responsible? Since these types of questions create a sense of ambiguity and uncertainty, most dietitians evaluate quality care by other means.

The second method of assessing quality of care is to evaluate the "process" or "what is done" by physicians or other health-care personnel. This approach requires a listing of what *should* be done in every condition and in every type of circumstance. Thus, the quality of care is measured by comparing the actual performance with the acceptable standard of activity. It is argued, however, that evaluation of "process" places emphasis on the health-care professional—not on the patient. When everything is done according to established procedures, quality of care may not be questioned even if the condition of the patient deteriorates. For example, if a dietitian has instructed a patient on a diabetic diet and the patient later goes to the vending machine for a candy bar, only the process of diet counseling will be examined—not the factors which motivated the patient to eat candy. To ameliorate these difficulties, most institutions write their standards in such a way that quality is based on a combination of professional practice and patient outcomes.

Quality of care is evaluated by comparing actual performance with established standards. Elaborate procedures and forms are prepared to collect information about what was done and how patients responded. The data are then summarized and analyzed to determine if guidelines and procedures have been followed and if anticipated outcomes were achieved. This process is known as an *audit* and is discussed in further detail as it applies to nutritional care.

**What components of quality care are measured?**  Anything can be measured as long as there are standards established, and conformance with the standards can be observed either directly or by using documentation in the medical record or other written material. Some components that are routinely measured are use of hospital beds, length of hospitalization, types of professionals involved in the care of patients, use of addictive medications, surgical complications, patient education, infection control, use of diagnostic tests, and compliance with standard procedures.

In addition to nutritional assessment and diet counseling, the quality of dietetic services includes such things as the type, amount, and service of food to patients. In this case, standards relate to nutrient composition of foods served, methods for assessing patient satisfaction, accuracy of tray service, and availability of food outside scheduled mealtimes. Comprehensive nutritional care is highly dependent on effective administration. Accordingly, dietary departments also maintain standards related to sanitation, recipe standardization, cost control, organizational effectiveness, and production of menu items that conform to established standards of food quality.

In summary, dietary department standards include definitions of quality for three areas: (1) the process of providing services related to the management of nutritional care to patients; (2) the system of food services to meet the unique and diverse needs of the patient population; and (3) the administration of a department that supplies quality food at minimum cost. These areas are discussed further under "Standards of Practice."

**Who decides what will be audited?**  Most hospitals have designated a committee that is responsible for maintaining a quality assurance program within the institution. Such committees may be known as "Professional Standards," "Peer Review," "Quality Assurance" or similar titles. The committee may actually carry out the evaluation process, or it may coordinate the efforts of other review committees at the institution. When total care provided by all professionals is being evaluated, interdisciplinary or multidisciplinary teams may be appointed by the quality assurance committee to be responsible for setting standards and conducting audits. Another approach is for a single group of professionals (nurses, physical therapists, or dietitians) to engage in a monodisciplinary audit to review and evaluate their performance and the contribution that they make to the total care of the patient. These monodisciplinary groups also report to the committee that coordinates all efforts to monitor and improve quality care within the institution.

**Who monitors quality assurance?**  Quality assurance programs are required by federal legislation for hospitals that receive Medicare and Medicaid funding. They are also required by the Joint Commission on Accreditation of Hospitals (JCAH).

The first quality assurance programs emerged in 1972 when Public Law 92-603 established Professional Standards Review Organizations (PSRO). The purpose of this legislation was to fund regional groups that would control the escalating costs of federal health programs by assuring that care is medically necessary, of acceptable quality, and delivered in the most economical setting. Quality assurance programs under PSRO seek answers for such questions as: "Does the patient *need* to be hospitalized? Were diagnostic and treatment procedures appropriate for the given symptoms? Are any problem areas reflected in long-term studies of patient profiles, such as unusual death rates, prolonged or unnecessary hospitalization, infections, surgical complications, or unjustified tests or treatments?" Even though PSRO encourages involvement of other health professionals, their administrative and medical care evaluations remain oriented primarily toward physicians.

Quality assurance programs required by JCAH are compatible with those of PSRO but their major concern is for the quality of health care provided by medical and health-care professionals in a specific hospital. Standards of accreditation require that each hospital has a quality assurance program that includes designation of a committee, defined standards of quality, schedule of audits, analysis of data to identify problems, and a procedure for taking corrective action when necessary.

The quality of health care is thereby assured through external controls of the government and hospital accreditation requirements, and internal controls of professionals who determine standards, evaluate the practice of their peers, and take corrective action that may be necessary to upgrade the quality of care.

All quality assurance programs are based on two major components: standards of practice and a systematic method by which practice is evaluated. These components are considered in detail as they relate to nutritional care.

# Professional standards of practice

### Rosita Schiller

### Background and definition

The concept of standard practice is not new in dietetics. What is new, however, is the establishment of standards for nutritional care as provided by clinical dietitians and the supportive personnel who assist them. To illustrate this point, one might study the 1963 listing of items deemed necessary for effective administration of a department of dietetics.[6] Of 71 standards given, only 9 relate directly to patient nutritional care, counseling, research, and participation of the dietitian as a member of the health-care team. Historically, the emphasis of dietetic standards has been on the service of quality food rather than on the delivery of nutritional care. Much of the work of clinical dietitians has revolved around the patient's getting a tray rather than on the management of care, including dietary assessment, patient education, and the integration of nutrition with other aspects of health care.

An effective system of quality assurance must include comprehensive standards of practice. These should elucidate components of the process of nutritional care, education, and research. They should also clarify processes necessary for management of systems that articulate nutrition, health, and the role of the clinical dietitian.

Standards of practice (or standards of performance) are short statements that delineate or define norms or expectations of nutritional care, education, research, or management. Because it is assumed that professionals know better than anyone else what their standards should be, these norms are generally defined and ratified by the respective professional group. Broad standards are often set at the national level and disseminated for general use. These general statements must be analyzed and defined in specific detail as the standards, objectives, and policies for a particular institution. For example, a standard may stipulate that individual and group diet instructions will be provided. At one hospital it may be the policy to begin instruction immediately following an assessment of educational needs. At another hospital it may be standard procedure to withhold instruction until it is prescribed by a physician. The frequency and types of group classes should also be spelled out at each hospital. The use of well-defined standards is one way to communicate to physicians, nurses, other health care professionals, and patients what dietetic services can be expected.

### Standards for nutritional care

As we have already seen, diverse responsibilities of the clinical dietitian require that standards be developed for three broad areas of practice.

First, standards should be established for *quality nutritional care* provided by the dietitian. These standards usually relate to the process of care or to the activities that contribute to the delivery of services.[7] Examples of these standards are shown in the list following. Although they are more difficult to write and evaluate, standards may also be defined in terms of patient outcomes. Standards of nutritional care for specific disease entities are usually defined as *criteria*. The development and use of criteria are considered later.

The second type of standards relates to *professional performance or productivity*.[8] Productivity of the dietitian is often measured by such things as numbers of instructions given, accuracy of trays served, or amount of time devoted to diet calculations or menu selections. Productivity in health care does not always lend itself to quantitative measures. Standards of productivity are more meaningful in health care when perceived broadly in terms of occupancy, effectiveness, and efficiency.

Occupancy refers to the amount of time spent working. Productivity is improved when less time is spent in such activities as waiting for work, going from one work area to another, or engaging in conversations and activities unrelated to work. Institutional standards or policies may be developed for expected levels of productive time.

Effectiveness of the task is an important aspect of productivity for dietitians. Is the task appropriate for the dietitian? In the order of priorities, is this the most essential task for the present moment? Should this task be

### Standards for Nutritional Care[1]

1. Screen each hospitalized patient within 72 hours of admission to ascertain the presence of nutritional risk.
2. Assess nutritional status of each patient who presents nutritional risk.
3. Assume responsibility for the nutritional care of all patients within sphere of responsibility.
4. Identify the need for nutritional care of each patient.
5. Set priorities for levels and types of nutritional care and delegate appropriate activities to supportive personnel.
6. Serve as a nutrition consultant by providing nutrition information and making recommendations for nutritional care.
7. Integrate nutritional with other aspects of medical care by frequent communication with other health-care professionals and by participating in medical rounds, case conferences, and multidisciplinary audits.
8. Provide effective coordination of nutrition services with the institutional food service system.
9. Maintain an effective system of recording, communicating, and integrating nutritional care with other departments and services.

delegated to supportive personnel? Should the activity be performed at all? Standards of practice that promote effectiveness can often be used to enhance the importance of nutritional care and the role of the clinical dietitian. The absence of such standards can serve as an excuse for the dietitian to spend valuable time performing routine activities, such as writing standard diets, making menu changes, or collecting selective menus in patient wards.

Efficiency, the third aspect of productivity, is related to accuracy and structure of the activity. Is the task being done in the right way? Is there a more cost-effective method that could be used? Work simplification methods and procedures can be developed to improve efficiency. It is necessary to update procedures and methods regularly to incorporate new techniques or instruments.

A third type of standards relates to the *management* of nutritional care. In past decades dietitians provided care. The present emphasis on team health care demands that the clinical dietitian assume a managerial role and take full responsibility for nutrition services. Management is often defined as "getting things done through others." Hence, the clinical dietitian should spend less time giving care and more time making sure that the right care is given by the appropriate person and in the correct way.

Standards need to be established for the functions of planning, organizing, directing, and evaluating the total system of nutritional care. Some examples of management standards for the clinical dietitian are given in the list below.

### Sample Standards for the Management of Nutritional Care

Planning: The goals of Nutrition Services are spelled out in writing and include statements that require
- Quality individualized nutritional care and counseling of hospitalized and ambulatory patients
- Nutrition education of health professionals
- Leadership in promoting nutrition as an integral component of health care and prevention of disease

Organizing: There is a clear definition of the relationship between Nutrition Services and Food Management showing
- Goals and objectives for each division
- A chart of organization with personnel assigned to each division
- A system of nutritional care differentiated from a system for production and service of food

Directing: There is an effective system of formal communication within nutrition services, including procedures for
- Coordination among members of nutritional care team
- Diet orders, changes, and discharges
- Nourishments, tube feedings, dietary supplements
- Individual patient requests
- Personnel directives
- Problem solving; shared decision making
- Providing information supportive of high morale, leadership, dedication to quality patient care, and cooperation with other divisions

Evaluating: Regular management audits of nutrition services are performed. Nutrition Service meetings are scheduled to take corrective action when needed, to review progress toward objectives, and to redefine goals and objectives as appropriate.

## The dietetic audit

The second major component of a quality assurance program is the analysis of performance to determine compliance with established standards. In recent years, the methodology for medical care audits has been adopted for use by other health-care groups. An audit consists of a series of defined steps that help to maintain objectivity in the process of evaluating group performance. It is an effective way to compare professional performance with expected standards of practice. The process includes the definition of criteria by which a

---

[1]For other standards, see Schiller R: Improving nutritional care: readers respond. Dietetic Currents (Ross Laboratories) 7:25, 1980

standard is to be evaluated; collection of specific data that show how the criteria are met; comparison of the data with the established criteria, standards, or expected levels of performance; identification of deficient or problem areas and development of plans to correct problems. Each step of the audit process is considered in detail. Application here is made to the direct care of patients, but it should be remembered that standards and criteria can be established for any aspect of nutritional care.[9]

### Setting criteria

Criteria are short statements that further define the standards of nutritional care for a specific group of patients. Each criterion must be clearly stated, measurable, relevant, given in behavioral terms, and must be achievable by the dietitian or the patient.

Criteria include only things that can be observed in practice or found written in the medical record or dietetic card file. When the criteria are drafted, they should indicate what documentation is to be used to show that the stated criteria have been maintained. The medical record is used for official documentation of total care, whereas the dietetic card file contains information that is useful to the dietitian or other dietary personnel. The patient care audit may be confined to either set of records, or it may include both the medical record and the dietetic card file. Information from the card file is used for concurrent audits that assess care while a patient is actually in the hospital. The medical record is often used for retrospective audits that are completed after patient discharge; it may also be used for some forms of peer review during patient hospitalization.

Criteria, like standards, may relate to the process of care or to patient outcomes. Process criteria relate to the activities of the dietitian. For example, criteria that elaborate the standard of documentation in the medical record might include entries for an assessment of nutritional status, verification of physician's diet order, calculation, and assessment of nutrient intake for a 3 to 5 day period, assessment of the patient's knowledge and ability to follow a diet, completion of diet instructions, an assessment of a patient's willingness and ability to follow the diet, and the potential need for follow-up care and referral.

Patient outcome criteria are infrequently used to assess nutritional care of hospitalized patients. Desired physical changes, such as weight loss or controlled levels of blood glucose, occur over long periods of time. Often they cannot be fully evaluated during the average hospital stay. Dietitians recognize that many factors outside their jurisdiction affect such things as weight loss, blood glucose levels, edema, serum protein, serum urea nitrogen, or the variety of other indices that reflect nutritional status. In specific instances, criteria may designate improvement in physical or biochemical indices. Otherwise it is simply assumed that if the dietitian performs her job as she should, her services will have a positive effect on patient behaviors and on the clinical manifestations that characterize the desired patient responses to nutritional care and counseling.

Patient achievement of learning objectives can be defined as *outcome criteria* and can be used as a way to evaluate the effectiveness of diet instructions. For example, the standard for providing individual and group diet instruction might include outcome criteria indicating that a patient can make appropriate food selections from a given menu, select an acceptable meal from a list of vending machine items, verbalize the types and amounts of an accepted daily food intake, and make appropriate food substitutions from available or preferred items. When the clinical dietitian in the hospital also is the one to conduct the follow-up counseling of the patient on visits to the outpatient department, the outcomes of nutrition intervention can be more accurately assessed.

Because an audit is essentially a peer review, dietetic standards and criteria must be ratified or accepted by dietitians who are expected to meet the standards of performance.

The level of expected conformance for each criterion should also be specified. This is usually done by stating the acceptable percentage of medical records or dietetic file cards which include the designated documentation. For example, one might expect to find verification of physician's diet orders on 100% of medical records but an analysis of complete nutritional assessment only 30% of the time.

Detailed and distinct criteria are usually established for each of the major diseases in which nutrition plays a significant part in diagnosis and treatment. Other criteria are defined to evaluate standards of overall professional performance or management of nutritional care. Once the criteria are established, they can be used repeatedly for successive audits and revised only when necessary.

### Data collection and analysis

Audit teams or committees are usually set up to provide leadership for individual audits. These committees decide what standards or disease entities are reviewed, when the audit will take place, how long it lasts, and how many records are examined. Forms are set up that include the criteria, expected levels of performance, and space for recording the information being collected.

During the dietetic audit, medical record personnel or audit team members investigate a specified number of medical records or file cards and note whether or not each record contains the required documentation.

After audit data are collected, the audit team examines the information to determine the number and percentage of records that include the specified documentation for each criterion. Although different audit topics may be reviewed at the same time, integrity must be maintained for each standard or the nutritional care of patients with a single disease. Results of each audit are analyzed and reported separately.

Problem areas become evident when actual data show that documentation or performance is significantly different from what is desired. Because the list of criteria is specific, the audit pinpoints areas of neglect in the completion or documentation of activities that are related to dietary assessment, planning nutritional care, providing and monitoring nutritional services, counseling patients and families, and evaluating care and education. The audit committee studies areas in which the greatest disparity exists between established criteria and actual performance. These discrepancies provide a base for problem solving.

### Problem solving

A successful audit helps to bring about needed changes in improving patient care. An audit is incomplete if it is terminated after the actual performance has been compared with the criteria or standards.

It is necessary for the audit team, along with the other dietitians, to study in detail the problem areas that have been identified through the audit. If there are numerous deficiencies, one or two of the more important areas should be selected for complete analysis and solution. Improved performance is more likely to occur if changes are suggested in only a few specific areas. For each problem area, the audit committee makes a list of all of the reasons why performance is below standard. It should be noted that audits do not evaluate the activities of individual professionals. They are used only to determine if the department as a whole is maintaining its standards. Performance appraisals are still needed to assess the contributions of each person.

A complete analysis of problem areas aids in clarifying underlying difficulties. It also aids in identifying feasible solutions, which attack roots rather than symptoms of the problem. The final result of the analysis is a list of optional solutions for specific problems that have been identified.

The audit committee studies all possible solutions, selects those that are most feasible, and recommends that they be implemented. Most solutions directly affect the dietitians. For this reason, dietitians should be actively involved in making decisions about changes in criteria, expected levels of conformance, procedures, or practices in their daily work.

Changes for improvement should be made soon after the audit is complete. Solutions often require the participation of dietetic administrators, clinical dietitians, dietetic technicians, supervisors, and other personnel. The complexity of proposed changes will determine the process that should be used for their implementation.

The effectiveness of changes can best be evaluated through a subsequent audit. Adequate time needs to be allowed so that solutions can be fully implemented before another audit is done on the same topic. Solutions often include educational programs, new policies, or changes in personnel responsibilities. At least 6 months should elapse before another audit is scheduled on the same topic. Results of the second audit are compared with the first to determine whether or not actual performance is more consistent with the stated standards and criteria.

### Benefits of quality assurance

Nutritional care audits provide a process through which dietitians can evaluate their own performance and assess changes that occur as a direct result of intervention by a dietitian. Many dietitians see the audit process as a tool to set meaningful objectives and strengthen their professional skills.[10] The development and use of standards helps to integrate nutritional services with other aspects of patient care. The results of an audit can be used to document productivity or to justify the need for additional professional and supportive services. Results may verify the effectiveness of patient education and nutrition counseling.

Patients will receive quality nutritional care if standards are established and maintained. The auditing process is designed to allow thorough evaluation of a situation in order to isolate those aspects of a system that need to be analyzed or corrected. The audit process requires that the parameters of high quality dietetic services be clearly defined. Nutrition is thus identified and documented as a necessary component of total medical care. The clinical dietitian's nutritional care and professional performance are likely to be most effective when these factors are integrated with a continuing program of quality assurance.

## Study questions and activities

1. Compare the menu selections of a group of patients on regular diets with the pattern dietary in Table 22-1. Will the selections of each patient provide adequately for his energy and nutrient needs?
2. Using the selective menu for a regular diet from any hospital in your community, check to determine whether or not any combination of meal selections for a day will provide an adequate nutrient intake for a 25-year-old postpartum mother who is breast-feeding her newborn infant.
3. Compare the soft diet in the diet manual your hospital uses with the soft diet in Table 22-2. Are there any major differences in the foods used in the two plans? With the help of your clinical instructor, identify the reasons for these differences.
4. With the assistance of your clinical instructor, obtain the diet history of a patient and record your findings in

his record. Did you use any judgmental words or phrases? Was your writing legible? Was your spelling correct? Did you write a SOAP note?

5. Obtain a record of the 24-hour intake of a patient on a clear liquid diet. Using the food composition tables in Part 4, estimate his calorie and nutrient intake. How adequate was this diet for him?

6. List five topics that could be used for a patient care or dietetic audit.

7. Using one of the topics listed above, state related standard(s) of practice and define criteria by which the topic could be evaluated.

8. List and describe the steps in the problem solving model used in the last phase of the audit process.

## References

1. Committee report. J Am Diet Assoc 64:661, 1974
2. Weed LL: N Engl J Med 278:593, 652, 1968
3. Mason M et al: The Dynamics of Clinical Dietetics, p 85–93. New York, John Wiley & Sons, 1977
4. Sorenson AW et al: Fam Community Health 1:91, 1978
5. International Classifications of Diseases, 9th Rev. Clinical Modification (10D.9.CM), Vol 1. Ann Arbor, Commission on Professional and Hospital Activities, 1978
6. Standards for effective administration of a hospital department of dietetics. J Am Diet Assoc 43:357, 1963
7. Scheel JP, McClusky KW: Standards of performance developed for clinical dietitians. Hospitals 52:157, Mar 16, 1978
8. Dahl T: Economics, management, and public health nutrition. J Am Diet Assoc 70:144, 1977
9. Schiller R, Behm V: Auditing dietetic services. Hospitals 53:105, May 1, 1979
10. Schiller R: Improving nutritional care: Readers respond. Dietetic Currents 7:25, 1980

## Supplementary readings

Altman JH et al: Sounding board: Patients who read their hospital charts. N Engl J Med 302:169, 1980

Eli-Beheri BB: Dietetic audit—A giant step for nutritional care. J Am Diet Assoc 74:321, 1979

Fifer WR: Quality assurance: Debate persists on goals, impact, and methods of evaluating care. Hospitals 53:163, Apr 1, 1979

Kaufman M, Vermeersch JA: Quality assurance in ambulatory nutritional care. I. Past, present, and future. J Am Diet Assoc 78:577, 1981

Maller O et al: Consumer opinion of hospital food and food service. J Am Diet Assoc 76:236, 1980

McLeroy MJ, Klover RV: Implementing problem-oriented medical records (POMR) in an out-patient clinic. J Am Diet Assoc 72:522, 1978

Miller B, Balsley M: JCAH revises dietetic service standards. Hospitals 54:102, Nov 1, 1980

Ohlson MA: Diet therapy in the U.S. in the past 200 years. J Am Diet Assoc 69:490, 1976

Reaburn JA et al: Social determinants in food selection. J Am Diet Assoc 74:637, 1979

Sadin RR: Impact on dietetics of PSROs (Professional Standards Review Organizations). J Am Diet Assoc 72:292, 1978

Sorenson AW et al: Dietitians: Contributing members of the health care team. Fam Community Health 1:91, 1978

Thomasma DC: Human values and ethics: Professional responsibility. J Am Diet Assoc 75:533, 1979

Vermeersch JA, Kaufman M: Quality assurance in ambulatory nutritional care. II. Field testing of criteria. J Am Diet Assoc 78:582, 1981

## Diet manuals

Air Force and Navy Diet Manual. Washington, DC, United States Government Printing Office, 1980

American Dietetic Association: Handbook of Clinical Dietetics. New Haven, Yale University Press, 1981

Diet Manual. New York, Memorial Sloan-Kettering Cancer Center and Hospital for Special Surgery, 1979

Diet Manual. Bronx, NY, Montefiore Hospital, Nutritional Department, 1979

Diet Manual: Utilizing a Vegetarian Diet Plan, 5th ed. Loma Linda, CA, Seventh-Day Adventist Dietetic Association, 1978

Franchi S: A Diet Manual for the Geriatric Center of Niagara Falls, N.Y. Niagara Falls, Niagara Geriatric Center, 1979

Grills NJ, Bosscher MV: Manual of Nutrition and Diet Therapy. New York, Macmillan, 1981

Pemberton CM, Gastineau GF (eds): Mayo Clinic Diet Manual, 5th ed. Philadelphia, WB Saunders, 1981

Phoenix Area Manual of Applied Nutrition, 2nd ed. Phoenix, Central Arizona District Dietetic Association, 1979

## Quality assurance manuals

Guidelines for Evaluating Dietetic Practice. American Dietetic Association, 1976

Patient Care Audit: A Quality Assurance Procedure Manual for Dietitians. American Dietetic Association, 1978

Professional Standards Review Procedure Manual. American Dietetic Association, 1976

Hospital Management Review. American Hospital Association, 1980

*For further references see Bibliography in Part 4.*

# Assessment of Patient Needs

## 23

**Cultural Factors**
**Psychological Influences**
**Physical Condition**
**Nutritional Assessment**
**Potential for Learning**

The first step in the quality assurance of nutritional care is the assessment of each patient's special needs. In the medical setting the assessment activity (see Chap. 13) takes on additional significance. The needs of the hospitalized patient whose diet is modified as part of the treatment of his acute or chronic disease may differ significantly from the needs of clients who are well. Together with all the factors in the patient's situation of which the dietitian must be aware, she must also try to discover his reaction to hospitalization and to understand his behavior in, for most people, an unfamiliar and anxiety-producing situation.

Hospitalization most often disrupts the life-style of a patient and forces him to interact with many unfamiliar people—physicians, nurses, dietitians, technicians—and, perhaps for the first time in his life, to share a room with a stranger. At the same time a patient may have very little time to think about and accept the diagnosis. For instance, between his noon and evening meal he may find he must change his food habits because the physician may have discovered after completing the glucose tolerance test that morning that the patient has diabetes mellitus.

As one seeks to help a patient accept a therapeutic modification of his food practices as part of the treatment of his disease, it must be kept in mind that his food habits are part of his social and cultural heritage. In addition, certain psychological factors and his physical condition influence his acceptance of food during his illness. Some of the factors that one needs to consider in assessing a patient's needs are discussed in the following paragraphs.

## Cultural factors

Cultural heritage, family background and status, religious customs, family methods of food preparation and service, emotional attitudes toward food, as well as exposure to nutrition education, food fads, and superstitions all contribute to a person's food habits and acceptance of food during hospitalization. A variety of ethnic food patterns may be encountered (see Chap. 14). The Orthodox

**AMC:** Arm Muscle Circumference
**BEE:** Basal Energy Expenditure
**CHI:** Creatinine Height Index
**SK-SD:** Streptokinase-streptodornase
**TIBC:** Total Iron-binding Capacity
**TSF:** Triceps Skinfold Thickness

Jewish, the Puerto Rican, the Mexican, the Polish, and the Italian patient may have food habits that differ from one another's and from those of other Americans. At the same time, care must be taken to avoid cultural patronage; for example, a patient whose surname identifies him as a member of an ethnic group may represent the third or fourth generation of his family. He may have been born and lived his whole life in the United States, and his food habits may be typically American.

In the United States, food patterns may vary widely by region, although modern transportation and communications media have modified these patterns to some extent. However, even today, a patient from the South who finds himself in a Northern hospital may feel that, because of the way vegetables are cooked, they are insipid and uninteresting, and he may refuse to eat them.

Most people live in families and eat their meals with others. To eat in bed and by oneself may accentuate his illness in the patient's mind. Some hospitals try to meet this problem by having as many patients eat together as possible, and here a room for four or six patients may actually be a better setting than a single room with its lone private patient. Even a sodium-restricted diet may be accepted when its restrictions are shared with a fellow patient.

## Psychological influences

Illness may change a person's psychological orientation to everyday occurrences and personal relationships; the need for the familiar and the customary is immeasurably increased. Because what, how, and with whom we eat is an everyday occurrence, illness, which interrupts this pattern, may have serious psychological repercussions. The fear, the worry, the insecurity, and the frustration that possess the patient as he changes from an independent, healthy individual to one dependent on others in illness is often expressed through regressive behavior. Fussiness, anorexia, or demands for extra attention are traits that may be exhibited by the worried patient. Babcock says that "it is easier to show discouragement through anorexia than it is to explain that one is feeling inadequate and depressed in the presence of a frightening disease or a disheartening experience."[1]

The apparent apathy or uncooperativeness of a patient may mean not that he does not want to eat, but that the food offered to him is unacceptable due to its emotional connotations. His food habits have developed slowly through the years and have become a personal and guarded part of himself, so that many foods may be associated with specific feelings and emotions separate from their nutritional significance. Such foods as milk, cocoa, custards, junket, creamed and strained foods, first met with in infancy, become associated with the dependency and the security of that period. Some adults refuse such foods despite their apparent nutritional value simply because they resent the dependency of illness. Due to the sense of security they convey, others may cling to using these same foods, even though they may not be desirable nutritionally or psychologically.

Desserts, sweets, and delicacies have become reward foods to many people because they first were received as a reward for cleaning one's plate or being a good child. It is not surprising that adolescents and older people, too, indulge in excessive intake of such foods when they are under stress and in need of psychological reward.

In the United States some foods have gained special status. Steaks, chops, green salads, and butter are four examples of these foods. Patients may resent suggestions to reduce the cost of food by substituting ground meat for steaks and chops, or margarine for butter. On the other hand, the homemaker who is well aware of the cost of food uses ground meat and margarine.

Tea, coffee, and alcoholic beverages may be thought of as adult foods by some patients because they were forbidden to them as children. Excessive use of these beverages, to the exclusion of milk, may be an expression of a desire to seem mature. On the other hand, some cultural groups use tea, coffee, and alcoholic beverages regularly as part of the daily diet for the whole family, including the children.

It must not be forgotten that the appearance of the food and the tray also produce a psychological effect that may determine acceptance or rejection of the meal. Hot food must be served *hot* and cold food *cold*. A pot of *hot* coffee or tea may make the remainder of a restricted diet acceptable. It tells the patient, as no words can, that those about him really care about him and are making every effort to make his food as palatable as possible.

The therapeutic diet itself may have meaning for the patient that is not evident to the professional staff. Everyone rejoices with the patient who progresses from a liquid diet to one containing solid food as concrete evidence that he is getting better. But, should that patient ask if he must follow a sodium-restricted diet for the rest of his life, are we aware that he may be inquiring in reality if he is going to have cardiac disease permanently, with all that this implies? The therapeutic diet that must be of long duration may give the patient a real sense of deprivation, with depressing overtones that are difficult to resolve.

All those concerned with nutrition need to be cognizant of what food means to people under various circumstances. Attempts to change long established and deeply ingrained patterns may be met with resistance. The overzealous nutrition counselor who is trying to teach a patient "what is good for him, nutritionally," may interpret the patient's response as "ignorance" or "lack of cooperation." Pumpian-Mindlin writes: "To accomplish the prime purpose of regulating and guiding what goes into a patient's mouth, one must learn to listen carefully to what first comes out of the same mouth. . . . Otherwise one may find himself in the position of having more than mere words thrown back in one's face."[2] We must be able to interpret what the patient says or does not say about food, what he does with food, and how he reacts to food service in the light of his emotional as well as his metabolic needs. Whatever dietary changes may be necessary for his therapy must be made within this framework if they are to be successful.

## Physical condition

Through observation, the physical characteristics of the patient that may influence his acceptance of food or ability to feed himself may be identified. Older patients may have lost some of their teeth, making chewing difficult if they are placed on a general house diet. Some patients use poor fitting dentures for cosmetic reasons and remove them at mealtime. The adolescent boy with a fractured jaw may complain bitterly of hunger because his liquid house diet has not been modified sufficiently in calorie content or frequency of feeding to satisfy his needs. Patients recovering from oral surgery do not appreciate the effects of citrus juices on a sore mouth. Assessment of the ability to swallow is critical for certain patients if aspiration and its adverse effects are to be avoided.

Patients with emphysema and other respiratory difficulties may be forced to eat and drink slowly and, therefore, may need their trays for a longer period of time than other patients. Providing adequate nutrients and fluids for these individuals may require four or five meals per day.

Many individuals with sight problems, including the blind, can and prefer to feed themselves. They need to be oriented to the placement of dishes and other articles on their trays. They may need help in pouring beverages, in opening milk cartons, and in removing protective coverings from foods. Patients with poor manipulative skills, such as the arthritic or the multiple sclerosis patient, may need the same kind of assistance. Assessing the ability of any handicapped person and providing the proper assistance not only reduces his frustrations and promotes his independence but also may help him to achieve a reasonable nutrient intake.

Every patient does not require the same size serving of food. "Appetite poor" recorded on the dietitian's Kardex after meal rounds may really mean that the patient was served too much food not, as this note is usually interpreted, that the patient did not eat enough food. A high-calorie diet for a woman who is 82 years old, 5 feet 1 inch, and chronically ill may be 2000 calories and for a man 27 years old, 6 feet 2 inches, after a hemorrhoidectomy, 3500 calories.

The long-term or chronically ill patient presents a special challenge to both the dietitian and the nurse. Cycle menus that repeat the same menus every 2 to 4 weeks are used in many hospitals. The long-term or chronically ill patient may experience two or three periods of a cycle menu plan; this may be a problem, even though the menu items are familiar and acceptable to him. Family members or friends can often be helpful when a patient becomes bored with the hospital's food by occasionally providing a favorite dish from home, although they need direction from the dietitian so that their contribution fits his diet plan.

Interval nourishments for the chronically ill patient need to be carefully planned. A 400-calorie milkshake at 10:30 A.M. may result in the patient's refusal of an 800-calorie meal at 12:00 noon. Four meals, with the last one served at 8:00 or 9:00 P.M., may be a more effective plan for providing for his nutrient needs, especially if he is accustomed to an evening snack at home.

The scheduling of treatments, diagnostic tests, and nursing care are often critical factors in obtaining a proper food intake. The best meal of the day for some of these patients is breakfast because they are rested or, for some of the older patients, because breakfast has always been an important meal. As the day progresses they may become increasingly tired and tend to eat less. Therefore, treatments should be planned so that the patient may rest before the noon and evening meals. Some of these patients may require only minimal assistance at breakfast and considerably more at the evening meal.

The patient restricted to prolonged bed rest benefits from nursing care procedures that promote the maximum movement by, or of, himself. Research has shown that immobilization, even with adequate food intake, promotes negative nitrogen and calcium balance, which may result in progressive muscular weakness. Turning and positioning the patient as ordered by the physician and providing passive exercise during personal care helps to prevent the adverse metabolic effects of immobility (see Chap. 25).

## Nutritional assessment

In the 1970s there has been a renewed interest in and concern for the nutritional status of acutely and chronically ill patients at the time of admission to the hospital, during hospitalization, and in follow-up after discharge. Surveys have demonstrated a relatively high degree of previously unrecognized malnutrition in children and adults on admission to the hospital,[3-5] and clinical studies have demonstrated a higher prevalence of morbidity and mortality in malnourished patients.[6,7] Both physicians and surgeons have come to the realization that new therapeutic agents and sophisticated technologies available for the treatment of complex medical and surgical problems are not effective unless the cells of the body have adequate quantities of energy, protein, and other nutrients as well as oxygen and fluid and electrolytes to support human metabolism.

Many major medical centers in the United States and Europe have established nutritional support teams that monitor the nutritional status of patients and recommend therapy. These teams usually consist of a physician, clinical dietitian, nurse specialist, clinical pharmacist, physical therapist, and social worker. The clinical dietitian on these teams must have a high degree of knowledge of, and skill in applying, the science and art of human nutrition and dietetics to the care of patients at risk for or with malnutrition,[8,9] and all clinical dietitians must apply the standards of practice to all patients to avoid the development of malnutrition during hospitalization.[10]

### Methodology for assessment

The methodology used to assess the nutritional status of the hospitalized patient has been adapted from that used to assess the nutritional status of population groups.[11-13] The subjective data as reported by the patient or a concerned person are recent usual weight and maximum lifetime weight; nutritional history, which includes the recent usual daily food intake, special diets, food aversions, intolerances, allergies, and any difficulty with chewing and swallowing or any nausea, vomiting, bloat-

ing, diarrhea, or steatorrhea; and an evaluation of daily physical activity.

The objective data that are usually collected for the assessment include: anthropometric data including height, weight, skinfold thickness, and arm muscle circumference; biochemical data, such as hemoglobin, hematocrit, serum transferrin, albumin, total lymphocyte count, and 24-hour nitrogen excretion; and skin test reactivity to common recall antigens. Figure 23-1 is an example of a data sheet used to record the assessment data of a patient. The form is filled in and kept up to date by the nutritional support team and filed in the patient's medical record.

Additional data that may also be collected are an estimation of the patient's 24-hour energy and nutrient intake during hospitalization, and such data as the 24-hour urinary creatinine excretion, thyroxin-binding protein, retinol-binding protein, lymphocyte response to phytohemaglutinin, and total iron-binding capacity from which the serum transferrin can be estimated.

### Types of malnutrition

The malnutrition that has been observed in patients at the time of admission or subsequent to admission to the hospital has been classified as marasmus, kwashiorkor,

**NUTRITIONAL ASSESSMENT**

THE OHIO STATE UNIVERSITY HOSPITALS

Primary Diagnosis:

Contributing Factors:

Initial Height/Weight Data

Recent Stable Body weight : _____Kg          Height          : _____cm

Present Weight          : _____Kg          Estimate Ideal Weight   : _____Kg

Percent Weight Change : _____%   Date

| | | | | |
|---|---|---|---|---|
| weight | | kg | kg | kg | kg |
| % ideal | | % | % | % | % |
| Triceps Skin Fold (TSF) | | mm | mm | mm | mm |
| % Standard | | % | % | % | % |
| Mid Arm Circumference | | cm | cm | cm | cm |
| Arm Muscle Circumference (AMC) | | cm | cm | cm | cm |
| % Standard | | % | % | % | % |
| Creatinine Excretion (24 hrs.) | | mg | mg | mg | mg |
| Creatinine/Height Index (CHI) | | % | % | % | % |
| Albumin | | g/100ml | g/100ml | g/100ml | g/100ml |
| Total Protein | | g/100ml | g/100ml | g/100ml | g/100ml |
| Total Iron Binding Capacity (TIBC) | | mcg/100ml | mcg/100ml | mcg/100ml | mcg/100ml |
| Transferrin | | mg/100ml | mg/100ml | mg/100ml | mg/100ml |
| White Blood Cell Count (WBC) | | /mm³ | /mm³ | /mm³ | /mm³ |
| Total Lymphocytes | | /mm³ | /mm³ | /mm³ | /mm³ |
| Skin Tests:   A | | | | | |
| B | | | | | |
| C | | | | | |
| D | | | | | |

Indications for Nutritional Support:

Nutritional Support Method:

Basal Energy Expenditure (Harris-Benedict Formula):

Energy Requirement : _____ Kcal          Nitrogen Requirement : _____gms

The Ohio State University
Form 9654   (466111)

**Fig. 23-1.** Nutritional Assessment form. (Nutrition Services, University Hospitals. The Ohio State University)

and marasmic-kwashiorkor,[14] the classical categories of malnutrition (see Chap. 21). The marasmic patient presents with a decrease in anthropometric measurements, such as a recent unintentional weight loss, which indicates a gradual loss of subcutaneous fat, and decreased arm muscle circumference, which indicates the erosion of muscle mass as a result of malabsorption or an inadequate intake of energy and nutrients. The serum levels of proteins are normal, indicating a reasonable maintenance of visceral protein.

Kwashiorkor, or kwashiorkor-type malnutrition, when applied to adults, is observed in patients who are in a severe catabolic state due to the injury complex (see Chap. 27) in combination with an inadequate intake of energy and nutrients. The anthropometric measurements are within the range of normal, but the serum levels of protein are depressed, indicating a decrease in visceral proteins. The patient is immune incompetent as demonstrated by a negative response to recall antigens and a depressed total lymphocyte count.

Marasmic-kwashiorkor indicates the presence of a decrease in both subcutaneous fat stores and the erosion of muscle mass combined with a deficiency of visceral protein and immune incompetency. This category of malnutrition presents the greatest risk for a poor response to nutritional rehabilitation.

## Data collection
### The nutritional history

The nutritional history should be comprehensive. The information obtained about the patient's usual food practices should be extensive enough for an estimation of the patient's recent average daily energy and protein intake, which is recorded in the medical record. Any significantly inadequate intake of vitamins and minerals and any specific food intolerances, any anorexia, nausea, vomiting, or protracted diarrhea, or recent modification of the consistency of food consumed should also be recorded together with the weight history, covering at least the preceding 3 to 6 months and preferably 1 year. It takes 30 to 45 minutes to collect a comprehensive nutritional history. This information should be recorded in the medical record within 24 hours after admission and should be followed by an estimate of the patient's 24-hour energy and protein intake of the food served to him in the hospital. If the patient's condition on admission makes it impossible to take a nutritional history, as much information as possible should be obtained from a family member or other person who might be knowledgeable about the patient's usual food practices.

Not every patient admitted to the hospital requires a comprehensive nutritional history. The clinical dietitian can identify the patient at risk for malnutrition by admitting diagnosis or laboratory data or both. Patients with any of the following admitting diagnoses can be suspected of being at high risk: cancer of any type; gastrointestinal

problems, such as malabsorption, peptic ulcer disease, pancreatic or hepatic disease, and inflammatory bowel disease; renal disease; endocrine diseases including patients receiving steroid therapy for inflammatory processes; and geriatric patients with organic brain disease. Visual inspection of the patient can often give the experienced clinical dietitian clues that a comprehensive nutritional history should be obtained. Clues from laboratory data on admission include the values for hemoglobin, hematocrit, serum albumin and transferrin, and the total lymphocyte count.

### Anthropometric data

The height and weight of each patient should be obtained on admission and recorded in the medical record (see Fig. 23-1). If the patient is unable to stand, a chair or bed scale can be used to obtain the weight.[15] In many instances adult patients are able to report their heights with a fair degree of accuracy. Without these two measurements a reasonable evaluation of weight status cannot be made on admission or weight changes monitored during hospitalization.

Triceps skinfold thickness (TSF) is used to estimate body fat stores and arm muscle circumference (AMC) in order to estimate muscle mass, bone size, and subcutaneous fat because height and weight measurements do not indicate body composition.

The TSF and the AMC are measured at the midpoint of the back of the upper right arm between the acromial process of the scapula and the olecranon of the ulna. The subject's forearm is positioned against his body perpendicular to the upper arm, the midpoint is measured with a flexible steel tape, and the point is marked with a fine tip ballpoint pen. At the dorsal midpoint of the arm hanging relaxed, the TSF is measured to the nearest 10th of a millimeter with a Lange skinfold caliper having a pressure of 10 g/mm² of contact surface area (see Fig. 23-2). If the patient must lie in bed, the measurement can be taken with the forearm comfortably folded across the chest.[16] The skinfold thickness is grasped between the left index finger and the thumb immediately above the dorsal midpoint and should include skin and subcutaneous fat but not muscle (see Fig. 23-2). The skinfold thickness is read from the caliper gauge after approximately a 3-second application of the caliper to the skinfold. Three readings are taken with the caliper pinch and finger-thumb grasp being released between each measurement. The mean of the three measurements is calculated and recorded. The arm circumference is measured at the midpoint in centimeters with a flexible steel tape in such a manner that the contour of the arm is not distorted.

The arm muscle circumference can be calculated from the arm circumference using the equation

Arm muscle circumference (mm) = arm circumference (mm) − 0.314 × triceps skinfold thickness (mm)

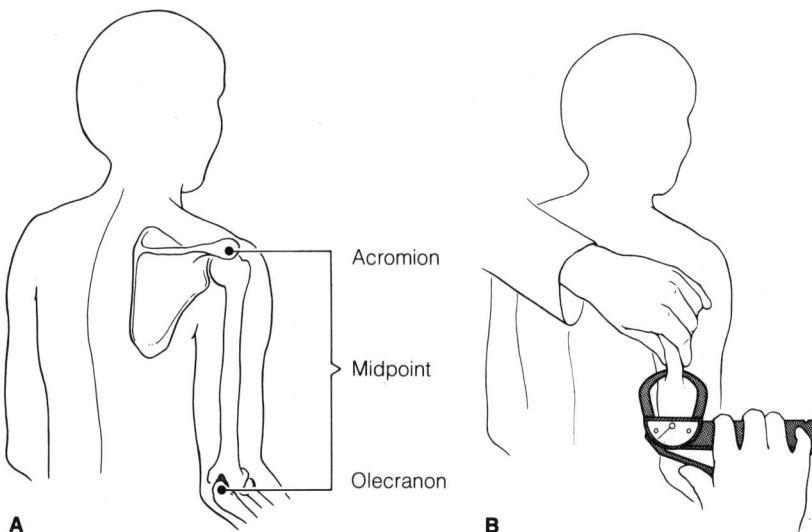

Acromion

Midpoint

Olecranon

**Fig. 23-2.** Arm Anthropometry. *A.* Measuring upper right arm midpoint. *B.* Applying caliper to measure skinfold thickness. (Courtesy Medical Illustrations, The Ohio State University)

A                                    B

The constant in this equation is pi ($\pi$). The arm muscle area and the arm muscle diameter can also be calculated from equations, using arm circumference and triceps skinfold thickness.[17]

One method that can be used to identify frame size (small, medium, or large) when using ideal body weight tables to evaluate weight status is to calculate the height to wrist circumference ratio. The wrist circumference is measured with a flexible steel tape just distal to the styloid process at the wrist crease on the right arm.[16] The formula for calculating the ratio is

$$r = \frac{\text{Height (cm)}}{\text{Wrist circumference (cm)}}$$

Frame size can be estimated as follows:

|         | Males        | Females      |
|---------|--------------|--------------|
| small   | r > 10.4     | r > 11.0     |
| medium  | r = 9.6–10.4 | r = 10.1–11.0 |
| large   | r < 9.6      | r < 10.1     |

### Biochemical data

The measurement of selected serum proteins is used to estimate the visceral protein status.[14,16] The laboratory analyses of serum albumin and transferrin provide an indirect measurement of the availability of protein (amino acids and nitrogen) to support the metabolic activity of liver cells and the cells of the gastrointestinal tract, pancreas, and other visceral tissues with a high degree of mitotic activity. The total lymphocyte count and recall skin antigen testing are also used to estimate visceral-protein status.[14]

Serum albumin is usually depressed during stress—surgical, septic, or traumatic. In the chronically ill pa-

tient, severely depressed levels occur in those with advanced hepatic cirrhosis, renal failure, and cardiac failure. Serum albumin is not a reliable indicator of very early protein depletion due to the relatively long half-life (20 days) of albumin and also the relatively large pool of body albumin.[16] A depressed level for more than 7 days in the stressed patient suggests a nutritional deficiency and with nutritional rehabilitation the serum level will return to normal slowly.

Serum transferrin can be measured directly in the laboratory or calculated from the determination of total iron-binding capacity (TIBC). The equation is

Serum transferrin = (0.8 × TIBC) − 43

Thyroxin-binding prealbumin and retinol-binding protein are also used to assess visceral protein status. Retinol-binding protein which has a half-life of 10 hours is probably the most sensitive indicator of visceral-protein depletion.[16]

The 24-hour creatinine excretion analysis is another indirect measure of lean body mass. The excretion of creatinine decreases in proportion to skeletal muscle depletion. A healthy man with normal kidney function excretes 23 mg creatinine per kilogram of body weight per 24 hours; a healthy woman, 18 mg per kilogram. The creatinine excretion index (CEI) can be calculated, using the equation[16]

$$\text{CEI} = \frac{\text{Actual 24-hour creatinine excretion}}{\text{Predicted 24-hour creatinine}} \times 100$$

The creatinine height index (CHI), which is also used to estimate lean body mass, is calculated from the 24-hour creatinine excretion, using the equation

$$\text{CHI} = \frac{\text{Actual urinary creatinine}}{\text{Ideal urinary creatinine}} \times 100$$

The ideal urinary creatinine values are derived from a table of ideal creatinine values by height[18] (see Table 23-1). Driver and McAlvey[19] question the use of the ideal creatinine excretion tables because they have observed that in 548 healthy men the urinary creatinine excretion values showed a decline with age, and the CHI declined by 20% by age 65 to 74. Therefore, the CHI may not be a valid indicator of lean body mass in older patients.

## Immune competence

Total lymphocyte count and skin tests with recall antigens (antigens with which most individuals have had previous experience) are used to evaluate cellular immunity. Three antigens commonly used are mumps, candida, and streptokinase-streptodornase (SK-SD). The antigen is administered intradermally, and the reaction is considered positive (immune competent) if the induration is 5 mm or more 24 to 48 hours after injection.[16] Patients with PEM will have low lymphocyte counts and depressed or no skin test reactivity.

## Evaluation of assessment data

With the exception of the height and weight tables (Table 10, Part 4) the criteria generally used to evaluate the nutritional assessment data[20] were derived from those published by WHO in 1966.[12] These criteria were compiled from the assessment of diverse, worldwide healthy population groups. At the time of writing there is considerable controversy[21-24] about whether or not the WHO criteria, especially the anthropometric ones, should be applied to people in the United States, specifically to hospitalized patients.

In place of the WHO criteria some investigators are recommending the use of criteria for anthropometric measurements that have been derived from the data collected in the Ten-State Nutrition Survey[16,22] or the National Health Survey, 1960 to 1961.[22] These criteria appear to be more applicable to patients in the United States than the WHO criteria. As Gray and Gray[21] demonstrate, the WHO data may lead to an overestimation of the number of severely malnourished patients entering United States hospitals. In the future the most appropriate anthropometric criteria may be those that are derived from the Health and Nutrition Examination Surveys (Round 1, 1971–1974, and Round 2, in the 1980s). In the meantime, a nutrition support team should select and agree upon a set of criteria and apply them equally to all patients. Any publication by the team or any of its members should state explicitly the criteria used.

## Nutritional history

The validity of the data obtained by diet history of the patient's usual food intake is open to question, and any analysis of energy and nutrient intake recorded in the medical record should be carefully labeled an *estimate*. The estimate of the first 24-hour intake of the patient after

## Table 23-1. Expected 24-hr Urine Creatinine Excretion of Normal Adult Men and Women of Different Heights

| Men* | | | | Women† | | | |
|---|---|---|---|---|---|---|---|
| Height‡ | Ideal Weight | Creatinine Coefficient | 24-hr Urine Creatinine | Height‡ | Ideal Weight | Creatinine Coefficient | 24-hr Urine Creatinine |
| in    cm | kg | mg/kg | gm | in    cm | kg | mg/kg | gm |
| 62    157.5 | 56.0 | 23 | 1.29 | 58    147.3 | 46.0 | 17 | 0.782 |
| 63    160.0 | 57.6 | | 1.32 | 59    149.9 | 47.2 | | 0.802 |
| 64    162.5 | 59.0 | | 1.36 | 60    152.4 | 48.6 | | 0.826 |
| 65    165.1 | 60.3 | | 1.39 | 61    154.9 | 49.9 | | 0.848 |
| 66    167.6 | 62.0 | | 1.43 | 62    157.5 | 51.3 | | 0.872 |
| 67    170.2 | 63.8 | | 1.47 | 63    160.0 | 52.6 | | 0.894 |
| 68    172.7 | 65.8 | | 1.51 | 64    162.6 | 54.3 | | 0.923 |
| 69    175.3 | 67.6 | | 1.55 | 65    165.1 | 55.9 | | 0.950 |
| 70    177.8 | 69.4 | | 1.60 | 66    167.6 | 57.8 | | 0.983 |
| 71    180.3 | 71.4 | | 1.64 | 67    170.2 | 59.6 | | 1.01 |
| 72    182.9 | 73.5 | | 1.69 | 68    172.7 | 61.5 | | 1.04 |
| 73    185.4 | 75.6 | | 1.74 | 69    175.3 | 63.3 | | 1.08 |
| 74    188.0 | 77.6 | | 1.78 | 70    177.8 | 65.1 | | 1.11 |
| 75    190.5 | 79.6 | | 1.83 | 71    180.3 | 66.9 | | 1.14 |
| 76    193.0 | 82.2 | | 1.89 | 72    182.9 | 68.7 | | 1.17 |

*See reference 7 in Bistrian.

†Unpublished observations.

‡Creatinine: height index is defined as the 24-hr creatinine excretion of the patient divided by the expected 24-hr creatinine excretion of a normal adult of the same height.

(Bistrian BR: J Am Diet Assoc 71:393, 1977)

admission may, in some instances, validate the diet history. However, if many meals are omitted for diagnostic tests, a common occurrence, this may not be possible. The clinical dietitian should have obtained some information about daily energy expenditure while taking the nutritional history. For example, prior to admission, was the patient living a bed-to-chair existence, or was the patient hyperactive? Present weight status can only be evaluated with a knowledge of both energy intake and energy expenditure.

### Weight status

Weight status is evaluated by one of two methods—the percentage of ideal body weight or percentage of usual body weight. If the first method is used, the patient's present weight is evaluated using Table 23-2, *Ideal Weights (kg) for Height (cm), Adults.* These are practically the same data as Table 10, *Desirable Weights for Men and Women Aged 25 and Over,* Part 4, except that the values are given in centimeters and kilograms, rather than in inches and pounds. Also, many hospitals are using the metric system for all measurements. The height and weight tables are presently under revision.[25] The height-wrist circumference should be calculated to estimate frame size.

Some nutritional support teams prefer to use percentage of recent weight loss (within the past 3–6 months) as an indicator because a recent unintentional change from what is usual weight for the patient is more informative.[16] The patient is being compared with himself, not with some "ideal" standard. Also, in the obese patient a recent, unintentional yet critical loss is more readily identified.

It is generally agreed that any patient who has had a recent, unintentional weight loss of 10% is at risk for malnutrition. Any patient who is 30% below any ideal weight standard is at very high risk for survival. Each patient's past weight status should be obtained by the clinical dietitian whether or not a comprehensive nutritional history is being taken.

### Skinfold thickness

Table 23-3 gives Bistrian's criteria for interpreting the triceps skinfold thickness values. The standards are the 50th percentile values for 30-year-old men and women derived from the Ten-State Nutrition Survey data.[17] Using Bistrian's criteria, 80% of the standard TSF indicates a mild, 70% a moderate, and 60% a severe depletion of body fat stores. Bistrian's criteria do not apply to older patients due to the age change in skin compressibility[26] nor to the well-trained athlete with low fat stores.

### Arm muscle circumference

Table 23-3 also gives Bistrian's criteria for arm muscle circumference calculated from the equation on page 403. The standards are the 50th percentile for 30-year-old men and women derived from the Ten-State Survey data. As with TSF, 80% of standard indicates a mild, 70% a

moderate, and 60% a severe loss of body protein and fat stores excluding visceral protein. Bistrian's criteria must be applied with caution to the elderly patient due to the decrease in lean body mass with age.

Collins and co-workers,[27] using *in vivo* neutron activation analysis to measure body nitrogen, have concluded that anthropometric measurements are not sensitive enough to assess protein stores in an individual patient and that there is no justification for the use of anthropometry in following total body nitrogen in individual patients over short periods of time (2 wk). However, Moore[28] questions the validity of measuring total body nitrogen by neutron activation analysis. Blackburn and Thornton[18] recommend that follow-up assessments using anthropometrics, other than body weight, be conducted every 21 to 30 days after the initial assessment; and the follow-up assessment of body weight should be conducted at least 3 times per week. Also, Grant[16] points out that there are no standards for triceps skinfold thickness and arm circumference for adults derived from United States populations beyond the age of 44, and that the standards should be applied with caution to elderly patients.

### Serum albumin

There is considerable agreement that a serum albumin level of 3.0 g per deciliter to 3.5 g per deciliter is associated with mild visceral protein depletion, and 2.1 g per deciliter to 3.0 g per deciliter is associated with severe depletion.[18] Grant[16] uses 2.8 g per deciliter to 3.5 g per deciliter as indicative of mild depletion and 2.1 g per deciliter to 2.7 g per deciliter as moderate depletion. The recommended interval for the follow-up of serum albumin is every 10 to 14 days because repletion of serum albumin is a relatively slow process.

### Serum transferrin

The range of normal concentrations of serum transferrin is 250 mg per deciliter to 300 mg per deciliter. As calculated from the TIBC, a serum transferrin value of 150 mg per deciliter to 200 mg per deciliter is considered indicative of mild visceral protein depletion, between 100 mg per deciliter and 150 mg per deciliter moderate depletion, and any value less than 100 mg per deciliter severe depletion.[16]

Serum protein levels must be interpreted cautiously in order to differentiate low levels due to primary nutritional deficiencies from low levels due to disease. Serum protein levels are depressed in advanced hepatic cirrhosis, chronic renal failure, congestive heart disease, and chronic inflammation.

### The Creatinine-height index (CHI)

The CHI in mild body cell mass depletion is 90% of normal, moderate is 60% to 90%, and severe is less than 60%. The recommended follow-up assessment of CHI is every 21 to 30 days.[18]

### Immune competence

The normal total lymphocyte count is 2500 mm.³ The total lymphocyte count may be reported by the laboratory as mm³ or as a percentage of total leucocytes (white blood cells). The value for total lymphocytes in mm³ can be derived by multiplying the total leucocyte count by the percentage of lymphocytes. A total lymphocyte count between 1200 mm³ and 2000 mm³ indicates mild, 800 mm³ to 1200 mm³ moderate, and 800 mm³ or less as severe depression of the immune system.[16]

An immune-competent person has a positive response (> 5 mm induration at the site of injection) to two

**Table 23-2. Ideal Weight (kg) for Height, Adults**

| cm | Males | | | Females | | |
|---|---|---|---|---|---|---|
| | Small Frame | Medium Frame | Large Frame | Small Frame | Medium Frame | Large Frame |
| 142 | | | | 41.8 | 45.0 | 49.5 |
| 143 | | | | 42.3 | 45.3 | 49.8 |
| 144 | | | | 42.8 | 45.6 | 50.1 |
| 145 | | | | 43.2 | 45.9 | 50.5 |
| 146 | | | | 43.7 | 46.6 | 51.2 |
| 147 | | | | 44.1 | 47.3 | 51.8 |
| 148 | | | | 44.6 | 47.7 | 52.3 |
| 149 | | | | 45.1 | 48.1 | 52.8 |
| 150 | | | | 45.5 | 48.6 | 53.2 |
| 151 | | | | 46.2 | 49.3 | 54.0 |
| 152 | | | | 46.8 | 50.0 | 54.5 |
| 153 | | | | 47.3 | 50.5 | 55.0 |
| 154 | | | | 47.8 | 51.0 | 55.5 |
| 155 | 50.0 | 53.6 | 58.2 | 48.2 | 51.4 | 55.9 |
| 156 | 50.7 | 54.3 | 58.8 | 48.9 | 52.3 | 56.8 |
| 157 | 51.4 | 55.0 | 59.5 | 49.5 | 53.2 | 57.7 |
| 158 | 51.8 | 55.5 | 60.0 | 50.0 | 53.6 | 58.3 |
| 159 | 52.2 | 56.0 | 60.5 | 50.5 | 54.0 | 58.9 |
| 160 | 52.7 | 56.4 | 60.9 | 50.9 | 54.5 | 59.5 |
| 161 | 53.2 | 56.8 | 61.5 | 51.5 | 55.3 | 60.1 |
| 162 | 53.7 | 57.2 | 62.1 | 52.1 | 56.1 | 60.7 |
| 163 | 54.1 | 57.7 | 62.7 | 52.7 | 56.8 | 61.4 |
| 164 | 55.0 | 58.5 | 63.4 | 53.6 | 57.7 | 62.3 |
| 165 | 55.9 | 59.5 | 64.1 | 54.5 | 58.6 | 63.2 |
| 166 | 56.5 | 60.1 | 64.8 | 55.1 | 59.2 | 63.8 |
| 167 | 57.1 | 60.7 | 65.6 | 55.7 | 59.8 | 64.4 |
| 168 | 57.7 | 61.4 | 66.4 | 56.4 | 60.5 | 65.0 |
| 169 | 58.6 | 62.3 | 67.5 | 57.3 | 61.4 | 65.9 |
| 170 | 59.5 | 63.2 | 68.6 | 58.2 | 62.2 | 66.8 |
| 171 | 60.1 | 63.8 | 69.2 | 58.8 | 62.8 | 67.4 |
| 172 | 60.7 | 64.4 | 69.8 | 59.4 | 63.4 | 68.0 |
| 173 | 61.4 | 65.0 | 70.5 | 60.0 | 64.1 | 68.6 |
| 174 | 62.3 | 65.9 | 71.4 | 60.9 | 65.0 | 69.8 |
| 175 | 63.2 | 66.8 | 72.3 | 61.8 | 65.9 | 70.9 |
| 176 | 63.8 | 67.5 | 72.9 | 62.4 | 66.5 | 71.7 |
| 177 | 64.4 | 68.2 | 73.5 | 63.0 | 67.1 | 72.5 |
| 178 | 65.0 | 69.0 | 74.1 | 63.6 | 67.7 | 73.2 |
| 179 | 65.9 | 69.9 | 75.3 | 64.5 | 68.6 | 74.1 |
| 180 | 66.8 | 70.9 | 76.4 | 65.5 | 69.5 | 75.0 |
| 181 | 67.4 | 71.7 | 77.1 | 66.1 | 70.1 | 75.6 |
| 182 | 68.0 | 72.5 | 77.8 | 66.7 | 70.7 | 76.2 |
| 183 | 68.6 | 73.2 | 78.6 | 67.3 | 71.4 | 76.8 |
| 184 | 69.8 | 74.1 | 79.8 | | | |
| 185 | 70.9 | 75.0 | 80.9 | | | |
| 186 | 71.5 | 75.8 | 81.7 | | | |
| 187 | 72.1 | 76.6 | 82.5 | | | |
| 188 | 72.7 | 77.3 | 83.2 | | | |
| 189 | 73.3 | 78.0 | 83.8 | | | |
| 190 | 73.9 | 78.7 | 84.4 | | | |
| 191 | 74.5 | 79.5 | 85.0 | | | |

This table corrects the 1969 Metropolitan Life Insurance Co. standards to height without shoes and nude weight.[192] (From Grant JP: Handbook of Total Parenteral Nutrition. Philadelphia, WB Saunders, 1980)

or more recall antigens (candida, mumps, SK-SD). A moderately malnourished patient responds to only one antigen, whereas a severely malnourished patient has no response to any antigen.[18] Depressed skin test reactivity has been observed when serum albumin is less than 3.0 g per deciliter or the percentage of ideal body weight is less than 85%.

### Abbreviated assessment methods

A number of investigators have recommended abbreviated assessment methods to screen high risk patients. Copeland and co-workers[6] define nutritional depletion as a recent unintentional body weight loss of 10 lb or more, a serum albumin level of less than 3.4 g per deciliter, and a negative reaction to skin test antigens.

Mullen and co-workers[5] have reported that the most accurate prognostic indicators of postoperative morbidity and mortality in malnourished patients are serum albumin level of less than 3 g per deciliter, a serum transferrin level of less than 220 mg per deciliter, and depressed skin test reactivity (no reaction to three recall antigens).

Seltzer and co-workers[29] have described a method of instantly assessing the nutritional status of the hospitalized patient as an early warning system applicable to all patients admitted to the hospital. Their data indicate that less than normal serum albumin levels and total lymphocyte counts are associated with increased morbidity and mortality. In most hospitals both tests are done routinely on admission.

## Setting and monitoring goals for nutritional care
### Energy

The first goal that the clinical dietitian sets for the nutritional care of the patient who is at risk for malnutrition or is malnourished or is in a hypercatabolic state due to the stress of trauma, surgery, or infection is establishing the level of energy intake needed daily. The NRC-RDA is not used to estimate this energy need. The basal energy expenditure is estimated using the Harris-Benedict[30] equations for men and women, which use the patient's height, weight, and age. These equations were first published in 1919. Recently Long[31] has demonstrated that they are applicable to the clinical setting today. The equations are

$$BEE\ (men) = 66.47 + (13.75 \times W) + (5.0 \times H) - (6.74 \times A)$$
$$BEE\ (women) =$$
$$665.10 + (9.56 \times W) + (1.85 \times H) - (4.68 \times A)$$

where W = weight in kg, H = height in cm, and A = age in years. Grant[16] has simplified the equations as follows:

$$BEE\ (men) = 66 + (13.7 \times W) + (5 \times H) - (6.8 \times A)$$
$$BEE\ (women) = 665 + (9.6 \times W) + (1.9 \times H) - (4.7 \times A)$$

In addition to calories needed for basal energy expenditure, calories are needed for activity and the metabolic stress of injury where applicable. From metabolic balance studies with hospitalized patients Long recommends multiplying the BEE by a factor of 1.2 for patients confined to bed or a factor of 1.3 for patients who are out of bed. Long's[31] injury factors are 1.20 for minor operations, 1.35 for skeletal trauma, 1.60 for major sepsis, and 2.10 for severe thermal burns. The rationale for increased energy in injury are discussed in Chapter 27, *Nutritional Care—Surgery and Burn Therapy.* The final calculation of energy needs is

Total energy needs = basal calories × activity factor or, if injury is present, total energy needs = basal calories × activity factor × injury factor.

### Table 23-3. Standards for Arm Muscle Circumference and Triceps Skinfold

| *Sex* | *Standard** | *90% of Standard* | *80% of Standard* | *70% of Standard* | *60% of Standard* |
|---|---|---|---|---|---|
| | | ←————————————*mm*————————————→ | | | |
| *Upper arm muscle circumference* ‡ | | | | | |
| Male | 270 | 243 | 216 | 189 | 162 |
| Female | 213 | 192 | 170 | 149 | 128 |
| *Triceps skinfold* | | | | | |
| Male | 11 | 10 | 9 | 8 | 7 |
| Female | 19 | 17 | 15 | 13 | 11 |

*Standard is 50th percentile of thirty-year-olds.

†See reference 6 in Bistrian.

‡Where upper arm muscle circumference = upper arm circumference − ($\pi$) (triceps skinfolds).

(Bistrian BR: J Am Diet Assoc 71:393, 1977)

## Protein

The protein needs for the malnourished or hypercatabolic patient depend on the amount of erosion of the body cell mass. Because protein synthesis uses energy (ATP), the energy intake must be adequate to support the synthesis of cellular proteins as well as the other energy needs of the body. The recommended kilocalorie to nitrogen ratio is 150 kcal per gram nitrogen.[31] The range of recommendations is 120 kcal to 180 kcal per gram nitrogen. There is also the recommendation of 1.2 g to 1.5 g of protein per kilogram of body weight.[32]

For example, a woman aged 63, weight 52 kg, and height 170 cm is admitted to the hospital for minor surgery. She is 10% below ideal body weight but has maintained this weight for the past 3 years on an average daily intake of 1600 kcal to 1800 kcal. The assessment of her visceral protein status indicates a mild protein deficit: albumin, 3.4 g per deciliter, and transferrin, 190 mg per deciliter. She is out of bed immediately after surgery. Her daily total energy and protein needs are

Energy:
BEE = 665 + (9.6 × 52) + (1.9 × 170)
− (4.7 × 63) = 1191

Total energy = 1191 × 1.3 (activity factor) = 1548.3 × 1.2 (injury factor) = 1858 kcal per day.

Protein: kilocalories: 1 g nitrogen
1858 kcal ÷ 150 kcal = 12 g N
12 g N = 75 g protein (N × 6.25 g)

Protein: grams per kilogram
52 kg × 1.2 g = 62 g protein
52 kg × 1.5 g = 78 g protein

## Mineral and vitamin

The mineral and vitamin needs vary with the patient's problem. Many patients require supplementary mineral and vitamin preparations to correct any significant deficits.

## Monitoring nutritional care

As a member of the nutritional support team, the clinical dietitian's single most important contribution is to help those patients who can be fed by mouth to consume food and fluids. The clinical dietitian is responsible for monitoring the daily energy and protein intake of the patient. Bistrian[33] recommends that daily energy and protein intake be calculated once or twice a week. Two to three times a week is preferable. The estimates are recorded the next day in the appropriate space in the medical record. Together with changes in body weight the clinical dietitian uses these estimates to validate the appropriateness of the calculated needs for energy and adjusts the calculated goal if necessary. Changes in fluid gain or loss must be considered when evaluating weight changes. During rehydration the severely dehydrated pa-

tient may show a significant weight gain in 24 to 48 hours, whereas during diuresis the edematous patient may show a significant early weight loss.

A crude method for calculating nitrogen balance can be used to validate the estimated protein need. Nitrogen balance can be estimated from the nitrogen intake compared to the urinary urea nitrogen excretion for the same 24-hour period because urea nitrogen accounts for approximately 85% of the daily nitrogen excretion. A factor of 2 g nitrogen is added to the value for urea nitrogen to cover other daily nitrogen losses from the body, such as feces.[16] The equation used to calculate nitrogen balance is:

$$\frac{\text{Protein intake (g)}}{6.25} = \text{Nitrogen intake (g)}$$

$$\frac{\text{Nitrogen intake (g)}}{\text{Urinary urea nitrogen (g)} + 2 \text{ g}} = \pm \text{ N Balance}$$

If there is proteinuria, the nitrogen in this protein must be added to the value for urinary urea nitrogen (1 g protein in urine ÷ 6.25 = 0.16 g nitrogen). If there is protein-losing enteropathy, excessive drainage from gastrointestinal fistulas or abscesses, or exudates from large burn surface areas, the factor of 2 g will not be adequate to cover the total nitrogen losses from the body.

## Potential for learning

As early as possible in her interaction with a patient, the dietitian should attempt to discover through observing, listening, and interviewing what he knows about nutrition and diet; his attitudes toward his diet and illness; and his readiness for learning, when necessary, how to manage his diet.

Studies tell us that, as our nutrition education programs in elementary and secondary schools have been improved, we have a better educated young adult population today than in the past. If one is to avoid boring patients by giving them nutrition information they already have, one needs to find out what they know and how they use their knowledge. In this way one can discover the problem, if any, and focus his teaching on the patient's real need (see Chapt. 13).

As one listens to the patient, his vocabulary gives numerous clues about the words and kinds of explanations that one needs to use in teaching him. For example, if the patient is a newly diagnosed diabetic who is an organic chemist, he may expect the nutrition counselor to use the word, *carbohydrate*, whereas, the mother of six children who reads and understands at the sixth-grade level needs to be approached quite differently. In helping her to understand diabetes and her diet one would more likely use the word, *sugar*.

With the increasing use of programmed instruction, any member of the health-care team should watch for clues whether or not a patient is literate, in English or any other language. Dietitians have not always been aware of this in the past as they used printed instructions, as children, friends, or other patients may have interpreted such instructions for the patient.

The dietitian who begins diet instruction as early as possible during the patient's hospitalization can use the trays served each day to demonstrate the kinds and amounts of food he will be eating at home. At the same time, she can involve him or a member of his family in the planning of his daily menu. The wife of a patient who will require a sodium-restricted diet for the years ahead may demonstrate her understanding of the dietitian's instructions and her skill in adjusting her methods of food preparation by bringing her husband the "fruits" of her labors. At the same time, she may feel a certain satisfaction from participating in her husband's care. This approach to patient education not only prepares the patient and his family for his discharge but also, in many instances, stimulates the patient's interest in learning about his diet.

## Study questions and activities

1. Select a patient who has been identified as a "feeding problem." With the assistance of your clinical instructor, determine what the patient's problem really is and with your instructor's guidance attempt to work toward a solution to the problem.
2. In the supine position with only *one* pillow to elevate your head, have someone feed you ½ cup of *hot* broth, two crackers and ½ cup of pudding or clear gelatin. Record the time it took you to consume all the food and fluids and your reaction to this experience. Write an outline of what you would use when instructing an individual responsible for feeding a hospitalized patient in the same position.
3. With your clinical instructor select a patient whose name identifies him as a member of some ethnic group. Interview this patient to find out what foods he commonly eats. Was his name a valid or an invalid clue to his usual food practices? In conference discuss this clinical encounter with your classmates.
4. With your clinical instructor using a form comparable to Figure 23-1, complete the nutritional assessment of a patient who is at high risk for malnutrition and formulate your care plan for meeting this patient's nutritional needs.

## References

1. Babcock CG: J Am Diet Assoc 28:222, 1952
2. Pumpian-Midlin EJ: J Am Diet Assoc 30:576, 1954
3. Parsons HG et al: Am J Clin Nutr 33:1140, 1980
4. Weinsier RL et al: Am J Clin Nutr 32:418, 1979
5. Mullen JL et al: Arch Surg 114:121, 1979
6. Copeland EM et al: Cancer 43:2108, 1979
7. Irvin TT: Surg Gynecol Obstet 146:33, 1978
8. Chernoff R: J Parent Ent Nutr 3:89, 1979
9. Wade JE: J Am Diet Assoc 70:185, 1977
10. Tobias AL, Van Itallie TB: J Am Diet Assoc 71:253, 1977
11. Bigwood EJ: Guiding Principles for Studies of the Nutrition of Populations. Geneva, League of Nations, 1939
12. Jelliffe DB: The assessment of the nutritional status of the community. WHO Monogr Ser, no. 53. Geneva, World Health Organization, 1966
13. Plan and Operation of the Health and Nutrition Examination Survey, U.S., 1971–1973. DHEW Publ. No. (HSM) 73-1310, 10 (A&B)
14. Dudrick SJ et al: Nutritional support: Assessment and indications. In Deitel M (ed): Nutrition in Clinical Surgery, 19–28. Baltimore, Williams & Wilkins, 1980
15. Reed ML et al: J Am Diet Assoc 72:409, 1978
16. Grant JP: Handbook of Total Parenteral Nutrition, pp 7–46. Philadelphia, WB Saunders, 1980
17. Frisancho AR: Am J Clin Nutr 27:1052, 1974
18. Blackburn GL, Thornton PA: Med Clin North Am 63:1103, 1979
19. Driver AG, McAlvey MT: Am J Clin Nutr 33:2057, 1980
20. Bistrian BR et al: JAMA 230:858, 1974
21. Gray GE, Gray LK: J Am Diet Assoc 77:534, 1980
22. Burgert SL, Anderson CF: Am J Clin Nutr 32:2136, 1979
23. Jelliffe DB, Jelliffe EFP: Am J Clin Nutr 33:2058, 1980
24. Bistrian BR: Am J Clin Nutr 33:2211, 1980
25. Build and Blood Pressure Study. Chicago, Society of Actuaries, 1980 (in press)
26. Brozek J, Kinzey W: J Gerontol 15:45, 1960
27. Collins JP et al: Am J Clin Nutr 32:1527, 1979
28. Moore FD: J Parent Ent Nutr 4:228, 1980
29. Seltzer MH: J Parent Ent Nutr 3:157, 1979
30. Harris JA, Benedict FG: Publ. No. 279. Carnegie Institute of Washington, 1919
31. Long CL et al: J Parent Ent Nutr 3:452, 1979
32. Blackburn GL et al: J Parent Ent Nutr 1:11, 1977
33. Bistrian BR: J Am Diet Assoc 71:393, 1977

## Supplementary readings

Blackburn GL, Thornton PA: Nutritional assessment of the hospitalized patient. Med Clin North Am 63:1103, 1979

Burgert SL, Anderson CF: A comparison of triceps skinfold values as measured by the plastic McGaw Caliper and the Lange Caliper. Am J Clin Nutr 32:1531, 1979

Butterworth CE Jr: Nutritional support for hospitalized patients: How do we cope? How should we cope? J Am Diet Assoc 75:227, 1979

Carson JAS: Nutrition in a team approach to rehabilitation of the patient with cancer. J Am Diet Assoc 72:407, 1978

Heymsfield SB et al: A radiographic method of quantifying protein–calorie undernutrition. Am J Clin Nutr 32:693, 1979

Mahalko JR, Johnson LK: Accuracy of predictions of long-term energy needs. J Am Diet Assoc 77:561, 1980

Meakins JL et al: Delayed hypersensitivity: Indicator of acquired failure of host defenses in sepsis and trauma. Ann Surg 186:241, 1977

Merritt RJ, Suskind RM: Nutritional survey of hospitalized pediatric patients. Am J Clin Nutr 32:1320, 1979

Page CP, Clibon U: Man the meal-eater and his interaction with parenteral nutrition. JAMA 224:1950, 1980

Shapiro LR: Streamlining and implementing nutritional assessment: The dietary approach. J Am Diet Assoc 75:230, 1979

Steffee WP: Malnutrition in hospitalized patients. JAMA 244:2630, 1980

Warnold I et al: Energy intake and expenditure in selected groups of hospital patients. Am J Clin Nutr 31:742, 1978

Winborn AL et al: A protocol for nutritional assessment in a community hospital. J Am Diet Assoc 78:129, 1981

Young GA, Hill GL: Assessment of protein–calorie malnutrition in surgical patients from plasma proteins and anthropometric measurements. Am J Clin Nutr 31:429, 1979

Young GA, Hill GL: Evaluation of protein–energy malnutrition in surgical patients from plasma valine and other amino acids, proteins and anthropometric measurements. Am J Clin Nutr 34:166, 1981

*For further references see Bibliography in Part 4.*

# Food Composition—
# A Basic Tool of
# Diet Therapy

# 24

Food Composition and Therapeutic
   Diets
Exchange System of Diet Calculation

The dietary modifications prescribed for any patient must be translated into the foods and serving sizes he is familiar with and into a meal pattern similar to that of his family's. This ensures a greater probability that the diet will be accepted and used and, as a result, succeed in its therapeutic goals. At the same time, one may encounter a patient whose usual food practices require drastic changes, not just modification, due to the complexity of his problem. Such a patient needs special support and understanding as he struggles to change his food practices (see Chap. 13).

To be able to design simple or complex therapeutic diet plans, the nutrition counselor must have extensive knowledge of both the kinds and amounts of nutrients in food (see Chap. 11). She must be familiar with the effect of food processing on the nutrient composition of foods and, with today's increasingly complex manipulation of nutrient intake in the treatment of certain diseases, she needs to know the composition of specially formulated foods and supplementary feedings used to implement various therapeutic diet plans. She should be an expert in food preparation and know how the adjustment of ingredients in a recipe may modify the dish.

Most nutritional misinformation among members of the health-care team today is due to a lack of quantitative, not qualitative, knowledge of the energy and nutrient composition of food. For example, a physician who orders a 1500-calorie diet, may complain strenuously when his patient has two slices of toast for breakfast, although the patient, perhaps a farmer, has been used to a substantial breakfast. Within the limits of his diet order the patient chose two slices of toast for his breakfast meal plan. When questioned the physician said: "Bread is fattening." He did not realize that one slice of bread contains approximately 70 calories and that two slices (140 calories) could be included in the breakfast plan for this patient's 1500-calorie diet. Many lay people share the same lack of infor-

PKU: Phenylketonuria

mation, such as the banker who says: "Potatoes and bread are fattening," while munching a glazed doughnut with his midmorning coffee.

The clinical dietitian, or any other nutrition counselor, may use the Daily Food Guide (Chap. 11) as a standard for assessing the adequacy of a person's nutritional intake. However, this standard may not be adequate in all situations. Life-styles vary in our society, and food practices that differ from the Food Guide can supply adequate intakes of nutrients. The diet of an adolescent boy who will not eat dark green or deep yellow vegetables in any form can still supply adequate vitamin A because of the amount of fortified skim milk he is drinking each day.

In addition, the clinical dietitian responsible for the calculation of therapeutic diets cannot approach the nutrient content of foods in the traditional way, such as milk for calcium, meat for protein, liver for iron. She must be aware of the significance of the total energy and nutrient content of a food. For example, 1 pint of milk (16 oz) contributes approximately $\frac{1}{3}$ of the protein, $\frac{3}{4}$ of the calcium, and $\frac{1}{2}$ of the riboflavin recommended daily by the NRC for the 23 to 50 year old man, whereas $3\frac{1}{2}$ oz of broiled hamburger contributes approximately $\frac{1}{2}$ of the protein, $\frac{1}{3}$ of the iron, and $\frac{1}{3}$ of the niacin for the same person. Together the pint of milk and $3\frac{1}{2}$ oz of broiled hamburger contribute almost $\frac{1}{4}$ of this man's daily energy needs when whole milk is used; or less, if he drinks skim milk.

At the same time the clinical dietitian must be prepared to answer questions on the spot from other members of the health-care team about both the qualitative and quantitative nutrient composition of foods. On rounds in the clinical setting with the renologist and his co-workers, the clinical dietitian can expect to be asked: "Is there potassium in tomato juice?" or: "How much potassium is in 100 ml of tomato juice?"

The clinical dietitian cannot be a walking food composition table. However, with a knowledge of general nutritional composition she can readily answer questions about the qualitative aspects of foods. By repeatedly using the nutrient values of common foods, she can evaluate the nutrient content of a food with a reasonable degree of accuracy without constant reference to food composition tables. The knowledge of qualitative and quantitative nutrient composition of foods is the dietitian's unique contribution to the health-care team, and she cannot expect the other members of the team to develop expertise in this area comparable to hers.

This chapter presents special resources for planning and a system for the calculation of diet patterns for therapeutic diets. The reader is urged to review at this point the discussions on food composition tables and the general information about the nutrient composition of foods in Chapter 11, *Meeting Nutritional Norms*. Additional information pertinent to planning modified diets is given in this chapter.

## Food composition and therapeutic diets
### Basic food composition tables

The food composition tables discussed in Chapter 11 and Tables 1 to 7 in Part 4 of this book are the primary resources for calculating the majority of modified diet patterns. Frequently, additional resources are required for more extensive information than is included in the tables in Part 4 and for calculating some of the more complex diet patterns; for example, values for the naturally occurring simple sugars in fruits and vegetables. A discussion of these special resources follows.

### Special food composition tables
#### Sugars

Only limited data on the mono-, di-, and polysaccharide content of foods are available because no standardized analytical method has been formulated until recently. Also, the free sugar content of fruits and vegetables varies by variety and stage of maturity; for example, a partially ripe banana contains significantly more starch than a ripe one (8.8 g vs. 1.2 g per 100 g edible portion).[1]

The most readily available information about the sugar that occurs in foods has been published by Hardinge and co-workers.[1] Table 1 in Hardinge's work is a tabulation of the data in the literature prior to 1965 and gives values for the sugars in fruits, vegetables, legumes, milk and milk products, and nuts and nut products. Table 2 gives limited data on less common sugars, such as arabinose, raffinose, stachyose, and sorbitol. In 1970 Yee, Shallenbarger, and Vittum[2] published the results of their own analyses of free sugars in fruits, vegetables, and legumes. They give values for glucose, fructose, sucrose, raffinose, and stachyose.

The figures for sugars in foods are used to calculate diets limited in simple sugars for the treatment of carbohydrate-induced hyperlipidemia and to identify foods that should be avoided in lactose intolerance or other disaccharide malabsorption problems and in galactosemia, fructosuria, or any other condition where the intake of a specific sugar must be avoided or limited.

#### Amino acids

Table 3 in Part 4 of this book was derived from *Amino Acid Content of Foods, USDA Home Economics Research Report, No. 4.* Unfortunately, values for the amino acid composition of all commonly used foods are not available in Research Report No. 4. The new USDA Handbook No. 8 Series (see Chap. 11) contains the amino acid composition of each item. When completed, the Handbook No. 8 Series will give the amino acid composition of a wide variety of foods.

The amino acid composition of diets may be modified for persons with inborn errors of intermediary metabolism. When the error occurs in the metabolism of an essential amino acid, such as phenylalanine or the branched chain amino acids, leucine, isoleucine, and valine, the intake is monitored to provide the person's needs for these essential nutrients without an excess. In planning diets for patients in renal failure or in impending hepatic coma, it is necessary to calculate amino acid values so that adequate essential amino acids and limited amounts of nonessential amino acids are provided.

### Lipids

The fatty acid values in Table 2 of Part 4 were derived from USDA Handbook No. 8, revised 1963, and the cholesterol figures from the recent findings of Feeley, Criner, and Watt.[3] Some manufacturers of soft margarine give the amounts in grams of the saturated and polyunsaturated fatty acids and cholesterol found in a specified quantity of their product. The USDA Handbook No. 8 Series also contains the fatty acid and cholesterol composition of each item.

The values for the fatty acid and cholesterol contents of foods are used to calculate diet patterns for patients with hyperlipidemias or elevated blood cholesterol levels or both.

### Electrolytes

Tables 1 and 4, Part 4, gives figures for the sodium, potassium, and magnesium content of foods. Values for a limited number of foods may also be found in recent issues of professional journals.

In addition to food, drinking water may, or may not be a significant source of sodium. This depends on the geological characteristics of an area and on the method used to treat water supplies. In some areas of the United States, local water supplies contain a significant amount of naturally occurring sodium (more than 2 mg per 100 ml). In some instances the equipment used to soften home water supplies adds sodium to the water.

## Convenience foods

Uncertainty about the energy, protein, fat, and carbohydrate contents of convenience foods, as well as their sodium and potassium content, make these foods unusable in therapeutic diet plans requiring complex manipulation of energy and nutrient content, for example, diets limited in energy, protein, electrolytes, or gluten. The administrator of dietetic services in the general hospital is faced with the same dilemma. Convenience food items served to patients on regular diets are rarely appropriate for therapeutic diets unless the suppliers of the foods prepare them according to rigid specifications set by the dietitian.

## Dietetic foods

Foods for special dietary use have been on the market in the United States for many years. The most commonly available ones have been fruits canned without the addition of sugar; bread made without salt, vegetables canned without sodium; and artificially sweetened pudding mixes, gelatin dessert powders, cookies, jellies, candy, gum, and carbonated beverages. The labels of these products state the energy and nutritive value of a specified serving of the contents of the container as required by the Food and Drug Administration regulations.

### Artificial sweeteners

Prior to 1969 when the Food and Drug Administration prohibited the use of cyclamate because research showed it to cause bladder tumors in rats, it was the most widely used nonnutritive sweetener. Before the ban went into effect, approximately half of the carbonated beverages sold in the United States were artificially sweetened with cyclamate or a combination of cyclamate and saccharin. Today sodium or calcium saccharin and sorbitol are the most widely used nonnutritive sweeteners, but the taste of the products in which they are used is not as acceptable as the taste of those sweetened with cyclamate.

There are a variety of sweeteners on the market that contain saccharin combined with small amounts of mono- or disaccharides and, therefore, cannot be classified as nonnutritive. Each product must be evaluated before use, especially if the diet is restricted not only in calories but also in simple sugars.

In 1981 FDA approved the use of the artificial sweetener, *aspartame,* a dipeptide composed of the amino acids, phenylalanine and aspartic acid. The product will bear a warning to phenylketonurics (PKU) who must restrict their intake of phenylalanine. See the discussion of PKU in Chapter 36, *Inborn Errors of Metabolism in Infancy and Childhood.*

### Diet breads and margarines

Both of these products contain fewer calories per serving than the regular products. One slice of diet bread weighing approximately 18 g contains approximately 45 kcal to 50 kcal, while one slice of regular bread weighing approximately 23 g contains 70 kcal. Three teaspoons of the diet margarines contain approximately the same number of calories as 1 teaspoon of regular margarine. The energy content of diet margarines vary by brand; the nutrition label of a brand should be checked for energy content per serving.

Before any dietetic products are recommended, the energy and nutrient content per serving must be estimated and the serving quantities carefully defined to avoid serious errors. Two slices of diet bread (90 kcal–100 kcal) cannot be substituted for one slice of regular bread (70 kcal). Also, many patients are confused about dietetic foods. They think that any food labeled dietetic may or must be used on their diets. For example, a woman who was restricting her energy intake because she was obese used canned vegetables without sodium added even though she did not have to restrict her sodium (salt) intake. Because the vegetables were labeled "dietetic," she thought she must use them in her low calorie diet.

## Medium-chain triglycerides (MCT)

Fat in the ordinary diet contains mainly the long-chain fatty acids, palmitic (C16:0), stearic (C18:0), and oleic (C18:1). The products of absorption of these fats are transported by the lymphatic system as chylomicrons to the thoracic duct and into the general circulation (see Chap. 9). Digestion and absorption depend on the availability of bile salts and pancreatic lipase. In several malabsorption syndromes (see Chap. 26) it is the long-chain fatty acids that are frequently not absorbed but are excreted in the feces.

About 5% of naturally occurring fat contains short- and medium-chain fatty acids, C6:0 to C12:0. Hashim and co-workers[4] showed that these are hydrolyzed to glycerol and fatty acids by the mucosal enzymes and are absorbed directly from the villi into the capillary bed without reesterification; they are then transported through the portal vein to the liver.

The synthesis of a fat containing only medium-chain fatty acids was accomplished by the hydrolysis of coconut oil and the distillation of the fatty acids. The short- and medium-chain fatty acids, C6:0 to C12:0, came off first, as they are the lightest. They were reesterified with glycerol to form a fat (an oil) that can replace regular fat in the diet. This product, containing almost entirely caprylic (C8:0) and capric (C10:0) fatty acids, is called medium-chain triglyceride or MCT.

Greenberger and Skillman[5] reviewed the use of MCT in the treatment of malabsorption syndromes and pointed out that it is effective as a substitute for ordinary dietary fats in reducing steatorrhea and the loss of sodium, potassium, and calcium in the feces in cystic fibrosis, celiac disease, intestinal lymphangiectasia, chylothorax, and small bowel resection. It has not proved effective in inflammatory bowel disease, massive bowel resection, or impending hepatic coma.

Medium-chain triglycerides yield 8.2 kcal to 8.4 kcal per gram and are available as MCT oil* or in a powdered-formula diet (Portagen).* MCT oil can be substituted for regular cooking oils. The powdered-formula diet is used as a food for infants and as a beverage by adults.

## Protein-free wheat starch products

These products are essentially free of protein and provide a source of energy in protein-restricted diets used to treat renal and hepatic disease. They are also gluten-free and can be used in the treatment of gluten-induced enteropathy. Their availability, use, and the problems encountered with them in food preparation are discussed in detail in Chapter 26, *Diet in Gastrointestinal Disease* and Chapter 32, *Renal Disease*.

---

*Mead Johnson Laboratories, Evansville, Ind, 47721.

## Food supplements

There are a variety of products available that can be used to supplement energy or energy and protein intakes. These products vary widely in availability, energy and nutrient density, acceptability, and cost. Some of them are used as beverages while others may be added to reinforce commonly used beverages and foods. The food and nutrient contents are supplied by the producer and should be carefully evaluated for the individual patient before use because in some instances the ingredients or electrolyte content may not be appropriate (see Chap. 27, *Nutritional Care—Surgery and Burn Therapy*).

## Exchange system of diet calculation

Therapeutic diet orders that prescribe a quantitative modification in nutritive intake require the calculation of a dietary pattern for the patient's use in selecting food each day. These dietary patterns may be calculated from food composition tables, by a system using composite figures for food groups (the Exchange System), or by programming the computer properly.

By the 1940s, dietitians and physicians were aware that food composition tables used to calculate therapeutic diets, especially diets for the diabetic patient, were cumbersome, time consuming, and needlessly precise, and that patients did not have the time or inclination to calculate for each day the energy and nutrient composition of the food required to fulfill his dietary prescription.

After careful study, a committee of the American Dietetic Association, working cooperatively with the Committee on Education of the American Diabetes Association and representatives of the Diabetes Branch of the United States Public Health Service, published a simplified system of diet calculation for diabetic patients known today as the *Exchange System.*[6] In 1976 the American Dietetic Association and the American Diabetes Association modified the 1950 Exchange System,[7] particularly the amount and type of lipids in the various food lists. Although originally planned for the calculation of dietary patterns for patients with diabetes, this Exchange System, or modifications of it, are widely used to calculate other therapeutic diets—for example, energy-restricted or fat-restricted diets.

The term, *exchange*, reflects the problems that a patient with diabetes encountered in the management of his diet prior to 1950. Frequently his instructions focused on menus, not dietary patterns. A breakfast menu might be ½ cup of orange juice, ½ cup of cooked oatmeal, 1 cup of milk, 1 slice of toast, and 1 teaspoon of butter. After 2 or 3 weeks of this meal he would ask, "Can't I have something in place of orange juice?" He would be offered ½ cup of grapefruit juice in "exchange" for ½ cup of orange juice. As a solution to this problem, foods of similar nutritive composition were grouped together for "exchanges" and formalized into the Exchange System.

The groups in the 1976 revision are milk, whole, skim, and evaporated; meat, lean, medium-fat and high-fat, including fish and poultry and such meat substitutes as eggs and cheese; fruits; vegetables; bread, including cereals and cereal products, legumes and starchy vegetables; and fats, including seed oils, margarine, and butter.

The food groups in the Exchange System are similar to, yet differ to some extent, from the groups in the Daily Food Guide. Table 24-1 illustrates the similarities and differences between these two classifications. The milk, meat, and bread-cereal groups of the Daily Food Guide are also in the Exchange System. The vegetable-fruit group of the Daily Guide becomes two items in the Exchange System—vegetable exchanges and fruit exchanges. Fat exchanges are included in the Exchange System but not in the Daily Food Guide.

Table 24-2 gives the average protein, fat, carbohydrate, and energy values for each exchange. These values are averages of the nutrient values of the foods in a group weighted by frequency of use. Table 24-3 gives the lists of the foods included in each exchange group. With the exception of the meat serving, which is 1 oz, the serving sizes of the items within each exchange are average servings. The average serving of meat for an adult is approximately 3 oz or 4 oz or three or four times the protein, fat, and energy values given in Table 24-2 for a meat exchange. Whenever the term, *cup*, is used to define a serving in dietetics it must be remembered that it means the standard 8-oz measuring cup, and a teaspoon or tablespoon refers to standard measuring spoons.

## Table 24-1. Daily Food Guide Compared with Exchange System

| *Daily Food Guide* | *Exchange System* |
| --- | --- |
| Milk group | Milk exchange |
| Meat group | Meat exchange |
| Vegetable fruit group | Vegetable exchanges Fruit exchanges |
| Bread cereal group | Bread exchanges Fat exchanges |

Each list of foods in Table 24-3 should be studied carefully, and any special directions should be noted; for instance, when whole milk is substituted for the skim milk calculated in the diet pattern, two fat exchanges should be subtracted to account for the fat in the whole milk. The nutrient values of each exchange apply only to the serving size of the food as described, not, for example, to fruits canned or frozen with sugar added, or to cooked meat served with gravy. It must also be noted that certain vegetables are listed with the bread exchanges. These contain 15 g of carbohydrate per serving as listed, such as $\frac{1}{3}$ cup of corn. The items in the fruit exchanges are listed by serving size that yields 10 g of carbohydrate. Bacon and nuts are listed in the fat exchanges, not in the meat exchanges, as might be expected. Their primary contribution to the diet in this system is fat rather than protein.

Wyse[8] analyzed the energy and nutrient composition of each list in the 1976 revision of the Exchange System. The foods in each list were entered into a computer pro-

## Table 24-2. Nutrient Composition of Food Exchanges

| Group | Amount | Weight (g) | Protein (g) | Fat (g) | Carbohydrate (g) | Energy (kcal) |
| --- | --- | --- | --- | --- | --- | --- |
| Milk, non-fat | $\frac{1}{2}$ pt (8 oz) | 240 | 8 | | 12 | 80 |
| Vegetables | $\frac{1}{2}$ cup | 100 | 2 | | 5 | 25 |
| Fruit | As defined* | | | | 10 | 40 |
| Bread | As defined* | | 2 | | 15 | 70 |
| Meat, lean | 1 oz | 30 | 7 | 3 | | 55 |
| Meat, medium fat | 1 oz | 30 | 7 | 5 | | 75 |
| Meat, high fat | 1 oz | 30 | 7 | 8 | | 100 |
| Fat | 1 tsp | 5 | | 5 | | 45 |

*See exchange lists.

(Adapted from Exchange Lists for Meal Planning, American Dietetic Association, 1976)

## Table 24-3. Exchange Lists

### Foods That Need Not Be Measured
(Insignificant carbohydrate or energy)

| | |
|---|---|
| Diet carbonated beverages | Parsley |
| Coffee | Nutmeg |
| Tea | Lemon |
| Clear broth | Mustard |
| Bouillon without fat | Chili powder |
| Unsweetened gelatin | Onion salt or powder |
| Salt and pepper | Horseradish |
| Red pepper | Vinegar |
| Paprika | Mint |
| Garlic | Cinnamon |
| Celery Salt | Lime |
| Unsweetened pickles | Other herbs and spices |

### List 1. Milk Exchange—Non-Fat, Low-Fat, and Whole Milk

One non-fat milk exchange contains 8 g protein, trace of fat, 12 g carbohydrate, and 80 kcalories.

*Non-fat fortified\* milk*

| | |
|---|---|
| Skim or non-fat milk | 1 c |
| Powdered (non-fat dry before adding liquid) | 1/3 c |
| Canned, evaporated skim milk (undiluted) | 1/2 c |
| Buttermilk made from skim milk | 1 c |
| Yogurt made from skim milk (plain, unflavored) | 1 c |

*Low-fat fortified\* milk*

| | |
|---|---|
| 1% fat, fortified milk (103 kcalories) (omit 1/2 fat exchange) | 1 c |
| 2% fat, fortified milk (125 kcalories) (omit 1 fat exchange) | 1 c |
| Yogurt made from 2% fat, fortified skim milk (plain, unflavored) (125 kcalories) (omit 1 fat exchange) | 1 c |

*Whole milk (170 kcalories) (omit 2 fat exchanges)*

| | |
|---|---|
| Whole milk | 1 c |
| Canned, evaporated whole milk (undiluted) | 1/2 c |
| Buttermilk made from whole milk | 1 c |
| Yogurt made from whole milk (plain, unflavored) | 1 c |

\* Fortified with vitamins A and D.

### List 2. Vegetable Exchanges

One vegetable exchange contains about 2 g protein, 5 g carbohydrate, and 25 kcalories. One exchange is 1/2 c.

| | | |
|---|---|---|
| Asparagus | Green pepper | Okra |
| Bean sprouts | Greens:* | Onions |
| Beets | Beet | Rhubarb |
| Broccoli | Chard | Rutabaga |
| Brussels sprouts | Collard | Sauerkraut |
| Cabbage† | Dandelion | String beans, yellow or green |
| Carrots* | Kale | Summer squash |
| Cauliflower | Mustard | Tomatoes† |
| Celery | Spinach | Tomato juice† |
| Cucumbers | Turnip | Vegetable juice cocktail |
| Eggplant | Mushrooms | Zucchini |

The following raw vegetables may be used as desired (not to exceed a total of 1 1/2 c per day).

| | |
|---|---|
| Chicory | Lettuce |
| Chinese cabbage | Parsley |
| Endive | Radishes |
| Escarole | Watercress |

*Good source of Vitamin A.

†Good source of Vitamin C.

### List 3. Fruit Exchanges

One fruit exchange contains 10 g carbohydrate and 40 kcalories

(This list shows the different amounts of fruits, fresh or processed without the addition of sugar, to use for one fruit exchange.)

| Fruit | Amount to Use |
|---|---|
| Apple | 1 small |
| Apple juice | 1/3 c |
| Applesauce (unsweetened) | 1/2 c |
| Apricots, fresh* | 2 medium |
| Apricots, dried* | 4 halves |
| Banana | 1/2 small |
| Berries | |
| Blackberries | 1/2 c |
| Blueberries | 1/2 c |
| Raspberries | 1/2 c |
| Strawberries† | 3/4 c |
| Cherries | 10 large |
| Cider | 1/3 c |
| Dates, dried | 2 |
| Figs, fresh | 1 |
| Figs, dried | 1 |
| Grapefruit† | 1/2 |
| Grapefruit juice† | 1/2 c |
| Grapes | 12 |
| Grape juice | 1/4 c |
| Mango | 1/2 small |
| Melon | |
| Cantaloupe† | 1/4 small |
| Honeydew† | 1/8 medium |
| Watermelon | 1 c |
| Nectarine | 1 small |
| Orange† | 1 small |
| Orange juice† | 1/2 c |
| Papaya† | 3/4 c |
| Peach | 1 medium |
| Pear | 1 small |
| Persimmon, native | 1 medium |
| Pineapple | 1/2 c |
| Pineapple juice | 1/3 c |
| Plums | 2 medium |
| Prunes | 2 medium |
| Prune juice | 1/4 c |
| Raisins | 2 tbsp |
| Tangerine† | 1 medium |

*Good source of Vitamin A.

†Good source of Vitamin C.

### List 4. Bread Exchanges

One bread exchange contains about 2 g protein, 15 g carbohydrate, and 70 kcalories.

(This list shows the different amounts of foods to use for one bread exchange.)

| Bread, Cereal and Others | Amount to use |
|---|---|
| Bread | |
| White (including French and Italian) | 1 slice |
| Whole wheat | 1 slice |
| Rye or pumpernickel | 1 slice |
| Raisin (unfrosted) | 1 slice |
| Bagel | 1/2 small |
| English muffin | 1/2 small |
| Plain roll, bread | 1 |
| Frankfurter roll | 1/2 |
| Hamburger roll | 1/2 |
| Dried bread crumbs | 3 tbsp |
| Tortilla | 1 (6") |

# Table 24-3. Exchange Lists (Continued)

## List 4. Bread Exchanges (Continued)

Cereals

| | |
|---|---|
| Bran flakes | $^1/_2$ c |
| Other ready-to-eat unsweetened cereal | $^3/_4$ c |
| Puffed cereal (unfrosted) | 1 c |
| Cereal (cooked) | $^1/_2$ c |
| Grits (cooked) | $^1/_2$ c |
| Rice or barley (cooked) | $^1/_2$ c |
| Pasta (cooked) | |
|   Spaghetti, noodles, macaroni | $^1/_2$ c |
| Popcorn (popped, no fat added) | 3 c |
| Cornmeal (dry) | 2 tbsp |
| Flour | $2^1/_2$ tbsp |
| Wheat germ | $^1/_4$ c |

Crackers

| | |
|---|---|
| Arrowroot | 3 |
| Graham ($2^1/_2''$ sq) | 2 |
| Matzo ($4''$–$6''$) | $^1/_2$ |
| Oyster | 20 |
| Pretzels ($3^1/_8''$ long, $^1/_8''$ diam) | 25 |
| Rye wafers ($2''$–$3^1/_2''$) | 3 |
| Saltines | 6 |
| Soda ($2^1/_2''$ sq) | 4 |

Dried beans, peas, and lentils
(omit one meat exchange)

| | |
|---|---|
| Beans, peas, lentils (dried and cooked) | $^1/_2$ c |
| Baked beans, no pork, canned | $^1/_4$ c |

High-carbohydrate vegetables

| | |
|---|---|
| Corn | $^1/_3$ c |
| Corn on the cob | 1 small |
| Lima beans | $^1/_2$ c |
| Parsnips | $^2/_3$ c |
| Peas, green (canned or frozen) | $^1/_2$ c |
| Potato, white | 1 small |
| Potato, mashed | $^1/_2$ c |
| Pumpkin | $^3/_4$ c |
| Winter acorn or butternut squash* | $^1/_2$ c |
| Yam or sweet potato* | $^1/_4$ c |

Prepared foods (omit one fat exchange)

| | |
|---|---|
| Biscuits ($2''$ diam) | 1 |
| Cornbread, ($2'' \times 2'' \times 1''$) | 1 |
| Corn muffin ($2''$ diam) | 1 |
| Crackers, round butter type | 5 |
| Muffin, plain small | 1 |
| Potatoes, French fried ($2''$–$3^1/_2''$ long) | 8 |
| Pancake ($5'' \times ^1/_2''$) | 1 |
| Waffle ($5'' \times ^1/_2''$) | 1 |

Potato or corn chips
(omit two fat exchanges) | 15

*Good source of Vitamin A.

## List 5. Meat Exchanges

### Lean Meat

One lean meat exchange contains 7 g protein, 3 g fat, and 55 kcalories.

(This list shows the different amounts of foods to use for one lean meat exchange.)

| Meat | Amount to Use |
|---|---|
| Beef | 1 oz |
|   Baby beef (very lean) | |
|   Steak, chuck, flank, tenderloin, plate ribs, round (bottom or top), rump, spare ribs, tripe) | |
| Lamb | 1 oz |
|   Leg, rib, sirloin, loin, shank, shoulder | |

## List 5. Meat Exchanges (Continued)

| Meat | Amount to Use |
|---|---|
| Pork | 1 oz |
|   Leg, whole rump, center shank, ham, center slices | |
| Veal | 1 oz |
|   Leg, loin, rib, shank, shoulder, cutlets | |
| Poultry (without skin) | 1 oz |
|   Chicken, turkey, cornish hen, guinea hen, pheasant | |
| Fish | |
|   Any fresh or frozen | 1 oz |
|   Canned salmon, tuna (water packed) | $^1/_4$ c |
|   Canned mackerel, crab, lobster | $^1/_4$ c |
|   Clams, oysters, scallops, shrimp | 5 or 1 oz |
|   Sardines, drained | 3 |
| Cheese | $^1/_4$ c |
|   Cottage cheese, dry and 2% butter fat | |
| Dried beans and peas (omit one bread exchange) | $^1/_2$ c |

### Medium-Fat Meat

One medium-fat meat exchange contains 7 g protein, 5 g fat, and 75 kcalories.

(This list shows the different amounts of foods to use for one medium-fat meat exchange.)

| Meat | Amount to Use |
|---|---|
| Beef | 1 oz |
|   Ground (15% fat) | |
|   Corned beef, canned | |
|   Ribeye | |
|   Round, ground (commercial) | |
| Pork | 1 oz |
|   Loin, all cuts | |
|   Shoulder arm, picnic | |
|   Shoulder blade | |
|   Boston butt | |
|   Canadian bacon | |
|   Boiled ham | |
| Organ Meats | 1 oz |
|   Liver | |
|   Heart | |
|   Kidney | |
|   Sweetbreads | |
| Cheese | |
|   Cottage cheese, creamed | $^1/_4$ c |
|   Mozzarella | 1 oz |
|   Ricotta | 1 oz |
|   Farmer's | 1 oz |
|   Neufchatel | 1 oz |
|   Parmesan | 3 tbsp |
| Egg | 1 |
| Peanut butter (omit two fat exchanges) | 2 tbsp |

### High-Fat Meat

One high-fat meat exchange contains 7 g protein, 8 g fat, and 100 kcalories.

(This list shows the different amounts of foods to use for one high-fat meat exchange.)

| Meat | Amount to Use |
|---|---|
| Beef | 1 oz |
|   Brisket | |
|   Corned beef, brisket | |
|   Ground beef, more than 20% fat | |
|   Hamburger, commercial | |

## Table 24-3. Exchange Lists (Continued)

| List 5. *Meat Exchanges (Continued)* | | List 6. *Fat Exchanges (Continued)* | |
|---|---|---|---|
| *Meat* | *Amount to Use* | *Fat* | *Amount to Use* |
| Ground chuck, commercial | | French dressing* | 1 tbsp |
| Rib roast | | Italian dressing* | 1 tbsp |
| Club and rib steaks | | Mayonnaise* | 1 tbsp |
| Lamb | 1 oz | Salad dressing*, mayonnaise type | 2 tsp |
| Breast | | Walnuts | 6 small |
| Pork | 1 oz | | |
| Spare ribs | | Monounsaturated fats | |
| Pork, ground | | Avocado, 4″ diam | ⅛ |
| Ham, country style | | Oil | 1 tsp |
| Deviled ham | | Olive | |
| Veal | 1 oz | Peanut | |
| Breast | | Olives | 5 small |
| Poultry | 1 oz | Almonds | 10 whole |
| Capon | | Pecans | 2 large whole |
| Duck, domestic | | Peanuts | |
| Goose | | Spanish | 20 whole |
| Cheese | 1 oz | Virginia | 10 whole |
| Cheddar types | | Nuts, others | 6 small |
| Cold cuts | 4½″ × ⅛″ slice | | |
| | | Saturated fats | |
| Frankfurter | 1 small | Margarine, regular stick (hard) | 1 tsp |
| | | Butter | 1 tsp |
| **List 6. *Fat Exchanges*** | | Bacon fat | 1 tsp |
| One fat exchange contains 5 g fat and 45 kcalories. | | Bacon, crisp | 1 strip |
| (This list shows the different amounts of foods to use for one fat exchange.) | | Cream, light | 2 tbsp |
| | | Cream, heavy | 1 tbsp |
| | | Cream, sour | 2 tbsp |
| *Fat* | *Amount to Use* | French dressing† | 1 tbsp |
| Polyunsaturated fat | | Italian dressing† | 1 tbsp |
| Margarine, tub or stick (soft) | 1 tsp | Lard | 1 tsp |
| Oil | 1 tsp | Mayonnaise† | 1 tsp |
| Corn | | Salad dressing,† mayonnaise type | 2 tsp |
| Cottonseed | | Salt pork | ¾″ cube |
| Safflower | | | |
| Soy | | *If made with polyunsaturated oils. | |
| Sunflower | | †When made with saturated oils such as olive or peanut oil. | |

(Adapted from Exchange Lists for Meal Planning (revised 1976), American Dietetic Association, 430 N. Michigan Avenue, Chicago, IL 60611)

gram (USDA revised 1972 computer tape) by serving size. The results of the analysis showed that the nonfat milk items provided an average of 97 kcal rather than the 80 kcal assigned to that list (see Table 24-2), and that the computer analysis agreed well with the energy and nutrient values assigned to the other lists. However, there is a wide range of values within each Exchange List. For example, one Bread Exchange (see Table 24-2) provided 70 kcal, but the dried beans, peas, and lentils in the bread list averaged approximately 104 kcal per serving.

Average values for minerals and vitamins have not been calculated for the Exchange System because of the wide variations within each exchange. For example, whole milk contains vitamin A, whereas skim milk, unless fortified with vitamin A, does not. Therefore, giving a vitamin A value to a milk exchange would imply that all items listed in the exchange contain vitamin A. When a diet pattern is calculated by the Exchange System, care must be taken to ensure proper mineral and vitamin composition.

The dietitian uses the Exchange System to calculate a diet pattern that translates the physician's diet order into the kinds and number of servings of food (exchanges) to be consumed by the patient each day. She uses the nutrient values in Table 24-2 to calculate this pattern. The patient then selects the specific foods he wants to eat at each meal using the foods listed in Table 24-3. Sample dietary patterns calculated by the Exchange System are found in subsequent chapters, for example, a 1500-calorie diabetic dietary pattern in Chapter 29.

By using the food composition tables and noting the frequency of food usage within each group, a dietitian can calculate an Exchange System for an individual patient and in this way satisfy his usual food choices. In other words, the nutrient composition of the Exchange System can be adjusted to the food likes and dislikes of each patient within the constraints set by his diet order.

Although this Exchange System and any other reflect average and not specific energy and nutrient values, the therapeutic successes that result when the values are used to calculate diet patterns demonstrate that the method is accurate enough to serve this purpose. The only method for determining the actual energy and nutrient intake of a patient is the laboratory analysis of an aliquot of the foods actually consumed by him. This technique is used in metabolic studies and requires a highly skilled research team, including the dietitian. In this setting she plans the diet described in the research protocol, prepares the aliquots for laboratory analyses, and closely monitors the serving and the patient's consumption of food and beverages.

## Study questions and activities

1. Weigh 1 level standard tablespoon of each food on a gram scale: granulated sugar, powdered sugar, corn syrup, instant potatoes, dry skim milk powder, infant cereal, and margarine. Is there a difference in the weights?
2. Weigh ½ standard measuring cup of each food on a gram scale: cooked carrots, cooked string beans, applesauce, orange juice, milk, and ginger ale. Are there differences in weight? What does this tell you about the accuracy of using volume as a measure of food composition?
3. Select what you think is a 3-oz serving of each one of the foods listed below and then weigh it on a gram scale: American cheese, cottage cheese, sliced bologna, hamburger patty, frankfurter, lettuce, raw carrot strips, potato chips, and jelly beans.
4. Using the data in Table 1, Part 4, calculate the gram weight of each item in the fruit exchanges which contains 15 g carbohydrate. Translate the gram weight for each item into portion size (volume).
5. Using the information obtained from a patient about the frequency with which he consumes the items in the meat exchanges, calculate the weighted values for protein, fat, and energy of his usual choices. Are these values similar to or different from those in Table 24-2? Would you use the values in Table 24-2 or those which reflect his food choices in calculating a diet pattern for him?

## References

1. Hardinge ME et al: J Am Diet Assoc 46:197, 1965
2. Yee CT et al: Free Sugars in Fruits and Vegetables. Food and Life Sciences Bulletin No. 1. Ithaca, Cornell University, 1970
3. Feeley RM et al: J Am Diet Assoc 61:134, 1972
4. Hashim SA et al: J Clin Invest 43:1238, 1964
5. Greenberger NJ, Skillman TC: N Engl J Med 280:1045, 1969
6. Caso EK et al: J Am Diet Assoc 26:575, 1960
7. Revision of the exchange lists. J Am Diet Assoc 69:15, 1976
8. Wyse BA: J Am Diet Assoc 75:238, 1979

## Supplementary readings

Ahrens EH Jr, Boucher CP: Composition of a simulated American diet: Comparison of chemical analysis and estimates from food composition tables. J Am Diet Assoc 73:613, 1978

Bieri JG, McKenna MC: Expressing dietary values for fat-soluble vitamins: Changes in concepts and terminology. Am J Clin Nutr 34:289, 1981

Fabietti LG: Method for converting food volume to weight. J Am Diet Assoc 60:135, 1972

Hertzler AA, Hoover LW: Development of food tables and use with computers. J Am Diet Assoc 70:20, 1977

Parham ES: Comparison of responses to bans on cyclamate (1969) and saccharin (1977). J Am Diet Assoc 72:59, 1978

Revision of exchange lists. J Am Diet Assoc 69:15, 1976

Wyse BA: Nutrient analysis of exchange lists for meal planning. I. Variation of nutrient levels. J Am Diet Assoc 75:238, 1979

## Food composition resources

Anderson BA et al: Comprehensive evaluation of fatty acid in food. II. Beef products. J Am Diet Assoc 67:35, 1975

Anderson BA: Comprehensive evaluation of fatty acids in foods. XIII. Sausages and luncheon meats. J Am Diet Assoc 72:48, 1978

Composition of Foods: Raw, Processed and Prepared. USDA Handbook No. 8 Series: 8-1, Dairy and Egg Products, 1976; 8-2, Spices and Herbs, 1977; 8-3, Baby Foods, 1978; 8-4, Fats and Oils, 1979; 8-5, Poultry Products, 1979; 8-6, Soups, Sauces, and Gravies, 1980

Exler J et al: Comprehensive evaluation of fatty acids in foods. XI. Leguminous seeds. J Am Diet Assoc 71:412, 1977

Exler J, Weihrauch JL: Comprehensive evaluation of fatty acids in foods. XII. Shellfish. J Am Diet Assoc 71:518, 1977

Freeland JH, Cousins RJ: Zinc content of selected foods. J Am Diet Assoc 68:526, 1976

Haeflein KA, Rasmussen AI: Zinc content of foods. J Am Diet Assoc 70:610, 1977

Koehler HH et al: Tocopherol in canned entrees and vended sandwiches. J Am Diet Assoc 70:616, 1977

Perloff BP, Butrum RA: Folacin in selected foods. J Am Diet Assoc 70:161, 1977

Walsh JH et al: Pantothenic acid content of 75 processed and cooked foods. J Am Diet Assoc 78:140, 1981

Weihrauch JE et al: Comprehensive evaluation of fatty acids in foods. VI. Cereal products. J Am Diet Assoc 68:335, 1976

Weihrauch JL, Gardner JM: Sterol content of foods of plant origin. J Am Diet Assoc 73:39, 1978

Wong NP et al: Mineral content of dairy products. I. Milk and milk products. J Am Diet Assoc 78:288, 1978

Wong NP et al: Mineral content of dairy products. II. Cheeses. J Am Diet Assoc 72:608, 1979

*For further references see Bibliography in Part 4.*

# Handicapping Problems— Self-Feeding, Chewing, Swallowing

# 25

## Physically handicapping conditions

Feeding difficulties due to physical handicaps may occur during any period of the life cycle. No matter what the timing and etiology, such difficulties should alert the health care professional to the possibility of consequential nutritional problems. The normal infant or child is fed and learns to feed himself in a "normal" developmental sequence. The child with a physical handicap may deviate from this sequence; feeding problems arise when a child has difficulty sucking, swallowing, or chewing or later, in maintaining the sitting balance and attaining the upper extremity motor control necessary for feeding himself. The adult with a handicapping condition may have an oral or upper extremity dysfunction that leads to feeding difficulties and is associated with weakness, paralysis, or incoordination due to accident or disease. Different concepts must be borne in mind when dealing with adults in contrast to children, although in some areas the approaches to remediation may be similar.

This chapter is an introduction to feeding problems, methods for remediation of difficulties, and implications for nutritional care.

## Assessment

A complete assessment of the strengths, needs, and problems of each handicapped individual should be made before a plan of care is developed. Primary areas of assessment include nutritional status and needs, physical capacities and limitations, and psychosocial considerations. This would optimally be carried out by an interdisciplinary team composed of a nurse, a dietitian or nutritionist,

This chapter was written in cooperation with Marian F. Chase, M.A., L.P.T., Chief of Physical Therapy, The Ohio State University, Nisonger Center and Associate Professor, School of Allied Medical Professions and Patricia A. Lubas, M.S., R.D., Nutritionist, The Ohio State University, Nisonger Center and Adjunct Instructor, Department of Human Nutrition and Food Management.

**CVA:** Cerebrovascular Accident

423

and an occupational or a physical therapist. The team might also include a speech therapist, a dental hygienist, a dentist, a physician, a psychologist, and a social worker.

### Nutritional status and needs

Nutritional assessment includes consideration of dietary, laboratory, and clinial information, just as it would for the nonhandicapped (see Chap. 23). However, particular aspects deserve special attention among the handicapped population.

The RDA (see Chap. 11) are not intended specifically for the physically handicapped population. This fact should not lead to an assumption that the dietary requirements of a handicapped person cannot be estimated or that attempts to assess his needs would be futile.

To assess nutritional needs, consideration should be given to the person's age, sex, body size and composition, growth history, physical health and health history, medications, nutritional history, and physical activity level, as well as to the type, extent, and duration of the handicapping condition. Energy expenditure may be either increased or decreased as the result of a physical handicap. Factors to consider include muscle tone, mobility, and the use of prostheses or appliances (such as braces, crutches, and wheelchairs).

The person with a physical handicap often is a person with multiple problems, some of which may have nutritional implications unrelated to the obvious feeding difficulties. For example, vitamin metabolism may be altered by anticonvulsant drug therapy in a handicapped person with a seizure disorder;[1] nutritional needs may be increased for the person who must undergo a series of surgical procedures (see Chap. 27).

### Dietary assessment

In addition to the information obtained by the usual methods (see Chap. 23) about amounts and types of food in the diet, information should be gathered about factors that influence the actual food consumption of the infant, child, or adult. Some of these factors are the textures of food in the diet, food loss from utensils or from the oral cavity due to limited motor control, the physical effort required for eating and the time required to complete a meal (recurrent fatigue during mealtimes may compromise the total food intake), mealtime behavior, and the attitudes, knowledge, and skills of those upon whom the person depends for feeding.

### Clinical assessment

Anthropometric measurements (see Chap. 23) of physically handicapped persons may, at times, be difficult to obtain or to interpret. Persons may have unusual body composition, abnormal body proportions, missing limbs, or other gross anatomical defects. Children may have growth disturbances of unknown etiology. Comparison of data with standard height-weight tables or growth charts (see Chap. 35) has limited value in many cases.[2,3] Nevertheless, serial measurements of a person, taken at regular intervals, provide a useful picture of how the body is growing, developing, and changing (or being maintained) over time. This information is essential for even minimum nutritional assessment.

Clinical assessment ordinarily involves a search for physical signs and symptoms of malnutrition. Among handicapped persons, clinical findings may, in addition, reveal physical problems that suggest the possibility of a feeding difficulty that could lead to malnutrition. Such problems are discussed in the following sections; they include neuromuscular dysfunction, malformed or missing limbs, and abnormal or diseased oral structures (including the teeth). Impairment of the senses also may lead to feeding difficulty because vision, hearing, smell, taste, and touch are all ordinarily involved in the experience of eating.

## Common physical performance problems of infants and young children

The most common problem of the young infant with a neuromuscular handicap is the limitation in the ability to suck. Initially, the parent can be taught to stroke the infant's cheek and oral area lightly to stimulate the sucking reflex. In some cases, a severely affected infant may need to be tube fed during the first few months to ensure adequate fluid, electrolyte, and nutrient intake (see Chap. 35). Oral stimulation and some oral feeding should be maintained even though tube feeding is necessary. Initially, the child must be totally fed by the caretaker, but gradually he develops skills in the areas necessary for self-feeding. These areas include sitting and head balance, sufficient upper extremity control to bring hand to mouth, utensil and cup grasp without help, ability to sip and take liquids from a cup, ability to bite, chew, and swallow with a minimum of drooling, and ability to remove food from the spoon with the lips. For a child to begin to learn to feed himself, it is not necessary that all these preskills be completely mastered, but some evidence of skill or readiness is necessary in all of these areas. Special or adaptive equipment may be used in the beginning in order to inititate skills in self-feeding. The environment, equipment, and choice of foods are very important to successful independent feeding.

### Positioning

In the beginning, the infant is usually held to be fed and later may be fed while lying in an infant recliner. As the child gains more head control, he may be positioned in a highchair or child's seat. The normal feeding position for humans is upright and requires the ability to sit up and control the head and trunk. Developmentally, this occurs normally at about 6 to 8 months of age. In the event that the child cannot completely control his head and trunk, secure positioning must be provided so that the child can concentrate on the feeding process without being distracted by a fear of falling. Secure positioning might include head support, side supports (small pillows or rolled towels work well), a seat belt and positioning feet securely on the floor, and a footstool or foot rest (see Fig. 25-1).

Binders should not be placed tightly around the chest in such a way that the child can slip down and "hang" from the strap. Children with handicaps often have respiratory limitations that are exacerbated through this kind of restriction.

### Upper extremity control, utensil and cup grasp

Reaching and grasping are facilitated through proper and secure positioning. The ability to bring the hand to the mouth in a smooth movement pattern is important to self-feeding. Development of this skill usually begins with the child's sucking his fingers, which is important in the development of the sensory-motor learning necessary for self-feeding and speech. Handicapped children who do not spontaneously bring their hands to their mouth should be encouraged to do so. Peanut butter, mashed potatoes, or pudding on the fingers may assist in encouraging this activity. Finger feeding is a preliminary step toward using utensils.

When the child is ready to use a spoon, it is important to give him foods that stick to the spoon easily, such as cooked cereal and mashed potatoes, vegetables, or fruits. At times it is helpful to guide the child's arm through the motions of scooping the food onto the spoon and bringing it to the mouth. Many handicapped children try to stabilize their arm by holding it close to their body and bringing their head down to the spoon. Repetition, gentle encouragement, giving only the required amount of help, and knowing when the child does not need assistance are important in feeding training.

There are many products commercially available that can assist the child. These include spoons with a built-up or looped handle, a bent or swivel spoon, and scoop dishes or plate guards that facilitate getting food onto the spoon. The child who has severe weakness in the upper extremities, as in Duchenne's muscular dystrophy, may benefit from use of swivel feeders (see Fig. 25-2).

Taking fluids is sometimes difficult for the neurologically handicapped child and often results in prolonged used of the bottle, which interferes with normal development and function of the oral structures. For drinking liquids, it is wise to place small quantities in the container to avoid spilling and to minimize the weight of the cup. Handles on the cup, cutout cups, or small plastic cups may work better. The need for good head position is important to avoid "pouring" the fluid when the child has

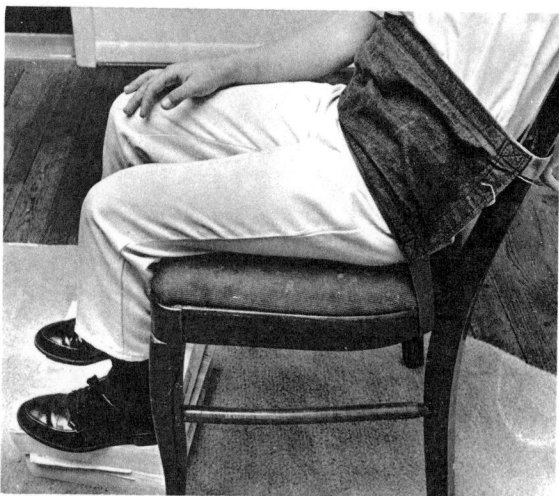

**Fig. 25-1.** A child with poor trunk control stabilized by a binder at the pelvis and feet supported. (Note use of telephone directories as a footstool)

his head thrown back. Drinking through a straw—a form of sucking—can be introduced when the child can purse his lips, suck, and swallow. Learning to drink through a straw may help with breath control, lip closure, and drooling. Some adaptations that can be used are a plastic straw with a 2-inch piece of rubber tubing on the end to avoid crushing the straw (see Fig. 25-3), bent plastic straws, and paper flex-straws. The shorter and narrower the diameter of the straw, the less sucking pressure

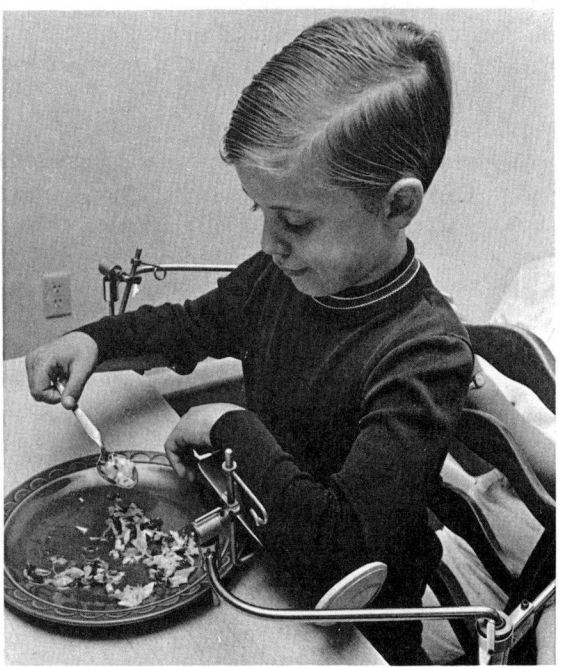

**Fig. 25-2.** Swivel feeder for child with very weak upper extremities.

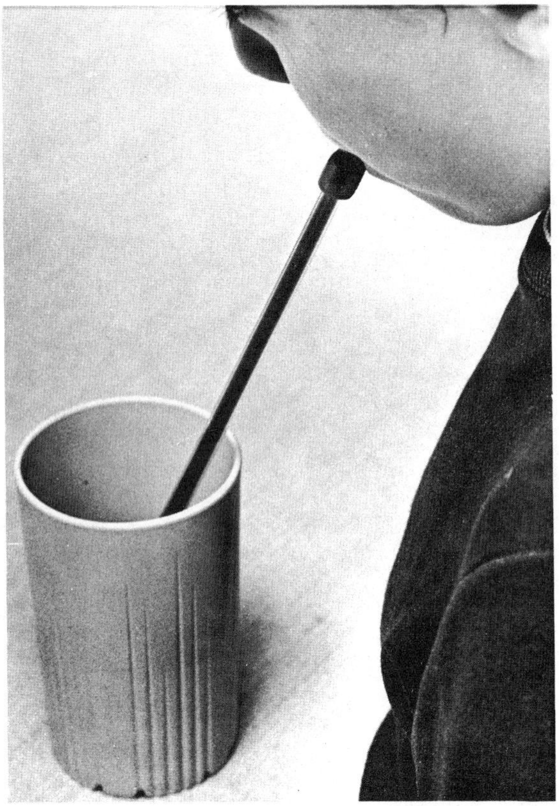

**Fig. 25-3.** Plastic straw with rubber tip to prevent crushing of the end of straw.

needed to bring the liquid to the mouth. As the child progresses in his ability to suck through a straw, the length and diameter may be increased, allowing him to take thicker fluids, which usually contain more nutrients.

### Biting, chewing, and swallowing

The child who has the ability to bite and chew can be offered food of various textures and, therefore, a greater variety of foods in the diet. Children who have neurologic problems and difficulty in biting and chewing but can take food without choking should be encouraged to bite off small amounts of soft or semisoft foods, for example, a small amount of boiled potato or a bite of well cooked carrot strip. The food should be placed in or directed to alternate sides of the mouth, and the patient encouraged to use his tongue to move the food in his mouth. The child should chew and swallow each bite before he takes more food. Food may become lodged between the teeth and inside the cheeks. This food may need to be dislodged carefully with the spoon, taking care not to elicit the gag reflex. In some cases the food may be dislodged with the finger; however, some children with cerebral palsy have a bite reflex, and caution should be exercised to avoid being bitten. Swallowing occurs after inhalation in order to

avoid choking. In feeding liquids to the severely palsied child, it may be wise to observe the breathing pattern before offering liquids. Swallowing is easier with the head and trunk in an upright position. The head may need to be supported either with a head support or with the caretaker's hand cupping the head at the base of the skull.

## Adults with physical performance problems

Adults who have had a cerebral vascular accident, an accident resulting in quadriplegia, rheumatoid arthritis (see Fig. 25-4), or other physically handicapping conditions have somewhat different problems from children. Adults are maintaining the skill or relearning the process of feeding themselves. Most often the problems involve paralysis, weakness, or incoordination. The psychological impact on the patient who must relearn this very basic function must be considered, and he must be treated as an adult. The individualized proper diet, the disease entity, activity level, and physical strengths and weaknesses must be assessed and an appropriate remedial program planned if the patient is to reach and maintain optimal feeding skills. Many of the techniques described for children also work well for adults, and the goals may be very similar. Particularly in the adult population, one should consider the possibilities of soreness in the mouth, lack of teeth, or poorly fitting dentures as deterrents to normal eating patterns. If the person must be fed, care should be taken to direct the food to each side of the mouth, permit time for chewing and swallowing of each bite before introducing another bite, and create a relaxed atmosphere to make the eating process as pleasant as possible.

### Proper positioning

Positioning in a normal upright position is the ultimate goal. The position should be comfortable as well as secure so that the patient can concentrate his efforts upon the process of eating. The following are some common errors in positioning: (1) The patient is slumped to one side. This may be rectified by using pillows, a rolled blanket, or foam wedges at his side. Sometimes a seat belt provides the needed trunk stability. A solid seat or wooden seat insert in the wheelchair provides better stability than a very soft seat or the canvas sling seat of the wheelchair. (2) The feet are not securely placed on the floor or on the wheelchair foot rests. A foot stool, telephone books, or blocks of wood can assist in more stable foot placement (Fig. 25-1). (3) The table height is incorrect, either too high or too low. If the table height cannot be adjusted, a table placed over the bed, adjusted to the correct height, or a lap board with a raised edge may be used with the wheelchair. Finally, look at the patient—does he look comfortable? Is he in as normal a position as possible?

## Adaptive feeding equipment

A careful evaluation of the patient's abilities and limitations must precede the selection of specialized equipment. Many adaptive feeding devices are commercially available, and proper selection is extremely important. The ultimate goal should be for the patient to be as independent and as normal-looking as possible with the least amount of adaptive equipment possible. Consultation with an occupational or a physical therapist experienced in feeding retraining can be very helpful both in assessing the patient for self-feeding and in selecting or designing specialized equipment. Adaptive devices are available to assist the patient with upper extremity control in the case of paralysis, weakness, or incoordination (see Fig. 25-5). Specialized equipment enhances the ability to suck or take liquids from a cup. There are modifications that enable the patient to grasp utensils and enable the patient to obtain the food on the utensil better (see Fig. 25-6). The handicapped homemaker can find many aids available to assist in kitchen and household tasks when

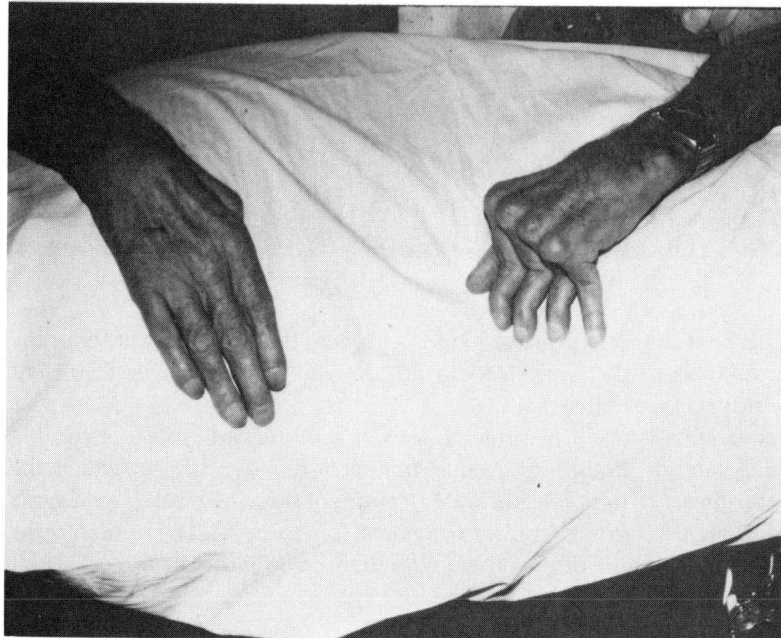

**Fig. 25-4.** Right hand, minimal rheumatoid arthritis; left hand, severe rheumatoid arthritis. (The Ohio State University, Dodd Hall, Nancy Snyder, with permission)

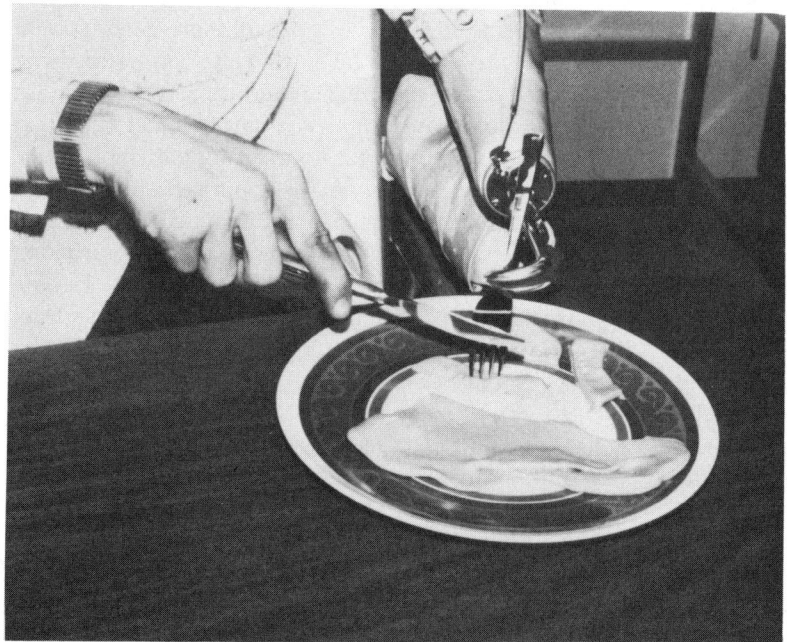

**Fig. 25-5.** Use of prosthesis in self-feeding. (The Ohio State University, Dodd Hall, Nancy Snyder, with permission)

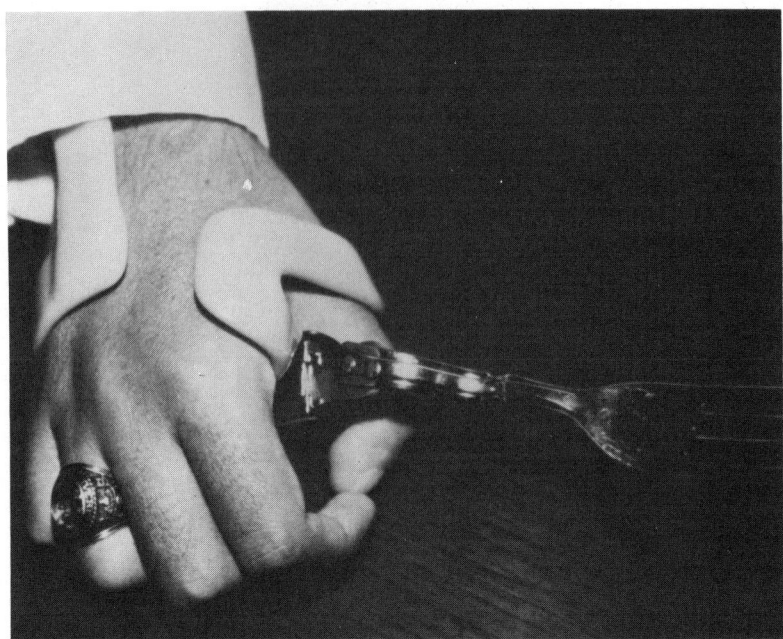

**Fig. 25-6.** Adapted fork commonly used in paralysis of the hand and limited grasp. (The Ohio State University, Dodd Hall, Nancy Snyder, with permission)

there is weakness in an upper extremity or when, perhaps, only one extremity can be used, which is often the case after a CVA. Examples of these devices include jar openers, one-handed can opener, bowl holders, one-handed rolling pin, one-handed mixer, rocker knives, and self-wringing mops. Many of these products are commercially available, some must be special ordered from a medical rehabilitation outlet, and some, with a little ingenuity, can be easily constructed at home.

## Common nutritional problems
### Infants

Because much of the early parent–infant interaction centers around the feeding process, problems in feeding an infant with a physically handicapping condition may interfere with the establishment of a mutually satisfying parent–child relationship. This difficulty can eventually lead to the development of behavior patterns that adversely affect the feeding situation and ultimately influence nutrient intake (see Chap. 35 for a discussion of the psychosocial aspects of infant feeding).

When the development of feeding skills in a handicapped infant does not seem to be progressing according to the "normal" timing and sequence, a parent may be uncertain how or when to introduce new types of foods, food textures, and methods of feeding. In some cases, the uncertainty results in the prolonged use of puréed foods of low caloric or nutrient density. This can lead to protein-energy malnutrition in the older child who continues to receive infant-sized servings of the types of foods usually used for infant feeding.

Another type of problem may arise when the caloric intake is adequate, but the only foods given are those that seem easiest to feed. A severe limitation of variety in the diet may lead to the development of isolated nutrient deficiencies.

The prolonged use of a bottle and nipple for feeding liquids to a child may create a situation in which the upper teeth are in continual contact with a cariogenic liquid (milk or fruit juice, for example). The result may be the development of "nursing bottle caries."[4]

### Adults
#### Fluid intake

Handicapped adults, especially those who can take only sips of fluids slowly by mouth, present a special problem. Care must be taken that they do not become dehydrated or overhydrated if they are also receiving intravenous fluids. Accurate records of fluid intake and output are a very important part of the nutritional care plan. If the patient cannot help himself, he must be offered fluids frequently. If he can manage himself, care must be taken that his glass, cup, or an adapted drinking device is conveniently placed within his reach. Adequate fluid intake is important in the prevention of urinary tract infection and, for some patients, the prevention of nephrolithiasis (see Chap. 32).

#### Activity and nutrient utilization

Immobility even in healthy people with adequate energy and protein intakes promotes a negative nitrogen balance. The loss of nitrogen is primarily from the muscle mass. Immobility in healthy people also promotes a negative calcium balance with calcium loss primarily from the long bones. Negative nitrogen and calcium balances also occur in immobilized patients; for example, a patient immobilized by the application of a cast, or one immobilized after a cerebral vascular accident. Muscular activity combined, whenever possible, with weight bearing on the long bones reverses the negative balances in both the healthy and the sick person. Therefore, the physically handicapped person requires a daily activity program for the effective utilization of his nutrient intake.

### Consistency of food

Two concerns should be kept in mind about the consistency of food offered the handicapped patient—its nutritional value and the progression from semiliquid to more solid foods as the patient progresses.

Generally, it is difficult to keep a reasonable proportion of protein, fat, and carbohydrate in semiliquid diets. Also, if milk is used extensively as a beverage, with mashed potatoes and cereals, and in other foods, the daily calcium intake may be excessive while the iron intake may be inadequate. At this time the relationship of calcium intake to the formation of kidney stones in the relatively immobile patient is not well understood, but it is probably advisable that daily calcium intake not exceed the NRC's Recommended Dietary Allowance (see Chap. 11).

Continuous evaluation of a patient's progress is necessary if he is to be helped to progress from semisolid to solid foods. It has been observed that patients may not progress because they are not encouraged and assisted to try more solid foods.

### Weight control

Weight control is a very important aspect of the nutritional care of the handicapped patient. Persons with paralysis or other motor dysfunctions that permanently limit physical activity require fewer calories to meet their energy needs. In these situations the diet pattern must be carefully planned so that adequate nutrients, without excessive calories, are consumed each day. The patient who is obese when he acquires his handicapping condition should be helped to lose weight for his own benefit and for the benefit of those who give him physical care (see Chap. 28, *Weight Control*).

### Constipation

Persons with paralysis or hypotonia often become constipated due to immobility and a diet low in roughage. Regular bowel movements may be encouraged by as much physical movement as possible and a diet with adequate roughage (see Chap. 26).

## Special programs
### Feeding training of the neurologically handicapped infant

In a number of centers in the United States, intensive study of the training of the neurologically handicapped infant and child is in progress to assist these children in learning to participate fully in the activities of daily living.

The feeding training of this program is concerned not only with the nutritional needs of these children but also with the development of self-feeding skills, so they can eat with their families at home and with others when away from home.

The staffs of these centers recognize that the key to success in the feeding training programs is repeating the activity, giving gentle yet consistent encouragement, giving only the required amount of help, and knowing when the child does not need assistance.

When the neurologically handicapped child who has been carefully trained to achieve his potential for self-feeding is admitted to a pediatric unit for an acute illness, the personnel should seek the help of the mother so that he can maintain the skills he has acquired and not regress.

### Rehabilitation teams in the general hospital

Various clinical services, such as head and neck surgery and neurology, have organized rehabilitation teams which are responsible for preparing patients with feeding problems for discharge from the acute care hospital. These teams usually include a nurse specialist, a physical or occupational therapist, a social worker, and a clinical dietitian who design the feeding training program and work closely with the patient during hospitalization and after discharge. Helping the patient learn new feeding skills is usually the responsibility of the physical or occupational therapist. The clinical dietitian monitors the patient's nutritional status; provides food of appropriate consistency and nutrient content to meet the patient's needs; and counsels patients and their families on how to manage the food preparation in the home. The social worker can often help the family to obtain any equipment needed for special foods preparation, such as a blender.

### Conclusions

The goals in any feeding program are an optimal dietary intake both in nutrition and consistency, and a person who can function in the feeding process in as near normal a manner as possible. In summary, important concepts include:

1. Assessment of patients' abilities and disabilities
2. Determination of the program of training
3. Assistance from other professionals who have expertise in working with the handicapped in the feeding process
4. Consideration of the role of the feeding process in the development of parent–child relationships and the psychological aspects underlying the relearning of a basic skill for adults
5. Assurance that the mother of an infant, the relations or friends of an adult, or the employees of an institution, are capable of and can tolerate the frustrations of assisting in the development or rehabilitation of self-feeding skills in handicapped persons

## Study questions and activities

1. Have a classmate or friend feed you a semisolid (*i.e.*, applesauce) while you are lying on your back without your head raised. What difficulties did you encounter?

2. While sitting, with your head back, have someone give you a sip of liquid from a cup. Try to swallow with your head back. What other problems did you have?

3. Visit a rehabilitation center during mealtime. Observe the patient's positioning. What adaptations did they use? What kinds of handicaps did you observe? Did the individual consume a reasonable energy and nutrient intake at this meal (one-quarter to one-half of his daily needs)?

4. Once a day for a week observe a skilled therapist work on developing self-feeding skills in a handicapped child. What were the problems? What type of diet was being used? What adaptive equipment was used? Did the child make progress?

5. Analyze one day's energy and nutrient intake of a handicapped person in a hospital or skilled nursing facility. Was the intake adequate to meet this person's needs?

## References

1. Reynolds EH: Epilepsia 16:319, 1975
2. Garn SM, Weir HF: Am J Clin Nutr 24:853, 1971
3. Roche AF: Kidney Int 14:369, 1978
4. Shelton PG et al: Pediatrics 59:777, 1977
5. Rickard K et al: J Am Diet Assoc 68:546, 1976

## Supplementary readings

Calvert SD et al: Dietary adequacy, feeding practices, and eating behavior of children with Down's syndrome. J Am Diet Assoc 69:152, 1976

Cornelius MS: Feeding handicapped patients. J Am Diet Assoc 67:136, 1975

Cronk CE: Growth of children with Down's syndrome: Birth to age 3 years. Pediatrics 61:564, 1978

Dufton-Gross NA: Nutrition intervention in a preschool for handicapped children. J Am Diet Assoc 75:154, 1979

Gaffney TW, Campbell RP: Feeding techniques for dysphagic patients. Am J Nurs 74:2194, 1974

Green KB: Coping daily with the handicapped and the elderly. J Home Econ 70:15, Fall, 1978

Gresham GE: Residual disability in stroke survivors—The Framingham study. N Engl J Med 293:954, 1975

Jones AM: Overcoming the feeding problems of the mentally and the physically handicapped. J Hum Nutr 32:359, 1978

Manning AM, Means JG: A self-feeding program for geriatric patients in a skilled nursing facility. J Am Diet Assoc 66:275, 1975

Nutrition and Feeding Techniques for Handicapped Children. Developmental Disabilities Program, California Department of Health, Sacramento, CA 95814, 1974

Ogg HL: Oral–pharyngeal development and evaluation. Phys Ther 55:235, 1975

Pipes PL, Holm VA: Feeding children with Down's syndrome. J Am Diet Assoc 77:277, 1980

Rickard K et al: Care of children with conditions characterized by high nutritional risks. J Am Diet Assoc 68:546, 1976

Roche AF: Growth assessment of handicapped children. Dietetic Currents 6:Nov, 1979

Wainwright H: Feeding problems in elderly disabled patients. Nurs Times 34:542, 1978

Weaver AW, Fleming SM: Partial laryngectomy: Analysis of associated swallowing disorders. Am J Surg 136:486, 1978

Webb Y: Feeding and nutrition problems of physically and mentally handicapped children in Britain: A report. J Hum Nutr 34:281, 1980

Weber B: Eating with a trach. Am J Nurs 74:1439, 1974

Zickefoose M: Feeding the child with a cleft palate. J Am Diet Assoc 36:129, 1960

## Patient resources

Adaptations and Techniques for the Disabled Homemaker. Sister Kenny Institute, Minneapolis MN 55407

Do It Yourself Again—Self-Help Devices for the Stroke Patient. American Heart Association, Dallas, TX, 75231

Goldbery RZ: So what if you can't chew, eat hearty! Recipes and a guide for the healthy and happy eating of soft and pureed foods. Springfield, IL, Charles C Thomas, 1980

Mealtime Manual for People with Disabilities and The Aging. Campbell Soup Co, Camden, NJ, 08101

Pershe R et al (eds): Mealtimes for Severely and Profoundly Handicapped Persons. Baltimore, University Park Press, 1977

Roueche JR: Dysphagia: An assessment and management program for adults. Minneapolis, Sister Kenny Institute, 1981

Smith, MAH (ed): Feeding the Handicapped Child. Memphis, University of Tennessee Child Development Center, 1976

*For further references see Bibliography in Part 4.*

# Diet in Gastrointestinal Disease

# 26

**BAO:** Basal Acid Output
**BE:** Barium Enema
**ERCP:** Endoscopic Retrograde
Cholangiopancreatography
**L-BHT:** Lactose Breath Hydrogen Test
**LTT:** Lactose Tolerance Test
**MAO:** Maximum Acid Output
**UGI:** Upper Gastrointestinal Series
**UGI-SBFT:** Upper Gastrointestinal Series
with Small Bowel Follow-through

Diet therapy in gastrointestinal disease is concerned with problems that may occur in the esophagus, at the lower esophageal sphincter, and in the stomach; in the small bowel, including the duodenum, jejunum, and ileum; in the large bowel (the colon), including the rectum and anus; and in the appendages to the tract—the liver, gallbladder, and pancreas. There is good evidence that dietary modifications are effective in the treatment of a number of malabsorption problems due to the lack of or inadequate amounts of specific pancreatic or intestinal enzymes required to hydrolyze certain constituents of food; the lack of conjugated bile salts from the liver to form a microemulsion of fat to facilitate its absorption in the small intestine; or a structural or functional defect of the villi of the small intestine, particularly in the distal duodenum, proximal jejunum, and terminal ileum, which interferes with the hydrolysis or transport of nutrients.

There is also good evidence that certain chemical constituents of beverages, such as the caffeine in coffee, theobromine in tea and chocolate, and alcohol enhance the secretion of hydrochloric acid by the parietal cells in the antrum of the stomach.

Otherwise the significance of diet therapy in the treatment of a variety of gastrointestinal diseases, such as peptic ulcer and ulcerative colitis is not clear. There are limited data on the effects of the chemical and physical characteristics of the nutrients in foods consumed in meals on the structure and functions of the gastrointestinal tract. At the same time there is no consensus about the definition of the term, *bland diet*, a diet widely used in the treatment of peptic ulcer.

This confusion in diet therapy in peptic ulcer disease reflects to some extent the confusion at present about its etiology. The problems encountered in working with physicians treating patients with peptic ulcer are best described by Fein's observation that "opinion regarding diagnosis and treatment of stomach disease may vary from locality to locality and from gastroenterologist to gastroenterologist."[1]

Also, the lay public has many misconceptions. Foods are said to be "hard to digest," which is equated with the rate at which food leaves the stomach. Or, foods may be classified as "irritating" or "gas forming." There is no question that certain foods may cause gastrointestinal discomfort in some people. This may be due to a specific substance in food, such as the lactose in milk in a lactase-deficient patient, or it may be an allergic response to a food protein.

Because food carries many emotional overtones, it is to be expected that the emotional state of a person can affect his digestion. The layman often attributes his "indigestion" or diarrhea to anger or anxiety; and in a 3 or 4 year old child the excitement of a birthday party or the anticipation of a trip to a favorite relative can initiate vomiting. Similarly, many neuroses and even psychoses may give rise to gastrointestinal symptoms.

Symptoms ascribed to disorders in the gastrointestinal tract may be due to pathologic conditions in other systems of the body. For example, severe congestive heart failure, chronic renal disease, space-occupying lesions in the central nervous system, such as brain tumors, and infections, such as pneumonia, bacteremia, and pulmonary tuberculosis, are often accompanied by symptoms of gastrointestinal distress.

Succeeding sections of this chapter present diet therapy in diseases of the esophagus and stomach, the small intestine, and the colon. The reader is advised to review the anatomy and physiology of the gastrointestinal tract and its appendages, including the neurohormonal control of the cephalic, gastric, and intestinal phase of digestion, and the structure and function of the absorptive cells of the small intestine. In this book he should review Chapter 9, *"Nutrient Utilization,"* and Chapter 25, *"Handicapping Problems,"* particularly the sections on chewing and swallowing. Malabsorption caused by cystic fibrosis and certain disaccharides that occurs primarily in infants and children is discussed in Chapter 35; the surgical removal of sections of the intestine or the colon presents problems in diet therapy that are discussed in Chapter 27. Liver disease is discussed in Chapter 33.

# Diagnostic procedures in gastrointestinal disease

Five common procedures used in the diagnosis of gastrointestinal disease are indirect visualization of the gastrointestinal tract by fluoroscopy or x-ray photographs after a barium meal has been ingested; direct visualization of the esophagus, stomach, duodenum, and colon by an endoscope; analysis of gastric secretions for the quantity of hydrochloric acid being produced; examination of intestinal tract tissue obtained by peroral suction biopsy; and absorptive function tests.

## Roentgenography

Roentgenography of the gastrointestinal tract is an important diagnostic procedure. It is done by x-ray photography. By this means the progress of an opaque "meal" of barium sulfate may be followed through the entire upper digestive tract; motility (including peristalsis), emptying time, general tonus, defects of outline indicative of ulcer or carcinoma, and other signs of abnormalities can be studied in detail. The barium meal is given in the morning, or at least 12 hours after the taking of food or drink. This test is known as an upper gastrointestinal series (UGI) or upper gastrointestinal series with small bowel follow-through (UGI-SBFT).

A barium enema (BE) is used to visualize the large bowel. The patient is prepared by enemas or by a clear liquid diet for 48 to 72 hours and enemas so that the bowel is free of fecal material. This procedure is used when cancer, diverticula, ulcerative colitis, or aganglionic megacolon is suspected.

## Endoscopy

The mucous membranes of the esophagus, stomach, duodenum, and the colon can be visualized directly by an endoscope, a flexible tube with a light at the end and an eyepiece through which the physician can examine the tissue. In upper gastrointestinal endoscopy the gastroscope is inserted through the mouth into the esophagus, stomach, and duodenum. In addition to visualizing the tissue the gastroscope is also capable of taking biopsy samples. The scope can also be passed through the papilla of Vater and a dye instilled to visualize the pancreatic and bile ducts radiographically. This procedure is known as *endoscopic retrograde cholangiopancreatography* (ERCP). The colonoscope is used to visualize the tissues of the colon from the anus to the ileocecal valve. Patients for endoscopy are prepared in the same way as those for UGI or BE.

## Gastric Analysis

This test is carried out in the morning, before the patient has received any food. A tube is passed from the mouth into the stomach, and any gastric secretion present is withdrawn. For the next hour the basal or nonstimulated gastric secretions are withdrawn. The patient is given an injection of histamine, a drug that stimulates gastric secretion, or pentagastrin, the last four amino acids of the C-terminal end of gastrin (Trp-Met-Asp-Phe-$NH_2$) stabilized with a fifth amino acid (Ala). The gastric contents are withdrawn at intervals, for an hour or longer. All samples, including the fasting one, are examined for the presence of undigested food, bile, and blood, and tested for the quantity of free and total hydrochloric acid each contains. Basal acid output (BAO) is derived from the analysis of the hydrochloric acid in the gastric secretions collected in the first hour and the maximum acid output (MAO) from the secretions in the second hour.

In the healthy person no remnants of a previous meal or of blood should be present. A small amount of bile is sometimes regurgitated from the duodenum. The amount of acid present in the fasting specimen in a normal person is 2.0 ± 1.8 mEq per hour for women and 3.0 ± 2.0 mEq per hour for men. After stimulation the commonly accepted normal values are 16 ± 5 mEq of acid per hour for women and 23 ± 5 mEq of acid for men.

If a higher range of acid is found, the condition is called *hyperchlorhydria* and may indicate the presence of an ulcer in the duodenum. If the range is much below normal, it is termed *hypochlorhydria*. It may indicate gastric disease in the presence of other findings. *Achlorhydria* denotes that no hydrochloric acid is present. It may occur in gastric disease and is often found in patients with pernicious anemia.

## Peroral suction biopsy

The peroral biopsy tube is used to obtain tissue specimens from the duodenum, jejunum, and ileum. These specimens can be analyzed for structural defects, such as the flattened villi in gluten-induced enteropathy, or functional defects, such as the level of disaccharidases in suspected deficiency.

## Absorptive tests

Various absorption tests are used to diagnose small bowel problems, such as the quantitative fecal fat test, the d-xylose absorption-excretion test, the lactose tolerance test, and the vitamin $B_{12}$ absorption test. During the collection of stool for the quantitative fecal fat test the adult patient must consume a diet of 100 g of fat per day. The absorption of less than 95% of the ingested fat is indicative of malabsorption. The other absorptive tests are well described in Davidsohn Todd-Sanford Clinical Diagnosis by Laboratory Methods, edited by Henry.[2]

# The upper gastrointestinal tract— peptic ulcer
## Terminology

The term, *gastric ulcer*, denotes an eroded lesion in the stomach, usually occurring along the lesser curvature or near the pylorus. A duodenal ulcer is the same type of lesion, but is found in the first part of the duodenum. It is much more common than a gastric ulcer. Whether an ulcer occurs in the stomach or in the duodenum, the treatment is similar. Both types are considered together here under the term, *peptic ulcer*. Peptic ulcer disease may be acute with bleeding and other complications or chronic with periodic recurrences of the acute phase.

The diagnosis of ulcer is commonly made by gastros-copy or by roentgenography. Hyperacidity and hypersecretion of gastric juice are usually found in examination of the stomach contents in patients with duodenal ulcer.

## Symptoms
### Pain

Pain in the epigastrium, occurring more or less regularly from 1 to 3 hours after meals, is characteristic of peptic ulcer. It is usually of a burning or gnawing type and is relieved by food, histamine$_2$ antagonists, or nonabsorbable antacids. The pain complained of by the peptic ulcer patient when the stomach is empty is due to the action of the highly acidic gastric juice on the open lesion because no food or antacid is present to neutralize the gastric acid.

### Hemorrhage and perforation

Sometimes hemorrhage is the first indication of the presence of an ulcer, or hemorrhage may occur if the ulcer goes untreated. Sudden weakness and tarry stools, the latter due to the presence of blood, are the outstanding symptoms, and the patient is usually hospitalized at once. If perforation of the gastric or the duodenal wall accompanies the hemorrhage, the situation is extremely serious and the patient is subjected to emergency surgery.

## Etiology

The etiology of peptic ulcer is presently under intensive investigation. It is not clear whether both types of ulcers, duodenal and gastric, are caused by similar or different problems. However, there is general agreement that there are three factors involved in the development of all peptic ulcers. These are the presence of gastric acid and pepsin, usually but not always, in amounts greater than normal; decreased mucosal resistance to the action of gastric acid and pepsin; and a higher degree of reaction to emotional stress and a higher level of anxiety in patients with peptic ulcer compared to people who do not develop ulcers.[3]

Gastric acid and pepsin must be present for the development of a peptic ulcer. It has been observed that in the absence of gastric acid and pepsin ulcers do not develop. However, the converse is not true, that is, in the presence of elevated levels of gastric acid and pepsin, ulcers occur. A small percentage of hypersecretors do not develop peptic ulcers. Also, not all people who develop ulcers have elevated levels of gastric acid and pepsin. Although the mechanisms are not well understood, the lesion in peptic ulcer appears to be caused by a combination of two factors—the presence of gastric acid and pepsin, and decreased mucosal resistance to the action of acid and pepsin.

The role of emotional stress is also not well understood. It is possible that stress may stimulate gastric acid and pepsin secretion or may reduce mucosal resistance in some way.

## Principles of Diet Therapy

The goal of the medical treatment of peptic ulcer is to reduce the secretion of gastric acid and pepsin and to neutralize the gastric acid that is secreted, to protect the ulcerated area from irritation, and to promote healing. Anticholinegeric drugs, nonabsorbable antacids, or histamine₂ antagonists are used to reduce secretions and to neutralize gastric acid. For many years, dietary programs have been an integral part of the medical treatment of peptic ulcer. These programs have varied from a severely restricted milk and cream regimen to a bland diet regimen or to a liberal regimen of frequent feedings of those foods that the patient tolerates. A number of clinical research studies have been conducted in an attempt to identify the best therapeutic diet plan for the treatment of peptic ulcer, but as yet there is no firm evidence for one specific approach to diet therapy in ulcer disease.[4] In the following discussion an attempt is made to analyze and summarize the major controversies of diet in peptic ulcer disease.

### Protein

When any food is ingested, it distends the antrum of the stomach. This process initiates the release of the hormone, *gastrin*, which in turn stimulates gastric acid secretion. As it enters the antrum, the protein in food buffers the gastric acid. Later, the products of the gastric digestion of protein and other gastric secretagogues (see later) are major stimulators of gastric acid secretion.[5] In healthy people when the $pH$ of the contents in the pyloric area drops to approximately 2.0 or less, gastrin release is inhibited. In the patient with active peptic ulcer disease the early buffering of gastric acid by protein relieves the pain, while the later drop in $pH$ due to stimulation by the products of gastric protein digestion causes the pain that many ulcer patients experience 1 to 3 hours after meals. To neutralize the gastric acid, the patient with an active ulcer takes an antacid 1 hour after a meal. However, if the $pH$ of the gastric contents does not drop to 2.0 or less, gastrin release is not inhibited and gastric acid secretion continues. Therefore, anticholinergic drugs are included in the therapeutic plan to reduce the vagal stimulation of gastrin release.

Recently a histamine₂ antagonist, cimetidine, has been used in the treatment of active peptic ulcer disease to inhibit histamine₂ stimulation of gastric acid secretion by the oxyntic (parietal) cells of the fundus and body of the stomach.[6] The use of cimetidine is under intensive study (see *Supplementary Readings* at the end of this chapter and the Bibliography in Part 4), and may replace antacids and anticholinergic drugs in the treatment of peptic ulcer disease.[7] There is evidence that its use may interfere with the absorption of vitamin B₁₂, and patients need to be monitored carefully to avoid B₁₂ deficiency.[8]

Although the protein in all foods stimulates gastric acid secretion, there is some evidence that the protein in milk may be a less potent stimulant than the protein in meat. This could be related to the fat in milk. However, the excessive use of milk is not recommended (see discussion on fat in this section).

Even though the products of protein digestion are major stimulators of gastric acid secretion, protein is included in the diet of the patient with peptic ulcer disease. The daily diet should provide at least 0.8 g per kg of body weight. If extensive blood loss has occurred, it is advisable to include 1 g to 1.5 g per kg to support red blood cell synthesis and maturation.

### Gastric secretagogues

In addition to the products of gastric protein digestion, it has been demonstrated that the methyl xanthines, caffeine and theobromine, cause an increase in gastric acid secretion. Alcohol is a mild stimulant of acid secretion but also is damaging to the mucosal barrier. Although not a secretagogue, aspirin (salicylic acid) damages the mucosal barrier.

Alcohol and beverages containing caffeine or theobromine, such as coffee, tea, chocolate, and cola beverages, are omitted from the diets of patients with ulcer disease. Decaffeinated coffee stimulates gastric acid secretion and is also omitted from the diet.[9] Meat extractives in meat-based soups and in meat drippings used to make gravies are also classified as gastric secretagogues and, therefore, are omitted from the diet.

### Fat and carbohydrates

Fat inhibits gastric secretion while carbohydrates neither stimulate nor inhibit it. Partly because fat inhibits gastric secretion, hourly feedings of a mixture of milk and cream have been used in the early phase of treatment of acute peptic ulcer disease. The hourly feedings of approximately 3 oz to 4 oz of the milk and cream mixture are combined with between-feeding doses of antacid to neutralize the gastric acid stimulated by the products of the digestion of the protein in the milk. This regimen was designed by Sippy in 1915 and became known as the Sippy diet. The milk and cream mixture was commonly referred to as *gastric mixture*. Between-meal feedings of milk and cream were continued during the convalescent phase.

This regimen is still used occasionally in the early treatment of the acute phase of peptic ulcer disease. However, with increasing knowledge of the relationship of the type of dietary fat to the level of serum cholesterol and development of atherosclerosis (see Chap. 20), the effects of a diet high in milk fat have been questioned. Sandweiss, in a study of 180 ulcer patients, found the mortality from heart disease 14% higher than in the general population.[10] Recently, when the Sippy regimen is ordered, whole or skim milk is used in place of milk and cream.

It is generally agreed that the diet for the treatment of

peptic ulcer disease should be moderate in fat, 80 g to 100 g per day, and contain sufficient carbohydrate to provide an adequate energy intake.

### Roughage

Raw fruits and vegetables, especially those with skins and small seeds, such as strawberries and tomatoes, and unrefined cereals and flours have been excluded from diets for peptic ulcer due to their fiber content, commonly referred to as *roughage.* From limited research it was suggested that the roughage in these foods was mechanically irritating to the ulcer in acute peptic ulcer. More research is needed to document whether or not roughage does irritate the ulcer crater.

### pH of beverages

There has been considerable controversy about citrus juices and other beverages with a *p*H of 4.0 or less. Some diet programs have included them, whereas others have excluded them. Further research by Castell and colleagues (see Reflux Esophagitis) may demonstrate that orange juice may be contraindicated in the diets of those patients with peptic ulcer who report distress after drinking it.

### Spicy foods

Spices are often excluded from diet programs for peptic ulcer. One group of investigators has shown that the use of considerable amounts of cinnamon, allspice, thyme, sage, paprika, clove, and other spices produced no increase in gastric secretions in patients with gastric ulcers. In 5 out of 50 patients in this study, some difficulty was encountered with chili, black pepper, mustard seed, and nutmeg.[11] This work and the more recent work of Castell and colleagues suggest that spices may be tolerated, although there may be some individual differences.

### Size of meals

Distention of the antrum stimulates gastric acid secretion. Therefore, in acute peptic ulcer, feedings of small to moderate volume may be used in an attempt to avoid excessive distention of the antrum. In such cases, frequent feedings are required to achieve a reasonable energy and nutrient intake. For the patient with a healed ulcer, Fordtran suggests that frequent small meals are contraindicated due to the repeated stimulus by food to gastric secretion, especially in duodenal ulcer patients who are hypersecretors.[3]

### Summary

The diet for the patient with peptic ulcer should meet each person's energy needs and provide adequate amounts of protein and moderate amounts of fat. Because blood loss may occur, special attention must be given to foods that are high in iron. If necessary, an iron supplement is prescribed. Future research may demonstrate more clearly whether or not there are individual intolerances to citrus juices and spicy foods. If citrus fruits and juices are not tolerated, a vitamin C supplement can be prescribed.

Today there is firm evidence that gastric secretagogues, commonly referred to as *gastric stimulants,* should be avoided by the patient with peptic ulcer. There is limited evidence and considerable controversy about the effectiveness of frequent "bland" meals in the treatment of ulcer disease. Because of this controversy, the American Dietetic Association published the association's position paper on the bland diet in the treatment of chronic duodenal ulcer disease, given in Table 26-1.[12] Section III of this paper states the generally, but not completely, accepted guidelines for planning diets for patients with peptic ulcer. That the guidelines in Table 26-1 have not been well accepted has been documented by Welsh. His survey in 1976 of 326 hospitals in the United States revealed that 77% used a "bland" diet for patients with peptic ulcer disease, while only 5% reported using the ADA guidelines.[4]

## Diet plans

In this section the traditional diet plans and the liberal plan for the treatment of peptic ulcer are presented for the reader's convenience. The bland diet is frequently used in the treatment of gastrointestinal diseases other than peptic ulcer. The affected patients may be receiving certain medications, such as steroids, or have hiatus hernia, or be recovering from acute gastritis.

### Progressive peptic ulcer routine—acute phase

The diet plan for the acute phase of peptic ulcer disease is given in Table 26-2 and is a modification of the original Sippy regimen, which restricted the acutely ill patient to hourly servings of milk and cream for 21 days. Then limited servings of refined cereals, eggs, and custard were added. Later this plan was reduced to 14 days with the addition of other simple foods, such as toast, cottage cheese, and milk-based soups. It is used today by some physicians for a short period of time in the early treatment of the patient who is bleeding on admission to the hospital.

### Progressive peptic ulcer routine—convalescent phase

The convalescent peptic ulcer diet plan in Table 26-3 is a further modification of the Sippy regimen, using bland foods and restricting roughage and condiments. As the patient progresses from the acute to the convalescent stage, the hourly feedings of milk are discontinued and six small meals or three meals with between-meal feedings are served. Table 26-4 shows a menu of three meals and three between-meal feedings for a convalescent peptic ulcer patient.

## Table 26-1. American Dietetic Association Position Paper on Bland Diet in the Treatment of Chronic Duodenal Ulcer Disease

I [The ADA] recognizes that the rationale (chemically and mechanically non-irritating) for the bland diet is not sufficiently supported by scientific evidence.

A. Spices, condiments, and highly seasoned foods are usually omitted on the basis that they irritate the gastric mucosa. However, experiments have indicated that no significant irritation occurs, even when most condiments are applied directly on the gastric mucosa. Exceptions are those items which do cause gastric irritation, including black pepper, chili powder, caffeine, coffee, tea, cocoa, alcohol, and drugs.

B. Milk has been the basis of diets for duodenal ulcer for many years. One of the primary aims in dietary management of duodenal ulcer disease is to reduce acid secretion and neutralize the acid present. While milk does relieve duodenal ulcer pain, the acid neutralizing effect is slight. Its buffering action could be overweighed by its ability to stimulate acid production. Most foods stimulate acid secretion to some extent; protein provides the greatest buffering action and is also the most powerful stimulus to acid secretion. The use of milk therapy has been greatly reduced over the past decade, owing to a better knowledge of its side effects and allergic reactions. The controversy regarding the use of milk still continues. There are those who still advocate the regular use of milk, primarily during the active stage of acute duodenal ulcer; however, strict insistence on its use during remission is unwarranted.

C. Roughage, or coarse food, has been excluded from the diet on the basis that it aggravates the inflamed mucosal area. There is no evidence that such foods as fruit skins, lettuce, nuts, and celery, when they are well masticated and mixed with saliva, will scrape or irritate the duodenal ulcer. Grinding or puréeing of foods is necessary only when the teeth are in poor condition or missing.

D. The effect of a bland diet on the healing of duodenal ulcer has been studied extensively. Investigations have compared various bland diets with regular or free-choice diets. The results indicate that a bland diet made no significant difference in healing the ulcer. One such study demonstrated that the acidity of the gastric contents was frequently lower when a free-choice diet was taken. Many foods have been incriminated as the cause of gastric discomfort and are subsequently eliminated from a patient's diet. Studies done on patients with and without documented gastrointestinal disease indicate that those with gastrointestinal disease cannot be distinguished by food intolerance. Symptoms of intolerance were more related to individual response than to intake of specific food or the presence of disease.

II. Believes that scientific investigation supports the validity of frequent, small feedings in the management of patients with duodenal ulcer disease. These have been found to offer the most comfort to the patient; additionally, acidity of the gastric contents is lower with small-volume, frequent feedings. It must also be recognized that rest, preferably in bed, rapidly reduces duodenal ulcer symptoms. This is a specially important factor in the healing of the ulcer.

III. Believes the following points should be of major consideration in developing a dietary plan for duodenal ulcer patients.
   A. Individualization of the dietary plan, since patients differ as to specific food intolerances, living patterns, life styles, work hours, and education.
   B. Utilization of small-volume, frequent feedings.
   C. Provision of educational materials relative to dietary support.

IV. Advocates the continued pursuit of current research and recommends that valid information be utilized in up-dating dietary regimens.

V. Suggests that dietetic practitioners be cognizant of the possible harmful effects of a milk-rich bland diet in patients who have a tendency towards hypercalcemia and/or atherosclerosis.

*Approved by the Executive Board, May 21, 1971, as Position Paper Number 0000H. (J Am Diet Assoc 59:243, 1971)

## Table 26-2. Progressive Peptic Ulcer Routine—Acute Phase

Milk and cream, half and half, or milk, or skim milk 3 oz every hour alternating with nonabsorbable antacid on the half hour

Supplements (given in 3 small meals, adding 2 or 3 foods each day as tolerated, in addition to hourly milk feedings):

Eggs
   Soft cooked or poached

Cereal
   Refined, cooked cereals only

Toast and crackers
   White, refined bread and crackers

Cottage and cream cheese
   May be substituted for an egg

Strained cream soup
   Made of bland, low-residue vegetables such as asparagus, corn (cream), peas, spinach, and strained before serving

Baked or soft custard, gelatin, junket

Purée fruits and vegetables
   Those available as infant foods are suitable

### Bland diet

Table 26-5 lists the foods included in a bland diet that may be used by some physicians as soon as the acutely ill patient with a peptic ulcer has improved. The convalescent ulcer diet plan in Table 26-3 is then omitted. The bland diet plan, which is somewhat less restrictive than the convalescent diet plan, may also be used after discharge from the hospital. Table 26-6 gives a typical day's menu using a bland diet. Most convalescent ulcer patients are advised to distribute this food into three small meals and three between-meal feedings to avoid gastric distention (see Table 26-4). For example, the canned pears and the bread and butter in the noon meal menu may be eaten at 3:00 P.M.

### Liberal diets

Some clinicians advocate a liberal diet in the treatment of peptic ulcer. The diet plan is usually based on the patient's usual dietary practices provided that his food choices provide an adequate nutrient intake. He should be counseled to omit any food that has regularly caused

## Table 26-3. Progressive Peptic Ulcer Routine—Convalescent Phase

*Foods Used*

Milk
  Milk, cream, buttermilk

Cheese
  Cottage, cream; other mild, soft cheeses. Cheddar cheese may be added later.

Fats
  Butter or margarine

Eggs
  Soft or hard cooked, poached, scrambled

Meats
  Tender beef, lamb, veal; sliced chicken; liver; fish, poached, broiled or baked; crisp bacon; smooth peanut butter

Soups
  Cream soups, using only vegetables listed below

Vegetables
  Well-cooked or canned: asparagus, beets, carrots, peas, green or wax beans, spinach; mashed squash or pumpkin; mashed or baked white and sweet potato (no skins)

Fruits
  Applesauce, baked apples without skin, ripe or baked bananas, diluted fruit juices, stewed or canned pears, peaches and peeled apricots, purée of all dried fruits except figs

  It is advisable to take citrus fruit juices after eating some of the other foods of the meal, or to dilute them half and half with water.

Breads, cereals, macaroni products
  Enriched wheat bread, fine whole wheat or light rye bread; refined cereals; all ready-to-eat cereals except those containing bran; oatmeal; macaroni, spaghetti, noodles

Desserts
  Ice cream, plain; custard; simple puddings of rice, cornstarch, tapioca or bread without fruit or nuts; gelatin desserts (with fruit as permitted above); sponge and other plain cakes, sugar cookies

Beverages
  Milk, cream, buttermilk. Postum, and decaffeinated coffee if allowed by physician

Condiments
  Moderate amounts of sugar, jelly and salt; others if permitted by physician

*Foods to be Avoided*

Fats
  All fried foods

Meats and fish
  Smoked and preserved meats and fish; pork; meat gravies

Soups
  All meat soups; all canned soups

Vegetables
  All raw vegetables; all gas-forming vegetables, including cabbage, cauliflower, brussels sprouts, broccoli, cucumbers, onions, turnips, radishes

Fruits
  All raw fruits except orange juice and ripe banana

Breads and cereal
  Coarse breads and cereals; hot breads

Desserts
  Pastries, nuts, raisins, currants, and candies

Beverages
  Coffee, tea, alcoholic, and carbonated beverages

Condiments
  All condiments except salt, unless permitted by physician

---

gastric distress. He may be advised to eat frequently—midmorning, midafternoon, and before retiring, together with three small meals—and to avoid excessive use of alcoholic beverages, tea, and coffee.[13] Other clinicians are of the opinion that the bedtime feeding should be omitted because it may result in an excessive secretion of gastric acid and, therefore, gastric distress in the early morning hours.[3]

The total calories in the diet of the patient of normal weight should be as many as are required to maintain weight. The obese patient should be assisted to lose weight.

## Table 26-4. Menu for Progressive Peptic Ulcer Routine—Convalescent Phase

| *Breakfast* | *Dinner* | *Supper* |
|---|---|---|
| Orange juice | Chicken, sliced | Cream of spinach soup |
| Eggs, scrambled | Baked potato (no skin) | Cottage cheese |
| White-bread toast | String beans purée | White-bread toast |
| Butter or margarine | White bread | Butter or margarine |
| Jelly | Butter or margarine | Milk |
| Milk | Milk | |
| *10 A.M.* | *3 P.M.* | *9 P.M.* |
| Cornflakes with milk | Canned peaches | Applesauce |
| Milk | Plain cookies | Milk |
| | Milk | |

## Table 26-5.  Bland Diet

### Principles

1. Low in fiber and connective tissue
2. Little or no condiments or spices, except salt in small amounts
3. No highly acidic foods
4. Foods simply prepared

### Foods Used

Milk
    Milk, cream, buttermilk, yogurt

Cheese
    Cream, cottage and other soft, mild cheeses

Fats
    Butter or margarine

Eggs
    Boiled, poached, scrambled in Teflon pan or top of double boiler

Meat, fish, fowl
    Roast beef and lamb; broiled steak, lamb or veal chops; stewed, broiled or roast chicken; fresh tongue; liver; sweetbreads; baked, poached or broiled fish

Soups
    With milk or cream-sauce foundation

Vegetables
    Potatoes, peas, squash, asparagus tips, carrots, tender string beans, beets, spinach. (In severe cases these vegetables are puréed.)

    Orange juice, ripe bananas, avocados, baked apple (without skin), applesauce, canned peaches, pears, apricots, white cherries, stewed prunes

Bread, cereals, macaroni products
    White bread and rolls, crackers, all refined cereals; macaroni, spaghetti, noodles

Desserts
    Custard, junket, ice cream, tapioca, rice, bread or cornstarch pudding, gelatin desserts, junket, sponge cake, plain cookies, prune, apricot or peach whip

Beverages
    Milk, buttermilk, malted milk, fruit juices (if tolerated)

### Foods to be Avoided

Fats
    Fried or fatty foods

Meat, fish
    Smoked and preserved meat and fish; pork

Vegetables
    All raw; all cooked, except those listed above

Fruits
    All except those listed above

Desserts, sweets
    Pastries, preserves, candies

Beverages
    Alcoholic beverages; carbonated drinks, unless prescribed by the doctor

Condiments
    Pepper, other spices, vinegar, ketchup, horseradish, relishes, gravies, mustard, pickles

## Counseling the patient

The physician's diet order determines the approach to dietary counseling. The personality of the patient may be a factor in the diet the physician chooses. A patient with an ulcer often expects some dietary restrictions.[14] If he is a worrisome, overanxious person, he may find a carefully controlled regimen, such as a bland diet, more to his liking than to be told he can eat what he wants. On the other hand, the patient who is able to take his diagnosis in stride or who finds dietary restrictions irksome may do very well on a liberal dietary regimen.

Patients who are employed may need some suggestions about what to eat at coffee breaks, at noontime in a cafeteria or restaurant, or what to include in a bag lunch. The homemaker responsible for preparing a bland diet may need some assistance in modifying food preparation methods.

## Surgical treatment

Peptic ulcer tends to be recurrent. If the ulcer proves to be resistant to medical treatment, or if it recurs fairly frequently, surgery is usually necessary. (For the dietary regimen following surgery for peptic ulcer, see Chap. 27.)

## Table 26-6.  Typical Menu for Bland Diet

| Breakfast | Noon Meal | Evening Meal |
|---|---|---|
| Banana, ripe | Roast lamb | Cream of potato soup |
| Farina with milk | Mashed potatoes | Cheese soufflé |
| 1 egg, poached | Peas | Fresh spinach |
| White-bread toast | White bread | White bread |
| Butter or margarine | Butter or margarine | Butter or margarine |
| Coffee substitute | Canned pears | Applesauce with sugar cookies |
| Cream | Milk | Milk |
| | Cream | Small glass orange juice* |
| | Small glass tomato juice* | |

*If tolerated.

# Other disorders of the upper gastrointestinal tract

## Achalasia

Achalasia or cardiospasm is a motor disorder of the esophagus in which the lower esophageal sphincter (LES) is constricted and impedes the flow of food and fluid into the stomach. At the same time, the normal peristaltic action of the upper part of the esophagus is inadequate. Difficulty in swallowing (dysphagia) is the most common symptom. As the problem progresses, food and fluid do not pass from the esophagus into the stomach and are regurgitated. As a result weight loss occurs. Dilatation of the upper part of the esophagus and inflammation of the lower end of the esophagus may also result.

The patient may be treated by a series of mechanical dilations of the stricture of the lower esophageal sphincter or, if necessary, by surgery. When the patient has recovered from the dilation procedure clear liquids are offered and, if the patient does not experience dysphagia, a regular or bland diet is ordered. Frequent small feedings may be better tolerated than three regular meals. Daily food intake should be closely monitored, especially in those patients who have experienced significant weight loss prior to treatment, or who may be apprehensive about their ability to swallow food.

## Reflux esophagitis

Esophagitis occurs when the gastric contents reflux into the lower esophagus. The condition may be mild, or it may be severe enough to cause bleeding and ultimately esophageal stenosis. It is often complicated by the presence of hiatus hernia. The primary function of the lower esophageal sphincter is to prevent the reflux of gastric contents into the esophagus, and it is generally agreed that reflux esophagitis is caused by a hypotensive and, therefore, incompetent lower esophageal sphincter. The most common clinical symptom is "heartburn" (pain high under the sternum). Regurgitation of gastric contents into the mouth, usually during the night or when bending over, also occurs.

Esophagitis is treated by vigorous antacid therapy and by the prevention of reflux by gravity. Cimetidine is also being used. The patient is advised to remain in an upright position after eating meals and to elevate the head of the bed to reduce reflux during sleep. A bland diet, excluding coffee, tea, and alcohol, in combination with antacid therapy has been used to treat reflux esophagitis. Also a regular diet, excluding coffee, tea, and alcohol and limited in fat, has been recommended with meals equal in size and moderate in quantity to minimize gastric distention.

Recent research indicates that in normal subjects a test meal of fat significantly decreases esophageal sphincter pressure; carbohydrate increases pressure only slightly.[15] Further research demonstrates that slight but significant decreases in lower esophageal sphincter pressure occurred with whole milk in contrast to a significant increase in pressure with skim milk.[16] A chocolate syrup with only 1.25% fat also lowered sphincter pressure. The investigators attribute these results to the caffeine and theobromine in chocolate. A tomato mixture representing spicy foods and orange juice produced considerable variation in pressure and frequent secondary esophageal contractions. Further research has substantiated these findings.[17] The investigators suggest the use of skim milk in the treatment of "heartburn" from gastric reflux and the avoidance of spicy foods, orange juice, and chocolate. Because of the caffeine content of coffee and of theobromine in tea, these beverages should also be excluded.

Although the evidence is limited, it would seem advisable that patients with reflux esophagitis eat regular meals of equal size and avoid coffee, tea, alcohol, chocolate, citrus juices, and spicy foods and limit the quantity of fat at each meal. Although the mechanism is not well understood, reflux esophagitis frequently occurs in the obese person and improves with weight reduction. Therefore, the diet may also be restricted in energy content. If both tomato and orange juices are omitted from the diet, a vitamin C supplement should be prescribed to ensure an adequate intake.

## Hiatus hernia

The terms *hiatus* and *diaphragmatic hernia*, refer to herniation of the cardiac portion of the stomach into the thoracic cavity. The esophagogastric junction slides up and down through the herniation depending on body posture, abdominal distention, and gastric filling. Hiatus hernias are usually asymptomatic. However, when the lower esophageal sphincter is incompetent, gastric reflux occurs and the patient develops reflux esophagitis (see previous discussion).

If bleeding occurs in hiatus hernia, the clinician may order a bland or convalescent ulcer diet, described earlier in this chapter. However, excessive fat intake should be avoided. In severe cases which do not respond to medical therapy, surgery may be advised.

## Hemorrhagic gastritis

Hemorrhagic gastritis is essentially an inflammation, which may be localized or diffuse, of the gastric mucosa. It is characterized by bleeding from superficial lesions compared with the deeper, localized lesions of peptic ulcer. The glands that secrete gastric acid and pepsin are not involved. It may follow the ingestion of aspirin, alcohol, or toxic substances; be associated with staphylococcal food poisoning or with infection; or be the terminal event in the uremia of renal disease.

The treatment varies with the cause. For example, if toxic substances have been ingested in an attempt to commit suicide, gastric lavage is used; or if aspirin or alcohol has caused the bleeding, ingestion of these is eliminated. When the bleeding is controlled, vigorous antacid therapy is used to neutralize the gastric acid in order to protect the gastric mucosa.

When tolerated, a full liquid diet (see Chap. 22) with frequent small feedings is usually offered. Depending on the problem, solid foods, such as dry toast, crackers, cooked cereals, and soft cooked eggs may be added to the diet. The patient may progress to a bland or regular diet as tolerated.

## Atrophic gastritis

Compared with hemorrhagic gastritis, in which the gastric glands are not involved, atrophy of the gastric glands in atrophic gastritis leads to the hyposecretion of gastric acid (hypochlorhydria). Most patients are asymptomatic, while some complain of indigestion. Atrophic gastritis may accompany organic diseases, such as cancer, pernicious anemia, iron deficiency anemia, and chronic infection like syphilis. There is also evidence that bile reflux from the duodenum into the stomach may cause chronic gastritis. The treatment consists of discovering and treating the underlying cause.

## Indigestion

Indigestion, characterized by "heartburn," regurgitation of gastric contents, frequent belching, and a sense of fullness, is symptomatic of various gastric and other organic diseases. When no organic disease is found, the indigestion is said to be functional. Functional indigestion may be due to poor food habits and hurried and irregular meals; to food idiosyncrasies and possible allergies; or to tension and anxiety.

People who live for much of the day on doughnuts and pastries accompanied by frequent cups of coffee or carbonated beverages, with a proper meal only in the evening, are good candidates for indigestion. Overeating, especially of very sweet and fatty foods, may be the cause of indigestion. Rapid eating, particularly when under pressure, resulting in "bolting" of food, cannot avoid causing gastric discomfort. For all these, the treatment consists of making time for rest and relaxation and adopting more moderate food habits. These patients may have to be persuaded of the necessity for such changes and reassured that it is their food habits and not organic disease that has caused their discomfort.

Certain foods have been considered difficult to digest, although the reason is not always clear. Such foods as lobster, crab, sardines, peanuts and nuts, raw apples, garlic, and pickles are in this group. The gas-forming vegetables and fruits may cause discomfort, either because of coarse cellulose or their volatile oils. Common gas-forming foods are cabbage and its relatives—brussels sprouts, broccoli, and cauliflower, dried peas and beans, onions, turnips, green peppers, radishes, cucumbers, and melons. If any of these foods are found to be troublesome, they should be omitted from the diet. True food allergies are discussed in Chapter 34.

Disturbed or anxious patients whose gastric distress is an outcome of their emotional problems are in need of medical guidance and help. They should be given sympathetic support and reassurance. A bland diet may be found to help in treatment.

## Cancer of the stomach
### Delayed diagnosis

Because the onset usually is very gradual and there are no distressing symptoms in the early stages of cancer of the stomach, it is frequently overlooked until too late to cure. For this reason, any continued abdominal discomfort should be investigated, even though seemingly inconsequential.

### Symptoms and diagnosis

Lack of appetite over a considerable period of time with loss of weight and strength are symptoms suggestive of carcinoma. Vomiting, particularly of food eaten many hours before, may occur and sometimes newly acquired constipation is a symptom. The absence of free hydrochloric acid in the gastric contents is suggestive, although in the earlier stages it may be increased. Occult blood is frequently present in the stools. The most important methods used in diagnosis are roentgenography and endoscopy. The early discovery of this condition, when surgical intervention is more likely to be successful, is of utmost importance.

### Dietary adaptations

When either a subtotal or a total resection of the stomach has been performed, the diet should follow that outlined in the chapter on preoperative and postoperative diets for peptic ulcer surgery (see Chap. 27).

Often in inoperable carcinoma of the stomach, patients feel that if only they could eat they would get well; therefore, the diet is difficult to prescribe. A bland or a convalescent ulcer diet is indicated, or even a liquid diet, particularly if there is obstruction or bleeding. However, the patient's morale may be benefited most by serving a regular house diet as long as possible and letting him choose from his tray what appeals to him.

## Zollinger-Ellison (Z-E) syndrome

This relatively rare syndrome is characterized by markedly excessive hypersecretion of gastric juice and hydrochloric acid due to gastrin-secreting tumors of the non-beta islet cells of the pancreas or of the duodenum, which results in extensive ulceration of the gastric mucosa. It is often accompanied by fat malabsorption and diarrhea. Total gastrectomy has proven more effective for these patients than removal of the tumor (see Chap. 27 for postoperative dietary treatment). Recently the use of cimetidine has been shown to be effective in the treatment of these patients for at least a year.[6] Further research is needed to prove its long-term effectiveness.

## Disorders of the small intestine

### Malabsorption

Intestinal malabsorption is any disturbance in the net absorption of any constituent in the gastrointestinal tract—fluid, electrolytes, or nutrients—across the intestinal mucosa, from the mucosal to the serosal side. There may also be excessive secretion of fluids and electrolytes into the lumen of the tract from the serosal to the mucosal side.[14] In practice the term also encompasses the problem of maldigestion of food nutrients as well as their absorption.

The final digestion (hydrolysis) and absorption of nutrients takes place primarily in the cells of the distal duodenum and the jejunum and, to a lesser extent, in the ileum, with the exception of vitamin $B_{12}$, which is absorbed only in the ileum. Maldigestion results when there are insufficient amounts of pancreatic enzymes and fluids entering the duodenum, an inadequate flow of bile from the liver to emulsify fats, or insufficient amounts or a deficiency of the digestive enzymes on the membranes of the cells of the small intestine. Maldigestion can also occur when there are structural defects in the small intestine, such as flattened villi or when there is increased peristaltic activity (peristaltic rushes). Maldigestion results in a decrease in net absorption of protein, fat, and carbohydrate because they have not been hydrolyzed to substances that can be absorbed—hexoses, di- and tripeptides, amino acids, fatty acids, and monoglycerides. The undigested nutrients, modified to some extent by intestinal bacteria, are excreted by the large bowel.

Malabsorption may be primary, such as lactose malabsorption due to a hereditary lack of lactase, or secondary, such as lactose malabsorption due to lactase deficiency following gastrointestinal infection.[15] The common symptoms of malabsorption are weight loss in adults or growth retardation in infants and children, abdominal distention and cramping, and diarrhea or steatorrhea.

### Diarrhea

In diarrhea the stools are fluid or semifluid and increased in number. In addition to water, the stool also contains sodium and potassium and frequently undigested food. With significant fluid and electrolyte losses dehydration and weight loss result. In infants and children the fluid and electrolyte losses may be critical.

### Steatorrhea

Steatorrhea means excessive fat in the stools. Massive maldigestion of fats results in stools that are frothy, large, foul smelling, and shiny in appearance. The number of stools per day is increased; they also contain significant amounts of water and electrolytes.

### Disaccharide problems—lactose malabsorption (lactose intolerance)

Malabsorption of lactose, the sugar of all commonly used mammalian milks, is due to an insufficiency of the disaccharidase lactase, which is found in the greatest quantity in the outer membrane of the mucosal cell of the jejunum. The degree of lactase insufficiency in individual people varies. Sahi[18] classifies a very low level of lactase activity as *hypolactasia* and moderate lactase activity as *lactase persistence*. Lactase deficiency implies a total lack of lactase, a condition that probably never occurs.[18] Lactose malabsorption is characterized by varying degrees of intestinal distention, cramps, increased flatus, and diarrhea due to unhydrolyzed lactose. Severe diarrhea can result in excessive fluid and electrolyte losses with hypovolemic shock.

Lactase deficiency in the newborn infant has been reported in the literature. However, recent research questions this diagnosis. More commonly, problems of lactose malabsorption occur in children after age 1 year, and in adolescents and adults whose derivation is Asian or African. It is estimated that 60% to 90% of adult American blacks and Orientals have lactose malabsorption compared with 5% to 15% of white American adults of northern European extraction.[19] Research indicates that lactase insufficiency is transmitted through an autosomal recessive gene.[18]

There are secondary causes of lactose malabsorption. There can be a reduction in jejunal lactase activity due to enteric infections. For example, infants and adults[20] are often intolerant of lactose during and for a period of time following infectious gastroenteritis. Lactose malabsorption may also occur in patients with celiac sprue, tropical sprue, cystic fibrosis, ileitis, and colitis as a result of structural damage to jejunal mucosa. Gastrointestinal surgery, such as a gastrojejunostomy, can cause lactose malabsorption because the area of the jejunum with the greatest concentration of lactase is bypassed by the gastric chyme as it leaves the stomach.

### Diagnostic tests

The lactose tolerance test (LTT) and the lactose breath hydrogen test (L-BHT) are the two tests most commonly used to diagnose lactose malabsorption. Also, jejunal tissue can be obtained by peroral suction biopsy for the quantitative analysis of lactase in mucosal membrane.

A rise in fasting blood glucose of 20 mg to 25 mg or

*more* per 100 ml, depending on the analytical method used, in the 1½ to 2 hours after ingestion of 50 g of lactose, indicates the presence of adequate quantities of lactase to hydrolyze the disaccharide resulting in the absorption of the glucose moiety of lactose. Colonic bacteria release hydrogen from lactose when it enters the colon unhydrolyzed due to insufficient lactase in the small intestine. Part of the hydrogen is absorbed from the colon into the blood and expired in the breath. During an LTT samples of breath can be collected for a total of 6 hours. A rise of *less* than 20 ppm above the baseline data indicates the presence of adequate quantities of lactase.

There can be wide variations in test results. For example, one person who is suspected of having lactose malabsorption may have a positive LTT with a fasting blood glucose rise of 16 mg per 100 ml, whereas another person may have a blood glucose rise of 4 mg per 100 ml. Both are lactose malabsorbers but to different degrees. Also, some people in high-risk populations who have a positive LTT report symptoms of lactose malabsorption, whereas others with a positive test are unaware of any symptoms.

### Dietary treatment

The lactose-restricted diet is used in the treatment of lactose malabsorption, and the level of restriction for each patient depends on the level of lactase activity. A very low level of lactase activity and severe gastrointestinal symptoms may require a diet essentially free of lactose while the patient with moderate levels of lactase activity and no symptoms may tolerate a moderate intake of lactose.[21] As the first step in planning with the patient, the clinical dietitian should take a comprehensive diet history to identify the level of lactose intake the patient can usually tolerate. After establishing an acceptable dietary pattern with the client, the clinical dietitian should estimate the average daily calcium and riboflavin intake provided by the pattern. This estimate should be recorded in the patient's medical record so that supplementary calcium and riboflavin can be prescribed if needed, since milk is the major source of these two nutrients.

The major source of lactose in the American diet is cow's or goat's milk, and foods made with milk, such as milk chocolate, ice cream, cream pies, puddings, custards, cream soups, and such dishes as casseroles and soufflés. Yeast breads, with few exceptions such as French or Italian bread, are made with approximately 4% milk solids. Biscuits, muffins, rolls, and such other doughs as doughnuts and sweet rolls are also made with milk. Bagels and many crackers and cookies are made without milk. Most cheeses have only traces of lactose per serving, that is, 0.2 g to 0.5 g per ounce.[22] The list of ingredients on the labels of all food packages must be read carefully because milk in some form is widely used in convenience foods and many other products. Also, lactose is an ingredient of some medications.

Research has demonstrated that people with moderate levels of lactase activity tolerate some milk (8 oz–16 oz per day) as a beverage with meals or in foods although milk consumed without a meal may cause symptoms. Also, it has been reported that fermented dairy products, such as buttermilk, cottage cheese, and yogurt are tolerated by some patients. This is possibly due to the modification of lactose in these products by bacterial fermentation during processing.

For people with very low levels of lactase activity Lact-Aid,* lactase enzyme, can be added to milk to hydrolyze the lactose. Unless 90% or more of the lactose is hydrolyzed, the milk so treated may cause symptoms in some patients. The enzyme-treated milk is somewhat sweeter to taste than untreated milk, but studies have shown good acceptance of the product.[23] Lact-Aid might also be used by those (such as adolescent boys), who have a moderate level of lactase activity and want to drink at least a quart of milk a day. For infants there are lactose-free formulas that can be used as a beverage at meals after weaning (see Table 35-4, Chap. 35).

## Celiac sprue (gluten-induced enteropathy, celiac disease, nontropical sprue)

Although the term *celiac disease* was originally applied only to children who exhibited this malabsorption syndrome, it is generally accepted today that what formerly was called *nontropical sprue* is in reality adult celiac disease and may be referred to as celiac sprue. It has been observed that a number of patients who developed celiac disease in adult life had a history of the disease in childhood. With the discovery that the gluten in cereal grains is the toxic agent, the syndrome is now also known as gluten-induced enteropathy. Celiac sprue is a classic example of malabsorption due to structural and functional defects of the small bowel, particularly the jejunal villi.

### Symptoms

Celiac sprue is characterized by steatorrhea, with the passing of at least two to three stools a day. These are described as bulky, foamy, light colored, and foul smelling. They contain a high percentage of fat, fatty acids, and calcium soaps, resulting from incomplete digestion and absorption of fat in the intestinal tract.

Because of the loss of fat and other nutrients in the stool a whole complex of symptoms results. There is often marked weight loss, muscle wasting, anorexia, and debilitation; in infants and sometimes in adults there is a typical "pot belly"; there is anemia due to poor absorption of iron and folic acid; there may be tetany, bone pain, and fractures resulting from the poor absorption of calcium and vitamin D; and hypoprothrombinemia and roughening of the skin may be present because fat-soluble vi-

*SugarLo Co., P.O. Box 1017, Atlantic City, N.J. 08404

tamins K and A are not absorbed. Occasionally, patients have glossitis and peripheral neuritis, possibly due to an inadequate absorption of the B vitamins. More recent findings suggest that there may also be a deficiency of vitamin E due to faulty fat absorption and of vitamin $B_6$.

## Diagnosis

The finding of unabsorbed fat and fatty acids in the feces and the history and appearance of the patient give the first clue to the diagnosis. A jejunal biopsy, viewed under the electron microscope, reveals marked changes in the jejunal mucosa. Instead of the fingerlike projections of the villi with their brushborder, the mucosa is flat and thickened and appears to have varying degress of epithelial cell atrophy, now recognized as characteristic of celiac disease (see Figs. 26-1 and 26-2). It is suspected that an immunological reaction in the tissues of the villi causes the changes in the jejunal mucosa.

In 1953 three Dutch investigators Dicke, Weijers, and van de Kamer reported that wheat, rye, and oat cereals were responsible for the steatorrhea and other symptoms of celiac disease in children.[24] When they excluded these cereals from the diets of their patients there was prompt and marked improvement. In a subsequent report these same authors showed that the two major components of wheat protein, glutenin and gliadin, which are also present in rye protein and, to a lesser extent, in oat protein, were the offending substances.[25] They indicated that the specific substance in the cereal gluten is the amino acid, glutamine, when it is bound in a peptide (a partial breakdown product of protein digestion). When they tested their treated patients with bound glutamine the symptoms recurred. This did not happen when they tested these same patients with glutamine alone. The more recent work of Cornell and Townley supports these findings.[26]

Glutamine, the amide of glutamic acid, occurs widely in all food proteins but the greatest concentration is found in the gluten of wheat, rye, barley, and, to a lesser extent, in oats. Although rice and corn also contain glutamine—but in smaller amounts than the other cereals— they are well tolerated in patients with celiac sprue.

## Dietary treatment

From the work of the Dutch investigators with children, and of others with adults with nontropical sprue, a *gluten-free* diet, which excluded the use of wheat, rye, barley, and oats, was begun and soon proved to be successful in controlling the disease. Foods used in the gluten-free diet are presented in Table 26-7. In the patient with severe diarrhea, the diet may be restricted in residue until the diarrhea is controlled.

The exclusion of all cereal grains except corn and rice from the diet may seem to be an easier matter than it actually is. Wheat flour and wheat bread products are used in such a variety of ways in food preparation that

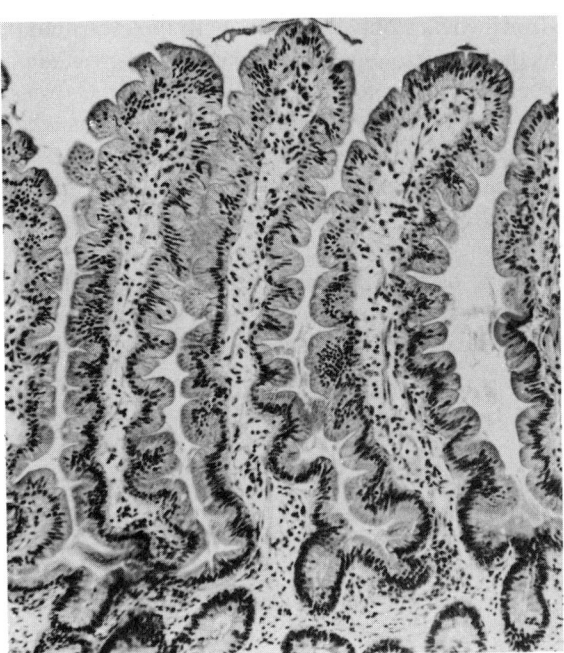

**Fig. 26-1.**  Jejunal biopsy. Normal jejunum. The villi are slender and of uniform size. The epithelial cells are intact in all areas. (Benson GD, Kowlessar OD, Sleisenger MH: Adult celiac disease with emphasis upon response to the gluten-free diet. Medicine 43:1, 1964)

their elimination poses many problems. Not only must all wheat bread and rolls be omitted, both white and whole wheat, but all breaded products, bread stuffing, gravies and cream sauces thickened with wheat flour, macaroni, spaghetti, noodles, biscuits, crackers, cakes, and cookies

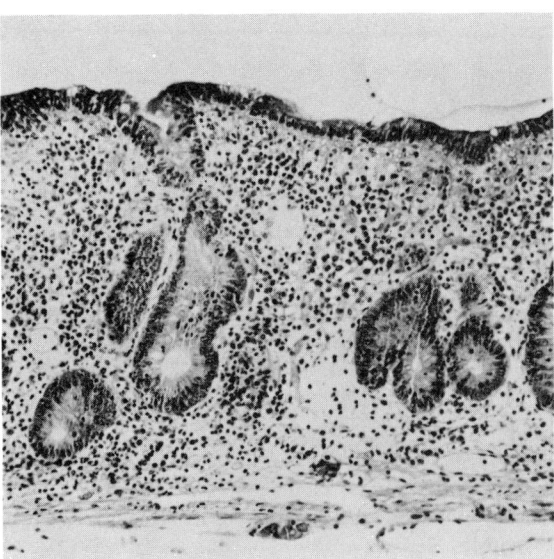

**Fig. 26-2.**  Jejunal biopsy. Adult celiac disease. Pretreatment biopsy showing severe changes. There is complete absence of villi, thinning of the mucosal surface, and disorganization of the epithelial cells. (Benson GD, Kowlessar OD, Sleisenger MH: Adult celiac disease with emphasis upon response to the gluten-free diet. Medicine 43:1, 1964)

made from wheat flour. Rye grain, with the exception of rye breads, pretzels, bagels, and Ry-Krisp, is less commonly used and, therefore, omitted more easily. Oatmeal is excluded, as it caused a recurrence of symptoms when reintroduced into the diet. Barley and buckwheat are also excluded, as their effect in the intestinal tract in this disease is not known. For adults, beer and ale must be omitted because they may contain cereal grain residues.[27]

In place of the cereals, which must be excluded, bread, biscuits, and cookies made from rice, corn, and soy flour, and wheat starch are used* (see Chap. 32 for wheat

*Gluten-Free Bread Mix, Chicago Dietetic Supply House, LaGrange, IL 60525; and dp Low Protein Baking Mix, Henkel Corporation, Minneapolis, MN 55435

starch products). Cornflakes, corn meal, hominy, rice, Rice Krispies, puffed rice, and precooked rice cereals may be used. Cornstarch and potato flour can be used to thicken gravies and cream sauces. Because wheat flour is in such common use, it is good to check the labels on commercially prepared foods for content before using them in this diet to be sure that no wheat flour or modified wheat starch has been used in their preparation. Postum, malted milk, and Ovaltine are examples of commercial products made from or containing cereal grains. Where such content is not included in the label, the food had better be omitted if there is a question.

The physician may augment the diet with mineral and vitamin supplements to correct deficiencies and

## Table 26-7. Gluten-Free Diet

### Characteristics

1. All forms of wheat, rye, oatmeal, buckwheat, and barley are omitted, except gluten-free wheat starch.
2. All other foods are permitted freely, including fats and starches.
3. The diet should be high in protein and calories. Mineral and vitamin supplements may be needed if malnutrition is present. After that, the diet should be sufficient to maintain normal growth and development in children, and normal weight in adults.

### Foods Used

Milk
2 glasses or more. Flavored if desired. More for children

Cheese
As desired. Cottage and pot cheese only for very young children

Fats
Butter and other fats as desired. (Note restrictions under "Foods To Be Avoided.")

Eggs
1 to 2 a day

Meat, fish, fowl
1 or 2 servings daily (not breaded, creamed, or served with gravy thickened with wheat flour; no bread dressings). Otherwise prepared as desired

Soups
All clear and vegetable soups; cream soups thickened with cream, cornstarch, or potato flour only

Vegetables
As desired. Include 2 servings of green or yellow vegetables and at least 1 raw vegetable daily. (The last may be omitted for very young children.) Rice may be substituted occasionally for potato. Cream sauce made with cornstarch.

Fruits
As desired; 2 or 3 servings daily. Include citrus fruit once a day.

Bread and cereals
Bread made from rice, corn, or soybean flour and gluten-free wheat starch only

Cornflakes, corn meal, hominy, rice, Rice Krispies, Puffed Rice, precooked rice cereals, and rice noodles

Desserts
Any of the following: Jello, fruit Jello, ice or sherbet, homemade ice cream, custard, junket, rice pudding, or cornstarch pudding (homemade)

Beverages
Milk, fruit juices, ginger ale, cocoa. (Read label to see that no wheat flour has been added to cocoa or cocoa syrup.) Coffee (made from ground coffee), tea, carbonated beverages

Condiments and sweets
Salt; sugar, white or brown; molasses; jellies and jams; honey; corn syrup

### Foods to be Avoided

Fats
Cream sauces made with wheat flour; commercial salad dressings, except pure mayonnaise. (Read labels.)

Meat, fish, fowl
Meat patties or meat, fish, or chicken loaf and pies made with bread or bread crumbs; croquettes; breaded meat, fish, or chicken. Chili con carne and other canned meat dishes. Cold cuts unless guaranteed pure meat. Bread stuffings

All gravies or cream sauces thickened with wheat flour

Soups
All canned soups except clear broth. All cream soups unless thickened with cream, cornstarch, or potato flour

Vegetables
Any prepared with cream sauce or breaded

Bread, cereals, macaroni products
All bread, rolls, crackers, cake and cookies made from wheat or rye; Ry-Krisp; muffins, biscuits, waffles, pancake flour and other prepared mixes; rusks, Zwieback, pretzels; any product containing oatmeal, barley, or buckwheat

Breaded foods, bread crumbs

All wheat and rye cereals; wheat germ, barley, oatmeal, buckwheat, kasha

Macaroni, spaghetti, noodles, dumplings

Desserts
Cakes, cookies, pastry; commercial ice cream and ice cream cones; prepared mixes, puddings. All homemade puddings thickened with wheat flour

Beverages
Postum, malted milk, Ovaltine. For adults: beer, ale

Sweets
Commercial candies containing cereal products. (Read labels.)

WARNING: Read labels on all packaged and prepared foods.

hasten recovery. Although fat excretion persists to some extent, fat is well tolerated and there is no need to limit it in the diet. However, some patients may require a moderate restriction (80 g–100 g per day).

***Results and prognosis.*** The response of the patient with celiac disease to the elimination of the offending cereal grains is often dramatic, and may occur within 24 hours to a week. The appetite returns, the patient begins to regain lost weight, the stools become less fatty and less frequent, and a sense of wellbeing is quickly apparent.

The long-term effects of adherence to the gluten-free diet are equally striking. Benson and co-workers, reporting on 32 patients with adult celiac disease followed for a number of years, found that there was improvement in every diagnostic finding, including in most cases a return to normal mucosal structure.[28] The degree of improvement was in direct proportion to the careful adherence to the diet. That the diet does not cure the disease is shown by the fact that symptoms recur if the patient consumes food containing gluten.

***Other findings.*** In untreated celiac sprue the structural defect in the villi reduces the quantity of disaccharidases available to hydrolyze disaccharides.[29] Weser and Sleisenger and others have reported that lactase deficiency and the absorption of undigested lactose occurred in some patients in whom celiac disease was untreated or who did not follow their diets carefully.[30] Symptoms were abdominal cramps, distention, and diarrhea, and were relieved when lactose and gluten were omitted from the diet. That this is not a permanent defect is shown by the fact that patients who had maintained a strict gluten-free diet for 2 years or more had no symptoms of lactase deficiency.

Persons with dermatitis herpetiformis, a skin disease of the extensor surfaces of the body, may have jejunal biopsies typical of those in patients with celiac sprue, but they do not have severe malabsorption. With a gluten-free diet the villous structure of the jejunum improves, but the dermatitis does not.[31]

## Tropical sprue

Tropical sprue, another malabsorption syndrome, is endemic in the native populations of some tropical and subtropical areas in the world, notably Puerto Rico and Southeast Asia. Military personnel as well as other residents from temperate countries who are stationed in these areas also may develop tropical sprue, either during their stay in the host country or on their return home.

The symptoms are diarrhea, with loss of nutrients, especially fat, weight loss, and macrocytic anemia. If the disease is of long standing, there will be severe malnutrition, megaloblastic bone marrow changes, and villous atrophy of the jejunal mucosa, eventually leading to the typical flat mucosa of celiac disease.

The syndrome responds dramatically to the administration of folic acid and antibiotics. In some patients, despite continuance of therapy, the megaloblastic anemia recurs due to deficient absorption of vitamin $B_{12}$. There is prompt response to vitamin $B_{12}$ therapy. The response to a gluten-free diet is minimal, and an ordinary, nutritionally adequate diet, increased in calories and protein to counteract malnutrition and weight loss, is sufficient. With treatment, patients become asymptomatic and eventually the intestinal mucosa returns to normal.

The etiology of tropical sprue is still in doubt. It has been thought to be due to a diet deficient in folic acid or to an interference with its absorption, but there is no basis for this hypothesis other than the response to treatment with folic acid. There is some evidence of the presence of an infective agent, because of the response to antibiotic therapy, but no pathogens have been demonstrated.[32]

## Pancreatitis
### Etiology

Pancreatitis, or inflammation of the pancreas, may be acute or chronic; the acute form may or may not progress to the chronic one. The etiology of pancreatitis is poorly understood at present. Three hypotheses are proposed to explain the disease: obstruction of the pancreatic duct; regurgitation of bile from the common duct up the pancreatic duct; and the reflux of duodenal contents into the pancreatic duct. The role of pancreatic enzymes in the pathogenesis of pancreatitis is also under investigation.

It has been observed that pancreatitis is associated with other diseases. Acute pancreatitis may occur with biliary tract disease, infection, alcohol ingestion, and hyperlipoproteinemia Types 1, 4, or 5. Chronic pancreatitis is associated with chronic alcoholism, untreated biliary tract disease, and familial abnormalities of the sphincter of Oddi.

The most common symptom of pancreatic disease is abdominal pain. Nausea, vomiting, and steatorrhea due to a deficiency of pancreatic lipase also occur. Hypovolemia, leading to circulatory failure, and paralytic ileus frequently accompany severe, acute pancreatitis.

### Dietary treatment

The presence in the duodenum of dilute hydrochloric acid and the products of protein digestion normally stimulate the flow of pancreatic juices and enzymes, while the presence of fat stimulates the flow of bile. The dietary treatment of pancreatitis is derived from these principles.

In severe acute pancreatitis the patient is maintained on total parenteral nutrition (see Chap. 27) until fluid and food by mouth is tolerated without pain. When oral feedings are tolerated, liquids containing primarily carbohydrate are offered because it is the nutrient that has the least effect on pancreatic exocrine excretion. During recovery, and with milder attacks, frequent small feedings that contain carbohydrate and protein and are limited in fat are given. Antacid therapy is used to neutralize gastric acid secretion. The diet is limited in fat because pancreatic lipase is deficient and with concurrent biliary disease bile may also be deficient. If hyperlipoproteinemia is present, the diet may be modified to treat this problem (see Chap. 30).

Chronic pancreatitis may be treated by a regular or bland diet limited in fat. When necessary, pancreatic extracts are given orally and are taken with each meal and snack. Medium chain triglycerides can be used as a source of energy because they do not appear to require pancreatic lipase or bile for digestion (see discussion of MCT oil in Chap. 24). If glucose intolerance develops due to lack of insulin because of fibrotic changes in the pancreatic beta cells, the diet may be restricted in carbohydrate (see Chap. 28).

Providing an adequate energy and nutrient intake for the patient with pancreatitis is difficult. The diet tends to be low in energy due to the fat restriction, and the patient's food intake is poor due to constant pain. Supplementary vitamins may be required. Every effort should be made to give the patient the foods that he can tolerate, and in such quantity that his nutritional needs continue to be met. In all cases of pancreatitis alcohol is prohibited.

## Gallbladder disease
### Etiology

The most common form of gallbladder disease is cholelithiasis (gallstones) complicated by cholecystitis (inflammation of the gallbladder), and it occurs more frequently in women over 40 years of age than in any other group. The largest proportion of stones are composed of cholesterol. It is known that the cholesterol in bile precipitates to form cholesterol stones when the amount of bile salts and lecithin in bile is inadequate to keep the cholesterol in solution. Conditions commonly associated with bile cholesterol saturation are obesity, ileal disease of the gastrointestinal tract, and estrogens and progestins, both endogenous and exogenous.[33]

### Symptoms

The major symptom of gallbladder disease is acute or intermittent epigastric pain. Indigestion, intolerance to fatty and spicy foods, and nausea and vomiting may also occur. If the flow of bile into the duodenum is decreased or the cystic duct is obstructed, jaundice and steatorrhea can occur. The pain cannot be attributed solely to fatty food ingestion because amino acids and gastric acid as well as fat stimulate cholecystokinin, the hormone that is the major mediator of gallbladder contraction.

### Treatment

Cholesterol gallstones can be treated medically or surgically. The oral administration of chenodeoxycholic and ursodeoxycholic acids dissolves cholesterol stones by reducing the bile cholesterol saturation in patients with functioning gallbladders. Patients who do not respond to medical treatment and those with other types of gallbladder disease are treated surgically by cholescystectomy (removal of the gallbladder).

### Dietary treatment

The obese patient with cholelithiasis who does not respond to medical treatment and who does not require emergency surgery is counseled to lose weight to avoid the risk of operative and postoperative complications of the obese. As a group, these patients require 1200 to 1400-calorie restricted diets (see Chap. 28).

Those patients with gallbladder disease who relate the intake of fatty and spicy foods to attacks of pain or who have steatorrhea due to inadequate bile flow into the duodenum for micelle formation require a fat-restricted diet (40 g to 60 g per day) preoperatively. Table 26-8 lists the foods containing significant amounts of fat, which must be used in limited quantities, and foods high in fat, which must be omitted. If the patient reports gastric distress from eggs, eggs should be omitted. Table 26-9 gives a low-fat bland diet menu. A fat-restricted bland diet is usually well tolerated. Following cholecystectomy, patients usually tolerate moderate amounts of fat (80 g to 100 g per day). If obese, the patient is counseled to achieve and maintain an appropriate weight status.

## Regional ileitis (Crohn's disease)
### Etiology

Regional ileitis is a chronic, progressive disease of the ileum of unknown etiology. It may first involve the terminal segment of the ileum proximal to the ileocecal valve, but, eventually, it will spread along the ileum and may involve the jejunum. It may also involve the esophagus and colon. For this reason the disease is sometimes called regional enteritis. The term *regional* refers to the fact that healthy areas of the bowel may alternate with diseased ones. Despite occasional remissions, the disease is progressive.

### Symptoms

The condition is characterized by hyperplasia (enlargement due to cell increase) of the lymphatics, which eventually interferes with the blood supply of the mucosa of that section of the intestinal tract which is affected. This in turn gives rise to edema and ulceration, scarring of the mucosa, thickening of the intestinal wall with narrowing of the lumen of the bowel, and obstruction. The most common symptoms are persistent diarrhea and pain.

Because of the persistent diarrhea, there may be marked malnutrition. If the disease is extensive, there is poor absorption of food nutrients, further accentuating the poor nutrition. A chronically ill patient may be markedly underweight and show signs of protein depletion. Anemia may be present due to blood loss and to poor absorption of iron and vitamin $B_{12}$. There may be insufficient absorption of fat-soluble vitamins as evidenced by hypoprothrombinemia and roughened skin. If medical treatment fails to restore the patient's nutritional status, or if there is obstruction, surgery may be indicated. See Chapter 27 for dietary care in the latter case.

### Dietary treatment

On admission to the hospital all patients with regional ileitis require an extensive assessment of nutritional status (see Chap. 23). Many have had a significant recent weight loss and have eliminated numerous foods from their diets that they feel have caused pain or diarrhea. Their food intake should be monitored daily with the energy and protein intake for the previous 24 hours recorded in the medical record each morning.

The diet in regional ileitis should be high in protein and calories and low in residue, as described in the next section of this chapter. High-residue diets can cause obstruction in the affected segments of the bowel. The patient may eat better when the diet is divided into six meals during the day and evening, and if he is given some choice. Seasonings and cold fluids are not well tolerated and should be omitted. Vitamin supplements should be given as additions to the diet. Vitamins K and $B_{12}$ and, possibly, iron should be given as parenteral medications, since they are not sufficiently absorbed from the intestinal tract. The restrictions for lactase insufficiency discussed earlier in the chapter should be observed in cases where the diagnosis has been established. Critically ill patients may be treated with total parenteral nutrition for 10 days to 2 weeks to rest the bowel (see Chap. 27).

## Disorders of the large bowel
### Dietary residue

Patients with problems in the terminal ileum and large bowel may require a low-residue diet. These patients may have regional ileitis, ulcerative colitis, malignant or nonmalignant lesions of the colon or rectum, or hemorrhoids. Regional ileitis and ulcerative colitis are

### Table 26-8. Restrictions and Omissions on a Low-Fat Diet

***Foods Limited***

Milk to 1 pint daily
Eggs to 1 daily
Butter or margarine to $1/2$ tablespoon daily
Lean meat, fish or fowl to 1 serving daily
(If skim milk is used, meat may be increased to 2 servings without altering the fat limitation.)

***Foods Omitted***

Cream; cheese other than pot or cottage cheese
All fried foods
Salad oils; salad dressings; gravies
All meat high in fat, such as pork, bacon, ham, goose, duck, fatty fish
Pastry; cake; cookies; ice cream
Nuts, olives, avocados

generally treated medically. Progression of the disease may lead to surgery—ileostomy in regional ileitis, and colostomy or ileostomy in ulcerative colitis. In all situations the low-residue diet is generally used as part of medical treatment or in preparation for surgical treatment of the patient.

### Residue in foods

The foods used in the residue-restricted diets are low in vegetable fiber to decrease the volume of fecal material. The elastin fibers of meat are restricted for the same reason. Fiber is that portion of food (cellulose, hemicellulose, and lignin) that is not enzymatically digested in the digestive tract (see Table 2-2, *Components of Dietary Fiber by Structure and Possible Physiologic Function*). Fruits, vegetables, nuts, and whole grains are the major contributors of fiber. The term *roughage* is also used to refer to fiber.

It is generally agreed that meats free of elastin fibers, fats such as butter and margarine, and highly refined carbohydrates such as flour, spaghetti, macaroni, noodles, rice, and sugar add minimal residue to the fecal

### Table 26-9. Very Low-Fat, Bland Diet Menu in Six Meals

| *Breakfast* | *Lunch* | *Dinner* |
|---|---|---|
| Stewed prunes | Cottage cheese | Sliced chicken |
| Cream of Wheat | Toast, lightly buttered, 2 slices | Baked potato |
| Milk, whole, $1/2$ c | Jelly or honey | Soft-cooked string beans |
| Postum | Applesauce | Canned apricots |
| Sugar | Tea, sugar | Tea, sugar |
| *10 A.M.* | *3 P.M.* | *8 P.M.* |
| Toast, lightly buttered, 2 slices | Junket made with skim milk | Crackers |
| Jelly or honey | Crackers | Jelly or honey |
| Skim milk, 1 glass | Jelly or honey | Skim milk, 1 glass |

This diet will contain approximately 70 g protein, 25 g fat, 325 g carbohydrate, and 1750 calories.

contents of the large bowel. Bananas and potatoes, which are low in residue, are exceptions among fruits and vegetable which are classified as high in residue (see Table 2-3, *Dietary Fiber in Foods*).

Limited evidence exists that indicates that milk may add residue to the fecal contents. As a result there is controversy about the use of milk in residue-restricted diet plans. It has been observed that some adult ulcerative colitis patients have insufficient amounts of lactase and respond favorably to a moderate lactose restriction[13] (see discussion of lactose malabsorption earlier in this chapter).

Tea, coffee, meat extractives, condiments, spices, and carbonated beverages are usually not excluded from the residue-restricted diet. Fruit and vegetable juices may be excluded in some situations, not because of residue, but because the organic acids in these beverages may stimulate peristaltic action.

### Residue-restricted diets

Residue-restricted diets may be ordered at various levels of restriction. Table 26-10, *Diets Varying in Residue*, presents different levels of residue-restricted diets.

The Minimal Residue Diet in Table 26-10 may be used to prepare a patient for bowel surgery or immediately after surgery. It is seen that the foods used in this diet are limited and that this diet can be inadequate in calcium and vitamins A and C. If used for any period of time, it should be supplemented with mineral and vitamin preparations.

The Moderate Residue Diet in Table 26-10 may be used as the patient progresses afer bowel surgery, in the early medical treatment of regional ileitis or ulcerative colitis, or for the symptomatic control of diarrhea. The Residue-Restricted Diet in Table 26-10 is usually the one used over a period of time by patients with regional ileitis or ulcerative colitis.

## Ulcerative colitis
### Etiology

Ulcerative colitis is an inflammatory disease of the colon, encountered in all age groups from very young children to the elderly. The etiology is unknown. No organism has been isolated as a cause of the disease. It has been ascribed to allergy, especially to milk, wheat, and eggs. In addition, there are indications that colitis may occur on an emotional basis, because these patients are often very painstaking and meticulous and seem to have more that an ordinary dependence on others.

### Table 26-10. Diets Varying in Residue

| Foods | Residue-Restricted Diet | Moderate-Residue Diet | Minimal-Residue Diet |
|---|---|---|---|
| Milk* | Milk, buttermilk, yogurt, cream | Same | Same |
| Cheese | Cottage, cream*, Cheddar | Same | Cottage, cream only* |
| Fat | Butter, margarine | Same | Same |
| Eggs | Cooked, poached, scrambled in double boiler | Same | Same |
| Meat, fish, fowl | Tender chicken, fish, sweetbreads, ground beef, and lamb | Same | Ground, tender meat; minced chicken and fish |
| Soups and Broths | Broth, strained meat-based soups | Same | Broth only |
| Vegetables | Cooked vegetables, asparagus, peas, string beans, spinach, carrots, beets, squash; potatoes—boiled, mashed, baked | Vegetable juice; vegetable purée, cooked asparagus tips, carrots; potatoes—boiled, mashed, baked | Unseasoned vegetable juices in limited amounts* |
| Fruits | Fruit juices, cooked and canned fruits (without skins, seeds or fiber), bananas | Fruit juice, fruit purée, ripe bananas, cooked, peeled apples, apricots, peaches, pears, plums | Fruit juices, preferably citrus in limited amounts* |
| Bread, cereals | Refined, enriched bread and cereals; macaroni, spaghetti, noodles, rice, crackers | Refined, enriched bread and cereals only, macaroni, spaghetti, noodles, rice, white crackers | As in moderately low residue |
| Desserts | Ices, ice cream*, junket*, cereal puddings*, custard*, gelatin, plain cake, and cookies; all without fruit and nuts | Same | Same |
| Beverages | Tea, coffee, carbonated beverages | Same | Tea, coffee as permitted |
| Condiments | Salt, moderate amounts of pepper, other mild spices, sugar | Salt and sugar | Salt and sugar |

*If tolerated.

## Symptoms

The disease is characterized by friability and hyperemia of the mucosa, leading to many small areas of bleeding ulceration. This may involve only a part of the rectum or the colon, but in advanced stages of the disease it usually involves the entire area of the large bowel. The stools, which may be as frequent as 15 to 20 a day, are semiliquid and contain blood and mucus. The patient suffers from the discomfort of the frequent stools and the accompanying cramps, and he is usually malnourished, often to an extreme degree. Anemia may be present due to blood loss, and the patient may be severely underweight. The disease is usually treated conservatively by medical means, but in advanced cases surgery may be resorted to and a colostomy or ileostomy performed. See Chapter 27 for dietary care in the latter case. 463

## Dietary treatment

In the critically ill patient total parenteral nutrition may be used to rest the bowel or to rehabilitate the patient nutritionally pre- and postoperatively (see Chap. 27). All ulcerative colitis patients require an extensive assessment of nutritional status (see Chap. 23). Their fluid and food intake should be monitored daily with the energy and protein intake for the previous 24 hours recorded in the record each morning.

Dietary treatment in the patient with chronic colitis is supportive rather than curative. A patient previously well controlled by diet and medication may have diarrhea when emotionally upset, even though he is adhering to his prescribed diet.

The frequency of the stools, the degree of bleeding and ulceration of the colon, and the general malnutrition present in all patients with severe colitis demand the use of a diet low in residue and as high in protein and calories as the patient can tolerate. The omission of roughage prevents irritation of the inflamed colon, and the high-protein, high-caloric diet helps to restore the patient to a better nutritional status. Vitamin and iron supplements should be given.

Either the moderate residue diet or the minimal residue diet listed in Table 26-10 is suitable for the very ill colitis patient. It should be served in six small meals at first. Unfortunately, the diet is not very palatable or colorful, and care must be taken to serve the food as attractively as possible. As his condition improves, the patient progresses to a residue-restricted diet. Lactose malabsorption may further complicate the dietary treatment of the patient with ulcerative colitis. Buttermilk or yogurt may be tried, but if they are not tolerated even these dairy products should be omitted.

Because colitis seems to have strong emotional components, a self-selected diet may be used to help the patient to achieve some degree of independence. The doctor may allow him to choose his own diet and encourage him to try whatever food appeals to him, even those that would seem to be contraindicated, such as foods high in residue. All members of the health-care team must be supportive as well as permissive, giving the patient confidence and encouraging him to make his own decisions. As the patient's feeling of security increases, he will eat larger and more nutritious meals, resulting in the subsequent healing of the colon and a gain in weight and strength.

## Food acceptance

Patients with colitis are fussy about their food and often extremely hard to please. They wish others to make choices for them, yet refuse to eat the food when it appears on the tray. They have the irritability of the badly nourished patient and need much understanding and encouragement. Fortunately, most patients recover, at least for a time, and can return to a more or less normal diet.

## Diverticulosis

Diverticulosis occurs primarily in the sigmoid colon and is characterized by herniations of the colonic mucosa through the muscular layer of the bowel wall. The greatest prevalence of the disease occurs in people over 50 years of age living in Western societies. Epidemiologic evidence suggests that diverticulosis is due to Western diets from which the natural fiber or roughage has been removed by food processing (see Chap. 2).

There are two types of diverticulosis, asymptomatic and symptomatic.[34] The asymptomatic type is usually discovered when a barium enema or colonoscopy is done to investigate other problems of the colon. In the symptomatic type, in addition to demonstrating the presence of diverticulosis by barium enema or colonoscopy, the patients experience moderate to severe lower abdominal pain and distention. On further workup, symptomatic, but not asymptomatic, patients demonstrate increased colonic intraluminal pressure, hypersegmentation, and hypertrophy of the colonic muscles. In some situations symptomatic diverticulosis may be complicated by diverticulitis and rectal bleeding.

## Dietary treatment

Traditionally, diverticulosis was treated with a residue-restricted diet (Table 26-10). Recently a diet high in fiber, especially unprocessed wheat bran of large particle size, which increases fecal bulk, has been used to treat symptomatic diverticulosis. The results of clinical trials with bran to treat diverticulosis have been conflicting.[35,36] Some investigators have reported improvement but others have not. As Kelsay[37] points out, the studies have not been well controlled and the quantity of unprocessed wheat bran added to the subjects' diet has varied from approximtely 16 g to 30 g per day. Coarse bran rather than fine bran has the capacity to absorb significant amounts of fluid, which increases stool softness. When unprocessed wheat bran was added to the diet some patients have reported clinical improvement in the form of an increase in fecal bulk and decreases in abdominal distention and pain.

At this point there are limited data on the type and quantity of fiber in commonly used food.[37] To increase total fiber, the diet should contain whole grain breads and cereals, raw and dried fruits, raw vegetables, and legumes in addition to unprocessed wheat bran. The quantity of unprocessed bran usually recommended is 6 teaspoons (16 g) per day added to food. The daily intake should begin at 2 teaspoons and increase slowly to 6 teaspoons in order to avoid colonic distention. The product should be as free as possible from endosperm to avoid the adverse effects of uncooked starch on the gastrointestinal tract.

During an attack of diverticulitis with bleeding from the mucosa of the colon, a moderate- or minimal-residue diet is used. If the diverticula perforate, surgery is usually required.

There is only limited evidence that a high-fiber diet may prevent diverticulosis. Gear[38] has compared the incidence of diverticulosis by x-ray diagnosis in a group of subjects 45 years of age and older who consumed the usual British diet with that in a group of people in the same age group who had been vegetarians for 10 years or more. His study showed that asymptomatic diverticular disease was more common in the nonvegetarian group of patients than in the vegetarians, and that the fiber of cereal grains appears to be the most important component of the diet in the prevention of diverticulosis.

## Cancer of the bowel

In all cases of constipation, or of constipation alternating with diarrhea, particularly if these symptoms are of short duration and if living habits are otherwise normal, there is the possibility of neoplastic growth of some section of the colon or the rectum. If this diagnosis is established by the use of proctoscopic and roentgenographic examinations, the patient is subjected to surgery. See Chapter 27 for postoperative diets.

## Constipation

A common disturbance of the digestive tract is *constipation*. However, there is considerable confusion as to what is meant by this term. Although a daily bowel movement has been stressed as desirable, there are many people for whom an evacuation every other day or even every third day is normal. Moreover, evacuation may occur regularly until an emotional upset occurs, in which case there may be either an increased number of bowel movements—almost diarrhea—or retention of the feces for a day or two, resembling constipation. The matter usually straightens itself out when the strain is relieved. However, if the person becomes anxious when no daily bowel movement occurs and begins to resort to cathartics or enemas, a vicious pattern is set up, and it may be difficult to effect a return to normal habits.

Chronic constipation may be due to a person's dietary and living habits. Insufficient rest, hurried irregular meals, a food intake that does not meet the nutritional needs of the body, and too sedentary a life all may contribute to poor bowel function. The problem here is to help the patient to accept a more regular mode of living, including a diet that meets all his nutritive requirements and a reasonable amount of exercise.

Elderly patients may suffer from constipation because muscle tone is relaxed, the dietary intake is inadequate for nutritional needs, and activity is diminished.

### Dietary treatment

In the hospitalized patient no dietary treatment for constipation begins until the diagnostic workup to exclude colon cancer or other lesions has been completed. In most cases of so-called constipation, a normal diet (see Chap. 11) containing roughage in the form of fresh and cooked fruit and vegetables and including whole grain bread and cereals provides sufficient bulk to maintain regular bowel evacuation. Where such regularity needs to be reestablished—for instance, following an illness in which the mobility of the patient has been greatly limited—the addition of stewed fruit and of fruit juices to the ordinary diet is found helpful. Prune juice, particularly, taken at bedtime or the first thing in the morning, is usually effective.

Elderly patients should not use foods with a high bran content for fear of impaction. Cooked fruits and vegetables are often better tolerated by the older patient than raw ones, except for bananas.

### Laxative abuse

The abuse of laxatives can lead to structural changes in the terminal ileum and colon. On roentgenography the terminal ileum appears tubelike in structure and the ileocecal sphincter becomes wide and gaping. The colon becomes dilated and loses its normal mucosal pattern. Hypokalemia (low blood potassium) also occurs with laxative abuse.[39] Laxative abuse, like any problem involving substance abuse, such as abuse of alcohol or drugs, can result in long-term chronic ill health. People who take excessive amounts of laxatives need consistent help to accept and use corrective diet therapy.

## Study questions and activities

1. Which components of gastric juice are thought to be responsible for the development of a peptic ulcer? What are some possible causes for these increases in gastric juices?
2. Of what symptoms does the patient with peptic ulcer usually complain?
3. Explain the principles underlying the dietary treat-

ment of peptic ulcer. What is the purpose of the antacid medication?

4. Is the Sippy diet in the early stages adequate for normal nutritional needs? What nutrients are likely to be low?

5. Why may the Sippy regimen contribute to the development of atherosclerosis?

6. Write out the dietary instructions for a secretary with achalasia who has been placed on a bland diet.

7. Name some of the causes of gastritis. Plan a menu for a day for a patient with hemorrhagic gastritis. Is it adequate for normal nutritional needs?

8. What are some of the causes of *indigestion* that are not due to an organic lesion? Write a diet for a homemaker who complains of heartburn and gastric discomfort. What are some of the questions you would ask her before giving her instruction?

9. What does the term, *malabsorption syndrome* mean?

10. Which two tests are most frequently done to determine disaccharidase deficiency?

11. Name six foods or food groups which must be omitted in lactose malabsorption.

12. What is the older term for adult celiac disease?

13. What are the symptoms of celiac sprue? What does the term *steatorrhea* mean? What pathologic changes are found in the jejunal mucosa?

14. Why is the so-called gluten-free diet used in celiac sprue? Which cereals must be omitted?

15. Plan a diet for an adult patient with celiac-sprue who eats at home; for a secretary with this disease who eats her lunch at a fast food restaurant.

16. What is the difference between celiac sprue and tropical sprue? How is the latter treated?

17. What is a medium chain triglyceride? Why may it be used effectively in some diseases of the small intestine?

18. Why does a patient with gallbladder disease have pain on the ingestion of fat?

19. Which foods should be avoided, which limited, on a low-fat diet?

20. Write a low-fat general diet for a patient with gallbladder disease who is 20 pounds overweight. Use Chapter 28.

21. Why may a low-fat bland diet be ordered for a patient with pancreatitis? Which foods must be omitted? Which severely restricted?

22. Why should a patient with ileitis have a residue-restricted diet? Can such a diet meet all the patient's nutritional requirements? How may additional calories and proteins be included?

23. Why may hospitalized patients develop constipation? Which groups are especially vulnerable? Name some simple remedies by which the problem may be corrected without the aid of cathartics.

24. Plan a diet for a working man with diverticulosis, using a diet high in fiber.

## References

1. Fein HD: In Goodhart RS, Shils ME (eds): Modern Nutrition in Health and Disease, 5th ed, p 770. Philadelphia, Lea & Febiger, 1973
2. Henry JB: Todd, Sanford, Davidsohn, Clinical Diagnosis and Management by Laboratory Methods, 16th ed. Philadelphia, WB Saunders, 1979
3. Peterson WL, Fordtran JS: In Sleisenger MH, Fordtran JS (eds): Gastrointestinal Disease, Vol 1, 2nd ed, pp 891–913. Philadelphia, WB Saunders, 1978
4. Welsh JD: Gastroenterology 72:740, 1977
5. Davenport HW: Physiology of the Digestive Tract, 4th ed. Chicago, Year Book, 1977
6. Finkelstein W, Isselbacher KJ: New Engl J Med 229:992, 1978
7. Steinberg WM et al: Dig Dis Sci 25:188, 1980
8. Ippoliti AF et al: Ann Intern Med 84:286, 1976
9. Cohen S, Booth GH Jr: N Engl J Med 293:897, 1975
10. Sandweiss SJ: Am J Dig Dis 6:929, 1961
11. Schneider MA et al: Am J Gastroenterol 26:722, 1956
12. J Am Diet Assoc 59:243, 1971
13. Spiro HM: Clinical Gastroenterology, 2nd ed. New York, Macmillan, 1977
14. Caron HS, Roth HP: J Am Diet Assoc 60:306, 1972
15. Nebel OT, Castell DO: Gastroenterology 61:778, 1972
16. Babka JC, Castell DO: Am J Dig Dis 18:391, 1973
17. Price SF et al: Gastroenterology 75:240, 1978
18. Sahi T: Gut 19:1074, 1978
19. Welsh JD: Am J Clin Nutr 31:592, 1978
20. Rayfield EJ et al: N Engl J Med 289:618, 1973
21. Garza C, Scrimshaw NS: Am J Clin Nutr 29:192, 1976
22. Adams CF: Nutritive Value of American Foods in Common Units. Agriculture Handbook No. 456. Washington, DC, USDA, Agriculture Research Service, 1975
23. Payne-Bose D et al: Am J Clin Nutr 30:695, 1977
24. Dicke WK et al: Acta Paediatr 42:34, 1953
25. Van de Kamer JH et al: Acta Paediatr 42:223, 1953
26. Cornell HJ, Townley RRW: Gut 15:862, 1974
27. Sleisenger MH et al: J Am Diet Assoc 33:1137, 1957
28. Benson GD et al: Medicine 43:1, 1964
29. McNicholl B et al: Gut 20:126, 1979
30. Weser E, Sleisenger MH: Gastroenterology 48:571, 1965
31. Cooper BT et al: Gut 19:754, 1978
32. Klipstein FA et al: Lancet 2:342, 1978
33. Bennion LJ, Grundy SM: N Engl J Med 299:1161, 1221, 1978
34. Almy TP, Howell DA: N Engl J Med 302:324, 1980
35. Brodribb AJM: Lancet 1:664, 1977
36. Søltoft JE et al: Lancet 1:270, 1976
37. Kelsay JL: Am J Clin Nutr 31:142, 1976
38. Gear JSS et al: Lancet 1:511, 1979
39. Cummings JH: Gut 15:758, 1974

## Supplementary readings
### Peptic ulcer disease

Arvanitakis C: Diet therapy in gastrointestinal disease: A commentary. J Am Diet Assoc 75:449, 1979

Finkelstein W, Isselbacher KJ: Cimetidine. N Engl J Med 299:992, 1978

Grimes DS, Goddard J: Gastric emptying of whole-meal and white bread. Gut 18:725, 1977

Jick H, Porter J: Drug-induced gastrointestinal bleeding. Lancet 2:87, 1978

Malagelada J-R et al: Different gastric, pancreatic, and biliary responses to solid-liquid or homogenized meals. Dig Dis Sci 24:101, 1979

Rune SJ et al: Recurrence of duodenal ulcer pain after treatment with cimetidine for four and eight weeks. Gut 21:151, 1980

Thomas J et al: Chronic gastric ulcer and life events. Gastroenterology 78:905, 1980

Welsh JD: Diet therapy in peptic ulcer disease. Gastroenterology 72:740, 1977

## Other upper gastrointestinal disease

Bennion LJ, Grundy SM: Risk factors for the development of cholelithiasis in man. N Engl J Med 299:1161, 1978

Blacklow NR, Cukor G: Viral gastroenteritis. N Engl J Med 304:397, 1981

Capron J-P et al: Evidence for an association between cholelithiasis and hiatus hernia. Lancet 2:329, 1978

Castell DO: Dysphagia. Gastroenterology 76:1015, 1979

Chernoff R, Dean JA: Medical and nutritional aspects of intractable diarrhea. J Am Diet Assoc 76:161, 1980

Cohen S, Booth GH: Gastric acid secretion and lower esophageal sphincter pressure in response to coffee and caffeine. N Engl J Med 293:897, 1975

Insogna KL et al: Osteomalacia and weakness from excessive antacid ingestion. JAMA 244:2544, 1980

King CS, Toskes PP: Small intestinal bacterial overgrowth. Gastroenterology 76:1055, 1979

Pitchumoni CS et al: Nutrition in the pathogenesis of alcoholic pancreatitis. Am J Clin Nutr 33:631, 1980

Price SF et al: Food sensitivity in reflux esophagitis. Gastroenterology 75:240, 1978

Roberts SH et al: Bacterial overgrowth syndrome without "blind loop": A cause for malnutrition in the elderly. Lancet 2:1193, 1977

Thomas FB et al: Inhibitory effect of coffee on lower esophageal sphincter pressure. Gastroenterology 79:1262, 1980

Thorpe CJ, Caprini JA: Gallbladder disease: Current trends and treatments. Am J Nurs 80:2181, 1980

Vantrappen G, Hellemans J: Treatment of achalasia and related motor disorders. Gastroenterology 79:144, 1980

## Lactose malabsorption

Cheng AHR et al: Long-term acceptance of low-lactose milk. Am J Clin Nutr 32:1989, 1979

Debongnie JC et al: Absorption of nutrients in lactase deficiency. Dig Dis Sci 24:225, 1979

Kilara A, Shahani K: Lactose activity of cultured and acidified dairy products. J Dairy Sci 59:2031, 1976

Simoons FJ et al: Perspectives on milk-drinking and malabsorption of lactose. Pediatrics 59:98, 1977

Welsh JD: Diet therapy in adult lactose malabsorption: Present practices. Am J Clin Nutr 31:592, 1978

## Celiac sprue

Caldwell KA: In vitro digestion of gliadin by gastrointestinal enzymes and pyrrolidinecarboxylate peptidase. Am J Clin Nutr 33:293, 1980

Cornell HJ, Rolles CJ: Further evidence of a primary mucosal defect in coeliac disease. Gut 19:253, 1978

Henry CL: Patients' view at a gluten-free diet. J Hum Nutr 34:50, 1980

Kumar PJ et al: Reintroduction of gluten in adults and children with treated coeliac disease. Gut 20:743, 1979

McNicholl B et al: Mucosal recovery in treated childhood celiac disease. J Pediatr 89:418, 1976

McNicholl B et al: Variability of gluten intolerance in treated childhood coeliac disease. Gut 20:126, 1979

Nishita KD: A yeast-leavened, rice-flour bread, J Am Diet Assoc 70:397, 1977

## Dietary fiber

Achord JA: Irritable bowel syndrome and dietary fiber. J Am Diet Assoc 75:452, 1979

Brodribb AJM, Groves C: Effect of bran particle size on stool weight. Gut 19:60, 1978

Connell AM: The effects of dietary fiber on gastrointestinal function. Am J Clin Nutr (Suppl)31:S152, 1978

Eastwood MA, Kay RM: An hypothesis for the action of dietary fiber along the gastrointestinal tract. Am J Clin Nutr 32:364, 1979

Eastwood MA: Fiber in the gastrointestinal tract. Am J Clin Nutr (Suppl)31:S30, 1978

Kang JY, Doe WF: Unprocessed bran causing intestinal obstruction. Br Med J 1:1249, 1979

Kelsay JL: A review of research of effects of fiber intake on man. Am J Clin Nutr 31:142, 1976

Mendeloff AI: Dietary fiber and human health. N Engl J Med 297:811, 1977

## Large bowel

Almy TP, Howell DA: Diverticular disease of the colon. N Engl J Med 302:324, 1980

Mallett SJ et al: Living with disease: Colitis. Lancet 2:619, 1978

Mekhjian HS et al: Clinical features and natural history of Crohn's disease. Gastroenterology 77:898, 1979

Sitrin MD et al: Nutritional and metabolic complications in a patient with Crohn's disease and ileal resection. Gastroenterology 78:1069, 1980

Sutalf LO, Levitt MD: Follow-up of a flatulent patient. Dig Dis Sci 24:652, 1979

## Patient resources

American Celiac Society, 45 Gilford Ave., Jersey City, NJ 07304

Celiac Disease Recipes. Hospital for Sick Children, 555 University, Toronto, Ontario, Canada

Hartsook EI: Gluten Intolerance Group Cookbook. Kent, WA 26604

Sheedy CB, Keifetz N: Cooking for Your Celiac Child. New York, Dial, 1969

Wood MN: Delicious and Easy Rice Flour Recipes. Springfield, IL, Charles C Thomas, 1972

Wood MN: Gourmet Food on a Wheat Free Diet. Springfield, IL, Charles C Thomas, 1972

*For further references see Bibliography in Part 4.*

# Nutritional Care— Surgery and Burn Therapy

# 27

Good nutritional status is an asset for patients who are to undergo surgery. This is relatively easy for those undergoing elective surgery for problems that do not interfere with eating an adequate diet, such as gynecological or orthopedic surgery or surgery for uncomplicated cholelithiasis, hernia, peptic ulcer disease, thyroid disease, and tonsillitis. Patients who are to undergo cardiac surgery or kidney transplantation need the appropriate dietary treatment prior to surgery to reduce operative risks (see Chaps. 31 and 32).

The obese surgical patient is a particular risk, especially for the anesthesiologist, because inhalant anesthesias may be sequestered in the fat depots and impede normal recovery from anesthesia postoperatively. When possible, the obese patient should be counseled to lose weight before surgery (see Chap. 28).

Patients with cancer of the oral cavity, esophagus, larynx, stomach, small intestine, or colon may come to surgery in a nutritionally debilitated state. The nutritional rehabilitation of these and certain other patients can be done before surgery with parenteral or enteral hyperalimentation. Research has demonstrated that, when emergency surgery is not required, nutritional rehabilitation preoperatively by hyperalimentation may reduce postoperative morbidity and mortality in the malnourished surgical patient.[1]

The key factors in nutritional care of the surgical patient are maintenance of energy, fluid, and electrolyte balance; adequate energy-protein intake; and adequate total nutrient intake to promote wound healing and the resumption of normal activities.

The orders for general surgical patients without underlying metabolic or endocrine disorders are usually regular, soft, or liquid diets. It is the clinical dietitian's responsibility to interpret the diet order to meet the energy and protein needs of the individual patient according to age, sex, height, and weight; to determine the quantity of food and the frequency of feeding for each patient; and to monitor and report daily food intake. The surgeon is working closely with the clinical dietitian to design and carry out the appropriate nutritional care plan for the malnourished surgical patient. He is concerned with the provision of biochemical substrates, enterally or parenterally, in the quantities and ratios that are required for intracellular function, and he views the clinical dietitian as the resource person on the nutritional support team.[2]

Principles of postoperative nutritional care, postoperative oral feeding routines, tube feedings, diet therapy used after surgery of the gastrointestinal tract, and the nutritional care of the severely burned patient are discussed in this chapter.

## Principles of nutritional care
### Metabolic responses to surgery and trauma

Surgical intervention, acute skeletal or muscle trauma due to accidents, thermal burns, infection, and sepsis elicit a hypermetabolic response; the more complex the surgical procedure, especially in the abdomen or the chest, or the more severe the trauma, the more intense the metabolic response. The purpose of the response is to provide glucose for the glucose-requiring cells of the body, such as the central and peripheral nervous systems, and the red blood cells; and the energy and substrates required for the synthesis of substances for wound healing as well as maintaining the other tissues and organs of the body. The metabolic responses may be categorized as the catabolic phase, the anabolic phase, and the fat gain phase.

### Catabolic phase

The sensory input of surgery or trauma activates the neuroendocrine system. The first responses are the release of glucocorticoids from the adrenal cortex, and the catecholamines, epinephrine and norepinephrine. The catecholamines stimulate the release of glucose from liver and muscle glycogen, while the glucocorticoids stimulate gluconeogenesis in the liver from lactate and alanine from the muscle mass. At this point the patient is hyperglycemic because insulin release from the pancreas is suppressed, and glucagon release is stimulated by the neuroendocrine response. Wilmore's work suggests that in addition to supplying glucose to the glucose-dependent tissues, the glycolytic pathway supplies energy for wound healing, at least in the burn wound, and the lactate formed is recycled to glucose through the Cori cycle in the liver. Both the catecholamines and the glucocorticoids stimulate the release of free fatty acids from the adipocytes by suppressing insulin release. At the same time antidiuretic hormone secreted by the pituitary gland and aldosterone secreted by the adrenal cortex work together to maintain the plasma volume and osmolality.

As a result of the neuroendocrine responses there is an erosion of body cell mass primarily in muscle tissue, which results in a negative nitrogen and potassium balance; retention of extracellular fluid associated with the retention of sodium; a decrease in adipose tissue and the mobilization of fatty acid as an energy source for the liver and other tissues; and alterations in blood *p*H and cardiac output. After serious trauma, such as burns or most surgery, the peristaltic and absorptive functions of the gastrointestinal tract, especially the sigmoid colon, are reduced. In uncomplicated surgery, the patient's catabolic response is minimal and decreases in three to five days, while in the severely burned patient or the patient with sepsis, catabolism may continue for 3 to 4 weeks accompanied by a critical loss of body cell mass.

### Anabolic phase

Anabolism does take place during the catabolic phase, probably at a reduced rate. The anabolic phase is characterized by a decrease in the catabolic hormones and the increased release and effectiveness of the anabolic hormones, insulin and growth hormone. Nitrogen balance becomes more positive until the nitrogen lost during the catabolic phase is restored. Restoration of the nitrogen balance is accompanied by the retention of potassium. There is a loss of sodium and water by diuresis, and gastrointestinal peristalsis returns to normal. At this time there is a significant improvement in the patient's appetite. However, total weight gain is slow as energy is used to synthesize cellular proteins, and water is lost by diuresis. The anabolic phase begins 5 to 7 days or earlier after most surgery or at what Moore calls the *turning point.*[3]

### Fat gain phase

This final metabolic phase, during which the fat lost during the catabolic phase is regained, may last for 2 or 3 months. Any degree of immobility may lead to the patient's becoming obese if counseling is not initiated to prevent it.

### Nutritional needs
#### Energy

For the majority of patients in the immediate postoperative period, the needs for energy, fluids, and electrolytes are supplied by intravenous solutions of 5% dextrose, combined if necessary with electrolytes and water-soluble vitamins. It is estimated that after trauma an adult requires 40 kcal to 70 kcal per kilogram[4] (2800 kcal–4900 kcal for a 70-kg man). There are 170 kcal in each 1000 ml of 5% dextrose, and no more than 2500 ml to 3000 ml (415 kcal–510 kcal) can be administered safely in 24 hours. Therefore, the total energy needs of an adult cannot be met by a 5% dextrose solution. More concentrated solutions of dextrose cannot be used since they cause thrombosis in peripheral veins. During this period stores of body fat serve as the primary energy supply, and the dextrose administered intravenously spares body proteins to some extent.

In general the average patient is able to take food and fluid orally in 1 to 3 or 4 days after surgery. For some patients it may be necessary at this point to supply energy, nutrients, and fluids by nasogastric, gastric, or jejunal tubes. As soon as the patient can tolerate fluids and foods, he is offered a diet adequate in energy and nutrients to meet his needs to ensure proper wound healing and a return to his normal activities. (See the discussion about monitoring food acceptance in this section.)

When the gastrointestinal tract cannot be used for any extensive period of time after surgery or the patient cannot eat enough to supply energy and nutrient needs, *e.g.*, after massive bowel resection after a mesenteric infarct, hyperalimentation through a catheter inserted into the superior vena cava during surgery is used.[2] The *hyperalimentation* solution contains fluids, electrolytes, minerals, vitamins, dextrose, and a source of nitrogen and is prepared under sterile conditions in the pharmacy; its administration is monitored by the nutrition support team.

### Protein

The loss of body cell mass accompanied by a negative nitrogen balance during the catabolic phase is poorly understood. In severe trauma as much as 30 g of nitrogen, equivalent to 2 lb of muscle tissue, can be lost in 1 day.[4] Significant losses of protein can also occur as a result of blood losses during surgery or trauma and because of atrophy of bone and muscle in the immobilized patient.

The negative nitrogen balance of the catabolic phase is generally attributed to the breakdown of amino acids to supply substrate for the gluconeogenic pathway with the urinary excretion of nitrogen as urea and ammonia. However Waterlow and co-workers[5] and O'Keefe and Sender[6] suggest that the reaction to moderate stress involves a decrease in the rate of cellular protein synthesis without an acute rise in the rate of protein breakdown.

Protein metabolism during the catabolic phase of the metabolic reactions to surgery and trauma is presently under intensive study. The focus of this research is on whether or not intravenous solutions of amino acids, alone or in combination with dextrose, administered in the immediate postoperative period are effective in reversing the negative nitrogen balance of the stress reaction.[7] However, Moore writes that an early intravenous source of amino acids is not required for wound healing in the catabolic phase.[3] The critical factor is the return to adequate oral alimentation in a reasonable period of time postoperatively. On the other hand, a prolonged period of time postoperatively without adequate energy and nutrient intake (starvation) does have adverse effects on all aspects of recovery from surgery or trauma. Therefore, the postoperative patient must be monitored carefully by the medical team for his readiness for, and his acceptance of, oral fluids and foods to support a positive nitrogen balance during the anabolic phase. Otherwise, enteral or parenteral alimentation must be used to support the patient's metabolic needs.

### Minerals and vitamins

Wound healing requires adequate supplies of minerals, trace elements, and vitamins as well as energy and amino acids. For example, the synthesis of collagen, which is a basic process of wound healing, requires vitamin C. Protein synthesis, in general, requires a variety of trace elements and vitamins as well as amino acids (see Chap. 8, *Water-soluble Vitamins*, and Chap. 9, *Nutrient Utilization*).

## Monitoring nutritional care and food acceptance
### Preoperative routines

Whenever possible a careful and extensive diet history and the specific food and fluid likes and dislikes of the patient should be obtained prior to surgery. The diet history is an important component of the assessment of nutritional status before surgery, and the patient's likes and dislikes can be used in menu planning postoperatively (see Chap. 23).

### Postoperative routines

After the return of normal peristalsis, the first oral feeding offered is a clear liquid diet. Clear liquids, such as broth and gelatin, are used to test the patient's tolerance for fluids by mouth. Clear liquids are also less hazardous if vomiting with aspiration occurs. If clear liquids are well tolerated, the patient may progress to a full liquid diet and then to a soft and finally a regular diet (see Chap. 22 for a description of these diets). For some patients the progression is directly from clear liquids to a regular diet.

It must be remembered that the clear liquid diet is nutritionally inadequate in calories, protein, and other nutrients; therefore, such patients should be observed carefully so that they may progress to an adequate diet as soon as it is tolerated. Because of cultural expectations of food for illness, an older patient who could be offered a regular diet after clear liquids may accept a soft diet more readily before progressing to a regular diet. Patients with a concurrent disease, such as diabetes mellitus or heart disease should be returned to their appropriate therapeutic regimen. Serious postoperative complications can occur if the appropriate diet is not offered (see also the section in this chapter on diet therapy after gastrointestinal surgery).

The acceptance of food and fluid by the postoperative patient must be monitored at each feeding to ensure that he achieves an adequate intake of energy and all nutrients to support his metabolic needs in order to avoid postoperative malnutrition and its sequelae. Whenever necessary, an estimate of the patient's energy and nutrient intake for the previous 24 hours should be recorded in his medical record each morning. This information should be available as part of the assessment of the patient's progress toward recovery.

## Preparation for discharge

Before discharge it should be ascertained that the postoperative patient is selecting and consuming a diet totally adequate to promote full recovery; and he should be counseled to continue these practices at home without gaining excessive weight during the fat gain phase.

Because many patients become fatigued easily for a period after surgery, attention should be given to the home situation. Special care should be taken to identify the mother with a large family or the person who lives alone. Such patients may need assistance after discharge with food buying and preparation at home (see *Meal Management*, Chap. 12). Otherwise, their recovery may be delayed. If relatives or friends are not available to assist them, a home health aide can be requested to help 2 or 3 times a week, or daily if required. For the patient over 65 this service is provided by Medicare. Some of these patients may need to transfer to an extended-care facility before returning to their own homes. The social worker can assist the nurse and the dietitian in these situations.

## Tube feedings

Enteral feeding can be accomplished by a nasogastric tube or a variety of tube enterostomies—pharyngostomy, esophagostomy, gastrostomy, duodenostomy, and jejunostomy—when it is not possible for patients to take food by the usual oral route.[8] This may occur after head and neck surgery for oral or esophageal cancer; when the esophagus and in some cases the tissue of the stomach have been injured by strong alkali solutions in attempted suicide; after gastric or small or large bowel surgery for cancer, for mesenteric infarct, or for inflammatory bowel disease; or when the patient is unconscious due to trauma to the head or a cerebral vascular accident (stroke). In addition, patients with neurological disorders, the profoundly mentally retarded, or the senile elderly may require tube feeding. This mode of feeding may be only a temporary measure, or it may be the method of feeding for the remainder of a patient's life.

The feeding must be liquid with a viscosity that permits it to pass easily through the tube by gravity flow; it must also be free of bacterial contamination and contain reasonable proportions of protein, fat, and carbohydrate, and the minerals, electrolytes, and vitamins needed to meet the individual patient's needs without causing dehydration or fluid overload.

## Types of feedings

There are three types of tube feedings—blenderized, polymeric, and monomeric (see Table 27-1). Blenderized feedings are usually milk-based with suspended solids from strained or blenderized foods, such as meats, vegetables, and fruit. Only pasteurized egg products are used. In the hospital raw eggs are never used in tube feedings because of the potential for contamination with salmonellae and the hospital's liability for nosocomial infections.

Polymeric (low residue) tube feedings contain protein, polysaccharides or a mixture of poly-, di-, and monosaccharides and a source of triglycerides.[9] The protein may be supplied by whole milk, nonfat dry milk solids, milk proteins (sodium or calcium caseinate), or soy protein or soy protein isolate. The triglycerides are supplied by various vegetable oils or milk fat when whole milk is used. A few polymeric formulas contain MCT oil. The carbohydrate sources vary from glucose polymers (Polycose*, maltodextrin, corn syrup solids) to disaccharides, such as sucrose and lactose (if milk is used), and the monosaccharide glucose. These feedings may be practically lactose-free when caseinate or soy protein isolate or a combination of both is the source of protein rather than whole milk or nonfat dry milk solids. As a group, these formulas are moderate to low in residue. The monomeric (elemental) diets contain either hydrolyzed casein or crystalline amino acids as the source of nitrogen (protein), vegetable or MCT oil, and mixtures of mono-, di-, and oligosaccharides. The blenderized formulas are the most viscid, and the monomeric ones the least viscid.

## Tube feeding products

Before the mid 1970s the majority of tube feedings were prepared by hospital dietary departments from ingredients on hand and a variety of nonstandardized or untested recipes. Today, commercial products are bacteriologically safe, are standardized in nutrient density per volume and are of a consistency that can be used with nasogastric tube feeding methods commonly used in most hospitals and other patient-care institutions. Many of these products are palatable and highly acceptable as beverages and are used as supplementary feedings by patients who cannot or will not consume enough regular food to meet their nutritional needs.

Table 27-1 lists some of the commercial tube feeding products commonly used in 1980. A comprehensive table of liquid formulas for oral and tube feeding prepared at the Memorial Sloan-Kettering Cancer Center[10] is listed in the Supplementary Materials at the end of this chapter. This publication gives information on a variety of formulas for special problems as well as on standard products. Under *Major Ingredients* in Table 27-1 only the sources of protein, fat, and carbohydrate are listed. Where lactose is listed as a source of carbohydrate, it reflects the

---

*Ross Laboratories, Columbus, OH 43215.

# Table 27-1. Commercial Tube Feeding Products

| Product | Producer | Major Ingredients | Nitrogen Kcalorie Ratio | Osmolality (mOsm/kg H$_2$O) |
|---|---|---|---|---|
| *Blenderized Formulas* | | | | |
| Compleat-B | Doyle Pharmaceutical Co. Minneapolis, MN 55417 | Beef purée, hydrolyzed cereal solids, green bean purée, pea purée, nonfat dry milk, corn oil, maltodextrin, peach purée, orange juice | 1:156 | 390 |
| Formula 2 | Cutter Laboratories Inc. Berkeley, CA 94710 | Nonfat milk, beef, corn oil, egg yolk, sucrose, vegetables, orange juice, wheat flour | 1:166 | 435–510 |
| *Low Residue (Polymeric)\** | | | | |
| Meritene Liquid | Doyle Pharmaceutical | Skim milk, sodium caseinate, corn oil, lactose, corn syrup solids, sucrose | 1:96 | 690 |
| Nutri-1000 | Cutter Laboratories | Skim milk, sodium caseinate, corn oil, corn syrup solids, sucrose, lactose | 1:166 | 503 |
| *Low Residue, Low Lactose (Polymeric)* | | | | |
| Nutri-1000 LF | Cutter Laboratories | Soy protein isolates, sodium and calcium caseinates, corn oil, soybean oil (partially hydrogenated) corn syrup solids | 1:166 | 381 |
| Precision LR | Doyle Pharmaceutical | Maltodextrin, pasteurized egg white solids, sucrose, MCT oil | 1:264 | 525 (Orange flavor) |
| Precision High Nitrogen | Doyle Pharmaceutical | Maltodextrin, pasteurized egg white solids, sucrose, MCT oil, partially hydrogenated soybean oil | 1:150 | 557 (Citrus) 500 (Vanilla) |
| Precision Isotonic | Doyle Pharmaceutical | Glucose oligosaccharides, pasteurized egg white solids, sucrose, partially hydrogenated soybean oil, sodium caseinate | 1:208 | 300 |
| Sustacal Liquid | Mead Johnson Laboratories Mead Johnson & Co. Evansville, IN 47721 | Sodium and calcium caseinate, soy protein isolate, partially hydrogenated soy oil, sucrose, corn syrup solids | 1:102 | 640 (Vanilla) |
| Isocal | Mead Johnson | Glucose oligosaccharides, soy oil, calcium caseinate, sodium caseinate, MCT oil, soy protein isolate | 1:194 | 350 |
| Ensure | Ross Laboratories Division of Abbott Laboratories Columbus, OH 43216 | Sodium and calcium caseinate, soy protein isolate, corn oil, corn syrup solids, sucrose | 1:178 | 450 |
| Ensure Plus† | Ross Laboratories | Sodium and calcium caseinate, soy protein isolate, corn oil, corn syrup solids, sucrose | 1:171 | 600 |
| Ensure Osmolite | Ross Laboratories | Sodium and calcium caseinate, soy protein isolate, corn oil, soy oil, MCT oil, glucose polymers | 1:178 | 300 |
| *Elemental Low Lactose (Monomeric)‡* | | | | |
| Vivonex | Eaton Laboratories Division, Morton-Norwich Products, Inc. Norwich, NY 13815 | Pure crystalline amino acids, safflower oil, glucose, oligosaccharides | 1:333 | 645 (Flavored) 550 (Unflavored) |
| Vivonex High Nitrogen | Eaton Laboratories | Pure crystalline amino acids, safflower oil, glucose, oligosaccharides | 1:125 | 870 (Flavored) 810 (Unflavored) |
| Vital | Ross Laboratories | Soy, meat, whey hydrolysates, free amino acids, sunflower oil, glucose, oligo- and polysaccharides, sucrose | 1:164 | 450 |
| Flexical | Mead Johnson | Corn syrup solids, hydrolyzed casein, partially hydrogenated soy oil, tapioca starch, MCT oil, crystalline amino acids | 1:279 | 550 |

\*Polymeric—protein, polysaccharides, and triglycerides.

†1.5 kcal/ml

‡Monomeric—free amino acids, oligo- and monosaccharides, and small amounts of triglycerides.

Nutrient analysis available from producer.

naturally occurring lactose in milk as a source of protein, not the addition of lactose to the formula. The mineral, electrolyte, and vitamin content contributed by the ingredients plus any supplementation by the producer can be obtained from the label on the product or any other source of up-to-date information supplied by the producer. The formulation of these products is modified frequently by the producer. Further supplementation of minerals, electrolytes, and vitamins may be required to meet the needs of individual patients. Some of the products are available in both liquid and powdered form and in a variety of flavors or unflavored with flavor packets. The monomeric products containing free crystalline amino acids are available only in powdered form. All powdered products should be reconstituted according to the producer's instruction under bacteriologically safe conditions.

The lactose-free formulas should be used when there is any possibility of lactose malabsorption. A careful diet history should rule out this possibility before the institution of tube feeding. Also, a patient who has had or is having a gastrojejunostomy or has a jejunostomy tube should be given a lactose-free formula because the greatest concentration of lactase in the gastrointestinal tract is in the distal duodenum and proximal jejunum. Products containing milk should be avoided by patients with an allergy to milk protein. This may also include products with sodium or calcium caseinate. Patients with allergies to corn protein may not be able to tolerate products with corn oil because the oil appears to be contaminated with traces of corn protein, which can cause reactions in highly sensitive patients.

The caloric density of the majority of these products at normal dilution is one kcal per milliliter or 100 kcal per deciliter. Table 27-1 demonstrates that there is some variation in the kilocalorie to nitrogen ratio. The osmolality (mOsm/kg $H_2O$) varies widely. For certain patients those formulas with an osmolality of 300 to 600 are better choices than those with a higher osmolality.

### The feeding tube

The most frequently used tubes are made of a very pliable silicone elastomer (Silastic), which is well tolerated by patients. There are significant variations in the caliber of these tubes—the larger the number, the larger the inside diameter (see Fig. 27-1). The caliber of the tube inserted determines the type of feeding (blenderized or solution) that can be used. The Number 8 tube is the most comfortable nasogastric tube for the patient, and only polymeric or monomeric formulas can flow freely through the tube without plugging it. Gastrostomy tubes that permit the use of blenderized products are usually Number 16 or larger.

### Selection of the formula

The standard tube feeding formulas (1 kcal per milliliter) are used with medical and surgical patients who do not have any complex gastrointestinal tract problems, and the size of the tube determines the type—blenderized or polymeric. Some of the medical patients who require tube feeding are those with advanced neurological disease that interferes with chewing and swallowing, moderately malnourished patients with cancer, and semicomatose or unconscious patients. Surgical patients include those who have had head and neck surgery or those who are moderately malnourished pre- and postoperatively and are at risk for sepsis or other postoperative complications.

Depending on the patient's nutritional needs, the standard formula (1 kcal per milliliter) or the more calorically dense formula (1.5 kcal per milliliter) is used. If it is anticipated that the patient will progress from formula by tube to formula as beverage or if the formula is used as a supplementary dietary beverage, the patient should be given the opportunity to taste a number of standard formulas with varying flavors to select the one that is most acceptable.[11]

Patients with complex problems of the gastrointestinal tract, such as extensive resection of the small bowel for inflammatory bowel disease (short bowel syndrome), postoperative or gastrointestinal tract fistulas, or severe malnutrition pre- or postoperatively usually require enteral or parenteral hyperalimentation (see next section).

### The administration of tube feedings
#### The first feeding

Food is required to maintain the structural and functional integrity of the small bowel. The majority of patients who require tube feeding have either not been eating or not consuming enough food to maintain the integrity of the bowel. Therefore, all tube feedings begin with limited quantities of a formula containing 0.5 kcal per milliliter or less to avoid substrate overload and resulting osmotic diarrhea. In general, the first feeding consists of 50 ml of dilute formula per hour for 12 to 18 hours administered by continuous drip. Bolus feeding is not recommended for the first feeding, although bolus feeding may be used when the patient has adjusted to the feeding process. Jejunostomy feedings can be administered only by the drip method. Monomeric formulas

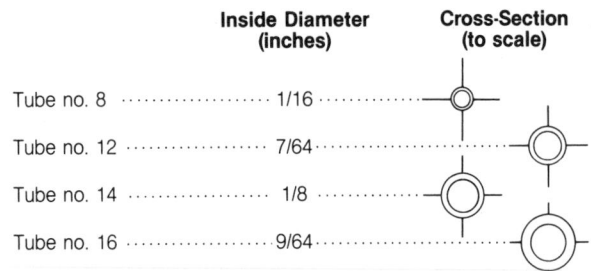

|  | Inside Diameter (inches) | Cross-Section (to scale) |
|---|---|---|
| Tube no. 8 | 1/16 | |
| Tube no. 12 | 7/64 | |
| Tube no. 14 | 1/8 | |
| Tube no. 16 | 9/64 | |

**Fig. 27-1.** Diameters of commonly-used nasogastric tubes. (Dietetic Currents, May-June 1975. Courtesy of Ross Laboratories, Columbus, OH)

with high osmolality are administered only by continuous drip, *never* by bolus feeding.

If the first feeding is tolerated without adverse reactions, such as nausea, vomiting, epigastric fullness, cramping, and diarrhea, the total quantity of formula is gradually increased during the next 24 hours. If this is tolerated, full-strength formula (1 kcal per milliliter) is introduced on the third day. If there are any adverse reactions to this change, the dilute formula is reinstituted with subsequent trials of the undiluted formula. Depending on the patient's problems, the continuous drip method of feeding may be continued, or bolus feeding may be instituted.

### Total fluid and nutritional intake

When tolerance has been established, the total quantity of formula fed per 24 hours depends on the patient's energy and nutrient needs. The clinical dietitian should calculate the 24-hour intake of energy, nitrogen, minerals, electrolytes, and vitamins to be certain that the quantity of formula consumed is providing the patient's nutritional needs. If any excesses or deficiencies of nutrients exist, these should be recorded in the medical record so that the health-care team can adjust the intake, if necessary.

The average tube feeding formula (1 kcal per milliliter) contains 85% to 88% water. Unless contraindicated, the adult patient requires approximately 2500 ml of fluid per day. The tube feeding does not supply the patient's total fluid intake. For example, if a patient requires 2000 kcal per day, this quantity of formula, 2000 ml, supplies 1760 ml of water. Therefore, the patient requires an additional 740 ml of water per day. This quantity of water is used to flush the tube to avoid any clogging of the catheter by the feeding and to give any necessary medications.

### Monitoring patient progress

Nursing personnel are responsible for administering tube feedings or supervising patients who are capable of administering it to themselves. Nurses are instructed to record the total milliliters of formula administered each 24 hours. Care must be taken to ensure that the recordings are for formula only and not for a combination of formula plus any water used to flush the tube. The clinical dietitian is responsible for recording the 24-hour energy, protein, sodium, and potassium intake, as well as any other nutrient(s) critical for a patient. The 24-hour nutrient intake, the patient's weight, and any other critical data (see *Nutritional Assessment*, Chap. 23) are used by the staff to assess a patient's progress.

The clinical dietitian is strongly advised to prepare a table of the total nutrient composition per 100 ml and the osmolality of the tube feedings most commonly used in the institution. This table will need constant revision as product formulations are modified. The table should be readily available to all staff—medical and nursing, as well as dietary—for ready reference.

### Hazards of tube feeding

There are four major hazards of tube feeding—contamination of the feeding, leading to gastrointestinal infection; too concentrated a feeding (hypertonic), particularly in protein and sodium, leading to diarrhea, dehydration, and an elevated blood urea nitrogen (BUN) level; diarrhea and other gastrointestinal problems due to lactose intolerance; and regurgitation leading to pulmonary aspiration of the gastric contents.

To avoid contamination any tube feeding reconstituted or prepared by the dietary staff should be prepared daily with carefully sanitized equipment and put in sterile containers. Immediately after preparation it should be delivered to the patient areas and refrigerated. To open commercial tube feeding products that are packaged in cans, the top of the can should be washed with sterile water and the can opened with an opener that is sterilized daily. After the appropriate amount of feeding has been measured out, the supply of feeding should be immediately refrigerated. With the exception of an unopened can of a commercial product, all tube feedings that have been in the refrigerator for 24 hours are discarded. Commercial products are available in 8-oz bottles for use with the equipment designed to administer feedings by the continuous drip method.

An excessive intake of protein and sodium without adequate fluid intake can lead to dehydration, hypernatremia, and an elevated BUN level. This is particularly hazardous for older patients with impaired renal function. Therefore, when a tube feeding for an older patient provides more than $1\frac{1}{2}$ g to 2 g of protein per kilogram of body weight per day, the fluid intake and output should be carefully measured and recorded daily, and the intake of protein in grams per kilogram of body weight should also be recorded daily in the patient's chart. Too concentrated a feeding can also result if the commercial products that come in powdered or concentrated form are not reconstituted according to the manufacturer's directions.

If watery diarrhea occurs in a patient receiving a tube feeding that has been administered correctly, it may be due to the carbohydrate content. Excessive amounts of milk and, therefore, lactose may cause diarrhea in some patients. In this case a feeding that is lactose-free should be used.

Regurgitation with pulmonary aspiration is a hazard for patients with incompetent lower esophageal sphincters or for those who are semicomatose or unconscious. For patients who are at risk for regurgitation, the continuous drip method of administering tube feeding is preferable to bolus feeding.

## Modular formulas

For some patients a nutrient or a combination of nutrients contained in the commercial formulas, which have a fixed nutrient composition, may not be appropriate. For example, the patient receiving corticosteroids and retaining salt and water requires a formula containing less sodium than the amount in the standard products. Therefore, a formula, which has the appropriate amount of sodium, must be designed for this patient.

Products that contain only protein, fat, or carbohydrate are available for use in preparing modular formulas (see Table 35-4). Protein hydrolysates, such as Casec,* can be used as the protein source; Polycose† as the carbohydrate; and MCT oil* or other oils as the fat source. These products contain only limited amounts, if any, of minerals, electrolytes, or vitamins. The modular formula requires the addition of minerals, electrolytes, and vitamins according to the requirements of the individual patient. The caloric density, viscosity, and osmolality of the formulation must also be considered.

One recommended approach to designing a modular formula is to 1) estimate the energy and total nutrient requirements of the patient (see Chap. 23); 2) ascertain the number of milliliters of fluid to be provided by the feeding in a 24-hour period; 3) determine the amount of each ingredient required to provide the energy, protein, fat, and carbohydrate to meet the patient's needs; 4) estimate the quantity of minerals, electrolytes, and vitamins contributed by the products used to supply the protein, fat, and carbohydrate and the amount of each nutrient that is needed as a supplement to achieve the estimated requirements of the patient (see No. 1 above); 5) mix the formula to the volume required (see No. 2 above); test its viscosity (ease of flow through the feeding tube being used) and have the chemistry laboratory in the hospital determine its osmolality; and 6) present the estimation of kilocalories per milliliter, the grams of protein per kilogram of body weight, the kilocalorie to nitrogen ratio, the mineral, electrolyte, and vitamin composition, the estimated supplementation requirements, and the osmolality of the formula to the nutritional support team. They then can evaluate the appropriateness of the energy and protein content and the osmolality and determine the appropriate addition of minerals, electrolytes, and vitamins to be given to the patient or, if the osmolality permits, added to the formula.

The preparation of modular formulas must be monitored continually by the clinical dietitian to ensure that the ingredients are weighed accurately and that accurate amounts of any mineral, electrolyte or vitamin that is required to be added during preparation are available and added to the final product. The method of preparation must also be monitored for bacteriologic safety. It is strongly recommended that modular formulas be prepared by the personnel in a clinical study kitchen or a pediatric formula preparation room; or, if these facilities

are not available, the preparation should be assigned to the personnel in the hospital pharmacy. If additional minerals, electrolytes, and vitamins are not being included in the formula, the nutritional support team is responsible for the provision of these nutrients.

## Enteral and parenteral hyperalimentation

Hyperalimentation is used for the nutritional rehabilitation of the severely malnourished medical or surgical patient; it is also used to maintain the flow of substrate for cellular metabolism in those patients at high risk for developing malnutrition as a result of the treatment required for complex medical or surgical problems. The goal of hyperalimentation is to reduce morbidity and mortality in the hospitalized patient and after discharge to sustain the patient who cannot return to regular enteral feedings.

Nutritional repletion of the malnourished patient or maintenance of the hypermetabolic adult patient (surgery, trauma, sepsis) requires an intake of 2700 kcal to 3500 kcal or more per 24 hours. A patient with extensive thermal burns or a patient with cancer cachexia may require 4000 kcal to 5000 kcal per 24 hours. This very high intake can be achieved through hyperalimentation in critically ill patients who, because they are usually anorectic, are unable to consume an equivalent quantity of energy and nutrients as foods and fluids by mouth. It is generally accepted that enteral hyperalimentation is used when there is adequate absorptive surface and function in the gastrointestinal tract to ensure a supply of energy and nutrients for intermediary metabolism. The parenteral route through an indwelling venous catheter is used when the gastrointestinal tract cannot support the metabolic needs of the patient.

### Enteral hyperalimentation

Enteral hyperalimentation may be done with a small catheter Silastic nasogastric tube or a tube enterostomy. The feeding may be administered by gravity flow or by a constant infusion pump to avoid gastric distention.[12] The patient's ability to tolerate the feeding depends on the rate of flow and the osmolality of the feeding. The feeding is usually administered for 24 hours. As the initial flow rate does not exceed 50 ml per hour, the full flow rate of the feeding to meet the patient's needs is not achieved for 36 or more hours. If total needs cannot be met by enteral hyperalimentation, peripheral fluids containing amino acids or intravenous lipid solutions can be used to augment the enteral feeding.[12]

Whenever possible a low viscosity, polymeric formula is preferred. The low viscosity formula is less apt to clog the tube and, therefore, requires less frequent

---

*Mead Johnson Co., Evansville, Indiana 47721.

†Ross Laboratories, Columbus, Ohio 43215.

changes of nasogastric tubes. The change of an enterostomy tube is a surgical procedure, which must be avoided if possible in the critically ill patient. The choice of a polymeric formula is based on research on protein digestion and absorption.[13] The work of Adibi and other investigators has demonstrated that the rate of amino acid uptake by the gastrointestinal tract is greater from di- and tripeptides and partially hydrolyzed protein than from solutions of pure crystalline amino acids. At the same time, monomeric formulas have a higher osmolality than polymeric ones (see Table 27-1).

### Clinical dietitian's responsibility

The first responsibility of the clinical dietitian is to calculate the total energy and protein needs of the patient (see *Nutritional Assessment*, Chap. 23). These are recorded on the patient's record together with an estimation of the number of milliliters of formula at 1.0 kcal per milliliter and at 1.5 kcal per milliliter per 24 hours to meet them. Subsequently, the dietitian is responsible for estimating and recording the intake of kilocalories, protein, sodium, and potassium per 24 hours from enteral feeding, as well as the contribution of peripheral feeding, if any. When full feeding has been achieved, the average 24-hour intake of minerals, electrolytes, vitamins, and total milliliters of fluid from the formula should be recorded on the patient's record. The intake of minerals and vitamins is recorded so that the nutritional support team can assess the adequacy of intake and avoid excessive supplementation with the fat-soluble vitamins. Unless the pharmacy is responsible for obtaining and dispensing enteral feedings, the dietary department is responsible for maintaining in the patient care unit a 24-hour supply of formula of the correct dilution.

### Parenteral alimentation

Parenteral alimentation, or, more appropriately, total parenteral nutrition (TPN), is a method of providing substrate for the metabolic needs of the patient who cannot be maintained by the oral route, such as the patient who has undergone extensive gastrointestinal surgery, one with extensive inflammatory bowel disease, or the severely nutritionally depleted patient. The TPN solution,[14] a hyperosmolar solution (1500 mOsm to 1800 mOsm per kilogram $H_2O$) is administered continuously each 24 hours through a subclavian catheter inserted into the superior vena cava. Twenty-five hundred kcal to 3500 kcal or more can be administered daily by this method. The high osmolality of the solution is tolerated because of the high rate of blood flow in the superior vena cava, which readily dilutes the solution.

The catheter is inserted by the surgeon under sterile conditions, and its maintenance is the joint responsibility of the surgeon and the nurse specialist on the nutrition support team.[15] TPN solutions are prepared in the pharmacy under sterile conditions, and their daily administration is monitored by the nursing staff.[16]

### TPN solutions

The standard TPN solutions, normal dilution, provide 1 kcal per milliliter, 6 g to 6.6 g of nitrogen per liter and a nonprotein kilocalorie to nitrogen ratio of 120 to 180:1. The solution is 20% to 25% anhydrous glucose, approximately 200 g to 250 g per liter. If necessary, regular insulin is infused to maintain normal serum glucose levels. There is no source of essential fatty acid in the present formulations of TPN solutions, and intravenous lipid solutions are administered approximately twice a week to provide essential fatty acids. Electrolytes, minerals, and vitamins are added during preparation in the pharmacy according to the needs of the patient.

The hypermetabolic patient's utilization of energy and nutrients introduced directly into the systemic circulation by TPN rather than from the gastrointestinal tract through the portal circulation to the liver is under intensive study. Still to be answered are such questions as the most appropriate ratio of essential to nonessential nitrogen (amino acids),[17,18] the most effective nonprotein kilocalorie to nitrogen ratio,[19] the quantity of trace elements required to prevent deficiencies or toxicities, and the requirements for electrolytes, minerals, and vitamins.

The nitrogen in the commonly used TPN solutions is provided by crystalline amino acids. The quantity of essential amino acids usually reflects the recommendation of Rose for the amino acid requirements of healthy young adults (see Chap. 4). However, the work of Waterhouse[17] and co-workers and other researchers indicates that the proportions of the amino acids in the present TPN formulations need further study. The research of Peters and Fischer[19] suggests that the most effective kilocalorie to nitrogen ratio in TPN solutions to promote nitrogen equilibrium in their study patients was 163:1.

### The clinical dietitian's role

In most but not all major medical centers the clinical dietitian is a member of the core team for nutritional support services (see Chap. 23). When it is suspected that a patient requires TPN or is on TPN, the responsibilities of the clinical dietitian are estimating recent daily energy and nutrient intake; taking the anthropometric measurements for the assessment of nutritional status; collating the patient's assessment data (see Fig. 23-1); and estimating the patient's daily requirements of energy and protein. As the patient progresses the clinical dietitian is responsible for the reassessment of nutritional status at the appropriate times (see Chap. 23) and for calculating nitrogen balance at least once a week. When the patient returns to oral feedings, the clinical dietitian is responsible for managing the patient's intake and reporting progress to the nutritional support team.

### Return to oral intake

The administration of TPN cannot be terminated abruptly. Even with a rapid fall in serum insulin upon the termination of TPN, instances of reactive hypoglycemia have been reported. This can result in central nervous system damage and death. The rate of infusion is tapered by daily decrements of approximately 1000 ml, followed by an infusion of 5% dextrose for 12 to 24 hours before the catheter is removed.

Some patients report a lack of hunger sensations during parenteral nutrition while others do not. Also, some patients have an increase in appetite as TPN is decreased, while others report early satiety on the resumption of oral intake. Grant[14] recommends that parenteral nutrition be continued at 1500 ml to 2000 ml (1500 kcal–2000 kcal) per day until 1500 kcal to 1800 kcal are consumed orally.

It is strongly recommended that oral intake begin with 400 kcal to 500 kcal per day to avoid adverse gastrointestinal reactions, such as diarrhea, even though the patient may be willing to try more to be free of the TPN catheter. Greene and co-workers[20] have demonstrated that the sucrase and maltase activity of the gastrointestinal tract decreases significantly when no carbohydrate is consumed orally for a period of 3 days or longer. An excessive intake of oral carbohydrate by the TPN patient could result in osmotic diarrhea with fluid and electrolyte losses. Patients should be helped to progress from 400 kcal to 500 kcal to 1500 kcal or more over a period of 3 to 5 days. The oral intake of fluid, kilocalories, protein, sodium, and potassium during this period should be estimated and recorded every 24 hours so that the nutrition support team can monitor total intake, oral and parenteral, as the patient is weaned from TPN. In some instances it may be necessary to change from parenteral nutrition to nasogastric or enterostomy tube feeding. The first tube feedings should contain no more than 0.5 kcal per milliliter administered by drip and 500 kcal per day, with progression toward full formula as tolerated.

### Complications of TPN

There are a variety of septic and metabolic complications in patients receiving total parenteral nutrition that are under intensive study by numerous investigators in large medical centers. The major complication of concern to the clinical dietitian is fluid overload in those patients who are taking fluids and food orally as well as TPN fluids by venous catheter.

Whenever the patient on TPN is permitted to take fluids orally, the physician should order a maximum quantity of fluid intake allowed in a 24-hour period rather than leave an order for fluids *ad lib (ad libitum)*. Although

the potential for fluid overload is lower with a central venous catheter than with a peripheral venous catheter, the potential does exist if the patient on TPN is permitted fluid intake orally. In addition to recording the milliliters of fluid intake daily, the clinical dietitian should also record daily an estimate of the nitrogen, sodium, and potassium in the fluids, as well as that in any food consumed. In this way, the total daily intake of nitrogen, sodium, and potassium can be estimated to avoid electrolyte imbalance as well as fluid overload.

### Home TPN

Some patients may require TPN for extended periods of time (6–30 mo) whereas others may require it for the remainder of their lives. Home TPN has been instituted to reduce the cost of long hospitalizations and to return the patient to the more familiar environment of the home. The social worker and nurse specialist are responsible for evaluating the patient's home environment and financial resources and the total nutritional support team is responsible for educating the patient and the family to manage the administration of TPN in the home and for providing follow-up care, including the supplies required to mix the TPN solution daily.

A study of nineteen patients[21] demonstrated that anxiety, depression, and fear were predictable and universal reactions in all patients being prepared for discharge on TPN. The greatest problem of adjustment was the loss of the ability to eat. How successful the patients in this study were in adjusting to the home TPN was related to family and hospital support systems, the degree of restoration of physical health, and the patient's own strength of ego. Home TPN forces major alterations in a patient's lifestyle.

## Diet therapy after gastrointestinal surgery
### Diet after gastric and duodenal surgery

The patient whose gastric or duodenal ulcer does not respond to medical treatment is the most common candidate for gastric surgery. He may have a vagotomy and pyloroplasty or partial gastrectomy and vagotomy.

### Principles of postoperative diet therapy

There are various approaches to the feeding of patients after gastric surgery. Two principles appear to apply to all routines—the restriction of the total volume of any feeding during the immediate postoperative period, with gradual increases as tolerated; and the restriction of concentrated carbohydrate, particularly excessive amounts of sucrose, and in some situations, lactose.

After peristalsis has returned and the patient has tolerated clear fluids by mouth—beginning with 30 ml per feeding on the first day and increasing to 60 ml on the second day—the patient is offered six to eight small feedings of soft or solid foods, neither very hot nor very cold.[22]

A small feeding in this situation may be limited to 3 or 4 oz increasing gradually to 8 oz to 10 oz. For example, one poached egg and one slice of buttered toast is approximately 3 oz of food.

Fluids including milk may or may not be included in the small frequent feedings. After gastric surgery the contents of the stomach may pass into the small intestine before it is in proper solution and cause distention of the jejunum. When this happens, the patient complains of nausea, cramps, diarrhea, lightheadedness, and extreme weakness. This occurs 15 min to 30 min after meals and is known as *early dumping syndrome.* It has been observed that this occurs less frequently if the patient avoids too much fluid with his meals.[23]

It has also been observed that excessive amounts of carbohydrate, especially sucrose and in some patients lactose, cause the early dumping syndrome. Therefore, sucrose is usually restricted in the diet of the patient immediately after gastric surgery. Candies, jams, jellies, frosted cakes, and beverages sweetened with sucrose are not used. After recovery from gastric surgery many patients tolerate moderate amounts of sugar.

Some but not all patients, after gastric surgery, develop lactose intolerance; therefore, some clinicians exclude milk after surgery. However, other clinicians exclude milk only after the patient has experienced distention and diarrhea that are relieved by the exclusion of milk.

### Nutritional care of the patient after gastric surgery

Table 27-2 lists the foods used after gastric surgery. These foods can be used in six to eight small meals. If any of the foods listed are not well tolerated by the patient before surgery, it is advisable to avoid them in the postoperative period.

Patients' food acceptance should be observed closely so that the volume of food in a meal can be increased as tolerated. Most patients after recovery from gastric surgery eventually eat normal amounts of food at a meal, but they should be advised to increase the amount of food at each meal slowly after discharge. As the volume consumed at each meal increases, the number of meals can be decreased from 6 to 8 meals to 4 to 5.

One dietitian who works closely with patients after gastric surgery tests each one's tolerance for concentrated carbohydrate before discharge. She serves a sweet, such as cake, ice cream, or jelly with toast at one meal and observes the patient's tolerance carefully.

### Late dumping syndrome or postgastrectomy hypoglycemia

A few patients develop severe dumping syndrome after gastric surgery. After taking sugar by mouth they have an elevated blood glucose level (hyperglycemia). This is followed by a precipitous drop of blood glucose to below normal levels (hypoglycemia) at which time the patient is dizzy, feels faint, and is nauseated. These pa-

tients usually have diarrhea and lose weight. They find it difficult to maintain a normal weight status.

A high-protein, high-fat, low-carbohydrate diet is usually well tolerated by these patients. One diet plan that has been used successfully contains 20 meat exchanges, 20 fat exchanges, 4 bread exchanges, 3 fruit exchanges, and 2 vegetable exchanges[24] (see Chap. 24). The food is served in six meals without fluids. One cup of coffee or tea with 40% cream is served 1 hour before breakfast, lunch, and dinner. If possible, medications requiring water should also be given 1 hour before meals.

The dietitian plans the diet with these patients daily, and the nurse should report to her any symptoms of the dumping syndrome the patient may have.

After the severe symptoms of the syndrome are controlled, individual patients may tolerate an increase in complex carbohydrate, such as bread, potatoes, and other starches, but may need to avoid sugar in any form. These patients may also be lactose-intolerant and need to exclude all milk from their diets.

### Bowel surgery

Many patients require surgery in other sections of the gastrointestinal tract, such as small or large bowel resection, hemorrhoidectomy, ileostomy, or colostomy.

#### Postoperative nutritional care

Postoperatively, after testing with clear liquids, these patients are usually given a residue-restricted diet. They progress from a minimal to a moderate residue diet (see the residue-restricted diet plans in Table 26-10).

### Table 27-2. Foods Used After Gastric Surgery

Milk*

Eggs and Cheese
  Eggs—boiled, poached, scrambled, or omelets
  Cottage cheese

Meat, Fish, Poultry
  Any type—baked, broiled, boiled, or in simple mixed dishes

Potato, Rice, Macaroni, Spaghetti, Noodles
  Plain or in simple mixed dishes

Bread, Crackers
  Enriched white bread and rolls toasted or plain in sandwiches
  Saltines and other plain crackers

Vegetables†
  Soft cooked vegetables

Fruits
  Cooked or well-drained canned fruit

Fat
  Butter, margarine, mayonnaise, bacon, and cream cheese

Desserts
  Cooked or well-drained canned fruit
  Baked custard or plain vanilla pudding*

---

*If tolerated.

†Avoid gas-forming vegetables (cabbage, cauliflower, brussels sprouts, broccoli, cucumbers, onions, turnips, and radishes).

Most patients with colostomies are able before long to return to their regular food practices, provided that these are adequate for their nutritional needs. They should omit foods that were not well tolerated before surgery, but no food is contraindicated once the patient has recovered from the operation.

The ileostomy patient may present a special problem. If a significant portion of the terminal ileum has been removed, there is a decrease in vitamin $B_{12}$ absorption because it is absorbed in the terminal ileum. In this case it may be necessary to give vitamin $B_{12}$ parenterally. After recovery from surgery, the ileostomy patient is able to tolerate a regular diet, although he may be advised to avoid excessive roughage, which has in some patients obstructed the stoma.

### Short bowel syndrome

In some situations a large portion of the ileum may be removed at surgery. Because of a decrease in the amount of absorptive surface, these patients often have difficulty maintaining a reasonable nutritional status. Depending on the extent of the bowel surgery, the nutritional needs of these patients may be met postoperatively by venous hyperalimentation, or by enteral hyperalimentation with a monomeric formula, because the nutrients in these feedings are absorbed primarily in the terminal duodenum and the proximal jejunum. Dilute feedings administered by drip are used first, followed by an increase in concentration as tolerated by the individual patient (see section on tube feedings). These patients are prone to develop hypersecretion of gastric acid and are given an $H_2$ receptor antagonist, such as cimetidine.[25]

It has been observed in some patients with extensive small bowel resection that, with time, there is hypertrophy of the remaining mucosa of the small intestine resulting in a larger absorptive surface. At this point these patients may respond to a diet of *small* frequent feedings high in protein and carbohydrate and relatively low (60 g–80 g) in fat. Medium chain triglycerides* have been used in such diets to supply energy, but in general the results have not been satisfactory.

### Nutrition following burns

Patients with extensive burns present nutritional problems much more far-reaching even than those who have undergone major surgery. As a result of the stress reaction there is massive loss of fluids and electrolytes, and serum proteins are lost by exudation from the burned areas. There is extensive tissue breakdown, lasting for periods of weeks as evidenced by tremendous losses of nitrogen and potassium in the urine. Such nitrogen losses continue for the first 30 days, then gradually diminish as healing takes place. Energy expenditure is markedly increased to supply the energy required for healing the burn surface area.[26]

The early part of treatment consists of the intravenous administration of dextrose and electrolyte solutions and blood plasma to replace the fluid being lost from the burn surface area. When the patient can take oral feeding, he is given a high-calorie, high-protein diet or tube feeding or both. Greatly increased amounts of ascorbic acid (to aid in wound healing) and the B vitamins (to meet tremendously increased metabolic demands) and two times the allowance of the fat-soluble vitamins should be given as medication.

If flames or fumes have been inhaled, injuring the respiratory and the gastrointestinal tracts, or if there are burns about the mouth and the face, it may be impossible at first to use the oral route for feeding. Oral or tube feeding may be further contraindicated, as badly burned patients frequently have gastrointestinal atony the first few days after injury. Some patients require TPN to meet their metabolic needs during the early recovery period.

If tube feeding is used for the first oral feeding, excessive protein without adequate water intake, especially in children, should be avoided (see *Hazards of Tube Feeding* in this chapter).

When food can be eaten in adequate quantities, between-meal feedings of high-calorie, high-protein beverages or the products in Table 27-1 are used. Because the burn patient may develop gastric hemorrhage, it is advisable to give tube feedings spread evenly over the 24-hour period or serve frequent small meals and between-meal beverages.

To estimate the energy needs of adults, Curreri and co-workers recommend 25 kcal times weight in kilograms plus 40 kcal times percent of total body surface burned.[27] Using this formula a 70-kg man with a 40% burn would require 3350 kcal per day ($25 \times 70 + 40 \times 40 = 3350$ kcal). The kilocaloric needs of an adult can also be calculated using the Harris-Benedict formula and Long's injury factor of $2.10$[28] (see Chap. 23). Depending on the severity and extent of the burn and on age, a child may require 70 to 100 calories per kilogram and 3 g to 5 g of protein per kilogram of body weight.

There is a tremendous need for supportive care of severely burned patients by nurses, doctors, dietitians, and all others with whom they come in contact. The importance of the greatly increased need for food must be carefully explained to the patient. The diet particularly must be individualized to meet his needs and desires, and close cooperation by all who care for him is essential to meet his nutritional and emotional needs.

### Study questions and activities

1. With the help of members of the nursing team, keep a record of the kinds and amounts of clear liquids consumed in a 24-hour period by a postoperative patient.

---

*MCT Oil, Mead Johnson Laboratories, Evansville, Ind. 47721

Using Table 1 in Part 4, estimate this patient's 24-hour energy and nutrient intake. Was it nutritionally adequate for him?

2. Using Table 27-2, plan eight small meals for a patient who has had gastric surgery. Describe the size of serving of each food item.

3. What food may be poorly tolerated after gastric surgery? Why?

4. What are some possible causes of diarrhea in the tube-fed patient? How may it be prevented?

5. Obtain from the dietitian the kinds and nutrient composition of the high-calorie, high-protein beverages served to burn patients or any other patient receiving a similar beverage. Estimate how much these beverages cost per serving.

# References

1. Mullen JL et al: Arch Surg 141:121, 1979
2. Dudrick SJ et al: J Parent Ent Nutr 3:444, 1979
3. Moore FD: In Sabiston DC Jr (ed): Davis-Christopher Textbook of Surgery, 11th ed, pp 27–64. Philadelphia, WB Saunders, 1977
4. Dudrick JS, Rhoads JE: In Sabiston, Davis-Christopher Textbook, pp 150–177
5. Waterlow JC et al: Am J Clin Nutr 30:1333, 1977
6. O'Keefe SJD et al: Lancet 2:1035, 1974
7. Elwyn DH et al: Am J Clin Nutr 32:1597, 1979
8. Torosian MH, Rombeau JL: Surg Gynecol Obstet 150:918, 1980
9. Bethel RA et al: Am J Clin Nutr 32:1112, 1979
10. Shils ME et al: Liquid Formulas for Oral and Tube Feedings, 2nd ed. New York, Sloan-Kettering Cancer Center, 1979
11. Harrah JD: Am J Clin Nutr 4:303, 1980
12. Heymsfield SB et al: Ann Intern Med 90:63, 1979
13. Sleisenger MH, Kim YS: N Engl J Med 300:659, 1979
14. Grant JP: Handbook of Total Parenteral Nutrition, pp 92–117. Philadelphia, WB Saunders, 1980
15. Grant, Handbook of Parenteral Nutrition, pp 47–69
16. Grant, Handbook of Parenteral Nutrition, pp 118–124
17. Waterhouse C et al: Am J Clin Nutr 32:2423, 1979
18. Wassner SJ et al: Am J Clin Nutr 32:1497, 1979
19. Peters C, Fischer JE: Surg Gynecol Obstet 151:1, 1980
20. Greene HL et al: Am J Clin Nutr 28:1122, 1975
21. Price BS, Levine EL: J Parent Ent Nutr 3:48, 1979
22. Malt RA: Nutr Today 6:30, 1971
23. Gulsrud PO et al: Gastroenterology 78:1463, 1980
24. Spiro HM: Clinical Gastroenterology, 2nd ed. New York, Macmillan, 1977
25. Weser E et al: Gastroenterology 77:579, 1979
26. Wilmore DW, Aulick LH: J Parent Ent Nutr 4:147, 1980
27. Curreri PW et al: J Am Diet Assoc 65:415, 1974
28. Long CL et al: J Parent Ent Nutr 3:452, 1979

# Supplementary readings

Alberti KGMM et al: Relative role of various hormones in mediating the metabolic response to injury. J Parent Ent Nutr 4:141, 1980

Buzby GP et al: Prognostic nutritional index in gastrointestinal surgery. Am J Surg 139:160, 1980

Chernoff R: The team concept: The dietitian's responsibility. J Parent Ent Nutr 3:89, 1979

Curreri PW, Luterman A: Nutritional support of the burned patient. Surg Clin North Am 58:1151, 1978

Dionigi R et al: Nutrition and infection. J Parent Ent Nutr 3:62, 1979

Fagawa-Busby KS et al: Effects of diet temperature on tolerance of enteral feedings. Nurs Res 29:276. Sept-Oct, 1980

Goodgame JT Jr: A critical assessment of the indications for total parenteral nutrition. Surg Gynecol Obstet 151:433, 1980

Guidelines for essential trace element preparations for parenteral use: A statement of the Nutrition Advisory Group. J Parent Ent Nutr 3:263, 1979

Heymsfield SB et al: Enteral hyperalimentation: An alternative to central venous hyperalimentation. Ann Intern Med 90:63, 1979

Hoover HC Jr et al: Nutritional benefits of immediate postoperative jejunal feeding of an elemental diet. Am J Surg 139:153, 1980

Long CL et al: Contribution of skeletal muscle protein in elevated rates of whole body protein catabolism in trauma patients. Am J Clin Nutr 34:1087, 1981

Multivitamin preparations for parenteral use: A statement by the Nutrition Advisory Group. J Parent Ent Nutr 3:258, 1979

Newmark SR et al: Home tube feeding for a long-term nutritional support. J Parent Ent Nutr 5:76, 1981

Nutrition in Trauma and Stress: Reference Manual. Doyle Pharmaceutical Co., Minneapolis, MN 55416

Padilla GV et al: Subjective distress of nasogastric tube feeding. J Parent Ent Nutr 3:53, 1979

Price BS, Levine EL: Permanent total parenteral nutrition: Psychological and social responses of the early stage. J Parent Ent Nutr 3:48, 1979

Ruppin H et al: Effects of liquid formula diets on proximal gastrointestinal function. Dig Dis Sci 26:202, 1981

Seltzer MH et al: Instant nutritional assessment in the intensive care unit. J Parent Ent Nutr 5:70, 1981

Sleisenger MH, Kim YS: Protein digestion and absorption. N Engl J Med 300:659, 1979

Timmons KN et al: Protein quality and the cost of selected commercial protein supplements. J Am Diet Assoc 78:606, 1981

Weser E et al: Short bowel syndrome. Gastroenterology 77:579, 1979

# Patient resources

Mullen BD, McGinn KA: The Ostomy Book. Palo Alto, CA, Bull, 1980

*For further references see Bibliography in Part 4.*

# Weight Control

# 28

Weight Norms
Obesity
Underweight
Anorexia Nervosa

The *achievement* and the *maintenance* of an appropriate weight status for height, sex, age, and activity throughout the life span are positive approaches to avoiding or delaying many of the health problems associated with obesity. It is estimated that 50 million of the 220 million people in the United States are above desirable weight due to overfatness. Some of these individuals are mildly obese, while others are moderately to grossly obese. It has been observed that diabetes mellitus and hypertension occur more frequently in those who are obese than in those of normal weight. Although there is not a clear association between obesity and coronary heart disease, the obese person is apt to experience elevated blood levels of triglycerides and cholesterol. The grossly obese as a group are poor risks for surgery due to adverse reactions to anesthesia. They also experience a variety of skin and skeletal problems. In addition, the analysis of mortality data indicates that the obese have a shorter life expectancy than the nonobese.[1] Inappropriate weight status during childhood and adolescence appears to be associated not only with physical problems but also with problems of psychosocial development, and the obese adult in our society faces many social pressures. The magnitude and the complexity of the problems of obesity make it readily apparent that the obese comprise a major portion of the clients served by the nutrition counselor (see Fig. 28-1).

At any point in the life span the achievement and maintenance of an appropriate weight status is client-managed (see Chap. 13). During infancy and childhood weight control is the responsibility of the parents, and throughout the remainder of the life span it is the responsibility of each individual. When one considers the prevalence and incidence of obesity in our society, it is evident that the major task of the nutrition counselor is to influence the food choices of clients so that they can achieve and maintain an appropriate weight status.

## Excess Mortality*

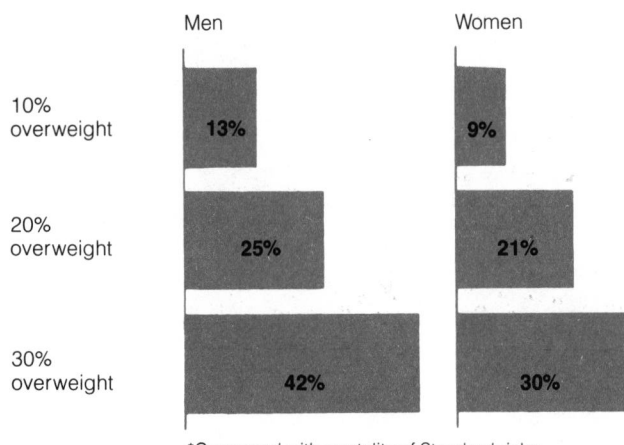

*Compared with mortality of Standard risks
(Mortality ratio of Standard risks = 100%)

**Fig. 28-1.** Overweight shortens life. (From Overweight—Its Significance and Prevention. Metropolitan Life Insurance Company. Derived from The Build and Blood Pressure Study, Society of Actuaries, 1959)

From the formulas and baby foods fed to infants to the meals served older adults in a congregate meals program, the energy value of food is the primary focus of proper weight status. It is also the primary focus in the dietary treatment of clients with excessive adipose tissue—that is, people who are obese with or without diabetes mellitus or hyperlipidemias. As pointed out in Chapter 11, the energy value of a food varies primarily according to differences in carbohydrate and fat content. In addition to monitoring the total carbohydrate and lipid content of food, the diet therapy for some obese clients requires modifications in the types of carbohydrates and lipids (mono-, di-, and polysaccharides; saturated and polyunsaturated fatty acids; and cholesterol) ingested.

Weight norms, obesity, underweight, and anorexia nervosa are discussed in this chapter. Diabetes mellitus and aberrations of lipid metabolism, particularly hyperlipoproteinemia, are presented in Chapters 29 and 30. The reader is advised to review *Energy*, Chapter 10, and *Nutrient Utilization*, Chapter 9, particularly the section on the glucose-fatty acid cycle and its hormonal control.

## Weight norms

The concept of what constitutes correct weight at any point in the life span has undergone marked revision in recent years. Even today the definition of the term *normal* or *desirable* weight, is sharply debated. To assess the weight status of each person height-weight tables have been traditionally used as weight norms and continue to be used while a number of investigators attempt to find more precise methods to assess body composition and its relation to weight status.

## Height-weight tables

The first tables for adults were based on the heights and weights for age of men and women who were life insurance policyholders. The figures in these tables reflected the average weights for height and age of the people measured. Since the data showed an increase in weight with age, the recommended weight for height in the tables increased with each age group. For example, it was recommended that a woman 5 ft 4 in tall weigh 131 lb at age 30, and 144 lb at age 55.[2]

In recent years the height-weight tables have been reevaluated and revised. It is now recognized that, when growth in height has been achieved by about age 20, there is no biological need to gain weight in excess of that which is satisfactory for each person. Also, the best health prognosis is found in those who have achieved and maintained a reasonable weight status throughout the life span.

It must be remembered that body weight is made up of a number of components: fat, muscle, organs, bone, and fluids. In evaluating a person's weight status, the percentage of the weight each one of these components contributes to the total weight is critical. One approach to this problem has been to classify people by body build (frame), using the terms *small*, *medium*, and *large*. These terms reflect Sheldon's somatotypes: the small frame, ectomorphy; the medium frame, mesomorphy; and the large frame, endomorphy.[3] However, as yet there are no commonly accepted clinical criteria for estimating precisely each person's frame size to identify his body build. Given two men of the same height, the one with a large frame normally weighs more than the one with a small frame.

The revised height-weight tables in current use reflect the concern for maintaining over the life span the weight appropriate for a person at age 25. The Metropolitan Life Insurance Company's Desirable Weight Tables, published in 1960, give desirable weight ranges for heights for men and women 25 years of age and over, while allowing for differences in body frame, designated as small, medium, and large. The range for a 5 ft 4 in woman with a small frame is 108 lb to 116 lb; with a medium frame, 113 lb to 126 lb; and with a large frame, 121 lb to 138 lb (see Table 10, Part 4).

In clinical practice height-weight tables must be used judiciously. For example, a professional football player may be overweight for height due to the size of his muscle mass, while a 50 year old woman who is at the correct weight for height and estimated frame may actually be overfat. The measuring equipment must be well maintained and measurements must be taken accurately under standardized conditions (with a minimum of clothes and without shoes). The assessment of weight status of infants and children is presented in Chapter 35, *Nutrition in Diseases of Infancy and Childhood*.

## Skinfold thickness

Brozek and co-workers, Behnke and co-workers, and other investigators are studying a variety of sophisticated techniques, such as measurements of body density, total body water, or total body potassium to determine body composition.[4] In general these investigations are directed to identifying the nonfat component of the body—the component that is the major determinant of energy and nutrient needs. At present the majority of the techniques used in this research are not adaptable to routine clinical use.

Fat is the component of body composition that has the greatest effect on variations in total body weight during growth in infants and children and after the adult has attained his full growth status. The fat content of people of normal weight varies, according to sex, age, and activity, from 14% to 30% of total body weight. A number of studies have shown that skinfold thickness measurements can be used to estimate the fat content of the body, particularly in adults.

Skinfold thickness measurements are discussed in Chapter 23 in the section on *nutritional status assessment.* Bray and co-workers[5] question the advisability of using calipers in assessing and following obese patients. For example, in some patients the fatfolds are greater than the calipers can accommodate. Their work also suggests that circumferences, especially of the biceps, may be better predictors of obesity. However, this work needs further study.

## Visual inspection

In many clinical settings the weight status of a person can be evaluated by visual inspection. During a physical examination the physician or nurse can observe excessive accumulations of body fat or the lack of body fat. The nutrition counselor can visually identify the client who is overfat or too thin as he sits beside the desk.

# Obesity

## Definition

Although at present there is no general agreement, the following descriptions of overweight and obesity are being used.

*Overweight* is "overheaviness" and the term does not carry any direct implication with regard to fatness. *Obesity* is described as a bodily condition marked by excessive generalized deposition or storage of fat in adipose tissue.

Many investigators define a person as obese who is 20% above the weight for age and sex in the weight tables. Others may use 5% to 10% as a criterion. These criteria do not differentiate overfatness from overheaviness. However, until the skinfold thickness measurements are better standardized so that one can estimate the number of pounds or the percentage of total body weight that is fat, weight will continue to be used to define obesity.

## Prevalence and incidence

Obesity is considered a major public health problem today, although there are limited statistics for its general prevalence and incidence in the total population. The prevalence appears to be increasing. The data from the National Center for Health Statistics show that both men and women examined in the data collection period 1971 to 1974 weighed more than those examined in the 1960 to 1962 period.[6]

Mayer observed a 20% prevalence of obesity in schoolchildren in a middle class suburban community.[7] The Ten-State Nutrition Survey reported that the percentage of obese adolescents varied from 11% to 39% for white men and from 5% to 33% for black men; and from 9% to 19% for white women and from 5% to 33% for black women.[8]

The highest prevalence of obesity in the Ten-State Nutrition Survey occurred in adult women. Fifty percent of the black women 45 to 55 years of age and 40% of the white women 45 to 55 years of age were obese. Obesity was less prevalent in adult men, although 20% of white men were found to be obese.

Excessive weight gain occurs more frequently at certain ages or periods in the life span. As the Ten-State Nutrition Survey indicates, obesity frequently occurs at adolescence in both boys and girls and after age 45 in women.

The Health and Nutrition Examination Survey data, 1971 to 1974, estimated that among women 20 to 74 years of age 4.5 million were severely obese (67 lb above reported average weight) and about 1.2 million of these women were between 45 to 54 years of age.[6]

The prevalence of obesity would also appear to be related to social class. The data of Stunkard and co-workers indicate that there is less obesity among the higher socioeconomic levels, particularly in women, than at a lower socioeconomic level.[20]

It has also been observed that there are two types of obese adults—those who became obese during childhood and adolescence and those who became obese later in life. The time of onset of obesity has implications for therapy and will be discussed later.

## Etiology

In previous editions of this book, obesity was attributed with a high degree of confidence to excessive food intake. Today, with the extensive research being reported on ATP utilization and other aspects of energy metabolism,[10] one is less sure of a direct relationship between food intake and obesity. However, if one studies the energy value of the preliminary 1979 figures from the USDA of the food available for civilian consumption (Chap. 11) it is reasonable to equate obesity with food intake.

From the evidence available today it appears that the etiology of obesity is multifactorial. In addition to energy imbalance, derangement of glucose and fat metabolism, genetics, and psychological processes may all contribute to the development of obesity.

### Energy imbalance (food intake and physical activity)

Obesity is the result of a positive energy balance and can be due to a daily calorie intake that exceeds a person's energy needs. It is generally accepted that a pound of body fat contains approximately 3500 calories. Theoretically an intake in excess of need of even 100 calories a day will add up to 3000 calories a month, or almost one pound of body weight. Over a year this will amount to a weight gain of 10 pounds.

However, not every obese client reports an excessive calorie intake. Energy expenditure is as important as food intake in the development of obesity. In the past 25 to 50 years, life in the highly developed areas of the world has undergone great changes. Work hours have been shortened, laborsaving machinery has been installed in homes and factories, transportation is easier, homes are well heated, and even our leisure-time activities are sedentary rather than active. This has reduced the energy needs of the body markedly, but, by and large, food habits have not changed sufficiently to offset the decreased need. Although the American breakfast is considerably smaller today than that which our ancestors were accustomed to eating, the coffee break, morning and afternoon, the increased use of sugar, the ubiquitous candy bar, and the "TV snack" (see Table 28-1) have more than compensated for the change in breakfast patterns. Perhaps the energy

crises and the inflation of the 1980s will reverse these trends to some extent (see Fig. 28-2).

A number of investigators have observed that the obese person, and particularly the obese child or adolescent, is less active than his counterpart of the same age. Whether this is due to his inability to keep pace with other children or to apathy born of emotional conflict, the inactivity lowers the energy needs of the body and in this way contributes to the overweight. This situation is also true of obese women compared to women of normal weight. In obese men the difference in activity is less striking but still of significance.

### Metabolic and endocrine aberrations (hypercellularity and hyperinsulinism)

In the past many attempts have been made to relate obesity to a disturbance of function of one or more of the endocrine glands, such as the thyroid or the pituitary. Patients with insufficient thyroid function (hypothyroidism) are usually overweight. However, part of the excess weight is due to the accumulation of hydrophilic mucopolysaccharides in the skin and other tissues. These patients contribute only a small percentage to the total number of overweight persons, and their condition responds to treatment with thyroid hormone. Truncal obesity is usually due to adrenal hyperplasia or the use of glucocorticoid therapy for a variety of diseases.

Following the work of Winick on the effect of an inadequate intake of energy and nutrients on cell division and cell size during infancy (see Chap. 16), Hirsch and Knittle studied the number and size of adipose cells in obese and nonobese children.[11] They have demonstrated that at all ages obese children have larger and more numerous adipose cells compared to the adipose cells in

### Table 28-1. Energy Values for Common "Snack" Foods

|  | *Amount or Average Serving* | *Energy (kcal)* |
|---|---|---|
| ***"Just a Little Sandwich"*** |  |  |
| Hamburger on bun | 3-in patty | 330 |
| Peanut butter sandwich | 2 tbsp | 330 |
| Cheese sandwich | 1 oz cheese | 280 |
| Ham sandwich | 1 oz ham | 320 |
| ***TV Snack*** |  |  |
| Pizza (cheese) | $\frac{1}{8}$ of 14-in diam pie | 185 |
| Popcorn with oil and salt | 1 c | 40 |
| Pretzel, thin, twisted | 1 | 25 |
| Cheese fondue | $\frac{1}{2}$ c | 265 |
| Dips (sour cream) | $\frac{1}{2}$ c | 248 |
| Chippers | 10 | 150 |
| ***Beverages*** |  |  |
| Carbonated drinks, soda, root beer, and so on | 6-oz glass | 80 |
| Cola beverages | 12-oz glass (Pepsi) | 150 |
| Club soda | 8-oz glass | 5 |
| Chocolate malted milk | 10-oz glass ($1\frac{3}{4}$ c) | 500 |
| Ginger ale | 6-oz glass | 60 |

## Table 28-1. Energy Values for Common "Snack" Foods (Continued)

| | Amount or Average Serving | Energy (kcal) |
|---|---|---|
| **Beverages (Continued)** | | |
| Tea or coffee, straight | 1 c | 0 |
| Tea or coffee, with 2 tablespoons cream and 2 teaspoons sugar | 1 c | 90 |
| **Alcoholic Drinks** | | |
| Ale | 8-oz glass | 155 |
| Beer | 8-oz glass | 110 |
| Highball (with ginger ale—ladies' style) | 8-oz glass | 185 |
| Manhattan | Average | 165 |
| Martini | Average | 140 |
| Wine, Muscatel or Port | 2-oz glass | 95 |
| Sherry | 2-oz glass | 75 |
| Scotch, bourbon, rye | $1\frac{1}{2}$-oz jigger | 130 |
| **Fruits** | | |
| Apple | 1  3-in | 75 |
| Banana | 1  6-in | 130 |
| Grapes | 30 medium | 75 |
| Orange | 1  $2\frac{3}{4}$-in | 70 |
| Pear | 1 | 65 |
| **Salted Nuts** | | |
| Almonds, filberts, hazelnuts | 12–15 | 95 |
| Cashews | 6–8 | 90 |
| Peanuts | 15–17 | 85 |
| Pecans, walnuts | 10–15 halves | 100 |
| **Candies** | | |
| Chocolate bars: | | |
| Plain, sweet milk | 1 bar (1 oz) | 155 |
| With almonds | 1 bar (1 oz) | 140 |
| Chocolate-covered bar | 1 bar | 270 |
| Chocolate cream, bon bon, fudge | 1 piece 1-in square | 90–120 |
| Caramels, plain | 2 medium | 85 |
| Hard candies, Lifesaver type | 1 roll | 95 |
| Peanut brittle | 1 piece $2\frac{1}{2} \times 2\frac{1}{2} \times \frac{3}{8}$ in | 110 |
| **Desserts** | | |
| Pie: | | |
| Fruit—apple, and so on | $\frac{1}{6}$ pie 1 average serving | 410 |
| Custard | $\frac{1}{6}$ pie 1 average serving | 265 |
| Mince | $\frac{1}{6}$ pie 1 average serving | 400 |
| Pumpkin pie with whipped cream | $\frac{1}{6}$ pie 1 average serving | 460 |
| Cake: | | |
| Chocolate layer | 3-in section | 350 |
| Doughnut, sugared | 1 average | 150 |
| **Sweets** | | |
| Ice Cream: | | |
| Plain vanilla | $\frac{1}{6}$ qt serving | 200 |
| Chocolate and other flavors | $\frac{1}{6}$ qt, $\frac{2}{3}$ c | 260 |
| Orange sherbet | $\frac{1}{2}$ c | 120 |
| Sundaes, small chocolate nut with whipped cream | Average | 400 |
| Ice-cream sodas, chocolate | 10-oz glass | 270 |
| **Midnight Snacks for Icebox Raiders** | | |
| Cold potato | $\frac{1}{2}$ medium | 65 |
| Chicken leg (fried) | 1 average | 88 |
| Milk | 7-oz glass | 140 |
| Mouthful of roast | $\frac{1}{2}$ in × 2 in × 3 in | 130 |
| Piece of cheese | $\frac{1}{4}$ in × 2 in × 3 in | 120 |
| Leftover beans | $\frac{1}{2}$ c | 105 |
| Brownie | $\frac{3}{4}$ in × $1\frac{3}{4}$ in × $2\frac{1}{4}$ in | 140 |
| Cream puff | 4 in diam | 450 |

(Adapted from Smith Kline and French Laboratories)

**The Nibble**    **Approximate mileage to "walk it off"**

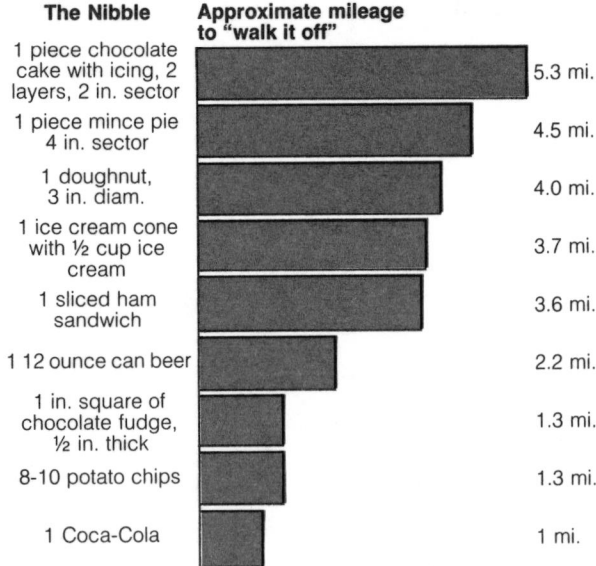

| The Nibble | mileage |
|---|---|
| 1 piece chocolate cake with icing, 2 layers, 2 in. sector | 5.3 mi. |
| 1 piece mince pie 4 in. sector | 4.5 mi. |
| 1 doughnut, 3 in. diam. | 4.0 mi. |
| 1 ice cream cone with ½ cup ice cream | 3.7 mi. |
| 1 sliced ham sandwich | 3.6 mi. |
| 1 12 ounce can beer | 2.2 mi. |
| 1 in. square of chocolate fudge, ½ in. thick | 1.3 mi. |
| 8-10 potato chips | 1.3 mi. |
| 1 Coca-Cola | 1 mi. |

**Fig. 28-2.** Mileage to walk off that nibble. (Peyton AB: Practical Nutrition, 2nd ed. Philadelphia, JB Lippincott; adapted from Hauck HM: How to control your weight. Ithaca, N.Y., New York State College of Home Economics)

nonobese children. In similar work with adults Hirsch and Knittle have shown that those subjects with onset of obesity in childhood had significantly more adipose cells than adults who were not obese and who had never been obese at any time in their lives. Some but not all of these subjects also had more lipid per cell. These researchers have also demonstrated that with significant weight loss there is a significant decrease in adipose cell size due to loss of lipid, but there is not a concomitant loss in numbers of adipose cells.

The data of Hirsch and Knittle are less clear as to whether or not the onset of obesity in adulthood results in an increase in adipose cell size only or an increase in both size and number. The data of Sims and co-workers suggest that the onset of obesity in adults results in an increase in adipose cell size but not in cell number.[12] More recent work indicates that an increase in adipose cell number (hyperplasia) as well as an increase in cell size (hypertrophy) may also occur in adults.[13]

The quantity and quality of adipose tissue in obese children and adults have important metabolic consequences. Many obese adults experience elevated blood glucose levels and excessive quantities of insulin in the blood (hyperinsulinemia) in the fasting and postprandial state.[14] The same metabolic aberrations have also been observed in obese children.[15] The prevalence of these occurrences is not known at this time.

It appears that a significant number of obese subjects with hyperinsulinemia also experience glucose intolerance. Knittle and other investigators suggest that the glucose intolerance is due to an unresponsiveness or resistance to insulin by the muscle and adipose cells. The pathophysiology of this unresponsiveness to insulin is not well understood. The size of the adipose cell in the obese person may be the cause. There is some evidence that the number of insulin receptor sites on the adipose cell membrane of obese people is decreased. Other research suggests that the impairment in insulin action is due to an alteration in intracellular glucose metabolism.[16]

It has been observed that following significant weight loss with reduction of adipose cell size due to loss of lipid the glucose intolerance improves and the blood levels of insulin return to normal. Sims and co-workers observed the development of glucose intolerance and hyperinsulinemia in a group of healthy men of normal weight after a period of high calorie feeding, which led to weight gain and measurable deposition of body fat.[12] When Sims' subjects returned to their usual food practices and lost weight the blood glucose and insulin levels returned to normal.

### Genetics

Genetic factors responsible for the development of obesity have been established in animals but not in humans. It has been observed that identical twins reared in the same environment differ less in weight than do fraternal twins. However, studies show that overweight and obesity tend to exist as a family pattern. Mayer found that 8% to 9% of children of normal weight parents became obese.[17] When one parent is obese, the likelihood of the child's becoming obese is 40%; this proportion rises to 80% when both parents are obese. Also, analysis by Garn and co-workers[18] of the Tecumseh Project data (Examination Round No. 1) indicates that the weight status of adopted children in the population sample is similar to the weight status of the adoptive parents.

### Emotional problems

The contribution of psychological factors to the etiology of obesity varies with each person. In some situations psychological characteristics play little or no role, while in others they are a major factor. In the latter case it is difficult to discover whether the psychological factors cause the obesity or the obesity causes the psychological problems. For example, does the obese adolescent feel worthless because he is obese or does he become obese because he feels worthless? The most comprehensive presentation of the emotional problems of obesity is found in Bruch's book, *Eating Disorders*.[19]

Stunkard and his co-workers have described a so-called night-eating syndrome, which occurs in some gravely obese patients.[20] Such patients eat little during the day, but in the evening and in the early night hours they consume large quantities of food. Some of these patients exhibit symptoms of severe emotional stress when an attempt is made to reduce their weight. The investigators concluded that it might be wiser to allow such patients to remain obese than to precipitate an emotional illness with a weight reduction program.

## Balance between hunger and satiety

In recent years there has been renewed interest in the physiological control of hunger and satiety. Many people maintain a balance between food intake and energy expenditure that keeps their weight comparatively stable over a period of many years. The work of Schachter indicates that eating is triggered by a different set of signals in the obese than in people of normal weight.[21] His experience seems to indicate that in the obese there is no relationship between the state of hunger and eating behavior. Instead, such external factors as smell, sight, taste, and other people's actions determine what and when the obese eat.

Campbell, Hashim, and Van Itallie have studied the responses of lean and obese young adults to variation in the nutrient density of a machine-dispensed liquid diet.[22] They observed that the lean subjects adjusted their intake to maintain weight when, unknown to the subjects, the energy content of the diet was adjusted. In contrast, the obese subjects were not able to adjust intake to physiological need when the nutrient density varied. They consumed the same amount of the diet whether it was diluted or concentrated.

For many years it has been accepted that the lateral and the ventromedial hypothalamus were the regulators of food intake and body weight. The lateral hypothalamus was identified as the "feeding" center and the ventromedial hypothalamus as the "satiety" center, with damage to the feeding center causing aphagia and to the satiety center, hyperphagia. The work of Stricker[23] and of other researchers questions this model. Their work suggests that the neurotransmitters norepinephrine and dopamine are involved in the arousal of hunger and that serotonin is involved in the cessation of hunger.

## Prevention

Successful weight reduction and the maintenance of weight loss are not easily achieved. It is hoped that as more is learned about the causes of obesity, health workers will focus their attention on its prevention at all stages in the life span.

## Infants and children

Prevention of obesity begins with the careful supervision of the feeding of infants and children. The physician and other health workers involved with infants and children can all play a role in prevention. The plotting of accurate weights and lengths on a growth chart combined with a dietary interview of the mother gives clues to the development of weight problems in infants and children. During the first year of life weight and length should be plotted on the infant growth chart every 6 weeks to 2 months, and at least every 6 months during childhood.

Effective nutrition counseling of the mother can correct the problem in its earliest stages. At the same time it must be remembered that the weight status of a child may reflect a problem of mother–child interaction and may not be solely a nutrition problem. Overfeeding in infancy may reflect a mother's inability to differentiate between fussiness and hunger in her infant (see Chap. 35).

For the school aged child the physical education programs in elementary and secondary schools and in youth groups should be directed to helping all boys and girls develop a lifetime pattern of physical activity. The present emphasis on team sports, which provide activity for only a few students, does not always help a person to be active in his adult years. Hiking, bicycle tours, cross-country skiing, tennis, and swimming are just five examples of individual activities (see Table 28-2).

Nutrition education including home economics courses can also focus on the prevention of obesity. The recipes used in foods classes should reflect society's need to control the intake of fats and refined sugar. And biology courses that introduce the role of DNA and RNA in human metabolism should also introduce cellular energy metabolism.

## Adolescents

The adolescent presents a special challenge. This is a period in life when peer group behavior competes with parental advice; food plays an important role in the adolescent's socialization. Overly weight-conscious adolescent girls are prone to try crash dieting to control their weight, while others establish a lifelong pattern of obesity during this period.

## Adults

As adults settle into a routine of daily living in their late 20s and early 30s, if physical activity is limited because of the demands of their employment, a conscious effort should be made to limit energy intake. For many adults this means decreasing their intakes of fats and sugars in such foods as gravies and sauces and high-calorie desserts and snacks, and carefully monitoring their intakes of alcohol and sweetened carbonated bev-

## Table 28-2. Kilocalorie Expenditure for Some Types of Activity

|  | 70-kg Man kcal/hr | 58-kg Woman kcal/hr |
| --- | --- | --- |
| Painting furniture | 200 | 160 |
| Walking (3 mi/hr) | 240 | 190 |
| Skating | 340 | 285 |
| Swimming (2 mi/hr) | 685 | 570 |

erages. For example, a man who maintained his normal weight at age 20 with a daily intake of 3000 calories may find at age 30 he will maintain his weight on 2500 calories (see NAS-NRC RDA, Table 11-1). The Pattern Dietary (Table 22-1) with reasonable additions of food to maintain weight provides a guide.

Both the activity and the time devoted to exercise must be taken into consideration when combined with food intake to control body weight. It is a consistent daily pattern of physical activity rather than occasional vigorous activity that is effective in controlling weight. Table 28-2 shows the calories expended by the 70-kg man (154 lb) or the 58-kg woman (128 lb) in a few activities. It must be noted that these figures apply to a *full* hour of continuous activity. For many adults in our society it is difficult to devote 1 hour every day to some form of physical activity. A conscious effort to increase activity throughout the day may be possible; for example, walking to a nearby grocery store or newspaper vending machine instead of driving the car, or walking up one or two flights of stairs instead of taking the elevator. In the 1980s to conserve one form of energy, one might expend another form of energy by using public transportation, bicycling, or walking. In our society today, however, finding a safe place to walk is often a real problem; many suburban areas have no sidewalks. And bicycling in heavy traffic may also be hazardous.

Controlling weight by diet and exercise is a family affair. Parents have the responsibility for planning and carrying out family activities that promote exercise. The homemaker is often the one who bears the major responsibility for food. If her family has a tendency to gain weight easily or has a family history of diabetes mellitus or coronary artery disease, she will have to pass up the recipes in gourmet cookbooks or in the daily newspaper that require $\frac{1}{2}$ pt of whipping cream, 1 pt of sour cream, 12 oz of cream cheese, or $\frac{1}{2}$ to $\frac{3}{4}$ lb of butter combined with 1 to 2 c of sugar. She can, on the other hand, control calories behind the scene by reducing the fat she uses in food preparation by substituting skim milk for whole milk in sauces and puddings and by broiling rather than frying meat with added fat.

The nutrition counselor in a health maintenance organization or any other health-care agency that focuses on preventive health-care services is responsible for reviewing annually the height, weight, and skinfold thickness status of all adults who entered the health-care plan at their desirable weights. Any adult whose measurements show an increase in body weight of 5 lb or more due to fat during the course of a year should be scheduled for either individual or group counseling and be helped to lose the excess weight. This approach may uncover problems other than excessive food intake, such as emotional problems or the beginning phase of alcoholism.

Whenever a patient enters the hospital for any reason, his height and weight should be measured and recorded as one item in his admission data (see Chap. 23).

Whenever the weight is 5% above ideal weight, the dietitian should identify the cause for this discrepancy in height and weight and, if appropriate, assist this patient to lose weight.

## Dietary treatment

The discussion of the dietary treatment of obesity in this section refers to the adult patient only. Obesity in infants and children is discussed in Chapter 35, *Nutrition in Diseases of Infancy and Childhood*.

## Designing the diet order

The diet order is prescribed by the physician and is designed for the patient. It reflects metabolic needs by height, sex, age, and life-style whenever possible. When life-style *per se* is the cause of obesity it will have to be modified.

### Principle

Since obesity represents the storage of an excess of energy as lipid in adipose cells, the energy intake must be less than the actual daily expenditure of energy if the body is to draw upon and reduce its surplus of energy stores. To maintain the weight loss, *continuous surveillance* of energy intake is required, or the adipose cells will be refilled with excess lipid.

### Determination of present practices

The first step in designing the diet order for an obese patient is to determine how he lives his day, specifically his food and beverage intake and his pattern of physical activity. With the hospitalized patient this information can be obtained, usually by the clinical dietitian, through individual interview (see Chap. 13). The interviewer should schedule $\frac{1}{2}$ to $\frac{3}{4}$ of an hour to collect the information required to appraise the patient's present practices. During the interview, the interviewer can also discover the patient's past experiences with energy-restricted diets, his knowledge of the energy value of foods, and his decision about losing weight. In some hospitals the patient is given a self-administered diet history, which the nutrition counselor reviews with the patient for clarification. This method cannot be used by patients with visual handicaps or by patients who are functional illiterates.

In the ambulatory care setting, more complete information can be obtained by having the patient who is able keep a detailed diary for 1 or 2 weeks. In this diary he should record all his activities of daily living—what he does each hour, when he eats, what and how much he eats, where he eats, with whom he eats, and what he does during mealtime. For example, does he read? watch television? On the patient's return to the ambulatory care facility the nutrition counselor should carefully review the diary with the patient.

With the information gained through the interview combined with a self-administered diet history or diary, one can estimate the energy value of the patient's usual food practices and the level of his physical activity. These estimates of energy intake and physical activity are used to design a diet that should promote weight loss.

## Calories

Considerable difficulty may be encountered in determining the appropriate level of reduced energy intake for a patient. His previous intake may have been underestimated, or his energy expenditure overestimated. Because it is difficult to estimate correctly the quantity of fat in meals or the amounts added to season food, 200 to 300 calories should be added to the estimate of a patient's usual calorie intake to prevent underestimation. For example, if the appraisal of a patient's usual food intake is 2300 calories per day, it is probable that his actual intake is 2500 to 2600 calories.

In theory, without an increase in activity, a deficit in intake of 500 calories per day, compared with previous intake, should promote a weight loss of approximately 1 lb per week. (500 calories × 7 = 3500 calories = 1 lb of fat.) A relatively sedentary obese woman 55 years old and 5 ft 4 in tall, who has been consuming approximately 1700 calories per day, should lose weight on a 1200-calorie diet, while a sedentary obese business executive 35 years old and 6 ft tall, who has been consuming 2500 to 3000 calories should lose weight on a 2000-calorie diet. Unfortunately, the rate of weight loss tends to decrease with the duration of a restricted energy intake because reduced energy intake produces some loss of lean body mass as well as fat. At this point energy expenditure tends to equal energy intake. Therefore, it can be anticipated that a patient may need to reduce his energy intake further to reach his goal.[24]

A deficit of 1000 calories per day should promote a loss of 2 lb per week. It is considered unwise for a person to lose more than 2 pounds per week unless he is under the close supervision of the physician. It is also considered unwise for a patient to attempt to maintain a diet of less than 1000 calories per day unless he is hospitalized.

Some physicians calculate the level of calorie restriction for a patient by multiplying the patient's ideal weight, obtained from a height-weight table, by a factor of 10 calories. For example, the physician would prescribe a 1500-calorie diet for a patient whose ideal weight is 150 pounds.

Regardless of the level of calorie restriction prescribed by the physician, it must be recognized that, through variations in daily food selection and serving size, the actual calorie intake at home will not equal exactly the number of calories ordered. For example, a 1200-calorie diet may vary by chance from 1000 to 1400 calories. Also, physical activity varies from day to day.

## Protein

For adults, 20% of calories from protein is recommended to supply the body's needs for this nutrient in 1000- to 1500-calorie diets (50 g–75 g of protein). Or, the diet may be planned to provide 1 g to $1\frac{1}{2}$ g of protein per kilogram of body weight. In the diet pattern this allows for a more liberal, and usually more satisfying, use of very lean meat, poultry, and fish, and low-fat cheeses.

## Fat and carbohydrate

Since these two nutrients constitute the greatest source of energy in the average diet, they are limited in amount in the energy-restricted diet. The 1200-calorie diet pattern in Table 28-3 derives approximately 20% of its calories from protein, or 68 g of protein; 35% from fat, or 45 g of fat; and approximately 45% from carbohydrate, or 124 g of carbohydrate. The usual 2400-calorie diet with 35% of its calories from fat would contain about 95 g of fat; and with 50% of its calories from carbohydrate, it would contain 300 g of carbohydrate.

There is considerable difference of opinion today whether carbohydrate or fat should be reduced to a minimum in an energy-restricted diet. People have reported significant weight losses in the first few days on a practically carbohydrate-free diet.[25] This is probably a loss of body water since Keys and Grande estimate that each gram of glycogen binds 3 g to 4 g of water.[4] Without carbohydrate in the diet the glycogen stores in the body are reduced and used to maintain normal blood glucose levels, while the bound water and electrolytes are excreted by the kidneys.

## Table 28-3. Nutrient Composition of a 1200-Kilocalorie Diet Pattern

| Food Exchanges* | Number | Household Measure | Protein (g) | Fat (g) | Carbohydrate (g) | Energy (kcal) |
|---|---|---|---|---|---|---|
| Milk, non-fat | 2 | 1 pint | 16 | | 24 | 160 |
| Vegetables | 2 | 1 c | 4 | | 10 | 50 |
| Fruit | 3 | Varies | | | 30 | 120 |
| Bread | 4 | Varies | 8 | | 60 | 280 |
| Meat, lean | 6 | 6 oz | 42 | 18 | | 330 |
| Fat | 5 | 5 tsp | | 25 | | 225 |
| Totals | | | 70 | 43 | 124 | 1165 |

*See Table 24-2.

Practically carbohydrate-free and, therefore, high-protein and high-fat reducing diets, consisting mainly of meat, poultry, fish, eggs, and butter, have been in and out of vogue since Banting published his "Letter on Corpulence" in 1860.[19] Up to the present time no carefully controlled studies have been conducted to prove their worth. The Council of Foods and Nutrition of the American Medical Association reminds us of the hazards of the intake of excessive amounts of saturated fatty acids and cholesterol from a diet of meats and eggs[26] (see Chap. 30). Until well controlled research has proven otherwise, the energy-reduced diet should contain a reasonable distribution of protein, fat, and carbohydrate, so that the energy-controlled diet can serve as a basis for the maintenance diet after weight loss has been achieved.

### Minerals and vitamins

Care should be taken to see that the energy-restricted diet plan provides all the other essentials of a normal diet, such as minerals and vitamins, in quantities at least equivalent to the Recommended Dietary Allowances. If the calorie intake is very restricted (less than 1000 calories), vitamin and mineral supplements are needed.

### Alcohol

One gram of alcohol provides 7 calories. Also, in some alcoholic beverages, such as beer and wines, carbohydrate contributes calories. If these beverages are to be used, their calorie value must be calculated in the energy-restricted diet plan. For some patients the calories from the alcoholic beverages they consume may be the difference between losing and not losing weight (see Table 7, Part 4).

### Water

Water and other nonnutritive fluids are not restricted unless there are heart or kidney complications. Sometimes there is fluid retention prior to menstruation, which may temporarily mask the real loss of body fat in women.

### Food selection and preparation for energy-restricted diets

The following discussion on food selection and preparation is organized around the Exchange System of food groups (see Chap. 24, Tables 24-2 and 24-3) and applies primarily to 1000- to 1500-calorie diets for adults. Much of the information is also applicable to the planning of diets for patients with diabetes or hyperlipoproteinemia (Chaps. 29 and 30), and it will not be repeated in subsequent chapters. Rather, additional information will be given where necessary. In the following discussions of the exchange food groups, the reader is advised to refer to Table 28-3, an example of the food used in a 1200-calorie diet pattern.

### Milk exchange

In the milk exchange group, skim milk (nonfat dried milk solids or fluid) fortified with vitamins A and D is the only item that can be used in a 1000- to 1500-calorie diet pattern. If a patient chooses to have more limited or no fat exchanges calculated in his pattern (see Table 28-3), then 2% or whole milk may be included. One pint of milk should be included to ensure an adequate calcium and riboflavin intake unless the patient selects adequate amounts of leafy green vegetables from vegetable exchange and low-fat cheese from the medium-fat meat exchange food groups. In this case a minimum of $\frac{1}{2}$ pt of skim milk should be included in the diet pattern.

Buttermilk made from skim milk is a possible choice but, if the information is not printed on the carton, the patient must check with local dairies to be sure it is made from skim milk. One-half pint (8 oz) of yogurt made from skim milk can be substituted for $\frac{1}{2}$ pt (8 oz) of skim milk. Sweetened flavored yogurt cannot be substituted for skim milk.

The milk exchanges included in a 1000- to 1500-calorie diet can be used as a beverage, in tea and coffee, as whipped topping sweetened with an artificial sweetener, or in mixed dishes (see section on mixed dishes).

### Vegetable exchange

Vegetables in this food group can be used in amounts as desired by the patient. At levels of 1000 to 1200 calories the amount should be limited to 2 c because amounts in excess of this could contribute an excess of 100 to 150 calories per day depending on the items and amounts selected.

These vegetables may be used raw, as garnishes or in salads, or cooked. Salt, pepper, herbs, low or no-calorie salad dressings, vinegar, or lemon juice may be used to flavor them. Any fat added for flavoring must be the fat included in the diet pattern. The low caloric density of the items in this food group can easily be changed to a higher density by the addition of fat. (1 tsp fat equals 45 calories.) For example, four spears (60 g) of asparagus contains 60 calories, while the same amount of asparagus with 1 tsp of margarine contains 105 calories. It should be pointed out to the patient that corn, a very popular vegetable, lima beans, pumpkin, winter squash, parsnips, and potatoes are listed in the bread exchange food group because of their higher carbohydrate content.

### Fruit exchange

The serving size of the items in the fruit exchange food group identifies the amount of fruit that contains 10 g of carbohydrate. These are fresh fruits served or processed without added sugar. Most of the canned fruits in the diet section of supermarkets today have been canned in unsweetened fruit juice and contain approximately 12 g of carbohydrate per serving, not the 10 g as listed in Table 24-3. Depending on frequency of use, fruits canned in light syrup can be used if they are well drained and the syrup is not used. However, the sugar penetrates into the fruit, and these fruits contain more carbohydrate per serving than either fresh or dietetic canned fruit. Many older patients prefer canned fruits, and in some small communities a wide variety of fresh fruits is not available throughout the year. Also, the cost of fresh fruits at certain times of the year often prohibits the use of three or four servings per day.

At least one serving of fruit should be included in the diet pattern with emphasis placed on the selection of a fruit that is a good source of vitamin C. If the patient prefers vegetables and selects two or three items, such as tomatoes and cabbage, from the vegetable exchange and potatoes from the bread exchange food group each day, he may have an adequate intake of vitamin C without a serving of fruit.

## Bread exchange

The serving sizes of the items listed in the bread exchange food group vary considerably. One slice of bread refers to the usual slice, which weighs approximately 23 g. One and one-third slices of diet bread, which weighs 18 g per slice, are equal in calories to one slice of bread weighing 23 g.

The biscuits, muffins, and cornbread listed in the bread exchanges are products made from standard home-style recipes, not the mixes widely available in the supermarket. The recipes used by patients who frequently make these hot breads should be checked for the amount of fat and sugar included. Some cooks make tender biscuits, muffins, or cornbread because they add more fat than stated in the recipe.

The use of a wider variety of crackers than listed in the bread exchange food group may be possible if the package includes a nutrient label. However, the amount of fat listed on the nutrient label must be checked in order to avoid a daily intake of fat in excess of 35% of the total calories.

The vegetables, potatoes, dried beans, and pasta listed in the bread exchange food group are prepared and served without added fat. If any fat is added to these items, it must be some of the fat included in the diet pattern. Some patients use part of the milk and margarine in their diet patterns to season mashed potatoes. Others remove the contents of a baked potato, mix it with some of their milk and margarine, return the mixture to the shell, and reheat the stuffed baked potato. French fried, pan fried or hash brown potatoes are excluded because these methods of preparation call for more fat than can be included in a 1000- to 1500-calorie diet pattern.

## Meat exchange (medium-fat)

Any serving of meat, poultry, or fish must be prepared and served without the addition of *any* fat, and no visible fat should be eaten. Only lean meats should be selected, for example, ground beef with less than 20% fat. The patient must be counseled to bake, broil, braise, or pan fry meat, poultry, and fish without adding fat and to drain off carefully all fat after cooking. If lean meat exchanges rather than medium-fat meat exchanges (see Table 24-3) are used, $\frac{1}{2}$ fat exchange may be added to the 3 fat exchanges calculated in the 1200-kcal diet pattern in Table 28-3.

The most efficient way to remove fat from the juices that collect when meat is roasted is to add a small amount of water to dissolve all the material in the bottom of the pan, put this fluid in a container, and to refrigerate overnight. The next day the hardened fat can be removed and discarded and the remaining juice, now fat-free, can be seasoned and heated to be served with meat or to season vegetables. This juice can also be used to make a gravy thickened with flour but without added fat. Two and one-half tbs of flour are equivalent to one bread exchange. Two and one-half tbs of presifted flour thicken 1 to 2 c of liquid. One-fourth c of this gravy contains approximately 20 calories compared with 100 or more calories in $\frac{1}{4}$ c of gravy made with flour and fat.

Eggs, cottage cheese, and low-fat cheese, but not cheddar or processed cheese or cheese spread, can be used as meat exchanges unless blood lipid levels indicate that their use should be restricted. For example, in a person with an elevated blood cholesterol level, eggs may be excluded or limited to no more than three per week.

## Fat exchange

For many obese clients the items selected from this food group should be limited to those made from oils and fats with a significant amount of polyunsaturated fatty acids. The items in the fat exchange list that fit this criterion are margarine and mayonnaise or French dressing made with vegetable oils—safflower, soy, or corn oils. This limitation is recommended since many obese persons demonstrate abnormalities of lipid, as well as of glucose, metabolism (see Chap. 30).

## Mixed dishes

The amounts of food in a diet pattern may be combined in mixed dishes. For example, if a person selected three meat exchanges, one vegetable exchange, and one bread exchange for his evening meal, he could combine in a casserole dish 3 oz cooked lean stew beef, $\frac{1}{2}$ cup mixed onions and carrots, and $\frac{1}{2}$ cup cooked rice. Herbs and other seasoning can be added as desired.

A number of cookbooks that give the exchange values of one serving of a recipe are available. Patients who are interested and skilled in food preparation often find that these cookbooks help relieve the monotony of an energy-restricted diet. A list of these cookbooks is included at the end of this chapter.

### Convenience foods

The majority of convenience foods, such as TV dinners, precooked frozen meats in gravy, and frozen vegetables in butter or other sauces cannot be used in energy-restricted diets. Exceptions to this list are the calorie-restricted TV dinners, which give the calorie and nutrient value per dinner on the label; they are available in most supermarkets.

It is possible that in the future with the increasing use of nutrient labeling by food manufacturers more convenience foods can be used. However, one is cautioned to check the distribution of nutrients in these products so that the total fat in the diet does not exceed 35% of the total calories in the diet order, even though calories in excess of the diet order are not consumed.

### Dietetic foods

With the exception of saccharin for sweetening beverages and other foods and an unsweetened gelatin dessert (D'Zerta), there are very few other "diet foods" that can be used in an energy-restricted diet. (See the discussion of dietetic foods in Chapter 24.)

### Planning the energy-restricted diet pattern

The clinical dietitian will need a form on which to calculate a client's diet pattern. Figure 28-3 is one example of a form for calculation. A copy of the calculation should be included in the client's medical record and a new one added whenever the pattern is revised so that other members of the health-care team have access to the plan.

### Step 1

The first step in calculating an energy-restricted diet pattern is to identify those items from the client's diet history which can be included in the pattern. For example, if a client usually has fruit juice, toast, and coffee for breakfast, his energy-restricted diet pattern will contain fruit and bread exchanges in the breakfast pattern.

The serving size or method of preparation of the foods as reported in the diet history may need to be modified when calculated in the energy-restricted diet pattern. Eight ounces of orange juice may be modified to 4 oz; French toast served with butter and syrup may be modified to one egg poached in water and served on unbuttered toast; and coffee with sugar and cream may be modified to coffee with saccharin and some of the skim milk calculated in the pattern.

### Step 2

The second step is to complete the calculation of the energy-restricted pattern with the client. The calories should be distributed reasonably in three meals. If the client wishes, a bedtime snack can be calculated. A pattern that provides one-half or more of the calories in one meal should be avoided, especially if the individual has hyperinsulinemia, because the quantity of insulin secreted is related to the quantity of food consumed at a meal.

Table 28-4 illustrates the nutrient composition of a 1200-calorie diet pattern, and Table 28-5 shows how the 1200 calories were distributed in three meals and a bedtime snack. This pattern was calculated with a 50 year old woman who was 30 lb above her ideal weight and who was limited in activity because of arthritis in one hip. This client preferred fruit juice and cereal with milk at breakfast; a salad and fruit at noontime; and meat, vegetables,

| PT. NAME _____ DIET_____ | | | | | | | | | | | | | | | |
|---|---|---|---|---|---|---|---|---|---|---|---|---|---|---|---|
| INSULIN _____ | | | | | | | | | | | | | | | |
| MEALS: | AMT. | P | F | C | kcal | AMT. | P | F | C | kcal | AMT. | P | F | C | kcal |
| MILK | | | | | | | | | | | | | | | |
| VEG. | | | | | | | | | | | | | | | |
| FRUIT | | | | | | | | | | | | | | | |
| BREAD | | | | | | | | | | | | | | | |
| MEAT | | | | | | | | | | | | | | | |
| FAT | | | | | | | | | | | | | | | |
| SUB-TOTAL | (M) | | | | | (N) | | | | | (E) | | | | |
| BETWEEN MEALS | | | | | | | | | | | | | | | |
| | | | | | | | | | | | | | | | |
| SUB-TOTAL | (IO) | | | | | (2) | | | | | (HS) | | | | |
| TOTALS    P          F          C          kcal | | | | | | | | | | | | | | | |

**Fig. 28-3.** Form for calculating diet patterns (8 x 5 Kardex card).

and salad at the evening meal, which she eats with her husband. The major modifications in her usual food practices were the omission of desserts, frequent snacks of cookies and candy during the day, and a sandwich at bedtime.

Table 28-6 shows a 1500-calorie diet pattern calculated with a young businessman who was 20 lb overweight. In addition to decreasing his daily energy intake, he also increased his energy expenditure by walking 10 blocks to work each morning.

## Counseling the obese individual

### Approaches to the patient

In 1960, Feinstein reviewed the literature of the treatment of obesity published in professional journals from 1940 to 1959.[27] He carried out a critical analysis of the methods used and the results obtained by numerous investigators. From his analysis of various approaches to the treatment of obese patients, he concluded that successful weight reduction involves the interaction of three sets of factors: the patient himself; the therapeutic relationship between patient and clinician; and the dietary program. The patient himself and the therapeutic relationship appeared to be the most significant factors, while the type of energy-restricted diet program was of lesser significance in promoting successful weight reduction.

The evidence available to Feinstein demonstrated that any obese patient could lose weight on an energy-restricted diet with varying proportions of protein, fat, and carbohydrate, with or without therapeutic adjuncts, such as appetite-depressant drugs, in an environment that restricted the patient's access to food, usually the hospital environment. Comparable success was not observed in patients being treated in an ambulatory care setting.

Since the restriction of the obese patient to hospitalization for treatment is unrealistic and expensive, Feinstein pointed out the patient characteristics that are related to success in any setting. A few obese patients are capable of losing weight when they decide to do so and are provided with the information that helps them to control their food intake. On the other hand, the majority of obese patients, even though they are knowledgeable about the energy value of foods, are unable to resist food intake. Within this category of obese patients there are two subgroups—one, the smaller of the two, requires psychiatric help because they are truly compulsive eaters; and the

## Table 28-4. 1200-Kilocalorie Diet Pattern (3 meals and a bedtime snack)

| Meal | Food Exchanges | Number | Protein (g) | Fat (g) | Carbohydrate (g) | Energy (kcal) |
|------|----------------|--------|-------------|---------|------------------|---------------|
| Morning | Fruit | 1 | | | 10 | 40 |
| | Bread | 1 | 2 | | 15 | 70 |
| | Milk, non-fat | 1 | 8 | | 12 | 80 |
| | Fat | 1 | | 5 | | 45 |
| | Total | | 10 | 5 | 37 | 235 |
| Noon | Meat, lean | 2 | 14 | 6 | | 110 |
| | Vegetable | 1 | 2 | | 5 | 25 |
| | Bread | 1 | 2 | | 15 | 70 |
| | Fruit | 1 | | | 10 | 40 |
| | Fat | 1 | | 5 | | 45 |
| | Total | | 18 | 11 | 30 | 290 |
| Evening | Meat, lean | 4 | 28 | 12 | | 220 |
| | Vegetable | 2 | 4 | | 10 | 50 |
| | Bread | 1 | 2 | | 15 | 70 |
| | Fruit | 1 | | | 10 | 40 |
| | Fat | 2 | | 10 | | 90 |
| | Total | | 34 | 22 | 35 | 470 |
| Bedtime | Milk, non-fat | 1 | 8 | | 12 | 80 |
| | Bread | 1 | 2 | | 15 | 70 |
| | Fat | 1 | | 5 | | 45 |
| | Total | | 10 | 5 | 27 | 195 |
| | Totals | | 72 | 43 | 129 | 1190 |

## Table 28-5. Suggested Menu— 1200 Kilocalorie Diet

**Breakfast**

½ cup unsweetened orange juice
½ cup cornflakes
½ cup non-fat milk
Coffee, black or with non-fat milk and saccharin

**Noon Meal**

Tuna salad plate
    2 ounces water-packed tuna
    1 teaspoon mayonnaise
    ½ cup mixture of cucumber wedges marinated in
      herb vinegar, tomato wedges, and celery curls
    salad greens
6 rye rounds
1 cup fresh strawberries
Coffee, black or with non-fat milk and saccharin

**Evening Meal**

4 ounces lean roast beef
½ cup carrots flavored with 1 teaspoon margarine
½ cup green salad with no-calorie dressing
Fruit cup parfait—½ cup of fruit cup canned
  without sugar in D'Zerta with whipped
  unsweetened non-fat milk topping

**Bedtime Snack**

8 ounces non-fat milk
6 rye rounds
1 teaspoon margarine

other, the majority of obese patients, do not have severe psychiatric problems yet have difficulty depriving themselves of food.

Feinstein points out that an external source of motivation may be the decisive factor in assisting the majority of obese patients to lose weight. The external source of motivation for many of these individuals is a continuing therapeutic relationship with a clinician. Feinstein identified the clinician as the physician or other person with an adequate knowledge of the energy values of foods and the ability to establish a positive relationship with the client. Feinstein emphasized that the clinician must see the patient frequently, or, as it is described today, there must be "continuity of care;" and that the clinician must be accepting of the patient's needs and problems.

Regarding the third factor, the dietary program, Feinstein pointed out that his data demonstrate that any patient will lose weight if he controls energy intake adequately and that some patients are more successful with unusual diet programs, such as liquid formulas or limited choices of foods.

Bruch's book, *Eating Disorders*, reinforces many of Feinstein's conclusions. Bruch points out:

> Among the many factors that need to be evaluated before a reducing regimen is prescribed, there is no one aspect more important than the patient's motive for wanting to lose weight, or conversely, for not being interested in it.[28]

In addition, Bruch shows from her experience that there are those patients who prefer to be obese and who meet the stresses of daily living more successfully when they are obese.[29]

Since Feinstein's review of the literature, self-help organizations such as TOPS (Take Off Pounds Sensibly) and Weight Watchers have been organized. The participants in these groups have had varying success in achieving and maintaining weight reduction, but this approach has not proved any more effective than the client-clinician approach.

Behavior modification as an approach to helping obese patients was first reported in the literature in the early 1970s.[30] The researchers view excessive eating leading to obesity as an overlearned habit, which is a strongly conditioned response to external and internal stimuli. The stimuli are emotional factors, such as loneliness, boredom, and anxiety-producing interpersonal relationships, not hunger. The goal of behavior modification is to extinguish the stimuli that lead to overeating and to enable patients to respond to the physiological stimulus of hunger to achieve an appropriate food intake.[31] The approach appears to be more effective in changing eating patterns than traditional nutrition counseling. However, there are people who do not respond,[31,32] and more research is needed.

## Table 28-6. Nutrient Composition of a 1500-Kilocalorie Diet Pattern

| Food Exchanges* | Number | Household Measure | Protein (g) | Fat (g) | Carbohydrate (g) | Energy (kcal) |
|---|---|---|---|---|---|---|
| Milk, non-fat | 2 | 1 pint | 16 | | 24 | 160 |
| Vegetable | 1 | ½ c | 2 | | 5 | 25 |
| Fruit | 3 | Varies | | | 30 | 120 |
| Bread | 7 | Varies | 14 | | 105 | 490 |
| Meat, medium fat | 6 | 6 oz | 42 | 30 | | 450 |
| Fat | 6 | 6 tsp | | 30 | | 270 |
| Totals | | | 76 | 60 | 164 | 1515 |

*See Table 24-2.

From the evidence available today, the person who is most likely to lose weight successfully:

1. Is slightly to moderately above a desirable weight for him, due to excess adipose tissue
2. Gained weight as an adult
3. Never attempted to lose weight as an adult
4. Is well adjusted emotionally
5. Accepts weight reduction as a realistic goal.[33]

### The nutrition counselor's role

The first responsibility of the nutrition counselor, as in any counseling situation, is to establish communication with the client so that together they can explore all aspects of the problem, and he can arrive at his own decision to lose weight and maintain his weight loss. This implies that the counselor must accept the client and his problem and be willing to help, not ridicule, him. In other words, the counselor must establish a helping relationship with the client (see Chap. 13). If the clinical dietitian wants to use behavior modification with obese patients, either individually or in groups, it is strongly advised that a clinical psychologist with expertise in this methodology work closely with the dietitian.

Within this relationship the counselor is responsible for assisting the patient to plan a diet pattern compatible with his life-style and the constraints of the diet order, thus enabling him to achieve a level of knowledge of the energy composition of foods so that his food choices will be consistent with his goal to lose weight. This includes such instructional aids as pamphlets, cookbooks, and, if necessary, a scale to help him become familiar with the weights of portions of food. Together with the physician and physical therapist, the clinical dietitian should help the client design and establish an exercise program compatible with the client's health status and life-style.

## Other approaches to weight reduction
### Starvation regimens

In 1964 Drenick and co-workers reported on the use of starvation to promote weight reduction.[34] Water and other noncaloric fluids together with vitamin and mineral supplements are used during the starvation period. The body conserves glucose to meet the metabolic needs of the brain by using adipose triglyceride and muscle protein to meet its energy needs. Ketoacidosis rarely occurs, but the increase in purine degradation to uric acid when muscle protein is used for fuel can result in gout, an abnormality of uric acid metabolism.

During fasting, weight loss is rapid, averaging 1 lb to 3 lb per day. Hospitalized patients appear to tolerate this approach for periods of 30 days or more. However, long-term follow-up reports of patients who have used this regimen indicate that weight loss is not easily maintained, and that it is no more effective than other approaches to the treatment of obesity.[35] It should never be self-administered and should be carried out only in a hospital setting where medical personnel can monitor the patient's clinical progress. Episodes of hypoglycemia with loss of consciousness can occur.

### Formula diets

Liquid formula diets fortified with vitamins and minerals are now available in most supermarkets. They contain approximately 225 calories per 8-oz serving; and four 8-oz servings per day yield 900 calories. Their advantage lies in the fact that they provide a specific number of calories per serving; their disadvantage lies in the monotony of a bland liquid diet.

Some people have found it helpful to use the formula diet for one meal a day and to eat a calorie-restricted diet at other meals. These formulas, generally made from nonfat dry skim milk with vitamins and minerals added, are relatively expensive.

### Protein-sparing modified fasts

This method of weight reduction is based on the theory that the consumption of protein alone reduces the loss of lean body mass, which occurs in total starvation and forces the body to mobilize fat from the adipose tissues for energy.[36] Theoretically the decrease in weight is due to the loss of water and adipose tissue, not lean body mass. However, metabolic balance studies do not support the theory that body protein is spared. For example, Lantigua and co-workers[37] reported that during a protein-sparing modified fast of 40 days their subjects lost an average of 2.25 g of nitrogen per day. Protein-sparing modified fast clinics, using proteins of high biological value to provide 300 to 400 calories per day, were established throughout the United State in the mid 1970s and reported[38] that under careful professional guidance obese persons were successful in losing significant amounts of weight on this regimen, averaging a loss of 2 lb to 3 lb per week. At the same time liquid and powdered protein products became available in drug and other stores. Although the producers strongly advised the consumer to use these products under the supervision of a physician, many people used them without professional guidance.

In 1977 the Center for Disease Control[39] reported the occurrence of 40 deaths associated with the use of very low protein diets for weight reduction. All had died suddenly of cardiac irregularities. Analyses of the consumer products showed that they contained an unbalanced amino acid distribution or had a low chemical score or both.[40] In 1978 the American Dietetic Association[41] stated that the liquid protein modified fast products should not be recommended for general use. Deaths due to cardiac irregularities have also been reported in patients on protein-sparing modified fasts under professional guidance.[42]

Lantigua[37] using a widely available, commercial liquid protein product, observed potentially life-threatening cardiac irregularities in subjects who were carefully monitored in a clinical research unit. These metabolic balance studies failed to reveal a cause of the irregularities. These workers strongly "recommend that the use of liquid protein diets should be terminated pending further investigation of the causes and the prevention of the cardiac toxicity."[37]

### Anorexigenic agents

The amphetamines and other drugs have been used to promote weight loss. They depress appetite, but it has been observed that their effectiveness decreases after about 6 weeks of use. In increasing doses they have unpleasant side effects. In the obese person who also has cardiac disease these drugs are dangerous. Anorexigenic drugs should be taken only under the supervision of the physician. With the recent abuse of amphetamines, physicians today rarely prescribe these drugs for obese patients.

### Hormones

Thyroid hormone has been used as an adjunct to diet therapy on the grounds that obese patients are in a hypometabolic state and need this metabolic stimulant if weight loss is to be accomplished. When a person has hypothyroidism, hormone preparations are required to achieve a weight loss. For obese patients with normal thyroid function—the majority of patients—thyroid hormone can be dangerous.

Injections of human chorionic gonadotrophin, a glycoprotein hormone produced by the trophoblasts of the placenta, have been used to treat obese women. In work with rats it has been observed that this hormone decreases the level of enzymes involved in fatty acid synthesis. The reports of clinical trials with humans are equivocal, and its future as an agent in the treatment of obesity is uncertain at this time.

### Diuretics and laxatives

The indiscriminate use of diuretics and laxatives, which promote fluid loss, may give the patient a false sense of accomplishment when he weighs himself. His weight loss reflects a water loss, not a decrease in adipose tissue. Only when the physician observes abnormal fluid retention in a patient should a diuretic be part of the patient's therapy.

Obese patients have used excessive amounts of laxatives to promote malabsorption of nutrients. This is usually achieved by taking a laxative after every meal. This practice not only interferes with the absorption of nutrients by increasing the transit time of food in the gastrointestinal tract but also can lead to fluid and electrolyte imbalance due to the diarrhea-type stools caused by the laxative.

### Surgical treatment in morbid obesity

Morbid obesity refers to a weight status of two to three times the ideal weight (200 lb to 300 lb or more), which has been maintained in spite of all efforts to reduce it by conventional treatment. The four surgical procedures presently used are jejunoileal bypass;[43] gastric bypass;[44] gastroplasty;[45] and gastric partitioning.[46] The first procedure reduces the absorptive surface of the small intestine and produces weight loss by malabsorption. The other three procedures reduce the size of the gastric reservoir to approximately 50 ml and produce weight loss by restricting the amount of food and fluid that can be consumed at any one feeding.

In the jejunoileal bypass, approximately 14 in of the proximal jejunum is anastomosed to the terminal 4 in of the ileum; the remainder of the jejunum and ileum is left *in situ*[47] so that continuity of the small intestine can be reestablished if necessary. Approximately 85% of the patients who have jejunoileal bypass operations lose about 35% of their preoperative weight[48] and reach a plateau at this level in 2 to 3 years postoperatively. All patients have diarrhea, which can be controlled by reducing fat intake, avoiding excessive quantities of sucrose and sometimes lactose, and taking calcium carbonate daily. Generally, patients seem to control the diarrhea by consuming less food postoperatively than preoperatively, avoiding snacking throughout the day, and distributing intake equally among three meals.[49,50]

Although the actual frequency is not known,[51] numerous metabolic complications have been reported in patients who have had jejunoileal bypass surgery. The most common complications appear to be fluid and electrolyte imbalance caused by the diarrhea, hepatic disease,[52] hyperoxaluria with renal calculi,[53] and bone disease probably due to mineral and vitamin malabsorption.[54] Low serum vitamin $B_{12}$ levels and deficiency of trace metals have also been reported.[55]

Reduction of the gastric reservoir is being studied in the hope that it will result in weight loss without the complications of the bypass procedure. Upon resumption of oral intake postoperatively, fluids restricted to 60 ml per feeding are used to avoid perforation of the stomach with peritonitis due to acute dilation.[44] The feedings then progress to restricted quantities of blenderized foods and then to solid foods, still in restricted volume per serving. Further research is needed to evaluate the efficacy of the gastric reservoir procedures.

## Underweight

*Underweight*, like overweight, is a relative term, being based on the ideal weight for a given height, build, and sex. Weight more than 10% below the ideal is usually considered to be abnormal, especially in persons under 25, and is worthy of medical investigation.

Leanness or underweight may be due to an inadequate energy intake, to excessive bodily activity, or to both; it may also be familial. Physical disease, such as malignancy, gastrointestinal disorders, chronic infectious disease, or such endocrine disturbances as hyperthyroidism, may be a cause of progressive weight loss (see Chap. 34).

Underweight due to an inadequate caloric intake may be a serious condition, especially in the young. Resistance to infection, particularly to tuberculosis, may be lowered; and the occurrence of the complications of pregnancy in young women may result from malnutrition due to an inadequate energy intake.

### Nutritional care of the underweight patient

Table 28-7 shows the kinds of foods used to increase calorie intake. Reasonable goals that take into consideration the person's age, height, and previous weight status must be set with each underweight patient. For example, a high-calorie diet for a 5 ft 4 in 40-year-old woman may be 2500 calories, while a high-calorie diet for a 6 ft 3 in 19-year-old boy may be 3500 calories.

The diet must be built up gradually or else the person may not be able to tolerate the sudden increase. Care must be taken to ascertain his likes and dislikes and to prepare and serve the food as appetizingly as possible. Above all, he must be encouraged to accept the necessity for his cooperating by consuming all food served to him.

Some guidelines for assisting the underweight person are

1. An adequate diet as described in Chapter 11.
2. Adequate energy intake that may be obtained by increasing the quantity of food eaten at each meal; increasing the carbohydrate and, to some extent, the fat intake; and adjusting the frequency of feedings. For some this last recommendation may be achieved by offering nourishments between meals, for others it may be more appropriate to offer a hearty bedtime snack of a sandwich or a dessert plus a beverage.
3. One g to 1.5 g of protein per kilogram of body weight to combat any previous inadequate intake.
4. Adequate intake of vitamins and minerals.
5. Reduction in bulk from excessive servings of fruits and vegetables in favor of foods with more concentrated energy value. Low-calorie soups, salads, and beverages should not be eaten at the beginning of a meal, as they tend to give temporary satiety and to diminish appetite for the more substantial part of the meal.
6. Easily digested foods. Carbohydrate is both easily digested and quickly converted into body fat. Foods rich in fat may be used to increase the energy value without unduly increasing bulk, but they must be used with discretion. Fat-rich foods lessen the appetite of many patients because they delay gastric emptying, and too much fat in any form is frequently distasteful unless cleverly disguised. The uncooked fats, such as cream, butter, and salad oils, are usually better tolerated than the fat in fried foods.

## Anorexia nervosa

Anorexia nervosa is a physiological disorder that derives from psychological problems. It occurs most frequently but not exclusively in adolescent girls, and in the past few years the incidence has been increasing rapidly.[56] It manifests itself as self-induced starvation resulting in marked cachexia and severe metabolic defects. If not treated, the starvation leads to death. The term, *anorexia*, is not truly descriptive of the problem. The patient does not lose her appetite. Rather she does not permit herself to eat. At the same time there is a tendency towards compulsive physical activity and a preoccupation with food. Amenorrhea is also a frequent finding in the anorexic patient. Many of the patients are expert calorie

### Table 28-7.  Kinds of Foods Used for Increased Energy Intake

*Principles*

1. High in caloric value: 25–50% above normal
2. High in protein: 90–100 g for adults
3. High in vitamins, especially in the vitamin B complex
4. Nourishment may be served between meals and before retiring

*Foods Used*

Milk
  Milk and yogurt
Cheese
  All kinds
Fats
  Butter and margarine; all other fats
Eggs
  Cooked in all ways
Meats, fish, and fowl
  All varieties; bacon and fat meats are indicated if the patient tolerates them
Soups
  Preferably creamed or thick soups
Bread, cereals, macaroni products
  All kinds; preferably whole grain or enriched
Vegetables
  All vegetables, including potatoes
Salads
  All kinds; oil dressings especially desirable
Fruits
  All fresh and cooked fruits and juices, jellies, jams, and marmalades
Desserts
  Ice cream, custards, tapioca and rice puddings, cake, fruit desserts, other desserts
Beverages
  Tea, coffee, cocoa; served with cream and sugar; fruit juices; malted preparations
Vitamin concentrates
  If ordered by the physician

counters and frequently place themselves on 600- to 900-calorie diets. For example, one 16 year old high school girl whose ideal weight was 104 lb consistently consumed 900 calories per day. She weighed 76 lb when seen by the physician.

The typical patient is a teenage girl. Prior to the onset of their illness many have been overweight and were teased or ridiculed about their weight status by family, friends, or teachers. Parents usually report that in the past the patient was cooperative and easy to get along with. Silverman describes the behavior of these patients at the time they come to medical treatment for significant weight loss as greedy, envious, narcissistic, and with desire to control the family.[57] Dally has noted in his series of patients that the major emotional problem is a poor mother–daughter relationship.[58] Patients may also exhibit binge eating, self-induced vomiting, a distorted body image, and a fear of physical maturation.

In addition to marked underweight (10%–50% of previous weight), Silverman has observed that a significant number of his 29 subjects exhibited dry, scaly skin, abnormal glucose tolerance tests (either a diabetic type or a flat curve), and elevated blood urea nitrogen (BUN) levels. The elevated BUN probably reflects an inadequate fluid intake in most instances, and the flat glucose tolerance curve probably functional malabsorption.

The treatment of the anorexia nervosa patient requires the intensive intervention of both medical and psychiatric personnel. The representatives of these two disciplines must work closely together. They establish their approach to treatment and must orient the other health disciplines, such as nursing and dietetics, to their treatment plan because these patients act in a manipulative way toward all staff. For the benefit of the patient, all the staff involved must consistently exhibit the same behavior in their contacts with her. For example, for the care of his patients when they are admitted to the hospital, Silverman has a very precise routine, which the staff together with him must implement without any variations. One of his requirements is that the patient drink a minimum of 1 liter of calorie-containing fluids each day.

In some situations it is necessary to institute tube feeding as a first step in treatment in order to correct fluid and electrolyte imbalance and to begin nutritional rehabilitation. One should begin with a dilute feeding and increase the caloric density as tolerated (see discussion of tube feedings, Chapter 27). An estimation of energy and nutrient intake should be recorded daily in the patient's medical record. It is interesting to note that Dally has observed that as these patients improve they talk freely about food and frequently request recipes and other instruction in food preparation.

Anorexia nervosa is an example of a nutritional problem that is secondary to another problem—in this case an emotional one. As Silverman has demonstrated, psychiatric as well as medical therapy is required if these patients are to achieve and maintain a reasonable weight status. Recently success has been reported with an approach that focuses on the use of family therapy and early intervention.[59]

## Study questions and activities

1. In conversation with adult patients ask each patient to recall what he or she weighed at age 12, 18, 25, 35, 45, and 55. For some patients it will be easier for them to relate weight to some event in their lives—for example, graduation from high school, the time of marriage, induction into the armed forces, or, the time of birth of the first baby. Do any of these patients illustrate: normal weight over their life span thus far; obesity throughout their life span; obesity which developed during their adult years?

2. In conversation with adult patients discover what foods they consider "fattening." In clinical conference with your classmates and instructor discuss these ideas.

3. Calculate a 1500-calorie diet pattern for yourself. For 3 days, use this pattern to select your foods for each meal. Record all food and beverages you consume each day. Appraise the caloric value of each day's intake. In clinical conference with your instructor discuss the problems you met and your feelings about "counting" calories each day.

4. Make an appointment to accompany the clinical dietitian when she conducts the diet interview and when she gives diet instruction to an obese patient. Observe and talk with this patient at one mealtime for at least 3 days and report your observations to the dietitian. Summarize this experience and with the dietitian report to your classmates in clinical conference.

5. How were today's weight tables established? What criteria were used?

6. Why is obesity considered a public health problem?

7. What is the direct cause of overweight? What are some of the factors which play a role in the development of obesity?

8. What role does exercise play in weight control? What factors militate today against maintaining desirable weight?

9. What are the criteria for successful weight reduction?

10. In teaching a patient, what should be the attitude of the nutrition counselor?

11. What are some methods of weight control besides food limitation? Why are most of these considered dangerous?

12. How can an underweight patient be helped to gain weight?

## References

1. Van Itallie TB: Am J Clin Nutr (Suppl)32:2723, 1979

2. Cooper LF et al: Nutrition in Health and Disease, 7th ed. Philadelphia, JB Lippincott, 1940

3. Sheldon W et al: Varieties of Human Physique. New York, Harper, 1940

4. Keys A, Grande F et al: In Goodhart RS, Shils ME (eds): Modern Nutrition in Health and Disease, 5th ed. pp 1–27. Philadelphia, Lea & Febiger, 1973

5. Bray GA et al: Am J Clin Nutr 31:769, 1978

6. National Center for Health Statistics: Dietary Intake Findings, United States 1971–1974. Series 11, No. 202. DHEW Publ. No. (PHS) 77-1647, 1977

7. Mayer J: In Goodhart and Shils, Modern Nutrition, pp 625–644

8. Ten-State Nutrition Survey, 1968–1970. III. Clinical Anthropometry, Dental. DHEW Publ. No. (HSM) 72-8131, 1972

9. Abraham S, Johnson CL: Am J Clin Nutr (Suppl)33:364, 1980

10. Webb P et al: Am J Clin Nutr 33:1287, 1299, 1980

11. Hirsch J, Knittle JL: Fed Proc 29:1516, 1970

12. Sims, EAH et al: Annu Rev Med 22:235, 1971

13. Hirsch J, Batchelor B: Clin Endocrinol Metab 5:299, 1976

14. Olefsky JM: Am J Med 70:151, 1981

15. Martin MM, Martin LA: Pediatrics 82:192, 1974

16. Salans LB: In Bray GA (ed): Obesity in America, pp 69–102. DHEW-NIH Publ. No. 80-359, 1980

17. Mayer J: Am J Clin Nutr 9:530, 1961

18. Garn SM et al: Am J Clin Nutr 29:1067, 1976

19. Bruch H: Eating Disorders. New York, Basic Books, 1973

20. Stunkard A et al: Am J Med 19:78, 1955

21. Schachter S: Science 161:751, 1968

22. Campbell RG et al: N Engl J Med 285:1402, 1971

23. Stricker EM: N Engl J Med 298:1010, 1978

24. Stuart RB et al: J Am Diet Assoc 75:258, 1979

25. Van Itallie TB, Yang MU: N Engl J Med 297:1158, 1977

26. Council on Food and Nutrition: JAMA 224:1415, 1973

27. Feinstein A: J Chronic Dis 11:349, 1960

28. Bruch H: Eating Disorders, p 325

29. Bruch H: Am J Clin Nutr 5:192, 1957

30. Jordan HA, Levitz LS: J Am Diet Assoc 62:27, 1973

31. Leon GR: Am J Clin Nutr 30:785, 1977

32. Stunkard AJ: In Bray, Obesity in America, pp 206–240

33. Young CM: Am J Clin Nutr 8:896, 1960

34. Drenick EJ et al: JAMA 187:100, 1964

35. Johnson D, Drenick EJ: Arch Intern Med 137:1381, 1977

36. Flatt JP, Blackburn GL: Am J Clin Nutr 27:175, 1974

37. Lantigua RA et al: N Engl J Med 303:735, 1980

38. Vertes V et al: JAMA 238:2151, 1977

39. Center for Disease Control: Morbidity and Mortality Weekly Report 26:383, 1977

40. Marable NL et al: J Am Diet Assoc 77:270, 1980

41. American Dietetic Association: Statement on diet protein products. J Am Diet Assoc 73:547, 1978

42. Isner JM et al: Circulation 60:1401, 1979

43. O'Leary JP: Am J Clin Nutr (Suppl)33:389, 1980

44. Mason EE et al: Am J Clin Nutr (Suppl)33:395, 1980

45. Gomez CA: Am J Clin Nutr (Suppl)33:406, 1980

46. Pace WG et al: Ann Surg 190:392, 1979

47. Palmer JA, Marliss EB: In Deitel M (ed): Nutrition in Clinical Surgery, pp 281–292. Baltimore, Williams & Wilkins, 1980

48. Iber FL, Cooper M: Am J Clin Nutr 30:4, 1977

49. Rauen MN, Tseng RYL: J Am Diet Assoc 75:454, 1979

50. Bray GA et al: Am J Clin Nutr 33:376, 1980

51. Andersen T et al: Am J Clin Nutr 33:440, 1980

52. Holzbach RT: Am J Clin Nutr 30:43, 1977

53. Stauffer JQ: Am J Clin Nutr 30:64, 1977

54. Compton JE et al: Lancet 2:1, 1978

55. Faloon WW et al: Am J Clin Nutr 33:431, 1980

56. Bruch H: The Golden Cage. Cambridge, Harvard University Press, 1978

57. Silverman JA: J Pediatr 84:68, 1974

58. Dally P: Anorexia Nervosa. New York, Grune & Stratton, 1969

59. Virgersky R (ed): Anorexia Nervosa. New York, Raven Press, 1977

## Supplementary readings
### Hazards of obesity

Drenick EJ et al: Excessive mortality and causes of death in morbidly obese men. JAMA 243:443, 1980

Kannel WB et al: Obesity, lipids, glucose intolerance: The Framingham Study. Am J Clin Nutr 32:1238, 1979

Van Itallie TB: Obesity: Adverse effects on health and longevity. Am J Clin Nutr (Suppl)32:2723, 1979

### Weight loss

Bray GA et al: Use of anthropometric measures to assess weight loss. Am J Clin Nutr 31:769, 1978

Franklin BA: Losing weight through exercise. JAMA 244:377, 1980

Garn SM et al: Effect of remaining family members on fatness prediction. Am J Clin Nutr 34:148, 1981

Konishi F, Harrison SL: Body weight-gain equivalents of selected foods. J Am Diet Assoc 70:365, 1977

Olefsky JM, Kolterman OG: Mechanisms of insulin resistance in obesity and noninsulin-dependent (type II) diabetes. Am J Med 70:151, 1981

Parham ES, Parham AR Jr: Saccharin use and sugar intake by college students. J Am Diet Assoc 76:560, 1980

Pirie P et al: Distortion in self-reported height and weight data. J Am Diet Assoc 78:601, 1981

Ravey MJR: Dietetic food diarrhea. JAMA 244:270, 1980

Stricker EM: Hyperphagia. N Engl J Med 298:1010, 1978

Stuart RB et al: Weight loss over time. Concomitants and consequences of a decreasing rate. J Am Diet Assoc 75:258, 1979

Van Itallie TB, Yang MU: Current concepts in nutrition: Diet and weight loss. N Engl J Med 297:1158, 1977

Volkmar FR et al: High attrition rates in commercial weight reduction programs. Arch Intern Med 141:426, 1981

Zifferblatt SM, Wilbur CS: Dietary counseling: Some realistic expectations and guidelines. J Am Diet Assoc 70:591, 1977

### Protein-sparing modified fast

American Dietetic Association: Statement on diet protein products. J Am Diet Assoc 73:547, 1978

DeHaven J et al: Nitrogen and sodium balance with sympathetic-nervous-system activity in obese subjects treated with a low-calorie protein or mixed diet. N Engl J Med 302:477, 1980

Jones AOL et al: Elemental content of predigested liquid protein products. Am J Clin Nutr 33:2545, 1980

Marable NL et al: Protein quality of supplements and meal replacements: Amino acid and calculated indicators of protein quality. J Am Diet Assoc 77:270, 1980

Van Itallie TB: Editorial: Liquid protein mayhem. JAMA 240:144, 1978

## Surgery in morbid obesity

Bray GA et al: Eating patterns of massively obese individuals: Direct vs indirect measurements. J Am Diet Assoc 72:24, 1978

Bukoff M, Carlson S: Diet modifications and behavioral changes for bariatric gastric surgery. J Am Diet Assoc 78:158, 1981

Rauen MN, Tseng RYL: Some dietary and food selection changes of jejunoileal bypass patients. J Am Diet Assoc 75:454, 1979

Rodin J: Changes in perceptual responsiveness following jejunoileostomy: Their potential role in reducing food intake. Am J Clin Nutr (Suppl)33:457, 1980

Rogers EL et al: Deficiency of fat soluble vitamins after jejunoileal bypass surgery for morbid obesity. Am J Clin Nutr 33:1208, 1980

Updegraff TA, Neufeld NJ: Protein, iron, and folate status of patients prior to and following surgery for morbid obesity. J Am Diet Assoc 78:135, 1981

## Anorexia nervosa

Bruch H: The Golden Gage. Cambridge, Harvard University Press, 1978

Dally P, Gomez J: Obesity and Anorexia Nervosa. Salem, NH, Faber & Faber, 1980

Schwabe AD et al: Anorexia nervosa. Ann Intern Med 94:371, 1981

## Patient resources

American Diabetes Association/American Dietetic Association Family Cookbook. Englewood Cliffs, NJ, Prentice-Hall, 1980

Better Meals for You with Low Calorie Count Gourmet Recipes. Cleveland, Diabetes Association of Greater Cleveland, 1980

Claiborne C, Franey P: Craig Claiborne's Gourmet Diet. New York, New York, Times Books, 1980

Cutler C: The Woman's Day Low-Calorie Dessert Cookbook. Boston, Houghton Mifflin, 1980

Katch FI, McArdle WD, Boylan BR: Getting in Shape: An Optimum Approach to Fitness and Weight Control. Boston, Houghton Mifflin, 1979

Stern JS, Denenberg RV: How to Stay Slim and Healthy on the Fast Food Diet. Englewood Cliffs, NJ, Prentice-Hall, 1980

*For further references see Bibliography in Part 4.*

# Diabetes Mellitus

**29**

**IDDM:** Insulin-dependent Diabetes Mellitus
**IGT:** Impaired Glucose Tolerance
**NDDG:** National Diabetes Data Group
**NIDDM:** Noninsulin-dependent Diabetes Mellitus
**NPH:** Neutral Protamine Hagedorn
**OGTT:** Oral Glucose Tolerance Test
**PG:** Plasma Glucose
**TAG:** Total Available Glucose
**UGDP:** University Group Diabetes Program

Diabetes mellitus is a chronic, hereditary disease characterized by an abnormally elevated level of blood glucose (hyperglycemia) and by the excretion of the excess glucose in the urine (glycosuria). The basic defect appears to be an absolute or relative lack of insulin or a decrease in insulin receptors on the membrane of the target cells,[1] which leads to abnormalities in carbohydrate (glucose) metabolism as well as in the metabolism of protein[2] and fat. Therefore, any patient with diabetes mellitus needs help in planning and accepting a daily diet containing the appropriate amounts of carbohydrate, protein, and fat, together with adequate amounts of vitamins and minerals. In severe, untreated diabetes mellitus abnormalities of fluid and electrolyte metabolism may also occur.

The history of diabetes mellitus goes back many centuries. The word *diabetes* was derived from the Greek word meaning "to siphon; to pass through," and *mellitus* came from the Latin word "honey." Thus two characteristic symptoms, copious urination (polyuria) and glucose in the urine (glycosuria), gave the name to the disease. It was not until 1921 that Banting and Best, working in Canada, demonstrated that the substance, insulin, extracted from the pancreas, lowered blood sugar in their experimental animals. Following this research, insulin extracted from the islet cells of the pancreas of animals became available for the treatment of diabetes mellitus in humans.

Today it is generally agreed that the hormone, insulin, secreted by the beta cells (islets of Langerhans) of the pancreas, controls glucose metabolism by mediating the transfer of glucose from the spaces around the cell (extracellular) into the cell interior (intracellular), particularly the cells of adipose tissue and muscle. Insulin also appears to mediate the transfer of amino acids from the extracellular spaces into the cells, especially in muscle. Present research indicates that in some patients with diabetes mellitus there is an absolute lack of insulin or an insufficient amount secreted by the beta cells of the pancreas. In other patients, such as the obese hyperglycemic, there is an elevated amount of insulin secreted but tissue resistance interferes with the action of insulin, which leads ultimately to hyperglycemia and glycosuria. The work of Unger and his associates[3] indicates that a relative excess of another pancreatic hormone, glucagon, is involved in the incidence of hyperglycemia in diabetes.

## Epidemiology

### Predisposing factors

It is generally accepted that diabetes mellitus is an inherited disease, although there has been no agreement on a single mode of transmission.[4] Recent research suggests that environmental factors, such as viruses, initiate the expression of the genetic potential for insulin-dependent diabetes mellitus in genetically predisposed individuals,[5] who may also have some immunological abnormality. On the other hand, excessive food intake resulting in hyperinsulinemia with a decrease in insulin receptors in obese people may initiate the expression of noninsulindependent diabetes mellitus in those who are genetically predisposed.

### Prevalence and incidence

It is estimated that approximately 10 million, or about 5% of the population of the United States, may have diabetes mellitus.[6] At present, there is no mechanism for reporting the national annual incidence of diabetes mellitus; however, it is estimated that between 200,000 and 300,000 new cases are diagnosed each year.[6] The World Health Organization has observed signs of the increasing prevalence of diabetes mellitus around the world, particularly in areas where there has been economic improvement due to industrialization and a more generous food supply.

Diabetes occurs in all age groups from young infants to the elderly. The greatest incidence occurs in middle or older aged adults. It is estimated that 80% to 85% of all patients with diabetes mellitus are 45 years of age or older. In the United States as a whole there appears to be a sex difference in the incidence of the disease. More women than men, and more women over 45 years of age who have had children have the disease. The higher incidence in women who have had children may reflect factors related to pregnancy. Today's longer life expectancy and the reduced mortality rate for infants of diabetic mothers results in the "seeding" of the diabetic potential; for this reason, the number of people who will develop the disease is expected to increase.

### Detection and preventive intervention

Screening programs conducted by health departments and the local chapters of the American Diabetes Association seek to discover people who have glycosuria or hyperglycemia and to guide them to medical care for confirmation of abnormal tests. Relatives of known diabetics are strongly advised to be tested by their physicians

each year; in this way, if they do develop the disease they can be identified and treated early enough to retard possible complications. Also, members of families with a history of diabetes are advised to maintain their weight at desirable or slightly below desirable levels throughout the life span because of the association of obesity with the disease.

### Classification by types

Diabetes mellitus has been and will probably continue to be classified by some as growth or juvenile onset and maturity or adult onset. The National Diabetes Data Group[7] (NDDG) has proposed a new classification without regard to age. The two primary types are insulindependent, ketosis prone diabetes mellitus and noninsulin-dependent, nonketosis prone diabetes mellitus.

#### Insulin-dependent diabetes mellitus (IDDM)

IDDM usually, but not always, occurs in people 40 years of age or younger. It rarely occurs under 1 year of age, and there appears to be no special frequency of occurrence by age in the younger group. About 10% of all diabetic patients have IDDM.

The onset of the disease is sudden, and the patient is frequently in ketoacidosis at the time of diagnosis. The majority of patients have lost weight prior to diagnosis due to glucose wastage (glycosuria) and most are underweight to some degree. Insulin secetion by the pancreas is minimal or lacking and, therefore, these patients are *insulin-dependent* and require diet plus insulin to control the disease. The course of the disease can be unstable, characterized by episodes of hypoglycemia (low blood sugar), hyperglycemia, and their sequelae.

#### Noninsulin-dependent diabetes mellitus (NIDDM)

NIDDM usually occurs in people over age 40 and most frequently in the older age group, 55 and over. These people may or may not be obese. In the oldest group the age-related increase in normal fasting blood glucose levels must be differentiated from the elevated blood glucose levels of diabetes mellitus.

The onset of the disease is gradual and may not be diagnosed until years after onset. The course of the disease in many instances is stable, and the patients are not prone to develop ketoacidosis except during a severe illness such as a myocardial infarction (heart attack) or a cerebral vascular accident (stroke). Approximately 85% of patients with NIDDM are obese at the time of diagnosis. Although adequate insulin may be produced by the pancreas, the secretion of insulin may be delayed in response to a glucose challenge, or there may be peripheral resistance (muscle and adipose cell) to the action of insulin with overproduction by the islet cells of the pancreas. It is possible that, over time, the ability of the pancreas to secrete insulin may decrease and, as a result, some patients may require exogenous insulin to control glucose metabolism. Otherwise, NIDDM can be controlled by diet or diet plus oral agents.

## Impaired glucose tolerance (IGT)

The National Diabetes Data Group[7] has proposed this classification for those who suffer from asymptomatic diabetes. The blood glucose level is mildly elevated with levels between normal and those which are clearly diagnostic for diabetes mellitus. Those affected may or may not progress to IDDM or NIDDM, and in some the blood glucose returns to normal.

## Other types

Diabetes mellitus can occur secondary to other disease states, such as pancreatitis, cirrhosis of the liver, cystic fibrosis of the pancreas, tumors of the pancreas (insulinomas), or disorders of other endocrine glands, for example, the pituitary, the adrenals, or the thyroid. It can also occur in patients receiving pharmacological doses of glucocorticoids.

## Metabolic aberrations

In Chapter 9, *Nutrient Utilization*, it was pointed out that insulin may be regarded as the hormone of energy storage. In the immediate postprandial (postfed) state it mediates the synthesis of glycogen and the glycolysis of glucose-6-$PO_4$ in the liver to provide substrate for the tricarboxylic acid cycle (TCA) or for triglyceride synthesis. Insulin also mediates the translocation of glucose and amino acids into muscle cells, where glucose can be synthesized into glycogen. Further, it mediates the translocation of glucose and triglycerides into the adipose cells, where the glucose provides substrate for further triglyceride synthesis.

### Metabolic consequences of insulin deficiency

Without insulin the synthesis of glycogen in the liver is depressed, and there is an increase in glucose synthesis through the gluconeogenic pathway. At the same time there is a decreased uptake of glucose by the muscle and adipose cells and an increased catabolism of glycogen in muscle cells. An increase in proteolysis also occurs, with the release of amino acids from muscle cells and an increase in lipolysis, with the release of fatty acids and glycerol from the adipose cells. Certain amino acids and the glycerol released from the cells serve as substrate for gluconeogenesis in the liver. Therefore, hyperglycemia and hyperlipemia occur in the absence of insulin (Fig. 29-1); such hyperglycemia may result in part from excessive amounts of glucagon.

Without insulin, fatty acids become the major fuel for energy metabolism in the TCA cycle. However, when an excess of acetyl CoA accumulates due to the lack of other substrate required by the TCA cycle, cholesterol and ke-

tone bodies are synthesized in the liver. The ketone bodies are acetoacetic and betahydroxy butyric acids and acetone. Acetoacetic acid and betahydroxy butyric acids can be metabolized for energy to some extent by brain and muscle cells. However, in the absence of insulin the quantity in the circulation exceeds the body's capacity to metabolize them, leading to ketonemia.

When the amount of glucose filtered by the glomeruli of the kidney exceeds the capacity of the renal tubules to reabsorb it, it is excreted in the urine. This usually occurs at blood glucose levels of 160 mg per 100 ml or higher. Since glucose requires water for excretion, an increase in urine volume results, with the loss of body water and the electrolyte sodium.

At the same time, there is an increase in the amount of urea nitrogen to be excreted due to the deamination of amino acids, so that their carbon structures can serve as substrate for gluconeogenesis. Also, when cellular proteins are catabolized and their amino acids transported to the liver for gluconeogenesis, potassium is lost from the cells. The increasing amounts of both urea and potassium in the circulation again require water for excretion by the kidneys.

Finally the ketone bodies, betahydroxy butyric acid, acetoacetic acid, and acetone, in excess of what the body can use require water for excretion by the kidney. Acetone is volatile and is also excreted by the lungs. This attempt by the kidney to excrete an abnormal quantity of metabolites leads to cellular dehydration and the depletion of body water and electrolytes. At the same time there is an increase in blood hydrogen ion concentration (metabolic acidosis). All of these metabolic events lead to circulatory failure. If treatment is not instituted promptly to reestablish carbohydrate metabolism and fluid and electrolyte balance, death may ensue.

Patients with noninsulin-dependent diabetes do not usually develop ketoacidosis. It appears that, since these patients frequently have hyperinsulinism, and insulin is antilipolytic, excessive amounts of fatty acids are not released from the adipose cell. However, this does not mean that these diabetics do not experience hyperlipemia. In the presence of insulin and excessive amounts of glucose, there is an increase of triglyceride synthesis in the liver with secretion into the circulation.

### Other metabolic problems

It has been observed that disease of the small and large blood vessels occurs more frequently in diabetics than in nondiabetics. Hypertriglyceridemia is a common finding in the untreated patient. In the diabetic there is a tendency to recurrent myocardial infarction with an increase in the incidence of congestive heart failure. Small blood vessel diseases, such as retinopathy, peripheral vascular disease, and nephropathy, also occur more frequently than in the nondiabetic. Diabetic retinopathy is a major cause of legal blindness or visual impairment in the

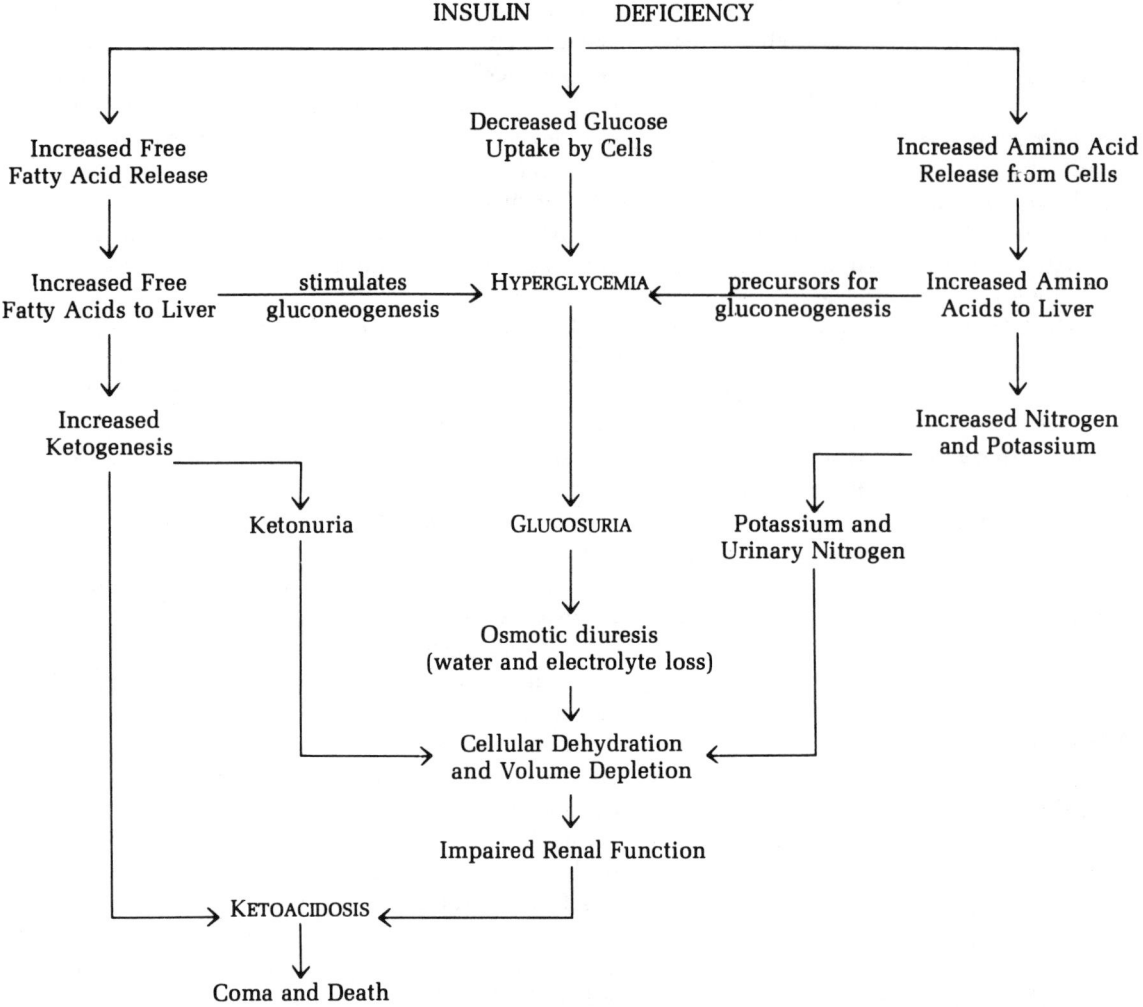

INSULIN    DEFICIENCY

**Fig. 29-1.** Metabolic consequences of insulin deficiency. (Adapted from Tepperman J: Metabolic and Endocrine Physiology, 4th ed. Chicago, Year Book Medical Publishers, © 1980)

United States. Diabetic nephropathy and atherosclerosis are the major causes of death among diabetics. Siperstein[8] has observed a thickening in the capillary basement membrane in diabetics, and Spiro[9] has identified an abnormality in the mucopolysaccharides in the basement membrane, which may account for the vascular complications of diabetes. The polyol pathway of glucose metabolism is also involved in some of the complications of the disease.

### Capillary basement membrane

The glomerular membranes of the kidney have been extensively studied because of the serious complications of the renal disease associated with long-standing diabetes mellitus.

Spiro[9] has observed that the normal glomerular basement membrane consists of a glycoprotein material made up of peptide chains to which carbohydrate is attached. An important unit in the membrane consists of a disac-

charide containing glucose and galactose linked to hydroxylysine. In the glomerular basement membrane of diabetics Spiro has observed a significant increase of the glucosylgalactose units attached to hydroxylysine with a proportional decrease in lysine. This change in composition changes the structure and function of the basement membrane.

At the present time the implications of this aberration on the treatment of diabetes mellitus are not clear. However, future research in this area may identify the real hazards of hyperglycemia and have a significant effect on therapy, including diet.

### Polyol pathway of glucose metabolism

Polyols are organic compounds containing multiple alcohol groups that are derived from sugars by the reduction of their aldo or keto groups. Sorbitol is the polyol that results from the reduction of glucose in mammalian tissues.

There seems to be some evidence that the cataracts that are associated with diabetes mellitus may result from an increased concentration of sorbitol in the lens. The lens does not require insulin for the intracellular transport of glucose. The presence of hyperglycemia, therefore, increases the concentration of sorbitol. The polyol pathway of glucose metabolism may also be involved in the neuropathy of diabetes mellitus.

### Symptoms

The onset of the symptoms of the metabolic aberrations in IDDM is usually abrupt. Ketoacidosis with nausea, vomiting, and lethargy is present at the time of diagnosis. Two to 3 weeks before this, the classical symptoms—polydipsia, polyphagia, polyuria, and weight loss—are observed. Usually an infectious disease or other illness occurs just before the onset of symptoms.

The onset of symptoms in NIDDM[10] is usually slow and the disease may go undetected for as long as 10 years. Although many of these patients have glycosuria, they are not aware that they are experiencing polydipsia and polyuria with nocturia. If they are hyperinsulinemic, they may also experience the symptoms of reactive hypoglycemia, such as sweating, tremor, and palpitation 3 to 4 hours after a meal. They do not often lose weight or develop spontaneous ketoacidosis. However, with a severe infection ketoacidosis may develop. The disease is often detected when patients participate in a community screening program, or when they seek medical care for the symptoms of diseases associated with diabetes, such as obesity, hypertension, heart disease, visual difficulties, and skin infections.

### Screening and diagnostic tests

The diagnosis of diabetes mellitus can be made with a fair degree of confidence in those with the classical symptoms of the disease and elevated fasting or postprandial levels of blood glucose and glycosuria. Ketonemia and ketonuria may or may not be present. In others, a glucose challenge administered under defined conditions is used for the clinical diagnosis of the disease. It can be anticipated that if an inexpensive clinical laboratory method is developed, the determination of blood insulin levels will also be used in the diagnostic workup of patients who are suspected diabetics.

### Tests

The most commonly used screening tests are the determination of the fasting blood glucose level or the 2-hour postprandial (after a meal) blood glucose level, while the most common diagnostic one is the oral glucose tolerance test (OGTT).

The normal levels for fasting plasma glucose vary between 65 mg to 115 mg per deciliter of blood (ferri-

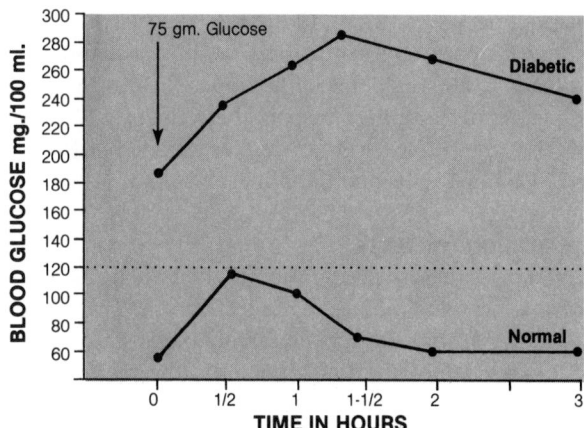

**Fig. 29-2.** Results of glucose tolerance tests in a normal person and a diabetic.

cyanide auto-analyzer method). For both the fasting and 2-hour postprandial tests levels in excess of 140 mg of glucose per deciliter of blood are indicative of diabetes mellitus, while values between 115 mg to 140 mg are equivocal. Plasma glucose (PG) values are 14% higher than values determined on whole blood. In the untreated diabetic patient without complications, the fasting level ranges from 180 mg to 300 mg per deciliter; and in a patient approaching or in ketoacidosis, the fasting blood glucose level exceeds 300 mg.

When the fasting or 2-hour postprandial blood glucose levels are equivocal, an oral glucose tolerance test is done. Following an overnight fast of not less than 10 hours or more than 16 hours, the patient is given a solution of glucose to drink. This contains 75 g of glucose for adults and less for children, depending on body size (1.75 g per kilogram ideal body weight not to exceed 75 g). Just prior to drinking the glucose solution, blood is drawn and a specimen of urine is collected. Blood and urine samples are obtained at $\frac{1}{2}$, 1, $1\frac{1}{2}$, 2, and 3 hours after the glucose solution is consumed. In some instances blood and urine are also obtained at 4 and 5 hours. In a normal person the blood glucose values will not exceed 100 mg per deciliter at zero time, 140 mg at $\frac{1}{2}$ hour, and will return to the fasting level at 2 hours (see Fig. 29-2). The urine will be free of glucose.

Table 29-1 gives the minimum criteria and interpretation of the oral glucose tolerance test formulated by the United States Public Health Service (USPHS) and by Fajans and Conn at the University of Michigan. Note that the USPHS uses a point system, while Fajans and Conn use specific blood glucose levels to identify diabetes mellitus.

The NDDG[7] criteria for the diagnosis of diabetes mellitus in the adult who does not have the classic symptoms of the disease are a fasting plasma glucose concentration greater than or equal to 140 mg per deciliter on more than one occasion; or in those who have a fasting plasma glucose less than 140 mg per deciliter but have a plasma glucose concentration at 2 hours equal to or greater than 200 mg per deciliter and a plasma glucose of 200 mg per deciliter at some point between 0 and 2 hours. Note that the NDDG levels are higher than either those of the USPHS or Fajans and Conn in Table 29-1.

### Preparation for tests

There is dietary preparation of the patient for the 2-hour postprandial blood glucose test and the oral glucose tolerance test, but not for the fasting blood glucose test. For 3 days before the first two tests, the patient must consume an adequate diet containing at least 150 g of carbohydrate daily. An inadequate carbohydrate intake prior to the test can influence the results. A person consuming a low- or no-carbohydrate diet would have an increase above normal limits in blood glucose after ingestion of the glucose challenge for either test, which would reflect previous intake, not the presence of diabetes. The patient should be carefully instructed in preparation for these tests, especially if he has restricted his carbohydrate intake because he suspects he has diabetes. The OGTT is done only on an outpatient basis with maintenance of the usual level of activity.

## Therapy

The goals of the treatment of diabetes mellitus are to prevent excessive postprandial hyperglycemia and, therefore, the symptoms of glucose wastage; prevent hypoglycemia if the patient is using insulin or an oral agent; achieve and maintain ideal body weight in adults and normal growth and development in children; return serum triglycerides and cholesterol to normal levels; and prevent or delay large and small blood vessel disease.

Depending on the needs of the patient, the goals of therapy may be achieved by *diet; diet* plus insulin; or *diet* plus oral hypoglycemic agents. In the obese diabetic without symptoms both the hyperglycemia and hyperinsulinemia may be corrected by an energy-restricted diet

resulting in weight loss. The insulin-dependent diabetic requires a diet appropriate to maintain ideal weight status or growth combined with daily insulin injections. The obese diabetic with symptoms usually responds to an energy-restricted diet to promote weight loss and an oral hypoglycemic agent. However, some of the patients in this last group may finally require insulin to treat their disease.

### Insulin

Since the discovery of insulin, many advances have been made in its commercial preparation from the pancreas of animals, primarily cattle and swine. Its production is carefully controlled to ensure the number of units of insulin per volume when the product is purchased by the diabetic patient. Insulin can be administered only hypodermically because it is a protein; if taken orally, it would undergo enzymatic digestion in the gastrointestinal tract, which would absorb its constituent amino acids, not the intact, active hormone.

#### Types of insulin

There are several types of insulins available for the treatment of the insulin-dependent diabetic patient. They differ primarily in the rate of onset and duration of action, which is reflected in the three classifications—rapid, intermediate, and long-acting (see Table 29-2). The most commonly used insulins today are the two intermediate acting ones, Lente and NPH (Neutral Protamine Hagedorn). They are stable solutions of insulin that possess the desirable properties of relatively rapid onset (2 to 8 hours) and moderately prolonged duration of action (24–28 hr). Regular insulin is used in the treatment of ketoacidosis because its rapid onset of action permits the physician to monitor blood glucose levels and adjust insulin injections to the need of the patient.

It must be recognized that the action of exogenous insulin injected hypodermically, usually once a day, is not the same physiologically as that of endogenous insulin released by the beta cells of the pancreas in response to the

### Table 29-1. Minimum Criteria and Interpretation of Oral Glucose Tolerance Test (Glucose Values in mg Percent)

| | United States Public Health Service* | | | Fajans and Conn† | |
| --- | --- | --- | --- | --- | --- |
| | *Whole Blood* | *Serum or Plasma* | | *Whole Blood* | *Serum or Plasma* |
| Fasting | 110 | 130 | 1 point | | |
| 1 hour | 170 | 195 | ½ point | 160 | 185 |
| 1½ hours | | | | 140 | 165 |
| 2 hours | 120 | 140 | ½ point | 120 | 140 |
| 3 hours | 110 | 130 | 1 point | | |

*Two or more points is definite diabetes, one point is possible diabetes.

†One- and two-hour levels at or exceeding the stated values represent diabetes; 1½-hour level must be reached or exceeded in borderline cases.

(Skillman TG, Tzagournis M: Diabetes Mellitus. Kalamazoo, Upjohn, 1973)

ingestion of food. Exogenous insulin is continuously available in the bloodstream and, therefore, the patient must adjust to it by consuming properly spaced meals. Although the mechanism that causes this is not understood, it has been observed that exercise enhances glucose utilization in the diabetic. The research of Pederson[11] and co-workers indicates that postprandial exercise was associated with a significant rise in insulin binding receptor sites on the cells that they studied—erythrocytes and monocytes. Therefore, if an insulin-dependent diabetic patient increases his activity significantly on any one day, he must increase his food intake or decrease his usual insulin dose for that day.

The stable IDDM patient usually requires one injection before breakfast of intermediate acting insulin to achieve reasonable control of blood sugar. However, some labile insulin-dependent diabetics require two injections to achieve reasonable control during the day and to avoid nocturnal hyperglycemia. One injection is given in the morning before breakfast and the second one preceding the evening meal or a feeding at bedtime. The quantity of insulin injected varies with each patient. Presently a continuous subcutaneous insulin infusion pump and an artificial pancreas are being tested in the hope of controlling the daily excursions in blood glucose levels that occur with the usual injections of insulin once or twice a day.[12]

## Insulin reactions

Hypoglycemic episodes in the diabetic due to excess insulin are to be avoided because prolonged and repeated insulin reactions lead to irreversible damage to the cortical neurons. Most of these reactions occur because the patient has not properly spaced his food intake or has omitted a meal entirely. They can also occur because of an unplanned increase in activity or the injection of the wrong dose of insulin.

Intermediate- and long-acting insulins in excess produce a gradual decrease in blood glucose levels. The patient experiences headache, blurred or double vision, fine tremors, uncontrollable yawning, mental confusion, and incoordination. If these symptoms are not treated, unconsciousness ensues. The insulin reaction in a patient who is conscious can be treated by an oral glucose solution, such as fruit juice and sweetened carbonated beverages or with sugar. Diabetic patients using intermediate- or long-acting insulin are advised to carry with them at all times a source of glucose, such as sugar cubes, candy, or a special tube of concentrated glucose.

Whenever the ability of the patient to swallow without aspiration is in question or he is unconscious, the hormone glucagon is injected subcutaneously to stimulate gluconeogenesis. When conscious, the patient is offered an oral glucose solution. If the patient is in a hospital, the glucagon injection may be followed by intravenous dextrose in water.

## Hypoglycemic hyperglycemia

Episodes of mild hypoglycemia followed almost immediately by hyperglycemia have been observed in patients using intermediate-acting insulin. Hypoglycemia, a reaction occurring at the peak time of insulin action, activates a counter-regulatory hormonal response characterized by the release of epinephrine, adrenal corticosteroids, and growth hormone. This hormonal release is a strong stimulus to gluconeogenesis, with the result that rebound hyperglycemia occurs. In other words, "hypoglycemia begets hyperglycemia." This swing in blood glucose is also known as the Symogyi effect. The problem is caused by too much insulin and is treated by slowly reducing the daily dose of insulin.

## Oral hypoglycemic agents

Four types of sulfonylureas—tolbutamide, tolazamide, acetohexamide, and chlorpropamide—can enhance glucose utilization in NIDDM patients who secrete reasonable amounts of insulin. They are not effective in the treatment of IDDM patients. The biguanides, another group of synthetic compounds with hypoglycemic effects, have been removed from the market by FDA because they promote lactic acidoses in diabetic patients.

The sulfonylureas stimulate the release of insulin from the beta cells of the pancreas. These drugs can be taken by mouth, which relieves the NIDDM patient of taking daily insulin injections when diet alone cannot control the blood glucose level. However, it has been observed that after effecting an initially good response, the drugs are not effective in the control of blood glucose in some NIDDM patients and, as a result, insulin therapy must be used. Shen and Bressler[13] estimate that only 20% to 30% of patients can use the oral hypoglycemic agents successfully for long periods of time and point out that these agents do not lower plasma lipids. Elevated plasma lipids are a risk factor in atherosclerosis (see Chap. 30).

The University Group Diabetes Program (UGDP) study indicates that patients using oral agents appear to experience a greater number of deaths from atherosclerosis than patients treated with insulin.[14] There is consider-

### Table 29-2. Insulin Action

| Type | Action | Peak action (Hours) | Duration (Hours) |
|------|--------|---------------------|------------------|
| Regular | Rapid | 1–2 | 5–6 |
| Semilente | Rapid | 1–2 | 12–16 |
| Globin | Intermediate | 2–4 | 18–24 |
| NPH | Intermediate | 2–8 | 24–28 |
| Lente | Intermediate | 2–8 | 24–28 |
| PZI | Long-acting | 8–12 | 36 |
| Ultralente | Long-acting | 8–14 | 36 |

(Adapted from Skillman TG, Tzagournis M: Diabetes Mellitus. Kalamazoo, Upjohn, 1975)

able controversy about the outcomes of the UGDP study. Some clinicians hesitate to use oral hypoglycemic agents, while others have continued to use them in the treatment of maturity onset diabetes.

Patients using oral hypoglycemic agents must space their meals properly because hypoglycemic reactions can occur, although not as commonly as they do in those using insulin. Hypoglycemia can occur in patients with uremia who are taking sulfonylureas because the drug is excreted by the kidney, and in uremia (kidney failure) excretion is limited due to decreased kidney function. Alcohol intolerance has also been observed in patients using the sulfonylureas.

### Approaches to therapy

There is a sharp controversy among physicians in the United States as to the best method of treating the patient with diabetes mellitus. The disagreement centers on the control of blood glucose levels. A group of conservative physicians believes that blood glucose levels higher than normal, resulting in the presence of glucose in the urine, contribute to the onset and the severity of vascular disease in diabetes. Hence, diet and insulin or oral hypoglycemic therapy are regulated carefully so that the blood glucose levels are kept within normal limits, without episodes of hypoglycemia. This careful treatment of diabetes is known as chemical regulation; it is achieved by the use of a weighed diet, repeated urine testing throughout the day, and frequent adjustments in the dose of insulin or oral agents.

A group of liberal physicians believe, from the evidence available to them, that careful regulation does not delay the onset of vascular disease. They treat their patients with insulin, if needed, and a liberal diet as long as no symptoms of diabetes other than glycosuria, without ketonuria and weight loss, are present. The physicians who advocate this approach to treatment claim that the patient lives a more nearly normal and satisfying life. This regimen is called the clinical method of regulation. The patient is placed on an unmeasured or "free" diet, restricting only sugar and foods high in sugar.

A third group, the majority of physicians who treat diabetic patients, have adopted a middle-of-the-road approach. Their treatment plan is neither as limiting as the chemical method nor as liberal as the clinical method. They use the Exchange Method of diet planning, a somewhat liberal yet moderately accurate method, which is based on standard household measures (see Chap. 24, Tables 24-2 and 24-3).

Regardless of the approach to therapy, the diet is an integral part of the treatment of any patient with diabetes mellitus. Every diabetic patient must consume daily the quantity of energy and nutrients he needs. There cannot be wide variations in intake from day to day. At the same time he must space his meals properly whether his treatment is dietary or dietary combined with insulin or the oral agents. To avoid variations in blood glucose levels, sugar and foods high in sugar content must be excluded from the diet. For some patients the diagnosis, diabetes mellitus, requires a drastic and unavoidable change in life-style if they are to achieve a reasonable degree of control.

## Diet therapy

The diet prescription for a patient with diabetes mellitus must be translated into a diet pattern acceptable to the patient. The diet must be nutritionally adequate; maintain, in so far as possible, normal blood glucose levels throughout 24 hours; and promote desirable weight status in the adult and normal growth and development in children and adolescents. This applies even to those situations where the diet prescription is regular (free) diet without added sugar or, as for children, diet-for-age without added sugar.

### The diet prescription
#### Energy

The energy requirement for the nonobese adult diabetic is the same as that for normal adults of the same sex, age, height, and activity. However, the diabetic is cautioned to maintain weight status slightly below his desirable weight. If his daily energy expenditure is significantly less than normal, his calorie prescription may be somewhat less. For example, a 55 year old woman who is a secretary may require 25 calories per kilogram, not the 30 calories per kilogram recommended for a more active woman. It is recommended that the Harris Benedict formula and Long's activity factors (see Chap. 23) be used to estimate the energy need of an adult of ideal body weight. The calorie prescription for an obese adult diabetic is designed to promote weight loss and is based on the criteria used to establish the calorie level of any energy-restricted diet (see Chap. 28). With experience and any change in the patient's life-style, the calorie level of the diet may need to be adjusted.

The energy requirement for a child or an adolescent diabetic who is not usually obese is the same as for others of his age group. The energy requirements for growth must be met to prevent growth retardation. Since insulin is lipogenic, it has been observed that energy intake may need to be reduced after adolescence to avoid an increase in body fat, especially in girls.

#### Carbohydrate

The American Diabetes Association[15] recommends that 50% to 60% of one's total calories should be derived from carbohydrate. For example, at 50% a 1500-calorie diet contains 187 g of carbohydrate.

$$\frac{50 \times 1500}{100} = 750 \text{ calories}{:}4 = 187 \text{ g carbohydrate}$$

However, for patients with carbohydrate-induced hyperlipidemia, it is recommended that carbohydrate be restricted to 40% of total calories (see Chap. 30).

The type of carbohydrate to be used, simple or complex, has to be considered. The simple carbohydrates are mono- and disaccharides, and the complex ones, polysaccharides. The disaccharide, sucrose, is excluded as a source of carbohydrate in any diabetic diet because it is readily hydrolyzed and absorbed in the gastrointestinal tract, especially when consumed without other foods, and has an adverse effect on blood glucose levels.

Although the American Diabetes Association did not take a position on fiber in the 1979 report,[15] the work of Jenkins[16] and co-workers in England and of Anderson[17] and co-workers in the United States indicates that diabetic diets with high fiber content may alter the absorption of carbohydrate and reduce postprandial hyperglycemia and glycosuria with a decrease in insulin requirements in IDDM patients and the withdrawal of sulfonylureas in NIDDM patients. These diets also contain more than 60% of the total energy from carbohydrate.[16] Pectins and storage polysaccharides such as gums and mucilages, which can form gels in the small intestine probably resulting in slower absorption of carbohydrate, appear to be more effective than structural food fibers, such as bran.[17]

Drash[18] has recommended 55% of total calories from carbohydrates for children, with 65% of the total carbohydrate to be derived from complex carbohydrates and 35% of the total carbohydrates from simple carbohydrates. The complex carbohydrate is derived from cereal grains, root vegetables, and dried seeds, while the simple carbohydrate is derived from the lactose in milk and the naturally occurring mono- and disaccharides in fruits and vegetables.

### Protein

The American Diabetes Association recommends that 12% to 20% of the total calories should be derived from protein. For example, at 15% a 1500-calorie diet contains 56 g of protein.

$$\frac{15 \times 1500}{100} = 225 \text{ calories}:4 = 56 \text{ g protein}$$

This is greater than the average protein intake of nondiabetics, which varies from 10% to 13% of total calories from protein. Drash recommends 15% protein for children.

For diabetic patients with chronic renal failure (Kimmelstiel-Wilson or other renal disease) the protein is limited to a limit that they can tolerate, and the total calories derived from carbohydrate will be increased (see Chap. 32, *Renal Disease.*)

### Fat

The remainder of the dietary energy requirements is supplied by fat. The American Diabetes Association[15] recommends that polyunsaturated fatty acids should supply up to 10% of the total dietary energy. It is advisable that no more than 35% of the total energy should be supplied by

fat. For example, at 35% a 1500-calorie diet contains approximately 58 g fat.

$$\frac{35 \times 1500}{100} = 525 \text{ calories}:9 = 58 \text{ g fat}$$

The quantity of cholesterol in the diabetic diet may also be restricted (see Chap. 31). For children, Drash recommends 30% of total calories from fat.[18]

### Daily distribution of energy intake

The diabetic patient who is dependent on exogenous insulin or an oral hypoglycemic agent to control blood glucose must distribute his energy intake in some reasonable fashion. Table 29-3 shows a commonly recommended distribution of energy intake by type of patient, using intermediate-acting insulin or diet with or without an oral agent.

Observe that both stable and labile insulin-dependent diabetic patients using intermediate-acting insulin must consume approximately one-half their energy intake during the hours of peak action of the insulin (2 to 8 hours after injection or between 7 to 8 A.M. and 3 to 4 P.M.) and the remainder in the evening to provide for the total duration of insulin activity.

The stable, insulin-dependent diabetic type is usually the nonketosis prone, patient and the labile insulin-dependent is most apt to be the ketosis prone patient. For this latter type, frequent snacks in addition to meals are customary for the preschool child and, fortunately, the same pattern of eating can be established for children and adolescents attending school.

The NIDDM patient is also advised to distribute his energy intake reasonably throughout the day to avoid an excessive challenge to the beta cells of the pancreas. He may or may not be using oral hypoglycemic agents. Table 29-3 recommends a 2/7, 2/7, 3/7 distribution. Some clini-

### Table 29-3. Examples of Daily Distribution of Caloric Content of Energy Intake

| Type of Diabetic Patient | Time of Day and Fraction of Total Calories | | | | | |
|---|---|---|---|---|---|---|
| | Break-fast | Mid-morning | Noon | After-noon | Supper | Bed-time |
| *Stable, insulin-requiring* | 2/7 | | 2/7 | | 2/7 | 1/7 |
| *Labile, insulin-requiring* | 2/10 | 1/10 | 2/10 | 1/10 | 3/10 | 1/10 |
| *Stable, noninsulin-requiring* | 2/7 | | 2/7 | | 3/7 | |

(Skillman TG, Tzagournis M: Diabetes Mellitus. Kalamazoo, Upjohn, 1975)

cians recommend a 1/3, 1/3, 1/3 distribution for these patients. If desired, these patients can also use a 2/7, 2/7, 2/7, 1/7 distribution.

Because it has been shown that total energy intake determines insulin requirements more than carbohydrate *per se*, emphasis has been placed on the daily distribution of energy intake; a reasonable distribution of carbohydrate, protein, and fat to supply the energy should be included in each feeding. For example, a bedtime snack might consist of an apple and cheese, not just an apple or other food which is primarily carbohydrate.

In summary, the diabetic diet prescription for a man 60 years of age who requires 1500 calories per day would contain 56 g protein, 58 g of fat and 186 g of carbohydrate, or 15% of calories from protein, 35% from fat, and 50% from carbohydrate. If this man is a stable, insulin-dependent diabetic, his diet pattern would be planned to contain approximately 430 calories in the morning, noon, and evening meals, and 215 calories at bedtime (2/7, 2/7, 2/7, 1/7).

### Food selection and preparations for diabetic diets

The reader is advised to study the section on food selection and preparation for energy-restricted diets in Chapter 28, pp. 476–478. This information applies as well to energy-restricted diabetic diets and is not repeated here. The following discussions of the exchange food groups present additional information related to diabetic diets.

#### Milk exchanges

All the items in the milk exchange food group (Chap. 24, Table 24-3) can be used in planning a diabetic diet pattern. These lowfat milk exchanges help to control the daily intake of saturated fatty acids and cholesterol.

To accomplish Drash's recommendation that no more than 30% of the total calories in a diabetic diet for children should be derived from fat, milk with 2% butterfat* or skim milk must be used. Otherwise only very limited quantities of the fat exchanges such as margarine or vegetable oil can be used in the diet pattern. It is advisable that an adolescent boy who requires 3000 calories per day use milk with 2% fat, or skim milk, to provide his calcium and riboflavin allowances without an excessive intake of fat from milk.

#### Vegetable exchanges

If simple carbohydrates (mono- and disaccharides) are to be limited in the diabetic diet, only 1 to 2 $^1/_2$-cup servings can be calculated in the diet pattern since the carbohydrate in these vegetables is primarily mono- and disaccharides. For well-controlled diabetic patients who also have carbohydrate-induced hypertriglyceridemia and a limited energy intake due to obesity, the diet pattern may be limited to only 1 $^1/_2$-cup serving of vegetables.

---

*Whole milk, 3.5% butterfat.

#### Fruit exchanges

The serving size of the items in the fruit exchange food group specifies the amount of fruit, fresh, dried, or canned, without the addition of sugar, which contains 10 g of carbohydrate. When the intake of simple carbohydrates is restricted, the amount of fruit in the diet pattern is limited. However, the patient should be guided to select a fruit each day that is a good source of vitamin C. If the total carbohydrate allows it, fresh potatoes (complex carbohydrate) in large enough quantity can be relied on as a significant source of vitamin C. Fruit drinks with vitamin C added should be avoided because the first and, therefore, most important, ingredient on labels of these beverages is sugar.

#### Bread exchanges

Traditionally, the use of bread exchanges as a source of carbohydrate in the diabetic diet pattern has been limited. In addition to milk, emphasis was placed on using more servings of fruits and vegetables than is usually consumed by normal, healthy persons. With the present interest in the type of carbohydrate (simple and complex), as well as an increase in total energy from carbohydrate, more bread exchanges may be used in diabetic diet patterns than in the past. However, one may encounter some difficulty implementing this change, particularly in the older patient who has had a long exposure to the concept that, not only sugar, but also bread and potatoes must be excluded from a diabetic or energy-restricted diet. On the other hand, most adolescent diabetic boys readily accept bread and potatoes in preference to excessive quantities of fruits and vegetables.

Items in the bread exchange food group that contain sugar, such as muffins, pancakes, and waffles, should be restricted to occasional use. Sugar coated cereals and any cereal product where sugar is the first or second item in the list of ingredients on the package must be excluded from the diet.

Diet cookies and cakes made with artificial sweeteners in place of sugar are not recommended. They are not usually acceptable substitutes due to their flavor and texture, and gram for gram, may contain as much carbohydrate and energy as products made from standard ingredients.

#### Meat exchanges

The items in this food group contain primarily protein and fat. The one exception is dried beans and peas. When these are used as a meat exchange, a $^1/_2$-c serving is also equivalent to one bread exchange as calculated in the diet pattern. The carbohydrate in one serving of dried beans or peas is equal to that in one bread exchange.

It is advisable that diabetic patients make the majority of their selections from the lean meat exchanges and limit the use of eggs to three a week to control their intake of saturated fatty acids and cholesterol.

## Fat exchanges

The best choices in this food group are those items that contain a significant amount of polyunsaturated fatty acids—the margarines and vegetable oils. Diabetic patients should limit their selections of, or omit entirely, bacon, bacon fat, cream, and cream cheese because of the saturated fatty acid and cholesterol content of these items.

## Mixed dishes

Cookbooks that give the exchange values of one serving of the product are available for diabetic patients, and a selection of books and publications containing these recipes are listed at the end of this chapter. The exchange values of a serving of the patient's own recipes can also be calculated by the clinical dietitian.

## Convenience foods

Unless the nutrient label makes it possible to estimate the exchange values of a serving of the product, convenience foods cannot be used by the diabetic patient. The list of ingredients on the packages of many convenience foods indicates that a variety of food fats, lactose in milk solids, or various forms of sugar, such as refiners syrup and invert sugar and corn syrups, are used by the processors in formulating these foods. Unfortunately, unless the package also has a nutrient label stating the energy, protein, fat, and carbohydrate value of an average serving, it is impossible to tell whether or not fats and sugars are present in significant or insignificant amounts.

## Fast foods

Some of the fast food restaurant chains have published the energy and nutrient content of their food items, including the exchange values per serving. The clinical dietitian should have this information in order to assist patients in learning how to select foods that fit into their diet patterns.

## Artificial sweeteners

With the present uncertainty about the safety of saccharin, scientists are trying to find another noncaloric sweetener. Various attempts have been made to replace saccharin with fructose, an absorbable hexose, and three sugar alcohols—sorbitol, mannitol, and xylitol—which are poorly absorbed. At this point none of those substances can be recommended for use by diabetics. Sorbitol when consumed in excessive quantities causes diarrhea.[19] There is no research that indicates that fructose is a safe sweetener for diabetics,[20] and it should not be used. Since there is no known biologic need for sucrose, it is strongly recommended that all members of the health-care team help the diabetic patient to avoid any sweeteners. Patients who have achieved this dietary change report that foods and beverages sweetened with natural or artificial sweeteners nauseate them. They develop an aversion to very sweet-tasting foods.

## Alcohol

If alcohol is used by the diabetic patient, the energy value of the amount to be used is subtracted from the calorie intake defined in the diet prescription before the grams of protein, fat, and carbohydrate are calculated. For example, an 1800-calorie diet prescription that includes 150 calories from alcohol becomes a 1650-calorie diet. The decision to include alcohol in the diet plan rests with the physician. It should be remembered that patients using the sulfonylureas may be intolerant of alcohol. Also, alcohol should be excluded from the diets of some patients with hyperlipidemias (see Chap. 30).

Distilled spirits—scotch, rye, bourbon, vodka, and gin—do not contain carbohydrate, while fermented spirits—beer, ales and wines—contain carbohydrate. Therefore, when alcohol is used, the patient should be advised to use distilled spirits. If the energy prescription is 1500 calories or less, alcoholic beverages must be excluded because although they provide calories, they do not contribute the other nutrients that are necessary to meet the patient's daily nutrient needs.

## Planning the diabetic diet pattern with the patient
### Step I

The first step in planning the diet pattern with any newly diagnosed patient, either in the hospital or in an ambulatory-care setting, is to obtain a complete history of the patient's usual food practices and daily activities. At the time of diagnosis many maturity onset diabetics do not require hospitalization. Gathering the data base for assessment before planning the diet pattern will probably take from 1 to 1$\frac{1}{2}$ hours and may require more than one encounter with the patient before a suitable diet pattern can be planned.

The data gathered about food practices should cover the same information one gains from any patient requiring a modified diet—the *when, what, where,* and with *whom* the patient customarily eats. With the diabetic patient it is very important to identify any variation in his daily schedule that may occur on weekends or on his days off from employment. Insulin-dependent patients must establish and maintain a consistent meal schedule every day of the week.

The kinds and amounts of foods consumed at each meal or snack must be determined in detail (see Chap. 13). How foods are prepared and the basic ingredients in commonly used recipes should also be elicited at this time. Knowledge of the methods of food preparation is important because it may be necessary to make modifications. If the patient is a married man, information about his daily meal pattern and methods of home food preparation is generally obtained from his wife.

The frequency with which a patient's usual meal pattern varies should also be ascertained. For example, routine social engagements, such as "bowling night," may modify the patient's usual evening meal pattern and intake of alcoholic beverages. Some patients report that "bowling night" is also "beer night."

Where and with whom the patient eats is also important information. With the national trend toward eating more meals outside the home, it is important to know the restaurants in which the patient eats most frequently and the type of menus offered. Many patients can continue this practice, depending on their diet prescription and the food served by the restaurant. If the patient is the mother, father, or a child in a large family, it is advisable to modify, if necessary, the family's usual food practices because other members of the family may be at risk for developing diabetes mellitus.

If the diabetic patient is a child, the data is obtained from the mother and any other person who may be closely involved in the child's care. For example, if the mother works, the babysitter should be included in the interview.

During the interview one can also discover what the client knows about diet in the treatment of diabetes mellitus. Some newly diagnosed adult patients have had experience with the diet if another family member also has diabetes. This experience can have a positive or a negative effect on the patient's attitude, depending on a number of factors, such as the type of diet and the severity of the relative's condition.

## Step II

The second step is to plan the diabetic diet pattern. It should be planned within the constraints of the diet prescription and incorporate, whenever possible, the usual food practices of the patient. Table 29-4 illustrates the energy and nutrient composition of the quantities of food in a 1500-calorie diabetic diet. Fifteen percent of the total calories is derived from protein, 30% from fat, and 50% from carbohydrate. Approximately 35% is simple and 65% complex carbohydrate. Table 29-5 illustrates the distribution of the exchanges used in Table 29-4 in three meals and a bedtime snack. The food exchanges in each meal reflect the choices of a 55 year old homemaker who developed this diet pattern with her nutrition counselor. The reader is advised to translate the diet pattern into a day's menu using the *Exchange Lists* on Table 24-3 of Chapter 24, p. 418, and the additional information on food selection and preparation in Chapter 28 (p. 476) and in this chapter. A copy of the diet pattern (see Fig. 28-2) should be entered in the patient's record for use by the health-care team and in follow-up counseling sessions.

Because many Americans omit or eat a very small breakfast, one of the major adjustments in food practices that an adult patient may need to be guided toward is accepting an increase in the quantity of foods he consumes at breakfast. The patient who uses intermediate-acting insulin may have an insulin reaction during the morning if he does not have an adequate breakfast.

## Regular diet with no added sugar

If the diet prescription is regular (free) diet, or diet-for-age, with no added sugar, the energy and nutrient needs of the patient must be identified and translated into reasonable quantities of foods for the day. This information is used to assist the patient to establish a consistent daily meal schedule. If the mother of a newly diagnosed child is very anxious about her ability to feed her child at home, it may be wise to offer her a meal plan using the Exchange System. As the mother gains confidence in her ability to feed her child, she will need help to make the plan more liberal.

## Weighed diets

The physician who uses the chemical method to treat the diabetic requires his patients to purchase a scale that measures in grams. The patient must weigh each serving of food at each meal. The instructional materials for the patient gives the gram weight of each serving of food. The equivalent household measure may also be included. Many of these physicians have adapted the Exchange System or have constructed a similar system for this method of diet instruction. The nutrient values of foods used by physicians may vary to some degree from those used in the Exchange System; for this reason, the counselor needs to use the nutrient values of the physician's diet plan when calculating the diet pattern with a patient. As the patient acquires experience in weighing his food, he

## Table 29-4. Nutrient Composition of 1500-Kilocalorie Diabetic Diet (35% Simple and 65% Complex Carbohydrate)

| Food Exchanges | Amount | | Protein (g) | Fat (g) | Carbohydrate (g) | Energy (Kcal) |
| --- | --- | --- | --- | --- | --- | --- |
| | *Number* | *Household Measure* | | | | |
| Milk, non-fat | 1 | 8 oz | 8 | | 12 | 80 |
| Vegetables | 2 | 1 c | 4 | | 10 | 50 |
| Fruit | 3 | Varies | | | 30 | 120 |
| Bread | 9 | Varies | 18 | | 135 | 630 |
| Meat, lean | 6 | 6 oz | 42 | 18 | | 330 |
| Fat | 7 | 7 tsp | | 35 | | 315 |
| Totals | | | 72 | 53 | 187 | 1525 |

becomes expert in judging serving size and may be advised by his physician to weigh his food only 1 day a week to check his practices.

### Diet planning for associated diseases

In addition to modifying the diabetic diet in the treatment of elevated blood levels of triglycerides and cholesterol, discussed in Chapter 30, the diet may also be modifed if other diseases are present. The consistency of the diabetic diet may be modified if there is gastrointestinal disease (see Chap. 26). If hypertension, or cardiac or renal disease[21] is present, the diet may also be restricted in fluids and the electrolyte sodium and, if necessary, in protein and potassium (see Chaps. 31 and 32).

### Counseling the patient

The diabetic patient must be helped to accept the fact that his disease cannot be cured but that he can, with proper dietary care, and the use of insulin or oral hypoglycemic agents, if necessary, live a comfortable and productive life. Explaining to the patient in understandable terms the nature of the disease and why his dietary program is necessary is frequently the responsibility of the physician and the nurse. As soon as the hospitalized patient's diabetes is stabilized, actual dietary counseling should begin, with the physician, nurse, and nutrition counselor working closely together.[22] In many instances a social worker and clinical psychologist should also be members of this team. In the ambulatory care setting, the health-care team has an advantage in that the patient's disease is usually stable, and he is less anxious and, therefore, better able to learn.

Stone[23] has demonstrated that, given adequate instruction and the time to learn, the majority of diabetic patients can manage their diets successfully—they are capable of client-managed care. No patient can accept the diagnosis of diabetes mellitus and learn to manage its control during hospitalization (an average of 7 to 8 days) or during two visits to ambulatory care services. Therefore, the health-care team must accept and plan to meet his needs for continuity of care.[24]

**Table 29-5. 1500-Kilocalorie Diabetic Diet Pattern (68 g Protein, 53 g Fat, 187 g Carbohydrate; 35% Simple and 65% Complex Carbohydrate)**

| | Food Exchange | | Protein | Fat | Carbohydrate | Energy |
|---|---|---|---|---|---|---|
| *Meal* | *Number* | *Amount* | *(g)* | *(g)* | *(g)* | *(Kcal)* |
| Morning | | | | | | |
| Fruit | 1 | Varies | | | 10 | 40 |
| Bread | 2 | Varies | 4 | | 30 | 140 |
| Milk, non-fat | 1 | 8 oz | 8 | | 12 | 80 |
| Fat | 2 | 2 tsp | | 10 | | 90 |
| Total | | | 12 | 10 | 52 | 350 |
| Noon | | | | | | |
| Meat, lean | 2 | 2 oz | 14 | 6 | | 110 |
| Bread | 2 | Varies | 4 | | 30 | 140 |
| Fruit | 1 | Varies | | | 10 | 40 |
| Fat | 2 | 2 tsp | | 10 | | 90 |
| Total | | | 18 | 16 | 40 | 380 |
| Evening | | | | | | |
| Meat, lean | 3 | 3 oz | 21 | 9 | | 165 |
| Bread | 3 | Varies | 6 | | 45 | 210 |
| Vegetable | 2 | 1 c | 4 | | 10 | 50 |
| Fruit | 1 | Varies | | | 10 | 40 |
| Fat | 3 | 3 tsp | | 15 | | 135 |
| Total | | | 31 | 24 | 65 | 600 |
| Bedtime | | | | | | |
| Meat, lean | 1 | 1 oz | 7 | 3 | | |
| Bread | 2 | Varies | 4 | | 30 | |
| Total | | | 11 | 3 | 30 | 195 |
| Totals | | | 72 | 53 | 187 | 1525 |

Gathering the assessment data is the first step in the counseling process.[22] From her appraisal of this data the counselor can plan her program. Also, this process often helps the client identify for himself the adjustments he will need to make in his food practices.

The primary objective of nutrition counseling for the diabetic patient is to help him use his diet pattern correctly. He needs to be able to translate his pattern into daily menus and to identify the correct size portion of each item in his menu. To do this he is given a permanent record of the number of food exchanges in his diet pattern (see Table 29-5) and a copy of the Exchange Lists (see Table 24-3) from which to select his daily menu.

For the hospitalized patient his trays are an important teaching aid. With guidance he can learn the size of food portions and familiarize himself with the items in each exchange food group. The lack of certain foods that do not appear on the tray, such as sugar, jelly, pies, cakes, and other desserts, can be emphasized. As counseling progresses, the selective menu can be used as a "paper and pencil test" to evaluate the patient's understanding.

In the ambulatory care setting food models are a useful aid in helping patients visualize portion sizes. If a demonstration kitchen and food are available, portion sizes can be demonstrated with real food. It is helpful to have the patient keep a record of his food intake for 1 or 2 days between appointments. These records are used to formulate precise objectives for the counseling session.[25]

Whenever the patient's food choices differ for ethnic reasons from those included in the teaching materials, the materials should be modified to suit his choices.[26]

Other members of the family should be involved in counseling sessions with the patient so that they understand his care and can give him support.[22] If work or other schedules make it impossible for family members to be available during the day, counseling sessions should be scheduled at the convenience of the patient and the relative during a weekend or late in the day. Some ambulatory care facilities schedule clinics at least one evening a week in addition to Saturday morning.

## Special concerns
### Ketoacidosis and coma

Ketoacidosis and coma require emergency treatment to reestablish fluid and electrolyte balance and normal metabolism. If the patient is in coma, or if he is nauseated and vomiting, insulin and intravenous fluids are used to treat him. As his hyperglycemia and ketonemia decrease, and when he can tolerate it, he is offered a variety of fluids by mouth. When his condition is stabilized he is given a diabetic diet and insulin.

When the patient can tolerate fluids, it is advisable that, directly after each feeding, the amount and nutrient composition be recorded in his chart so that this information is readily available to the physician and nurse as they monitor the patient's progress. When a known diabetic is able to eat, he can assist with his menu selection. The newly diagnosed patient can share his food preferences with the dietitian but she is responsible for planning his meals until his condition improves to the point where the patient and the family can attend to diet instructions.

### Replacements

It is expected that diabetic patients receiving insulin or an oral hypoglycemic agent will consume all the food served at each meal to prevent the possibility of insulin reaction. When a patient refuses a food, he should be provided with a substitute equal in nutritional composition to the food refused.

If a patient refuses the major portion of a meal for any reason, the physician may require that the total available glucose of the meal be replaced. Carbohydrate, together with protein and fat, contribute to the total available glucose in a meal. The grams of carbohydrate yield an equal number of grams of glucose, or 100% glucose. It is estimated that 58% of protein and 10% of fat form glucose in intermediary metabolism. Therefore, to calculate the total available glucose (TAG) in a meal, one multiplies the grams of carbohydrate by 1.0, the grams of protein by 0.58, and the grams of fat by 0.10; the results are then added to obtain the total available glucose.

For example, a meal containing 30 g of protein, 30 g of fat and 60 g of carbohydrate has 80 g of available glucose.

30 g of protein × 0.58 = 17.4 g of glucose; 30 g of fat × 0.1 = 3 g of glucose; and 60 g of carbohydrate = 60 g of glucose.

This amount of carbohydrate may have to be given in several small feedings within the next 2 or 3 hours to prevent hypoglycemia.

### Surgery

Today diabetic patients undergo surgery with comparative safety. In emergencies, such as an acute appendicitis, there is usually no reason to delay surgery because of diabetes. In these situations the patient is given insulin and intravenous fluids and glucose.

When there is time to prepare for surgery, the status of the patient's diabetes is carefully evaluated and, if his disease is not well controlled, the proper diet and insulin treatment is instituted before he undergoes surgery. On the day of surgery breakfast is withheld. Part of the usual dose of moderate-acting insulin may be given before surgery. After the operation, glucose and fluids with sufficient insulin are given intravenously. Oral feedings of liquids, such as fruit juices, broth, tea, and ginger ale, are started as early as possible. Later, the patient's usual diet is resumed.

## Diabetes in pregnancy

Diabetes has always been a special hazard in pregnancy. There is increased fetal loss in the course of the pregnancy as well as an increased loss of infants carried to term compared with the nondiabetic patient. Also, it has been observed that the infants experience a greater number of problems in the neonatal period than do infants of nondiabetic mothers. In the past few years, however, by keeping close watch on the mother and infant, physicians have been able to secure a far greater number of successful pregnancies than formerly.[27]

Early prenatal care is an important factor in the salvage of these babies as well as in the maintenance of the mother's health. The diet during pregnancy must be adjusted to control the mother's diabetes and to provide for the nutritional needs of the developing fetus. As the woman progresses through pregnancy her insulin requirement increases steadily, and decreases dramatically to prepregnancy levels immediately after delivery.[28] In an obstetrical unit food acceptance by the postpartum woman must be closely monitored to avoid insulin reactions.

Throughout pregnancy and in the immediate postpartum period the diabetic patient needs frequent contact with the clinical dietitian to help her manage her diet in order to avoid both hyper- and hypoglycemia. The energy level of the diet needs adjustment to provide for her nutrient needs as well as that of the growing fetus. Women who present with gestational diabetes (the onset of diabetes during pregnancy) require intensive counseling sessions to help them manage both the pregnancy and the hyperglycemia. Most of these women have normal blood glucose levels about 1 month after delivery, but about 60% ultimately become overt diabetics.

## Diabetes in children

The outlook for children who develop diabetes has changed markedly from the preinsulin days when the disease invariably was fatal. White[29] reported on 1072 patients whose onset of diabetes occurred before the age of 15 and who had had the disease 20 years or more. Of these, 879 were living at the time of the study. Of the 879 patients, 71% had had diabetes from 20 to 29 years, 24% had had diabetes from 30 to 34 years, and 5% had had the disease for more than 35 years.

However, in a large percentage of such patients, complications develop after 15 to 20 years or more of diabetes. These include diminished vision and heart and kidney disease, all attributable to blood vessel changes. In

a later paper[30] White states that 90% of patients who developed diabetes before the age of 15 and had had the disease for 30 years or more could be shown to have such blood vessel changes. Thus, although gains have been made in increasing the lifespan of the young diabetic, much remains to be done in terms of halting the complications of the disease.

## Dietary management

The controversy over the best approach to treatment applies particularly to this younger age group of patients. Clinicians who advocate the "free" diet or diet-for-age without added sugar feel that it promotes a more positive attitude in the family and a more normal psychosocial development in the child. To avoid wide daily variations in blood glucose levels, however, the nutrition counselor is called on to assist the mother with meal planning so that there is a consistent daily intake of energy and nutrients. For example, a 4-year-old child cannot consume 1000 calories today and 1600 calories tomorrow and still maintain reasonable control. At the same time, food intake must be spaced throughout the day as with any patient using intermediate-acting insulin to avoid hyper- or hypoglycemic episodes. Sosenko and co-workers[31] have demonstrated that poor control of blood glucose in young IDDM patients is accompanied by elevated blood lipid levels. Elevated blood lipids may be one factor leading to excessive vascular disease in patients with diabetes.

## Achievement of genetic growth potential

Drash[18] reports that diabetic children attain an adult height that is well within the range of normal but below the mean for the population of the United States. English observers report that with the onset of diabetes prior to the adolescent growth spurt, full growth potential is not achieved. However, with the use of long- and intermediate-acting insulins and adequate food intake, the diabetic dwarfism of the past does not occur.

## Emotional adjustment

Coping with a chronic disease in childhood, such as diabetes mellitus, presents a major challenge to both the family and the child. A number of studies show that there is an increased incidence of emotional stress in children with diabetes compared with that in normal children. They tend to be dependent, anxious, hostile, and have impaired self-images. Acute emotional stress adversely affects diabetic control and can cause ketoacidosis. Rage and extreme anxiety can trigger epinephrine release from the adrenal medulla. Epinephrine stimulates gluconeogenesis, which can result in hyperglycemia. Also, emotional stress may lead to episodes of food gorging or omitting insulin injections entirely. The child with diabetes who experiences episodes of ketoacidosis due to emotional stress and his family may need the help of a psychiatrist or psychologist to establish an environment within the family that promotes the stabilization of the child's diabetes mellitus.

## Study questions and activities

1. Check the products on the "diet" shelf in a local supermarket or health food store. Compare the energy and nutrient composition of a dietetic product with the composition of the same amount of a standard product. For example 1 oz of a dietetic chocolate bar with 1 oz of a standard chocolate bar.

2. Discover by observation and interview how the mother of a well-controlled school-aged diabetic child (who has been hospitalized in a state of ketoacidosis due to overwhelming infection) manages his diet and activities of daily living. What resources has she used for guidance and counseling? What adjustment, if any, has the family made in its life-style since the child's diagnosis?

3. Mrs. A. is a 70 year old diabetic. Her major source of income is her monthly social security check of $250.00. She purchases food stamps to supplement her food budget. Her diet prescription is 1500 calories. Calculate her diet pattern, and write up a week's menu and a market order. Price the market order at a store in a neighborhood where many of the elderly in your community live. What percentage of her income would she spend on food?

4. Price U-40 and U-100 insulin and the equipment needed to inject insulin at a discount drugstore, an independently owned drugstore, and the hospital pharmacy. How much does it cost a diabetic patient to administer 35 units of insulin per day?

5. Collect menus from a variety of local restaurants. Select a noon and evening meal using the diet pattern which you planned for the diet prescription in question 3.

6. Find out the total number of adult diabetic patients in your hospital today. The therapeutic dietitian's records of diet orders can give you this information most readily. How many of these diets are also calorie-restricted (1500 or less)?

7. Record the 24-hour food and nutrient beverage intake of a patient with diabetes. Using the appropriate food value system, appraise his calorie and nutrient intake. Compare his actual intake of calories, protein, fat, and carbohydrate with the diet order prescribed by his physician. Compare his mineral and vitamin intake with guidelines appropriate for him. If there is any significant discrepancy between intake and order, seek the assistance of your instructors in identifying the reason and in solving the problem.

8. Give five substitutions that a diabetic can make for a slice of bread.

9. What is meant by the chemical regulation of diabetes? The clinical regulation? Why is there controversy over these two methods of regulation?

10. What is meant by a "free" diabetic diet? What advantages are claimed for it?

## References

1. Bar R, Roth J: Arch Intern Med 137:474, 1977
2. Felig P et al: Arch Intern Med 137:507, 1977
3. Unger RH, Orci L: N Engl J Med 304:1518, 1575, 1981
4. Foster DW: In Isselbacher et al (eds) Harrison's Principles of Internal Medicine, 9th ed, pp 1741–1755. New York, McGraw-Hill, 1980
5. Craighead JE: N Engl J Med 299:1439, 1978
6. Notkins AL: Sci Am 241:62, 1979
7. National Diabetes Data Group: Diabetes 28:1639, 1979
8. Siperstein MD: In Fajans, Sussman (eds): Diabetes Mellitus, Vol 3. New York, American Diabetes Association, 1971
9. Spiro RG: N Engl J Med 288:1337, 1973
10. Anderson TW: Diabetes 15:160, 1966
11. Pederson O et al: N Engl J Med 302:886, 1980
12. Rizza RA et al: N Engl J Med 303:1314, 1980
13. Shen SW, Bressler K: N Engl J Med 296:787, 1977
14. Diabetes (Suppl 2) 19:747, 1970
15. Nuttall FQ: Am J Clin Nutr 33:1311, 1980
16. Jenkins DJA et al: Am J Clin Nutr 33:1729, 1980
17. Anderson JW, Chen WJL: Am J Clin Nutr 32:346, 1979
18. Drash A: J Pediatr 78:919, 1971
19. Ravry MJR: JAMA 244:270, 1980
20. Brunzell JD: J Am Diet Assoc 73:499, 1978
21. Davis M et al: J Am Diet Assoc 75:265, 1979
22. Davidson JK: Postgrad Med 59:114, Jan, 1976
23. Stone DB: Am J Med Sci 241:436, 1961
24. Etzwiler DD: Med Clin North Am 62:857, 1978
25. Zifferblatt SM, Wilbur CS: J Am Diet Assoc 70:591, 1977
26. Goldsmith MP, Davidson JK: J Am Diet Assoc 70:61, 1977
27. Gugliucci CL et al: Am J Obstet Gynecol 125:435, 1976
28. Jouganatos DM, Gabbe SG: J Am Diet Assoc 73:168, 1978
29. White P: Diabetes 5:445, 1956
30. White P: Diabetes 9:345, 1960
31. Sosenko JM et al: N Engl J Med 302:650, 1980

## Supplementary readings
### Diabetes

Cahill GF Jr, McDevitt HO: Insulin-dependent diabetes mellitus: The initial lesion. N Engl J Med 304:1454, 1981
Levin ME et al: Prevention and treatment of diabetic complications. Arch Intern Med 140:691, 1980
Maurer AC: The therapy of diabetes. Am Sci 67:422, 1979
Paz-Guevara AT et al: Juvenile diabetes mellitus after 40 years. Diabetes 24:559, 1975
Uranic M, Berger M: Exercise and diabetes. Diabetes 28:147, 1979

### Diet planning

Fial AZ: Adding spice to sugar-reduced diets. J Am Diet Assoc 73:658, 1978
Flood JM: Diet and diabetes mellitus. Hosp Pract 15:61, Feb, 1979

Goldsmith MP, Davidson JK: Southern ethnic food preferences and exchange values for the diabetic diet. J Am Diet Assoc 70:61, 1977

Murphy EW et al: Nutrient content of spices and herbs. J Am Diet Assoc 72:174, 1978

Ravry MJR: Dietetic food diarrhea. JAMA 244:270, 1980

Southgate DAT et al: Free sugars in foods. J Hum Nutr 32:335, 1978

## Patient education

Belmonte MM et al: The problem of the "cheating" in the diabetic child and adolescent. Diabetes Care 4:116, 1981

Etzwiler DD: Education of the patient with diabetes. Med Clin North Am 62:857, 1978

Page P et al: Patient recall of self-care recommendations in diabetes. Diabetes Care 4:96, 1981

Slowie LA: Using the new Exchange Lists for instructing patients with diabetes. J Am Diet Assoc 70:59, 1977

Zifferblatt SM, Wilbur CS: Dietary counseling: Some realistic expectations and guidelines. J Am Diet Assoc 70:591, 1977

## Dietary fiber

Anderson JW et al: Mineral and vitamin status on high-fiber diets: Long-term studies of diabetic patients. Diabetes Care 3:38, 1980

Anderson JW, Chen WJL: Plant fiber. Carbohydrate and lipid metabolism. Am J Clin Nutr 32:346, 1979

Crapo PA et al: Comparison of serum glucose, insulin, and glucagon responses to different types of complex carbohydrate in noninsulin-dependent diabetic patients. Am J Clin Nutr 34:184, 1981

Miranda PM, Horwitz DL: High-fiber diets in the treatment of diabetes mellitus. Ann Intern Med 88:482, 1978

## The young diabetic

Farquhar JW, Campbell ML: Care of the diabetic child in the community. Br Med J 281:1534, 1980

Jackson RL: Education of the parents of the child with diabetes. Nutr Today 15:30, May-June, 1980

Jackson RL: Insulin-dependent diabetes in children and young adults. Nutr Today 14:26, Nov-Dec, 1979

Jackson RL: Management and treatment of the child with diabetes. Nutr Today 15:6, Mar-Apr, 1980

## Diabetes and pregnancy

Jouganatos DM, Gabbe SG: Diabetes in pregnancy: Metabolic changes and current managment. J Am Diet Assoc 73:168, 1978

Schulman PK: Diabetes in pregnancy: Nutritional aspects of care. J Am Diet Assoc 76:575, 1980

White P: Diabetes mellitus in pregnancy. Clin Perinatol 1:3331, 1974

## Special problems

Davis M et al: Dietary management of patients with diabetes treated with hemodialysis. J Am Diet Assoc 75:265, 1979

Feldman M et al: Abnormal gastric function in longstanding, insulin-dependent diabetes. Gastroenterology 77:12, 1979

## Patient resources

American Diabetes Association/American Dietetic Association Family Cookbook. Englewood Cliffs, NJ, Prentice-Hall, 1980

Brown A: The Diabetic Gourmet, rev ed. New York, Barnes and Noble, 1980

Claiborne C, Franey P: Craig Claiborne's Gourmet Diet. New York, New York Times Books, 1980

Finsand MJ: The Complete Diabetic Cookbook. New York, Sterling, 1980

Helsel J, Lansing E: The ABC's of Diabetic Cooking and Dining. New York, Dell, 1979

Krall LP (ed): Joslin Diabetes Manual, 11th ed. Philadelphia, Lea & Febiger, 1978

Middleton K, Hess MA: The Art of Cooking for the Diabetic. Chicago, Contemporary Books, 1978

Stern JS, Denenberg RV: How to Stay Slim and Healthy on a Fast Food Diet. Englewood Cliffs, NJ, Prentice-Hall, 1980

*For further references see Bibliography in Part 4.*

# Atherosclerosis

# 30

Prevalence and Incidence
Diagnostic Procedures
Diet Therapy
Patient Counseling
Hypolipidemic Drugs

**ILDL:** Intermediate Low-density
Lipoprotein
**MRFIT:** Multiple Risk Factor Intervention
Trial

**Therese A. Dolecek**

This chapter could appropriately be subtitled *Hyperlipidemia* or *Hyperlipoproteinemia* (Table 30-1, *Glossary of Terms*). From the available evidence the incidence of atherosclerosis is strongly associated with aberrations in the intermediary metabolism of cholesterol and triglycerides. Evidence is also available that the manipulation of the dietary intake of cholesterol and the type of fatty acids, saturated or polyunsaturated, can have a positive effect on the blood lipid abnormalities in hyperlipidemia, both in prevention and in therapy. Reference is made to these dietary manipulations in the previous chapters on obesity and diabetes mellitus (Chaps. 28 and 29), because hyperlipidemia is frequently associated with these metabolic problems. However, not all hyperlipidemic patients are obese or diabetic.

Before proceeding with the following discussion of atherosclerosis and the dietary modifications recommended for the prevention and treatment of hyperlipidemia, the reader is advised to review Chapter 3, *Fats and Other Lipids*, and Chapter 9, *Nutrient Utilization*, in this book, and the structures and functions of the cardiovascular system in a basic physiology textbook.

Although atherosclerosis is not the only disease state associated with hyperlipidemia, it is the one that occurs most frequently in the United States and in many other developed countries in the Western world. The term atherosclerosis is derived from two Greek words: *athēra*, meaning "porridge" or "mush," and *skleros*, meaning "hard." The atheromatous lesion, which develops in the arterial blood vessels, begins as a soft deposit and hardens as it ages. Essential to the initial atherosclerotic process is a weakening of the arterial wall due to aging, excessively high blood cholesterol, high blood pressure and cigarette smoking. As the lesion develops there is an accumulation of lipids, especially cholesterol and cholesterol ester; in some manner, these are brought into the lining of the artery by the plasma lipoproteins. With time these lesions,

### Table 30-1.  Glossary of Terms

*Hyperlipidemia:* an elevation of the concentration of any blood lipid constituent; usually implies elevated cholesterol or triglycerides or both.

*Hyperlipoproteinemia (HLP):* an elevation of the blood concentration of one or more lipoprotein families; nearly always accompanied by hyperlipidemia.

*Hyperlipemia:* a lactescent (milky) appearance of blood caused by increased concentration of triglyceride in either very low-density lipoproteins (VLDL) or chylomicrons.

*Hyperglyceridemia (or hypertriglyceridemia):* an elevation in the blood levels of glycerides, usually triglycerides.

*Hyperchylomicronemia:* an elevation in the blood levels of chylomicrons.

*Hypercholesterolemia:* an elevation in the blood level of total cholesterol.

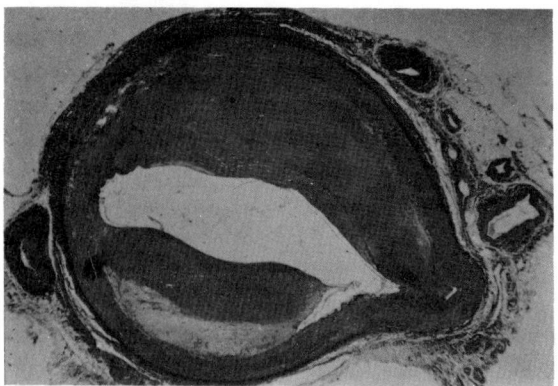

**Fig. 30-1.**   Atherosclerotic obliteration of the lumen of the iliac artery. (Bailey CP et al: Rheumatic and Coronary Heart Disease, Philadelphia, JB Lippincott, 1967)

known as *plaques*, gradually grow and thicken the intima of the arterial walls, thereby narrowing the lumen of the blood vessels (Fig. 30-1). The atherosclerotic plaque is composed of various substances that include cholesterol, fatty acids, lipoproteins (a complex molecule of protein and fat), calcium deposits, complex carbohydrates, fibrous scar tissue, and blood.[1] How and why these plaques develop is not well understood, and numerous theories have been under intensive study.

Myocardial infarction, commonly called heart attack, occurs when a blood clot forms suddenly and occludes the lumen of a coronary artery already narrowed by

### Table 30-2.  Factors Known to Increase the Risk of Coronary Heart Disease

GROUP 1.  *(Not amenable to preventive intervention)*
    Maleness
    Age (increased risk with increased age)
    Family history (positive for premature vascular disease)
    Certain somatotypes
    Particular behavior patterns and personality types

GROUP 2.  *(Associated disease entities)*
    Hyperlipoproteinemias
    Arterial hypertension
    Obesity
    Diabetes mellitus
    Hyperuricemia and gout

GROUP 3.  *(Primarily due to culture and environment)*
    Dietary practices (high intake of cholesterol, saturated fats, sucrose* and energy)
    Sedentary living habits (lack of physical exercise)
    Cigarette smoking
    Excessive coffee drinking†
    Soft water for drinking‡

*Ahrens RA: Am J Clin Nutr 27:403, 1974

†Jick H et al: N Engl J Med 289:63, 1973

‡Perry HM Jr: J Am Diet Assoc 62:631, 1973

(Adapted from Brusis OA, McGandy RB: Fed Proc 30:1417, 1971)

an atheromatous plaque. This event deprives the surrounding tissue of its blood supply. Depending on the extent of damage to the tissue of the heart in the area of the occlusion, the patient may survive or may die suddenly. If the occlusion of a blood vessel occurs in the brain, the result is a cerebral hemorrhage, or "stroke." Other arterial blood vessels in the body may also be occluded, causing serious disease or death.

## Prevalence and incidence

Atherosclerosis is a major public health problem because the sequelae to the formation of atheroma—coronary artery disease and cerebral hemorrhage—are the leading causes of disability and death in the United States and Canada. Although there has been a major downward trend over the last 15 years in cardiovascular disease mortality in the United States, the prevalence of these diseases remains a serious concern. In 1972 more than 600,000 persons in the United States and 77,000 in Canada died of coronary heart disease. It is estimated that over 160,000 of the deaths in the United States occurred in persons under 65 years of age, predominantly males in this age group. According to the National Health Examination Survey data, 5 million Americans have atherosclerosis, which makes it the second most prevalent cardiovascular disease (the most prevalent cardiovascular problem is hypertension).

### Coronary risk factors

After 30 years of intensive epidemiologic and laboratory research, the etiology of atherosclerosis is still equivocal. However, there is relatively general agreement that the causation is multifactorial, that is, a number of factors interact in determining the inception, rate of progression, and ultimate clinical course of atherosclerosis. Table 30-2 lists the factors that appear to increase the risk of coronary heart disease, but not all investigators would agree that each item in the table is a risk factor. For example, there is considerable controversy about the role of excessive caffeine consumption. However, there is consensus that the three major risk factors in coronary heart disease, which can be modified, are increase in the level of blood cholesterol, excessive cigarette smoking, and blood pressure levels above normal.

In 1972 the Heart, Lung, and Blood Institute of the National Institutes of Health established the Multiple Risk Factor Intervention Trial (MRFIT) to assess the effectiveness of measures to reduce elevated blood cholesterol, high blood pressure, and cigarette smoking in preventing first heart attacks and reducing death rates from cardiovascular disease.[2] Twenty clinical research centers around the country each recruited approximately 600 men, ages 35 to 57, who were at above average risk for coronary heart disease due to various combinations of these three factors. Half of the men participate in a special intervention program to reduce their risk factors; the other half were referred to their usual source of medical care for treatment and are seen only annually by clinic staff. Included in the staff of each study center to assist the special intervention group are nutritionists to counsel the subjects in modifying their diets, behavioral scientists to help reduce smoking, and physicians to direct the medical procedures to reduce blood pressure.

Another clinical trial currently in progress and sponsored by the National Heart, Lung, and Blood Institute is being carried out through the Lipids Research Clinics to test the efficacy of reducing blood cholesterol levels in relation to coronary primary prevention.[3] This trial uses both diet and hypolipidemic drugs to lower blood cholesterol.

### Nutritional research

The relationship to coronary heart disease of the dietary intake of cholesterol, total fat and fatty acids, carbohydrate, and energy has been and continues to be under intensive investigation.

#### Blood cholesterol

The majority of patients with coronary artery disease have an elevated blood cholesterol level, and researchers are attempting to relate the occurrence of this elevation in cholesterol to dietary intake in order to design therapeutic as well as preventive nutritional care. Both epidemiologic and clinical research have been used to study this problem.

#### Dietary fats, fatty acids, and cholesterol

The Seven Countries Study showed that the incidence of coronary heart disease in the populations studied seemed to be related to the amount of saturated fat in the national diet.[4] For example, Japan, Greece, Italy, and Yugoslavia, countries with low saturated fat diets, had a

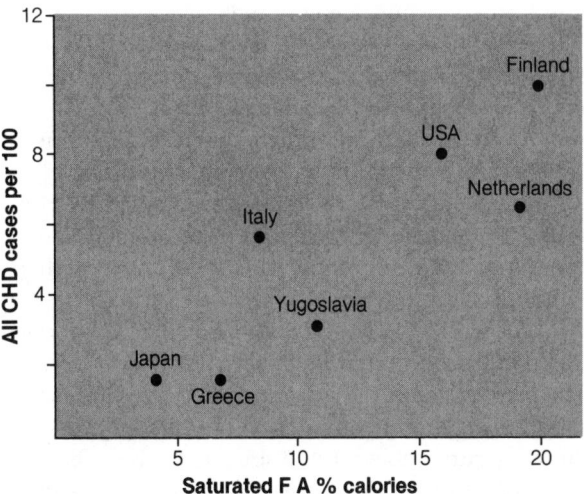

**Fig. 30-2.** Rates for all diagnoses of new coronary heart disease in seven countries studied by Keys, compared to percentage of total calories provided by saturated fatty acids in the diet. (Feldman UB: Nutrition and Cardiovascular Disease. New York, Appleton-Century-Crofts, 1976)

low incidence of coronary heart disease, whereas Finland, the United States, and the Netherlands, countries consuming high saturated fat diets, had very high rates of coronary heart disease (see Fig. 30-2).

Following these population studies, extensive research was done to determine the effect of fatty acids on serum cholesterol levels in humans and animals. The results of these investigations indicate that saturated fats tend to increase serum cholesterol, while fats containing primarily polyunsaturated fats tend to decrease serum cholesterol.[5] Monounsaturated fats appear to have no effect. There is, as yet, no agreement on the mechanisms by which the degree of saturation of fats affects serum cholesterol levels.

The role of dietary cholesterol as a contributor to blood cholesterol level was investigated in the late 1960s. Findings from these studies indicate that blood levels do reflect in part the dietary intake of cholesterol. Hegsted estimated that every 100 mg of dietary cholesterol would increase blood cholesterol level by 5 mg per deciliter.[6]

It has been shown that the usual American diet contains an average of 600 mg to 800 mg of cholesterol per day. The major sources of dietary cholesterol are meat, eggs, and milk products. Table and cooking fats and commercial baked goods also contribute dietary cholesterol. Depending on food choices, a person can easily consume more than 1000 mg per day. For example, one egg contains about 250 mg of cholesterol. Two or three eggs per day contribute 500 mg to 750 mg of cholesterol.

It must be remembered that the cholesterol absorbed from food is not the only source of blood cholesterol. It is synthesized endogenously by the cells of the liver and gastrointestinal tract from the two carbon structure acetate formed in intermediary metabolism (see Chap. 9). Therefore, hexoses, glycerol, fatty acids, and certain de-aminized amino acids can contribute carbon atoms for the endogenous synthesis of cholesterol.

At the same time, other investigators studied the effects of modifying the fatty acid composition of usual diets on blood cholesterol levels. They studied individuals, primarily men, under metabolic research conditions, and groups of men living and eating at home with their families.

The work of Page and Brown and their co-workers in Cleveland is one example of the first type of research.[7] These investigators have determined critical limits for the fat and cholesterol composition of a diet effective in reducing serum cholesterol. Table 30-3 shows that a diet with 30% to 40% of calories from fat was effective in lowering serum cholesterol when less than 14% of total calories was provided by saturated fatty acids, more than 14% of total calories was from polyunsaturated fatty acids (linoleic), and the diet contained less than 350 mg of cholesterol. A diet containing 25% to 30% of calories from fat was effective when less than 11% of total calories was provided by saturated fatty acids, more than 13% by polyunsaturated fatty acids, and the diet contained less than 300 mg of cholesterol.

The National Diet-Heart Study was designed to study the effect of dietary control on blood cholesterol levels in a free-living population.[8] Approximately 1000 men in five American cities were enrolled in a program to consume specially prepared foods for a 1-year period. The foods included were developed to meet the specifications of three diets outlined in Table 30-4. An average cholesterol drop of 26 mg per deciliter below the baseline level of 230 mg per deciliter was observed in each of the two test diet groups studied.

Christakis and his group in New York have studied 814 men ages 40 to 59 who were placed on a diet low in saturated fat and cholesterol and relatively rich in polyunsaturated fatty acids.[9] This diet resulted in a significant decrease in serum cholesterol levels, and the decrease was maintained for as long as 5 years. A control group of 463 men on nonrestricted diets was also studied. Compared with the control group, the diet group suffered less morbidity from new coronary heart disease.

No population has ever consumed a diet high in polyunsaturates. Several studies have shown an increase in the incidence of cancer in people consuming a high polyunsaturated fat diet.[10] However, other studies do not confirm this observation.[11] The relation of a high polyunsaturated fat intake to increased gallstone formation is

### Table 30-3. Critical Limits of Dietary Fat Composition for Serum Cholesterol Reduction

| Component | Diet with 30–40 Percent Fat Calories | Diet with 25–30 Percent Fat Calories |
|---|---|---|
| Saturated fatty acids | Less than 14% calories | Less than 11% calories |
| Polyunsaturated fatty acids (linoleic) | More than 14% calories | More than 13% calories |
| Cholesterol | Less than 350 mg | Less than 300 mg |

(Brown HB, Farrand ME: J Am Diet Assoc 49:303, 1966)

### Table 30-4. Planned Test Diets of the National Diet–Heart Study

| Component | Diets | | |
| | Test 1 | Test 2 | Control |
|---|---|---|---|
| *Total fat (% total cal)* | 30 | 40 | 40 |
| *Saturated fatty acids (% total cal)* | <9 | <9 | ≤18 |
| *Polyunsaturated fatty acids (% total cal)* | ≥15 | 18–20 | ≤7 |
| *Cholesterol (mg/day)* | 350–450 | 350–450 | 650–750 |

(From National Diet–Heart Study Research Group: National Diet–Heart Study Report. Circulation (Suppl 1) 37:I, 1968. By permission of the American Heart Association, Inc.)

less equivocal. Although polyunsaturated fats have a lowering effect on blood cholesterol levels and replace foods containing saturates in the diet, excessive intake should not be encouraged as the issue of toxicity is still in question.

Current research focuses on the effect of lowering blood cholesterol level on the atherosclerotic lesions. Blankenhorn and associates in Los Angeles have compared femoral angiograms over time to evaluate the severity, regression, or progression of atherosclerosis. In a recent study 25 hyperlipidemic men and women were placed on a fat-controlled diet and received lipid-lowering drugs to reduce blood lipid levels. After 13 months an evaluation using femoral angiography indicated a regression of lesions in those patients who demonstrated a significant reduction in blood lipid levels.[12] These studies are encouraging as they seem to indicate that through blood lipid lowering atherosclerosis may be reversible.

### Energy intake

There has been conflicting evidence about the role of obesity *per se* as a risk factor in coronary heart disease. Bagdade has observed that hyperlipidemia, especially hypertriglyceridemia, frequently occurs in the obese.[13] The data from the Framingham Heart Study, a continuing study of the development of coronary heart disease in a community, show that moderately large changes in serum cholesterol and blood pressure were proportional to changes over time in relative body weight.[14] Levy and co-workers have shown that, with restricted total energy intake leading to weight reduction, the cholesterol and triglyceride levels can be kept at normal levels in almost all patients with abnormal blood lipid levels.[15]

### Carbohydrates

It appears that carbohydrates, simple or complex, as part of the diet have little effect on blood lipid levels. However, when carbohydrates are substituted for fat in the diet a small transient rise in fasting plasma triglyceride level may be observed in some people.[16] Carbohydrates can add excess calories to the diet, particularly sucrose, which contributes to the development of obesity and indirectly to blood lipid elevations.

### Alcohol

Hypertriglyceridemia is the lipid abnormality most often associated with excessive alcohol intake. Alcohol also provides an appreciable amount of calories and may contribute to the development of obesity.

### Other dietary factors

The role of other dietary factors, including fiber, caffeine, trace minerals, hardness of water, and vitamins is currently being studied. The relationship of these factors to atherosclerosis is not well understood.

### Lipoproteins

Fredrickson, Levy, and Lee at the National Institutes of Health demonstrated that measurements of the lipoproteins *per se* were better indicators of blood lipid abnormalities than analyses of the concentrations of total blood lipid values. In Chapter 3 it is pointed out that lipids are transported in the blood by chylomicrons, very low-density lipoproteins (VLDL), low-density lipoproteins (LDL), and high-density lipoproteins (HDL) (see Table 3-3). An intermediate low-density lipoprotein (ILDL) that is a catabolic product of VLDL has also been identified.

The National Institutes of Health's original classification of the hyperlipoproteinemias (HLP) into Types I, II, III, IV, and V has been modified to Type I, hyperchylomicronemia (normal or elevated cholesterol with markedly elevated triglyceride); Type IIa, hypercholesterolemia (increased LDL); Type IIb or Type III, hypercholesterolemia with endogenous hyperglyceridemia (Type IIb, increased LDL and VLDL and Type III, increased ILDL); Type IV, endogenous hyperglyceridemia (increased VLDL); and Type V, mixed hyperglyceridemia (increased chylomicrons and VLDL).

They have also demonstrated that HLPs are of two classes: primary or familial with genetic transmission; and those secondary to other diseases, such as diabetes, hypothyroidism, obstructive liver disease, pancreatitis, and alcoholism. Premature atherosclerosis occurs frequently in people with primary Type IIa, IIb, or IV lipoprotein patterns[17] (Table 30-5). This work also lends support for family history (genetics) as an important risk factor in the development of coronary heart disease. By manipulating the intake of cholesterol, fatty acids, and carbohydrate, as well as the total energy when the patient is obese, researchers showed that the blood lipid abnormalities could be modified.

Recently, the role that each of these fractions plays in the development of atherosclerosis has become more evident. Epidemiologic evidence indicates that increased levels of HDL cholesterol are associated with reduced incidence of coronary heart disease. Increased coronary heart disease is observed when LDL levels are elevated. This relationship is shown in Figure 30-3, which illustrates the Cooperative Lipoprotein Phenotyping Studies Pooled Data.[18] It can be seen that for this group of men aged 50 to 69 as LDL cholesterol increased, the incidence of coronary heart disease increased. The reverse was true for HDL cholesterol.

Biochemical research has also helped to clarify the role of lipoproteins in the atherogenic process. From the work of Brown and Goldstein it has been shown that the LDL fraction enters the arterial lining and causes increased smooth muscle cell proliferation and, ultimately, over time, atherosclerosis. HDL removes cholesterol from the tissues and appears to interfere with the binding of

## Table 30-5. Five Types of Primary Hyperlipoproteinemia

| Features | Type I | Type II a | Type II b or III | Type IV | Type V |
|---|---|---|---|---|---|
| Incidence | Very rare | Common | Relatively uncommon | Common | Uncommon |
| Appearance of plasma | Cream layer over clear infranatant fluid on standing | Clear | Clear, cloudy, or milky | Slightly turbid to cloudy, unchanged with standing | Cream layer over turbid infranatant on standing |
| Cholesterol | Normal or elevated | Elevated | Elevated | Normal or elevated | Elevated or normal |
| Triglyceride | Markedly elevated | Normal or slightly elevated | Usually elevated | Elevated | Elevated to markedly elevated |
| Lipoprotein family | Elevated chylomicrons | Increased LDL | II b—Increased LDL and VLDL III—Increased ILDL | Increased VLDL | Increased chylomicrons and VLDL |
| Clinical presentation | Lipemia retinalis, eruptive xanthomas, hepatosplenomegaly, abdominal pain | Xanthelasma, tendon and tuberous xanthomas, juvenilis corneal arcus, accelerated atherosclerosis | Xanthoma planum; tuberoeruptive and tendon xanthomas; accelerated atherosclerosis of coronary and peripheral vessels | Accelerated coronary vessel disease, abnormal glucose tolerance, hyperuricemia | Lipemia retinalis, eruptive xanthomas, hepatosplenomegaly, abdominal pain, hyperglycemia, hyperuricemia |
| Origin; possible mechanism | Genetic recessive; deficiency in lipoprotein lipase | When genetic, dominant, sporadic; decreased catabolism of beta-lipoprotein | When genetic, recessive; sporadic? | When genetic, dominant, sporadic; excessive endogenous glyceride synthesis or deficient glyceride clearance? | Probably genetic, dominant, sporadic |
| Age of detection | Early childhood | Early childhood (in severe cases) | Adulthood (over age 20) | Adulthood | Early adulthood |
| Conditions to be excluded* | Dysgammaglobulinemia, insulinopenic diabetes | Dietary cholesterol excess, porphyria, myxedema, myeloma, nephrosis, obstructive liver disease | Myxedema, dysgammaglobulinemia | Diabetes, glycogen storage disease, nephrotic syndrome, pregnancy, Werner's syndrome | Myeloma, dysproteinemias, diabetic acidosis, nephrosis, alcoholism, pancreatitis |

*Secondary hyperlipoproteinemias.

(Adapted from Levy RI: Fed Proc 30:829, 1971, and N Engl J Med 290:1295, 1974)

LDL at the cell membrane, thus having a protective effect.[19]

The role that VLDL cholesterol plays in the process is not clear. Currently, it is thought that this fraction does not significantly influence atherogenesis.

Research has shown that specific dietary substances have definite effects upon plasma lipid and lipoprotein concentrations. Saturated fats and dietary cholesterol increase the LDL cholesterol and to some extent the VLDL and IDL fractions. Chylomicrons are affected by total fat, whether saturated, monounsaturated, or polyunsaturated. Weight gain due to excessive caloric intake results in increases in the VLDL and the IDL fractions.[20] The effect of diet on HDL is currently under investigation. It has been hypothesized that weight loss and the fat-controlled diet may increase HDL levels. However, research to date has not produced substantial evidence showing this to be true.

### Recommendations for the prevention of CHD

In recent years, recommendations to change dietary practices for the prevention of coronary heart disease have been directed toward the public. It has been estimated that 5% or less of the American population has severe and genetically determined hyperlipidemia.[21] The majority of Americans who develop coronary heart disease have moderately elevated blood cholesterol levels (220 mg–280 mg per deciliter), which are induced by diet and only partially caused by genetics.[22] For this reason, the American Heart Association has advocated a fat-controlled dietary plan intended for the general population to lower lipid levels and thereby to decrease risk for coronary heart disease.[16] In 1977 the Select Committee on Nutrition and Human Needs, United States Senate, published *Dietary Goals for the United States*, based on current scientific evidence.[23] The purpose of these goals is "to provide nutrition knowledge with which Americans can begin to take responsibility for maintaining their health and reducing their risk of illness." Each of the seven goals includes recommendations that apply to the prevention of atherosclerosis. In 1980, the United States Department of Agriculture published dietary guidelines for Americans titled *Nutrition and Your Health*.[24] These guidelines are intended for use by already "healthy" citizens and stress good eating habits based on moderation and variety to help maintain and improve health, including the prevention of coronary heart disease. (See Chapter 1.)

## Diagnostic procedures
### Blood lipids

Blood is drawn after a 12- to 14-hour fast for analysis of blood lipids. Correlations of blood cholesterol with the incidence of premature coronary heart disease show that there is an increasing risk when the cholesterol is higher than 220 mg per 100 ml of blood. A fasting triglyceride of greater than 150 mg is also considered elevated.

### Lipoprotein analysis

Lipoprotein analysis is a complex procedure; the reader is referred to a discussion of the method presented in *Hyperlipidemia Diagnosis and Therapy*.[25] The conditions for the preparation of the subject for drawing blood for lipid analysis are of concern to the nutrition counselor. The subject must fast for 12 to 14 hours; for the preceding 2 weeks, he must consume his usual diet and neither gain nor lose weight; he must not be taking any medication known to affect plasma lipids; and he must not consume alcoholic beverages or take any other medication in the preceding 24 hours.

## Diet therapy

Dietary modification is the primary means of managing hyperlipidemia once diagnosis and classification have been made. Improvement occurs with appropriate dietary change almost without exception whether or not the abnormality is partially or completely genetic. As described by Connor, the objective of the dietary management of hyperlipidemia is the achievement of normal plasma cholesterol and triglyceride levels in order to prevent and treat atherosclerosis of the coronary arteries and of the aorta and its other branches, to prevent episodes of abdominal pain and pancreatitis, and to correct and prevent xanthomatous deposits in the skin and tendons.[20]

The current trend in the management of hyperlipidemia is initially to use a basic diet that incorporates the recommendations of the American Heart Association (AHA), which recommends that energy intake should be adjusted to achieve and maintain ideal weight; no more than 30% to 35% of total calories should be contributed by fat; saturated fatty acids should be restricted to less than

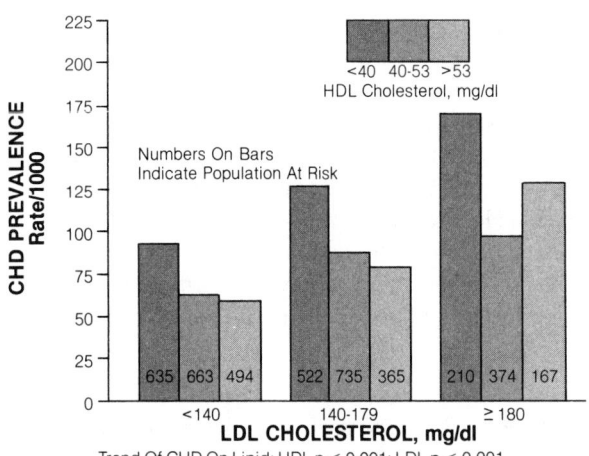

**Fig. 30-3.** Prevalence of CHD by levels of LDL-C and HDL-C in men aged 50 to 69. Pooled data from Cooperative Lipoprotein Phenotyping Studies. (Castelli WP et al: HDL Cholesterol and Other Lipids in Coronary Heart Disease. The Cooperative Lipoprotein Phenotyping Study. 55:767, 1977. Reproduced by permission of the American Heart Association, Inc.)

10% of total calories and polyunsaturated fatty acids should comprise up to 10% of total calories; and dietary cholesterol should be restricted to less than 300 mg per day. Pamphlets are available through the American Heart Association directed toward dietary control of hyperlipidemia (see *Patient Resources* at end of this chapter).

Table 30-6 summarizes the recommendations of Fredrickson and co-workers for the dietary management of hyperlipoproteinemias. Note that in addition to recommendations for energy, fat, and cholesterol, this table includes recommendations for protein, carbohydrate, and alcohol. The dietary recommendations of the American Heart Association and of Fredrickson and co-workers for the prevention and treatment of various types of HLPs share many characteristics. The National Heart, Lung, and Blood Institute has also published a series of pamphlets for patients (see *Patient Resources* at end of chapter).

Achieving and maintaining ideal body weight through calorie restriction and increasing energy expenditure often corrects hyperlipidemia in overweight or obese patients. Many of the patients who have premature atherosclerosis or coronary heart disease or diabetes or both are overweight or obese. Hypercholesterolemia usually responds to a diet that incorporates the AHA recommendations for total fat, saturated fat, polyunsaturated fat, and dietary cholesterol. Some very resistant patients (Type IIa) may require further reductions in total fat, saturated fat, and cholesterol. Hyperlipidemic conditions that are characterized by hypertriglyceridemia (Types IIb, III, IV) may require reduction of total carbohydrate to approximately 50% of calories. Triglyceride elevations are often corrected by weight loss. Sugar, particularly sucrose, has been reported to increase blood triglyceride and, for this reason, is restricted in diets aimed at correcting hyper-triglyceridemia. Treatment of chylomicronemia (Type I) requires a very low total fat diet. A diet providing about 12% calories from fat is usually recommended. Patients with elevated VLDL levels in addition to chylomicronemia (Type V) require a low total fat diet, less than 30% calories as well as less carbohydrate, approximately 50% calories. Patients with hyperlipidemia should be followed closely so that the effect of prescribed diets on blood lipid levels can be monitored and diets modified accordingly.

## Planning diet patterns

A reduced calorie diet is frequently the first diet prescription in the treatment of hyperlipidemias because many of these patients are overweight. The achievement and maintenance of ideal weight status can correct the hyperlipidemia in most of these patients. In these situations one can use the information in Chapter 28 for planning diets with special emphasis on fat modification.

Food may be classified as fat-containing or low in fat. Fat-containing foods are listed in Table 30-7 according to

## Table 30-6.  Summary of Diets for Type I–V Hyperlipoproteinemias

|  | Type I (Diet 1) Hyperchylo-micronemia | Type IIa (Diet 2) Hypercholes-terolemia | Type IIb or III (Diet 3) Hypercholes-terolemia and endogenous hyper-glyceridemia | Type IV (Diet 4) Endogenous hyperglycer-idemia | Type V (Diet 5) Mixed hyper-glyceridemia |
|---|---|---|---|---|---|
| Diet Prescription | Low fat (25–35 g) | Low cholesterol, increased polyunsaturated fat | Low cholesterol, approximately 20% calories from protein, 40% calories from fat, 40% calories from carbohydrate; restricted cholesterol | Controlled carbohydrate, approximately 45% of calories. Moderately restricted cholesterol | Restricted fat, 30% of calories; controlled carbohydrate, 50% of calories; moderately restricted cholesterol |
| Energy | Calories not restricted | Calories not restricted | Achieve and maintain "ideal" weight. (Reduction diet if necessary) | Achieve and maintain "ideal" weight. (Reduction diet if necessary) | Achieve and maintain "ideal" weight. (Reduction diet if necessary) |
| Protein | Total protein not limited | Total protein not limited | 1½–2 g per kg of body weight or 18%–21% total calories | Total protein not limited | 1½–2 g per kg of body weight or 21%–24% total calories |
| Fat | Restricted to 25–35 g per day, type of fat not important | Increased polyunsaturated fatty acid. Limited saturated fat | 40% of total calories (polyunsaturated fatty acid in preference to saturated fatty acid) | Not limited unless reduction diet needed (polyunsaturated fatty acid in preference to saturated fatty acid) | 0.9–1.3 g per kg body weight. Polyunsaturated fatty acid in preference to saturated fatty acid |
| Cholesterol | Not restricted | Less than 300 mg per day (as low as possible, 100–200 mg preferred) | Less than 300 mg per day | 300–500 mg per day | 300–500 mg per day |
| Carbohydrate | Not limited | Not limited | Controlled—sucrose and concentrated sweets are restricted | Limited to 4–5 g per kg body weight Sucrose and concentrated sweets are restricted | Limited to 5 g per kg body weight Sucrose and concentrated sweets are limited |
| Alcohol | Not recommended | May be used with discretion | Limited to 2 oz of gin, rum, vodka, or whisky | Limited to 2 oz of gin, rum, vodka, or whisky | Not recommended |

(Adapted from Dietary Management of Hyperlipoproteinemia. A Handbook for Physicians and Dietitians, NIH rev. Bethesda, MD, National Heart, Lung and Blood Institute, 1973)

their source—animal or vegetable—and by the fat component present. Saturated fatty acids are primarily found in meat and dairy or butter fat and the vegetable sources, cocoa butter, coconut oil, and palm oil. Cholesterol is present *only* in animal products. No cholesterol is found in any product of vegetable origin. Polyunsaturated fatty acids are provided by fish oil and fat, most oils, soft margarines, and walnuts. Food sources of monounsaturated fatty acids are also listed. Egg yolk contains primarily monounsaturated fat but also contains 250 mg of

cholesterol; because this represents almost all of one day's allowance when the goal is to restrict cholesterol to less than 300 mg per day, eggs should be used sparingly. Low-fat food items include bread, cereal, pasta, fruit, and vegetables.

Food selection for the fat-controlled diet should be based on the principles that provide a nutritionally sound diet that meets individual needs. Table 30-8 gives guidelines for daily food selection that meet the AHA recommendations previously described. Fat modification

### Table 30-7. Grouping of Fat-containing Foods by Source and Fat Component

| Fat Component | Animal Products | Vegetable Products | Hydrogenated Products |
|---|---|---|---|
| Saturated fatty acids | Fat in meat and poultry<br>Butter fat | Cocoa butter<br>Coconut oil<br>Palm and palm kernel oil | |
| Monounsaturated fatty acids | Egg yolk fat | Olives<br>Olive oil<br>Nuts<br>Peanut butter | Margarine<br>Shortening<br>Soybean oil (hydrogenated) |
| Polyunsaturated fatty acids | Fish oil and fat | Salad oils<br>Cottonseed<br>Corn<br>Walnuts<br>Safflower<br>Soya<br>Sunflower | Soft margarine<br>Soybean oil (hydrogenated) |
| Cholesterol | Butter fat<br>Meat<br>Poultry<br>Fish<br>Shellfish<br>Egg yolk<br>Organ meats | | |

(Brown HB: Practical Cardiology, April, 1976)

### Table 30-8. Daily Food Selection

| Food Item | Amount |
|---|---|
| Lean meat, poultry, fish | 6–8 ounces lean meat, fish, or poultry |
| Egg yolks | 2 or less per week |
| Dairy products<br>  Skim, low fat | 3 or more cups for children 12 years or under<br>4 or more cups for teenagers<br>2 or more cups for adults |
| Polyunsaturated vegetable fats and oils | 2–4 tablespoons* |
| Low-fat nutritious foods<br>  Bread, cereal, pasta | 4 servings or more (whole grain or enriched)* |
| Fruit and vegetables | 4 servings or more (1 serving = $\frac{1}{2}$ cup)* |
| Nonessential foods<br>  Sugar, sweets, low-fat desserts, alcohol | Limited or eliminated* |

*Amount adjusted to food pattern and caloric requirement.

is achieved by using only lean meat that is well trimmed of visible fat, using more poultry and fish, and controlling meat portions. Egg yolks are limited to no more than two per week. Dairy products should be nonfat or low fat. Polyunsaturated oils and margarines should be substituted for saturated fats, such as butter, lard, and hydrogenated shortenings. Low-fat foods including breads, cereals, fruits, and vegetables may be used freely unless the control of calories is necessary. Nonessential foods, such as sugars, sweets, and alcohol, should be limited as these foods provide substantial calories without contributing other essential nutrients.

### Nutrient composition of fat-controlled exchange system

When planning fat-controlled diets, a tool that provides a means for the nutrition counselor to individualize diet patterns is an exchange system. A fat-controlled exchange system and exchange lists are presented in this section. This exchange system is based on Table 24-2 in Chapter 24.

Table 30-9 gives the energy and nutrient composition of the exchange food groups that can be used to calculate a fat-controlled diet pattern. Note that in addition to pro-

tein, fat, carbohydrate, and energy, values are given for cholesterol and saturated and polyunsaturated (linoleic) fatty acids. The figures are derived from the 1977 NHLBI Nutrition Coding Center Food Table.[26] The fatty acid figures for meat reflect weighted averages derived from values for lean red meat, poultry without skin, and fish. Red meat contributed 50% to the fatty acid and cholesterol values; poultry and fish each contributed 25%.

Note that, in comparison with the other food groups in Table 30-9, the 1 oz of lean meat and the $2/_7$ of an egg make the most significant contributions to the saturated fatty acid and cholesterol values. On the other hand, the vegetable oils and margarine contribute the most significant quantities of the polyunsaturated fatty acid, linoleic acid. The fatty acid values for meat, egg, and vegetable oils and margarine demonstrate the quantitative differences between the types of fatty acids in animal fats and vegetable oils. Table 30-10 also demonstrates this difference.

To satisfy the recommendation of polyunsaturated fatty acids in preference to saturated ones (see Table 30-6) vegetable oils and margarine are the only food fats that can be used as fat exchanges in the diet patterns. The fatty acid values in Table 30-9 may be used to plan a diet pattern with a specific ratio of linoleic to saturated fatty

**Table 30-9. Nutrient Composition of Exchange System for Fat-controlled Diets**

| | | | | Fat | | | | | |
| | | | | Total Fat (g) | Saturated Fatty Acids (g) | Linoleic Fatty Acid (g) | Cholesterol (mg) | Carbohydrate (g) | Energy (Kcal) |
| Food Group | Amount | Weight | Protein | | | | | | |
|---|---|---|---|---|---|---|---|---|---|
| Non-fat milk (<1% fat) | 1 c (8 oz) | 240 | 8.0 | tr | 0.1 | 0.0 | 4 | 12 | 80 |
| Vegetables | ½ c | 100 | 2.0 | | | | | 5 | 25 |
| Fruit | Varies | | | | | | | 10 | 40 |
| Bread and cereal | Varies | | 2.0 | 1.0 | 0.2 | 0.2 | | 15 | 75 |
| Meat, lean | 1 oz | 30 | 7.0 | 3.0 | 0.7 | 0.4 | 24 | | 55 |
| Eggs, whole | 2/wk | 14 | 2.0 | 2.0 | 0.5 | 0.2 | 72 | | 25 |
| Fat (polyunsaturated margarines and oils) | 1 tsp | 5 | | 5.0 | 0.6 | 2.1 | | | 45 |

(Compiled from NHLBI Nutrition Coding Center Food Table, Minneapolis, 1977)

**Table 30-10. Fatty Acid and Energy Composition of Selected Foods**

| Food | Measure | Weight (g) | Total Fat (g) | Saturated Fatty Acids (g) | Linoleic Fatty Acid (g) | Energy (Kcal) |
|---|---|---|---|---|---|---|
| Margarine* | 1 tbsp | 14 | 11 | 2.6 | 6.3 | 100 |
| Vegetable oil†‡ | 1 tbsp | 14 | 14 | 2.0 | 7.7 | 120 |
| Butter‡ | 1 tbsp | 14 | 12 | 6.3 | 0.3 | 100 |
| Milk, whole‡ | 1 c | 240 | 9 | 4.7 | 0.2 | 160 |
| Beef, rib with fat‡ | 1 oz | 30 | 12 | 5.8 | 0.2 | 135 |

*Fleischmann's Tub Margarine.

†Corn, cottonseed, safflower, soybean oils.

‡From Adams CF: Nutritive Value of Americn Foods in Common Units. Agriculture Handbook No. 456, pp 27, 39, 97, 102, 183, 190, 225, 228, 229. Washington, DC, USDA, United States Government Printing Office, 1975

acids (P:S ratio). The calculation of a 1500-calorie, fat-controlled diet pattern with a P:S ratio of 1.7:1 is shown in Table 30-11.

### Exchange lists

The Fat-Controlled Exchange Lists are presented in Table 30-12 and should be compared to the Exchange Lists in Table 24-3 in Chapter 24.

***Milk exchange.*** Only nonfat milk products are used because the fat-controlled diets restrict total fat or recommend polyunsaturated fatty acids in preference to saturated fatty acids. The fat-controlled diets also restrict cholesterol. For example, 8 oz of whole milk contains 34 mg of cholesterol, while 8 oz of skim milk contains 5 mg. Yogurt and buttermilk should be made from skim milk.

***Vegetable exchange and fruit exchange.*** The items in the vegetable and fruit exchange lists in Table 24-3, Chapter 24, are used to plan daily menus for fat-controlled diets and are not reproduced in Table 30-12. If the patient is not obese and the diet is not restricted in sucrose, fruits canned or frozen with sugar may be used, but vegetables frozen in butter sauce or any other sauce must not be used. Any fat exchanges calculated in a diet pattern can be used to season cooked vegetables or in salad dressings. The number of servings of vegetables and fruits is limited in the diet pattern if the diet prescription limits the amount of simple carbohydrates (see discussion of simple and complex carbohydrates in Chapter 29, *Diabetes Mellitus*).

***Bread exchange.*** This list is less extensive than the bread exchange list in Table 24-3, Chapter 24. The breads in Table 30-12 are limited to those made with a minimum amount of added fat. One gram of fat has been added to the bread exchange value to reflect the fat used in breadmaking and the quantity of fat in cereal products. Therefore, the energy value of one exchange is 75 calories.

Prepared foods, such as one biscuit (2-in diameter), one muffin (plain, small), one pancake (5-in diameter), or one waffle (5-in diameter) can be substituted for one bread exchange and one fat exchange (1 tsp), provided they are made with skim milk and vegetable oil or margarine. Muffins, pancakes, and waffles may not be used if sucrose or simple carbohydrates are limited by the diet prescription because sugar is an ingredient in the recipes for these products.

Only the fat exchanges calculated in the diet pattern can be used as a spread on bread or to season the other items in this list, such as the pasta, rice, potatoes, and corn.

***Meat exchange.*** In order to control the total fat, saturated fatty acid, and cholesterol contributed to the diet pattern, only items included in List 5A Lean Meat are included in the Fat-Controlled Meat Exchange List. Only well trimmed, lean meat, poultry without skin, and fish can be used. The skin of poultry is excluded because of the amount of fat it contains. Luncheon meats, frankfurters, sausage, bacon, and other high-fat cuts of meat are also excluded because of their fat content. If available, uncreamed (dry curd) cottage cheese or cheeses containing less than 5% butter fat can be used as meat exchanges.

***Egg exchange.*** It should be carefully noted that eggs are limited to 2 per week and that a list of substitutions for eggs is given. This restriction on the use of eggs reflects their cholesterol content. Table 30-13 lists the cholesterol content of selected foods. Whole milk cheeses are not included in the meat or egg exchange food groups because of their saturated fatty acid content.

Since eggs and liver are significant sources of dietary iron and are limited or excluded from the diet patterns, the counselor should check the iron content of a patient's usual menu selections. Iron medication may be required to meet the daily needs for this mineral, especially for children and women of childbearing age.

***Fat exchange.*** The items in the fat exchange list include only vegetable oils, salad dressing made with vegetable oils, and margarines because of the amount of

### Table 30-11. Nutrient Composition of a 1500 Calorie Fat-controlled or Hyperlipoproteinemia Type IV Diet (P/S Ratio 1.7:1)

| Food Group | Amount | Weight (g) | Protein (g) | Total Fat (g) | Saturated Fatty Acids (g) | Linoleic Fatty Acid (g) | Cholesterol (mg) | Carbohydrate (g) | Energy (Kcal) |
|---|---|---|---|---|---|---|---|---|---|
| Non-fat milk (<1% fat) | 1 pt (2 c) | 480 | 16 | tr | 0.2 | | 8 | 24 | 160 |
| Vegetables | ½ c | 100 | 2 | | | | | 5 | 25 |
| Fruit | 3 servings | Varies | | | | | | 30 | 120 |
| Bread and cereal | 7 servings | Varies | 14 | 7 | 1.4 | 1.4 | | 105 | 525 |
| Meat, lean | 6 oz | 180 | 42 | 18 | 4.2 | 2.4 | 144 | | 330 |
| Eggs, whole | 2/wk | 14 | 2 | 2 | 0.5 | 0.2 | 72 | | 25 |
| Fat (polyunsaturated margarines and oils) | 7 tsp | 35 | | 35 | 4.2 | 14.7 | | | 315 |
| Totals | | | 76 | 62 | 10.5 | 18.7 | 224 | 164 | 1500 |

## Table 30-12. Food Exchange Lists for Fat-controlled Diets

### Milk Exchanges

One serving contains 8 g protein, 12 g carbohydrate, 4 mg cholesterol, and 80 kcalories.

| | |
|---|---|
| Skim milk | 1 c |
| Non-fat dried milk | $^1/_3$ c |
| Canned, evaporated skim milk (undiluted) | $^1/_2$ c |
| Buttermilk (made from skim milk) | 1 c |
| Yogurt (made from skim milk) | 1 c |

### Vegetable Exchanges

One serving contains 5 g carbohydrate, 2 g protein, and 25 kcalories. See Table 24-3.

### Fruit Exchanges

One serving contains 10 g carbohydrate and 40 kcalories. See Table 24-3.

### Bread Exchanges

One serving contains 2 g protein, 1 g fat, 15 g carbohydrate, and 75 kcalories.

Bread

| | |
|---|---|
| White (including French and Italian) | 1 slice |
| Whole wheat | 1 slice |
| Rye or pumpernickel | 1 slice |
| Raisin (unfrosted) | 1 slice |
| Bagel | $^1/_2$ small |
| English muffin | $^1/_2$ small |
| Plain roll, bread | 1 |
| Frankfurter roll | $^1/_2$ |
| Hamburger roll | $^1/_2$ |
| Dried bread crumbs | 3 tbsp |
| Tortilla | 1, 6″ |

Cereals

| | |
|---|---|
| Bran flakes | $^1/_2$ c |
| Other ready-to-eat-unsweetened cereal | $^3/_4$ c |
| Puffed cereal (unfrosted) | 1 c |
| Cereal (cooked) | $^1/_2$ c |
| Grits (cooked) | $^1/_2$ c |
| Rice or barley (cooked) | $^1/_2$ c |
| Pasta (cooked) | |
|   Spaghetti, noodles, macaroni | $^1/_2$ c |
| Popcorn (popped, no fat added) | 3 c |
| Cornmeal (dry) | 2 tbsp |
| Flour | $2^1/_2$ tbsp |
| Wheat germ | $^1/_4$ c |

Crackers

| | |
|---|---|
| Arrowroot | 3 |
| Graham ($2^1/_2$″ sq) | 2 |
| Matzo (4″–6″) | $^1/_2$ |
| Oyster | 20 |
| Pretzels ($3^1/_8$″ long, $^1/_8$″ diam) | 25 |
| Rye wafers (2″–$3^1/_2$″) | 3 |
| Saltines | 6 |
| Soda ($2^1/_2$″ sq) | 4 |

Dried beans, peas, and lentils
(Omit 1 meat exchange)

| | |
|---|---|
| Beans, peas, lentils (dried and cooked) | $^1/_2$ c |
| Baked beans, no pork, canned | $^1/_4$ c |

High-carbohydrate vegetables

| | |
|---|---|
| Corn | $^1/_3$ c |
| Corn on the cob | 1 small |

### Bread Exchanges (Continued)

High-carbohydrate vegetables (Continued)

| | |
|---|---|
| Lima beans | $^1/_2$ c |
| Parsnips | $^2/_3$ c |
| Peas, green (canned or frozen) | $^1/_2$ c |
| Potato, white | 1 small |
| Potato, mashed | $^1/_2$ c |
| Pumpkin | $^3/_4$ c |
| Winter acorn or butternut squash | $^1/_2$ c |
| Yam or sweet potato | $^1/_4$ c |

### Meat Exchanges

1 oz contains 7 g protein, 3 g fat, 24 mg cholesterol, and 55 kcalories. Lean meats only.

| | |
|---|---|
| Beef | 1 oz |
|   Baby beef (very lean) | |
|   Steak, chuck, flank, tenderloin, plate ribs, round (bottom or top), rump, spare ribs, tripe | |
| Lamb | 1 oz |
|   Leg, rib, sirloin, loin shank, shoulder | |
| Pork | 1 oz |
|   Leg, whole rump, center shank, ham center slices | |
| Veal | 1 oz |
|   Leg, loin, rib, shank, shoulder cutlets | |
| Poultry (without skin) | 1 oz |
|   Chicken, turkey, cornish hen, guinea hen, pheasant | |
| Fish | 1 oz |
|   Any fresh or frozen | |
|   Canned salmon, tuna (water packed) | $^1/_4$ c |
|   Canned mackerel, crab, lobster | $^1/_4$ c |
|   Clams, oysters, scallops | 5 or 1 oz |
| Cheese | |
|   Cottage cheese, dry and 2% butter fat | $^1/_4$ c |
|   Cheeses containing less than 5% butterfat | 1 oz |
|   Dried beans and peas (omit 1 bread exchange) | $^1/_2$ c |

### Egg Exchanges

2 eggs per week contain 2 g protein, 2 g fat, 72 mg of cholesterol, and 25 kcalories. Limit to 2 per week.

2 oz of one of the following may be substituted for 1 egg: Shrimp, sardines, liver, or other organ meats.

### Fat Exchanges

1 teaspoon of vegetable oil contains 5 g fat, .6 g saturated fatty acid, 2 g linoleic fatty acid, and 45 kcalories.

| | |
|---|---|
| Polyunsaturated fat | |
|   Margarine, tub or stick (soft) | 1 tsp |
| Oil | 1 tsp |
|   Corn | |
|   Cottonseed | |
|   Safflower | |
|   Soy | |
|   Sunflower | |
| French dressing* | 1 tbsp |
| Italian dressing* | 1 tbsp |
| Mayonnaise* | 1 tsp |
| Salad dressing*, mayonnaise type | 2 tsps |
| Walnuts | 6 small |

*If made with polyunsaturated oils.

## Table 30-12. Food Exchange Lists for Fat-controlled Diets (Continued)

**Sugar and Dessert Exchanges**
One serving contains about 12 g of carbohydrate and 50 kcalories.

Sugars
| | |
|---|---|
| White, brown, or maple | 1 tbsp |
| Corn syrup or maple syrup | 1 tbsp |
| Honey | 1 tbsp |
| Molasses | 1 tbsp |
| Jelly, jam, or marmalade | 1 tbsp |

Desserts
| | |
|---|---|
| Tapioca or cornstarch pudding (made with fruit and fruit juice or with skim milk from milk calculated in diet plan) | 1/4 c |
| Gelatin dessert | 1/3 c |

**Sugar and Dessert Exchanges (Continued)**
Desserts (Continued)
| | |
|---|---|
| Fruit whip (made with egg whites, no cream) | 1/4 c |
| Water ice | 1/4 c |
| Sweetened canned or frozen fruit (equals 1 fruit exchange and 1 tbsp sugar) | |
| Angel food cake, plain | 1 small piece |
| Sweetened carbonated beverages | 6 oz |

Candies
| | |
|---|---|
| Gumdrops | 3 medium or 14 small |
| Marshmallows | 3 large |
| Hard fruit drops | 4 |

(Adapted from Exchange Lists for Meal Planning, American Dietetic Association, 1976)

the polyunsaturated fatty acid, linoleic, which they contain (see Table 30-14). Butter, lard, hydrogenated shortening, and bacon are excluded.

**Sugar and dessert exchanges.** This list is included to show the types of sugars and desserts that can be used to meet energy needs when total fat and cholesterol are severely restricted, but total energy is not restricted, in the diet pattern. If simple carbohydrates are also restricted for any reason, the items in this exchange list cannot be used. Note that only egg whites, which do not contain fat or cholesterol, and skim milk are used to make desserts.

**Mixed dishes.** Many items included in a fat-controlled diet pattern can be combined in mixed dishes. For example, a white sauce can be made with skim milk and flour without the addition of any fat, and gravy can be made with fat-free broth or fat-free meat drippings and flour. Tomatoes, tomato juice, or tomato paste can be used in combination with pasta or rice, meat, or uncreamed cottage cheese and other vegetables to make casserole dishes.

**Convenience foods.** Unless the nutrition label defines the types and amounts of fatty acids and the cholesterol content of a serving of the food, these products cannot be used on fat-controlled diets. In some cases the quantity of sucrose in the product may also restrict its use.

**Dietetic foods.** Various egg and cheese products and meat substitutes made from soy protein isolate that are modified in cholesterol and fatty acid composition in comparison with the usual foods are now available in most supermarkets. For example, Cheez-ola* is a filled pasteurized processed cheese that contains corn oil in place of milk fat and has a 4.5:1 P:S ratio. However, the sodium content of this product limits its use since the diets for patients with hypertension and edema or for those recovering from myocardial infarction are also restricted

*Fisher Cheese Co., Wapakoneta, Ohio.

## Table 30-13. Cholesterol Content of Foods (Per Exchange Serving)

| Food | Household Measure | Weight (g) | Cholesterol (mg) |
|---|---|---|---|
| Whole milk | 8 oz | 240 | 34 |
| Egg | 1 | 50 | 242 |
| Meat, fish | 1 oz | 30 | 21 |
| Chicken (with skin) | 1 oz | 30 | 24 |
| Liver | 1 oz | 30 | 131 |
| Sweetbreads | 1 oz | 30 | 140 |
| Shrimp | 1 oz | 30 | 45 |
| Lobster | 1 oz | 30 | 25 |
| Crab | 1 oz | 30 | 30 |
| Oysters, clams | 1 oz | 30 | 15 |
| Cheese, cheddar | 1 oz | 30 | 28 |
| Butter | 1 tbsp | 14 | 35 |
| Margarine (all vegetable oil) | 1 tbsp | 14 | 0 |

(Calculated from Feeley RM et al: J Am Diet Assoc 61:134, 1972)

## Table 30-14. Approximate Fatty Acid Composition of Vegetable Oils

| Vegetable Oil | Saturated Fatty Acids* | Monounsaturated Fatty Acids* | Polyunsaturated Fatty Acids* |
|---|---|---|---|
| Coconut | 87 | 6 | 2 |
| Cocoa butter | 60 | 33 | 3 |
| Olive | 14 | 74 | 8 |
| Peanut | 17 | 46 | 32 |
| Cottonseed | 26 | 18 | 52 |
| Soy | 14 | 23 | 58 |
| Corn | 13 | 24 | 59 |
| Safflower | 9 | 12 | 75 |

*Grams/100 g

(From Reeves JB, Weihrauch JL: Composition of Foods. Fats and Oils: Raw, Processed and Prepared Agriculture Handbook No. 8-4. Washington, DC, USDA, United States Government Printing Office, 1979)

in sodium. Because 1 oz of Cheez-ola contains 480 mg sodium, it could not be used in planning a 1000- or 2000-mg sodium-restricted diet pattern (see Chap. 31). However, a low sodium Cheez-ola product is now on the market. The egg and meat substitutes also contain significant amounts of sodium.

### Calculation of the fat-controlled diets

Table 30-11 shows the calculation of a 1500-calorie, fat-controlled diet using the exchange system. The diet calculated derives approximately 20% calories from protein, 35% from fat, and 45% from carbohydrate. Approximately 65% of the carbohydrate is derived from complex carbohydrates and 35% from simple carbohydrates. This diet is low in saturated fatty acids (less than 10% calories) and contains less than 300 mg of cholesterol per day. It meets the recommendations of the American Heart Association and would also be suitable for the treatment of Type IIb and Type IV hyperlipoproteinemia, the most common lipoprotein disorders seen.

A suggested menu for the sample diet pattern using the foods in the fat-controlled exchange lists is given in Table 30-15. Part of the skim milk in the breakfast menu could be reserved for making whipped topping from skim milk powder to garnish the fruit in the D'Zerta in the evening meal. One teaspoonful of margarine is used as an ingredient of the biscuit. Two teaspoonsful of margarine would be available to season the potatoes and peas.

### Table 30-15. Suggested Menu for 1500 Calorie Fat-controlled or Hyperlipoproteinemia Type IV Diet

*Breakfast*
4 ounces orange juice
½ cup cooked oatmeal
1 slice of toast
1 teaspoon margarine
8 ounces skim milk

*Noon Meal*
Chicken sandwich
  2 slices of bread
  2 ounces chicken
  2 teaspoons mayonnaise
  lettuce
Fresh peach
8 ounces skim milk

*Evening Meal*
4 ounces roast veal
½ cup mashed potatoes
½ cup green peas
Sliced tomatoes with 1 tablespoon French dressing
1 biscuit
  (made with 1 teaspoon allowed fat)
2 teaspoons margarine
½ cup fruit cup, made with fruit canned without sugar
  (in D'Zerta with skim milk whipped topping)

For the hospitalized patient, careful precautions must be taken to ensure that the patient who requires a fat-controlled diet is not served vegetables that have been seasoned with butter, meat that is well marbled with fat or from which the visible fat has not been removed, or hot breads made with other than vegetable oil shortening. At the same time, relatives and friends should be instructed to avoid offering the patient candies and ice cream or beverages made with whole milk and ice cream.

### Special considerations when planning hyperlipoproteinemia diets (see Table 30-6)
#### HLP diet 1

The fat in Diet 1 for patients with hyperchylomicronemia is restricted to 25 g to 35 g per day, or 12% of total calories. None of the items in the fat exchange food group can be included in the Diet 1 diet pattern because all long-chain fatty acids, other than those in the meat and bread exchange food groups, are excluded from the diet. For example, six meat exchanges and ten bread exchanges contain 28 g of fat, primarily long-chain saturated fatty acids. If the patient requires 2000 or more calories per day, he must make extensive use of dried beans, peas, and legumes and the sugar and dessert exchanges.

The physician may prescribe the use of medium-chain triglycerides (see Chap. 24) in the Diet 1 pattern because the medium-chain fatty acids in these triglycerides are absorbed into the portal circulation and do not require the synthesis of chylomicrons for transport. Medium-chain triglyceride oil (MCT) can be used in frying and in making hot breads and salad dressings. However, MCT oil is expensive and may not be acceptable to the patient as a substitute for regular food fats and oils.

#### HLP diet 2

In this diet the cholesterol is severely limited (preferably to 100 mg–200 mg per day) and the polyunsaturated fatty acid is increased. To achieve the cholesterol restriction, the egg exchange food group cannot be included in the diet pattern (see Table 30-9). Adequate amounts of vegetable oils and margarine must be used to ensure an increased intake of linoleic acid. Unless the patient is obese, energy and carbohydrate are not restricted. Therefore, the sugar and dessert exchanges can be included in the diet pattern.

#### HLP diet 3

This diet is restricted to less than 300 mg of cholesterol per day; 20% of total calories are derived from protein, 40% from fat, and 40% from carbohydrate. When the 1500-calorie, fat-controlled diet in Table 30-11 is used as a model to achieve the Diet 3 recommendations, the number of bread and fruit exchanges is reduced and the number of the fat exchanges increased. It is advisable to exclude egg exchanges from the diet pattern to control the cholesterol intake. The physician's diet prescription may exclude all sugar and dessert exchanges. Otherwise a sugar or dessert exchange may be substituted for a fruit or bread exchange two or three times a week.

## HLP diet 5

This diet restricts fat to 30% of total calories. Fifty percent of total calories is derived from carbohydrate and 20% from protein. Because blood triglycerides are markedly elevated, the sugar and dessert exchanges are usually excluded from the diet pattern.

## Patient counseling

The first step in nutrition counseling, as with any diet, is to gather extensive information about the patient's usual food practices. In some cases it is also important to know about the whole family's practices, particularly families of patients with primary HLP. For example, Glueck and co-workers have reported that in 70 families where one parent had a myocardial infarction before age 50, 31% of the children had Type IIa, IIb, or IV lipoprotein patterns. These investigators strongly recommend an early intervention program for these children.[27]

The patient receiving counseling in a fat-controlled diet needs careful, detailed diet instructions because these diets require extensive changes in the use of fats, and usually sugar, compared with the average American diet (see Chap. 11). Since the majority of patients who experience heart attacks are men, it is essential that the patient's wife be present for the diet history interview and during all diet instruction. Many of these patients and their wives are well motivated to learn how to adjust to the fat-controlled diet. Also, if the children in the family have been screened and are found to have positive lipoprotein patterns, the homemaker needs help in modifying the food practices of the whole family.

In her contact with the patient and his family, the nutrition counselor should determine how much and what kinds of fats are consumed by the family; the commonly used methods of food preparation, which may add fats to otherwise low-fat foods, and the amounts of simple carbohydrate and alcohol consumed daily. Information about snack foods, shopping practices, and frequency of eating outside the home, as well as the usual meal pattern, should be obtained.

The press, popular magazines, and television have all helped to make middle aged Americans conscious of the need for "polyunsaturates" in their diets. Unfortunately, some of these media have oversimplified the problem by emphasizing only one food—for example, changing from butter to "special" margarines and salad oils—without also stating the need to change to skim milk and skim milk products, lean meat, and reduced meat portions, and to monitor the number of eggs used each week.

It is possible that many purchasing practices and methods of food preparation need to be changed. For example, if a homemaker has always made fruit whip with whipped cream, she needs to be instructed to make it with egg whites. Or, if she has found it convenient to use frozen dinners frequently, she may need help in choosing suitable convenience food items and in planning the preparation of meals that require more of her time in the kitchen. If she has children, she needs help in planning meals and snacks to meet their energy and nutrient needs for growth, and at the same time modifying the types and amounts of fat and sugar in their diets.

Various kinds of cookbooks are available to patients. One of these has been published by the American Heart Association.[28] The recipes in some of the other books are not appropriate for every type of diet. Therefore, the counselor should review any cookbook before recommending it. It would also be advisable to test a few of the recipes in these cookbooks for ease of preparation and the quality and acceptability of the product. With the help of the counselor many homemakers can modify their own favorite recipes.

In recent years, educational programs have been developed to assist nutrition counselors in their efforts to teach those who require blood lipid lowering the principles necessary to achieve desired dietary change. One such program is the Heart Saver Program developed as part of the Nutrition Education Project (NEP). Mojonnier described the goal of this project to establish habitual food choices that would control the intake of nutrients associated with high incidence of coronary heart disease in a group of hyperlipidemic subjects.[29] Two hundred twenty four hyperlipidemic men and women participated in a program to change dietary habits for blood lipid lowering. The Heart Saver program consisted of six lessons recorded on color slides and synchronized magnetic tape cassettes with accompanying teaching materials. Four teaching methods, which included individual, group, self and multi (a combination of the first three methods described), were used to implement the program over a period of 6 to 9 months. The group that reviewed the program was compared to a control group of 69 similar men and women who had not received the program. After completion, the group participating in the program demonstrated reductions that were significantly greater than the control group in serum cholesterol; decreases in dietary cholesterol, percentage of total calories from saturated fat and caloric intake; and increases in the percentage of total calories from polyunsaturated fat. The Heart Saver Program materials may be ordered from the Chicago Heart Association (see *Patient Resources* at end of chapter). These materials are suitable for use in many patient education settings.

Resources for patient education, which the clinical dietitian can use to supplement her own educational material, are listed at the end of the chapter. However, as with any complex food modification, continuing contact with the nutrition counselor is necessary as patients learn to live with their problems. As the disease progresses in patients who have had a myocardial infarction, the clinical dietitian can also expect to help them restrict sodium intake as well as fat.

## Hypolipidemic drugs

Two types of hypolipidemic drugs may be used in conjunction with diet to treat hyperlipidemias.[30] One type decreases VLDL synthesis. The two most commonly used agents of this type are nicotinic acid, a B vitamin, and clofibrate, a branched-chain fatty acid. Both agents may cause nausea and diarrhea. The other type increases LDL catabolism. The two most commonly used agents of this type are the resins, cholestyramine and sitosterol. Cholestyramine frequently causes constipation in older patients and occasionally nausea, vomiting, abdominal distention, and cramps. Sitosterol may have a mild laxative effect or may sometimes produce nausea and diarrhea.

## Study questions and activities

1. Why is atherosclerosis a public health problem of major importance?
2. List the foods which contain the greatest percentage of linoleic fatty acid.
3. Is it correct to say that all plant oils contain only linoleic acid and that all animal fats contain only saturated fat (see Table 30-7)?
4. List some of the foods commonly used in the American diet that are omitted on the fat-controlled diets.
5. What epidemiologic study is being carried out to assess the effect of diet on elevated blood cholesterol levels in men?
6. Why should the prevention of coronary artery disease begin in childhood?
7. Can a diet without eggs be adequate in all nutrients?
8. Calculate a 2000-calorie, fat-controlled diet containing 35% fat, 10% linoleic fatty acid, less than 10% saturated fat, and less than 300 mg cholesterol.
9. Estimate the cholesterol in the food you consumed in one day (see Table 2, Part 4).
10. Check the supermarkets in your area for the availability and cost of special foods for fat-controlled diets.
11. Review the menu the next time you eat in a restaurant and note what items could be selected on a fat-controlled diet.

## References

1. Spain DM: Sci Am 215:48, 1966
2. Farrand ME, Mojonnier ML: J Am Diet Assoc 76:347, 1980
3. Rifkind BM, Levy RI: Arch Surg 113:80, 1978
4. Keys A (ed): AHA Monograph No. 29. Circulation (Suppl 1) 41:176, 1970
5. Mueller JF: J Am Diet Assoc 62:613, 1973
6. Hegsted DM et al: Am J Clin Nutr 17:281, 1965
7. Brown HB, Farrand ME: J Am Diet Assoc 49:303, 1966
8. National Diet–Heart Study Research Group: National Diet–Heart Study Final Report. Circulation (Suppl 1) 37:1, 1968
9. Christakis G et al: JAMA 198:129, 1966
10. Pearce ML, Dayton S: Lancet 1:464, 1971
11. Ederer F: Lancet 2:203, 1971
12. Blankenhorn DH et al: Circulation 57:355, 1978
13. Bagdade JD: Lancet 2:630, 1968
14. Hatch FT: Am J Clin Nutr 29:80, 1974
15. Levy RI et al: J Am Diet Assoc 58:406, 1971
16. Diet and Coronary Heart Disease. A Statement for Physicians and Other Health Professionals. Dallas, American Heart Association, 1978
17. Fredrickson DS et al: N Engl J Med 276:32, 94, 148, 215, 273, 1967
18. Castelli WP et al: Circulation 55:767, 1977
19. Goldstein JL, Brown MS: Annu Rev Biochem 46:897, 1977
20. Connor WE, Connor SJ: In Rifkind BM, Levy RI (eds): Hyperlipidemia Diagnosis and Therapy. New York, Grune & Stratton, 1977
21. U.S. National Center for Health Statistics: Vital and Health Statistics: Data from the National Health Survey. Series 11, No. 22. Serum Cholesterol Level of Adults, United States, 1960–62. Washington, DC, DHEW, 1967
22. Kannel WB et al: Ann Intern Med 74:1, 1971
23. U.S. Senate. Select Committee on Nutrition and Human Needs: Dietary Goals for the United States. Washington, DC, United States Government Printing Office, 1977
24. USDA, DHHS: Nutrition and Your Health. Washington, DC, United States Government Printing Office, 1980
25. Rifkind BM, Levy RI (eds): Hyperlipidemia Diagnosis and Therapy, pp 41–65. New York, Grune & Stratton, 1977
26. NHLBI Nutrition Coding Center Food Table. Minneapolis, 1977
27. Glueck CJ et al: Am J Dis Child 127:70, 1974
28. Eshleman R, Winston M: The American Heart Association Cookbook. New York, McKay, 1979
29. Mojonnier ML et al: J Am Diet Assoc 77:140, 1980
30. Levy RI et al: N Engl J Med 290:1295, 1974

## Supplementary readings

Albrink MJ: Dietary and drug treatment of hyperlipidemia in diabetes. Diabetes 29:913, 1974

Anderson JT et al: Cholesterol-lowering diets. J Am Diet Assoc 62:133, 1973

Birenbaum ML et al: Ten-year experience of modified diets of younger men with coronary heart disease. Lancet 1:1404, 1973

Blacket RB et al: Type IV hyperlipidemia and weight-gain after maturity. Lancet 2:517, 1975

Brown HB: Diet management of hyperlipidemia. Practical Cardiology April, 1976

Farrand ME, Mojonnier ML: Nutrition in the Multiple Risk Factor Intervention Trial (MRFIT). J Am Diet Assoc 76:347, 1980

Feeley RM et al: Cholesterol content of foods. J Am Diet Assoc 61:134, 1972

Gangl A, Ockner RK: Intestinal metabolism of lipids and lipoproteins. Gastroenterology 68:167, 1975

Glueck CJ et al: Hypercholesterolemia and hypertriglyceridemia in children: A pediatric approach to primary atherosclerosis prevention. Am J Dis Child 128:569, 1974

Gotto AM: Is atherosclerosis reversible? J Am Diet Assoc 74:551, 1979

Hackett TP, Cassem NH: The psychologic reactions of patients in the pre- and post-hospital phases of myocardial infarction. Postgrad Med 57:43, 1975

Hulley SB et al: Plasma high-density lipoprotein cholesterol level influence of risk factor intervention. JAMA 238:2269, 1977

Kritchevsky D: Fiber, lipids, and atherosclerosis. Am J Clin Nutr (Suppl) 31:365, 1978

Levy RI: The meaning of lipid profiles. Postgrad Med 57:35, 1975

Mandriota R et al: Nutrition intervention strategies in the Multiple Risk Factor Intervention Trial (MRFIT). J Am Diet Assoc 77:138, 1980

Mojonnier ML et al: Experiences in changing food habits of hyperlipidemic men and women. J Am Diet Assoc 77:140, 1980

Ostrander J et al: Egg substitutes: Use and preference—With and without nutritional information. J Am Diet Assoc 70:267, 1977

Remmell PS et al: Assessing dietary adherence in the Multiple Risk Factor Intervention Trial (MRFIT). I. Use of a dietary monitoring tool. J Am Diet Assoc 76:353, 1980

Scott LW et al: Are low-cholesterol diets expensive? J Am Diet Assoc 74:558, 1979

Stamler J: Major coronary risk factors before and after myocardial infarction. Postgrad Med 57:25, 1975

Comprehensive Evaluation of Fatty Acids in Foods. In J Am Diet Assoc. Dairy, 66:482, May, 1975; Beef, 67:35, July, 1975; Egg, 67:111, Aug, 1975; Unhydrogenated Fats and Oils, 68:224, Mar, 1976; Nuts, Peanuts, Soups, 67:351, Oct, 1976; Cereal, 68:335, Apr, 1976; Pork, 69:44, July, 1976; Fowl, 69:577, Nov, 1976; Veal, 70:53, Jan, 1977; Leguminous Seeds, 71:412, Oct, 1977; Shellfish, 71:518, Nov, 1977; Sausage, Luncheon Meats, 72:48, Jan, 1978

## Patient resources
### Pamphlets

Dietary Management of Hyperlipoproteinemia. Bethesda, MD, National Heart and Lung Institute, NIH, revised, 1973. Diet 1 for Hyperchylomicronemia; Diet 2 for Hypercholesterolemia; Diet 3 for Hypercholesterolemia with Hyperglyceridemia; Diet 4 for Endogenous Hyperglyceridemia; Diet 5 for Mixed Hyperglyceridemia

Fats in Food and Diet. Washington, DC, USDA, United States Government Printing Office, 1974

Heart Saver Eating Style (A guide to planning nutritious meals low in satured fat and cholesterol to reduce the risk of heart attack and low in calories for weight control—while saving money). Chicago, Chicago Heart Association, 1978

A Maximal Approach to the Dietary Treatment of the Hyperlipidemias, New York, American Heart Association, 1973. Diet A—The Low-Cholesterol (100 mg) Moderately Low-Fat Diet; Diet B—The Low-Cholesterol (200 mg) Moderately Low-Fat Diet; Diet C—The Low-Cholesterol, High-Polyunsaturated-Fat Diet; Diet D—The Extremely Low-Fat Diet

Nutrition Education Project: The Heart Saver Eating Style. Chicago, Chicago Heart Association, 1977

Nutrition Education Project: Weight Control, the Heart Saver Way. Chicago, Chicago Heart Association, 1975

Planning Fat-Controlled Meals for 1200 and 1800 Calories, rev. New York, American Heart Association, 1966

Planning Fat-Controlled Meals for Approximately 2000–2600 Calories, rev. New York, American Heart Association, 1967

Programmed Instruction for Fat-Controlled Diet, 1800 Calories. New York, American Heart Association, 1969

The Way to a Man's Heart. New York, American Heart Association, 1972

### Books

Bennett I, Simon M: The Prudent Diet. New York, David White, 1973

Claiborne C, Franey P: Craig Claiborne's Gourmet Diet. New York, New York Times Books, 1980

Connor WE, Connor SL: The Alternative Diet Book. Iowa City, University of Iowa Press, 1976

Cutler C: Haute Cuisine for Your Heart's Delight. New York, Potter, 1973 (distributed by Crown)

Eshleman R, Winston M: The American Heart Association Cookbook. New York, McKay, 1979

Ferguson JM, Taylor CB: A Change for Heart. Palo Alto, Bull, 1978

Heart Saver Program (A complete package of materials for teaching the heart-saver eating style—including six slide tape units describing dietary recommendations with audio tapes adapted for use in individual counseling, self-teaching, or group teaching). Chicago, Chicago Heart Association, 1975

Heiss KB, Heiss CG: Eat to Your Heart's Content. San Francisco, Chronicle, 1972

Keys M, Keys A: The Benevolent Bean. New York, Farrar, 1972

Rosenthal S: Live High on Low Fat. Philadelphia, JB Lippincott, 1975

Salmon MB, Quigley AE (eds): Enjoying Your Restricted Diet. Springfield, IL, Charles C Thomas, 1972

Stead EA, Warren JV: Low-Fat Cookery, 3rd ed. New York, McGraw-Hill, 1975

Zane P: The Jack Sprat Cookbook. New York, Harper, 1973

*For further references see Bibliography in Part 4.*

# Cardiovascular Disease

*31*

The basic metabolic problem in cardiac disease and in the diseases discussed in Chapters 32 and 33, renal and liver disease, is fluid and electrolyte balance. From Chapter 5, *Water and Electrolyte Metabolism*, remember that the maintenance of the appropriate fluid volume in the vascular system, in the spaces surrounding the cell (interstitial), and within the cells (intracellular) is a function not only of the constituents of the blood and the integrity of the vascular tissue but also of the heart, kidneys, liver, and lungs. Moreover, all of these interrelated functions are mediated by a variety of hormones.

## Etiology

The focus on fluid and electrolyte metabolism in this chapter is determined by the problems presented by cardiac disease and vascular disease or cardiovascular disease. Cardiac disease may be primary or secondary. Congenital anomalies of the heart, many of which can be corrected by surgery, are the major cause of primary disease. Secondary cardiac disease is due to infections, such as rheumatic fever (streptococcal infection) or syphilis; or diseases of the vascular system, such as hypertension and arteriosclerosis, including atherosclerosis.

Arteriosclerosis is the generic term for any vascular disease characterized by induration or thickening of the arterial wall. Atherosclerosis, a form of arteriosclerosis, involves the intimal layer of the arteries, while arteriosclerosis involves primarily the medial layer. The etiology of primary hypertension, an elevation of arterial blood pressure due to peripheral resistance, cannot be defined at this time, although neurogenic mechanisms are suspected. The major causes of secondary hypertension are diseases of the kidney or the adrenal glands. Secondary hypertension has also been observed in some women taking oral contraceptive agents.

## Prevalence and incidence

In 1977 there were 1,898,000 deaths from all causes with over half of these deaths (960,000) due to all forms of cardiovascular disease.[1] It is the leading cause of death among people above 35, and over 90% of these deaths can be attributed to atherosclerosis and other forms of arteriosclerosis and hypertension. It is estimated that 15% to 20% of the adult population in the United States has hypertension, with the highest prevalence among blacks. Studies indicate that hypertension may occur in children more frequently than previously suspected.[2]

The morbidity and mortality from all forms of cardiovascular disease, especially in adults during the productive years from ages 35 to 65, have a major social impact on the individual, the family, and the public at large. The Social Security Administration has reported that cardiovascular disorders are the greatest cause of permanent disability.[1] If the patient is the wage earner, his income may be reduced as a consequence of his disability. Coronary care units in community hospitals are expensive to staff and maintain, and Medicare and Medicaid are used in addition to private medical insurance plans to finance the acute and continuing care of the patient with cardiovascular disease. In the United States today health agencies and organizations are urging early detection and treatment of cardiovascular disease to reduce the cost to society. It would appear that these efforts are meeting with success: between 1968 and 1977 there was a 23% decline in deaths due to all forms of cardiovascular disease.[1]

## Severity of involvement

The severity of cardiovascular disease depends on the degree to which the normal functions of the system are altered and the extent to which this alteration interferes with them. The onset may be sudden, with no previous history of problems, such as may occur in the patient with a myocardial infarction. Or the disease may be chronic, of long standing, with increasing loss of cardiac function, often referred to as cardiac reserve. If the problem is minimal and the heart is able to maintain adequate circulation to all tissues of the body, the disease is classified as mild or "compensated." The patients may have to avoid strenuous activity that increases the oxygen needs of the body, but otherwise they will be able to perform their daily tasks without discomfort.

Decompensation, or severe cardiac disease, is said to occur when the heart is unable to sustain adequate circulation of blood to the tissues. The blood flow to the lungs is slowed, and oxygen uptake and carbon dioxide excretion are inadequate. The patient suffers from shortness of breath and chest pain when he performs any sort of activity. As decompensation progresses, edema may appear in the dependent parts of the body and, some-

times, in the pleural and peritoneal cavities, and the kidneys and the liver may become involved. Severe cardiac disease of this magnitude is called congestive heart failure.

When patients are chronically ill with severe heart disease, their activities must be severely restricted, and they may even have to spend much of their time in bed so that the limited oxygen supply will be sufficient for whatever activity is allowed. Drugs to improve the function of the heart muscle or to reduce blood pressure are commonly prescribed. If edema is present, diuretic drugs to increase sodium and water excretion are usually given, and a diet restricted in sodium is prescribed.

## Edema

Braunwald defines edema as an increase in and retention of the extravascular component of the extracellular (interstitial) fluid volume.[3] Sodium is retained with the fluid. Edema in cardiovascular disease is caused primarily by an alteration of the pressure in the vascular system, which permits the outflow of fluids into the interstitial spaces but interferes with the return of the fluids into the vascular system. In addition, the blood flow to the kidney may be involved so that there is a reduction in the glomerular filtration rate with a decrease in the excretion of fluids and sodium. Aldosterone, the adrenal cortical hormone, which promotes sodium retention and potassium excretion by the kidney, and the pituitary antidiuretic hormone, which aids the kidney in the reabsorption of water, may also be involved. Hypernatremia, an elevated blood sodium level, may also occur.

Mild edema may cause some swelling of the ankles, puffiness around the eyes, or the tightness of a ring on a finger. The persistence of an indentation of the skin following pressure is known as pitting edema. Ascites and hydrothorax refer to the accumulation of excess fluid in the peritoneal and pleural cavities respectively, and anasarca refers to gross generalized edema.

## Rationale for restricting dietary sodium intake

The quantity of extracellular fluid volume is largely dependent on its sodium content (see Chapter 5, *Water and Electrolyte Metabolism*). The reduction of the extracellular fluid volume is dependent primarily on reducing total body sodium stores; the restriction of dietary sodium intake is one factor in reducing these stores.

Dietary restriction alone may be effective in reducing fluid volume in patients with mild heart failure. However, patients with moderate or severe heart failure also require diuretics and a digitalis compound to reestablish normal fluid volume. Diuretics are used to increase the rate of urine formation and to decrease sodium reabsorption by the kidney, which leads to increased fluid and electrolyte excretion.[4] High sodium intakes reduce the sodium-lowering effects of diuretics and, therefore, both diuretic and diet therapy are required for the best therapeutic results.[5] Digitalis compounds increase the force of myocardial contractions, which increases cardiac output. As a result of this action there is also an increase in fluid and electrolyte excretion.

Certain diuretics also promote potassium excretion, which can lead to hypokalemia (low blood potassium). This is hazardous for the patient with cardiovascular disease because hypokalemia results in disturbances in neuromuscular function, including the muscles of the heart. The dietary implications of hypokalemia are discussed in the section on special concerns in this chapter.

### Average sodium intake

It is estimated that the average adult in the United States consumes from 2000 mg to 7000 mg (100 mEq–300 mEq) of sodium per day, equivalent to 6 g to 18 g of salt (NaCl). However, salt is not the only source of dietary sodium. In addition to the salt added to food during preparation and at mealtimes, certain foods naturally contain some sodium. However, the major source of sodium in the diets of most Americans today is probably the salt and many sodium compounds added to foods during production and processing.

Except for the small amount of sodium needed by the body each day—estimated to be equivalent in the adult to the sodium in 1 g of salt (400 mg)—sodium intake in excess of need is excreted by the kidneys in urine or lost in perspiration. Dahl has shown that prolonged feeding of excessive salt to his experimental animals leads to hypertension.[6] However, there is no evidence to show that hypertension can be produced in normal humans by ordinary salt intake. On the other hand, the blood pressure in hypertensive people does respond to a restricted sodium intake.[7]

### Water intake

Most patients who require diuretics and a restriction of sodium intake do not require a restriction of water intake. As has been demonstrated, when sodium is excreted from the body, there is a corresponding water loss (see the discussion of the sodium content of water supplies later in the chapter). However, in most severe cases of congestive heart failure water as well as sodium may be restricted because of excessive secretion of antidiuretic hormone due to dilutional hyponatremia.[8]

### The diet prescription

Energy

The achievement and the maintenance of weight status slightly below the ideal are the first goals of diet therapy in the treatment of all patients with cardiovascular disease. Not only does this measure tend to reduce

basal metabolism and thus the work of the heart, but it also contributes to the reduction of hyperlipidemia and hypertension if they are also present.

Sodium

The level of sodium restriction in milligrams is stated in the prescription and reflects the patient's condition. An intake of 2000 mg to 3000 mg (90 mEq–130 mEq) of sodium per day is considered a mild restriction; 1000 mg to 2000 mg (43 mEq–90 mEq) a moderate restriction; and any amount less than 1000 mg (43 mEq) a severe restriction. With the effectiveness of the diuretics in current use, the most commonly prescribed restrictions vary from 1000 mg to 3000 mg.

In diet prescriptions that state the quantity of sodium in milliequivalents (mEq) rather than milligrams, mEq have to be converted to milligrams because food composition tables give the sodium content of foods in milligrams. One milliequivalent of sodium is 23 mg, the gram-atomic weight. For example, a diet prescription of 40 mEq sodium converts to 920 mg sodium. Sodium chloride is 39.3% sodium. Therefore, to convert a specified weight of sodium chloride to sodium, one multiplies the weight in grams by 0.393. For example, 5 g of sodium chloride contains 1.965 g, or 1965 mg of sodium, or 85.4 mEq.

Whenever necessary, the energy-restricted, fat-controlled, hyperlipoproteinemia (HLP), diabetic diets, and others can also be restricted in sodium. However, a high-protein diet (2 g to 3 g per kilogram of body weight) is not compatible with a restriction of 1000 mg or less of sodium, unless special sodium-free foods are used.

## Diet therapy
### Sodium in food

The *sodium* content of food depends on whether the food is from an animal or a plant source. Even when *produced, processed,* and *prepared without* the addition of salt (NaCl) or any other sodium compound, meat, fish and poultry, milk and milk products, and eggs contain *significant* amounts of sodium. The fluids surrounding the cells of meat are physiological saline solutions just as the fluids surrounding human muscle cells. Animal fats and seed oils contain no, or insignificant amounts of, sodium; cereal grains and fruits and vegetables contain *insignificant* amounts of sodium provided they are produced, processed, or prepared without the addition of salt or any other sodium compound.

If all the foods in the Pattern Dietary (Table 22-1) are produced, processed, or prepared without the addition of any sodium compound, and no salt is added at the table, the sodium content of this 1400-calorie diet pattern is approximately 500 mg. The pint of milk, one egg, and 4 oz of cooked meat contribute approximately 400 mg of sodium; and the cereal, bread, fruits, and vegetables contribute approximately 100 mg of sodium.

There are two other important sources of dietary sodium—the sodium in the various compounds *added* to foods during processing; and the salt or other flavor enhancers, such as monosodium glutamate, added to foods during preparation in the home, institution, or restaurant, or by the diner at the time of consumption of the food at the table. The sodium added to some foods during processing is obvious, for example, the salt on crackers and potato chips or the salt used to cure ham. However, some foods can contain a significant amount of added sodium without tasting salty, for example, frozen vegetables with monosodium glutamate added during processing.

### Sodium-restricted exchange systems

Table 31-1 gives the sodium composition of the exchange food groups that are used to calculate sodium-restricted diet patterns. The protein, fat, carbohydrate, and energy values in Table 24-2 in Chapter 24 also apply in this Exchange System and are not repeated in Table 31-1. The sodium values apply only to foods *produced*, *processed*, and *prepared without* the addition of salt or any other sodium compound and reflect the quantities of sodium that foods naturally contain.

Observe that the milk, meat, and egg exchanges contribute the most significant amounts of sodium, while vegetables, fruits, cereal grains, and fats contribute the least important amounts. The addition of salt or any sodium compound to any exchange will invalidate these figures. For example, 1 tsp of unsalted butter contains about $\frac{1}{4}$ mg of sodium, while 1 tsp of butter with salt added (regular butter) contains approximately 50 mg of sodium (see Table 4, Part 4).

### Sodium-restricted exchange lists

The Sodium-Restricted Exchange Lists are given in Table 31-2. The foods listed in each exchange group apply to the calculation of diet patterns containing 1000 mg of sodium or less. Some additions can be made to certain lists when the diet prescription for sodium is greater than 1000 mg, and these are included in the discussion of each exchange list.

### Table 31-1. Sodium-Restricted Exchange System

| Food Group | Household Measure | Weight (g) | Sodium* (mg) |
|---|---|---|---|
| Milk exchanges | 8 oz ($\frac{1}{2}$ pt) | 240 | 120 |
| Meat exchanges | 1 oz | 30 | 25 |
| Egg exchange | 1 | 50 | 70 |
| Vegetable exchanges | $\frac{1}{2}$ c | 100 | 9 |
| Fruit exchanges | 1 serving | Varies | 2 |
| Bread exchanges | 1 serving | Varies | 5 |
| Fat exchanges | 1 tsp | 5 | 0 |

*Food produced, processed, or prepared without the addition of any sodium compound.

### Milk exchanges

The items in this food group do not differ significantly from those in the milk exchange list in Table 24-3, Chapter 24. One cup (8 oz) of whole or skim milk contains 120 mg of sodium. Because salt is frequently added to buttermilk, one must check with the producer before using it. Due to its sodium content, any milk used in food preparation should be part of the milk exchanges calculated in the sodium-restricted diet pattern.

### Meat exchanges

One ounce (30 g) of the items in this list contains 25 mg of sodium after cooking without the addition of salt or any sodium-containing compound. This figure applies to meat, poultry, and fish that is fresh, frozen, or canned without the addition of sodium. The products canned without added salt or sodium in any form are referred to as "dietetic" canned. No meats or fish cured with salt, such as ham, bacon, chipped beef, smoked tongue, or smoked fish, or products, such as luncheon meat, frankfurters, or sausage, are included in the meat list.

Kosher meat and poultry may present a problem for Jewish patients who follow orthodox dietary laws. Under the conditions for koshering, freshly slaughtered meat or poultry is salted for 1 hour to remove the blood. Then the meat or poultry is washed thoroughly before it is cooked. Although this removes some of the added salt, a good deal will already have penetrated the inner portion of the meat. Kaufman states that meat so treated has from 334 mg to 375 mg of sodium per 100 g (90 mg–115 mg per 30 g), depending on the manner of cooking.[9] She suggests that Jewish patients be taught to salt their meat lightly and allow it to stand for the minimal amount of time. After it has been rinsed and soaked in water, it should be boiled in a generous amount of water and the broth should be discarded. Meat so treated has been found to contain 63 mg of sodium per 100 g (19 mg per 30 g). As an alternative, she suggests the use of ammonium chloride salt in place of sodium chloride for drawing out the blood. Ammonium chloride cannot be used by those with advanced cirrhosis of the liver (Chap. 33).

Only fresh or dietetic canned fish is included in the meat exchanges. Fresh fish must be rinsed thoroughly in water because it is sometimes kept in saltwater or temporarily frozen with salt before it reaches the market. Shellfish vary in sodium content. However, at prescriptions of sodium above 3000 mg, it may be possible to show patients how to include them in their diet pattern (see Table 4, Part 4 or other food composition tables).

Cheeses are not included in the meat exchange list in Table 31-2 because of their sodium content. For example, 1 oz of cheddar cheese contains approximately 210 mg of sodium. This amount reflects the sodium in the milk used to make cheese and the sodium in compounds added during processing. Low-sodium dietetic cheeses are available in some markets. The amount of sodium in milligrams per serving is listed on the label. These products are relatively expensive compared to regular cheese. However, some patients use them for variety in menu planning and need directions for calculating the amount of cheese they can substitute for 1 oz of meat. For example, Low-sodium Colby Cheese, produced by Pauly, a division of Swift and

Company, contains 20 mg per 100 g, or 6 mg per 30 g of cheese.* Because of the sodium content, 3 oz of this cheese can be substituted for 1 oz of meat, or 1 oz of cheese could be added to a hamburger patty without increasing sodium significantly.

———

*Label information, Low-sodium Colby Cheese, 1973.

## Table 31-2. Sodium-Restricted Exchange Lists

### Milk Exchanges

*1 cup (8 oz) contains 120 mg sodium.*

Whole milk
Skim milk
Evaporated milk
Unsalted buttermilk
6 oz plain yogurt

### Meat Exchanges

*Each ounce, cooked, contains 25 mg of sodium.*

*Fresh or Frozen Meat*

| | |
|---|---|
| Beef | Tongue |
| Lamb | Liver |
| Pork | Rabbit |
| Veal | |

*Fresh or Frozen Poultry*

Chicken
Cornish hens
Duck
Turkey

*Fresh or Dietetic Canned Fish*

| | |
|---|---|
| Cod | Bass |
| Flounder | Perch (lake) |
| Haddock | Pike |
| Halibut | Whitefish |
| Perch (ocean) | |
| Salmon | |
| Tuna | |

### Egg Exchange

*1 egg contains 70 mg sodium.*

### Vegetable Exchanges

*1 serving, ½ cup, contains about 9 mg sodium.*

*Fresh, frozen without any sodium compound, and low-sodium canned dietetic vegetables or vegetable juices.*

| | |
|---|---|
| Asparagus | Onions |
| Broccoli | Peas, green |
| Brussels sprouts | Peppers |
| Cabbage | Pumpkin |
| Cauliflower | Radishes |
| Chicory | Rutabagas |
| Cucumbers | String beans |
| Eggplant | Squash, summer |
| Escarole | Squash, winter |
| Green beans | Tomatoes |
| Lettuce | Tomato juice |
| Mushrooms | Wax beans |
| Okra | |

### Fruit Exchanges

*Each serving contains about 2 mg sodium.*

Fresh, frozen, canned, or dried fruit and fruit juices. See Table 24-3 for complete listing.

### Bread Exchanges

*Each serving contains about 5 mg sodium.*

Low-sodium bread, 1 slice
Low-sodium rolls, 1 medium
Crackers
    Low-sodium dietetic melba toast, 4 slices
Cereals, long cooking, ½ c
    Farina
    Hominy grits
    Oatmeal
    Rolled wheat
    Wheat meal
Dry cereals, ¾ c
    Puffed Rice
    Puffed Wheat
Pasta and other cereal products, ½ c cooked
    Macaroni
    Noodles
    Spaghetti
    Barley
Flour, white or whole wheat, 1 c
Dried beans and peas, ½ c cooked
Corn, ⅓ c cooked
Potato, white, 1 small or ½ c cooked
Sweet potatoes, ¼ c cooked

### Fat Exchanges

*1 tsp contains practically no sodium*

Unsalted butter and margarine
Vegetable oils
Shortenings
Low-sodium mayonnaise and salad dressings

### Miscellaneous Foods

*The following foods contain no sodium:*

| | |
|---|---|
| *Coffee, no instant* | *Limes* |
| *Tea, no instant* | *Gelatin* |
| *Sugar, white* | *Vinegar* |
| *Honey* | *Sodium-free* |
| *Calcium saccharin* |    *baking powder* |
| *Lemons* | *Yeast* |

The low-sodium dietetic cheeses are made from dialyzed milk, a process that removes the sodium. Unfortunately, during dialysis potassium is usually exchanged for the sodium. Since some patients who require sodium-restriction may also require potassium-restriction (see Chap. 32, *Renal Disease,*) not all patients should use these cheeses.

On the other hand, if the diet prescription is 2000 mg to 3000 mg of sodium, and the patient customarily uses cheese, he can be shown how to substitute regular cheese for the milk exchanges calculated in his diet pattern. The substitutes can be calculated from the figures for the sodium content of cheese from Table 4, Part 4, or items in USDA Handbook No. 8-1 series, or, if available, from the nutrition label on a package of cheese. If the diet is also fat-controlled, no whole-milk cheese can be used (see Chap. 30).

One-fourth cup (55 g) of unsalted dry curd cottage cheese contains approximately 30 mg of sodium, and $1/4$ c of creamed cottage cheese contains approximately 150 mg of sodium. The patient who prefers cottage cheese to milk can be shown how to substitute creamed cottage cheese for the milk exchanges calculated in his diet pattern. Low-sodium peanut butters are also available, and from the label information one can calculate the amount of peanut butter that can be substituted for meat.

### Egg exchange

One egg contains 70 mg of sodium. Therefore, it cannot be considered an exchange for meat. The major portion of the sodium in an egg is in the white. One egg yolk contains approximately 10 mg of sodium. However, all the fat and cholesterol in an egg are in the yolk. Therefore, if cholesterol and fat or saturated fatty acids are also restricted, eggs cannot be included in the diet pattern.

### Table 31-3. Sodium in Selected Fresh Vegetables

| Vegetable* | Sodium (mg per 100 g)† |
|---|---|
| Beets | 36 |
| Beet greens, cooked | 76 |
| Carrots | 33 |
| Celery, raw | 126 |
| Chard, cooked | 86 |
| Collards, cooked | 25 |
| Kale, cooked | 43 |
| Mustard greens, cooked | 18 |
| Spinach, cooked | 45 |
| Turnips | 34 |

*Cooked without added salt.

†Pennington JAT, Church HN: Bowes & Church's Food Values of Portions Commonly Used, 13th ed. Philadelphia, JB Lippincott, 1980

### Vegetable exchanges

One serving, $1/2$ c, of the items in this list contains approximately 9 mg of sodium if no salt or sodium compound is added during production, processing, or preparation. The items in the vegetable exchange list in Table 24-3, Chapter 24, which are not in this vegetable exchange list, are excluded because of their natural sodium content. For example, $1/2$ c of fresh spinach cooked without added salt contains 45 mg of sodium.

Frozen peas and lima beans cannot be used because during processing the vegetables are put in a brine solution and a significant amount of sodium is picked up. For example, 100 g of fresh green peas contain about 1 mg of sodium, while 100 g of frozen peas contain about 115 mg of sodium. Frozen vegetables in sauces or those labeled "lightly salted" or "monosodium glutamate added" cannot be used.

The use of low-sodium dietetic canned vegetables should be limited to those listed in Table 31-2. Low-sodium canned carrots are available. However, $1/2$ cup of this product contains approximately 36 mg of sodium.

When the diet prescription is 2000 mg of sodium or more, the vegetables that have been excluded from Table 31-2 because they contain more than 9 mg of sodium per $1/2$-c serving may be calculated in a diet pattern. Table 31-3 gives the sodium content of these vegetables. Observe that they are primarily leaves and roots. Ten grams of chopped raw celery could be added to the vegetable exchange list in Table 31-2 for those patients who enjoy this in tuna or other salads.

Also, at levels above 2000 mg of sodium, vegetables canned with salt added, such as string beans, peas, carrots, and beets can be used if the solids are well drained from the liquid in the can. The vegetables should then be rinsed with water in a strainer and heated for serving in unsalted water. This process significantly reduces the amount of sodium in the vegetables.[10]

### Fruit exchanges

Each serving, as described in Table 24-3, contains approximately 2 mg of sodium. The items in this food group, fresh, frozen, or canned, do not present problems regarding the addition of sodium. However, the labels on cans of synthetic fruit drinks should be carefully checked for food additives containing sodium.

### Bread exchanges

Each serving as described in this food group contains approximately 5 mg of sodium. The sodium figure applies to one slice of bread made without milk. When low-sodium bread is made with milk, the sodium content increases to approximately 30 mg per slice. One slice of regular bread contains approximately 150 mg of sodium, contributed by milk, salt, and other sodium compounds used to prevent staling or molding.

The instant forms of cooked cereals, such as instant oatmeal or farina (Cream of Wheat) cannot be used because disodium phosphate is used in the precooking process. Dry cereals, other than the two listed, are also excluded because of their sodium content. For example, $\frac{1}{2}$ c of wheat flakes contains approximately 200 mg of sodium. Quick-cooking rice and instant mashed potatoes cannot be used because they undergo the same precooking with added sodium as the instant cereals.

The common leavening agents used in batters and doughs, yeast and baking powder, differ significantly in the amount of sodium they contain. Yeast does not contain sodium, while baking powder does. Products made from yeast doughs, however, must not contain added salt or sodium compounds when used in planning sodium-restricted diets. A low-sodium baking powder* is available for making biscuits or muffins that can be substituted for bread. Any milk or egg used in making these products should be from the daily allowance calculated in the patient's diet pattern. (See Resources for Patients at the end of this chapter for a list of cookbooks with tested recipes using low-sodium baking powder.) Low-sodium baking powder contains significant amounts of potassium, which limits its use in diets restricted in potassium as well as sodium (see Chap. 32). It is not wise to substitute the low-sodium baking powder for regular baking powder in a recipe in a standard cookbook.

Low-sodium bread is not readily available in all communities and is usually more expensive than regular bread. Also, because the activity of many patients requiring sodium-restricted diets is limited, they are not able to expend their limited energy kneading bread dough. Therefore, whenever the sodium level of the diet permits, usually about 1000 mg, regular bread, containing 150 mg of sodium per slice, is calculated in the diet pattern. The sodium content of regular bread can also be applied to one hamburger or one frankfurter bun.

In addition to low-sodium dietetic melba toast, a variety of crackers with unsalted tops is available in most supermarkets. The list of ingredients on the labels of these products should be read carefully. Although salt has not been added to the tops of these crackers, some are made from a dough that usually contains some sodium compound. This type of cracker was originally called soda cracker.

## Fat exchanges

One *teaspoonful* of the items listed in this exchange contains practically no sodium. Both unsalted butter and unsalted margarine are widely available. If a blender is

*Cellu-Featherweight, Chicago Dietetic Supply, Inc., LaGrange, Ill.

available, low-sodium mayonnaise can easily be made in the home using a standard recipe but omitting the salt. However, various low-sodium salad dressings and mayonnaise may also be found in the supermarket.

Whenever the diet is also fat-controlled, only margarine and corn, cottonseed, safflower, or soybean oils are used in calculating the diet pattern.

## Mixed dishes

Any of the exchanges calculated in the diet pattern can be used to prepare mixed dishes. A variety of herbs and spices, instead of salt, can be used (see *Salt Substitutes and Seasonings*). Many patients requiring sodium-restricted diets become, with guidance, excellent gourmet cooks. However, wines and other alcoholic beverages, common ingredients in gourmet recipes, cannot be used because of their wide variation in sodium content.[11]

## Convenience and other processed foods

Since many sodium compounds are found in convenience and other processed foods, these cannot be used by patients requiring sodium-restricted diets unless the milligrams of sodium per serving are clearly stated on the nutrition label. The quantity of sodium in some convenience foods will vary from minimal to excessive. One frozen entree, a veal dish, contains 1200 mg of sodium for each 2-oz serving of the meat. The same item, if made at home without salt added, would contain approximately 75 mg of sodium.

A partial list of food additives containing sodium that are commonly used in food processing is given in Table 31-4. The function of the additive and the foods in which it is used are also given. Food additives may or may not be listed on the product label. The listing of ingredients on the label is not required for processed foods for which the Food and Drug Administration has established standards of identity. The standard specifies the kind and minimum content of each ingredient to be used in processing the product. Therefore, if salt or a food additive containing sodium is included in the standard of identity, it does not have to be listed on the package label.

The listing of the quantity of sodium per serving under the Nutrition Labeling Law is optional and is usually stated only on the labels of dietetic foods (see *Low-Sodium Dietetic Foods*).

Some of the commonly used convenience foods that must be excluded from any sodium-restricted diet are TV dinners and frozen entrees; frozen vegetables in seasoned sauces; biscuit, muffin, pancake, cake, and cookie mixes and self-rising flours; seasoned rice; packaged potato dishes; hamburger extenders and seasoned bread stuffings; meat substitutes made from textured soy isolate protein; and snack crackers.

## Low-sodium dietetic foods

Products offered as low-sodium dietetic foods come under the Food and Drug Administration's Nutrition Labeling Law (1973). Under the regulations, the milligrams of sodium per serving size, as defined by the producer, must be listed on the label.

In addition to those products already mentioned, such as low-sodium canned vegetables, cheeses, and melba toast, various low-sodium dietetic condiments, entrees, soups, and baked products are available in many supermarkets. Some of these products may not be permitted in diets restricted to 2000 mg or less of sodium because, although reduced in sodium compared with the regular food, they still contain too much sodium per serving. Each product needs to be evaluated before it is used, and patients must be instructed that the symbol Na, rather than the term sodium, may be used on some labels.

## Salt substitutes and seasonings

Many patients find a sodium-restricted diet unappetizing because of the flatness or blandness of foods served without added salt. It can be explained that they are experiencing the real flavor of food, but this does not make the food any more appealing to them. Salt substitutes and spices and herbs can be used to make the diet more palatable.

Salt substitutes are available in drugstores and some supermarkets. They usually contain potassium or ammonium in place of sodium. These substitutes are contraindicated if there is renal or liver disease. In the hospital they may be offered to patients on sodium-restricted diets routinely or only by order of the physician. Those patients who use a salt substitute need to be advised to use it sparingly because in excessive amounts some find the taste unpleasant. Also, it may be more acceptable when added to the food at the table, rather than during cooking. One of the substitutes, labeled "seasoned," has a variety of spices added and is very palatable. Lite-Salt* cannot be used in sodium-restricted diets because it contains about one-half the sodium chloride content of regular salt.

Various spices and herbs that can be used are listed in Table 31-5. Fortunately, most of these are low in sodium; however, some commonly used seasonings contain a large amount of salt. These are celery, garlic, and onion salt; dried parsley and onion flakes; prepared mustard, Worcestershire sauce, and soy sauce; and monosodium glutamate and meat tenderizers. Patients who have not previously used a variety of spices and herbs should be cautioned to use them sparingly until they are sure they enjoy the new flavors.

## Drinking water

In some areas of the country drinking water may present a special hazard because of its high sodium content. This may be due either to the sodium content of the soil from which the water is drawn or to the use of water softener. In one study of over 2000 local water supplies widely distributed throughout the United States and covering approximately 50% of the population, great variation in sodium content was found, as shown in Table 31-6.[12]

Note that only 58% or a little over one-half the water supply was within the range of none to 20 mg of sodium

---

*Morton Salt Co., Chicago, Ill.

## Table 31-4. Food Additives Containing Sodium (Partial List)

| Compound | Function | Food |
|---|---|---|
| Sodium bicarbonate | Leavening agent, adjust acidity | Baking powder, tomato soup, ices, sherbets, syrups for frozen products, confections, self-rising flours |
| Sodium carbonate | Neutralizer | Butter, cream, ice cream, processing olives, cocoa products |
| Sodium caseinate | Texturizer | Ice cream, frozen custard, ice milk, sherbet |
| Sodium hexametaphosphate | Emulsifier, sequestrant, texturizer | Breakfast cereals, angel food cake, flaked fish, ice cream, ice milk, bottled beverages, puddings, processed cheeses, artificially sweetened jellies |
| Sodium hydroxide | Glazing agent, peeling agent, neutralizer | Pretzels, tubers and fruits, sour cream, cocoa products, canned peas |
| Sodium pectinate | Stabilizer and thickener | Syrups for frozen products, ice cream, ice milk, confections, fruit sherbets, French dressing, other salad dressings, fruit jelly, preserves, jams |
| Sodium stearoyl-2-lactylate | Emulsifier, plasticizer, surface active agent | Bakery mixes, baked products, cake icings, fillings and toppings, dehydrated fruits and vegetables, frozen desserts, pancake mixes, precooked instant rice, pudding mixes |
| Monosodium glutamate | Flavor enhancer | Meats, condiments, pickles, soups, candy, baked goods, frozen vegetables |

## Table 31-5. Seasonings, Extracts, Herbs, and Spices

| Low in Sodium (May be Used Freely) | | High in Sodium (Do Not Use) |
|---|---|---|
| Allspice | Mint. | Bouillon cubes, regular |
| Almond extract | Mustard, dry, or mustard seed | Catsup |
| Anise seed | Nutmeg | Celery flakes, seed, salt |
| Basil | Onion, onion juice, or onion | Chili sauce |
| Bay leaf | powder | Garlic salt |
| Bouillon cube, low-sodium | Orange extract | Horseradish, prepared with salt |
| dietetic if less than 5 mg | Oregano | Instant vegetable broth |
| sodium per cube | Paprika | Meat extracts |
| Caraway seed | Parsley | Meat sauces |
| Cardamon | Pepper, fresh green or red | Meat tenderizers |
| Catsup, dietetic | Pepper, black, red, or white | Monosodium glutamate |
| Chili powder | Peppermint extract | Mustard, prepared |
| Chives | Pimiento peppers for garnish | Olives |
| Cinnamon | Poppy seed | Onion salt |
| Cloves | Poultry seasoning | Parsley flakes |
| Cocoa (1–2 teaspoonsful) | Purslane | Pickles |
| Coconut | Rosemary | Relishes |
| Cumin | Saffron, calcium (sugar | Saccharin, sodium (sugar |
| Curry | substitute) | substitute) |
| Dill | Saffron | **Salt** |
| Fennel | Sage | Salt substitutes, unless recom- |
| Garlic, garlic juice, or garlic | Salt substitutes, if recommended | mended by the physician |
| powder | by the physician | Soy sauce |
| Ginger | Savory | Tomato paste |
| Horseradish root or horseradish | Sesame seeds | Worcestershire sauce |
| prepared without salt | Sorrel | |
| Juniper | Sugar | |
| Lemon juice or extract | Tarragon | |
| Mace | Thyme | |
| Maple extract | Turmeric | |
| Marjoram | Vanilla extract | |
| Meat extract, low-sodium | Vinegar | |
| dietetic | Wine, if allowed | |
| Meat tenderizers, low-sodium dietetic | Walnut extract | |

(Adapted from "Your 1000-milligram Sodium Diet." By permission of the American Heart Association, Inc.)

per liter (approximately a quart). Water used for coffee and tea, for drinking, and for food preparation is estimated at $2\frac{1}{2}$ to 3 liters per person per day. When water contains more than 20 mg of sodium per liter, it can significantly increase the sodium content of the diet. The patient should obtain information about his community's water supply by contacting the department of health. Also, home water-softening systems should be checked to ensure that the sodium content of the water has not been increased. In the northern part of the United States there have been reports of an increase in the sodium content of water supplies. This has been attributed to the run-off of sodium chloride from streets and highways during the icy winter months.

## Soft drinks

Bottled soft drinks may be high in sodium due to the sodium content of the water in the area where they are manufactured. Low caloric beverages may have their sodium content increased still further by the substitution of sodium saccharin, an artificial sweetener, for sugar. They

are therefore omitted when careful sodium restriction must be maintained. Iannaccone and co-workers[13] report that 7 oz of Mountain Valley Water contains 1.5 mg of sodium and 6.6 oz of Perrier Water contains 2.5 mg of sodium.

## Table 31-6. Range of Sodium Ion in Drinking Water for a Sampling Period

| Range of Sodium Ion Concentration (mg/L) | Number of Samples | Percent of Total Samples |
|---|---|---|
| 0– 19.9 | 1194 | 58.2 |
| 20– 49.9 | 391 | 19.0 |
| 50– 99.9 | 190 | 9.3 |
| 100–249.9 | 178 | 8.7 |
| 250–399.9 | 74 | 3.6 |
| 400–499.9 | 10 | 0.5 |
| 500–999.9 | 14 | 0.7 |
| Over 1000 | 2 | 0.1 |

(From White JM et al: Sodium ion in drinking water. J Am Diet Assoc 50:32, 1967)

## Planning the sodium-restricted diet pattern

The first step in planning any sodium-restricted diet pattern is to estimate, from the patient's diet history, the sodium content of his usual food choices and the amount of salt he customarily adds to foods at the table. Special care should be taken to identify the kinds and amounts of processed and convenience foods eaten at home and the frequency with which meals are eaten in restaurants or in a social setting. This information helps to identify the magnitude of the adjustment facing the patient. Some hospitalized patients have been advised previously to "cut down on salt," while others may have had no previous diet counseling.

### The moderately sodium-restricted diet pattern, 1000 mg to 2000 mg (43 mEq to 86 mEq)

Table 31-7 shows a diet pattern calculated with Mr. A., a 55-year-old man in moderate congestive failure due to rheumatic fever in childhood. His diet prescription was

### Table 31-7. A 1000-mg (43 mEq) Sodium-Restricted, 1500-Calorie Diet Pattern

| Food Group | Amount | Sodium (mg) | Energy (Kcalories) |
|---|---|---|---|
| Milk, whole | 1 pt | 240 | 340 |
| Meat | 4 oz, cooked | 100 | 300 |
| Egg | 1 | 70 | 75 |
| Vegetables | 4 ½-cup servings | 36 | 100 |
| Fruit | 3 servings | 6 | 120 |
| Bread, unsalted | 3 servings | 15 | 210 |
| Bread, salted | 3 slices | 450 | 210 |
| Fat, unsalted | 3 tsp | | 135 |
| **Totals** | | 917 | 1490 |

### Table 31-8. A Day's Menu Selected by Mr. A.

*Breakfast*
½ cup of orange juice
1 soft poached egg
1 slice of regular bread, toasted
1 cup of decaffeinated coffee

*Noon Meal*
Sandwich
   1 oz of roast beef, unsalted
   lettuce
   2 slices of regular bread
8 oz of whole milk
1 peach

*Evening Meal*
3 oz of roast veal, unsalted
1 cup of mashed potato with 1 tsp of salt-free butter
1 cup of salt-free string beans with 1 tsp of salt-free butter
1 cup of salt-free broccoli with lemon juice

*Bedtime*
8 oz of whole milk
10 grapes
4 slices of unsalted melba toast

1000 mg of sodium and 1500 calories because he was 30 pounds overweight.

The six bread exchanges in his diet pattern consist of three unsalted ones and three slices of regular bread. The choice of regular bread made the diet more palatable for him. Occasionally he substituted 8 oz of skim milk for whole milk and added two unsalted fat exchanges. Table 31-8 is a day's menu selected by Mr. A., using his diet pattern in Table 31-7.

In four weeks, when Mr. A.'s condition had improved, his physician increased his sodium allowance to 1500 mg per day but continued the restriction in calories to 1500. Table 31-9 shows how his diet pattern was modified. The six bread exchanges now consisted of items with salt added. Mr. A. chose to have four slices of regular bread and 1 cup of mashed potatoes, which Mrs. A. made from potatoes cooked in lightly salted (less than ⅛ tsp of salt) water. The fat exchanges were now also salted ones.

Mr. A., with Mrs. A.'s help, readily accepted his sodium-restricted diets. Fortunately he had not added excessive amounts of salt to his food, and Mrs. A. used very few convenience or processed foods and salted food lightly during preparation. However, she frequently fried meats and potatoes with fat and had to modify this practice. Mr. A. had to give up three of his favorite foods, bacon, ham, and pretzels.

### The mildly sodium-restricted diet pattern, 2000 mg to 3000 mg (86 mEq to 130 mEq)

All highly salted foods and the addition of salt to food at the table are excluded from any mildly sodium-restricted diet. At 2000 mg, foods processed or cooked with moderate amounts of salt can be used. The processed foods include cottage cheese, regular breads without salt toppings, salted butter or margarine, and vegetables canned with added salt. During preparation meats and fresh vegetables can be lightly salted. Otherwise food choices should be restricted to those in the Exchange Lists, Table 31-2.

At 3000 mg of sodium, regular canned tuna, shellfish, all cereals, and biscuits and muffins made from standard recipes using baking powder can be used. If there is no restriction in energy, doughnuts, sweet rolls, fruit pies, sugar cookies, and ice cream can also be included. Catsup, but not chili sauce or pickles, can be used. The convenience foods previously mentioned and cured meats and fish are excluded at any level of mild sodium restriction.

When Mr. A. had achieved his normal weight status, he underwent surgery for a heart valve replacement. After surgery his physician prescribed a mildly sodium-restricted diet, 2500 mg to 3000 mg per day. Mr. A.'s diet was modified by the addition of salt to the preparation of meats and vegetables, and the occasional use of cheddar cheese, shellfish, and homemade biscuits and muffins in place of bread. He continued to monitor his weight status and on special occasions had fruit pies or ice cream for dessert.

### The severely sodium-restricted diet pattern, less than 1000 mg (43mEq)

Patients with gross edema due to severe congestive failure or with massive ascites due to hepatic failure usually require sodium restriction to 500 mg or less. These patients are hospitalized because they are critically ill and frequently have a very poor appetite. Their nutritional care at this point is primarily practitioner-managed (see Chap. 13).

Table 31-10 shows a 500-mg, sodium-restricted diet pattern. The same quantities of exchanges were used to calculate this pattern as the 1000-mg sodium-restricted diet pattern in Table 31-7. However, compared with the bread exchanges in Table 31-7, all the bread exchanges in Table 31-10 are salt free. Most critically ill patients will probably not want the vegetables calculated in this diet pattern and will prefer fruit juices to fruit, if their fluid intake is not restricted as well.

If the diet prescription were 250 mg of sodium in place of 500 mg, Lonalac,* a low-sodium milk, could be used in place of whole milk. One pint of Lonalac contains approximately 12 mg of sodium, which would reduce the sodium content of the diet pattern in Table 31-10 to 254 mg.

Severe restrictions of sodium for patients with cardiovascular disease are usually prescribed as an emergency measure. After fluid and electrolyte balance is reestablished, a more moderate restriction is usually prescribed. The planning and serving of the 500-mg, sodium-restricted diet to hospitalized patients must be carefully monitored so that errors are not made. If two slices of regular bread were served in place of two slices of salt-free bread, the patient would consume 300 mg, not 10 mg, of sodium, and his day's intake of sodium would be far in excess of the amount ordered due to this one error. At the same time, the clinical dietitian and those responsible for patient food preparation must demonstrate a high degree of creativity in menu planning and food preparation. Contrary to popular opinion, sodium-restricted diets *do not have to be unpalatable* (see *Patient Resources* at end of chap.).

## Counseling the patient

### Patient problems

The sodium-restricted diet is probably the most difficult therapeutic diet for the patient to accept. In addition to modifying his food choices, he is confronted with a major change in the taste of his food. For the patient who has always added salt liberally at the table, his food now

*Mead Johnson Laboratories, Evansville, Ind. 47721.

tastes flat and unappetizing. At the same time that he is coping with a sodium-restricted diet, he may also be advised by his physician to modify drastically his total lifestyle. For example, an aggressive businessman, who may require mild sodium restriction of a fat-controlled diet after a severe myocardial infarction, may encounter difficulty in accepting diet counseling.

As well as helping the patient and spouse to understand the purpose of the sodium-restricted intake, the counselor must also help them identify all dietary sources of sodium. Salt, because of its distinctive taste, is not difficult for the patient to understand. However, food additives with sodium are more difficult to interpret to the patient because many of them do not give a salty taste to food.

With the present progress in the United States in the adoption of the metric system, it can be anticipated that some patients will be able to understand instructions better about grams and milligrams of salt and sodium. The patient with a strong science background will readily understand the metric system. The patient who can understand grams and milligrams has an advantage in that he can interpret the information on labels and have a wider selection of foods or be able to avoid those that he cannot use. For the patient who cannot comprehend the metric system, food choices will be limited to the food lists

### Table 31-9. A 1500-mg (65 mEq) Sodium-Restricted, 1500-Calorie Diet Pattern

| Food Group | Amount | Sodium (mg) | Energy (Kcalories) |
|---|---|---|---|
| Milk, whole | 1 pt | 240 | 340 |
| Meat | 4 oz, cooked | 100 | 300 |
| Egg | 1 | 70 | 75 |
| Vegetables | 4 ½-cup servings | 36 | 100 |
| Fruit | 3 servings | 6 | 120 |
| Bread, salted | 6 servings | 900 | 420 |
| Fat, salted | 3 tsp | 150 | 135 |
| **Totals** | | 1502 | 1490 |

### Table 31-10. A 500-mg (21 mEq) Sodium-Restricted Diet Pattern

| Food Group | Amount | Sodium (mg) | Energy (Kcalories) |
|---|---|---|---|
| Milk, whole | 1 pt | 240 | 340 |
| Meat | 4 oz, cooked | 100 | 300 |
| Egg | 1 | 70 | 75 |
| Vegetables | 4 ½-cup servings | 36 | 100 |
| Fruit | 3 servings | 6 | 120 |
| Bread, unsalted | 6 servings | 30 | 420 |
| Fat, unsalted | 3 tsp | | 135 |
| **Totals** | | 482 | 1490 |

in the instructional materials which he receives, and he will need considerable assistance in making any additions to the lists.

People who eat frequently in restaurants will need help with menu selection. Plain broiled meats, baked potatoes, and green salad with oil and vinegar dressing are three items that can be served without salt added. Unfortunately meat tenderizers are used in many restaurants today. In congregate meal programs for the elderly no highly salted foods, such as ham should be served, and foods should be lightly salted during preparation because many of the participants in these programs may have mild cardiovascular disease.

Ethnic food practices also present some problems. Southern patients in the habit of cooking with bacon or salt pork must be warned about this. This is also true for people who eat "soul" foods. Jewish patients, following their dietary laws of heavily salting their meats before cooking (koshering) need help in readjusting their deeply ingrained convictions (see earlier in this chapter). Italian patients should be warned not to use commercially canned tomato paste, olives, Italian cheese, and Italian bread. Tomato paste can be made at home, omitting salt and spices containing sodium. Occasionally an Italian

## Table 31-11. Suggested Nutritional Pattern for a Coronary Care Unit

The following nutritional pattern for use in the Coronary Care Unit is suggested for short-term use (*i.e.,* the initial five- to ten-day period, following acute myocardial infarction).

(a) Nothing by mouth prior to evaluation by the physician. In most instances, intravenous solution started to facilitate administration of drugs required if arrhythmias and shock ensue.

(b) Patient to be reevaluated for dietetic progression after first 24 hr.

(c) For the first 24 hr, 500- to 800-kcal (1000 to 1500 ml) liquid diet, with only small amounts of liquid taken at a time. Foods that may be offered include clear soups, broth, skim milk, fruit juices, tea, ginger ale, and water.

(d) Caloric level of 1000 to 1200 kcal to meet patient's basal metabolic requirement. Nutritional proportions should be approximately 20% protein, 45% carbohydrate, and 30 to 35% fat (low saturated fat; polyunsaturates as the primary source of dietary fat) with cholesterol limited to 300 mg per day. Sodium restriction if indicated by patient's condition.

(e) Beverages and other liquids served at body temperatures. Non-caffeine and decaffeinated beverages are preferred. Stimulants and extremes in temperature to be avoided.

(f) Small, frequent meals consisting of foods that are easily digested, free of gastric irritants, soft, and low in roughage.

(g) Foods to be included: tender, lean cuts of meat; fish and poultry; tender, cooked or canned vegetables and fruits; plain breads; cooked cereals; simple puddings and gelatin desserts. Egg yolks limited to three a week.

(h) Nutritional plan to be individualized on basis of patient's clinical status and physiologic and psychologic needs. Areas usually requiring modification are carbohydrates, protein, fat, total calories, electrolytes, and fluids.

(Christakis G, Winston M: J Am Diet Assoc 63:233, 1973)

bakery makes low-sodium bread if there is sufficient demand for it. Japanese and Chinese patients must particularly be cautioned to omit monosodium glutamate and soy sauce, both of which are commonly used in the seasoning of their food. Greek patients and those coming from the Near East frequently use heavily salted olives as an accompaniment to meals.

Research has demonstrated that relatives of patients with essential hypertension are at risk for developing the disease.[14] Therefore, it is strongly advised that the family of a hypertensive patient monitor its sodium intake by avoiding highly salted foods and foods with significant amounts of sodium compounds added during processing.

### Instructional materials

In addition to the instructional materials developed by a hospital or other health agency for patients requiring sodium-restricted diets, three booklets have been published by the American Heart Association. They are available to the patient only through his physician, who may obtain them from the local heart association or, where there is no local association, from the national office.* The booklets were prepared by the American Heart Association in conjunction with the American Dietetic Association, the Council on Foods and Nutrition of the American Medical Association, the Nutrition Foundation, and the Public Health Service of the Department of Health, Education, and Welfare. The diets are constructed on the Exchange System similar to the one presented in this chapter. The three booklets are entitled, *Your 500 Milligram Sodium Restricted Diet; Your 1000 Milligram Sodium Restricted Diet;* and *Your Mild Sodium-Restricted Diet.* The first two booklets have also been issued as simplified leaflets.

Any instruction materials for patients on sodium-restricted diets should reflect as much as possible the usual food practices in the area and be reviewed and revised constantly as changes occur in food processing. "New and improved" products may contain more sodium than the original ones.

### The patient with an acute myocardial infarction

The nutritional care of the patients in a coronary care unit has been reviewed by Hemzacek[15] and by Christakis and Winston.[16] Table 31-11 presents the latter's recommendations. The nutritional care is usually given by the nursing staff in consultation with the clinical dietitian.

As soon as possible after admission, the patient's likes and dislikes of the fluids used should be ascertained, usually from a relative or close friend in order not to disturb the patient. Special care should be taken to determine if the patient has any intolerance to milk, such as

*American Heart Association, New York, N.Y.

gastric distress or diarrhea, so that this fluid can be avoided, if necessary. In some coronary units the physicians may exclude carbonated beverages since some patients experience epigastric distress after drinking them.

It is also advisable to be sure that fluids, and food when tolerated, are not too hot or too cold because extremes in temperature of fluids and foods may have an adverse effect on the function of cardiac muscle (cardiac arrhythmias). Coffee and tea are usually excluded because the stimulants they contain may increase heart rate. Decaffeinated beverages may be substituted. Many physicians advise their patients with heart disease to exclude or to limit strictly their consumption of any beverage containing caffeine or other stimulants (coffee, tea, cocoa, chocolate, cola beverages).

### Hypokalemia

Three types of diuretics, the thiazides, furosemide, and ethacrynic acid, can promote hypokalemia. In addition to oral intake of potassium chloride or the rotation of diuretics, foods with significant quantities of potassium can also be used to prevent hypokalemia. Potassium is present in all foods, but fruits and fruit juices are significant sources that can be recommended without, at the same time, increasing the sodium intake.

### Sodium in medications

The physician should avoid prescribing medications which contain sodium. The patient should be cautioned to take no medication, "patent" medicine, or home remedy without consulting his physician. Baking soda (sodium bicarbonate), a popular home remedy for indigestion or "heartburn," and many alkalizers, antacids, headache remedies, sedatives, and cathartics which are high in sodium should not be used.

### The debilitated patient

Since many patients with cardiovascular disease, especially arteriosclerosis, are in the older age group, they frequently present special nutritional care problems. A person may be confused and disoriented and require assistance in feeding himself at each meal or may need to be fed by a staff member in an institution or by a relative in his home. If he lacks teeth or has poorly fitting dentures, the consistency of his food should be modified so that he can chew. Not all patients require the same modification.

Appetite may vary during the day. In the morning, after a night's rest, patients may eat well at breakfast. As the day progresses, they may become progressively weaker and eat less well at the noon and evening meals. Five small meals a day may be helpful. It is well to avoid those foods that the patient reports give him gastric distress. Frequently these foods are milk, members of the cabbage family, and dried peas and beans.

## Study questions and activities

1. Why may the patient with cardiac disease develop edema?
2. Why will a diet restricted in sodium aid in preventing or eliminating edema in the cardiac patient?
3. Is low-sodium bread available in your community? How does its price compare with regular bread?
4. What is the sodium content of one slice of regular bread? of 1 tsp of salted butter or margarine? of 1 tbsp?
5. Make out a menu for a day for a patient with congestive heart failure whose diet order is 1000 mg sodium, soft diet, five meals.
6. Which foods used in planning the sodium-restricted diet contain the most sodium? Which the least?
7. Using Table 2, Part 4, make a list of common beverages which contain a significant amount of potassium for a patient taking a diuretic which promotes potassium excretion.
8. What should a patient on a sodium-restricted diet be taught about convenience foods and the labels on any food package?

## References

1. Levy RI: In Heart Disease: Public Health Enemy No. 1, pp 3–16. Washington, DC, Committee on Agriculture, Nutrition and Forestry, 1979
2. Goldring D: J Pediatr 91:884, 1977
3. Braunwald E: In Isselbacher KJ et al (eds): Harrison's Principles of Internal Medicine, 9th ed, pp 171–175. New York, McGraw-Hill, 1980
4. Ramirez A, Abelman WH: N Engl J Med 290:499, 1974
5. Tobian L: Am J Clin Nutr 32:2739, 1979
6. Dahl LK: J Exp Med 114:231, 1961
7. Morgan T et al: Lancet 1:227, 1978
8. Braunwald, In Isselbacher, Harrison's Principles, pp 1035–1044
9. Kaufman M: Am J Clin Nutr 5:676, 1957
10. Sinar LJ, Mason M: J Am Diet Assoc 66:155, 1975
11. Newberg B: Arch Intern Med 123:692, 1969
12. White JM et al: J Am Diet Assoc 50:32, 1967
13. Iannaccone ST et al: JAMA 244:436, 1980
14. Pietinen PI et al: Am J Clin Nutr 32:997, 1979
15. Hemzacek KI: J Am Diet Assoc 72:182, 1978
16. Christakis G, Winston M: J Am Diet Assoc 63:233, 1973

## Supplementary readings

Altschul AM, Grommet JK: Sodium intake and sodium sensitivity. Nutr Rev 38:393, 1980

Hemzacek KI: Dietary protocol for the patient who has suffered a myocardial infarction. J Am Diet Assoc 72:182, 1978

Iannaccone ST et al: Sodium content of bottled sparkling water. JAMA 244:436, 1980

Loggie JMH et al: Renal function and diuretic therapy in infants and children. J Pediatr 86:485; 657; 825; 1975

Porter GA: The role of diuretics in the treatment of heart failure. JAMA 244:1614, 1980

Ram CVS et al: Moderate sodium restriction and various diuretics in the treatment of hypertension: Effects on potassium wastage and blood pressure control. Arch Intern Med 141:1015, 1981

Report of the Joint National Committee on Detection, Evaluation and Treatment of High Blood Pressure. Arch Intern Med 140:1280, 1980

Robertson D et al: Effects of caffeine on plasma renin activity, catecholamines and blood pressure. N Engl J Med 298:181, 1978

Schlierf G et al: Salt and hypertension data from the "Heidelberg Study". Am J Clin Nutr 33:872, 1980

Seman DL et al: Effect of reduction and partial replacement of sodium on bologna characteristics and acceptability. J Food Sci 45:1116, 1980

Tobian L: The relationship of salt to hypertension. Am J Clin Nutr 32:2739, 1979

Williams GH et al: Hypertensive cardiovascular disease. In Isselbacher KJ et al (eds): Harrison's Principles of Internal Medicine, 9th ed, pp 1167–1178. New York, McGraw-Hill, 1980

Zifferblatt SM, Wilbur CS: Dietary counseling: Some realistic expectations and guidelines. J Am Diet Assoc 70:591, 1977

## Patient Resources

American Heart Association Cookbook, 3rd ed. New York, David McKay, 1979

Claiborne C, Franey P: Craig Claiborne's Gourmet Diet. New York, New York Times Books, 1980

Dosti R et al: Light Style: The New American Cuisine. San Francisco, Harper & Row, 1979

Jones J: Secrets of Salt-Free Cooking. San Francisco, 101 Productions, 1979

Margie JD, Hunt JC: Living with High Blood Pressure: The Hypertension Cook Book. Bloomfield, NJ, HLS Press, 1978

Margie JD, Levy RI, Hunt JC: Living Better: Recipes for a Healthy Heart. Bloomfield, NJ, HLS Press, 1980

Payne AS, Callahan D: Fat and Sodium Control Cookbook, 4th ed. Boston, Little, Brown, 1975

*For further references see Bibliography in Part 4.*

# Renal Disease: Nephrolithiasis

**32**

**BUN:** Blood Urea Nitrogen
**GFR:** Glomerular Filtration Rate
**MAO:** Monoamine Oxidase
**PTH:** Parathyroid Hormone

**Lois Schroeder**

The nutritional care of patients with renal diseases involves modification of the intake of calories, protein, fluids, and electrolytes appropriate to the level of kidney function. In the early stages of renal disease, manipulation of dietary intake may be moderate. However, as acute or chronic renal disease progresses to renal failure, nutritional care becomes one of the most critical components of the medical care plan. Appropriate diet prescriptions for patients in renal failure usually reflect significant modifications of the normal food intake of a healthy person. These modifications should be based upon a sound understanding of the varied metabolic changes induced by renal failure.

Before proceeding with the discussion of renal diseases and diet therapy, the reader is urged to review Chapter 4, *Proteins*; Chapter 5, *Fluid and Electrolyte Metabolism*; and the sodium-restricted diet in Chapter 31, *Cardiovascular Disease*.

## The kidneys' role in normal metabolism

The kidneys are the major organs involved in maintaining the body's internal environment by regulating fluid and electrolyte balance, acid–base balance, and the balance between intake of nutrients and excretion of the byproducts of metabolism. Although the kidneys are primarily thought of as excretory organs, they also have important metabolic and hormonal functions. Their task of maintaining a homeostatic environment in the body is accomplished by cleansing the blood through complex processes involving filtration, reabsorption, and secretion, leading to the production of urine. Any condition that interferes with these functions may alter both the intracellular and extracellular composition of many organs and, as a result, may have serious consequences for the whole organism.

### Excretory function

The nephron, which is the functional unit of the kidneys, is a structure approximately 6 cm in length with five major components: the glomerulus, proximal tubule, loop of Henle, distal tubule, and the collecting duct (see Fig. 32-1). It is estimated that each kidney contains approximately one million nephrons. The glomerulus is the filtering unit of the nephron. An afferent arteriole carries blood into a capillary network where a filtrate of plasma is forced by net hydrostatic pressure into a cup-like capsule, Bowman's capsule, which leads into the proximal tubule. The amount of filtrate formed, or the glomerular filtration rate, averages approximately 100 ml to 120 ml per minute in an adult human. This rate results in the formation of approximately 180 liters of filtrate per day. The filtrate resembles plasma except that it contains only

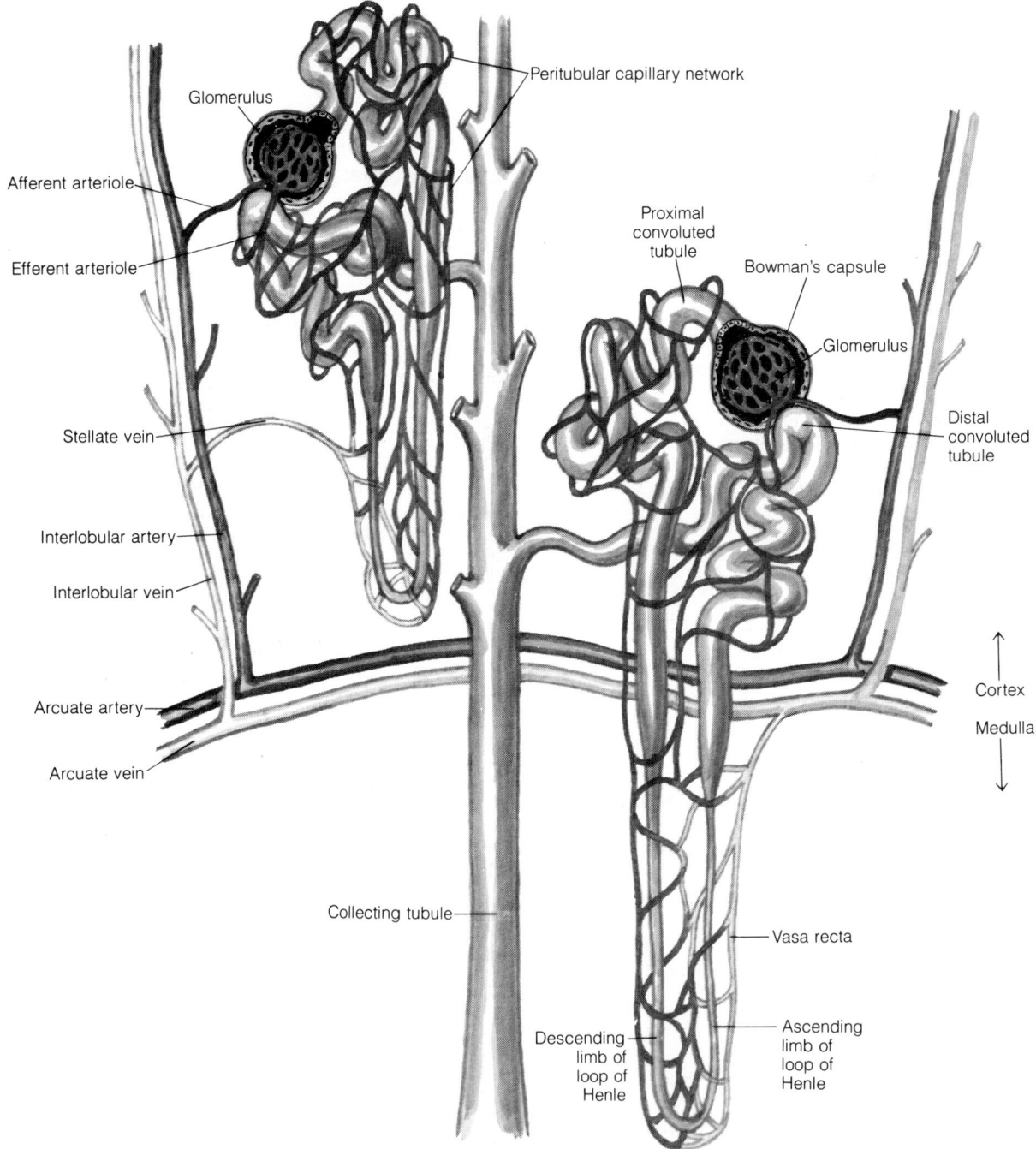

**Fig. 32-1.** Diagram of two nephrons and their blood supply. *Left,* nephron has a short loop of Henle; *right,* the other nephron has a long loop of Henle and a more extensive blood supply. (Chaffee EE, Lytle IM: Basic Physiology and Anatomy, 4th ed. Philadelphia, JB Lippincott, 1980)

small amounts of protein or other substances with molecular weights greater than 40,000 daltons. From Bowman's capsule the filtrate moves into a tubule that consists of three major sections. The first section, the proximal convoluted tubule, is the primary site for reabsorption of the bulk of the filtrate volume and for the selective reabsorption of certain filtered substances. Physiologically useful materials that are actively reabsorbed include amino acids, low molecular weight proteins, sodium, glucose, potassium, vitamins, and others. In addition, the bulk of filtered bicarbonate is reabsorbed in the proximal tubule in association with hydrogen ion secretion. Also, a large portion of the filtered water is passively reabsorbed into the blood vessels surrounding the proximal tubule as a result of active solute (sodium and chloride) transport. Certain substances are poorly reabsorbed and remain in the filtrate. These include the metabolic waste products: urea, uric acid, sulfates, phosphates, nitrates, and creatinine. Other substances, in particular many drugs and exogenous toxins, may be secreted into the proximal tubular fluid.

As the filtrate passes from the proximal convoluted tubule through the descending and ascending limbs of the loop of Henle, it is further reduced in volume and becomes more dilute. By the time the filtrate reaches the distal convoluted tubule from the ascending loop of Henle, its volume is approximately one-eighth of its original amount, and its solute concentration is reduced by half. From this point the kidney can concentrate the filtrate further by the passive reabsorption of water or can dilute the filtrate by selective reabsorption of solutes depending on the needs of the organism. The dilution-concentration process is dependent on the action of antidiuretic hormone on the distal tubule and collecting duct. Other major functions of the distal tubule include further secretion of hydrogen ions, secretion of potassium, and regulation of sodium reabsorption. Most of the secreted hydrogen ion is buffered by filtered phosphate and secreted ammonia. The excretion of potassium and reabsorption of sodium is controlled by hormonal mechanisms responsive to the body's needs. From the distal tubule the filtrate, or urine, moves through collecting ducts, which collect fluid from several nephrons, and from there to the ureter and the bladder.

Thus, the normal kidney achieves homeostasis of body fluids by processing a large amount of plasma ultrafiltrate and, through selective reabsorption and secretion, by reducing this to a small volume of fluid with a composition ideally suited to keeping the volume and content of the body fluids normal.

### Metabolic functions

In addition to its excretory function, the kidney is important in several metabolic schemes. It is an active site for nitrogen metabolism. Certain amino acids are deaminated in the kidney, producing ammonia and providing carbon skeletons for glucose synthesis. The ammonia so produced is a major buffer for hydrogen ions in the urine and is thereby important in determining the ability of the kidney to control body fluid acidity. Glucose production is another metabolic function of the kidney that can be significant during periods of acidosis or starvation. Also the kidney processes a variety of toxic organic substances into less toxic compounds, which can be excreted.

### Hormonal functions

The kidney is now recognized as important in several hormonal systems. The final conversion of vitamin D to its active form, 1,25-dihydroxycholecalciferol ($1,25-(OH)_2D_3$), takes place in the kidney. This active form of vitamin D, along with parathyroid hormone, plays an important regulatory role in calcium and phosphorus metabolism (see Chap. 7, *Fat-soluble Vitamins*). The kidney also plays an important role in the control of blood pressure through the regulation of extracellular fluid volume and the synthesis of prohypertensive (renin) and antihypertensive agents (certain prostaglandins). Synthesis of both renin and prostaglandins is apparently influenced by changes in blood pressure due to a reduction in plasma volume or changes in body sodium content or both. These two systems may act in concert to regulate intrarenal blood flow and to influence systemic blood pressure. Another hormonal role of the kidney is the synthesis of an erythropoietic factor that acts on bone marrow to stimulate the production of red blood cells.

## Renal terminology and physiologic aberrations

*Chronic renal failure* refers to any permanent reduction in overall renal function, usually expressed as the glomerular filtration rate (GFR). As the GFR decreases, nitrogenous waste products are no longer excreted at a normal rate and their concentration rises in the blood. The blood levels of urea nitrogen (BUN) and serum creatinine are commonly used to estimate the levels of nitrogenous waste products. The normal range for the blood urea nitrogen is 8 mg to 18 mg per deciliter. The level of BUN is a relatively insensitive index of renal function since it is affected by protein intake and the rate of protein breakdown. A mildly elevated BUN value may be associated with a fairly good GFR in a patient with a high protein intake, or it may represent a severely reduced GFR in a patient whose diet is low in protein. Another indicator of the filtration rate is the serum creatinine level. The normal serum creatinine range is 0.5 mg to 1.5 mg per deciliter. In contrast to the BUN, the serum creatinine level is independent of exogenous protein intake, and, therefore, the serum creatinine level is largely determined by the renal excretion rate, which correlates closely with the GFR. Using a calculation involving the serum creatinine level and timed urine creatinine excretion, a value termed *creatinine clearance* can be determined, which is an accurate estimate of the GFR and, thus, of overall renal function.

Chronic renal failure is often classified as "early" or "late" or "mild" to "severe" depending upon the level of reduction of the GFR. *Azotemia* refers to an elevated serum concentration of the end products of protein catabolism without the clinical symptoms of uremia being present. Renal failure usually becomes symptomatic when the blood biochemistry becomes significantly abnormal. This usually occurs at a GFR of approximately 30 ml per minute or less (normal GFR is approximately 120 ml per minute) or when the blood urea nitrogen (BUN) level approaches 100 mg per deciliter (normal is 8 mg–18 mg per deciliter). The term used to describe symptomatic renal failure is *uremia* or *uremic syndrome*. *End-stage renal disease* is an additional term referring to advanced chronic renal failure or the terminal stage of renal failure, usually when the GFR falls to less than 10 ml per minute and when dialysis or transplantation is necessary.

As kidney disease progresses and nephrons cease functioning, it is thought that the remaining working nephrons carry on the excretion process by increasing the volume of glomerular filtrate. The tubules hypertrophy in their effort to handle the extra filtrate. Polyuria (excess urine production) may develop when the tubular cells are no longer able to concentrate the filtrate. The patient may become increasingly thirsty and excess quantities of fluid and electrolytes are excreted as the kidney attempts to handle the usual solute load. Polyuria may reach a peak while the GFR decreases from 25 ml to 5 ml per minute and then the volume of urine no longer remains excessive, but may decrease to a state of oliguria (urine volume of less than 400 ml per day). With oliguria or anuria (urine volume of less than 100 ml per day), retention of sodium and potassium occurs. If the destruction of renal tissue has reached the point where the excretory and regulatory functions of the kidneys are severely compromised, death is imminent unless dialysis or transplantation is instituted.[1]

The hallmarks of renal failure include retention of urea, creatinine, and uric acid; progressive acidosis; inability to excrete a maximally dilute or a maximally concentrated urine; and blood electrolyte disturbances.[2] Renal insufficiency exists at varying levels of severity, and each patient is treated individually according to clinical and biochemical indices and symptoms. Advanced uremia may include many clinical symptoms, such as anorexia, nausea, vomiting, an ammonia-like taste in the mouth, hiccups, diarrhea, general weakness, and hypertension. This obviously influences dietary management since patients find it very difficult to maintain adequate food intake when they feel so ill.

*Acute renal failure* is characterized by a sudden decrease in glomerular filtration rate, sometimes to values of less than 1% to 2% of the normal rate, and is often accompanied by oliguria or anuria. The BUN, serum creatinine, uric acid, and phosphate may rise rapidly, and acute derangements in electrolyte concentrations may occur. It may be caused by trauma, such as burns, ingestion of toxic agents, hypotension associated with sepsis, surgery or myocardial infarction, urinary obstruction, or an obstruction to renal bloodflow. Because the possibility of acute renal failure can be anticipated in a variety of clinical situations, major emphasis should be directed toward prevention. Acute renal failure may last a few days or for several weeks and, unlike chronic renal failure, is considered reversible until proven otherwise. During acute renal failure, therapy is directed toward daily medical management of fluid-electrolyte and acid-base balance and toward minimizing protein catabolism. If the kidneys fail to recover within a few days and if response to conservative medical management is poor, dialysis may be instituted to control the effects of uremia.[3] The average length of renal "shutdown" in acute renal failure is 10 to 14 days. During the recovery phase, urinary volume may increase strikingly, and this may be associated with significant loss of sodium and potassium. Appropriate adjustments of intake of these solutes and water may have to be made at this time.

## Classifications of renal diseases

Renal diseases may be classified in several different ways. The most common classifications are based on both pathologic and physiologic findings. Initially the disease may involve primarily one segment of the kidney (such as glomeruli in glomerulonephritis) and may present with distinctive clinical and functional manifestations. If the disease progresses to cause advanced renal failure, however, these characteristic features may be obscured by the common features of uremia described above.

The kidneys may be involved primarily in diseases such as glomerulonephritis, pyelonephritis, or cystic diseases, or secondarily, usually as a result of vascular changes, in systemic diseases such as hypertension, diabetes, gout, or lupus erythematosus. The following discussion briefly describes salient features of some of the major disorders that might affect the kidneys.

### Glomerular diseases

A number of forms of glomerulonephritis (diseases involving primarily the glomeruli) account for half of the patients with renal failure and for two-thirds of the patients who are candidates for hemodialysis or transplantation. Since each glomerulus consists of highly specialized capillaries, glomerular disease can be regarded as a form of capillary disease. Inflammatory glomerular diseases are most commonly the result of antigen-antibody disorders. The principal clinical features that reflect glomerular injury include hematuria (presence of blood in the urine reflecting damage to the glomerular capillary wall) and proteinuria (presence of protein in the urine). Oliguria, azotemia, edema, and hypertension may also occur.

Glomerulonephritis can be subclassified as *acute* or *chronic*. Acute glomerulonephritis may be self-limited and resolve completely (as is often the case when associated with streptococcal pharyngitis in children) or may lead to chronic progressive destruction of renal function. In a small percentage of cases (less than 5%) the acute phase may be severe and may lead to rapid deterioration of renal function. This type is appropriately termed *rapidly progressive glomerulonephritis.*

In any of the types of glomerular injury, proteinuria may be significant, and this may lead to hypoalbuminemia, sodium retention, and generalized edema, the features of nephrotic syndrome. Hypoalbuminemia in nephrotic syndrome is often accompanied by elevation of cholesterol and blood lipids. In addition, sodium retention associated with glomerular injury may contribute to hypertension.

## Tubulo-interstitial nephritis

*Tubulo-interstitial nephritis* is the term used for a group of diseases that cause inflammation of the tubules and interstitial tissues in the kidney, usually sparing the glomeruli. They may present as acute or chronic processes and the former may progress to the latter. The inflammation may be due to an immune disorder, to an allergic-like reaction to drugs (particularly of the penicillin family), to toxins, or it may result from a systemic disease, such as gout. The most common cause in many Western countries is the chronic ingestion of phenacetin-aspirin–containing analgesics. In Australia this accounts for 20% of patients with end-stage renal disease. The severity of the disease relates to the cumulative dose ingested, and the renal deterioration may cease or reverse if the drug is discontinued.

## Pyelonephritis

Pyelonephritis is a form of tubulo-interstitial nephritis caused by bacterial infection. Bacterial infection of the bladder is called cystitis, and, in the great majority of cases, this type of infection remains confined to the bladder. In some cases, bacteria reach the kidneys through the ureters from the lower urinary tract, usually in association with some predisposing conditions, such as urinary obstruction from strictures or calculi (kidney stones) or reflux of urine from the bladder into the ureters. Paraplegics who require continuous indwelling catheters frequently develop chronic pyelonephritis. Diabetic patients with their increased susceptibility to urinary tract infections are also predisposed to developing pyelonephritis. The therapeutic management of pyelonephritis involves relief of obstruction, if that is a causative factor, and appropriate drug therapy. Patients are instructed to drink fluids generously and to void frequently. Patients suffering from recurrent episodes of acute pyelonephritis may gradually develop end-stage renal failure with severe hypertension.

## Polycystic kidney disease

Adult polycystic kidney disease is responsible for the renal failure of 5% to 7% of patients on dialysis or undergoing transplantation. It is transmitted as a mendelian dominant trait. Renal function is normal during the early decades of life, but progressive cyst formation results in renal failure by the fifth decade. The kidney in end-stage polycystic kidney disease is misshapen and enlarged, sometimes to the size of a football. The external surface is covered with numerous cysts, which, upon microscopic examination, appear to have compressed normal renal tissue. The renal failure that occurs in adult polycystic kidney disease is caused by this cyst expansion.

## Nephrosclerosis

The most common form of nephropathy is benign nephrosclerosis, which occurs in older patients. It is sometimes seen in younger age groups in association with hypertension and diabetes. It is the result of arteriosclerosis and mild to moderate hypertension of long standing. In general, these patients have lost an element of renal reserve and are prone to develop azotemia in the face of stress, such as gastrointestinal hemorrhage or surgery. Patients with severe prolonged benign nephrosclerosis can develop more profound renal functional changes, and when renal failure occurs, it is due to the development of an accelerated or malignant phase of hypertension.

# Dialysis and transplantation

The basic principle involved in dialysis is the diffusion of dissolved particles across a semipermeable membrane from one fluid compartment to another. Hemodialysis and peritoneal dialysis are the two types of dialysis in use. Hemodialysis involves circulating the patient's blood outside the body through a dialyzer with a semipermeable membrane separating the blood from dialysate fluid which has an electrolyte composition similar to normal serum. As the blood is pumped through the dialyzer, it is cleansed of waste products, electrolyte concentrations are restored to normal levels, and excess water is removed by processes of diffusion, osmosis, and ultrafiltration. This dialysis process is conducted for 4 to 6 hours, two to three times per week. It requires that a permanent access site into the patient's vascular system be surgically created in order to provide blood flow into the dialyzer. Hemodialysis is used extensively for long-term care of patients in renal failure. When performed in the hospital setting, hemodialysis costs approximately $25,000 per year. This procedure can be performed at about one-third to one-half the cost in the home if the patient has a willing dialysis partner.[4]

Peritoneal dialysis takes place in the patient's peritoneal cavity without the use of a dialyzer. The peritoneal membrane serves as the semipermeable membrane and a catheter is inserted into the abdomen for access. The dialysate is run into the patient's abdomen for a period of time and then drained. The removal of waste products takes place more slowly and more gently with this method. Numerous exchanges can be made in a 24-hour period. Great care must be taken to avoid infection, however. Peritoneal dialysis is used in acute renal failure in the hospital setting, but it is also being used increasingly for management of chronic renal failure in the non-hospitalized renal patient. When used in this manner, a permanent catheter is inserted. In some cases patients dialyze continuously using four to five exchanges per day. This process is called *continuous ambulatory peritoneal dialysis* (CAPD). The cost of chronic peritoneal dialysis is between $8000 and $10,000 per year.[5]

### Transplantation

Long-term dialysis therapy, although lifesaving for the patient in renal failure, is not a perfect substitute for actual kidney function. Transplantation of a kidney either from a live donor (parent or sibling) or from a cadaver is often preferable, particularly in the case of children. Renal transplantation is not without risks, however, because of the immunosuppressive therapy that accompanies the transplant in order to prevent the body from rejecting the new kidney. The immunosuppressive agents decrease resistance to infection and can cause side effects, such as hypertension, decreased glucose tolerance, obesity, and gastric ulcers. The possibility also exists that the transplanted kidney will not function well and that the patient will still have some degree of renal insufficiency. These patients and their families, as well as patients on long-term dialysis, need understanding and emotional support from all members of the health-care team.

### Diet therapy
### Principles of diet therapy

The basic objectives in the dietary treatment of renal disease are to lighten the excretory load of products of metabolism and to help the kidney maintain the normal equilibrium of the body's internal environment. At the point in progressive renal failure when clinical symptoms develop, diet modifications become an important aspect of treatment. Depending on the type and course of the kidney disease, progression of renal failure may even be delayed for a period of time by careful dietary measures.

The following discussion of the principles of diet therapy refers primarily to the metabolic problems of chronic and end-stage renal failure. However, many of the same principles apply in acute renal failure.

### Energy

All patients in renal failure, whether acute, chronic, or end stage, require an adequate caloric intake (approximately 35 kcal to 40 kcal per kilogram body weight for adults). Without adequate calories supplied by carbohydrate and fat, amino acids from food and body cells will be deaminized in intermediary metabolism to contribute to energy needs through the gluconeogenic pathway. This decreases the amount of protein available to compensate for the loss of protein in the urine (*e.g.*, proteinuria in nephrotic syndrome), or the catabolism of protein for energy increases the amount of nitrogen available for the synthesis of urea, thereby leading to an increase in the amount of urea to be excreted. Consideration of this critical relationship between energy and protein in intermediary metabolism is the first step in planning diet therapy for the patient with renal disease and is often not emphasized sufficiently. Kopple reported that approximately half of his patients had inadequate caloric intakes.[6]

Patients with chronic renal disease are not often obese. However, for those who are, a moderate restriction of caloric intake (1800 calories or less) may be prescribed. The energy intake of a child must be adequate to support normal growth as far as possible. Several studies have reported that growth failure in children with renal disease could be attributed in part to inadequate intakes of energy.[7,8]

### Protein

When symptoms of uremia occur or nitrogen retention is evident (BUN over 100 mg per deciliter) or both, protein in the diet is restricted to control the amount of nitrogen available for urea synthesis. At the same time the body's needs for essential amino acids must be met by proteins of high biologic value. Proteins of high biologic value have most of their nitrogen present in their essential amino acids; contain all the essential amino acids; and have a concentration of amino acids roughly proportional to Rose's minimum daily requirements (see Table 32-1). The foods that best satisfy these criteria are milk and eggs. Meats also satisfy these criteria except that they contain somewhat more nitrogen from nonessential amino acids than do milk and eggs.

The evidence that demonstrated the importance of restricting the intake to proteins of high biologic value in uremia was first published by Giordano in 1963.[9] He fed a group of uremic patients in Italy a diet adequate in energy, vitamins, and minerals with a mixture of synthetic essential amino acids as the sole source of nitrogen. The quantity of nitrogen was adequate to meet the needs of the patients. He reported that the patients came into positive nitrogen balance, their BUN levels decreased, and uremic symptoms such as nausea and vomiting decreased. He postulated that the nitrogen in the BUN was used for the synthesis of nonessential amino acids in the body.

In 1964, Giovannetti and Maggiore reported results similar to Giordano's when they used a mixture of the synthetic essential amino acids or two eggs (100 g) and an adequate energy intake from low-protein wheatstarch and cornstarch.[10]

In 1965, Shaw and his co-workers in England reported on their treatment of uremic patients using a modified Giovannetti diet.[11] Their diet, adequate in energy, minerals, and vitamins, contained 18 g to 20 g of protein, 12 g of which was supplied by the high biologic value protein in 50 g of egg (1 egg) and 200 ml of milk. These patients also experienced relief from uremic symptoms. Similar results with a modified Giovannetti diet were reported in the United States.[12] The diet contained 20 g of protein with 12 g to 13 g provided by 50 g of egg and 200 ml of milk. The remainder of the protein was obtained from low-protein cereals and vegetables and fruit. Wheatstarch, sugars, and fats were used to supply an adequate intake of energy.

Table 32-1 shows the essential amino acids in 200 ml of milk and 50 g of egg and in 100 g of egg compared with Rose's minimum requirements for the essential amino acids. Both the Giovannetti and the Shaw diets are in good agreement with Rose's figures with the exception of phenylalanine and methionine.

This low-protein regimen provided temporary relief of uremic symptoms. However, long-term use of a diet so low in protein may lead to progressive loss of weight and muscle mass. In addition, several complications of uremia may develop even though dietary management effectively controls the BUN level. Therefore, although protein restriction remains an important aspect of conservative management of renal failure, it is not always

clear at what point more aggressive treatment (dialysis or transplantation) should be instituted. Since clinical signs of uremic toxicity appear when the BUN level rises above 90 mg per 100 ml, nephrologists usually restrict dietary protein to prevent the BUN from reaching this level, preferring to keep it below 60 mg per 100 ml.

The amount of protein prescribed for the patient in chronic renal failure not on dialysis can be determined from the GFR. Restriction is rarely needed until the GFR is below 25 ml per minute. Below this level Kopple modifies the daily protein intake for a 70-kg man as follows: for a GFR of 20 ml to 25 ml per minute, a protein intake up to 90 g; for a GFR of 15 ml to 20 ml per minute, protein up to 70 g; and for a GFR of 10 ml to 15 ml per minute, protein up to 50 g. When the GFR is 4 ml to 10 ml per minute, a protein intake of 40 g (or 35 g for women and small men) is recommended. The 40 g protein level is based on a protein intake of 0.55 g to 0.60 g per kilogram body weight per day. A protein intake calculated to match a specific GFR usually maintains a patient in neutral or positive nitrogen balance provided the diet contains sufficient calories and 60% to 70% of the protein is of high biologic value. When the GFR drops below 4 ml to 5 ml per minute, diets providing less protein (16 g–20 g daily) and supplemented with essential amino acids or a mixture of essential amino acids and ketoacid analogs can be used. However, it has not been determined how favorably this regimen compares with regular dialysis therapy and higher protein intakes in keeping the patient in good nutritional status and free of uremic symptoms.[13]

Patients, particularly those who are anorectic, often find it difficult to consume low-protein diets because they are monotonous and unpalatable. For this reason nephrologists may prefer to initiate dialysis before the patient's GFR requires a protein intake below 40 g. It is thought that patients may commence long-term maintenance dialysis in better nutritional status before severe uremia and protein depletion develop.[14] If dialysis is not an option, the patient should be managed medically or

**Table 32-1. Comparison of Shaw and Giovannetti Diets with Rose's Proposed Minimum Requirements of Essential Amino Acids (Male)**

| Food | Weight (g) | Amino Acids (mg)* | | | | | | | | Protein (g) |
|------|------------|-------|------|------|------|------|------|------|------|---------|
| | | *Phe* | *Ile* | *Leu* | *Val* | *Met* | *Trp* | *The* | *Lys* | |
| Milk, whole† | 200 | 340 | 446 | 683 | 480 | 228 | 98 | 322 | 544 | 7 |
| Egg (1)† | 50 | 369 | 425 | 563 | 475 | 350 | 105 | 318 | 409 | 7 |
| Totals | | 709 | 871 | 1251 | 955 | 578 | 203 | 640 | 953 | 14 |
| Eggs (2)‡ | 100 | 739 | 850 | 1126 | 950 | 700 | 211 | 637 | 819 | 14 |
| Rose's Proposed Requirements§ | | 1110 | 700 | 1100 | 800 | 1100 | 250 | 500 | 800 | |

*See Table 3, Part 4.

†Shaw AB: QJ Med 34:237, 1965

‡Giovannetti S, Maggiore G: Lancet 1:100, 1964

§See Chapter 4.

conservatively by no less than 35 g to 40 g of protein per day as long as possible to prevent wasting. Good adherence to protein restriction during this period can enable the patient to lead a reasonably comfortable life with some relief from gastrointestinal symptoms.

Other measurements may be used to select optimal protein intake. It has been shown that the BUN to serum creatinine ratio correlates with protein intake in uremic patients.[15] As a result, the patient's serum creatinine level can be used to estimate the protein intake that maintains the BUN at the desired level. Calculation of urea nitrogen appearance is another method of determining recent protein intake in patients who are metabolically stable.[16] Sargent and Gotch calculated the net protein catabolic rate in both stable and unstable dialysis patients to estimate dietary protein intake and to determine clinically nitrogen balance.[17] These measurements allow the dietitian to direct the patient's protein intake into a range that will balance his protein catabolic rate (determined from the rate of urea generation). In the case of dialyzed patients, the length of dialysis therapy necessary to maintain the serum urea nitrogen within a certain range is then calculated by urea kinetic analysis, a calculation involving the patient's protein catabolic rate, remaining renal function, and size of dialyzer.[18]

Many studies have been conducted based on the Giordano-Giovannetti theory of using low-protein diets to control uremia symptoms. In one study Bergstrom and coworkers fed renal patients an unrestricted 20 g protein diet supplemented with essential amino acids. This diet offered patients greater variety in food selection and resulted in improved compliance. The patients were brought into positive nitrogen balance, kept free of uremic symptoms, and, in general, showed improved nutritional status.[19] Walser and his co-workers described feeding renal patients a low protein diet supplemented with the keto analogs of essential amino acids. It was believed that the analog could be transaminated by either ammonia derived from urea hydrolysis in the intestine or ammonia derived from urea precursors in the liver (glutamine and alanine). The study showed that the keto analogs reduced urea accumulation and deferred dialysis therapy for a period of time.[20] Although it has generally been accepted that keto acid analogs of some essential amino acids can be aminated *in vivo*, recent work has suggested that reutilizaton of urea nitrogen may not be the major mechanism of action of the keto acids.[21] Nevertheless, keto acid analogs and essential amino acid supplements are currently important means of investigating the role of diet therapy in the predialysis patient.[22,23]

During dialysis treatments, some amino acids, peptides, and small proteins pass into the dialysate and are thus removed from the body. It has been estimated that 6 g to 10 g of free amino acids are lost during a single hemodialysis, but there is apparently little protein loss in this type of dialysis. During peritoneal dialysis, however, there is little amino acid loss, but losses of 0.5 g to 2 g of protein per liter of dialysate have been reported. Total protein loss can run as high as 6 g to 12 g during each day of maintenance peritoneal dialysis. It is obvious that the protein allowance for the patient on maintenance dialysis must replace these losses to prevent wasting. The recommended daily protein intake for adult patients undergoing hemodialysis thrice weekly has been 1.0 g per kilogram body weight. Recently, however, this has been increased to 1.2 g of protein per kilogram of body weight. Patients on peritoneal dialysis may require 1.2 g to 1.5 g of protein per kilogram body weight daily because of greater nutrient losses into the dialysate. Individual protein requirements vary, depending on such factors as type of dialysis, length of dialysis treatments, and the nutritional status of the patient.[24-27]

### Sodium and fluid

People with normal kidney function can conserve or excrete sodium over a broad range. On a low-sodium intake the normal kidney conserves sodium, but if a diet contains 400 mEq of sodium, the normal kidney can excrete that amount easily. Patients with kidney disease, however, excrete or conserve sodium over a more restricted range. This range narrows as the GFR declines. The appropriate level of sodium intake for the patient with kidney disease depends, therefore, not only on the presence or absence of hypertension, heart failure, or edema, but also on the state of kidney function.

Some patients with interstitial nephritis or polycystic kidney disease may be renal "salt-losers" or "salt-wasters." These patients have little ability to conserve sodium. Dietary restriction of sodium in these patients leads to sodium depletion, a reduction in blood volume, and decreased glomerular filtration, which further aggravates the uremia. Anorexia, nausea, and even vomiting may develop, which inhibit sodium intake at the same time renal salt-wasting persists. Replacement of adequate amounts of sodium can break this depletion cycle.

In contrast, patients with chronic renal failure who are oliguric or anuric have limited ability to excrete a sodium load. When the GFR falls below 10 ml per minute in these patients, they retain sodium, become thirsty, and consequently consume and retain fluid. Sodium and water retention in these patients may then lead to edema, hypertension, and, eventually, congestive heart failure. Therefore, sodium and fluid are usually restricted in these patients.

In the nondialyzed uremic patient, fluid intake is usually maintained in a range of 1500 ml to 3000 ml per day. For the oliguric or anuric patient, however, fluid intake must be more restricted. For patients on maintenance hemodialysis who have some urine output, the fluid allotment is usually based on that output (determined from a 24-hour urine collection) plus an additional 500 cc to 600 cc for insensible loss. If sodium intake is controlled, the thirst mechanism may be an adequate indicator for fluid intake at a level to maintain water balance. If the patient consumes more fluid than the prescribed amount, and is retaining sodium, he may become edematous or hypertensive or both, as described above. Sodium excess and overhydration are partners in a pathologic sequence that causes an expanded vascular volume, hypertension, and eventual heart failure. Excessive sodium intake is indicated by rapid weight gain and a rise in blood pressure. Inadequate sodium ingestion, on the other hand, can lead to weight loss and a decrease in blood pressure. To determine if sodium and fluid intakes are appropriate, it is necessary to monitor body weight, serum sodium level, and blood pressure. Individual requirements vary greatly from one patient to another, however, and each patient should be evaluated separately as to the ability to handle sodium, using the blood pressure, weight, and degree of kidney function as guidelines.

### Phosphorus, calcium, and vitamin D

Impaired renal function is associated with metabolic and endocrine changes that affect mineralization of bone. Renal osteodystrophy (often called uremic bone disease) is a broad term that describes a number of skeletal syndromes resulting from the changes that occur in the metabolism of parathyroid hormone, calcium, phosphate, and vitamin D. The amount of phosphorus in the body is normally regulated through urinary excretion. Consequently, a fall in the GFR leads to phosphate retention (hyperphosphatemia), which in turn leads to low serum calcium levels since these two minerals share a reciprocal relationship in the blood. In an effort to raise the serum calcium level, parathyroid hormone (PTH) secretion rises, causing increased bone resorption and increased phosphorus excretion. When the GFR is less than 25 ml per minute, higher levels of PTH are no longer able to keep serum phosphorus and calcium levels normal. The renal patient remains hypocalcemic, the PTH remains elevated, and the patient is said to have hyperparathyroidism secondary to his renal disease.

Renal cells normally hydroxylate the inactive form of vitamin D, 25-OH-$D_3$, to its most potent form, 1,25-$(OH)_2D_3$. This metabolically active form of vitamin D enhances the intestinal absorption of calcium and under certain conditions, mobilizes calcium from bone.[28] Since the diseased kidney is unable to carry out this hydroxylation, patients develop a vitamin D resistant malabsorption of calcium recognized as a feature of chronic renal failure. Thus, uremic bone disease is the consequence of abnormal vitamin D metabolism and secondary hyperparathyroidism. To control the hyperphosphatemia, low phosphorus diets (800 mg–1200 mg per day) are prescribed, and phosphorus-binding antacids (aluminum carbonate and aluminum hydroxide) are consumed at mealtime by renal patients to sequester dietary phosphorus in the gastrointestinal tract and to prevent its absorption. It should be noted that it is difficult to develop low phosphorus diets for patients on dialysis who have relatively liberal protein intakes. Slatopolsky suggested that restricting dietary phosphorus and administering phosphate binders early in the course of renal insufficiency would prevent secondary hyperparathyroidism.[29] A recent study confirmed that early phosphorus restriction, calcium supplementation, and vitamin D administration are effective in preventing the development of both hyperparathyroidism and osteomalacia in patients with chronic renal failure.[30] Furthermore, there is clinical evidence that control of serum phosphate early in the course of chronic renal failure may greatly retard, and in some cases, halt progression of the disease.[31] Massry has shown that initiation of therapy with safe doses of 1,25-$(OH)_2D_3$ in patients with early to moderate renal failure may prevent the progression of renal osteodystrophy even if the patient's compliance with a phosphate-restricted diet is poor.[32]

There is evidence of an increased need for calcium in renal patients. Calcium balance studies have shown that calcium equilibrium was achieved in renal patients only when calcium intakes approached 1200 mg per day.[33] It is possible that the renal patient's requirement for calcium may be as high as 1.5 g to 2 g per day.[34] Unfortunately, the best sources of calcium in the diet—dairy foods—are high in phosphorus and potassium and, for this reason, are restricted. Since the calcium concentration in the dialysate has a major effect on the plasma calcium level, it can be manipulated to help maintain a normal plasma calcium level in dialysis patients.[35] Furthermore, if the renal patient is successful in keeping his serum phosphorus near normal with a phosphate-restricted diet and phosphorus binders, calcium supplementation (*e.g.*, calcium carbonate or lactate) can help prevent negative calcium balance. For patients with severe bone disease who do not respond well to calcium supplementation, the metabolically active form of vitamin $D_3$ may be prescribed.

### Potassium

Serum potassium levels are normally maintained in a narrow range, 3.5 mEq to 5 mEq per liter. Potassium values above (hyperkalemia) or below (hypokalemia) this range may be associated with cardiac and other systemic abnormalities. For much of the course of renal failure, plasma potassium remains normal or is only slightly elevated. In late renal failure, however, hyperkalemia becomes common. Hyperkalemia may develop without symptoms. Patients may experience some muscle weakness but in general may be unaware that they have dangerously elevated potassium levels until arrhythmias or cardiac arrest occurs. In late renal failure dangerous hyperkalemic peaks can result from acidemia, trauma, surgery, anesthesia, blood transfusions, or excessive dietary potassium intake. The usual adult intake of potassium is between 50 mEq and 150 mEq per day. Most patients in renal failure must restrict their potassium intake to 40 mEq to 70 mEq per day. This is difficult because eggs, milk, meats, and many fruits and vegetables contain large amounts of potassium. For patients who consistently have problems with hyperkalemia, even on potassium-restricted diet plans, an oral ion exchange resin (Kayexalate) can be prescribed. This material binds dietary potassium in the gastrointestinal tract in exchange for sodium and prevents its absorption. Its chronic use is discouraged because it leads to increased sodium absorption and decreases available calcium for absorption.

### Vitamins and minerals

Although there have been a number of studies of uremic patients in which blood levels of vitamins and minerals were measured, the dietary requirements for these nutrients in patients with renal failure have not been well defined. There is evidence that, in patients with renal disease, requirements for some nutrients may be different than in healthy persons because of the altered metabolism of the major nutrients, impaired mineral and vitamin metabolism, and vitamin losses that occur with dialysis treatments.[36,37]

The dietary restrictions imposed on patients with renal disease generally decrease the intake of water-soluble vitamins. In addition, since many of these compounds of relatively low molecular weight may not be protein bound in the aqueous phase of blood, dialysis treatments increase their loss. The metabolism of vitamin $B_6$ appears to be altered in renal failure, and the requirement for this vitamin may be increased.[38] Vitamin $B_6$ deficiency is of clinical importance to hemodialysis patients as a possible factor in their abnormal lipid metabolism. Data from one study suggest a beneficial effect of pyridoxine supplementation on high density lipoprotein levels in vitamin $B_6$-deficient dialysis patients.[39] Stone suggested 5 mg of pyridoxine daily for renal patients not on drugs, which would increase their $B_6$ requirements. Folate, being dialyzable, is usually supplemented at the level of 1 mg daily.[40] Thiamin and riboflavin are also dialyzable and are usually supplemented at the level of one U.S. RDA. Kopple recommended 100 mg per day of highly dialyzable vitamin C.[24]

Supplements of vitamin A should not be given as serum levels of this vitamin are frequently elevated in uremia.[41] Supplements of vitamins E and K need not be given generally. However, patients receiving antibiotics that suppress the intestinal flora may need vitamin K.[6]

Renal diets may be deficient in iron depending on their protein content. Furthermore, iron may not be absorbed normally from the intestine in renal patients.

These factors, in addition to there being less erythropoietin synthesized by the diseased kidney and frequent blood sampling, all contribute to the normochromic, normocytic anemia developed by such patients. Iron supplementation in the form of ferrous sulfate is routinely prescribed.

In general, most patients in renal failure receive supplements of iron, calcium, ascorbic acid, folic acid, and the remaining B vitamins. Table 32-2 summarizes the recommended dietary intakes for uremic patients on dialysis or for those being managed conservatively without dialysis.

### Hypertriglyceridemia in patients with renal failure

Approximately 40% to 60% of both dialyzed and undialyzed patients with chronic renal failure have elevated serum triglyceride levels (hypertriglyceridemia) due to abnormal fat metabolism.[42] These patients exhibit decreased efficiency in triglyceride removal from plasma. Since hypertriglyceridemia may contribute to the accelerated atherosclerosis associated with chronic renal failure, efforts have been directed to reducing this risk with dietary modifications. One study has shown that decreasing the dietary carbohydrate intake by 15% led to a significant fall in plasma triglyceride concentration.[43] Other studies have shown that, by restricting carbohydrate consumption and increasing polyunsaturated fat consumption, serum triglyceride levels may be significantly decreased in dialysis patients.[44,45] Such diet modifications pose a problem with an already complex renal diet. Saturated fats and simple sugars must be limited. These foods have traditionally been used as major energy sources in a diet that tends to be low in calories. However, use of polyunsaturated margarines, lean meats, and such complex carbohydrate foods as breads and cereals, at least for dialysis patients, are effective measures that can help control serum triglyceride levels without eliminating essential food groups.

### Diet therapy in acute renal failure

The preferred treatment of acute renal failure is early and frequent dialysis, either peritoneal or hemodialysis. With frequent dialysis, salt and water need not be severely restricted, and a good caloric intake (minimum of 1500 calories in an adult) and a moderate amount of protein (40 g–60 g) may be permitted.[46]

If dialysis is not available, water, sodium, and potassium must be strictly controlled to keep chemical and volume abnormalities of body fluids minimal. In a patient who is not dialyzed the amount of fluid usually allowed is 400 ml to 500 ml per day to replace insensible losses. Excess fluid in a patient with acute renal failure could cause hyponatremia and congestive heart failure and pulmonary edema.

If the patient is able to ingest food without being nauseated, Bricker recommends an intake of approx-

**Table 32-2.  Recommended Dietary Intakes for Uremic Patients Undergoing and Not Undergoing Maintanance Dialysis**

| Component | No Dialysis* | Hemodialysis (HD) or Peritoneal Dialysis (PD) |
|---|---|---|
| Protein | Men: ≥40 gm/day (0.55–0.60 gm/kg/day) (28 gm of high biologic value)<br><br>Women, small men: ≥35 gm/day (23–25 gm of high biologic value) | HD: 1.0 gm/kg/day<br>PD: 1.2–1.5 gm/kg/day<br>(>50% of high biologic value) |
| Calories | ≥ 35 kcal/kg/day unless patient is obese | |
| Vitamins | (Quantities to be Supplemented) | |
| Thiamine (mg/day) | 1.5 | 1.5 |
| Riboflavin (mg/day) | 1.8 | 1.8 |
| Pantothenic acid (mg/day) | 5 | 5 |
| Niacin (mg/day) | 20 | 20 |
| Pyridoxine hydrochloride (mg/day) | 5 | 10 |
| Vitamin B$_{12}$ (μg/day) | 3 | 3 |
| Vitamin C (mg/day) | 70–100 | 100 |
| Folic acid (mg/day) | 1 | 1 |
| Vitamin A | None | None |
| Vitamin D | Not established | Not established |
| Vitamin E (IU/day) | 15 | 15 |
| Vitamin K | None† | None† |
| Minerals | (Range of Total Intake) | |
| Sodium (mg/day) | 1000–3000 | 750–1000 |
| Potassium (mEq/day) | 40–70 | 40–70 |
| Phosphorus (mg/day)‡ | 600–1200 | 600–1200 |
| Calcium (mg/day) | 1000–2000§ | 1000–1500§ |
| Magnesium (mg/day) | 200–300 | 200–300 |
| Trace elements | Unknown | Unknown |
| Water | Up to 3000 ml/day as tolerated | Usually 750–1500 ml/day |

*Glomerular filtration rate >4–5 ml/min but <15–25 ml/min.

†May be needed in patients receiving antibiotics.

‡Phosphate binders (aluminum carbonate, aluminum hydroxide) usually needed as well.

§Dietary intake usually must be supplemented to provide these levels.

(Kopple JD: Postgrad Med 64:135, 1978)

imately 2000 calories essentially free of potassium, protein, and sodium to minimize catabolism.[47] Some clinicians, however, favor 20 g to 30 g of protein in addition, to meet minimal essential amino acid requirements. If parenteral alimentation is necessary, a minimum of 250 g of glucose and vitamins and minerals are administered daily; essential amino acids or their keto analogs and fat emulsions can be infused to help meet caloric and nutritional requirements. The glucose is usually prepared in a concentrated solution because of the fluid restriction. Caution is necessary to prevent venous thrombosis or infection with this method of feeding.

The patient in acute renal failure should be closely monitored to prevent development of hyperkalemia. Adequate caloric intake helps by preventing catabolism, promoting glycogen deposition, and aids in preventing acidemia. A potassium-binding resin, Kayexalate, may be administered by mouth or by enema when the serum potassium level is between 5.5 mEq and 6.5 mEq per liter. If the serum potassium level is dangerously high (over 6.5 mEq per liter) emergency measures are employed, but the potassium exchange resin and dialysis are usually also initiated to prevent recurrence.

During the early part of the recovery phase of acute renal failure (characterized by diuresis), careful monitoring of fluid and electrolyte balance is essential. Adjustments in fluid and electrolytes may have to be made as frequently as every hour.

**Diet therapy in nephrotic syndrome**

There is a lack of agreement concerning the appropriate treatment with diet therapy for nephrotic syndrome. High-calorie, high-protein diets have been traditionally used to raise blood protein levels.[48] A minimum of 1.5 g of protein per kilogram of body weight daily is recommended unless the glomerular filtration rate is less than 20 ml per minute. Some investigators state, however, that there is no way of increasing plasma albumin while protein losses continue, even though the cause of the edema is the low serum albumin concentration.[46] High protein diets occasionally bring about a marginal increase in plasma albumin levels, but often they simply increase urinary protein loss. Administration of intravenous protein produces only a transitory effect and is impractical for long-term treatment. Current treatment consists of judicious use of diuretics, starting with relatively gentle agents and progressing to more powerful diuretics if initial treatment fails to produce diuresis. Severe sodium restriction combined with diuretics hastens the disappearance of edema but is not often prescribed because a diet severely restricted in sodium is unpalatable. In general, nephrotic patients are encouraged to ingest a high-calorie, relatively high-protein diet, and, since nephrotic syndrome is usually a chronic state, they are encouraged to follow normal routines as much as possible. Guides to assessing the progress of the nephrotic patient include the presence or absence of edema, body weight, 24-hour urinary protein excretion, and serum albumin concentration. Dietetic therapy must be adjusted as these values are monitored.

## Planning the protein, phosphorus, sodium, and potassium-restricted diet for patients with chronic renal failure

A diet restricted in protein, phosphorus, sodium, and potassium may be used to treat moderate renal failure or to relieve the symptoms of uremia in end-stage renal disease before dialysis is started. It is one of the most complex therapeutic diets with which both the patient and the clinical dietitian must cope. With hemodialysis or continuous peritoneal dialysis the restrictions are lightened to some extent.

### Special problems in food composition
Phosphorus and protein

The first alteration in diet for the patient with renal failure should be the reduction of phosphorus intake. This restriction should occur early in the course of renal disease, often before there is a need for protein restriction. To achieve this, the intake of dairy products, meats, and milk, which are major sources of phosphorus in the diet, must be limited.

As discussed earlier, protein foods of high biologic value are emphasized on low-protein diets. The protein in cheese is of high biologic value, but cheese is usually not

### Table 32-3. Vegetables Grouped by Their Protein Content (Serving Size = ½ c)

| *1 g* | *2 g* | *3–4 g* |
|---|---|---|
| Beans, green or wax | Cauliflower | Asparagus |
| Beets | Mushrooms | Broccoli |
| Cabbage | Okra | Brussels sprouts |
| Carrots | Potato, white or sweet | Corn |
| Cucumbers | Spinach | Mixed vegetables |
| Eggplant | Squash, winter | Peas |
| Endive | | |
| Green peppers | | |
| Lettuce | | |
| Radishes | | |
| Squash, summer | | |
| Romaine | | |
| Rutabagas | | |
| Tomatoes | | |

### Table 32-4. Comparison of Low-Protein Bread and Regular White Bread

| | *Low Protein (½ in slice)\** <br> 32 g/slice | *Regular (½ in slice)* <br> 23 g/slice |
|---|---|---|
| Calories | 78 | 73 |
| Protein, g | 0.3 | 2 |
| Sodium, mg | 10 | 150 |
| Phosphorus, mg | 0 | 24 |
| Potassium, mg | 8 | 30 |

*Values for dp Low Protein Bread, Henkel Dietary Specialties, Minneapolis

included in the renal diet because of its high sodium and phosphorus contents. Grains and vegetables are used sparingly or not at all on the very low protein diets (20 g or 30 g protein), because their protein is of low biologic value. Table 32-3 groups vegetables by their protein content for ½-c servings. Vegetables in the 3 g to 4 g protein group should be eliminated on very low protein diets or used in very small amounts.

On 20- to 40-g protein diets it is necessary to use a bread made from deglutinized wheat flour since gluten in wheat is the source of low biologic value protein. Table 32-4 compares one slice of low-protein bread and one slice of regular white bread. The amount of protein in regular bread can represent a substantial amount of low-quality protein at the 40 g level if three slices are consumed daily with other starches that contribute additional low-quality protein.

Table 32-5 summarizes an Exchange System for calculating protein, sodium, phosphorus, and potassium-restricted diets. Energy values are not indicated because they vary widely within an exchange. It should be noted that ½ c or 4 oz of milk in renal diet therapy is considered one serving, not 8 oz. Even though it contains high biologic value protein, milk is used sparingly on all renal diets, because it is fluid and contains significant potassium and phosphate. Table 32-6 illustrates 20-, 30-, 40-, and 60-g protein diet plans using the protein exchange values for each food category listed in Table 32-5.

Dried beans, dried peas, and legumes are normally considered good sources of protein if they are supplemented with a complementary vegetable protein or an animal protein to ensure inclusion of all essential amino acids. These foods should be avoided on renal diets, however, because they contain large amounts of potassium.

### Table 32-5. Exchange System for Calculating Protein-, Sodium-, Phosphorus-, and Potassium-Restricted Diets

| Food Exchanges | Household Measure | Grams | Protein (g) | Sodium (mg) | Phosphorus (mg) | Potassium (mg) |
|---|---|---|---|---|---|---|
| Milk | ½ c | 120 | 4 | 60 | 100 | 175 |
| Meat | 1 oz | 30 | 7 | 25 | 75 | 90 |
| Egg, large | 1 | 57 | 7 | 60 | 100 | 65 |
| Bread | | | | | | |
| Regular | 1 serving | Varies | 2 | 150 | 40 | 40 |
| Low protein | 1 serving | 32 | 0.3 | 10 | 0 | 8 |
| Vegetables | | | | | | |
| Group I | ½ c | Varies | Varies | 7 | 25 | 100 |
| Group II | ½ c | Varies | Varies | 20 | 35 | 175 |
| Group III | ½ c | Varies | Varies | 20 | 40 | 280 |
| Fruit | | | | | | |
| Group I | ½ c | Varies | 0.5 | 2 | 15 | 85 |
| Group II | ½ c | Varies | 0.5 | 2 | 15 | 170 |
| Group III | ½ c | Varies | 1.0 | 5 | 25 | 300 |
| Fat, salted | 1 tsp | 5 | 0 | 50 | 1 | 0 |

### Table 32-6. Sample Diet Plans for 20-, 30-, 40-, or 60-g Protein Diets

| Foods | 20 g | | 30 g | | 40 g | | 60 g | |
|---|---|---|---|---|---|---|---|---|
| Milk | ½ c | (4) | ½ c | (4) | ½ c | (4) | ½ c | (4) |
| Vegetables | | | | | | | | |
| 1 g group | 2 servings | (2) | 2 servings | (2) | 2 servings | (2) | 2 servings | (2) |
| 2 g group | | | 1 serving | (2) | 1 serving | (2) | 1 serving | (2) |
| Fruits | 3 servings | (1.5) | 3 servings | (1.5) | 3 servings | (1.5) | 4 servings | (2) |
| Starches | 2 servings | (4) | 3 servings | (6) | 4 servings | (8) | 7 servings | (14) |
| Low-protein bread | 3 or more servings | (1) | 3 or more servings | (1) | 3 or more servings | (1) | | |
| Meat | | | 1 serving* | (7) | 2 servings* | (14) | 4 servings* | (28) |
| Egg, large | 1 serving | (7) | 1 serving | (7) | 1 serving | (7) | 1 serving | (7) |
| Fats | As desired | | As desired | | As desired | | As desired | |
| Miscellaneous | Selective | | Selective | | Selective | | Selective | |
| Total Protein | | 20 g | | 31 g | | 40 g | | 59 g |

*1 Serving of a meat exchange = 1 oz.

## Low protein products

To meet the recommended caloric intake of 35 kcal to 40 kcal per kilogram of body weight, carbohydrates and polyunsaturated fats should be provided in liberal amounts since their metabolic products, carbon dioxide and water, are not toxic. A patient on a low-protein diet should be encouraged to use ample amounts of simple carbohydrates, such as sugar, marmalade, jams, jellies, syrups, and honey, to increase caloric intake. Low-protein bread can serve as a carrier for generous amounts of polyunsaturated margarine and jams, jellies, or honey. Other sweets that are frequently used to increase calories because they contain no protein and are low in electrolytes include hard candies, sour balls, jelly beans, gum drops, ice pops, and fruit ices. The *Miscellaneous* category in the Exchange Lists, Table 32-7, contains a number of foods that can add calories; however, some of the foods in this list may be limited due to their electrolyte contents.

The *Miscellaneous* List, Table 32-7, includes a number of specially prepared, renal supplements that are high in calories, low in electrolytes, and protein-free. These may come in liquid or powder form, and include Controlyte* (a hydrolysate of cornstarch and vegetable oil), Hycal[†] (a deionized liquid glucose polymer), Cal Power[‡] (a deionized liquid glucose), Polycose[§] (a glucose polymer), and Lipomul-Oral[‖] (a corn oil emulsion). These supplements may be used in food preparation, as syrups, or in sauces, desserts, or beverages. In addition to low-protein bread (or low-protein bread mix), other high-calorie commercial products include low-protein baking mixes and wheat starches.[‡] These products can be used to make bread, biscuits, cookies, muffins, and pie crusts. Low-protein rusk, porridge, and imitation pasta products are produced in Italy and marketed in the United States under the name Aproten.[‡] These products are relatively expensive and are well accepted by patients. The structure, texture, and flavor of bread made from wheatstarch differ from bread made from regular flour. Some patients consider low-protein bread unpalatable. Toasting the bread and using liberal amounts of margarine and jelly with it make it more acceptable. Pies and cookies made from wheatstarch are well accepted. The companies that manufacture these special products provide recipes for their use. Another high-calorie supplement designed for use in renal failure is Amin-Aid.[¶] One packet of this supplement contains 6.6 g of essential amino acids, histidine, and approximately 700 kilocalories.

---

* Doyle Pharmaceutical Co., Minneapolis, Minn. 55416
[†] Beecham-Massengill Pharmaceuticals
[‡] Henkel Corporation, Minneapolis, Minn. 55423
[§] Ross Laboratories, Columbus, OH 43216
[‖] Upjohn Co., Kalamazoo, MI
[¶] McGaw Laboratories, Glendale, CA

## Potassium in food

Potassium is found in the cells of all living tissues and is, therefore, widely distributed in all foods with the exception of refined sugars and pure fats and oils. The average adult potassium intake varies from 50 mEq to 150 mEq daily. In advanced renal failure dietary potassium may be restricted to 40 mEq to 60 mEq per day. Since relatively large amounts of potassium are found in fruits, meats, milk, and vegetables, it is not difficult to restrict potassium in a diet if the protein level of that diet is low, but it becomes increasingly difficult to maintain the potassium level below 50 mEq when the diet contains ample protein, for example, in the case of diets for patients on maintenance hemodialysis.

The degree to which a food is processed affects its potassium content. Highly refined foods, such as white bread, rice, noodles, macaroni, spaghetti, and certain cereals, such as farina or Cream of Wheat, contain little potassium. Foods made from whole grains, however, have a much higher potassium content. For example, whole-wheat bread contains two to three times more potassium than white bread (see the *Bread, Cereal, Starch Exchanges*, Table 32-7). Brown sugar contains considerable potassium, while white sugar contains none (see *Sweets and Desserts* under *Miscellanous*, Table 32-7).

Fruits have a low-protein content but a relatively high fluid and potassium content. They make a menu appealing, however, so they must be carefully selected, the portion size must be controlled, and their method of preparation considered. Fresh fruits, especially those eaten with the peel or skin, contain the greatest amount of potassium. In canned fruits much of the potassium has shifted into the syrup during the canning process. For this reason, canned fruits should be drained when served to renal patients. Canned fruits are preferable to fresh fruits, not only because of their lower potassium content, but because of their higher caloric content due to added sugar. Renal patients should consume fruits packed in heavy syrup instead of those packed in juice or water. Whipped cream or nondairy products like Cool-Whip served on canned fruits also add calories and are low in electrolytes (see *Nondairy Products* in *Miscellaneous*, Table 32-7).

Certain vegetables are very high in potassium (see *Group III Vegetables* in Table 32-7). For example, 1 c of homefried potatoes contains approximately 33 mEq of potassium. To appreciate this potassium content, it should be remembered that some renal patients are restricted to 40 mEq of potassium for the entire day. However, if the potatoes are not fried but prepared by peeling and cutting them into thin slices, soaking them in a large quantity of water for several hours, discarding this water and then cooking them in fresh water, much of the potassium can be eliminated. In general, renal patients should be advised to consume cooked rather than fresh

## Table 32-7.  Protein, Phosphorus, Sodium, and Potassium Exchange Lists

*Dairy Exchanges* *

One serving contains 4 g protein, 100 mg phosphorus, 60 mg sodium, and 175 mg potassium.

| Item | G | Amount | Calories | Protein (g) | P (mg) | Na (mg) | K (mg) |
|---|---|---|---|---|---|---|---|
| Cream, half and half | 120 | ½ c | 161 | 3.8 | 102 | 55 | 154 |
| Cream, heavy | 120 | ½ c | 419 | 2.6 | 70 | 38 | 106 |
| Cream, light | 120 | ½ c | 253 | 3.6 | 96 | 52 | 147 |
| Ice cream (10% fat) | 67 | ½ c | 129 | 3.0 | 77 | 42 | 120 |
| Milk | | | | | | | |
|   Condensed | 77 | ¼ c | 245 | 6.2 | 105 | 86 | 240 |
|   Evaporated | 63 | ¼ c | 86 | 4.4 | 130 | 75 | 191 |
|   Whole, fresh | 120 | ½ c | 80 | 4.2 | 114 | 61 | 176 |
|   Low fat (2%) | 120 | ½ c | 68 | 4.3 | 117 | 63 | 178 |
|   Skim | 120 | ½ c | 44 | 4.4 | 117 | 64 | 178 |
| Yogurt, made from partially skimmed milk | 120 | ½ c | 62 | 4.2 | 115 | 63 | 175 |

*Meat Exchanges*

One serving contains 7 g protein, 75 mg phosphorus, 25 mg sodium, and 90 mg potassium.

| Item | G | Amount | Calories | Protein (g) | P (mg) | Na* (mg) | K (mg) |
|---|---|---|---|---|---|---|---|
| Beef, rump roast, 75% lean | 28 | 1 oz | 98 | 6.7 | 55 | 16 | 75 |
| Beef pattie, 90% lean | 28 | 1 oz | 62 | 7.7 | 65 | 19 | 81 |
| Chicken | | | | | | | |
|   Light meat, without skin | 28 | 1 oz | 52 | 9.1 | 77 | 19 | 120 |
|   Dark meat, without skin | 28 | 1 oz | 52 | 8.3 | 67 | 25 | 94 |
| Lamb, 83% lean | 28 | 1 oz | 79 | 7.0 | 59 | 18 | 80 |
| Organ meats | | | | | | | |
|   Beef heart | 28 | 1 oz | 53 | 8.9 | 51 | 29 | 66 |
|   Gizzard, chicken | 28 | 1 oz | 42 | 7.6 | 20 | 16 | 60 |
|   Tongue, beef | 28 | 1 oz | 69 | 6.1 | 33 | 17 | 47 |
|   Liver | | | | | | | |
|     Beef | 28 | 1 oz | 65 | 7.4 | 135 | 52 | 108 |
|     Calf | 28 | 1 oz | 74 | 8.3 | 152 | 33 | 128 |
|     Chicken | 28 | 1 oz | 47 | 7.5 | 45 | 17 | 43 |
| Peanut butter | 32 | 2 tbsp | 188 | 8.0 | 122 | 194 | 200 |
| Pork, 80% lean | 28 | 1 oz | 103 | 6.9 | 73 | 17 | 78 |
| Seafood | | | | | | | |
|   Flounder, baked | 28 | 1 oz | 57 | 8.5 | 98 | 67 | 166 |
|   Haddock, fried | 28 | 1 oz | 47 | 5.6 | 70 | 50 | 99 |
|   Halibut, broiled | 28 | 1 oz | 48 | 7.1 | 70 | 38 | 149 |
|   Lobster, northern | 28 | 1 oz | 27 | 5.3 | 54 | 60 | 51 |
|   Salmon, broiled or baked | 28 | 1 oz | 52 | 7.7 | 117 | 33 | 126 |
|   Shrimp, French fried | 28 | 1 oz | 64 | 5.8 | 54 | 53 | 65 |
|   Tuna, canned, in water | | | | | | | |
|     Without salt | 28 | 1 oz | 36 | 7.9 | 54 | 12 | 79 |
|     With salt | 28 | 1 oz | 36 | 7.9 | 54 | 212 | 79 |
|   Tuna, canned, in oil | | | | | | | |
|     With salt | 28 | 1 oz | 82 | 7.8 | 84 | 227 | 85 |
| Turkey, without skin | 28 | 1 oz | 54 | 8.9 | 71 | 37 | 104 |
| Veal, rump roast | 28 | 1 oz | 66 | 7.6 | 65 | 18 | 86 |
| Additional Values for Substitutions | | | | | | | |
|   Egg | 57 | 1 large | 82 | 6.5 | 103 | 61 | 65 |
|   Cottage cheese | 56 | ¼ c | 58 | 7.6 | 85 | 128 | 48 |

*This figure represents the average for meats cooked without salt.

(Continued)

## Table 32-7.  Protein, Phosphorus, Sodium, and Potassium Exchange Lists (Continued)

*Bread Exchanges*
One serving contains 2 g protein, 40 mg phosphorus, variable sodium, and 40 mg potassium.

| Item | G | Amount | Calories | Protein (g) | P (mg) | Na (mg) | K (mg) |
|---|---|---|---|---|---|---|---|
| Breads | | | | | | | |
| Biscuit, baking powder | 35 | 1 (2″ diam) | 129 | 2.6 | 61 | 219 | 41 |
| Bread | | | | | | | |
| White, regular | 25 | 1 slice | 68 | 2.2 | 24 | 127 | 26 |
| White, without salt | 25 | 1 slice | 68 | 2.2 | 24 | 5 | 26 |
| Whole wheat | 28 | 1 slice | 67 | 2.6 | 71 | 148 | 72 |
| Rye, American | 25 | 1 slice | 61 | 2.3 | 37 | 139 | 36 |
| Doughnut, cake type, plain | 25 | 1 small | 98 | 1.2 | 48 | 125 | 23 |
| Doughnut, yeast | 42 | 1 | 176 | 2.7 | 32 | 99 | 34 |
| Graham crackers | 14 | 2 (2½″ squares) | 55 | 1.1 | 21 | 95 | 55 |
| Hamburger or frankfurter bun | 40 | 1 | 119 | 3.3 | 34 | 202 | 38 |
| Muffin, plain | 40 | 1 (3″ diam) | 118 | 3.1 | 60 | 176 | 50 |
| Muffin, blueberry | 40 | 1 (3″ diam) | 112 | 2.9 | 53 | 253 | 46 |
| Pancake | 27 | 1 (4″ diam) | 61 | 1.9 | 70 | 152 | 42 |
| Saltines, unsalted tops | 14 | 5 | 62 | 1.3 | 13 | 5 | 17 |
| Cooked cereals | | | | | | | |
| Cream of rice, slow cooking | | | | | | | |
| With salt | 120 | ½ c | 62 | 1.0 | 16 | 216 | |
| Without salt | 120 | ½ c | 62 | 1.0 | 16 | 1 | |
| Cream of Wheat, slow cooking | | | | | | | |
| With salt | 120 | ½ c | 52 | 1.6 | 15 | 177 | 11 |
| Without salt | 120 | ½ c | 52 | 1.6 | 15 | 1 | 11 |
| Oatmeal, slow cooking, | | | | | | | |
| With salt | 120 | ½ c | 66 | 2.4 | 69 | 262 | 73 |
| Without salt | 120 | ½ c | 66 | 2.4 | 69 | 2 | 73 |
| Whole wheat, slow cooking | | | | | | | |
| With salt | 120 | ½ c | 55 | 2.2 | 64 | 260 | 59 |
| Without salt | 120 | ½ c | 55 | 2.2 | 64 | 2 | 59 |
| Dry cereals | | | | | | | |
| Cornflakes | 18 | ¾ c | 72 | 1.5 | 7 | 188 | 23 |
| Frosted Flakes | 30 | ¾ c | 115 | 1.4 | 8 | 200 | 21 |
| Frosted Mini-wheats | 30 | 4 biscuits | 105 | 2.6 | 97 | 5 | 55 |
| Puffed Rice | 11 | ¾ c | 45 | 0.7 | 11 | | 11 |
| Puffed Wheat | 11 | ¾ c | 40 | 1.7 | 36 | 1 | 38 |
| Raisin Bran | 38 | ¾ c | 108 | 3.2 | 110 | 160 | 116 |
| Rice Krispies | 23 | ¾ c | 88 | 1.4 | 21 | 212 | 22 |
| Shredded Wheat | 25 | 1 biscuit | 89 | 2.5 | 97 | 1 | 87 |
| Starches | | | | | | | |
| Enriched macaroni, cooked without salt | 70 | ½ c | 78 | 2.4 | 35 | 1 | 43 |
| Enriched noodles, cooked without salt | 80 | ½ c | 100 | 3.3 | 47 | 2 | 35 |
| Enriched rice, cooked | | | | | | | |
| With salt | 102 | ½ c | 112 | 2.0 | 29 | 384 | 29 |
| Without salt | 102 | ½ c | 112 | 2.0 | 29 | 1 | 29 |
| Enriched spaghetti, cooked without salt | 70 | ½ c | 78 | 2.4 | 35 | 1 | 43 |
| Popcorn, popped plain, large kernel | 6 | 1 c | 23 | 0.8 | 17 | | 30 |

*Vegetable Exchanges, Group I*
One serving contains variable protein, 25 mg phosphorus, 5 mg sodium, and 100 mg potassium.

| Item | G | Amount | Calories | Protein (g) | P (mg) | Na* (mg) | K (mg) |
|---|---|---|---|---|---|---|---|
| Asparagus, fresh, cooked, cut | 73 | ½ c | 15 | 1.6 | 73 | 1 | 133 |
| Beans, green or wax, fresh, cooked, cut | 63 | ½ c | 15 | 1.0 | 23 | 3 | 95 |

## Table 32-7. Protein, Phosphorus, Sodium, and Potassium Exchange Lists (Continued)

*Vegetable Exchanges, Group I (Continued)*
One serving contains variable protein, 25 mg phosphorus, 5 mg sodium, and 100 mg potassium.

| Item | G | Amount | Calories | Protein (g) | P (mg) | Na* (mg) | K (mg) |
|---|---|---|---|---|---|---|---|
| Beans, green or wax, canned, drained, cut | | | | | | | |
|   Regular | 68 | ½ c | 16 | 1.0 | 17 | 160 | 64 |
|   Special diet pack | 68 | ½ c | 16 | 1.0 | 17 | 2 | 64 |
| Beans, green or wax, frozen, cooked, cut | 68 | ½ c | 18 | 1.2 | 22 | 1 | 106 |
| Bean sprouts, mung, fresh | 53 | ½ c | 19 | 2.0 | 34 | 3 | 117 |
| Cabbage, raw, coarsely shredded | 35 | ½ c | 9 | 0.5 | 10 | 7 | 82 |
| Cabbage, cooked, shredded | 73 | ½ c | 15 | 0.8 | 15 | 10 | 118 |
| Cabbage, Chinese, 1″ pieces | 38 | ½ c | 6 | 0.5 | 15 | 9 | 95 |
| Carrots, raw, 1 oz | 28 | 6–8 strips | 12 | 0.3 | 5 | 13 | 97 |
| Carrots, canned, sliced, drained | | | | | | | |
|   Regular | 78 | ½ c | 24 | 0.6 | 17 | 183 | 93 |
|   Special diet pack | 78 | ½ c | 24 | 0.6 | 17 | 30 | 93 |
| Cauliflower, fresh, cooked | 63 | ½ c | 14 | 1.5 | 27 | 6 | 129 |
| Celery, pascal, fresh, 1 oz | 28 | 6–8 strips | 5 | 0.3 | 4 | 36 | 97 |
| Corn, fresh, cooked | 83 | ½ c | 69 | 2.7 | 74 | | 136 |
| Corn, canned, drained | | | | | | | |
|   Regular | 83 | ½ c | 70 | 2.2 | 41 | 195 | 80 |
|   Special diet pack | 83 | ½ c | 70 | 2.2 | 41 | 2 | 80 |
| Cucumber, fresh, pared, sliced | 70 | ½ c | 10 | 0.4 | 13 | 4 | 112 |
| Endive, fresh, cut in small pieces | 50 | ½ c | 5 | 0.5 | 14 | 4 | 74 |
| Lettuce, fresh, cut in chunks | 38 | ½ c | 5 | 0.4 | 9 | 4 | 66 |
| Onions, green, raw | 30 | 2 medium or 6 small | 14 | 0.3 | 12 | 2 | 69 |
| Onions, mature, dry, chopped | 85 | ½ c | 33 | 1.3 | 31 | 9 | 134 |
| Onions, cooked, drained | 105 | ½ c | 31 | 1.3 | 31 | 8 | 115 |
| Parsley, raw | 10 | 10 sprigs (2½″ long) | 4 | 0.2 | 6 | 3 | 37 |
| Peas, canned, drained | | | | | | | |
|   Regular | 85 | ½ c | 68 | 3.9 | 65 | 200 | 82 |
|   Special diet pack | 85 | ½ c | 68 | 3.9 | 65 | 3 | 82 |
| Peas, frozen, cooked | 80 | ½ c | 55 | 4.1 | 69 | 92 | 108 |
| Potato, leached, boiled | 100 | ½ c | 70 | 2.0 | 33 | 2 | 120 |
| Peppers, green, raw, cut into strips | 50 | ½ c | 11 | 0.6 | 11 | 7 | 107 |
| Radishes, raw | 25 | 5 medium | 4 | 0.3 | 7 | 4 | 73 |
| Squash, summer, yellow and zucchini, cooked, sliced, drained | 90 | ½ c | 21 | 2.7 | 23 | 1 | 127 |

*Values for vegetables canned with salt were excluded from calculation of this average.

*Vegetable Exchanges, Group II*
One serving contains variable protein, 35 mg phosphorus, 20 mg sodium, and 170 mg potassium.

| Item | G | Amount | Calories | Protein (g) | P (mg) | Na* (mg) | K (mg) |
|---|---|---|---|---|---|---|---|
| Asparagus, canned, cut | | | | | | | |
|   Regular | 117 | ½ c | 26 | 2.0 | 63 | 277 | 165 |
|   Dietary pack | 117 | ½ c | 26 | 2.0 | 63 | 5 | 165 |
| Asparagus, frozen, cooked, cut | 90 | ½ c | 20 | 2.9 | 58 | 1 | 198 |
| Beets, fresh, cooked, diced | 85 | ½ c | 27 | 1.0 | 20 | 37 | 177 |
| Beets, canned, diced | | | | | | | |
|   Regular | 85 | ½ c | 32 | 0.9 | 16 | 200 | 142 |
|   Special diet pack | 85 | ½ c | 32 | 0.9 | 16 | 39 | 142 |
| Broccoli, fresh, cooked | 78 | ½ c | 20 | 2.4 | 48 | 8 | 207 |
| Broccoli, frozen, cooked | 93 | ½ c | 24 | 2.7 | 52 | 14 | 196 |
| Carrots, fresh, cooked, sliced, drained | 78 | ½ c | 24 | 0.7 | 24 | 25 | 172 |
| Cauliflower, raw, flowerbuds | 50 | ½ c | 14 | 1.4 | 28 | 7 | 148 |

(Continued)

## Table 32-7.  Protein, Phosphorus, Sodium, and Potassium Exchange Lists (Continued)

*Vegetable Exchanges, Group II (Continued)*
One serving contains variable protein, 35 mg phosphorus, 20 mg sodium, and 170 mg potassium.

| Item | G | Amount | Calories | Protein (g) | P (mg) | Na* (mg) | K (mg) |
|---|---|---|---|---|---|---|---|
| Cauliflower, frozen, cooked | 90 | ½ c | 16 | 1.7 | 34 | 9 | 186 |
| Celery, fresh, diced | 60 | ½ c | 10 | 0.6 | 17 | 76 | 205 |
| Celery, cooked, diced | 75 | ½ c | 11 | 0.6 | 17 | 66 | 179 |
| Corn, frozen, cooked | 83 | ½ c | 65 | 2.5 | 60 | 1 | 152 |
| Eggplant, fresh, cooked, diced | 100 | ½ c | 19 | 1.0 | 21 | 1 | 150 |
| Mushrooms, raw, sliced | 35 | ½ c | 10 | 1.0 | 41 | 6 | 145 |
| Mushrooms, canned, solids and liquid | 100 | ½ c | 17 | 1.9 | 68 | 400 | 197 |
| Mustard greens, fresh, cooked | 70 | ½ c | 16 | 1.6 | 23 | 13 | 154 |
| Okra, fresh, cooked, sliced | 80 | ½ c | 23 | 1.6 | 33 | 2 | 139 |
| Peas, fresh, cooked | 80 | ½ c | 57 | 4.3 | 79 | 1 | 157 |
| Rutabaga, cooked, cubed | 85 | ½ c | 30 | 0.8 | 27 | 4 | 142 |
| Sweet potato, baked (2″ diam, 5″ long) | 73 | ½ potato | 81 | 1.2 | 33 | 7 | 171 |
| Turnips, raw, cubed | 65 | ½ c | 20 | 0.7 | 20 | 32 | 174 |
| Turnips, cooked, cubed | 78 | ½ c | 18 | 0.6 | 20 | 27 | 146 |

*Values for vegetables canned with salt were excluded from calculation of this average.

*Vegetable Exchanges, Group III*
One serving contains variable protein, 40 mg phosphorus, 20 mg sodium, and 280 mg potassium.

| Item | G | Amount | Calories | Protein (g) | P (mg) | Na* (mg) | K (mg) |
|---|---|---|---|---|---|---|---|
| Beet greens, fresh, cooked | 73 | ½ c | 13 | 1.3 | 18 | 55 | 240 |
| Brussels sprouts, fresh, cooked | 78 | ½ c (4 sprouts) | 28 | 3.3 | 56 | 8 | 212 |
| Brussels sprouts, frozen, cooked | 78 | ½ c (4 sprouts) | 26 | 2.5 | 48 | 11 | 229 |
| Chard, Swiss, cooked | 87 | ½ c | 16 | 1.6 | 21 | 76 | 281 |
| Collards, fresh, cooked | 95 | ½ c | 32 | 3.4 | 50 | 34 | 249 |
| Parsnips, cooked, diced | 78 | ½ c | 51 | 1.2 | 48 | 6 | 294 |
| Potato, mashed | 105 | ½ c | 99 | 2.2 | 51 | 5 | 263 |
| Potato, baked (2½″ diam, 4½″ long) | 100 | ½ potato | 73 | 2.0 | 51 | 3 | 391 |
| Pumpkin, canned, salt added | 120 | ½ c | 41 | 1.3 | 32 | 289 | 294 |
| Spinach, cooked, drained | 90 | ½ c | 21 | 2.7 | 34 | 45 | 292 |
| Squash, winter, acorn, baked | 103 | ½ c | 57 | 2.0 | 30 | 1 | 492 |
| Sweet potato, mashed | 128 | ½ c | 138 | 2.6 | 53 | 61 | 255 |
| Tomato paste, no salt added | 33 | 2 tbsp | 27 | 1.1 | 23 | 13 | 280 |
| Tomato, fresh, not peeled (2⅖″ diam) | 100 | 1 | 20 | 1.0 | 25 | 3 | 222 |
| Tomatoes, canned | | | | | | | |
|   Regular | 120 | ½ c | 25 | 1.4 | 23 | 157 | 261 |
|   Special diet pack | 120 | ½ c | 25 | 1.4 | 23 | 3 | 261 |
| Tomato juice, regular | 120 | ½ c | 23 | 1.1 | 22 | 243 | 276 |

*Values for vegetables canned with salt were excluded from calculation of this average.

*Fruit Exchanges, Group I*
One serving contains 0.5 g protein, 15 mg phosphorus, 2 mg sodium, and 85 mg potassium.

| Item | G | Amount | Calories* | Protein (g) | P (mg) | Na (mg) | K (mg) |
|---|---|---|---|---|---|---|---|
| Apple, raw, small | 115 | 1–2½″ diam | 61 | 0.2 | 11 | 1 | 116 |
| Apple juice, canned | 120 | ½ c | 59 | 0.1 | 11 | 1 | 125 |
| Applesauce | 120 | ½ c | 116 | 0.3 | 7 | 2.5 | 83 |
| Blackberries, fresh | 72 | ½ c | 42 | 0.9 | 14 | 0.5 | 123 |
| Blackberries, frozen | 72 | ½ c | 42 | 0.9 | 14 | 1 | 122 |
| Blueberries, fresh | 73 | ½ c | 45 | 0.5 | 10 | 0.5 | 59 |
| Boysenberries, frozen, sweetened | 72 | ½ c | 69 | 0.5 | 12 | 0.5 | 75 |
| Cranberries, raw | 48 | ½ c | 22 | 0.2 | 5 | 1 | 39 |
| Cranberry sauce | 138 | ½ c | 202 | 0.2 | 6 | 1.5 | 42 |

# Table 32-7.  Protein, Phosphorus, Sodium, and Potassium Exchange Lists (Continued)

*Fruit Exchanges, Group I (Continued)*
One serving contains 0.5 g protein, 15 mg phosphorus, 2 mg sodium, and 85 mg potassium.

| Item | G | Amount | Calories* | Protein (g) | P (mg) | Na (mg) | K (mg) |
|---|---|---|---|---|---|---|---|
| Cranberry juice | 127 | ½ c | 82 | 0.1 | 4 | 1.5 | 13 |
| Figs, raw | 65 | 1 large | 52 | 0.8 | 14 | 1 | 126 |
| Grapes, white seedless | 50 | 10 whole | 34 | 0.3 | 10 | 2 | 87 |
| Grape juice, frozen, sweetened | 125 | ½ c | 67 | 0.2 | 5 | 1.5 | 43 |
| Grapefruit sections | 88 | ½ c | 36 | 0.5 | 18 | 1 | 118 |
| Lemonade, frozen, diluted | 124 | ½ c | 54 | tr | 1.5 | 0.5 | 20 |
| Lime juice, fresh | 123 | ½ c | 32 | 0.4 | 14 | 1 | 128 |
| Limeade | 124 | ½ c | 51 | tr | 1.5 | tr | 16 |
| Peach, canned, with 1⅔ tbsp syrup | 76 | 1 half | 59 | 0.3 | 9 | 2 | 99 |
| Peach nectar | 125 | ½ c | 60 | 0.3 | 14 | 1 | 97 |
| Pear, raw, Bartlett (2½″ diam, 3½″ high) | 90 | 1 half | 50 | 0.6 | 9 | 1.5 | 107 |
| Pear, canned, with 1 tbsp syrup | 48 | 1 half | 36 | 0.1 | 3 | tr | 40 |
| Pear nectar | 125 | ½ c | 65 | 0.4 | 7 | 1.5 | 49 |
| Pineapple, fresh (¾″ thick, 3½″ diam) | 84 | 1 slice | 44 | 0.3 | 7 | 1 | 123 |
| Pineapple, canned, with 1½ tbsp syrup | 58 | 1 medium slice | 43 | 0.2 | 3 | 1 | 56 |
| Plums, raw, damson (1″ diam) | 33 | 3 | 21 | tr | 6 | 0.6 | 90 |
| Plums, raw, prune (1½″ diam) | 60 | 2 | 42 | 0.4 | 10 | tr | 96 |
| Strawberries, fresh, whole | 75 | ½ c | 28 | 0.5 | 16 | 0.5 | 122 |
| Tangerine | 136 | 1 large | 46 | 0.8 | 18 | 2 | 127 |

*Caloric values for canned fruit are based on fruits canned in heavy syrup.

*Fruit Exchanges, Group II*
One serving contains 0.5 g protein, 15 mg phosphorus, 2 mg sodium, and 170 mg potassium.

| Item | G | Amount | Calories* | Protein (g) | P (mg) | Na (mg) | K (mg) |
|---|---|---|---|---|---|---|---|
| Apricot nectar | 120 | ½ c | 72 | 0.4 | 15 | tr | 190 |
| Cherries, raw, sour | 78 | ½ c | 45 | 1.0 | 15 | 1.5 | 148 |
| Cherries, raw, sweet | 73 | ½ c | 51 | 0.9 | 14 | 1.5 | 139 |
| Cherries, sweet, canned | 129 | ½ c | 104 | 1.1 | 17 | 1.5 | 162 |
| Figs, canned | 130 | ½ c | 109 | 0.7 | 17 | 2.5 | 193 |
| Fruit cocktail | 128 | ½ c | 97 | 0.5 | 16 | 7 | 206 |
| Grapes, halves, all varieties | 88 | ½ c | 59 | 0.5 | 18 | 2.5 | 152 |
| Grapefruit, fresh | 184 | 1 half | 40 | 0.5 | 16 | 1 | 132 |
| Grapefruit juice | 123 | ½ c | 48 | 0.6 | 19 | 1 | 200 |
| Lemon juice, fresh | 122 | ½ c | 31 | 0.6 | 12 | 1 | 172 |
| Nectarine (2½″ diam) | 75 | 1 half | 44 | 0.4 | 17 | 4 | 203 |
| Peach, raw, pared (2½″ diam) | 115 | 1 | 33 | 0.5 | 17 | 1 | 177 |
| Pineapple juice | 125 | ½ c | 69 | 0.5 | 12 | 1.5 | 187 |
| Plums, canned | 136 | ½ c | 107 | 0.5 | 13 | 1.5 | 184 |
| Strawberries, frozen, sweetened | 128 | ½ c | 136 | 0.7 | 22 | 1.5 | 143 |
| Watermelon | 160 | 1 c | 42 | 0.8 | 16 | 2 | 160 |

*Caloric values for canned fruits are based on fruits canned in heavy syrup.

*Fruit Exchanges, Group III*
One serving contains 1 g protein, 25 mg phosphorus, 5 mg sodium, and 300 mg potassium.

| Item | G | Amount | Calories* | Protein (g) | P (mg) | Na (mg) | K (mg) |
|---|---|---|---|---|---|---|---|
| Apricots, canned | 129 | ½ c | 111 | 0.7 | 20 | 1 | 302 |
| Apricots, fresh | 114 | 3 whole | 55 | 1.1 | 25 | 0.5 | 301 |
| Banana | 88 | ½ medium | 50 | 0.7 | 16 | 0.5 | 220 |
| Cantaloupe | 160 | 1 c melon balls | 48 | 1.1 | 26 | 19 | 402 |

(Continued)

## Table 32-7. Protein, Phosphorus, Sodium, and Potassium Exchange Lists (Continued)

*Fruit Exchanges, Group III (Continued)*
One serving contains 1 g protein, 25 mg phosphorus, 5 mg sodium, and 300 mg potassium.

| Item | G | Amount | Calories* | Protein (g) | P (mg) | Na (mg) | K (mg) |
|---|---|---|---|---|---|---|---|
| Honeydew | 170 | 1 c melon balls | 56 | 1.4 | 27 | 20 | 427 |
| Orange (2⅝″ diam) | 180 | 1 | 64 | 1.3 | 26 | 1 | 263 |
| Orange juice | 124 | ½ c | 56 | 0.9 | 21 | 1 | 248 |
| Prunes, cooked and sweetened | 140 | ½ c | 205 | 1.0 | 36 | 4 | 312 |
| Prune juice | 128 | ½ c | 99 | 0.5 | 26 | 2.5 | 301 |
| Rhubarb, cooked and sweetened | 135 | ½ c | 190 | 0.7 | 21 | 2.5 | 274 |

*Caloric values for canned fruits are based on fruits canned in heavy syrup.

*Fat Exchanges*
One serving contains 0 g protein, 1 mg phosphorus, 50 mg sodium, and 1 mg potassium.

| Item | G | Amount | Calories | Protein (g) | P (mg) | Na (mg) | K (mg) |
|---|---|---|---|---|---|---|---|
| Butter, salted* | 5 | 1 tsp | 45 | 0 | 1 | 48 | 1 |
| Margarine, salted* | 5 | 1 tsp | 45 | 0 | 1 | 48 | 1 |
| Mayonnaise, salted | 5 | 1 tsp | 34 | 0 | 1 | 30 | 1 |
| Half and half | 30 | 2 tbsp | 40 | 1 | 26 | 14 | 38 |
| Whipping cream | 30 | 2 tbsp | 106 | 0.6 | 18 | 10 | 26 |

*Unsalted butter and margarine, and vegetable oil may be used as desired.

*Miscellaneous List*

| Item | G | Amount | Calories | Protein (g) | P (mg) | Na (mg) | K (mg) |
|---|---|---|---|---|---|---|---|
| Beverages | | | | | | | |
| Alcoholic (physician's permission) | | | | | | | |
| Beer | 240 | 8 oz | 100 | 0.7 | 72 | 17 | 60 |
| Gin, vodka, rum, whiskey | 90 | 3 oz | 210 | 0 | tr | 1 | 2 |
| Wine | | | | | | | |
| Dessert | 120 | 4 oz | 165 | 0.1 | tr | 5 | 90 |
| Table | 120 | 4 oz | 102 | 0.1 | 12 | 6 | 110 |
| Carbonated | | | | | | | |
| Coca-Cola | 240 | 8 oz | 96 | 0 | 40 | 0 | 0 |
| Ginger ale | 240 | 8 oz | 88 | 0 | 0 | 0 | 0 |
| Pepsi Cola | 240 | 8 oz | 110 | 0 | | 28 | 9 |
| Fanta Orange | 240 | 8 oz | 128 | 0 | 0 | 8 | 0 |
| Sprite | 240 | 8 oz | 96 | 0 | 0 | 40 | 0 |
| Bitter lemon | 240 | 8 oz | 104 | 0 | 0 | 16 | 0 |
| Coffee, tea, bouillon | | | | | | | |
| Coffee | 240 | 8 oz | 5 | 0.3 | 5 | 5 | 135 |
| Tea | 240 | 8 oz | 5 | | | 5 | 95 |
| Bouillon | | | | | | | |
| Salted | 4 | 1 cube | 5 | 0.2 | | 960 | 4 |
| Unsalted | 4 | 1 cube | 11 | 0.3 | | 2 | 500 |
| Fruit drinks | | | | | | | |
| Awake | 120 | 4 oz | 51 | tr | | 5 | 41 |
| Cranberry juice | 120 | 4 oz | 78 | 0.2 | 3.6 | 1 | 12 |
| Grape Tang | 120 | 4 oz | 61 | tr | 40 | 55 | 1 |
| Lemonade | 120 | 4 oz | 54 | tr | 2 | 1 | 22 |
| Orange Tang | 120 | 4 oz | 61 | tr | 60 | 13 | 45 |
| Kool-aid | 120 | 4 oz | 45 | tr | | 1 | 1 |
| Hawaiian Punch | 120 | 4 oz | 49 | 0.4 | | 2 | 11 |

## Table 32-7. Protein, Phosphorus, Sodium, and Potassium Exchange List (Continued)

*Miscellaneous List (Continued)*

| Item | G | Amount | Calories | Protein (g) | P (mg) | Na (mg) | K (mg) |
|---|---|---|---|---|---|---|---|
| **Fats** | | | | | | | |
| Bacon, fried | 7 | 1 slice | 48 | 1.5 | 16 | 76 | 17 |
| Butter, margarine | | | | | | | |
|   Salted | 14 | 1 tbsp | 102 | 0.1 | 2 | 140 | 3 |
|   Unsalted | 14 | 1 tbsp | 102 | 0.1 | 2 | 1 | 3 |
| Cream cheese | 14 | 1 tbsp | 53 | 1.1 | 13 | 35 | 11 |
| French dressing | 14 | 1 tbsp | 66 | 0.1 | 2 | 219 | 13 |
| Italian dressing | 14 | 1 tbsp | 83 | tr | 1 | 314 | 2 |
| Mayonnaise | | | | | | | |
|   Regular | 14 | 1 tbsp | 101 | 0.2 | 4 | 84 | 5 |
|   Low sodium | 14 | 1 tbsp | 105 | 0.4 | 4 | 3 | 5 |
| Roquefort dressing | 15 | 1 tbsp | 76 | 0.7 | 11 | 164 | 6 |
| Peanut butter | | | | | | | |
|   Regular | 16 | 1 tbsp | 94 | 4.0 | 61 | 97 | 100 |
|   Low sodium | 16 | 1 tbsp | 94 | 4.0 | 61 | 2 | 100 |
| Vegetable oil | 14 | 1 tbsp | 120 | 0 | 0 | 0 | 0 |
| Whipping cream | 15 | 1 tbsp | 53 | 0.3 | 9 | 5 | 13 |
| **Low-protein products** | | | | | | | |
| Cornstarch | 8 | 1 tbsp | 29 | tr | 0 | tr | tr |
| Low-protein bread—dp | | | | | | | |
| (Henkle Dietary Specialties) | 32 | 1 slice | 78 | 0.3 | 0 | 10 | 8 |
| Low-protein pasta, cooked | | | | | | | |
| (Aproten) | 100 | ½ c | 91 | 0.2 | 0 | 8 | 2 |
| Low-protein rusk (Aproten) | 12 | 1 slice | 48 | 0.1 | | 4 | 5 |
| Wheatstarch (Henkle) | 100 | 1 c | 360 | 0.4 | 45 | 60 | 10 |
| **Non-dairy products** | | | | | | | |
| Coffee-Rich, liquid | 60 | ¼ c | 94 | 0.2 | | 24 | 27 |
| Cool-Whip | 18 | ¼ c | 60 | 0.2 | | 4 | tr |
| Cremora powder (Borden) | 12 | 2 tbsp | 66 | 0.6 | | 1 | 10 |
| Mocha Mix | 60 | ¼ c | 86 | 0.2 | | 60 | 35 |
| Rich's Whip Topping, whipped | 23 | ½ c | 63 | 0 | | 13 | tr |
| Poly Perx | 60 | ¼ c | 84 | 0.44 | tr | tr | tr |
| **Spices, seasonings, condiments*** | | | | | | | |
| Garlic, fresh | 2 | 1 clove | 3 | 0.1 | 5 | 1 | 11 |
| Green pepper, fresh, chopped | 10 | 1 tbsp | 2 | 0.1 | 2.2 | 1 | 21 |
| Horseradish, prepared | 5 | 1 tsp | 2 | 0.1 | 1.6 | 5 | 16 |
| Lemon juice, fresh | 15 | 1 tbsp | 4 | 0.1 | 1.5 | 1 | 21 |
| Lime juice, fresh | 15 | 1 tbsp | 4 | 0.1 | 1.7 | 1 | 16 |
| Mustard | | | | | | | |
|   Low sodium (Cellu) | 5 | 1 tsp | 4 | 0.2 | | 1 | 21 |
|   Prepared yellow, regular | 5 | 1 tsp | 4 | 0.2 | 3.7 | 63 | 6.5 |
| Onion, fresh, chopped | 10 | 1 tbsp | 4 | 0.2 | 3.6 | 1 | 16 |
| Tabasco sauce | 2 | ½ tsp | tr | tr | | 11 | 2 |
| Tomato catsup | 15 | 1 tbsp | 16 | 0.3 | 7.5 | 156 | 54 |
| Tomato, chili sauce | 15 | 1 tbsp | 16 | 0.4 | 8 | 201 | 56 |
| Vinegar, distilled | 15 | 1 tbsp | 2 | | | 2 | 36 |
| Worcestershire sauce | 5 | 1 tsp | 4 | 0.1 | | 105 | 24 |

*All dry spices, herbs, and extracts may be used for flavoring.

vegetables to help reduce their potassium intake. Canned vegetables should be drained and then heated in fresh water since considerable potassium is contained in the canning juice. Methods of cooking, such as frying and baking, do not remove any potassium from the vegetables.

Because the broths and juices from cooking meats and poultry contain significant amounts of potassium, they are not used in potassium-restricted diet plans. As with vegetables, frying, roasting, or baking does not remove potassium from meats and poultry. Stewing these foods, however, does remove some potassium.

Coffee and tea, which contain potassium, are limited on these diets, not only for that reason, but also because of their fluid content.

Salt substitutes and sodium-free baking powder are contraindicated on potassium-restricted diets because potassium has been substituted for the sodium in these compounds. Low-sodium milk should never be used by the renal patient for the same reason. The sodium ions in the milk have been replaced by potassium ions. It is unlikely, however, that a renal patient would ever be so severely restricted in sodium that low-sodium milk would be required.

### Sodium

About 1% to 2% of patients with early chronic renal failure have significant renal salt-wasting and may become sodium depleted even on a normal salt intake. They are normotensive or hypotensive at rest and exhibit postural hypotension when sodium depleted. Treatment consists of cautious sodium repletion.

Sodium retention is more common than sodium depletion in chronic renal failure, however, and is the main factor in the development of hypertension in these patients. The sodium-restricted Exchange System and food lists presented in Chapter 31, *Cardiovascular Disease*, may be used to calculate sodium-restricted diet patterns. For patients not on dialysis, sodium balance is usually maintained in a range from 40 mEq to 130 mEq per day, depending on blood pressure, weight, and level of kidney function. Patients on dialysis are usually oliguric or anuric and are maintained on 60 mEq to 100 mEq per day. If the sodium-restricted patient develops vomiting or diarrhea, fluid and salt intake may have to be increased temporarily to prevent hyponatremia (low serum sodium level) or a state of fluid depletion.

### Fluid

In most patients urine output reaches a peak, while the GFR declines through the range 25 ml to 5 ml per minute, and then decreases to below normal in terminal renal failure. Thirst accompanies polyuria, and the patient usually maintains water balance in a normal state if he has free access to water. Thirst may be excessive in some patients due to dryness of the mouth, which is common in renal failure. In such cases, an upper limit of fluid intake should be stipulated. The oliguric patient has a more difficult, psychological battle to wage in his effort to maintain strict control of his fluid intake. Drinking is widespread in our society. "Drinking something" is a form of socialization (*e.g.*, the coffee break, the cocktail party, the glass of ice water in a restaurant). Magazine and television ads continually remind one to drink. Jokes about the coffee addict or the "six pack a day" beer drinker are common. The renal patient on fluid restriction has a difficult time in such an environment. The renal dietitian sometimes achieves success with the habitual overdrinker by using the technique of behavior modification, which forces the patient to identify the situation that caused him

to drink too much. It is sometimes helpful for a patient to fill a pitcher with water to the level of his fluid allowance for the day and then discard a comparable amount of the water every time he drinks. In this manner he can see how much of his fluid allowance he has left for the remainder of the day.

It is important for the patient to realize that an 8-oz cupful of retained fluid means a weight gain of $\frac{1}{2}$ lb. For the patient on hemodialysis, a weight gain of no more than 1 to 2 lb per day between dialyses is desirable. Another way of expressing this rate of weight gain would be to recommend an interdialytic weight gain of no more than 1 to 2 kg (2 lb to 4 lb) if the patient is being dialyzed three times weekly. The interdialytic weight gain allowed may vary, depending upon the ease with which fluid can be removed during each treatment. Rapid weight gain in a dialysis patient represents fluid weight, not real weight, and a gain of 3 or more kg (6 or more lb) between dialyses is cause for concern. That kind of weight gain requires immediate counseling from the dietitian. Patients should be instructed to weigh themselves each morning before breakfast. If their weight gain is excessive, they know they must restrict their fluid intake more closely that day.

The renal patient's caloric requirement must be considered when beverage choices are made. In general, such noncaloric beverages as coffee, tea, and diet soda should be avoided unless calories can be added (*e.g.*, cream and sugar in the coffee). Carbonated beverages and fruit drinks containing calories, but not large amounts of potassium, may be found in the *Miscellaneous List*, Table 32-7.

If the renal disease is secondary to diabetes, it is important to realize that elevated blood sugar causes excessive thirst. Good control of the diabetes is difficult to achieve in renal failure and requires close cooperation between the patient and all members of the health-care team.

Food items are classified as fluids if they are liquid at room temperature. Ice cream, sherbet, gelatins, ice pops, and fruit ices are accordingly calculated as liquids. The fluid content of fruit is acknowledged but is usually not calculated as part of the fluid on a fluid-restricted diet.

It is important that renal patients have a thorough understanding of fluid control and the consequences of fluid abuse. Aggressive dialysis to remove excess fluid can result in severe muscle cramps, headache, nausea, vomiting, and a sudden drop in blood pressure.

## Exchange system for diet planning
### Exchange lists

The Exchange System for calculating protein, sodium, phosphorus, and potassium-restricted diet patterns is given in Table 32-5. The protein and electrolyte values given for each exchange are averages derived from the values given in the Exchange Lists in Table 32-7. It should be noted that protein values for fruits are listed in the renal Exchange System and Exchange Lists. This differs from the customary exchange system used for calorie-controlled diet planning. Since specific quantities of milk, eggs, and meat are used to provide the essential amino acids, and the intake of nonessential amino acids is restricted, the protein in breads, fruits, and all vegetables must be calculated to avoid an excess of nonessential amino acids at the low-protein diet levels (see Table 32-6).

The fruit and vegetable lists shown in Table 32-7 have been subdivided into three groups according to their average potassium content. Groups I and II contain low and moderate amounts of potassium, respectively. Group III fruits and Group III vegetables, which contain large amounts of potassium, are generally avoided on potassium-restricted diet plans unless special means of preparation, such as soaking, are used to remove some of the potassium. The classification of starchy vegetables is also different from that of the calorie-controlled exchange lists where they are listed as bread exchanges. In the renal Exchange System they are placed in the vegetable lists and are classified by their potassium content. They are also classified in Table 32-3 by their protein content.

If the sodium restriction is in the range of 1500 mg to 2000 mg, some lightly salted foods may have to be used to meet the prescribed level, because the major contributors of natural sodium to the diet—milk, meat, and eggs—are limited. For that reason the fat exchanges are those with added salt. Salted butter or margarine increases the acceptability of the low-protein breads and pastas. If the sodium is severely restricted (less than 1000 mg), however, only unsalted fats are used. Well drained and rinsed vegetables canned with added salt can be used on moderately restricted sodium diets.

Figures for the low-protein Aproten products are

listed under *Miscellaneous*, Table 32-7. Spices and flavorings, also in the *Miscellanous List*, can be used to enhance the flavor of foods. For example, dry mustard, vinegar, or lemon juice can greatly improve the flavor of unsalted meat, fish, or poultry.

### Calculating the diet pattern

Table 32-8 demonstrates the calculation of a pattern for a diet prescription of 40 g protein, 1000 mg sodium, and 1500 mg potassium. The six slices of low-protein bread and the ten fat exchanges provide approximately 930 kcal. The remaining foods in the pattern provide approximately 850 kcal. By using sugar, jams, jellies, other wheatstarch products, or low-protein Aproten pastas, it would be possible to provide an additional 300 kcal to 400 kcal for a total of approximately 2000 kcal per day.

Foods containing high biologic value protein contribute about 60% of the total protein in the diet pattern. Additional wheatstarch products would add sodium and potassium to correct the discrepancies between the prescribed levels of electrolytes and the calculated levels.

Table 32-9 illustrates a day's menu using the calculated diet pattern shown in Table 32-8. This menu contains approximately 600 ml of fluid.

### Special problems

Many renal patients understandably find their diet and fluid restrictions difficult to follow. Members of the health-care team must appreciate the psychological stress and frustration that result from the changes in life-style imposed by these diets and other treatment therapies, such as dialysis. Some patients become totally preoccupied with thoughts of food or drink. Compliance with a treatment regimen is obviously a critical factor in determining their level of adjustment to the disease and their

### Table 32-8. Calculation of Meal Pattern for 40-g Protein, 1000-mg Sodium, 1500-mg Potassium Diet

| Food Group | Amount | Protein g | Sodium mg | Phosphorus mg | Potassium mg |
|---|---|---|---|---|---|
| Milk | ½ c | 4 | 60 | 100 | 175 |
| Meat | 2 oz | 14 | 50 | 150 | 180 |
| Egg, large | 1 | 7 | 60 | 100 | 65 |
| Vegetables | | | | | |
|   Group I (1 g) | 2 servings | 2 | 14 | 50 | 200 |
|   Group II (2 g) | 1 serving | 2 | 20 | 35 | 170 |
| Fruit | | | | | |
|   Group I | 2 servings | 1 | 4 | 30 | 170 |
|   Group II | 1 serving | 0.5 | 2 | 15 | 170 |
| Bread | | | | | |
|   Unsalted | 3 servings | 6 | 15 | 120 | 120 |
|   Low protein | 6 slices | 1.8 | 60 | | 48 |
| Fats, salted | 10 tsp | | 450 | 9 | |
| Totals | | 38.8 | 735* | 609 | 1298* |

*Does not include other foods made with wheatstarch (*i.e.*, fruit pies, cookies) which will increase sodium and potassium to the prescribed levels.

general sense of wellbeing. One study of patients on chronic hemodialysis examined the degree of dietary compliance, as indicated by serum potassium and phosphorus levels and interdialytic weight gains.[49] Compliance with potassium restriction was related to the length of time on dialysis and to the patient's gender. Women and those who were on dialysis for a short time tended to be more conscientious. The same held true for phosphate restriction. Compliance with interdialytic weight gain was greater in patients with lower levels of education. Seventy nine percent of the patients were considered to be compliant with potassium restriction, 62% with phosphorus restriction (involving not only compliance with the phosphorus-restricted diet but also the taking of prescribed phosphorus binders), and 40% were compliant with control of weight. Another study found a relatively strong relationship between compliance and the simple presence of another person in the home. Patients living alone showed significantly lower compliance rates.[50] In a review and analysis of compliance studies, compliance rates for renal diets were compared with those associated with other nutritional regimens. Renal diets had substantially poorer rates than those for gluten-free, low-phenylalanine, and modified fat diets, but compared favorably with compliance rates for insulin-dependent diabetics.[51] The complexity of renal diet regimens and their restrictiveness were cited as reasons for lack of compliance.

The dietitian–patient relationship is unique in renal diet therapy. No other chronic condition treated on an outpatient basis has as frequent or lengthy patient–dietitian encounters where predialysis blood chemistries allow the dietitian to confront the patient about his degree of compliance. From this position the dietitian can support and encourage the patient in his attempts to deal with his disease and treatment-related factors.

Close cooperation between dietary and nursing services is required to carry out fluid orders for hospitalized renal patients. Aside from water, which may or may not be a significant source of sodium and potassium, many fluids commonly offered to hospitalized patients contain substantial amounts of sodium or potassium or both. For example, orange juice and tea contain potassium; tomato juice canned with added salt contains large amounts of sodium and potassium. If a diet is severely restricted in electrolytes, a 4-oz to 8-oz serving of any one of these beverages could contribute to a serious error in therapy. A severe fluid restriction also presents a special problem. The nurse needs to give water with medications and the dietitian needs to provide fluids to enhance the palatability of the diet. Special arrangements must be made between these departments to prevent any errors from occurring.

### Diet therapy in peritoneal dialysis

Initially the use of peritoneal dialysis for treatment of chronic renal disease was associated with general wasting and malnutrition due to several factors: the great loss of protein and other nutrients into the effluent peritoneal dialysate; frequent peritonitis causing severe protein catabolism and increasing the risk of superimposed illness; persisting uremia due to inadequate dialysis; and insufficient dietary intake. Developments in recent years have changed this association, and the incidence of peritonitis has been markedly reduced. Implantable catheters and better techniques for delivery of peritoneal dialysis have permitted this treatment to be self-administered by patients. Protein losses during the dialysis have also been reduced. However, there are few data on nutritional requirements for chronic peritoneal dialysis patients. Most investigators today do not restrict protein in these patients. Recommended protein intake for patients on maintenance peritoneal dialysis is in the range of 1.2 g to 1.5 g per kilogram of body weight. Approximately 75% of this protein intake should be from foods of high biologic value.[52,53] Milk may be used as a meat substitute with 1 c or 2 c per day permitted depending on the patient's serum potassium and phosphorus levels. Serum albumin levels are closely monitored, and, if a downward trend in serum albumin is noted, the patient is again counseled about

### Table 32-9. Menu for 40-g Protein, 1000-mg Sodium, and 1500-mg Potassium Diet

*Breakfast*
½ cup cranberry juice
1 cup Puffed Wheat
½ cup milk
1 fried egg
2 slices low-protein bread
3 teaspoons salted margarine
2 tablespoons jam
½ cup coffee

*Noon Meal*
1 ounce tuna, special diet pack
2 slices low-protein bread
1 leaf lettuce
2 teaspoons salted mayonnaise
½ cup unsalted canned green beans seasoned with 1 teaspoon salted margarine
½ cup frozen strawberries
3 low-protein cookies
½ cup ginger ale

*Evening Meal*
1 ounce baked chicken
½ cup rice seasoned with 1 teaspoon salted margarine
½ cup cooked carrots seasoned with 1 teaspoon salted margarine
2 slices low-protein bread
2 teaspoons salted margarine
1 tablespoon honey
1 piece apple pie (wheatstarch crust)
½ cup lemonade

This menu provides 600 ml of a day's total fluid.

protein intake. This level of protein intake accompanied by sufficient caloric intake promotes anabolism in patients on continuous ambulatory peritoneal dialysis. A minimum of 35 calories per kilogram of body weight is prescribed for most patients. Peritoneal dialysate contains glucose; a considerable amount of this glucose is absorbed by the patient and provides an additional source of calories. Actually, obesity is now a problem for many chronic peritoneal dialysis patients.[54]

The hypertriglyceridemia commonly seen in patients with renal failure may be more of a problem in patients on peritoneal dialysis for two reasons. These patients do not receive heparin as do patients on hemodialysis. Heparin enhances triglyceride clearance. Secondly, there is loss into the peritoneal dialysate of a glycoprotein that is a cofactor for lipoprotein lipase, the enzyme responsible for clearing triglycerides from the blood. Serum triglyceride levels have been reported to average 340 mg per deciliter in patients who have undergone continuous ambulatory peritoneal dialysis for at least 10 months.[5] It should be remembered that patients who are being treated with this type of dialysis are never truly fasting, because they are continuously taking up glucose from the dialysate in their peritoneal cavity. Since cardiovascular disease is the most common cause of death in patients on dialysis, control of serum triglyceride levels in these patients may be important. Lowering of carbohydrate intake and increasing polyunsaturated fat intake lowered serum triglyceride levels in hemodialysis patients, but there are no data on the effects of diet on serum triglyceride levels in patients on peritoneal dialysis. Blumenkrantz[26] prescribed a carbohydrate intake for peritoneal dialysis patients of 30% to 35% of total calories with as many calories coming from polyunsaturated fats as possible. Meats, fish, and poultry protein sources should be low in fat.

Recommended daily intakes for vitamins and minerals for patients on either type of dialysis include 100 mg ascorbic acid, 1 mg folate, 10 mg pyridoxine, and the recommended allowances for the other water-soluble vitamins. Vitamin D should be prescribed if needed. The daily recommended intake of calcium is 2 g (see discussion in *Diet Therapy Principles for Chronic Renal Failure*). Oral iron supplements are routinely prescribed.[13]

Sodium and water balance and blood pressure improve on continuous ambulatory peritoneal dialysis, allowing the patients a more liberal intake of sodium and fluid. Patients training on this type of dialysis are taught to monitor their fluid status by weight, blood pressure, and the glucose concentration of the dialysate. The glucose concentration aids in removing excess fluid. Occasionally a patient needs a mild sodium restriction, but frequently additional sodium and fluid are prescribed to correct postural hypotension.

There appears to be an increased clearance of phosphorus in peritoneal dialysis, resulting in a decreased need

for phosphate binders.[55] It has been suggested that the occurrence of dialysis dementia (a central nervous system disorder seen in some patients on long-term maintenance dialysis) may be associated with chronic use of phosphate binders, such as aluminum hydroxide. Restriction of phosphorus intake is difficult in diets with relatively high protein intakes, but it may be warranted in view of the suggested association between long-term use of phosphate binders and the incidence of dialysis dementia.

Potassium restriction is not usually necessary in peritoneal dialysis even though the intake is greater due to increased protein intake. Patients are instructed about foods with high potassium contents (those over 250 mg of potassium per serving), however, and warned against overuse of these foods.[53]

### Diet posttransplant

The immunosuppressive therapy that accompanies transplantation can cause complications, some of which require diet manipulation. These complications include hypertension, decreased glucose tolerance, obesity, lipid disorders, and gastric ulcer. Cardiovascular disease is the second most common cause of death in transplant recipients and is exceeded only by infection. Since plasma levels of cholesterol and triglycerides are significantly higher in transplant patients than in normal controls, it is important to reduce these independent cardiovascular risk factors, if possible. In one study, hypocaloric diets, low in carbohydrate (130 g), were administered to stable transplant patients with persistent hypertriglyceridemia or mixed hypertriglyceridemia and hypercholesterolemia. When patients lost weight, plasma lipid concentrations returned to normal and remained stable as long as patients maintained their ideal body weights. It was determined that weight control and restriction of triglyceride precursors, carbohydrate and alcohol, were responsible for correction of these lipid abnormalities.[56]

The current diet recommended for a patient with a transplanted kidney that is functioning well is moderately restricted in sodium (approximtely 2 g), low in total carbohydrate (approximately 120 g), high in protein (approximately 1.5 g to 2 g per kilogram of body weight), and may be restricted in calories if weight loss is advisable. Use of polyunsaturated fats in place of saturated fats and a calcium intake of 1200 mg daily are advised. Some clinicians recommend a bland diet if gastrointestinal problems arise.[57]

## Nutritional assessment of the renal patient

It is important that techniques for the assessment of nutritional status of patients with renal failure be established since muscle wasting and malnutrition are problems in this population. The causes of wasting include inadequate intake of nutrients, loss of nutrients into dialysate, intercurrent illnesses, uremic toxins and endocrine abnormalities, such as insulin resistance. This altered state of wasting and malnutrition contributes in turn to the uremic syndrome due to increased susceptibility to infection, impaired wound healing, decreased strength and vigor, and poor quality of life in general. Techniques have been developed for evaluating nutritional status of healthy people, but the metabolic disorders that occur in renal failure may invalidate those techniques. Blumenkrantz showed that certain anthropometric and biochemical measurements of nutritional status were abnormal in a group of robust-appearing renal patients and concluded that factors in addition to nutritional intake lead to abnormal values in these patients.[58] It was determined that serial measurements of several nutritional parameters in the same patients over a period of time could increase the sensitivity and accuracy of assessment of body nutriture.

The nutritional problems that are most common in uremic patients are protein and calorie deficiency and excessive salt and water intake. Accurate diet histories (obtained by dietitians skilled in interviewing), anthropometric measurements (weight to height ratio, midarm muscle circumference, and triceps skinfold), and serum protein measurements (total protein, albumin, and transferrin) provide the data that are used to assess the nutritional status of the patient.

Renal diets present a unique challenge. They must include adequate protein to prevent wasting and malnutrition, but if protein intake is excessive, uremic toxicity will worsen. The serum urea nitrogen to serum creatinine ratio and the urea nitrogen appearance can be used to determine optimal protein intake. For renal patients with impaired gastrointestinal function due to superimposed organic diseases, such as diabetes mellitus, vascular disease, and inflammatory bowel disease, combinations of ways of providing nutriture may be necessary to prevent catabolism. Nutritional therapy for such patients may include formula feedings, tube feedings, or possibly total parenteral nutrition.[59]

## Counseling the patient

Diets for renal patients with regulated protein and sodium levels and restricted potassium, phosphorus, and fluid content are complex. Adherence by a patient to this kind of diet regimen requires support and encouragement from members of the medical team and the patient's family and friends.

The dietitian provides intensive instruction for the patient and his family over an extended period of time. If the patient is hospitalized, the tray is a visual aid for teaching not only what foods may be used, but also portion size. Providing appropriate recipes and information about where special foods may be obtained and describing what can be ordered in a restaurant, are ways through which the dietitian can develop a positive, concerned relationship with the renal patient. Since counseling the patient with kidney disease does not end with his hospital stay, the dietitian can help the patient adjust to the changes the diet imposes on his life-style. The diet regimen must be carefully taught, monitored, and periodically evaluated to ensure adequate nutrient intake and to prevent wasting in the adult renal patient or growth failure in the uremic child. Renal dietitians have been collaborating to develop criteria that will provide optimum nutritional care across the country and to ensure adequate and uniform patient education.[60]

## Nephrolithiasis

Kidney stones, or urinary or renal calculi, have a long medical history. Although the mechanisms responsible for their formation are under much investigation and progress has been made, nephrolithiasis remains a puzzling disease. Kidney stones vary in size from fine, sand-like particles to those that fill the pelvis of the kidney. They may form in the kidney, ureter, or the bladder. They are classified as calcium stones (oxalate or phosphate), uric acid, cystine, or struvite (magnesium ammonium phosphate) stones. Each type of stone has its own group of causes; therefore, treatment is individualized and directed toward management of the condition responsible for stone formation. All four stone types share a common pathogenesis, however, based on supersaturation of the urine with a poorly soluble material, modified in the case of calcium stones by crystallization inhibitors and sources of seed crystals.

Many patients with renal calculi are asymptomatic. Some calculi remain silent and are found incidentally during radiographic evaluation for nonrenal reasons. However, passage of a calculus into the ureter with resulting intense, severe pain (called renal colic) is the classic manifestation of calculus disease. It is not uncommon for small, sand-like stones to pass with relatively little pain. Not all stones traverse the ureter. Some remain at their location of origin and continue to grow. Clinical signs may consist of hematuria, urinary tract infections, or obstruction.

A combination of factors appears responsible for calculus formation. The occurrence and type of calculus disease is modified by geographic area, sex, race, and possibly diet. In the United States it is most prevalent in the Southeast. Several developing countries (*i.e.,* South Africa, parts of India, and southeast Asia) have unusually high occurrences. Calcium oxalate and calcium phosphate stones are uncommon in white women and rare in blacks of either sex. The higher incidence of calculi in white men is unexplained.

Patients who are immobilized due to trauma, paraplegia, or stroke have a high incidence of renal calculi. Immobilization for long periods causes excessive mineral loss from bones, which raises serum mineral levels, and which, in turn, the kidney must restore to normal. Urinary tract infections are also associated with immobilization for long periods. Significant decreases in stone occurrence have been achieved by prompt and effective treatment of these infections in paraplegic patients.

Approximately two-thirds of all kidney stones contain calcium. Cystine and uric acid stones together account for about 10% of all stones, and those composed of magnesium ammonium phosphate account for approximately 15%. The latter usually occur in patients with recurrent urinary tract infections and persistently alkaline urine.

## Calcium stones

Certain disorders, particularly primary hyperparathyroidism, predispose to stone formation and overcome the protective influence of gender or race. This can be a valuable diagnostic tool in searching for the cause of renal calculi in white women or blacks. Pure calcium phosphate stones may occur in primary hyperparathyroidism, but most patients form a typical mixed calcium oxalate-calcium phosphate or pure calcium oxalate stone.[61] In normal subjects the amount of dietary calcium used by the body is controlled by vitamin D and parathyroid hormone. If excess calcium is consumed, intestinal absorption adjusts, and less calcium is absorbed. In idiopathic nephrolithiasis, most patients have hypercalciuria (urinary excretion of greater than 300 mg in 24 hours), which appears due to increased intestinal absorption of dietary calcium. It is suggested that there is an increased production of $1,25\text{-}(OH)_2D_3$ in these patients with idiopathic hypercalciuria. Since idiopathic hypercalciuria is thought to be a defect in absorption from the intestine, nutritional therapy has consisted of reducing dietary calcium intake to approximately 600 mg per day.[62] However, there is a lack of agreement in the literature that this regimen is beneficial. Some think that a very low calcium diet could aggravate or cause a secondary hyperparathyroidism.[63,64] A moderate calcium-, phosphate-restricted diet should be advised if the patient has elevated plasma $1,25\text{-}(OH)_2D_3$ levels. Table 32-10 illustrates a diet plan moderately restricted in calcium and phosphorus.

## Table 32-10. Moderately Calcium- and Phosphorus-Restricted Diet Plan
### (This diet will contain from 500 to 700 mg of calcium and from 1000 to 1200 mg of phosphorus)

*Foods Used*

Milk
   Limited to 1 c (½ pint) a day. Cream may be substituted for part of the milk

Cheese
   Pot or cottage cheese only. Limited to 2 oz

Fats
   As desired

Eggs
   Limited to 1 a day; egg whites as desired

Meat, fish, fowl
   Limited to 4 oz daily of beef, lamb, pork, veal, chicken, turkey, fish. See those to be avoided.

Soups and broths
   All. Cream soups made with milk allowance only.

Vegetables
   At least 3 servings besides potato. One or 2 servings of deep green or deep yellow vegetables to be included daily. See list of those to be avoided.

Fruits
   All except rhubarb. Include citrus fruit daily.

Breads, cereals, Italian pastas
   White, enriched bread, rolls and crackers except those made from self-rising white flour. Farina (not enriched), cornflakes, corn meal, hominy grits, rice, Rice Krispies, Puffed Rice. Macaroni, spaghetti, noodles.

Desserts
   Fruit pies, fruit cobblers, fruit ices, gelatin. Puddings made with allowed milk and egg. Angel food cake. (Do not use packaged mixes.)

Beverages
   Coffee, Postum, Sanka, tea, ginger ale

Condiments
   Sugar, jellies, honey, salt, pepper, spices

*Foods to be Avoided*

Cheese
   All except pot or cottage cheese.

Meat, fish, fowl
   Brains, heart, liver, kidney, sweetbreads. Game (pheasant, rabbit, deer, grouse). Sardines, fish roe.

Vegetables
   Beet greens, chard, collards, mustard greens, spinach, turnip greens. Dried beans, peas, lentils, soybeans.

Fruits
   Rhubard

Breads, cereals, Italian pastas
   Whole-grain breads, cereals and crackers. Rye bread. All breads made with self-rising flour. Oatmeal, brown and wild rice. Bran, Bran Flakes, wheat germ. All dry cereals except those allowed.

Desserts
   All except those allowed.

Beverages
   Carbonated "soft" drinks, cocoa.

Miscellaneous
   Nuts, peanut butter, chocolate, cocoa. Condiments having a calcium or a phosphate base. (Read labels.)

(Adapted from Shorr E: Aluminum hydroxide gels in the management of renal stone. J Urol 53:507, 1945; © 1945 by The Williams & Wilkens Co., Baltimore)

This plan contains approximately 600 mg of calcium and 1100 mg of phosphorus.

It has been recognized for a long time that maintaining a urine volume above 2500 ml per 24 hours is beneficial for patients with nephrolithiasis. Patients are advised to drink large amounts of fluid, at least 3 to 4 liters daily.[65] Two recent studies reported that when those who formed idiopathic stones were treated with traditional therapy (a low calcium diet and high fluid intake), more than 50% of patients had a recurrence of stones within 3 years. However, there were no data on patient compliance with the low-calcium, high-fluid regimen.[66,67]

### Oxalate stones

Calcium oxalate stones are the most common type of renal calculi. They may occur in patients with no apparent abnormality in calcium or oxalate metabolism as well as in patients with hypercalciuria and hyperoxaluria. Calcium oxalate is relatively insoluble in urine, and urine is normally supersaturated with this compound. Small increases in oxalate concentration may increase the calcium oxalate activity, resulting in crystal formation. Therefore, oxalate-rich foods, such as almonds, cashews, chocolate, cocoa, citrus fruits and juices, cola drinks, rhubarb, spinach and tea, may increase the urinary excretion of oxalate and enhance stone formation. Dietary calcium normally combines with oxalate in the intestinal lumen preventing its absorption. Consequently, a low-calcium diet that is high in oxalate provides more oxalate for absorption and increases urinary excretion of oxalate.

There is an increased incidence of renal calculi in patients with small bowel disease, chronic pancreatitis or biliary disease, and in patients who have had ileal resections. Morbidly obese patients who have undergone jejunoileal anastomosis for weight control also tend to develop oxalate kidney stones. These patients usually exhibit malabsorption, steatorrhea, and hyperoxaluria. Evidence indicates that the hyperoxaluria is secondary to the steatorrhea. Calcium is bound by the unabsorbed fatty acids within the intestinal lumen permitting increased absorption of oxalate and resulting hyperoxaluria. Current treatment restricts dietary fat and high-oxalate foods and supplements with daily calcium to promote formation of insoluble calcium oxalate in the gut.[68] Recent British studies show a strong correlation between high levels of dietary animal protein and the occurrence of oxalate stones. The incidence of kidney stones was significantly lower in vegetarians than in the meat-eating population.[69]

### Uric acid stones

Uric acid is the end product of purine metabolism. Low urine $pH$ has been clearly implicated in patients with idiopathic uric acid calculi, but the mechanism is not fully understood. Increased urinary excretion of uric acid (hyperuricosuria) is another factor in the development of uric acid calculi. A high-protein diet and excessive ethanol consumption are two factors associated with an increase in uric acid excretion. Urate solubility increases dramatically as urine become alkaline. Foods that are high in purine content often have a high acid ash content, which not only tends to increase urinary excretion of uric acid, but also tends to acidify the urine, creating favorable conditions for stone formation. It is possible to reduce uric acid production and excretion by limiting foods with a high purine content (see discussion on gout, Chap. 34), but such a diet is not readily accepted by patients. Current management of uric acid stones includes high fluid intake, alkalinization of the urine, and administration of allopurinol, a drug that inhibits formation of uric acid. This therapy has successfully reduced uric acid concentration in urine with subsequent stone dissolution.[70]

### Cystinuria: cystine stones

Cystinuria is an inherited inborn error of metabolism that interferes with both the gastrointestinal and tubular transport of the amino acids, cystine, ornithine, lysine, and arginine. Of these, cystine is the least soluble naturally occurring amino acid, and it precipitates to form stones when its concentration in the urine is excessive. It is possible to lower cystine concentration by reducing methionine in the diet. However, this greatly restricts the protein content of the diet and is not well tolerated. Present therapy for patients with hyperuricemia, or cystine calculi, includes high fluid intake, alkalinization of the urine, and use of penicillamine, a drug that keeps cystine in solution. The side effects of this drug limit its use, however.[71]

### Acid and alkaline ash diets

The mineral elements in food are sometimes referred to as "ash" because they are not oxidized in metabolism. They form a residue that is eventually excreted either by the intestinal tract (most of the calcium and the iron) or in the urine. By changing the composition of the diet, the urine may be made either acid or alkaline. An acid urine may act to limit enlargement of already present alkaline stones, or prevent their further formation. Likewise, an alkaline urine may affect the less common acid stones in the same manner.

Most vegetables and fruits yield an alkaline ash and, therefore, aid in the formation of an alkaline urine. Meats, fish, fowl, eggs, and cereals give an acid ash when metabolized, causing the urine to be acid. Since much of the calcium of milk is excreted in the intestinal tract while the remainder of its mineral content is excreted in the urine, its effect on the acidity or the alkalinity of urine is problematical.

Although most physicians alter the $pH$ of the urine by prescribing the appropriate medication, occasionally a diet may be ordered to achieve a change in $pH$. On an alkaline ash diet, sometimes used for oxalate stones, vegetables and fruits should predominate, while meat, eggs, and cereals are somewhat restricted. Conversely, on an acid ash diet, which may be prescribed for calcium phosphate and calcium carbonate stones, meat, eggs, and cereals are liberally included and vegetables and fruits are restricted. On either diet milk is restricted to 1 pt. All foods should be sufficient in quantity for nutritional adequacy.

## Study questions and activities

1. What are the basic metabolic functions of the kidney? Using Figure 32-1, explain how they are accomplished.
2. What substances are filtered from the blood? Which are largely reabsorbed? Which are excreted?
3. Plan a day's menu for a 10 year old boy with acute glomerulonephritis whose diet prescription is 2000 calories, 30 g of protein, 800 mg of sodium, and 800 ml of fluid.
4. In which circumstances is protein usually restricted in the diet of a patient with nephritis? What is the purpose of this restriction? When may the protein in the diet be increased over normal needs? Why?
5. Why may sodium be restricted in kidney disease?
6. What is the danger of an increased potassium level in the blood?
7. What is meant by the sodium depletion syndrome? How may the physician treat it?
8. Why are fluids restricted in kidney failure? On what basis is the amount of fluid allowed calculated?
9. Using the Protein-, Phosphorus-, Sodium-, and Potassium-Restricted Diet Exchange Lists in Table 32-7, calculate a Pattern Dietary for a 16 year old boy who is receiving hemodialysis. His physician has ordered a diet containing 60 g of protein, 1500 mg of sodium, 2000 mg of potassium, and fluids restricted to 1000 ml. The boy is in school, continually hungry, and rather anxious.
10. Name some of the seasonings the boy's mother may use on the above diet to make it more palatable. How would you advise him to incorporate polyunsaturated fats into his diet?
11. Make out a menu for a day for a patient critically ill with nephrosclerosis and uremia. His physician has ordered 30 g of protein, 500 mg of sodium, 1500 mg of potassium, fluids restricted to 800 ml. The patient is anorectic and has some nausea. The diet should be bland and semisoft.
12. Look at Table 4 in Section 4. What foods are high in sodium? In potassium? Take average servings of foods into account.
13. Make out a menu for a day for a patient who has a calcium phosphate kidney stone, and who has been placed on a moderately low calcium and phosphorus diet. He is young and considers himself a gourmet.

## References

1. Kerr DNS: In Beeson PB, McDermott W, Wyngaarden JB (eds): Cecil's Textbook of Medicine, 15th ed, pp 1351–1367. Philadelphia, WB Saunders, 1979
2. Burton BT: J Am Diet Assoc 65:627, 1974
3. Flamenbaum W, Kaufman JS: The Kidney 9, No. 5:21, 1976
4. Freedman EA et al: N Engl J Med 298:368, 1978
5. Oreopoulos DG: Dial Transplant 8, No. 5:460, 1979
6. Kopple JD: In Massry SC, Sellers AL (eds): Clinical Aspects of Uremia and Dialysis, pp 453–489. Springfield IL, Charles C Thomas, 1976
7. Simmons JM et al: N Engl J Med 285:653, 1971
8. Holliday MA: Kidney Int 7:S-73, 1975
9. Giordano C: J Lab Clin Med 62:231, 1963
10. Giovannetti S, Maggiore Q: Lancet 1:1000, 1964
11. Shaw AB et al: Q J Med 34:237, 1965
12. Bailey GL, Sullivan NR: J Am Diet Assoc 52:125, 1968
13. Kopple JD: Postgrad Med 64:135, 1978
14. Ritz E et al: Am J Clin Nutr 31:1703, 1978
15. Kopple JD, Coburn JW: JAMA 27:41, 1974
16. Grodstein G, Kopple JD: Kidney Int 16:953, 1979
17. Sargent J et al: Am J Clin Nutr 31:1696, 1978
18. Bennett N: Council on Renal Nutrition News, National Kidney Foundation 4, No. 2:8, 1980
19. Bergstrom J et al: Clin Nephrol 3:187, 1975
20. Walser M et al: J Clin Invest 52:678, 1973
21. Varcoe R et al: Clin Sci Mol Med 48:379, 1975
22. Burns J et al: Am J Clin Nutr 31:1767, 1978
23. Walser M: Am J Clin Nutr 33:1629, 1980
24. Kopple J et al: Trans Am Soc Artif Intern Organs 15:302, 1969
25. Kluthe R et al: Am J Clin Nutr 31:1812, 1978
26. Blumenkrantz MJ et al: J Am Diet Assoc 73:251, 1978
27. Blumenkrantz MJ: In Diamond LH (ed): Proceedings of The Renal Physicians Association Symposium on Peritoneal Dialysis, Vol 3, p 9, New York, 1979
28. DeLuca HF: N Engl J Med 27:479, 1973
29. Slatopolsky E et al: Kidney Int 2:147, 1972
30. Maschio G et al: Am J Clin Nutr 33:1546, 1980
31. Llach F et al: Kidney Int 12:459, 1977
32. Massry SG: Am J Clin Nutr 33:1530, 1980
33. Kopple JD, Coburn JW: Medicine 52:597, 1973
34. Nortman DF, Coburn JW: Postgrad Med 64, No. 5:123, 1978
35. Johnson WJ: Nephron 17:241, 1976
36. Kopple JD, Swendseid ME: Kidney Int (Suppl 2) 7:S-79, 1975
37. Swendseid ME: J Am Diet Assoc 70:488, 1977
38. Stone WJ et al: Am J Clin Nutr 28:950, 1975
39. Kleiner MJ et al: Am J Clin Nutr 33:1612, 1980
40. Stone WJ: Dial Transplant 6, No. 6:51, 1977
41. Smith FR, Goodman DS: J Clin Invest 50:2426, 1971
42. Sanfelippo ML et al: Kidney Int 11:54, 1977
43. Reaven GM et al: Am J Clin Nutr 33:1476, 1980
44. Sanfelippo ML et al: Kidney Int 14:180, 1978
45. Gokal R et al: Am J Clin Nutr 31:1915, 1978
46. Wrong OM: In Beeson, McDermott and Wyngaarden, Cecil's Textbook of Medicine, 15th ed, pp 1386–1402
47. Bricker NS: In Beeson, McDermott and Wyngaarden, Cecil's Textbook of Medicine, 15th ed, pp 1367–1375
48. Glassock RJ: Hosp Pract 14:105, Nov, 1979
49. Blackburn SL: Am J Clin Nutr 70:31, 1977
50. Procci WR: Psychosomatics 19:16, 1978

51. Miller RW, St Jeor ST: Dial Transplant 9, No. 10:968, 1980
52. Blumenkrantz MJ et al: Kidney Int 16:882, 1979
53. Wells E: Dial Transplant 9, No. 3:224, 1980
54. Oreopoulos DG et al: Dial Transplant 9, No. 3:224, 1980
55. Moncrief JW, Popovich RP: In Controversies in Nephrology, Vol 1, p 35. Washington, DC, Georgetown University, 1979
56. Ponticelli C et al: Nephron 20:189, 1978
57. Liddle VR et al: Dial Transplant 6:9, 1977
58. Blumenkrantz MJ et al: Am J Clin Nutr 33:1567, 1980
59. Harvey KB et al: Am J Clin Nutr 33:1586, 1980
60. Walters FM, Crumley SJ (eds): Patient Care Audit: A Quality Assurance Procedure Manual for Dietitians. Chicago, American Dietetic Association Quality Assurance Committee, 1978
61. Broadus AE: In Coe FL (ed): Nephrolithiasis, pp 59–85. New York, Churchill Livingstone, 1980
62. Smith LH et al: N Engl J Med 298:87, 1978
63. Thomas WC: In Beeson, McDermott and Wyngaarden, Cecil's Textbook of Medicine, 15th ed, pp 1443–1447
64. Lemann J Jr: In Coe, Nephrolithiasis, pp 86–115
65. Ing TS, Kark RM: In Schreider HA, Anderson CE, Coursin DB (eds): Nutritional Support of Medical Practice, pp 367–383. New York, Harper & Row, 1977
66. Coe FL: Ann Intern Med 87:404, 1977
67. Ettinger B: Am J Med 61:200, 1976
68. Kopple JD: In Hodges RE (ed): Human Nutrition: A Comprehensive Treatise, Vol 4, Metabolic and Clinical Applications, pp 409–457. New York, Plenum Press, 1979
69. Welcome Trends in Urology 2, No. 6:4, 1980
70. Holmes EW: In Coe, Nephrolithiasis, pp 188–207
71. Halperin EC, Thier SO: In Coe, Nephrolithiasis, pp 208–230

## Supplementary readings

Burton BT: Nutritional implications of renal disease. I. Current overview and general principles. J Am Diet Assoc 70:479, 1977

Coe FL: Nephrolithiasis. The Kidney 12, No. 1:1, 1979

Gahl GM et al: Outpatient evaluation of dietary intake and nitrogen removal in continuous ambulatory peritoneal dialysis. Ann Intern Med 94:643, 1981

Giordano C: The role of diet in renal disease. Hosp Pract 12:113, 1977

Hamburger RJ: The management of uremia. Am Fam Physician 16, No. 3:125, 1977

Knochel RP: Pathogenesis of uremic syndrome. Postgrad Med 64:88, 1978

Kopple JD: Nutritional management of chronic renal failure. Postgrad Med 64:135, 1978

Massry SG, Ritz E: Pathogenesis of secondary hyperparathyroidism in renal failure. Is there a controversy? Arch Intern Med 138:853, 1978

Nortman DF, Coburn JW: Renal osteodystrophy in end-stage renal failure. Postgrad Med 64, No. 5:123, 1978

Popovich RP et al: Continuous ambulatory peritoneal dialysis. Ann Intern Med 88, No. 4:449, 1978

Walser M, Mitch W: Dietary management of renal failure. The Kidney 10, No. 3:13, 1977

Watson L: Dietary aspects of renal care. Dial Transplant 9, No. 5:459, 1980

Wineman RJ et al: Nutritional implications of renal disease. II. The dietitian's key role in studies of dialysis therapy. J Am Diet Assoc 70:483, 1977

## Patient resources

Aproten Low Protein Products. Henkel Corporation, Dietary Specialties, 4620 W. 77th Street, Minneapolis, MN 55435

Cost J: Dietary Management of Renal Disease. Charles B. Slack, Inc., 6900 Grove Road, Thorofare, NJ 08086

Diet Instruction for Diabetics with Kidney Disease. Council on Renal Nutrition of Michigan, Kidney Foundation of Michigan, 3378 Washtenaw Avenue, Ann Arbor, MI 48104

Greene M: Lenox Hill Hospital, The Gourmet Renal Nutrition Cookbook. 100 East 77th Street, New York, NY 10021

Jones W: Diet Guide for Patients on Chronic Dialysis. DHEW Publ. No. (NIH) 75-685. Washington, DC, United States Government Printing Office, 1975

Low Protein Baking Mix and Bread Mix. Cellu-Featherweight, Chicago Dietetic Supply, Inc., 405 E. Shawmut Avenue, La Grange, IL 60525

Low Protein Products (wheat starch, baking mix, bread, cookies). Henkel Corporation, Dietary Specialties, 4620 W. 77th Street, Minneapolis, MN 55435

Margie J et al: The Mayo Clinic Renal Diet Cookbook. New York, Western, 1974

The Renal Meal Pattern in Pictures. Greenville Dialysis Center, Doctors' Park, Building 6, Greenville, NC 27834

St Jeor S et al: Meal Planning for People with Kidney Disease. Salt Lake City, University of Utah Press, 1978

Understanding Your Renal Diet. Iowa Council of Renal Nutritionists, Kidney Foundation of Iowa, 8611 Hickman Road, Des Moines, IA 50322

*For further references see Bibliography in Part 4.*

# Liver Disease

**33**

The nutritional care in liver disease shares many of the characteristics of nutritional care in renal disease because the disease process can alter the structure and function of the liver so that its metabolic functions are impaired. These alterations, particularly in progressive chronic liver disease leading to end-stage hepatic failure, also require modifications in the dietary intake of energy, protein, fluid, and electrolytes. Liver disease may be acute or chronic, progressing to end-stage hepatic failure, and the acute phase may or may not progress to the chronic phase. Because the liver is unique in its ability to regenerate cells, the successful treatment (primarily dietary) of the early stages of liver disease usually results in the recovery of adequate liver function.

Many patients with liver disease present the same challenges to nutritional care as those with renal disease because they also experience nausea and vomiting, and fatigue due to anemia; and, in end-stage hepatic failure (hepatic coma), they are often disoriented. In one aspect the medical care of the patient with liver disease differs from the care of the renal patient. For those patients whose liver disease is due to alcoholism, the treatment is both medical and psychiatric because alcoholism is an addictive process.

Before proceeding with the discussion of liver disease and diet therapy, the reader is urged to review Chapter 9, *Nutrient Utilization*, as well as the metabolism of alcohol[1,2] and the structure and function of the liver.[3] Diseases of the gallbladder and pancreas, which are usually discussed with liver disease, are presented in Chapter 26, *Gastrointestinal Disease*, because the nutritional problems they present are more directly related to this pathology.

## Normal metabolic functions of the liver

Because of the diversity of its metabolic functions, the liver is one of the most important glandular organs in the body. All nutrients that are ingested and absorbed are transported directly to the liver by the portal circulation, with the exception of long-chain fatty acids and fat-soluble vitamins. Through the systemic circulation a portion of the long-chain fatty acids and the fat-soluble vitamins are also transported to the liver. The liver uses the nutrients in both synthetic and degradative metabolic processes and also stores nutrients, particularly the fat-soluble vitamins, vitamin $B_{12}$, and glucose, as glycogen.

### Amino acids

The liver regulates the distribution of the amino acids to the cells of the body where they are used in the synthesis of cellular proteins. It synthesizes many protein enzymes and the plasma proteins, fibrinogen, prothrombin, albumin, and most of the alpha and beta globulins. Urea, the end product of the degradation of all amino acid nitrogen, is synthesized in the liver (see Chap. 9).

### Carbohydrate

The liver converts glucose, fructose, and galactose to glycogen and through glycogenolysis provides glucose to maintain energy metabolism in the brain, muscles, adipose, and other body cells. An excess of the intermediary metabolites of glucose are converted to fats. Through the gluconeogenic pathway it also synthesizes glucose from the deaminated amino acids.

### Lipids

The liver converts fats to very low-density lipoproteins, which are transported to other tissues for storage as triglycerides. The liver synthesizes cholesterol from acetyl-CoA through the squalene pathway and is the only organ in the body that synthesizes ketone bodies.

### Minerals and vitamins

An important function of the liver is the storage of iron, as ferritin, and copper, which are made available for the synthesis of the hemoglobin in red blood cells. Other minerals, such as zinc and magnesium, are also present in the liver where they function as a part of many essential enzymatic reactions in intermediary metabolism. For example, alcohol dehydrogenase in the liver requires zinc for its activity.

Most of the vitamin A stored in the body is found in the liver. Although the major portion of ingested carotene is converted to vitamin A in the cells of the gastrointestinal tract, some carotene is also converted in the liver. The other fat-soluble vitamins, D, E, and K, are stored in the liver. The B vitamins are also found there in considerable amounts, where they function as parts of the enzyme systems in intermediary metabolism.

### Bile

Bile, which is composed of bile acids, pigments (bilirubin) and salts, cholesterol, and water, is synthesized by the cells of the liver and flows through the bile ducts to the cystic duct to be stored in the gallbladder (see Chap. 26 for the role of bile in digestion).

### Detoxification

A major degradative function of the liver is detoxification. It detoxifies many substances, such as hormones and drugs. For example, oral contraceptives, morphine, and barbiturates are inactivated by the liver to terminate their effect.

## Metabolic aberrations

It is not surprising that an organ that performs as many critical metabolic functions as the liver does should cause many aberrations in intermediary metabolism when it is diseased. The metabolic aberrations reflect primarily alterations in structure and function due to the disease processes. These alterations can be classified as fatty infiltration of hepatic cells; diffuse inflammation with hepatic cell necrosis and regenerative activity; and loss of functional liver cells due to necrosis accompanied by fibrosis of supporting tissues and the vascular bed and nodular regeneration of the remaining cell mass.

### Fatty infiltration

There is an excessive accumulation of lipids in the cytoplasm of the liver cells in fatty liver disease, which may result from an increased influx of fatty acids into the liver; an increase in fatty acid synthesis by the hepatic cells; a decrease in fatty acid oxidation; or, a decreased synthesis of protein for triglyceride transport out of the liver. Fatty livers occur in poorly controlled diabetes, obesity, acute and chronic alcoholism,[4] and energy-protein malnutrition in infancy and early childhood, and it is frequently a complication of long-standing heart failure. Severe acute fatty liver is produced by hepatotoxins, such as carbontetrachloride and DDT.

Removal of alcohol or hepatotoxins, treatment of the underlying disease, and appropriate diet usually result in a decrease in the accumulation of lipids in the hepatic cells. However, there may be some necrosis of liver cells produced by chronic alcohol ingestion or by hepatotoxins. Diet is determined by the underlying disease, for example, diabetes, obesity, and heart disease. An adequate diet appropriate for age is required for malnourished infants and children, and one appropriate for weight, sex, and age should be used for adults whose fatty liver is due to alcoholism.

### Diffuse inflammation (hepatitis)

There are two forms of hepatitis—acute and chronic. Viral infection is the most common cause of acute hepatitis although it may be induced by drugs, alcohol, and hepatotoxins. The infectious form of acute hepatitis is caused by two different agents, hepatitis A and hepatitis B, and both can be transmitted by the oral or parenteral route. Hepatitis A was formerly called *infectious hepatitis* and hepatitis B, *serum hepatitis.* There is a third form of hepatitis, non-A and non-B, but the specific virus that causes the disease has not been identified.[5] The cause of chronic hepatitis is unknown in most cases, although some people with hepatitis B do develop it.

In addition to the inflammatory process in hepatitis, there is necrosis and regenerative activity in the hepatic cells and, in some people, bile stasis with jaundice. There is an elevation of serum transaminase and bilirubin and a decrease in plasma prothrombin levels due to hepatic cell necrosis. In acute viral hepatitis the total serum proteins are usually normal or there may be a slight decrease in serum albumin, while in chronic hepatitis there is usually a decrease in serum albumin levels. Anorexia and fatigue followed by nausea, vomiting, and diarrhea are common symptoms with all types of hepatitis. In acute hepatitis the anorexia is often severe, resulting in a strong aversion to food.

During the nausea and vomiting phase, a full liquid diet as tolerated is prescribed or, if necessary, a standard tube feeding is used (see liquid diets and tube feedings, Chap. 27). When food is tolerated, a diet adequate in energy and nutrients is provided to support the regenerative activity of the hepatic cells and to meet the total metabolic needs of the body. For the adult the diet should contain 35 to 40 calories per kilogram of body weight with 12% to 15% of the energy from protein, about 35% from fat, and the remainder from carbohydrate. The diet contains 75 g to 90 g protein, about 80 g fat, and 300 g carbohydrate for an adult requiring 2500 calories per day. It should be adequate in minerals and vitamins. However, depending on the patient's problems, supplementary minerals and vitamins may be required. Davidson has observed that patients with acute hepatitis eat better if they consume frequent small meals rather than three meals a day.[6]

If massive necrosis of the liver cells occurs in severe hepatitis, a high or even normal intake of protein can induce hepatic coma with hyperammonemia (see discussion of protein in *Diet Therapy* in this chapter). Therefore, the protein in the diet may be severely restricted or excluded in this case until there is improvement in hepatic function.

## Loss of functional hepatic cells (cirrhosis)

Cirrhosis is a generic term used to describe all forms of liver disease characterized by a significant loss of cells.[7] The most common types are Laennec's, postnecrotic, biliary, and cardiac or congestive cirrhosis. Cirrhosis also occurs due to congenital anomalies of the liver, in hemachromatosis (abnormal iron metabolism) and in Wilson's disease (abnormal copper metabolism). Alcoholism is usually, but not always, a factor in the development of Laennec's cirrhosis, while viral hepatitis is a factor in many cases of postnecrotic cirrhosis.

Although regenerative activity occurs in cirrhosis, the progressive loss of liver cells exceeds cell replacement. At the same time there is also progressive distortion of the vascular system, which results in interference with the portal blood flow through the liver. In early cirrhosis there is a variable elevation in serum bilirubin and transaminase levels. The serum albumin and urea levels are usually depressed, and anemia is a common problem.

In severe advanced cirrhosis there are four major complications: portal hypertension, ascites, esophageal varices, and hepatic encephalopathy. The distortion of the vascular bed of the liver leads to portal hypertension and the shunting of portal blood into the portalsystemic venous collateral circulation. With portal hypertension ascites occurs; there is sodium retention, impaired water excretion, and decreased plasma oncotic pressure because of severe hypoalbuminemia. The shunting of portal blood into the systemic circulation causes engorgement of the lower esophageal veins (esophageal varices). When the varices rupture, severe hemorrhage occurs. At the same time there is a deficiency of prothrombin with poor blood clotting. The blood urea nitrogen, which is synthesized primarily in the liver, is low normal or low.

Hepatic encephalopathy occurs with portalsystemic shunting of blood. It is characterized by drowsiness, lethargy, fetor hepaticus (liver breath), asterixis (flapping tremors of the hands and tongue when extended), and disorientation.[7] These patients have a hypersecretion of glucagon, an elevation of the blood levels of the aromatic amino acids as well as ammonia (hyperammonemia), and a decrease in the blood levels of the branched chain amino acids. The relation of these metabolic aberrations to hepatic encephalopathy is under intensive investigation at present. Fischer and co-workers[8] theorize that the inability of the liver to synthesize urea leads to hyperammonemia. The excessive blood levels of ammonia in turn raise the concentration of aromatic amino acids in the brain. The aromatic amino acids, in turn, alter neurotransmitter metabolism, and the alteration in the metabolism of the neurotransmitters causes the encephalopathy. Untreated, the encephalopathy leads to coma and, ultimately, to death.

In the treatment of early cirrhosis the diet for adults should provide 35 to 40 calories or more and 1 g of protein of high biologic value per kilogram of body weight, with an adequate intake of minerals and vitamins. In biliary cirrhosis dietary fat is usually not well tolerated because of a significant decrease in bile flow, so that the intake should be restricted to 30 g to 40 g daily (see *Low-fat Diet*, Chap. 26). In hepatic encephalopathy, as the ability of the liver to synthesize urea decreases,[9] the dietary protein is restricted to tolerance and limited to proteins of high biologic value (see *Diet Therapy* section in this chapter). With ascites the sodium is restricted to 200 mg to 500 mg (10 mEq–20 mEq) per day, and fluid intake is restricted to the amount lost each day. The diet may also be restricted in roughage if esophageal varices are present but not bleeding. If esophageal bleeding occurs, a liquid diet restricted in fluid, protein, and sodium, if necessary, may be required.

# Alcohol and liver disease

In the United States the ingestion of alcohol is one of the most common causes of all categories of liver disease—fatty infiltration, hepatitis, and cirrhosis. It is estimated that there are 10 million people who can be classified as alcoholics.[10] Ten to twenty percent of chronic users of alcohol[7] develop cirrhosis; in those who do not abstain from alcohol, the cirrhosis can progress to end-stage hepatic failure. The development of alcoholic cirrhosis appears to be related to the duration of alcohol intake and the amount consumed daily. Research indicates that the mean duration of alcohol intake to produce cirrhosis is 10 years, and the dose is estimated to be in excess of 160 g of alcohol daily,[11] for example, 16 oz of Scotch whiskey.

For many years it was thought that all forms of alcoholic liver disease were not caused by alcohol *per se* but by the inadequate diets consumed by many chronic alcoholics, and it has been common practice to advise individuals who drink appreciable amounts of alcohol daily to eat an adequate diet to avoid liver disease. However, the current research of Rubin and Lieber[11] demonstrates that alcohol is the causative agent. Using baboons, which are phylogenetically closer to man than other laboratory animals, they have observed in their animals the development of fatty livers with progression to alcoholic hepatitis and cirrhosis when fed a nutritionally adequate diet with a daily isocaloric substitution for carbohydrate of 4.5 g to 8.3 g of alcohol per kilogram of body weight. They conclude that adequate nutrient intake with the continued intake of excessive quantities of alcohol will not prevent the development of fatty livers, alcoholic hepatitis, or cirrhosis.

Recent research has shown that alcohol and malnutrition are synergistic in their effects on the development of hepatic cirrhosis.[4] The consumption of alcohol directly damages the hepatocyte and increases the deposition of hepatic collagen, which promotes fibrogenesis in the supporting structures of the liver. Malnutrition in the alcoholic patient is caused by a number of factors. (1) The intake of energy and nutrients may be inadequate, as chronic alcohol intake can decrease food intake. Folic acid deficiency with megaloblastic anemia and thiamin, riboflavin, niacin, and pyridoxine deficiency is frequently observed in patients with alcoholic cirrhosis. (2) Alcohol consumption combined with folic acid deficiency can cause intestinal malabsorption. There is evidence that alcohol has a toxic effect on the absorptive cells of the small intestine and that folic acid deficiency adversely affects the functional capacity of the absorptive cells. (3) Alcohol *per se* interferes with hepatic cellular metabolism of vitamins such as folic acid, pyridoxine and thiamin. (4) Decreased storage and increased excretion of nutrients have been observed in the patient with cirrhosis. Decreased storage of vitamins is due to decreased storage

space with cellular necrosis and tissue fibrosis. Also, the increased urinary excretion of zinc and magnesium has been observed.

Alcoholic cirrhotic patients frequently have the polyneuritis of thiamin deficiency and the cheilosis and beefy red tongue of riboflavin deficiency. The Wernicke-Korsakoff syndrome, an acute form of thiamin deficiency, can also occur.[12] With abstinence from alcohol, adequate energy and nutrient intake corrects the malnutrition of chronic alcoholism and, at the same time, supports the regenerative activity of the liver cells provided the disease process has not progressed to end-stage hepatic failure.

## Diet therapy
### Principles of diet therapy

The following discussion focuses primarily on diet therapy in advanced cirrhosis, including the complication of ascites, esophageal bleeding, hepatic encephalopathy and coma.

### Energy

All patients with liver disease require an adequate energy intake (approximately 35–40 calories per kilogram for adults). Without adequate energy supplied by carbohydrate and fat, amino acids from food and body cells are deaminated in intermediary metabolism to contribute to energy needs through the gluconeogenic pathway. This decreases the quantity of amino acids available for liver cell regeneration and, in advanced cirrhotics, increases the amount of ammonia available for ureagenesis.

In advanced cirrhosis with a decrease in the number of functioning liver cells, 50% to 60% or more of the calories should be derived from carbohydrate. The research of Walker and his associates[13] suggests that in this situation carbohydrate is important, not only as a source of energy, but also as a depressor of glucagon and, therefore, gluconeogenesis. Walker's group supplemented the diets of five cirrhotics who were moderately intolerant of protein (40 g–60 g per day) with hourly feedings of glucose (20 g). Insulin blood levels increased significantly, and glucagon levels were significantly depressed; the blood ammonia level did not rise in any of the subjects. This research also suggests that the high carbohydrate diet patterns for advanced cirrhosis should include six to eight or more feedings daily.

### Protein

Hyperammonemia can develop in acute hepatitis or advanced cirrhosis. To reduce the blood ammonia levels in pre-coma, dietary protein is restricted to tolerance. The restriction may vary depending on the patient's situation from 0.3 g to 0.8 g of protein per kilogram of body weight (20 g–60 g of protein per day for a 70-kg man). In hepatic coma all protein is excluded from the feedings. A tube feeding of glucose or glucose and fat or intravenous glucose is used to provide energy. As the patient improves, small quantities of protein as tolerated are added to the diet. The first addition may be as little as 10 g of protein per day. Any patient with advanced cirrhosis who has experienced pre-coma or coma may need to restrict protein intake to tolerance for the rest of his life.

The work of Rudman and co-workers[14] suggests that the protein used in the diet of any patient with advanced cirrhosis should be primarily of high biologic value, not only to supply the essential amino acids but also to control blood ammonia levels. In both cirrhotic patients and in normal people, they tested the ammonigenicity of 18 of the 20 amino acids that occur in food. They did not test methionine and cystine, the sulfur-containing amino acids. Methionine is known to precipitate coma in cirrhotics with portal shunting even without hyperammonemia.[7] From the results of their study Rudman and co-workers classified the 18 amino acids into three groups based on the increase observed in blood ammonia levels when the acids were fed to the cirrhotic subjects. Group A, with the highest ammonigenic potency, contains seven amino acids—glycine, serine, threonine, glutamine, histidine, lysine, and asparagine. The other two groups, B and C, containing the other 11 amino acids tested, were significantly less ammonigenic than the seven acids in Group A. With the exception of threonine and lysine, the amino acids in Group A are nonessential amino acids. Rudman and co-workers concluded that the Group A amino acids have a greater ammonigenic potency than those in Groups B and C because they are deaminated, not transaminated, in body tissues, which releases ammonia into the circulation; and that the ammonigenicity of the Group A amino acids is directly dependent on the dietary intake. They recommended that, at least theoretically, the results of their study might be applied to planning diets limited in Group A amino acids yet otherwise nutritionally adequate.

Although the evidence is limited, it appears that a diet reduced in ammonigenicity can be achieved by applying the same principles as those used in planning the protein content in the protein-restricted diet for renal disease (see Chap. 32, *Renal Disease*). The amino acid content of selected foods is available (see Table 3, Part 4). However, there are limited data on the glutamine and asparagine content of foods. One major food source of glutamine is cereal protein, and of asparagine plant protein. For example, 40% of the amino acids in the gliadin fraction of the wheat protein, gluten, is glutamine.[15] A significant reduction in glutamine intake can be achieved by using low-protein wheatstarch products (see Chap. 26). The Group A amino acids, exclusive of glutamine and asparagine, in the quantity of milk, egg, and meat containing 7 g of protein are given in Table 33-1. Note that the total quantity of ammonigenic amino acids in milk is less

than in egg or meat. Therefore, the choice of milk or milk and egg appears to be the best when protein is limited to 20 g or less per day because of severe protein intolerance.

Although limited to the experience with three cirrhotic patients, Greenberger[16] achieved a reduction in blood ammonia levels in patients with chronic hepatic encephalopathy using a diet containing 40 g of vegetable protein. The vegetable protein diet contained lower amounts of the Group A amino acids and lower amounts of the aromatic amino acids than a diet containing comparable amounts of protein from meat, eggs, and milk. Further research is needed to document these findings.

Other measures are also used to control blood ammonia levels in advanced cirrhosis. It is estimated that approximately 25% of the blood urea nitrogen normally diffuses into the lumen of the gastrointestinal tract where it is hydrolyzed by urease, which is of bacterial origin. The ammonia released by this process is reabsorbed primarily in the colon. Other sources of ammonia in the gut are amino acids in the colon and, possibly, ammonia occurring naturally in foods.[7] If gastrointestinal bleeding is present, the digested blood may also be a source of ammonia. Neomycin, an antibiotic, is used to sterilize the colon to reduce urease. Lactulose, a nonabsorbable, nonmetabolized, synthetic disaccharide is also used in the treatment of hepatic coma. The lactulose is metabolized by colonic bacteria to organic acids, which lowers the $pH$ in the colon. The excess hydrogen ions convert ammonia ($NH_3$) to ammonium ($NH_4$), which is not readily absorbed.[7]

### Vitamins and minerals

With the restriction of protein, and, if low-protein wheatstarch products are used as a major source of calories, it is strongly recommended that nutrient intake from food be supplemented with vitamin and mineral preparations including all the B vitamins, iron, and trace minerals.

### Table 33-1. Milligrams of Group A Amino Acids in Foods Containing 7 Grams of Protein

| Amino Acids (mg) | Milk (Whole) * (200 g) | Egg * (55 g) | Meat † ‡ (44 g) |
|---|---|---|---|
| Glycine | 140 | 202 | 436 |
| Serine | 358 | 461 | 285 |
| Threonine | 298 | 298 | 311 |
| Histidine | 178 | 146 | 245 |
| Lysine | 522 | 410 | 615 |
| Totals | 1495 | 1517 | 1892 |

*Calculated from Composition of Foods—Dairy and Egg Products: Raw, Processed, and Prepared. Agriculture Handbook No. 8-1. Washington, DC, USDA, 1976.

†Hamburger.

‡Calculated from Amino Acid Content of Foods. Home Economics Research Report No. 4. Washington, DC, USDA.

## Electrolytes and fluids

If ascites is present, sodium intake is restricted to 200 mg to 500 mg (10 mEq–20 mEq) per day, and fluid is restricted to the amount lost each day. The limited sodium and fluid intake may also be combined with some level of protein restriction. Sodium-restricted diets are discussed in Chapter 31.

Potassium is usually not a problem in cirrhosis. However, renal failure commonly occurs in end-stage hepatic failure. When this occurs the potassium in the diet may also be limited. Potassium-restricted diets are discussed in Chapter 32.

## Frequency of meals

From the work of Walker and his associates[13] and the observations of Davidson,[6] the patient with advanced cirrhosis should consume frequent small feedings. Also, the patient with severe ascites needs frequent small feedings because the fluid collection in his abdomen makes it impossible for him to eat large quantities of food at a meal.

### Table 33-2. Protein–Sodium-Restricted Exchange System

| Food Group | Household Measure | Weight (g) | Protein (g) | Sodium* (mg) |
|---|---|---|---|---|
| Milk exchanges | 8 oz | 240 | 8 | 120 |
| Meat exchanges | 1 oz | 30 | 7 | 25 |
| Egg | 1 | 50 | 7 | 70 |
| Vegetable exchanges | ½ c | 100 | 2 | 9 |
| Fruit exchanges | 1 serving | Varies | 1 | 2 |
| Bread exchanges | Varies | Varies | 2 | 5 |
| Fat exchanges | 1 tsp | 5 | 0 | 0 |

*Foods produced, processed, or prepared without the addition of any sodium compound.

### Table 33-3. A 1500-Calorie, 75-g Protein, 500-mg Sodium Diet Pattern

| Food Group | Amount | Protein (g) | Sodium* (mg) | Energy (Kcalories) |
|---|---|---|---|---|
| Milk, whole | 1 pint | 16 | 240 | 340 |
| Meat | 4 oz, cooked | 28 | 100 | 300 |
| Egg | 1 | 7 | 70 | 75 |
| Vegetables | 4 ½-c servings | 8 | 36 | 100 |
| Fruit | 3 servings | 3 | 6 | 120 |
| Bread (unsalted) | 6 servings | 12 | 30 | 420 |
| Fat (unsalted) | 3 tsp | 0 | 0 | 135 |
| Totals | | 74 | 482 | 1490† |

*Foods produced, processed, or prepared without the addition of any sodium compound.

†Add sugar and additional unsalted fat, if tolerated, for 1800 to 2000 calories.

See Table 31-10, with protein calculation added.

## Summary

Diets for the treatment of advanced cirrhosis are adequate in energy, restricted to tolerance in protein using food proteins of high biologic value, usually restricted in sodium, and, if necessary, limited in fluids. If required, nasogastric feeding may be used in the absence of esophageal bleeding.

## Planning the diet pattern

### Protein-sodium-restricted exchange system

The protein values for the food Exchanges in Table 33-2 are the same as those in the basic Exchange System (see Table 24-2, Chapter 24) with the exception that a value of 1.0 g of protein per serving is given for fruit. As in the diet for patients with renal disease, the protein in fruit is calculated in the diet pattern of patients with cirrhosis to reflect the potential nitrogen in all foods. The sodium values in Table 33-2 are the same as those in Table 31-1, *Sodium-restricted Exchange System*, Chapter 31, and apply only to foods produced, processed, and prepared without the addition of any sodium compounds.

The Protein-Sodium Exchange System is used to calculate patterns for diet prescriptions ranging from 10 g to 60 g protein and 250 mg to 500 mg or more of sodium per day. If the diet prescription specifies only proteins of high biologic value, then the low-protein wheatstarch products are used as Bread Exchanges when the protein is restricted to 30 g or less (see Table 32-7, Chap. 32).

### Exchange Lists

The Sodium-restricted Exchange Lists in Table 31-2, Chapter 31, are used to plan the daily menus for protein- and sodium-restricted diets, and the table is not repeated in this chapter. The discussion in Chapter 31 on the foods used in these diets and the material on convenience foods and sodium in water supplies should be reviewed.

### Calculating the diet pattern

Tables 33-3, 33-4, and 33-5 demonstrate the calculation of a 1500-Calorie Diet Pattern with varying amounts of protein and sodium. The diet pattern in Table 33-3 is the same as the one in Table 31-10, Chapter 31. This diet pattern contains approximately 75 g protein and 500 mg of sodium. The energy can be increased to 1800 or 2000 calories by the addition of sugar to fruits and cereals and an increase in the quantity of unsalted fat, if tolerated.

Table 33-4 demonstrates a diet pattern containing approximately 60 g of protein and 500 mg of sodium, while Table 33-5 demonstrates a 1500-calorie diet containing approximately 35 g of protein and 250 mg of sodium. The diet pattern in Table 33-5 contains 1500 calories only if high-calorie, low-electrolyte supplements are used. If tolerated, additional unsalted fat can also be used to increase calories. However, the research of Walker and co-workers[6] suggests that patients with advanced cirrhosis might benefit more from the carbohydrate in the high-calorie, low-electrolyte supplements than the addition of unsalted fats.

If the diet for the patient with cirrhosis is limited in the Group A amino acids (see discussion of protein on p. 571), wheatstarch products are substituted for regular bread exchanges. In this situation the diet pattern is planned using the protein and sodium values in the exchange system in Table 32-6, Chapter 32. The exchange lists in Table 32-7 are used to plan menus. The potassium is not calculated in the diet pattern for the patient with cirrhosis unless renal as well as hepatic failure occurs.

### Parenteral and enteral feeding

A TPN product, F080,* which differs from the standard TPN formulas, is being used experimentally to treat the patient with severe hepatic failure complicated by encephalopathy. The quantity of the aromatic amino acids are reduced, and the branched chain amino acids are increased in F080 compared to the amino acid composition of the standard formulations. Fischer and co-workers[17] report that patients with hepatic encephalopathy due to Laennec's, postnecrotic, or biliary cirrhosis respond favorably to treatment with F080. The encephalopathy improves, the blood amino acid levels are normalized, and the blood ammonia levels decrease. The standard TPN solutions do not reverse the symptoms of encephalopathy in patients with severe hepatic failure.[18] As of 1981, F080 has not been released by FDA for general use.

A product for enteral or oral feeding, Hepatic-Aid,* is available for use with patients who can be tube fed or whose level of consciousness permits oral intake. The proportion of the aromatic to branched-chain amino acids is similar to that of F080. Per 1000 ml Hepatic-Aid contains 1670 kcal, 43.5 g amino acids, 37 g fat, and 293 g carbohydrate from maltodextrins and sucrose.[19] The osmolality is 900 mOsm. No vitamins or minerals have been added to the product. If used as a tube feeding, it must be administered by continuous drip to avoid the complications of a hyperosmolar solution. Freund and co-workers[20] report the use of Hepatic-Aid for 2 years by a patient with severe hepatic disease and chronic encephalopathy. The patient's daily diet was Hepatic-Aid equivalent to 24 g of amino acids, 20 g to 30 g food protein, and 2000 kcal. The patient's condition stabilized without any signs of encephalopathy.

### Special problems

Since the majority of hospitalized patients with liver disease are anorexic, their fluid and nutrient intake should be carefully monitored daily. Each morning an estimate of the patient's intake of energy, protein, and sodium for

the previous 24 hours should be recorded in his medical record. The physician needs this information so that he can correlate energy and nutrient intake with the patient's symptoms and laboratory data. Some appraisal of the mineral and vitamin intake should also be recorded so that supplementary preparations can be provided if necessary.

A record of the patient's food likes and dislikes should be obtained from the patient or a relative so that, so far as possible, he can be served foods and beverages that he will consume.

### Salt substitutes

Salt substitutes containing ammonia are not used to enhance the flavor of the sodium-restricted diets of patients with liver disease because the ammonia in the substitute can increase the quantity absorbed from the gastrointestinal tract. This is hazardous for patients prone to hyperammonemia.

**Table 33-4. A 1500-Calorie, 60-g Protein, 500-mg Sodium Diet Pattern**

| *Food Group* | *Amount* | *Protein* (g) | *Sodium** (mg) | *Energy* (Kcalories) |
|---|---|---|---|---|
| Milk, whole | 1 pint | 16 | 240 | 340 |
| Meat | 2 oz, cooked | 14 | 50 | 150 |
| Egg | 1 | 7 | 70 | 75 |
| Vegetables | 4 $\frac{1}{2}$-c servings | 8 | 36 | 100 |
| Fruit | 3 servings | 3 | 6 | 120 |
| Bread (unsalted) | 6 servings | 12 | 30 | 420 |
| Fat (unsalted) | 6 tsp | 0 | 0 | 270 |
| Totals | | 60 | 432 | 1475† |

*Foods produced, processed, and prepared without the addition of any sodium compound.

†Add sugar and additional unsalted fat, if tolerated, for 1800 to 2000 calories.

**Table 33-5. A 1500-Calorie, 35-g Protein, 250-mg Sodium Diet Pattern**

| *Food Group* | *Amount* | *Protein* (g) | *Sodium** (mg) | *Energy* (Kcalories) |
|---|---|---|---|---|
| Milk, whole | 8 oz | 8 | 120 | 170 |
| Meat | 0 | | | |
| Egg | 1 | 7 | 70 | 75 |
| Vegetables | 2 $\frac{1}{2}$-c servings | 4 | 18 | 50 |
| Fruit | 3 servings | 3 | 6 | 120 |
| Bread (unsalted) | 6 servings | 12 | 30 | 420 |
| Fat (unsalted) | 6 tsp | 0 | 0 | 270 |
| Totals | | 34 | 244 | 1105† |

*Foods produced, processed, or prepared without the addition of any sodium compound.

†Plus high-calorie, low-electrolyte supplement and additional unsalted fat, if tolerated, to supply 1500 or more calories.

*McGaw Laboratories, Irvine, CA 92714

### Esophageal bleeding

In patients with esophageal bleeding due to portal hypertension, surgical intervention may be required. A portacaval or other types of shunts[21] are made to relieve the pressure in the esophageal veins. If considerable liver damage has occurred before the surgery, the diet will continue to be restricted in protein and sodium after surgery.

## Counseling the patient

The patient with liver disease presents the nutrition counselor with a number of challenges, especially the patient with liver disease due to chronic alcoholism. Many of these patients have limited resources, little money, and inadequate living quarters; frequently they have alienated themselves from their families. At the same time, the health-care team often has difficulty in accepting them unconditionally.

If the patient has liver damage complicated by ascites, his diet will be severely restricted in sodium for 6 months or more to resolve the ascites. It may also be restricted in protein to some extent. Therefore, he needs help over time to learn how to manage his diet and information about where to buy sodium-restricted foods in his community (see *Counseling the Patient*, Chap. 32).

At the same time that the patient is accommodating himself to a restricted diet, he is also trying to learn to live without alcohol. If receptive, the patient can often be helped by a psychiatric counselor or by a community self-help group, such as Alcoholics Anonymous.

## Wilson's disease

Wilson's disease (hepatolenticular degeneration) is a degenerative disease characterized by the storage of excessive amounts of copper in the liver and other tissues. It is inherited as an autosomal recessive trait, and the disease is not detected until young adulthood, usually between 20 and 30 years of age. Approximately 98% of serum copper is bound normally to a specific protein, ceruloplasmin. It has been demonstrated that patients with Wilson's disease have a decreased amount of ceruloplasmin with which to bind serum copper, with the result that toxic amounts of copper are stored in the liver and other tissues.

Wilson's disease is treated with chelating agents to increase the urinary excretion of copper; the intake of dietary copper is also restricted to 1.0 mg per day. At this point there are limited data on the copper content of foods. Pennington and Calloway[22] have recently published a review of the factors affecting the copper content of food and have compiled a table showing the range of values for copper as reported by various investigators. The information in this publication may be useful in designing a copper-restricted diet pattern and exchange lists for a patient with Wilson's disease.

## Study questions and activities

1. How does the liver function in the metabolism of nutrients? As an organ of storage? In detoxification?
2. Why may a diet increased in protein be a source of danger to the patient with severe liver disease?
3. How may hepatic coma develop? Why is a diet devoid of or severely restricted in protein essential?
4. Calculate a diet pattern for a 2000-calorie, 20-g protein-restricted in Group A amino acids, 500 mg-sodium diet.
5. Calculate a diet pattern for an 1800-calorie, 60 g-protein, 1000-mg sodium diet. Plan menus, a weekly market order, and instructional materials for a man living alone who has a gas stove (top burners only), a sink, limited storage space, and shares a refrigerator with two other men. He has $20.00 a week for food and the nearest supermarket is five blocks from his house.
6. What are the resources in your community for helping the chronic alcoholic?

## References

1. Boeker EA: J Am Diet Assoc 76:550, 1980
2. Lieber CS: Gastroenterology 79:373, 1980
3. Jones AL, Schmucker DL: Gastroenterology 73:833, 1977
4. Mezey E: Am J Clin Nutr 33:2709, 1980
5. Dienstag JL et al: In Isselbacher KJ et al (eds): Harrison's Principles of Internal Medicine, 9th ed, pp 1459–1470. New York, McGraw-Hill, 1980
6. Davidson CS: J Am Diet Assoc 62:515, 1973
7. LaMont JT et al: In Isselbacher, Harrison's Principles, pp 1473–1484
8. James JH et al: Lancet 2:772, 1979
9. Galambos JT: Cirrhosis, p 164. Philadelphia, WB Saunders, 1979
10. Lieber CS: N Engl J Med 298:888, 1978
11. Rubin E, Lieber CS: N Engl J Med 290:128, 1974
12. Blass JP, Gibson GE: N Engl J Med 297:1367, 1977
13. Walker C et al: N Engl J Med 291:168, 1974
14. Rudman D et al: Am J Clin Nutr 26:190, 1973
15. Patey AE: Lancet 1:722, 1974
16. Greenberger NJ et al: Dig Dis 22:845, 1977
17. Fischer JE et al: Surgery 80:77, 1976
18. Grant JP: Handbook of Total Parenteral Nutrition, p 39. Philadelphia, WB Saunders, 1980
19. Kay RM et al: In Deitel M (ed): Nutrition in Clinical Surgery, pp 29–41. Baltimore, Williams & Wilkins, 1980
20. Freund H et al: JAMA 242:347, 1979
21. Malt RA: N Engl J Med 295:24; 80, 1976
22. Pennington JT, Calloway DH: J Am Diet Assoc 63:143, 1973

## Supplementary readings

Blass JP, Gibson GE: Abnormality of a thiamine-requiring enzyme in patients with Wernicke-Korsakoff syndrome. N Engl J Med 297:1367, 1977

Boeker EA: Metabolism of ethanol. J Am Diet Assoc 76:550, 1980

Borowsky SA et al: Continued heavy drinking and survival in alcoholic cirrhotics. Gastroenterology 80:1405, 1981

Gilberstadt S et al: Defective intellectual function in alcoholic cirrhotics and non-cirrhotic alcoholics: Relationship to severity of liver disease. Gastroenterology 74:1037, 1978

Hoyumpa AM et al: Clinical conference: Hepatic encephalopathy. Gastroenterology 76:184, 1979

Lindeman J, Roman MJ: Nutritional anemia in alcoholism. Am J Clin Nutr 33:2727, 1980

Mendelson JH, Mello NK: Biologic concomitants of alcoholism. N Engl J Med 301:912, 1979

Mezey E: Alcoholic liver disease: Roles of alcohol and malnutrition. Am J Clin Nutr 33:2709, 1980

Roe DA: Nutritional concerns in the alcoholic. J Am Diet Assoc 78:17, 1981

Tomaiolo PP, Kraus V: Nutritional status of hospitalized patients. J Parent Ent Nutr 4:1, 1980

*For further references see Bibliography in Part 4.*

# Cancer and Special Problems

# 34

## Cancer

*Cancer* is the term applied to a variety of malignant diseases that are characterized by the abnormal growth of cells (*neoplasia*). It is estimated that one in four Americans will develop cancer during his lifetime, and in the 1980s cancer will continue to be the second leading cause of death in the general population. It can occur in any cell, including the blood-forming cells, or tissue in the body. Certain types of cancer can be spread from the primary site in the body by the lymph or blood (*metastatis*). Although the exact etiology of cancer is not known, there is evidence that genetic predisposition, viruses, environmental factors, and therapeutic agents are involved. It also appears that immunologic factors may predispose a person to develop cancer.[1]

The malignant cell mass (tumor) can be considered a parasite in the host since it requires energy and nutrients to maintain and increase tumor mass. The Cori cycle (see Chap. 9) is the major source of energy for the tumor cell. As with any cell, the malignant cell requires nitrogen and other nutrients for cellular mitosis. In the early stages of the disease patients lose weight without any intentional decrease in daily energy intake. As the disease progresses many patients experience anorexia, which, combined with the hypermetabolic processes of the tumor cells, leads to severe weight loss, malnutrition, and, ultimately, cancer cachexia and death.[2-5]

There are three modes of treatment for cancer: surgery, radiation, and chemotherapy.[1] Any one mode or a combination of two or three modes of treatment may be used. For example, in some instances the tumor mass may be removed surgically, and radiation or chemotherapy or both may be used either pre- or postoperatively or both in an attempt to destroy all cancer cells. When surgery is not possible, only radiation and chemotherapy are used.

Depending on the location of the tumor cell mass, each mode of therapy can present numerous nutritional problems. The surgical removal of the stomach in gastric cancer may result in the postgastrectomy syndrome. Radiation of head and neck cancers can cause loss of the sense of taste and decreased salivary secretion. The most commonly used chemotherapeutic agents inhibit one or more metabolic steps in the synthesis of the elements required for all cell mitosis, such as purines, pyrimidines, DNA, and RNA. Therefore, the normal cells as well as malignant cells are affected. Because of their cytotoxic effects, radiation and chemotherapy treatments are scheduled intermittently to provide time for normal cells to recover.

## Nutritional problems in cancer and cancer therapy

### Weight loss

Weight loss is a common occurrence in the majority of cancer patients. This can occur without any change in appetite, usual daily energy intake, or physical activity patterns. It probably reflects the use of energy and nutrients by the cancer cells to promote their growth.[6] The major decrease in body mass is in the muscle tissue. As the disease progresses the weight loss can become critical (20%–30% of ideal weight) and is accompanied by hypoalbuminemia and anemia. The various modes of therapy can also lead to weight loss unless careful attention is given to supplying the nutritional needs of the patient by oral, enteral, or parenteral alimentation.

### Cachexia

Cachexia is a profound state of ill health and malnutrition. Cancer cachexia is characterized by severe weight loss, anorexia, early satiety, and anemia.[7] Morrison[3] stresses that anorexia is a late feature of cancer. Clinically, those patients who present with the most complex problems of food aversions are usually in the advanced or terminal stages of the disease. The food acceptance problems of those patients who have been diagnosed and treated early are engendered by the mode of therapy, particularly radiation or chemotherapy.

DeWys[6] points out that anorectic cancer patients can experience various changes in the senses of taste and smell. In some but not all patients there is an elevation of the taste threshold for sweetness and in some a significant lowering of the threshold for bitterness. The sense of smell may also be distorted, especially for the odors of food.

Radiation therapy may also alter the senses of taste and smell. Dysgeusia, the perversion of the sense of taste, commonly occurs with radiation therapy to the head and neck. With an altered sense of taste and a decrease in salivary secretions, cancer patients undergoing radiation therapy are often severely anorectic.

The taste problems of the patient undergoing chemotherapy may be related to the cytotoxicity of the agents. Pfaffman[8] states that the taste bud is a highly mitotic cell, since it has a life span of approximately 10 days. It is possible that in the periods between chemotherapy treatments the taste buds do not have the opportunity to recover sufficiently to maintain normal sensitivity.

The early satiety of the anorectic patient may be the result of decreased digestive secretions. The altered taste sensation may interfere with the cephalic phase of gastric digestion. Also, in the severely debilitated patient, the loss of muscle mass in the abdominal wall may delay gastric emptying.

There may also be a biochemical component of the anorexia and early satiety of cancer cachexia. Glucose intolerance, which is probably related to abnormal insulin production or peripheral resistance, is frequently observed in cancer patients.[9] Hyperglycemia delays gastric emptying[10] and, at the same time, may blunt the sensation of hunger.

### Food aversions

Conditioned food aversions often develop in the patient receiving radiation or chemotherapy or both.[6] If therapy is given shortly before or after food intake, patients may attribute any gastric distress with or without vomiting to the food consumed. Frequent episodes of distress related to intermittent therapy could result in multiple food aversions and, subsequently a very limited range of food items being acceptable to the patient. Bernstein and Sigmundi[11] raise the question whether or not learned food aversions also contribute to tumor anorexia.

### Malabsorption

Malabsorption can occur in the untreated cancer patient for two reasons: the lesion is in the mucosa of the gastrointestinal tract; or the integrity of the absorptive cells of the gastrointestinal tract is compromised by the generalized malnutrition that accompanies the malignant process at any site in the body. In either case the body is incapable of absorbing nutrients to meet its hypermetabolic needs.

Malabsorption is a concomitant of both radiation and chemotherapy. Abdominal radiation blunts the intestinal villi, leading to a decrease in absorptive surface. The effects of the chemotherapeutic agents on cell mitosis reduce the synthesis of the absorptive cells in the gastrointestinal tract. This results in alterations of the structure and function of the absorptive cells of the gut, which, in turn, leads to malabsorption and diarrhea.

### Hypercalcemia

Extensive bone involvement resulting in hypercalcemia occurs in patients with some cancers, such as breast or prostate carcinoma.[1] The blood calcium levels are elevated by immobilization with or without bony metastases. Also, some lung tumors may produce a parathyroid hormone-like substance that causes the hypercalcemia. Chronic hypercalcemia may lead to kidney stones (nephrocalcinosis) and impairment of kidney function. This form of hypercalcemia responds to treatment of the underlying disease.

## Nutritional care of the patient with cancer

Each cancer patient presents special nutritional care needs. There is no single feeding program or mode of feeding that can be applied routinely to all patients. However, the major challenges for the clinical dietitian are those patients with head and neck cancer that affects chewing and swallowing and the markedly cachectic patient with anorexia, nausea, vomiting, and distortion of the senses of taste and smell. There are many recommendations for feeding the cancer patient in general, but these suggestions must be adapted to the needs of each patient.[6,12-14] The first step is to develop a helping relationship with the patient and to avoid pressuring and constantly reminding the patient that he must eat. The patient is well aware that he must eat, and constant pressure may only heighten rather than decrease the anorexia.

### Assessment

On the patient's admission to either inpatient or ambulatory services, his nutritional status should be assessed. Copeland[15] recommends a screening process to identify the patient at risk for malnutrition based on the following factors: a recent, unintentional weight loss of 10% or more of usual body weight; a serum albumin of 3.4 g per deciliter or less; and a negative reaction to recall skin antigens. The clinical dietitian should collect a comprehensive nutritional history (see Chap. 23) on all patients at risk for malnutrition on admission and on those patients who it can be anticipated will be at risk for developing malnutrition from the physician's therapeutic plan—surgery, radiation, and chemotherapy. Any chewing and swallowing difficulties and food aversions should be identified at this time. When the patient is readmitted for intermittent chemotherapy or radiation, food likes and dislikes as well as the patient's readmission weight status should be checked and recorded in the clinical dietitian's records.

### Planning

The energy and nutrient needs of each patient should be estimated using the method described in Chapter 23. It is also advisable to estimate the patient's BEE using ideal weight as well as present weight to identify a long-term and an immediate goal for energy intake. At present there is no reliable method for estimating total energy needs for the cancer patient comparable with Long's injury factors (see Chap. 23). Since many patients will have elevated temperatures, the Long factor for sepsis can be used. The estimation of energy and nutrient need is used to set goals for oral, enteral, or parenteral alimentation, and continuous monitoring of the patient's status will indicate any need for adjustment.

The most appropriate diet order for the patient who does not require enteral or parenteral alimentation (see Chap. 27) is "diet as tolerated" or "catered diet." Concurrent medical problems or complications of the disease or therapy may require a diet modified in fluid and electrolytes or a nutrient, such as lipids or carbohydrate. Energy-restricted diets are not recommended for the overweight patient with cancer unless the patient is grossly obese and the obesity is a hazard should anesthesia be required for surgery. The overweight cancer patient will lose weight during therapy or with the progression of the disease if it does not respond to therapy.

The majority of patients receiving chemotherapy experience gastric distress with nausea and vomiting at the time of or shortly after the agent is given, usually by intravenous infusion. The health-care team should design a schedule for administering chemotherapy so that it is not given for *at least* 2 hours before or 2 hours after a meal. Patients with early cancer will not lose significant amounts of weight if this type of schedule is established. In one hospital no chemotherapy was given before 9:00 P.M., 3 hours after the evening meal. These patients usually accepted and consumed enough food during the day to maintain their weight status and feeling of well-being. Designing a therapy schedule within the constraints of the food service system and professional staffing patterns presents a real challenge to the health-care team.[16] However, research shows that the well-nourished patient has a more positive response to therapy than the malnourished one.[4,15]

Supplementary feeding products (see Chap. 27) are frequently recommended for patients who have had a significant weight loss and can consume food orally. If the patient is experiencing any symptoms of delayed gastric emptying, it is unwise to offer these products as nourishments between meals, since a 300-kcal supplement may interfere with the acceptance of a 900-kcal meal. Also, frequent offerings of food and beverages can be a depressing reminder to the patient who cannot eat but knows he should eat. For patients with delayed gastric emptying it would seem more reasonable to attempt to improve intake by spacing meals. For example, breakfast at 7:00 to 7:30 A.M., the noon meal at 12:30 to 1:00 P.M., the evening meal at 6:00 to 6:30 P.M. and a fourth meal (not a snack) at 10:00 to 10:30 P.M., with any supplement served at mealtime. Aker[16] has demonstrated the advantage to the patient when food service is available 18 hours a day, 7 days a week.

The severely cachectic patient requires enteral or parenteral alimentation. For some patients enteral or parenteral alimentation is the only method of nutritional support for the remainder of their lives (see Chap. 27).

### Implementation

The clinical dietitian together with her food service employees invests considerable time and effort in helping each cancer patient achieve a reasonable daily intake of foods and beverages. The staff must be prepared and willing to work with anorectic patients who select food one day for the next only to find it makes them nauseous when it is served. Family members can often help during prolonged hospitalizations by bringing food that the patient particularly likes. An 8-year-old boy with leukemia often prefers his favorite brand of hamburger and french fries to those prepared in the hospital.

Patients with a distorted sense of smell often find that cold foods are more acceptable than hot foods. It is hoped that the odor of hot food on the tray of the patient in the next bed can be controlled. Patients with a lowered threshold for bitter taste may avoid meats, such as beef and chicken, and accept the more bland protein foods, such as milk, eggs, cheese, and fish.[12] With an increased threshold for sweets, sugar can be added to hot or cold beverages and tart juices, such as grapefruit, lemon, and cranberry.

### Evaluation

Continuous *unobtrusive* appraisal of daily energy and nutrient intake must be carried out to document objectively a patient's intake. One can gain a false impression of a patient's intake from observing *one* meal or the patient's refusal of *one* between-meal snack. All food consumed, including that served by the hospital personnel, and any food provided by the family or friends should be evaluated as frequently as necessary to obtain a valid appraisal, and the data recorded in the patient's medical record. This information combined with other objective patient data (see Chap. 23) is used by the health-care team to monitor patient progress and to initiate enteral or parenteral alimentation if necessary. The dietary data can also be used to evaluate the schedule for giving medications for nausea and pain. Daily weighing is not recommended because it can discourage the patient who is gaining weight slowly or continuing to lose weight even though the intake is adequate.

### Follow-up

The patient who is receiving intermittent therapy should have access to resources and instructional materials (see *Patient Resources* at end of this chapter) to use at home so that nutritional status can be maintained or improved between treatments. Adequate food intake before or after each treatment is a very crucial aspect of therapy. As the gastrointestinal cells recover after a chemotherapy treatment, absorption improves, and the patient's appetite usually improves. The social worker, nurse specialist, and clinical dietitian should work closely with the patient to ensure that a reasonable daily intake of food can be achieved during this period. For example, a patient with limited physical energy who lives alone may need help with food purchasing and preparation, while another patient may need financial assistance to purchase food.

## Allergy

Allergy is described as an adverse physiological reaction in various tissues resulting from the interaction of an antigen with an antibody or lymphoid cells.[17] The tissues involved are the skin, mucous membranes, or vascular endothelium. The antibodies are immunoglobulins; of these immunoglobulin E (IgE) is the one most commonly involved. The allergic reactions in mucous membranes are attributable to the IgE antibodies synthesized by plasma cells located predominantly under mucosal surfaces, especially the respiratory and gastrointestinal tracts. There is a significant familial incidence, which may aid in diagnosis; and there may be a strong emotional component related to the severity of allergic manifestations.

### Causes

Allergic reactions are caused by a wide variety of substances and conditions. These include pollens, dust, cosmetics, and animal hair; poisonous plants; serums, vaccines, and drugs; physical agents, such as heat, cold, and sunlight; as well as a variety of foods. Reactions to a particular substance may occur in one person, and in another person a similar reaction may be caused by an entirely different substance. On the other hand, the same substance may cause two widely differing reactions in each of two people.

### Symptoms

The symptoms of allergy are as varied as the substances causing the reaction. Eczema is most common in infants and young children; rhinitis and asthma occur in both children and adults and are sometimes preceded by allergic eczema in infancy. Urticaria (hives), physical allergies, and angioneurotic edema are common in adults. Serum sickness and drug reactions are directly related to the administration of vaccines and drugs and may occur at any age.

## Foods and allergy

This discussion is chiefly concerned with food allergies, but it should be kept in mind that any allergy from any cause whatever, if severe, may interfere with the nutrition of a person due to the effect on appetite and, as a result, on general health. This is often the case with a child, whose growth and development may be retarded seriously unless his diet is evaluated carefully and made as attractive and nutritionally adequate as possible.

The protein component of a food is considered to be the causative factor in food allergy, even though foods that cause an allergic reaction may vary widely in protein content. Reaction to a food, such as honey, is associated with protein in the pollen grains mixed in the honey, for it has been shown that very minute amounts of a given protein may cause an allergic reaction. Also, allergic responses to a food may be either immediate or delayed.

Among the common allergy-producing foods, particularly in children, are oranges, milk, eggs, and sometimes wheat. Other common food allergens are fish and shellfish, chocolate, tomatoes, and strawberries. It has been found that members of the same botanic family may have a similar allergic effect. Lemons and grapefruit are likely to cause a reaction if oranges are allergenic. Likewise, if cabbage triggers an allergic reaction, so may broccoli, brussels sprouts, and cauliflower.

Whether or not an allergic disturbance follows the eating of a specific food depends largely upon a person's physical and often emotional state. This may make the search for the offending food or foods a difficult process. Moreover, no immunologic mechanisms specific to food allergy have been identified, and symptoms are sometimes ascribed to allergy when their cause is obscure.

## Diagnosis
### History

All investigators stress the need for a careful history. This is especially true for the older child and the adult, who eat a variety of foods. In the very young infant ingesting only a limited number of foods, the diagnosis may be more easily established. In all instances a detailed history of recent food intake, appearance of symptoms, and other events and conditions relating to the illness is of utmost importance.

### Skin tests

If a careful history does not reveal the cause of the allergic symptoms, the physician may resort to skin tests. Solutions, each containing a small quantity of a common allergen, are applied to a scratched portion of the skin and then covered with cellophane for 2 to 4 days. Interdermal injections of the suspected allergen may also be used.

In the event that welts, wheals, and redness develop from any of these tests, an allergic reaction is indicated. However, it has been observed that many foods may give a positive skin test without causing allergic symptoms.

### Food challenge

When a food is suspected of causing an allergic reaction, it is excluded from the diet for 7 to 10 days. Even though the exclusion results in improvement in symptoms, the food is reintroduced into the diet in large amounts for several meals. If the suspected food contains the allergen, symptoms will recur in a reasonable period of time, usually within 7 days. The testing should be done in a blind manner. For example, if milk is the suspected food, it can be hidden in mashed potatoes and breads.

### Elimination test diets

The Rowe[18] elimination test diets are also used by some physicians to identify food allergies. The foods included in these diets are considered unlikely to produce allergic reactions. Table 34-1 lists the foods used in Rowe's cereal-free elimination diet; and Table 34-2, Rowe's fruit-free, cereal-free elimination diet. Both diets exclude breast and cow's milk. Rowe recommends the use of soy milks

### Table 34-1. Rowe's Cereal-Free Elimination Diet

| Foods Used | |
| --- | --- |
| Tapioca (pearl or minute) | Apricots† |
| White potatoes | Grapefruit |
| Sweet potatoes | Lemons |
| Breads made with any combination of soy, lima, potato starch, and tapioca flour | Peaches |
| | Pineapples |
| Soy milk: Mull-Soy and Neo-Mull Soy* | Prunes |
| | Pears |
| Lamb | Cane or beet sugar |
| Chicken, fryers, roosters, capon (no hens) | Salt |
| | Sesame oil (not Chinese) |
| Bacon | Soybean oil |
| Liver (lamb, chicken) | Margarine‡ |
| | White vinegar |
| Peas | Vanilla extract |
| Spinach | Cornstarch-free baking powder |
| Squash | Baking soda |
| String beans | Cream of tartar |
| Tomatoes | |
| Artichokes | Maple syrup or syrup made with cane sugar flavored with maple |
| Asparagus | |
| Carrots | |
| Lettuce | |
| Lima beans | |

*Free of corn syrup solids and corn oil (Syntex Laboratories, Palo Alto, CA 94304).

†Fruits, fresh or canned in cane sugar.

‡Free of milk solids or corn oil.

(Adapted from Rowe AH: Food Allergy, 1972. Courtesy of Charles C Thomas, Publisher, Springfield, IL)

### Table 34-2. Rowe's Fruit-Free, Cereal-Free Elimination Diet

| Foods Used | |
| --- | --- |
| Tapioca (pearl only) | Cooked carrots |
| White potatoes | Squash |
| Sweet potatoes | Artichokes |
| Bread made with any combination of soy, lima, potato starch, or tapioca flour | Peas |
| | Lima beans |
| | String beans |
| Soy milk: Mull-Soy and Neo-Mull Soy* | Cane or beet sugar |
| | Soybean oil |
| Lamb | Margarine† |
| Chicken, fryers, roosters, capon (no hens) | Gelatin (Knox) |
| | Salt |
| Bacon | Syrup made from cane sugar (no maple syrup) |
| Liver (lamb, chicken) | Corn-free, tartaric acid-free baking powder‡ |

*Free of corn syrup solids and corn oil (Syntex Laboratories, Palo Alto, CA 94304).

†Free of milk solids and corn oil.

‡Tartaric acid is made from grapes.

(Adapted from Rowe AH: Food Allergy, 1972. Courtesy of Charles C Thomas, Publisher, Springfield, IL)

free of the sugars derived from cornstarch on the theory that corn sugars could be contaminated with corn protein.

The patient is placed on one of the test diets for a period of a week. If the symptoms do not abate, the other diet is tried for the same length of time. If, at the end of the second test diet, relief has not been obtained, it is evident that causes other than food should be sought as allergic agents.

On the other hand, if the patient is relieved of his symptoms on any one of the elimination test diets, he is kept on this diet for another week. Other foods, first chosen from the related test diets and then more generally, are added one by one, with wheat, eggs, and milk last, because these foods are most likely to produce allergy. If the patient shows allergic symptoms after the addition of any one food, that food may be suspected as the cause of the allergic reaction and must be omitted from the diet.

In infants or young children suspected of food allergy, the problem of eliminating the offending foods may be solved by placing the patient, if he is an infant, on nothing by mouth except a soy protein formula or on a simple elimination diet consisting of lamb, rice, carrots, pears, and a soy formula if he is older. If symptoms clear, other foods are added to the child's diet one at a time. As with adults, if there is no improvement on the elimination diet, it may be assumed that the allergic symptoms are due to causes other than food.

Hughes[19] has reported on the use of a chemically defined diet, Vivonex (see Chap. 27), as an elimination test diet. The subjects studied took only the chemically defined diet and water for 7 to 10 days. The next step was to test for food allergies by adding a suspected food to the basic chemically defined diet and observing the subject for possible allergic responses. For those patients who tolerated the Vivonex this method was successful in identifying specific food allergies.

### Dietary treatment
#### Milk allergy

Allergy to cow's milk protein appears to occur most commonly in children under 2 years of age and, in many of these children, tolerance to milk protein increases as they grow older. The lactoglobulin fraction is considered to be the most common allergen in cow's milk protein.

A variety of milk-free formulas are available for feeding these infants and children (see Table 35-4, Chapter 35). The soy-base formulas and those made with casein hydrolysate are commonly used in place of milk-based formulas. These preparations are equal in calorie and nutrient value to other commercial infant formulas and, when used as directed, are well-tolerated and support adequate growth.[20]

Evaporated goat's milk may be fed an infant who is allergic to cow's milk. However, some infants have the same reaction to goat's milk protein that they have to the protein in cow's milk. Also, because goat's milk is low in vitamins D, $B_{12}$, and folic acid, when it is used, it must be supplemented with preparations of these vitamins to supply the infant's needs.

When solid foods are included in the infant's diet, care must be taken to avoid foods that have milk or nonfat dry milk added during processing. The mother must be advised to read labels carefully so that she can avoid these products. The companies that market baby foods make available to the nutrition counselor lists of ingredients in their products.

If the child does not accept special milks when he is older, it is necessary to supplement his diet with calcium pills and riboflavin. Even the older child who tolerates limited amounts of milk, such as the 2% to 4% dry milk solids found in some bread, and the milk used in preparation of foods, such as cakes and cookies, needs calcium pills to meet his calcium need. It may also be advisable for the adult who is allergic to milk to use calcium supplements daily. Vitamin D supplements are also needed.

#### Wheat allergy

Because wheat bread and other products made with wheat cereal or flour are basic items in the American diet, the person who is allergic to wheat finds he cannot eat many common foods. He must learn that baker's rye bread contains some wheat flour; that practically all hot breads, pancakes, pastries, and crackers are made chiefly or partly from wheat products; that bran and gluten are wheat derivatives. Thickened gravies, cream soups, and sauces are to be avoided unless thickened with corn or rice starch. Even meat dishes, such as meat loaf, hamburger, bologna, and sausage may contain wheat flour or bread. All malted beverages must be avoided by the person who is wheat-sensitive.

For a complete description of the omissions necessary in wheat sensitivity, see Chapter 26, *Gluten-free Diet*. For the patient allergic to wheat only, the restrictions on rye flour and oatmeal do not apply, but the remaining material proves helpful in ensuring that all wheat products are eliminated from the diet.

#### Egg allergy

The patient who is allergic to egg must investigate carefully all commercial products before eating them. He must remember that even the baking powder used in baked goods may contain dried egg white, that egg white may be used in the preparation of foaming beverages, and that most desserts, especially cakes, cookies, pastries, puddings, and ice cream, contain eggs. These patients may also be allergic to chicken, which must then be omitted from the diet.

### Allergy to citrus fruit

The major problem for these patients is an adequate daily intake of vitamin C. Potatoes, other vegetables, and fruits can provide an adequate intake, although some patients may take 50 mg of ascorbic acid as medication each day to ensure an adequate intake.

### Resources for patients

At the end of this chapter is a list of sources of recipes for allergy patients. These recipes may help them discover new dishes because allergy diets can become monotonous and uninteresting.

## Desensitizing the patient

The difficulties inherent in strict avoidance of allergy-causing foods, especially in a child, may cause the physician to try to desensitize him to such food. This treatment should follow a period of complete abstinence from the offending food. Fortunately, it may be possible to desensitize by mouth; beginning with doses so minute that they cause no reactions in the person being treated, gradually the amount is increased until ordinary food portions can be tolerated.

To illustrate, one child sensitive to egg white was desensitized in this way over a period of 7 months by a dosage beginning with 1 mg of dry or powdered egg white. Another child could tolerate at first only such a small amount of egg white as that present in a teaspoonful of a dilution made by adding one drop of egg white to a pint of water. In 3 months, however, he was able to include eggs in his diet.

Often adults may desensitize themselves successfully. A man acutely but periodically sensitive to milk desensitizes himself every 3 or 4 years, in the following way. After eliminating milk, he takes daily an increasing number of drops of cream until he can resume the use of both cream and milk in his diet.

## Anemias

In addition to nutritional anemias the hospitalized patient often presents with anemias due to defective or decreased red cell production, decreased red blood cell life span, red blood cell hemolysis, or hemorrhagic blood loss.[21] These anemias are symptomatic of chronic disease, such as renal or hepatic failure; inflammation or infection; neoplasias and cancer therapies; and gastrointestinal bleeding, metrorrhagia, or trauma. The treatment of the primary disease may improve or correct many of these anemias, while dietary therapy plays a supportive role. However, in some instances where the anorexia of chronic diseases lead to malnutrition, dietary treatment is an important part of the total therapeutic plan and for many patients is supportive of treatment with iron medication.

The clinical dietitian is cautioned not to interpret any abnormal hemoglobin or hematocrit level as nutritional anemia before a definitive diagnosis of the patient's problem has been made by the physician. The lay person may interpret any undue emphasis on iron-rich foods as the best method of treatment and not comply with other treatment modes. The reader is referred to Chapters 6 and 35 for discussions of iron deficiency anemia and to Chapter 8 for a discussion of vitamin $B_{12}$ and pernicious anemia.

## Chronic infection and inflammation

Mild to moderate anemia develops in chronic infection, such as lung abcess, tuberculosis, pyelonephritis, and chronic inflammatory diseases, such as rheumatoid arthritis. Both defective red cell production and decreased red cell life span account for the anemia. It does not respond to an increased intake of iron, folic acid, or vitamin $B_{12}$ but does respond to the treatment of the underlying disease.

## Acute and chronic blood loss

Over 60% of the body's iron (approximately 2.5 g of iron in an adult) is in the hemoglobin of the circulating red cells, and in each milliliter of whole blood there is, on the average, 0.7 mg of iron. Therefore, the loss of 500 ml of blood results in the loss of 350 mg or about $\frac{1}{3}$ g of iron.

### Acute blood loss

Acute blood loss is seen most frequently in traumatized patients, patients with the massive hemorrhage of ruptured esophageal or gastric varices or bleeding peptic ulcer disease and women with long-standing untreated metrorrhagia. In severe hemorrhage the immediate treatment is restoration of blood volume by transfusion. The blood must be further restored by an increase in the production of red blood cells and hemoglobin. In an otherwise normal person, recovery is spontaneous, but the red cells are replenished more rapidly than is the hemoglobin. The latter will be restored gradually, but the speed of its restoration seems to depend largely on the diet. The necessary nutrients must be supplied in the diet in order that each of these red cells may contain the normal amount of hemoglobin.

### Chronic blood loss

Chronic blood loss may accompany such conditions as gastric ulcer, colitis, or long untreated hemorrhoids. The important aspect of treatment is to determine the cause of the blood loss and to control it. The anemia may be mild or moderate.

## Renal failure

The anemia of renal failure is proportional to the elevation of serum urea nitrogen; therefore, it can vary from mild to very severe with hemoglobin levels as low as 4 g per deciliter in patients with chronic renal failure.[21]

The red blood cell mass is decreased as a result of decreased red cell production because the kidneys cannot produce adequate amounts of erythropoietin to support erythrocyte synthesis. A minor red blood cell hemolysis also takes place.[22] There is a moderate improvement in the anemia with hemodialysis and a marked improvement with renal transplantation. Oral iron therapy is usually given to the patient in renal failure because the renal diet is inadequate in iron (see Chap. 32).

## Hepatic failure

A number of factors contribute to the anemia of hepatic failure. Alcohol *per se* inhibits heme synthesis,[23] and in advanced cirrhosis there is an impairment of folic acid utilization (see Chap. 33). In addition to a decrease in the red cell production there is some decrease in the red cell life span. Blood loss from esophageal or gastric hemorrhage may also contribute to the anemia of hepatic failure. In early alcoholic cirrhosis, with abstinence from alcohol coupled with an adequate intake of iron, folic acid, and vitamin $B_{12}$, the anemia will improve. In the late stages of cirrhosis, with extensive cell necrosis and tissue fibrosis, the anemia will not improve. These patients usually have a hemoglobin level of 9 g to 11 g per deciliter, which decreases with impending hepatic coma and death.

## Cancer

The first diagnostic symptom of cancer may be anemia from increased destruction of red cells or inadequate red cell production or both. Also, with some cancers there may be blood loss, such as in cancer of the colon, or there may be hemolysis of red cells.[24] Cancer chemotherapy and any extensive radiation therapy to the sternum or other important quantities of bone marrow also contribute to the anemia. For many of these patients blood transfusions are the only effective method of treatment.

# Diseases of the musculoskeletal system
## Arthritis

Arthritis is a chronic disease process that involves the joints. Perhaps due to its chronic nature and its accompanying discomfort and pain, many arthritics become the victims of food faddists, self-appointed "arthritis experts" or quacks, who advocate quick and miraculous cures with bizarre diets. At present there is no known dietary cause or cure for arthritis, and the medical treatment is palliative, not curative.

### Osteoarthritis

Osteoarthritis or degenerative joint disease occurs in the older age group, more frequently in women than in men. The disease is due to structural changes in the articular cartilage in the joints, usually those that are weight-bearing, such as the spine, hips, and knees. As the process progresses, the joints become stiff and often painful. For this reason activity may be curtailed, and there is a tendency to overweight in this group of patients, placing additional strain on the affected joints.

The nutritional requirements for the older person as described in Chapter 20 are equally important for the person with arthritis. Sufficient protein, calcium, iron, and vitamins are needed to maintain good health. Only the energy needs are somewhat reduced, since activity is lessened.

The overweight arthritic will benefit from a further decrease in calories. Sometimes a moderate reduction in energy intake accomplishes this purpose. A more controlled reduction regimen is detailed in Chapter 28. As weight approaches the normal range for height and build, the patient with osteoarthritis may well experience some relief from discomfort and pain, and achieve an increase in activity. Patients who are candidates for artificial hip or knee replacements for osteoarthritis should be at their "ideal" body weight or somewhat below for effective postoperative rehabilitation.

### Rheumatoid arthritis

Rheumatoid arthritis occurs more frequently than osteoarthritis. It may be seen in children, but usually appears between the ages of 25 and 50. It is three times more common in women than in men. The disease is due to an inflammatory process of the synovium or lining of the joints, accompanied by swelling and eventual deformity. It is a disfiguring, debilitating, and chronic disease, marked by exacerbations and remissions.

In contrast with the osteoarthritic, the patient with rheumatoid arthritis is frequently underweight. Also, many patients have such severe involvement of the joints of the fingers and hands that they have difficulty feeding themselves. In order to achieve an adequate energy and nutrient intake they often need to be trained to use the adaptive equipment presented in Chapter 25.

### Other treatment

Therapeutic doses of aspirin are used in the treatment of both types of arthritis. Because aspirin can cause gastric distress it is recommended that it be taken after meals. Occasionally corticosteroids are used in the treatment of rheumatoid arthritis. Since these medications promote sodium retention, the diet may be moderately restricted in sodium. Frequently the patient taking aspirin or steroids is advised to use a bland diet and antacids because both medications may cause gastric distress and occasionally gastritis (see Chap. 26).

## Gout

Gout or tophic arthritis is due to an inborn error of purine metabolism, characterized by an increase in blood uric acid levels and the deposition of urate crystals in the soft tissues and in the joints, particularly of the fingers and toes. Very occasionally it appears in children, but the incidence is greatest in men after the age of 30. It is relatively rare in women.

In primary gout the metabolic error in the majority of subjects results in overproduction of uric acid (hyperuricemia), underexcretion of uric acid or both. Secondary gout due to reduced excretion of uric acid occurs in chronic renal disease, hypertensive cardiovascular disease, and starvation in the treatment of obesity. For many years the excessive intake of alcohol has been associated with gout.

Normal blood levels of uric acid are from 2.5 mg to 5 mg per deciliter. A level of 6 mg per deciliter for men, and 5.5 mg per deciliter for women is considered hyperuricemia and is indicative of the presence of gout, although no overt symptoms may appear. The clinical course of gout may best be described as having three stages. The first is hyperuricemia without symptoms, perhaps discovered at a routine physical examination. The second is characterized by an acute and painful attack of gouty arthritis. The attack may subside spontaneously in anywhere from 2 days to 2 weeks, or respond to treatment with drugs that promote uric acid excretion. There may be a long interval before another attack occurs. Chronic tophaceous gout is the third and most severe form of the disease. Tophi, or accumulations of urate crystals, are present in and around one or more of the joints, causing destruction of bone and deformity (Fig. 34-1). Kidney stones or urate crystals may also occur (see Chap. 32).

### Medical treatment

The source of uric acid arises from the metabolism of purines, a constituent of nucleoproteins found in all cells. Purines are obtained from ingested food and from the breakdown of body protein. Purines are also synthesized in the liver from smaller metabolic fragments. Colchicine, a drug used in the treatment of gout for many years, is thought to inhibit the metabolic reactions by which uric

**Table 34-3.  Purine Content of Foods Per 100 Grams**

| *Group I* (0–15 mg) | *Group II* (50–150 mg) | *Group III* (150–800 mg) |
|---|---|---|
| Vegetables | Meats, poultry | Sweetbreads |
| Fruits | Fish | Anchovies |
| Milk | Seafood | Sardines |
| Cheese | Beans, dry | Liver |
| Eggs | Peas, dry | Kidney |
| Cereals, bread | Lentils | Meat extracts |
| Sugars, fats | Spinach | Brains |

(Adapted from Turner D: Handbook of Diet Therapy, 5th ed. Chicago, University of Chicago Press, 1971)

acid is derived from purine compounds. More recently, drugs have been available that facilitate the excretion of uric acid by the kidney. These two drugs help to lower the blood uric acid levels in patients with gout.

### Dietary treatment

In the past a purine-restricted diet was used as part of the treatment of gout but it is seldom used routinely today. In the purine-restricted diet, all foods in Group III in Table 34-3, *Purine Content of Foods*, were excluded and only limited amounts of those in Group II were used.

Today, some physicians restrict foods that are very high in purine content, such as liver, kidney, brains and sweetbreads. Otherwise the diet is adequate to meet the patient's needs. Patients with gout should be cautioned about fasting, whether to lose weight or, unintentionally, on an alcoholic spree, because it has been observed that fasting, even for 1 or 2 days, leads to an increase in blood uric acid.

## Diet–medication interrelationships

Hartshorn,[25] points out that diet–medication interactions are of two types: the medication may impair the absorption or utilization of nutrients or both; or the food

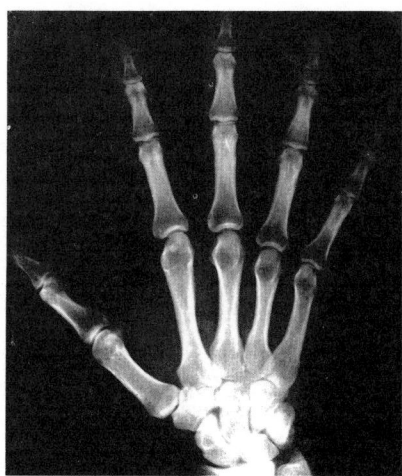
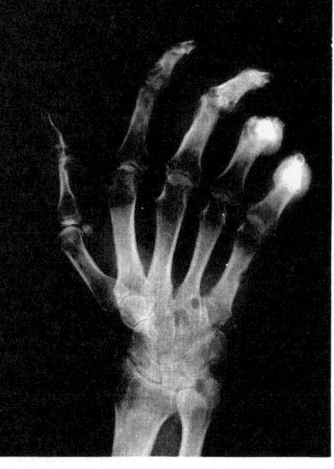

**Fig. 34-1.**  *Left,* bones of the hand of a normal person; *right,* far-advanced gout, showing marked skeletal changes. (The Department of Radiology, The New York Hospital)

consumed may alter the effects of a medication. Also, some medications may cause gastric distress, nausea, vomiting, and diarrhea, which can lead to a decrease in food intake. In most, but not in all situations, the nutritional problems result from long-term use of the medication and can be averted in some instances by nutritional supplements. Table 34-4 lists some of the nutritional problems produced by various types of commonly used classes of medications.

The clinical dietitian is strongly advised to work closely with the clinical pharmacologist and the pharmacy technician. Both of these professionals are relatively new members of the health-care team in most hospitals and outpatient facilities. Clinical pharmacologists are responsible for identifying adverse diet–medication and medication–medication interactions and bringing them to the attention of the other members of the health-care team. They are an important resource for the clinical dietitian, who cannot be both a nutrition specialist and a pharmacologist.

In this section commonly used medications, such as cancer therapeutic agents and steroids, which have widespread effects on nutritional status, are discussed together with specific food–medication interactions, such as tyramine and monoamine oxidase inhibitors.

## Table 34-4. Nutritional Problems Due to Various Types of Medications

| Nutritional Problem | Medications |
| --- | --- |
| Stomatitis | Cancer chemotherapeutic agents |
| | Antibiotics |
| Hyperplasia of gums | Anticonvulsants |
| Nausea, vomiting, gastritis, gastric hemorrhage | Cancer chemotherapeutic agents |
| | Antibiotics |
| | Salicylates |
| | Steroids |
| | Potassium and other electrolytes |
| | Anticonvulsants |
| Malabsorption with diarrhea or steatorrhea | Cancer chemotherapeutic agents |
| | Antibiotics |
| | Laxatives |
| | Clofibrate and cholestyramine |
| | Antacids |
| | Alcohol |
| Constipation | Anticholinergics |
| | Hypnotics, sedatives |
| Nutrient Utilization | |
| Glucose | Steroids |
| Protein | Cancer chemotherapeutic agents |
| | Steroids |
| Lipids | Steroids |
| Vitamins and minerals | Cancer chemotherapeutic agents |
| | Anticoagulants |
| | Anticonvulsants |
| | Sedatives |
| Electrolytes | Diuretics, digitalis |
| | Steroids |

## Cancer chemotherapeutic agents

The chemotherapeutic agents used in the treatment of cancer, frequently in combination with other modes of therapy, are cytotoxic drugs. They have an inhibitory effect on the mitotic processes of the cell nucleus and, therefore, inhibit the proliferation of cancer cells (see section on *Cancer* in this chapter). However, the action of the drugs is not limited to cancer cells. They also have adverse effects on other cell nuclei. In nutritional status, the most important cells, which can be classed as continuously mitotic, are the absorptive cells and other cells of the gastrointestinal tract and the bone marrow cells, the precursors of red blood cells.

The immediate effect of most chemotherapeutic agents is nausea and vomiting. Therefore, the medication is usually given late in the evening so that the patient is able to consume food during the day. Subsequently, a nonspecific malabsorption of nutrients occurs through the effect of the agents on the absorptive cells of the gastrointestinal tract. The intermittent use of the drugs reduces the severity of this problem. With some agents stomatitis occurs, making it difficult for the patient to eat. In this situation acid foods, such as citrus fruits and juices, vinegar, and very salty foods, are avoided.

In addition to the general inhibition of bone marrow cell formation by chemotherapy, one agent, methotrexate, is a folic acid antimetabolite. The use of this agent can lead to megaloblastic anemia. Therefore, folinic acid (citrovorum factor) is administered with methotrexate to avoid this type of anemia.

In addition to red blood cell problems, the use of cancer chemotherapeutic agents can also result in a deficiency of immunoglobulins, the blood proteins involved in combating infection. The patient, therefore, is readily susceptible to infection and, when hospitalized, is protected by reverse isolation. All hospital personnel, including food service workers, with upper respiratory or other infections must be excluded from any contact with these patients.

## Steroids

Steroids are anti-inflammatory agents that are used in the treatment of a wide variety of disorders. Gastric bleeding is a common complication. When large doses are administered orally, some clinicians advise taking the drug with meals and antacids between meals. Generally, gastric secretagogues are avoided (see Chap. 26).

The majority of steroid preparations promote sodium and, therefore, fluid retention. Depending on the problem, dietary sodium intake may be mildly or moderately restricted. In some situations the sodium intake may be severely restricted that is, to 10 mEq (see Chap. 31). Hypokalemia can result with some steroid preparations. If this occurs, potassium chloride is used to correct the deficit.

Glucose intolerance develops in some patients on

long-term steroid therapy. This may result in steroid-induced diabetes. These patients are treated by diet and an oral hypoglycemic agent or insulin (see Chap. 29). The steroid therapy is continued. Osteoporosis is also a frequent complication of steroid therapy. If it develops, therapy may be discontinued.

## Specific food–drug problems
### Tyramine and MAO inhibitors

Monoamine oxidase (MAO) inhibitors used in the treatment of depressed patients interact adversely with tyramine, an amine derived from the amino acid tyrosine. The MAO inhibitor-tyramine interaction results in the release of norepinephrine from the nerve endings, which causes a marked rise in blood pressure and other cardiovascular changes. Headache is a common symptom of the elevated blood pressure (hypertension). Intracranial bleeding and death due to the hypertensive crises have been reported.[25]

Tyramine occurs naturally in certain foods such as aged cheeses, liver, dried fish, and in fermented alcoholic beverages such as beer, ale, and some wines (see Table 34-5). The foods listed in Table 34-5 are excluded from the diets of patients taking MAO inhibitors, although yeast bread is not excluded from the diet unless symptoms occur.

### Salicylate-induced urticaria

Salicylate-induced urticaria (hives) responds not only to the avoidance of salicylates in medications (aspirin and other drugs containing salicylate) but also to the exclusion of naturally occurring salicylates in foods. Table 34-6 lists the foods that contain naturally occurring salicylates. These foods must be avoided by the patient with salicylate-induced urticaria. Noid and co-workers[26] give a list of processed foods free of salicylates. Fresh meat, fish and poultry, whole or skim milk, regular bread, unprocessed cereals, butter, sugar, and the fruits and vegetables *not* listed in Table 34-6 can be used. Because the fruits are limited, a vitamin C supplement is recommended.

### Monosodium glutamate

It has been observed that some people react adversely to monosodium glutamate, a flavor enhancer widely used in food processing. The reaction, known as the "Chinese restaurant syndrome," is characterized by headache, burning sensations of the extremities, facial pressure, and chest pain. It appears to be dose-related although the quantity of monosodium glutamate that stimulates the reaction varies from person to person. Dizziness, diarrhea, nausea, and stomach cramps have also been reported.[27] North Americans touring China are experiencing acute reactions to monosodium glutamate because of the quantities commonly used in Chinese food preparation.

## Miscellaneous metabolic problems
### Hyperthyroidism

The patient with untreated hyperthyroidism, a condition characterized by excessive secretion of the hormone, thyroxine, which regulates metabolism, experiences hunger and weight loss. Medical or surgical treatment reduces the hypermetabolic state. However, before treatment can effect this change, patients may require 4000 to 5000 calories a day (adequate in all nutrients) to meet their metabolic needs and prevent further weight loss. Supplementary vitamins and minerals may be prescribed, and all stimulants such as tea, coffee, alcohol, and tobacco are limited or omitted.

### Table 34-5. Food Rich in Tyramine

| *Dairy Products* | *Meats* |
|---|---|
| Yogurt | Liver |
| Aged cheeses | Game |
| Cheddar | Dried fish |
| Gruyere | Herring |
| Stilton | Cod |
| Emmentaler | Caplin |
| Brie | Pickled herring |
| Camembert | *Vegetables* |
| Gouda | Italian broad beans with pods |
| Mozzarella | (fava beans) |
| Parmesan | |
| Provolone | *Others* |
| Romano | Vanilla |
| Roquefort | Chocolate |
| *Alcoholic Beverages* | Yeast and yeast extracts |
| Beer and ale | Soya sauce |
| Wine | |
| Chianti | |
| Sherry | |
| Riesling | |
| Sauterne | |

(Reprinted from *Journal of Food Science*, Vol. 34, p. 22, Year 1969. © by Institute of Food Technologists)

### Table 34-6. Foods Containing Salicylates

| *Vegetables* | *Fruits (cont.)* |
|---|---|
| Potatoes | Grapes |
| Cucumbers | Lemons |
| Peppers (green, bell, | Melons |
| tabasco) | Nectarines |
| Tomatoes | Oranges |
| *Fruits* | Peaches |
| Apples | Plums |
| Apricots | Prunes |
| Blackberries | Raisins |
| Boysenberries | Raspberries |
| Cherries | Strawberries |
| Currants | *Nuts* |
| Dewberries | Almonds |
| Gooseberries | *Beverages* |
| Grapefruit | Root beer |

(Adapted from Noid HE et al: Arch Dermatol 109:866, 1974; © 1974, American Medical Association)

In addition to regular meal service sizable snacks of sandwiches and other items should be available to the hospitalized patients at their request to avoid hunger.

### Hypoglycemia

Functional hypoglycemia wihout demonstrable organic disease may occur in adults. The symptoms of an attack are almost identical to those produced by an overdose of insulin and are due to low blood sugar. There is weakness, trembling, sweating, and extreme hunger. In severe cases there may be convulsions, hysterical symptoms, and, eventually, unconsciousness. The attacks do not occur in the fasting state. They are caused by overstimulation of the pancreas resulting in the production of excess insulin following a meal, particularly one high in mono- and disaccharides. Abdominal discomfort, which is also characteristic, is sometimes ascribed to peptic ulcer because the symptoms are similar. Foa and co-workers have suggested that adult hypoglycemia may be due to pancreatic glucagon insufficiency.[28]

#### Dietary treatment

The objective of dietary treatment is to prevent a marked rise in the blood sugar, which stimulates the pancreas to overproduce insulin. For this reason the patient must avoid the quickly digested sugars and limit other carbohydrate foods. The more slowly digested proteins and fats may be ingested freely.

The diet should contain from 120 g to 150 g of protein, from 75 g to 100 g of primarily complex carbohydrate, and sufficient fat to meet caloric requirements. No candy, sugar, jellies, jams, desserts, and soft drinks containing sugar should be eaten. Saccharin may be substituted for sugar. The low carbohydrate vegetables and fruits (see Chap. 24), and limited quantities of bread, cereal, and potatoes should provide the carbohydrate of the diet. A generous serving of meat, fish, fowl, eggs, or cheese must be included at each meal. Because milk contains the sugar lactose, it must be limited to a pint a day in the adult. Butter or margarine, cream, bacon, mayonnaise, other oil dressing, and meat fats supply the fat needed for calories. It is best to divide the food intake into five to eight meals a day. The patient may find it useful to carry crackers and a cube of cheese with him to control attacks if they are frequent.

### Study questions and activities

1. What are some common allergenic foods?
2. Using the producers' literature, make a list of popular baby foods that cannot be fed to an infant who is allergic to cow's milk.
3. Plan an inexpensive dinner menu for a family of four—two adults and two children—with one child who is allergic to wheat.
4. At time of discharge from the obstetrical unit, Mrs. A who had a postpartum hemorrhage is advised to eat high-iron foods. She dislikes liver in any form. What foods would you suggest she eat to supply an adequate daily intake of iron (see Chap. 6)?
5. Why may a patient who needs large doses of aspirin also be taking an antacid medication?
6. Select a patient on cancer chemotherapy who has been readmitted to the hospital. Check the patient's readmission weight with the weight on discharge 3 weeks ago. Find out how much and what foods and beverages the patient has been consuming since discharge.

### References

1. Ultman JE, Golomb HM: In Isselbacher KJ et al (eds): Harrison's Principles of Internal Medicine, 9th ed, pp 1583–1597. New York, McGraw-Hill, 1980
2. Theologides A: Am J Clin Nutr 29:552, 1976
3. Morrison SD: Am J Clin Nutr 31:1104, 1978
4. Shils ME: Med Clin North Am 63:1009, 1979
5. Lawrence W Jr: Cancer 43:2020, 1979
6. DeWys WD: JAMA 244:374, 1980
7. Theologides A: Cancer 43:2004, 1979
8. Pfaffmann C: Am J Clin Nutr 31:1058, 1978
9. Theologides A: Cancer 43:2004, 1979
10. MacGregor IL et al: Gastroenterology 70:190, 1976
11. Bernstein IL, Sigmundi RA: Science 209:416, 1980
12. Carson JAS, Gormican A: J Am Diet Assoc 70:361, 1977
13. Dwyer JT: Cancer 43:2077, 1979
14. Fleming SM et al: J Am Diet Assoc 70:391, 1977
15. Copeland EM III et al: Cancer 43:2108, 1979
16. Aker SN: Cancer 43:2103, 1979
17. Belut D et al: Dig Dis Sci 25:323, 1980
18. Rowe AH: Food Allergy. Springfield, IL, Charles C Thomas, 1972
19. Hughes EC: Ann Allergy 40:393, 1978
20. Laupus WE: In Vaughan VC III, McKay RJ (eds): Nelson Textbook of Pediatrics, 10th ed, pp 146–162. Philadelphia, WB Saunders, 1975
21. Bunn HF: In Isselbacher, Harrison's Principles, pp 1530–1532
22. Anderson CF: In Knox FG (ed): Textbook of Renal Pathophysiology, pp 254–261. New York, Harper & Row, 1978
23. Lindenbaum J, Roman MJ: Am J Clin Nutr 33:2727, 1980
24. De Vita VT Jr: In Isselbacher, Harrison's Principles, pp 1597–1620
25. Hartshorn EA: J Am Diet Assoc 70:15, 1977
26. Noid HE et al: Arch Dermatol 109:866, 1974
27. Reif-Lehrer L: Fed Proc 36:1617, 1977
28. Foa PP et al: JAMA 244:2281, 1980

### Supplementary readings
#### Cancer

Carson JAS, Gormican A: Taste acuity and food attitudes of selected patients with cancer. J Am Diet Assoc 70:361, 1977
Costa G, Donaldson SS: Current concepts in cancer: Effects of cancer and cancer treatment on nutrition of the host. N Engl J Med 300:1471, 1979

DeWys WD: Nutritional care of the cancer patient. JAMA 244:374, 1980

Dwyer JT: Dietetic assessment of ambulatory cancer patients. Cancer 43:2077, 1979

Morrison SD: Origins of anorexia in neoplastic disease. Am J Clin Nutr 31:1104, 1978

Pfaffmann C: Neurophysiological mechanisms of taste. Am J Clin Nutr 31:1058, 1978

Remington JS, Schimpff SC: Occasional notes: Please don't eat the salads. N Engl J Med 304:433, 1981

### Allergy

May CD: Editorial: Food allergy—Material and ethereal. N Engl J Med 302:1142, 1980

Parker C: Food allergies. Am J Nurs 80:262, 1980

### Nutrient–medication interrelationships

Chabner BA et al: The clinical pharmacology of antineoplastic agents. N Engl J Med 292:1107, 1975

Hartshorn EA: Food and drug interactions. J Am Diet Assoc 70:15, 1977

Reif-Lehrer L: A questionnaire study of the prevalence of Chinese restaurant syndrome. Fed Proc 36:1617, 1977

Roe DA: Interactions between drugs and nutrients. Med Clin North Am 53:985, 1979

## Patient resources
### Cancer

Aker S, Lenssen P: A Guide to Good Nutrition During and After Chemotherapy and Radiation, 2nd ed. (Available from Research Dietary Services, Fred Hutchinson Cancer Research Center, 1124 Columbia St., Seattle, WA 98104)

Diet and Nutrition: A Resource for Patients of Children with Cancer. NIH Publ. No. 80-2038. Washington, DC, NIH, 1979

Eating Hints: Recipes and Tips for Better Nutrition During Treatment. NIH Publ. No. 80-2079. Washington, DC, NIH, 1980

Keith RL et al: Looking Forward: A Guidebook for the Laryngectomee. Rochester, MN, Mayo Foundation, 1977

Local Chapter of the American Cancer Society

Mullen BD: The Ostomy Book: Living Comfortably with Colostomies, Ileostomies and Urostomies. Palo Alto, CA, Bull, 1980

Rosenbaum SH et al: Nutrition for the Cancer Patient. Palo Alto, CA, Bull, 1980

### Food allergy

Allergy Recipes. (Available from the American Dietetic Association, 430 Michigan Ave., Chicago, IL 60611)

Baking for People with Food Allergies. Home and Garden Bulletin No. 147. Superintendent of Documents, United States Government Printing Office, Washington, DC 20402

Dietary Information for Allergy Patients. (Available from Chicago Dietetic Supply Inc., 405 E. Shawmut, LaGrange, IL 60525)

125 Great Recipes for Allergy Diets. (Available from Good Housekeeping, 959 Fifth Ave., New York, NY 10021)

Rudoff C: The Allergy Baker. Menlo Park, CA, Prologue, 1980

Thomas LL: Caring and Cooking for the Allergic Child, rev ed. New York, Sterling, 1980

### Diet-medication interrelationships

Graedon J: The People's Pharmacy—2. New York, Avon Books, 1980

*For further references see Bibliography in Part 4.*

# Nutrition in Diseases of Infancy and Childhood

## 35

**ADD:** Attention Deficit Disorder
**CF:** Cystic Fibrosis
**CNSD:** Chronic Nonspecific Diarrhea
**FTT:** Failure-to-thrive
**HRV:** Human Rotovirus
**LBW:** Low Birth Weight
**NEC:** Necrotizing Enterocolitis
**NICN:** Neonatal Intensive Care Nursery
**SGA:** Small-for-gestational-age
**TBSB:** Total Body Surface Burned
**TBW:** Total Body Weight
**VLBW:** Very Low Birth Weight

**Linda J. Boyne**

There are two major categories of illness presented by the infant or child admitted to the pediatric unit of a general hospital or to a pediatric hospital. The illness may be caused by extrinsic, or environmental factors; or it may be related to intrinsic factors, problems existing at or before birth. Some of the problems that derive from extrinsic factors are acute infections, especially those not controlled by immunization, such as respiratory or gastrointestinal infections; accidents either within or outside the home, including burns; child abuse, including physical injury or underfeeding; and emotional problems. Some of the intrinsic problems that may be present at birth or expressed at a later time are congenital anomalies of various structures, such as the heart, kidneys, palate, esophagus, intestines, skeleton, and neurologic system; and inborn errors of metabolism. Some of the malignancies of early childhood are also categorized as intrinsic in origin.

Whether they are at home or in the hospital, the majority of infants and children need a diet that supplies the energy and nutrients appropriate to the age and expected rate of growth of the individual child. This applies even to the acutely ill child after the treatment of the critical problem, such as the correction of dehydration due to infectious diarrhea, or to the child who has undergone surgery. Some children with a birth defect or long-term illness may need modifications in the consistency of food or in the feeding method, such as the child with a cleft palate or the child with cerebral palsy. Other children may need modifications in nutrient intake, such as a sodium-restricted diet for the child with a congenital anomaly of the heart or the restriction of phenylalanine, an essential amino acid, in phenylketonuria, an inborn error of metabolism. Normal diet for age is presented in Chapters 18 and 19. The information in these chapters should be reviewed for it applies to the sick infant or child as well.

Although the sick infant or child is the primary focus of the health-care team, the needs of the parents must also be met. During the acute illness of their child, parents are anxious and their anxieties can often be relieved if the health-care team takes time to communicate with them. When the child with either an acute or a long-term illness is hospitalized, many mothers want to be involved in their child's care, especially at meal times. These women need to be accepted as members of the health-care team. On the other hand a woman who cannot be at the hospital with her child because she has other children at home or has to work to support her family should not be slighted by the team. Rather, they should accept her situation and communicate with her whenever she is available. And, in some situations, it may be the father or grandparents who join the team.

The families of children with handicaps or chronic illnesses present special problems. Handicaps and chronic illnesses often demand major adjustments in a family's life-style. Special medications, foods, and equipment can use up a major portion of the family's income. For example, 1 qt (approximately 1 liter) of medium-chain triglyceride oil costs approximately eight times as much as 1 qt of vegetable oil. Other children may feel neglected because so much of the parents' time, effort, and money is spent on the ill child.

At the same time parents may have strong feelings of anxiety and guilt at having produced a child who is handicapped or has a chronic illness. As a result, they may overprotect or completely reject the child. They may also reject genetic counseling in applicable situations. As the child grows into adolescence, questions may arise in his mind about his future, about marriage, about supporting himself, and always, about being different.

These individual family dynamics must be dealt with by the health-care team. The team must be able to cope with the family's anxieties and guilt feelings, to counsel the parents on how to care for the child, and, very important, to build the parents' confidence in their ability to carry out the program of care. The family must also be informed of any financial assistance and community resources that are available to them. In many states Medicaid and other state or federal programs are available to assist families in meeting medical costs for chronically ill children.

Organizations of parents, professionals, and other interested people, such as the American Diabetes Association, the United Cerebral Palsy Association, and the National Cystic Fibrosis Research Foundation, among others, were founded to stimulate research and to promote knowledge of the disease and care of the affected child. Local chapters of the national associations are often of great help to parents by enabling them to share their anxieties and fears with others facing the same problems, and by channelling their feelings into constructive action.

## Feeding the sick child
### Food and illness

When children become ill they tend to regress to an earlier developmental level. A 13 month old baby who has been drinking from a cup may accept fluids only from a nursing bottle, or a $2\frac{1}{2}$ year old who has been doing a good job of feeding himsef may now want to be fed. Also, the type of food the sick child will accept is often limited. The wisest response in a short-term illness, such as a cold or minor gastrointestinal upset, is to let him have his way, but be sure his fluid intake is adequate. When he feels better, he will return quickly to his more recently acquired food practices and will make up, both in quantity and in quality, the nutrients that were missing in his diet during his illness.

Food intake may become a serious problem in the child who has a chronic illness. Enough food must be eaten to provide his nutritional needs for growth and development as well as additional energy to cover energy expenditures related to his disease, for example, in the child with cystic fibrosis. If a modified diet is not required as part of his treatment, he should be offered the normal diet for age (see Chaps. 18 and 19). If he has a poor appetite, it may be easier for him to eat smaller, more frequent meals, and occasional surprises may help him look forward to mealtimes. However, it may not be wise to offer the very young child who is ill a meal of totally unfamiliar foods or new combinations of his favorite foods. For the child restricted to bed at home, a picnic lunch with his family or a special afternoon snack with his friends in the neighborhood may stimulate him to eat more than he would otherwise. In some situations poor food acceptance by the child with a chronic illness may be a symptom of a poor relationship between the mother and child, and the mother may need counseling to solve the problem.

Some children with chronic illnesses that do not permit much physical activity, for example, myelomeningocele, may become obese because eating is their only form of recreation. These children need help developing hobbies and activities that, while adapted to their lack of mobility, provide new sources of recreation.

### The child in the hospital

The sick child who must be hospitalized finds himself in strange surroundings among strange people. In the midst of all this strangeness the one experience he may recognize and enjoy is eating. In this new setting the child must be given a great deal of freedom about his food, even to the point of being allowed to refuse it. Some children eat only bread and butter and drink milk for the first few days in the hospital, as these foods are most reminiscent of home. Children from homes with ethnic food patterns that differ from those of the community at large may have considerable difficulty accepting unfamiliar foods.

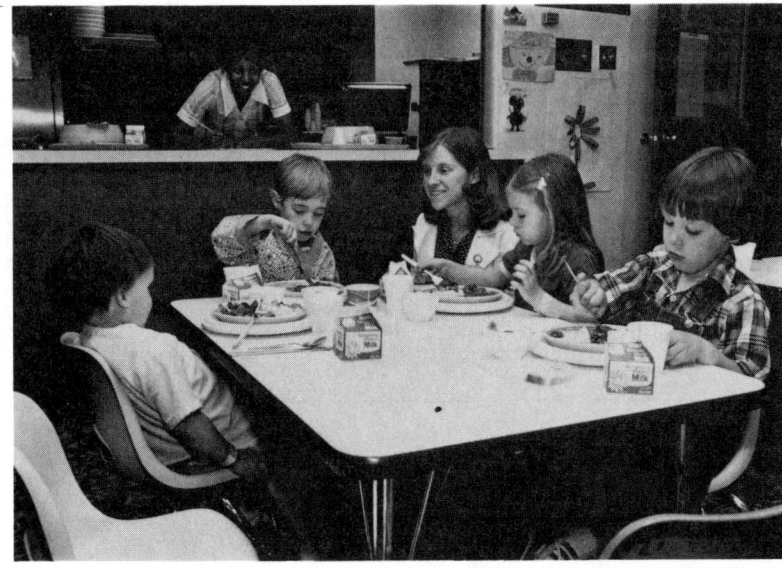

**Fig. 35-1.**   Meals taste better when they are eaten in company with other children in the hospital. (Columbus Children's Hospital, Columbus, Ohio, with permission)

In so far as possible, the food served by the dietary department should reflect the usual food practices of the community. It is helpful if, on admission or as soon as possible after admission, a staff member obtains from the mother of the young child or directly from the older child a list of his food preferences. This helps to avoid serving him foods that he dislikes even when well. Although this helps to bridge the gap between home and hospital, it does not solve the problem, however, because the methods of food preparation vary and the taste of a food prepared in the hospital may differ from the same dish prepared at home. Also, today's child may not be comparing the food served in the hospital with that served at home, but with his past experiences of eating away from home in fast-food service chains, or in preschool or school feeding programs.

Another way of helping the child to feel at home in the hospital is to have him eat at a table with other children of his age as soon as this is feasible (Fig. 35-1). Children often eat better around a table with other children. Also, it takes the time of only one staff member to help these children in a group compared with the number of staff members required to serve individual children in their rooms or at bedside in a ward. When a hospitalized child has a birthday, a birthday treat shared with other patients his age helps to relieve the unpleasantness of illness.

Most of all, it is important that mealtime be a happy time, with no pressures about cleaning up plates, drinking all the milk, or not being allowed dessert because not all the other food served was eaten. The dessert should be as important a source of nutrients as any other item on the menu. An illness is not the time for a child to have to learn to eat new foods or to acquire new skills in eating unless he does this on his own initiative. Also, mealtimes should

*never* be interrupted to draw blood, to change dressings, or to do other painful procedures; and treatments such as physiotherapy and postural drainage should be scheduled so that the child has a rest period before his meals.

The size of a serving offered the child is also important. "Appetite poor" recorded in the nursing notes may mean that a child was served too much food. A serving of 4 oz (120 ml) of soup and half a sandwich is adequate for many 2 to 3 year olds, while a 12 year old boy may need a "man size" serving. Table 35-1, using the Exchange System, illustrates the amount of food needed in a day to meet the energy needs of children 2 to 6 years old. When this food is distributed over three meals and two or three between meal feedings, the servings are small by adult standards. Another suggestion for determining serving sizes of meat, fruits, and vegetables is to use 1 tablespoon per year of age as a basis. For example, a 2-tbsp serving of green beans is sufficient for a 2 year old.

Finally, parents have rights. The mother who spends the day with her hospitalized child usually wants to contribute to his care. Choosing the food and feeding the child may be the only contribution she can make. This is especially true if the child has a terminal illness. These mothers may be demanding; they have a right to be demanding, and their demands should be met if possible.

## General principles of diet therapy in pediatric nutrition

Whenever the diet must be modified as part of the treatment of illness in an infant or child, the following general principles must be considered in each situation. In this way, the therapeutic diet plan not only contributes to the treatment of the specific problem but also promotes, so far as possible, the normal growth and development of the child.

**Table 35-1.  Daily Amounts of Foods to Meet Energy Needs of 2- to 6-Year-Old Children**

| | 2 to 3 Years | | 3 to 4 Years | | 4 to 6 Years | |
|---|---|---|---|---|---|---|
| *Food Exchanges* | *Amount* | *Energy (kcal)** | *Amount* | *Energy (kcal)* | *Amount* | *Energy (kcal)* |
| Milk | 3 c (750 ml) | 510 | 3 c (750 ml) | 510 | 4 c (1000 ml) | 680 |
| Meat | 1 oz (30 g) | 75 | 2 oz (60 g) | 150 | 2 oz (60 g) | 150 |
| Egg | 1 | 75 | 1 | 75 | 1 | 75 |
| Bread† | 4 exchanges | 280 | 4 exchanges | 280 | 5 exchanges | 350 |
| Fruit | 2 servings | 80 | 2 servings | 80 | 2 servings | 80 |
| Vegetables | 1 serving | 35 | 1 serving | 35 | 1 serving | 35 |
| Fat | 2 tsp | 90 | 3 tsp | 135 | 3 tsp | 135 |
| Dessert‡ | ⅔ serving | 100 | 1 serving | 150 | 1 serving | 150 |
| Totals | | 1245 | | 1415 | | 1655 |
| NRC-RDA | 1250 kcal | | 1400 kcal | | 1600 kcal | |

*See exchange system, Chapter 24.

†Includes bread, potatoes, crackers, and pasta.

‡Chocolate pudding. See Table 1 in Part 4.

### Energy-protein

In order to support normal growth, the energy and protein needs of the child must be met. For example, the dwarfism in children with diabetes that occurred in the 1930s was due more to inadequate energy intakes than to poor control of the disease with regular insulin.

Table 35-2 is a guide to the energy and protein needs per kilogram of body weight for infants and children by age; and for adolescents by age and sex. The energy figures in this table can be used to estimate reasonable goals for daily calorie intakes. The estimates may need to be revised because the rate of growth and the energy expenditure due to the level of activity vary with each infant and child. However, the energy intake should not be significantly less than recommended, since, without an adequate energy intake from fat and carbohydrate, the protein in the diet will be used for energy rather than for the synthesis of cellular proteins. One 7 month old infant boy was signifi-

**Table 35-2.  Guide for Calculating Energy and Protein Needs for Infants and Children**

| Age (Years) | Energy (Kcal/kg) | Protein (g/kg) |
|---|---|---|
| 0.0–0.5 | 115 | 2.2 |
| 0.5–1.0 | 105 | 2.0 |
| 1–3 | 100 | 1.8 |
| 4–6 | 85 | 1.5 |
| 7–10 | 85 | 1.2 |
| *Males* | | |
| 11–14 | 60 | 1.0 |
| 15–18 | 40 | 0.9 |
| *Females* | | |
| 11–14 | 50 | 1.0 |
| 15–18 | 40 | 0.9 |

(Calculated from Food and Nutrition Board: Recommended Dietary Allowances, 9th rev ed. Washington, DC, NAS-NRC, 1980)

cantly underweight due to a daily energy deficit of 400 kcal with no deficit in protein intake.

If the infant or child has experienced growth retardation due to his illness, the estimate of daily energy and total nutrient intake may need to be adjusted upward for a period of time to support catch-up growth. A formula containing 24 kcal per ounce (30 ml) may be used for an infant under 4 months of age, while increased quantities of a formula containing 20 kcal per ounce (30 ml) plus infant foods, such as cereal, may be adequate for the older infant. The older child needs larger servings of an adequate diet for age to catch up. Daily weighing of infants and weekly weighing of very young children are used to monitor the adequacy of energy intake.

When the protein is adjusted for therapeutic reasons, two important factors must be considered. If total protein intake is limited, proteins of high biologic value must be supplied to support the infant's or child's requirement of essential amino acids. For example, the order for 1.5 g of protein per kilogram of body weight for a 2 week old infant with an inborn error of metabolism in the urea cycle must provide the infant's requirement for the essential amino acids without an excessive quantity of nonessential nitrogen.

The essential amino acid requirements of infants 2 to 4 months of age as determined by Holt and Snyderman and co-workers are listed in Chapter 36, Table 36-1, in the section on inborn errors of amino acid metabolism. These investigators[1] have also shown that the infants they studied grew well on an intake of 1.3 g of cow's milk protein per kilogram of body weight with supplemental nitrogen. This quantity of milk protein supplied the amount of essential amino acids required by their subjects. In clinical practice one can determine the amount of cow's milk protein required to supply an infant's essential amino acid requirement and supplement this with cereal for an adequate nitrogen supply.

Although the infant and the young child require more protein per kilogram of body weight than do adults to support cellular growth, excessive intakes of protein can be hazardous. In early infancy an intake in excess of 4 g to 5 g of protein per kilogram of body weight per day should be carefully monitored because kidney, and possibly liver, function is immature at this age. Excessive blood levels of the end-products of protein catabolism, particularly ammonia, can be detrimental to the developing central nervous system. In any child excessive intakes of protein without adequate fluid intake can lead to dehydration.

### Fluids

Unless contraindicated by a medical problem, such as renal failure, the normal fluid requirements of the infant and child must be taken into consideration when therapeutic diets are planned. Table 35-3 gives the range of average fluid requirements for infants and children under ordinary conditions. An appropriate intake of formula or breast milk provides these fluid needs for the young infant, particularly the breast-fed infant. In the older child fluid needs can be met by water and a variety of other fluids, including milk and fruit juices. It is important to remember that water, not additional formula or milk, should be offered to the infant during hot weather to prevent dehydration.

### Fats

Fats supply approximately 50% of the total energy intake of the breast-fed infant. The energy from fat in the commonly used infant formulas varies from 45% to 50%. As the child grows older, fat usually supplies 35% to 45% of the total energy intake. The Committee on Nutrition of the American Academy of Pediatrics recommends that 3% of total calories for an infant or young child come from linoleic acid, the essential fatty acid (see Chap. 3, *Fats*). When medium-chain triglycerides (MCT) are used as the major source of fat in a formula for an infant with malabsorption problems, a source of linoleic acid must be included, since MCT oils do not contain linoleic acid. Corn oil, which contains linoleic acid, is added to special infant formulas that derive their fat content primarily from MCTs (see Table 35-4, *Special Infant Formulas*). The older child can use the appropriate amounts of margarine or mayonnaise made with corn oil if the diet pattern does not include linoleic acid from other sources.

If a child has a familial hyperlipoproteinemia, modification of his diet in the type of fatty acid or the cholesterol content or both may be recommended (see Chap. 30, *Atherosclerosis*).

### Carbohydrate

Carbohydrate usually supplies 45% to 50% of the total energy intake of infants and young children. Without a source of carbohydrate in the diet, infants will develop hypoglycemia. One formula, RCF,* is available for infants with carbohydrate malabsorption problems. The formula contains protein and fat, but a carbohydrate that is tolerated by the infant must be added to prevent hypoglycemia and ketosis.[2]

The amount of sucrose should be limited in any therapeutic diet, as in any normal diet for age, to prevent dental caries. In hyperlipoproteinemias and diabetes mellitus the type of carbohydrate (simple or complex) may also be modified.

### Electrolytes

With problems of excessive fluid and electrolyte loss in infancy and early childhood, oral solutions of electrolytes may be required (see discussion of diarrhea in next section). In other situations, especially in renal and cardiac disease, the intake of sodium and potassium may be modified.

### Vitamins

If the therapeutic diet cannot supply an adequate intake of vitamins, supplements are used. However, excessive intakes of vitamins, especially the fat-soluble ones, must be avoided. When fat malabsorption occurs, as in cystic fibrosis, water-miscible preparations of the fat-soluble vitamins are used.

### Minerals

Care must be taken to ensure that therapeutic diets for infants and children contain adequate amounts of minerals. It must be remembered that the quantity of a mineral required at one age may not be adequate as the child grows older. For example, at 1 month of age Fomon[3]

---

*Ross Laboratories, Columbus, OH 43216

**Table 35-3. Range of Average Daily Fluid Requirements of Infants and Children Under Ordinary Conditions**

| Age | Average Body Weight (kg) | Fluid Per kg of Body Weight (ml) |
|---|---|---|
| 3 days | 3.0 | 80–100 |
| 10 days | 3.2 | 125–150 |
| 3 months | 5.4 | 140–160 |
| 6 months | 7.3 | 130–155 |
| 9 months | 8.6 | 125–145 |
| 1 year | 9.5 | 120–135 |
| 2 years | 11.8 | 115–125 |
| 4 years | 16.2 | 100–110 |
| 6 years | 20.0 | 90–100 |
| 10 years | 28.7 | 70–85 |
| 14 years | 45.0 | 50–60 |
| 18 years | 54.0 | 40–50 |

(Adapted from Vaughan VC III, McKay RJ Jr, Behrman RE (eds): Nelson Textbook of Pediatrics, 11th ed, p 175. Philadelphia, WB Saunders, 1979)

## Table 35-4. Special Formulas with Vitamins and Minerals Added

| Product and Producer | Protein | Carbohydrate | Fat | Special Comments | Osmolality* per kg H₂O | Uses |
|---|---|---|---|---|---|---|
| *Soy-Based, Lactose Free* | | | | | | |
| Isomil (Ross Laboratories, Columbus, OH 43216) | Soy isolate | Corn syrup, sucrose | Coconut and soy oils | Concentrate or ready to feed Iron fortified only | 250 mOsm | Diarrhea, cow's milk allergy, lactase deficiency |
| Prosobee (Mead-Johnson Laboratories, Evansville, IN 47721) | Soy isolate | Corn syrup, solids | Soy and coconut oils | Concentrate, ready to feed Iron fortified only; now lactose and sucrose free | 180 mOsm | Cow's milk sensitivity, lactose or sucrose intolerance, galactosemia, diarrhea |
| Soyalac (Loma Linda Foods, Riverside, CA 92515) | Soybean solids and methionine | Corn syrup, solids, sucrose | Soybean oil | Concentrate | 273 mOsm | Cow's milk allergy |
| I-Soyalac (Loma Linda Foods) | Soy isolate | Sucrose, modified tapioca starch | Soy oil | Concentrate. Corn and lactose free | 206 mOsm | Cow's milk allergy, galactosemia |
| Nursoy (Wyeth Laboratories, Philadelphia, PA 19101) | Soy isolate, methionine added | Sucrose | Oleo, coconut, safflower, and soy oils | Concentrate, ready to feed | 296 mOsm | Cow's milk allergy |
| RCF (Ross) | Soy isolate | To be added | Soy and coconut oil | Carbohydrate must be added Concentrate | | Diarrhea, disaccharide intolerance |
| *Non-Soy, Lactose Free* | | | | | | |
| Nutramigen (Mead-Johnson) | Enzymatically hydrolyzed and charcoal treated casein | Sucrose, tapioca starch | Corn oil | Powder (9.5 g/2 oz H₂O = 20 kcal/oz) 15% calories from protein | 479 mOsm | Diarrhea, cow's milk allergy, intact protein sensitivity |
| MBF, meat-base formula (Gerber Products Co., Fremont, MI 49412) | Beef heart | Sucrose, tapioca starch | Sesame oil | Concentrate | 207.8 mOsm | Cow's milk allergies |
| Pregestimil (Mead-Johnson) | Casein hydrolysate, amino acids | Corn syrup solids, modified tapioca starch | Corn oil, medium chain triglycerides | Powder, (9.7g/2 oz H₂O = 20 kcal/oz) 14% calories from protein | 348 mOsm | Diarrhea, disaccharidase deficiency, steatorrhea |
| Lofenalac (Mead-Johnson) | Casein hydrolysate processed to remove most of phenylalanine, amino acids added | Corn syrup solids, tapioca starch | Corn oil | Powder (9.4 g/2 oz H₂O = 20 kcal/oz) 15% calories from protein Phenylalanine content approximately 0.08% | 454 mOsm | Infants with phenylketonuria |
| Phenyl-Free (Mead-Johnson) | Phenylalanine free food amino acids | Sucrose, corn syrup solids, modified | Corn oil | Powder (98.5 g/13.5 oz H₂O = 25 kcal/oz) 16 oz formula = 1 day intake 20% calories from protein | 420 mOsm | Children over 2 years with PKU |
| MSUD Diet Powder (Mead-Johnson) | Amino acids free of branched chain amino acids isoleucine, leucine, and valine | Corn syrup solids and modified tapioca starch | Corn oil | Powder (9 g/2 oz H₂O = 20 kcal/oz) | 358 mOsm | Maple syrup urine disease |

**Table 35-4. Special Formulas with Vitamins and Minerals Added (Continued)**

| Product and Producer | Protein | Carbohydrate | Fat | Special Comments | Osmolality* per kg H₂O | Uses |
|---|---|---|---|---|---|---|
| *Other Special Formulas* | | | | | | |
| Portagen (Mead-Johnson) | Sodium caseinate | Sucrose, corn syrup solids | Medium chain triglyceride oil, corn oil | Powder (9.5 g/2 oz H₂O = 20 kcal/oz) 14% calories from protein; 43% from fat | 158 mOsm | Fat malabsorption |
| Probana (Mead-Johnson) | Whole and non-fat cow's milk, banana powder, casein hydrolysate | Dextrose, lactose, banana powder | Corn oil, butterfat | Powder (9.8 g/2 oz H₂O = 20 kcal/oz) 24% calories from protein; 29% from fat | 592 mOsm | Diarrhea, steatorrhea |
| Similac PM60/40 (Ross Laboratories) | Partially demineralized whey, sodium caseinate | Lactose | Corn and coconut oils | Powder (8.56 g/2 oz H₂O = 20 kcal/oz) 60:40 lactalbumin:casein Electrolyte composition similar to human milk | 260 mOsm | Renal and cardiac disease |
| SMA, S-29 (Wyeth Laboratories) | Electrodialyzed whey | Lactose | Oleo, coconut, safflower, and soy oils | Powder (8.4 g/2 oz H₂O = 20 kcal/oz) Very low in electrolytes | 310 mOsm | Acute congestive heart failure, acute renal disease |
| SMA, S-14 (Wyeth Laboratories) | Non-fat milk | Lactose | Oleo, coconut, safflower, and soy oils | Powder (7.4 g/2 oz H₂O = 20 kcal/oz) 9% calories from protein; low in leucine (33 mg/oz) | 280 mOsm | Leucine-induced hypoglycemia |
| *Special Formulas for Preterm Infants* | | | | | | |
| Enfamil Premature (Mead-Johnson) | Demineralized whey, non-fat milk solids | Corn syrup solids | Medium chain triglyceride oils, corn and coconut oils | Available for hospital use only, ready to feed 12% calories from protein; 48% calories from fat; 24 kcal/oz | 300 mOsm | Growing low-birth-weight infants |
| Similac/Special Care Infant Formula | Whey and casein 60:40 | Lactose, corn syrup solids | Medium chain triglycerides, corn and coconut oils | Available in 4-oz bottles ready to feed, hospital use only 11% total calories from protein; 46% total calories from fat; 42% total calories from carbohydrate 24 kcal/oz | 300 mOsm | Growing low-birth-weight infants |
| *Other Products* | | | | | | |
| Casec (Mead-Johnson) | Dried, soluble calcium caseinate derived from skim milk curd | Trace | Butterfat | Powder (4.7 g/ contains 4 g protein, 75 mg calcium, 2.7 mg sodium, and 17 kcal) | | Protein supplement or for designing individualized formulas |
| MCT Oil (Mead-Johnson) | None | None | Triglycerides of medium chain fatty acids | Liquid (68% C₈ fatty acids, 24% C₁₀ fatty acids) | | Substitution for energy from long-chain fatty acids |
| Polycose (Ross Laboratories) | None | Glucose polymers derived from controlled hydrolysis of cornstarch | None | Powder (8 g = 30 calories; 9.2 mg sodium) Liquid (1 oz = 60 calories; 17.4 mg sodium) | 850 mOsm | Carbohydrate supplement for formulas |

*From manufacturer's information.

advises a daily iron intake of 7 mg and at 2 to 3 months 8 mg. The trace mineral composition of most synthetic formulas used in the treatment of inborn errors of amino acid metabolism has been adjusted to meet the recommended levels to support normal growth. The composition should be checked carefully to be sure, however.

### Special infant formulas

Special infant formulas that vary from the standard ones (see Table 18-4, Chap. 18) in the kinds and amounts of ingredients, are widely available to meet the nutrient needs of infants with metabolic problems. Although the majority of special formulas have the same energy density as the standard ones (20 kcal per 30 ml, normal dilution) the food sources of protein, fat, and carbohydrate differ. For example, some formulas have soy isolate as the source of protein for infants who are allergic to milk protein (see Table 35-4).

Special infant formulas can also be prepared from basic ingredients—casein, dextrin, sugars, and fats (see Table 35-4). Formulas prepared from basic ingredients must contain a distribution of protein, fat, and carbohydrate similar to standard formulas in order to support normal growth and development. The addition of minerals, vitamins, and electrolytes is usually necessary. All special formulas (concentrates or powders) must be mixed with water to normal dilution. The water used to prepare formulas need not be boiled as long as the safety of the water supply has been determined. The powdered formulas are easier to mix, however, if lukewarm water is used. People who obtain their water from a private well should have their water tested periodically by the local health department.

The bottles, nipples, caps, and can opener should be thoroughly washed, rinsed, and boiled before the formula is prepared. The can lid should be washed and rinsed. Bottles are easier to clean if cold water is added to the bottle after a feeding. The nipple may be put to soak in a clean container. Terminal sterilization may be used, if desired, with the exception of some protein hydrolysate formulas in which the protein is rendered undigestible during terminal sterilization.

## The acutely ill infant or young child
### Nutritional concerns in the high risk neonate
The neonatal intensive care nursery

An increasing number of neonatal intensive care nurseries (NICN) have been established recently in pediatric hospitals or pediatric units in major medical centers across the United States. These nurseries provide life-support systems for the newborn infant who has difficulty surviving the birth process. These infants present a variety of problems, such as congenital anomalies, respiratory distress syndrome, infection acquired *in utero* and an inappropriate weight status with or without congenital anomalies and other critical conditions. Because total or partial funding for these units is provided through grants from the Federal Government, numerous data are generated concerning the various aspects of treatment for these infants.

Team approach

The NICN is staffed by a team of highly specialized health professionals: the neonatologist, pediatric surgeon, pediatric cardiologist, nurse specialists, respiratory technicians, social workers, and the pediatric dietitian.

Special preparation in pediatric nutrition is needed by the dietitian who serves on this team. The dietitian is responsible for assessing the nutritional needs of each infant receiving care in the unit; planning and monitoring the nutritional care; counseling parents during the infant's hospitalization and providing follow-up care after discharge; and participating in staff and community educational programs on the high-risk infant.

The low-birth-weight and the small-for-gestational age infants

Many, although not all, of the infants admitted to NICNs are at risk because of their weight status at birth. The low-birth-weight (LBW) infant, who weighs less than 2500 g, may have had a shortened intrauterine period (less than 37 wk), a slower than expected rate of growth, or both. The terms *LBW*, *premature*, and *preterm* are often used interchangeably. LBW infants are frequently associated with a lower parental socioeconomic status, maternal undernutrition, inadequate prenatal care, and, to a lesser degree, teenage pregnancies. Small-for-gestational age (SGA) infants are those who, although they may be fullterm, are shorter in length, lighter in weight, and appear to have disproportionately larger heads relative to body size than is expected for their gestational age. These infants have suffered from intrauterine growth retardation. SGA infants may be associated with maternal toxemia, excessive maternal smoking, placental abnormalities, congenital heart disease, congenital rubella, and cytomegalovirus infection.

The clinical problems presented by the SGA infant are different from those of the LBW infant, who is developmentally appropriate for gestational age. The SGA infant has inappropriate neurologic development for gestational age as well as immature anatomic structure and physiological and biochemical functions. It can be anticipated that extrauterine growth rates will differ. The LBW infant may catch up to his fullterm counterparts by 2 years of age, whereas the SGA infant may narrow the gap but probably will not catch up. The SGA infant may also fail to achieve a normal level of mental ability. Both the

LBW and the SGA infant may or may not have congenital anomalies or other critical conditions.

Lubchenco and co-workers[4,5] in Denver have developed charts (see Fig. 35-2) that can be used to classify newborns based on maturity and intrauterine growth. These charts are useful in identifying the infant who has suffered intrauterine undernutrition and in monitoring the infant's rate of weight gain after birth.

## Feeding the LBW and SGA infant

Some of the complications that may be encountered in providing nutritional support to the LBW and SGA infant are immature gastrointestinal, renal, and respiratory systems. The smaller the infant the more frequently are the sucking and swallowing reflexes poorly developed. This leads to regurgitation with the possibility of aspiration of gastric contents into the lungs. Therefore, many of

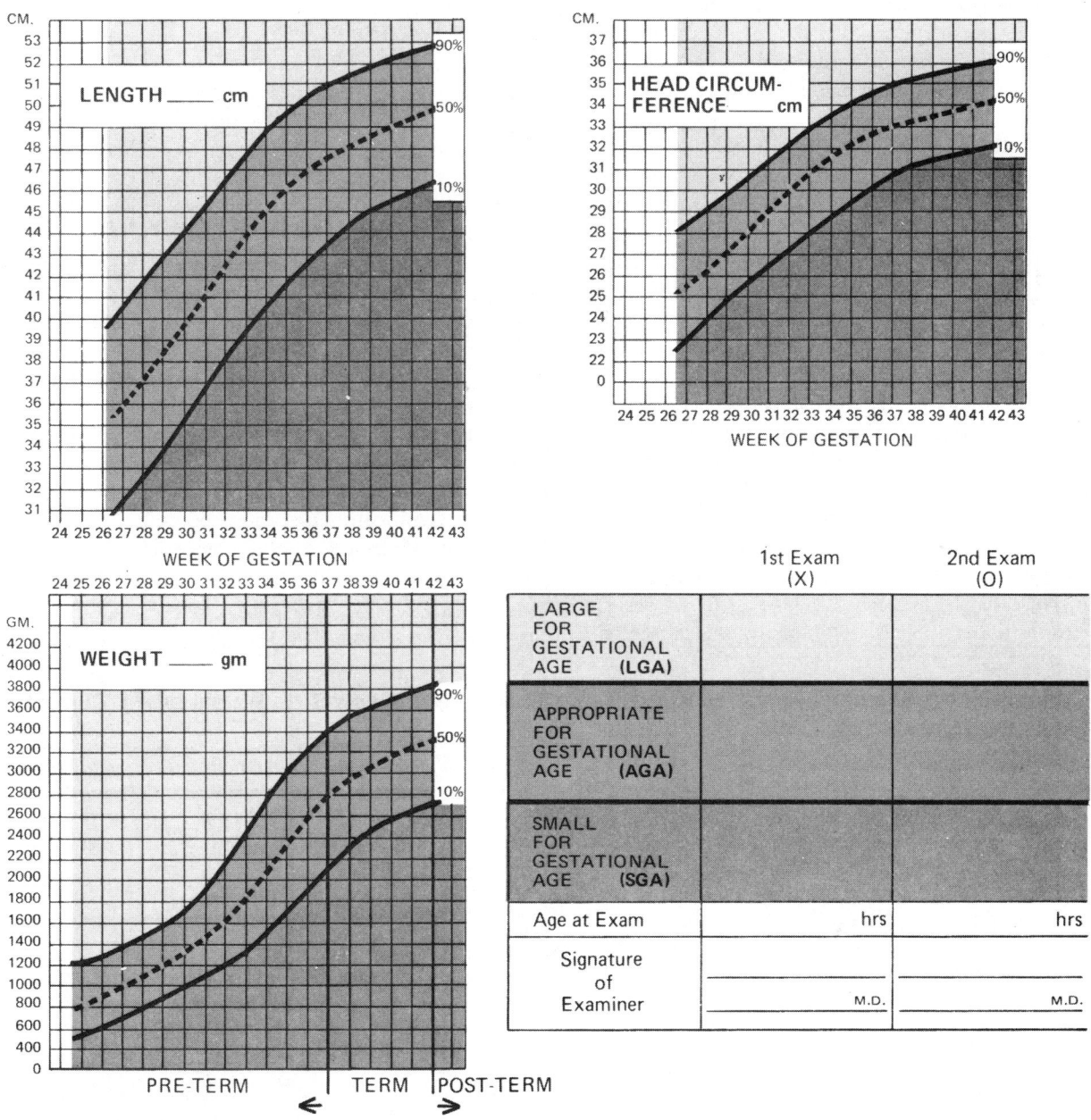

**Fig. 35-2.** Classification of newborns, based on maturity and intrauterine growth. (Lubchenco LC, Hansman C, Boyd E: Pediatr 37:403, 1966; Battaglia Lubchenco LC: J Pediatr 71:159, 1967)

the infants are fed by nasogastric tube. The metabolic enzyme systems of these infants may be immature, and there may be an unavailability of substrate for the gluconeogenic pathway, resulting in neonatal hypoglycemia. They may have an insufficient quantity of bile, which can result in decreased micelle formation with a decreased ability to absorb fat.

### Nutritional requirements

Factors that need to be considered when designing a feeding program for these infants are: estimation of nutritional requirements; type and distribution of protein, fat, and carbohydrates; other nutrient needs; the renal solute load; and the gastrointestinal osmotic load.

### Advisable intakes

The nutritional requirements for LBW and SGA infants differ from those of term infants because a larger intake is necessary to promote the tissue synthesis that did not take place *in utero*. The optimal rate of growth for these infants is not known. The Committee on Nutrition of the American Academy of Pediatrics states that the optimal diet supports a rate of growth approximating that of the third trimester of intrauterine life without causing stress on the developing systems.[6] However, perhaps the composition of this growth should differ from that expected during the third trimester. The increased percentage of fat deposition occurring during the last trimester of intrauterine life may not be desirable in extrauterine life.

Zeigler and associates[7] have designed a reference fetus using published data on the chemical analyses of human fetuses with gestational ages of 24 to 40 weeks. Body composition at various gestational ages is presented

and from this, weight gain and composition of the gain has been calculated. These calculations have been used to develop advisable intakes for the LBW infant[8] (see Table 35-5). This method, though imprecise, is the most satisfactory method currently available.

### Energy

When the LBW infant is fed enterally, the energy intake should be in the range of 110 kcal to 150 kcal per kilogram per day. SGA infants may have an even greater energy need. The energy distribution should approximate that of the term infant—protein 7% to 16%, carbohydrate 30% to 65%, and fat 40% to 55% of total calories.[9] The higher fat content is preferred to an increased protein content, which would increase the renal solute load. Calorically dense formulas, those that provide 81 kcal per 100 ml, may be needed to meet these needs because of the low volume that the infant is able to consume in a 24-hour period. Two formulas developed specifically to meet the needs of the growing LBW infant are currently available for hospital use only, Enfamil Premature Formula* and Similac Special Care Infant Formula† (see Table 35-5).

The suitability of human milk for the preterm infant is being questioned. In 1977 Fomon[10] suggested that even when supplemented with vitamins, mature human milk will probably be inadequate in protein, calcium, and sodium to promote a weight gain. However, there are new data that indicate that the milk of mothers who deliver preterm is significantly higher in sodium, chloride, and protein than the milk of mothers who deliver at term.[11]

---

*Mead Johnson Laboratories, Evansville, IN 47721
†Ross Laboratories, Columbus, OH 43216

---

### Table 35-5. Selected Nutrients Compared to Advisable Intakes* for the Low Birth Weight Infant (Current Information as of October 31, 1980)

| | *800–1200 g* *(26–28 wks)* | *1200–1800 g* *(29–31 wks)* | *Full Term Human Milk*† | *Similac 20‡ Enfamil§ SMA‖* | *Enfamil Premature Formula§* | *Similac Special Care Infant Formula‡* |
|---|---|---|---|---|---|---|
| Caloric Density | | | | | | |
| Kcal/100 ml | | | 67–75 | 67–68 | 81 | 81 |
| Kcal/oz | | | 22 | 20 | 24 | 24 |
| Protein (g/100Kcal) | 3.1 | 2.7 | 1.5 | 2.2–2.3 | 3.0 | 2.7 |
| Calcium (mg/100Kcal) | 160 | 140 | 45 | 66–81 | 117 | 160 |
| Sodium (mEq/100 Kcal) | 2.7 | 2.3 | 1.05 | 1.0–1.6 | 1.7 | 1.9 |
| Chloride (mEq/100Kcal) | 2.4 | 2.0 | 1.7 | 1.5–2.2 | 2.4 | 2.3 |
| Phosphorus (mg/100Kcal) | 108 | 95 | 21.0 | 49–69 | 58.5 | 89 |
| Calcium: Phosphorus Ratio | | | | | 2.0 | 1.8 |
| | | | Amount per 100 Kcal | | | |
| Vitamin E IU/day | 30 | 30 | .94 | 1.0–2.0 | 2.0 | 3.7 |
| Vitamin C mg/day | 60 | 60 | .45 | 8 | 8.5 | 37 |
| Folic acid µg/day | 60 | 60 | 7.8 | 8–16 | 7.8 | 37 |
| Osmolality (mOsm/kg H₂O) | | | 300 | 288–300 | 300 | 300 |

*Zeigler EE et al: Nutritional requirements of the premature infant. In Suskind RM (ed): Symposium on Pediatric Nutrition. New York, Raven Press (in press)
†Source: Fomon, SJ: Infant Nutrition, 2nd ed., pp 362–63. Philadelphia, WB Saunders, 1974
‡Ross Laboratories, Columbus, OH 43216
§Mead Johnson Laboratories, Evansville, IN 47721
‖Wyeth Laboratories, Philadelphia, PA 19101

The preterm milk is also lower in lactose concentration. Atkinson and associates[12] also demonstrated that the energy density of preterm milk was approximately 20% higher than that of fullterm milk, although Gross[11] found no difference between the two milks in energy content. It may be that the milk of an LBW infant's own mother may be acceptable, qualitatively and quantitatively, for meeting the nitrogen needs during the early weeks of life.

### Protein

A reasonable goal for protein intake is between 3 g and 4 g per kilogram per day. Impaired intellectual function has been reported in infants on protein intakes greater than 6 g per kilogram per day.[13] It is recognized that LBW infants need additional essential amino acids, compared to fullterm infants. Tyrosine and cystine are needed because of the reduced ability to catabolize phenylalanine and methionine. Taurine is also considered essential although it is not certain just what the metabolic significance of a taurine deficiency is.[9]

### Fat

Because of the relative inability of the LBW infant to absorb fat, particularly long-chain fatty acids, medium-chain triglyceride (MCT)* oils are commonly used as a primary source of fat in formulas for LBW infants. It must be remembered that MCT oil is not a source of essential fatty acids (EFA); therefore EFAs must be provided by adding corn oil to the formula. The Committee on Nutrition of the American Academy of Pediatrics suggests that 3% of the total calories for infants come from essential fatty acids.[6]

### Carbohydrates

Lactose is the main source of carbohydrate, although lactase activity is reduced in LBW infants the first few days after birth.[3] Some formulas for LBW infants (see Table 35-5) include Polycose† and decreased amounts of lactose, thereby reducing the possibility of lactose malabsorption due to the reduced lactase activity of the intestinal mucosa.

### Other nutrients

The LBW infant has an increased need for vitamin E due to poor absorption rates. In addition, the calorically dense formulas used for LBW infant feeding are relatively high in polyunsaturated fatty acids, which also affects the need for vitamin E. It is recommended that the diet of the LBW infant be supplemented with 30 IU of a water-miscible vitamin E preparation daily for the first 3 months of life to guard against hemolytic anemia.

Even though LBW infants are susceptible to iron deficiency anemia earlier in their postnatal life than their term counterparts because of low iron stores at birth, iron supplementation is generally not recommended before

the LBW infant is 2 months of age. The delay in iron supplementation is recommended because of the interaction of vitamin E and iron. When additional iron is provided the vitamin E is used as a reducing agent for the iron and is not available to protect the red blood cell from hemolysis. Therefore the American Academy of Pediatrics, Committee on Nutrition recommends beginning iron supplementation of 2 mg per kilogram per day (not to exceed 15 mg per day) at 2 months of age for LBW infants.[3]

Serum folate levels in LBW infants drop shortly after birth. Therefore supplemental folate is recommended for the first 3 months of life. It is not known if folate insufficiency affects somatic growth or neurologic development in the LBW infant.[14]

LBW infants, especially very low-birth-weight (VLBW) infants (less than 1500 g) are susceptible to hyponatremia early in life because of immature renal function. To offset these high urinary sodium losses, an intake of 3 mEq per kilogram per day is recommended.[15]

The VLBW infant is predisposed to hypocalcemia because significant amounts of calcium are deposited in the fetus during the last trimester of intrauterine life. These infants are at risk for developing the rickets of prematurity. It has been shown that infants who received a calcium lactate supplement had better defined bone texture and wider cortices than did unsupplemented infants receiving the same formula.

### Renal solute load

Renal solute load is the collective term for the nitrogenous end products of protein metabolism and the electrolytes sodium, chloride, and potassium, which must be excreted in the urine. As long as the LBW infant is growing, renal solute load should not present a problem because the nitrogenous end products are used for tissue synthesis. The obligatory water necessary to excrete the renal solute load needs to be carefully considered, however, when fluid intake is low, when there are high extrarenal losses and a decreased urine concentrating ability, and when renal solute load is high. The critically ill neonate may incur one or more of these problems at one time. Fluid intake and output must be closely monitored to prevent dehydration.

### Gastrointestinal osmotic load

A high gastrointestinal osmotic load may be a factor associated with the development of necrotizing enterocolitis (NEC) in the LBW infant. NEC is a diffuse or patchy necrosis of the mucosa or submucosa of the small or large bowel, usually in the ileocecal area.[16] The incidence of NEC is highest in the infant who weighs less than 1500 g and who has undergone a major crisis. Symptoms such as abdominal distention, temperature instability, Hematest-positive stools and gastric residual develop during the first week of life after oral feeding has begun. The pathogenesis of the disease is uncertain, but three factors are

---

*Mead Johnson Laboratories, Evansville, IN 47721

†Ross Laboratories, Columbus, OH 43216

necessary for its development: a mucosal injury; intestinal microflora; and the availability of a metabolic substrate (feeding). The increasing frequency of this disease has paralleled the increase in the number of NICNs and may be the result of better reporting added to the increased survival rates of the VLBW infant. The calorically dense formulas have been implicated in the increased frequency of NEC but as yet the etiology of the disease is unknown. Medical management, which includes having the infant NPO for approximately 10 days and feeding by hyperalimentation is frequently successful, but if an intestinal perforation or gangrene of the bowel occurs, surgery is indicated. Postsurgical management may also involve total parenteral nutrition (TPN), which is discussed later in this chapter, to meet the infant's nutritional needs.

Another problem that has been noted with increased frequency since the advent of the calorically dense formulas is the lactobezoar, a large, mobile mass in the stomach thought to be a calcium sodium caseinate curd. The symptoms of lactobezoar are similar to those of NEC and also occur after feeding has begun. The MCT oil as well as the increased calcium content of the special LBW formulas are thought to delay gastric emptying time, which may be a factor in lactobezoar development. (These factors are known to delay gastric emptying time in adults; they may be a factor in infants.) However, the cause is assumed to be multifactorial. It has been suggested that delaying the introduction of the calorically dense formula (81 kcal per 100 ml) until after 2 weeks of age may prevent formation of the lactobezoars.[17]

## Feeding methods

Many LBW infants, especially those less than 34 weeks gestational age, are unable to feed orally either because of immature sucking and swallowing reflexes or because of their precarious physical condition. Frequently the VLBW infant is unable to tolerate the volume of formula needed to supply adequate energy to sustain growth. Each infant should be assessed and an individual feeding method determined.

Continuous drip intragastric infusion of formula is often better tolerated in the LBW infant. For some infants, a nasojejunal feeding technique is used. The gastrostomy feeding technique is contraindicated for the LBW infant due to increased mortality rates associated with its use.[18]

## Hyperalimentation in the neonatal intensive care nursery

Indications for the use of TPN in the pediatric setting[19] are (1) a patient who is unable to take a significant amount of enteral feeding (a patient, such as a burn patient, with high energy needs may receive partial parenteral nutrition to provide additional intake above what can be tolerated orally); (2) a patient with a major anomaly of the gastrointestinal tract, such as short bowel syn-

drome, or one who has undergone gastrointestinal surgery; (3) infants with chronic intractable diarrhea (TPN allows complete rest of the gastrointestinal tract and, therefore, assists in breaking the diarrhea-malnutrition cycle); and (4) TPN may be indicated for the VLBW infant who is unable to tolerate enteral feeding. With TPN, satisfactory growth and a positive nitrogen balance can be achieved without undue risk. However, the long-term outcome of this use of TPN has not yet been evaluated.

TPN may be administered either peripherally (through a scalp vein) in an infant or directly into the superior vena cava through the internal or external jugular vein to provide a central line infusion. Deciding which method to use depends primarily upon the length of time TPN will be necessary. Problems with peripheral TPN include difficulty maintaining infusion sites, and the amount of infusate required may exceed the infant's fluid tolerance level. However, it is the preferred method unless it is known that enteral feeding cannot be tolerated for a long time. A central line infusion permits the use of a hyperosmolar infusate, and it is better able to meet the infant's nutritional needs over an extended period of time.

## Composition of the infusate

At present there is no ideal TPN solution for pediatric use. The actual requirement for vitamins, minerals, and trace elements when TPN is used are unknown. It is generally agreed that the newborn on TPN needs a minimum of 80 kcal per kilogram per 24 hours to promote normal growth. Protein in a TPN solution is generally provided by a crystalline amino acid mixture. A 10% or 15% glucose solution is used as the source of carbohydrate. A Multi Vitamin infusion* (MVI) and minerals are added to the solution.

Until recently these ingredients were the only source of nutrients available and approved for pediatric use in the United States. Problems occurred because LBW infants develop essential fatty acid deficiencies very easily. Their adipose stores are less than those of term infants, and mobilization of EFA from triglyceride stores is partially blocked during hyperalimentation because of high insulin levels accompanying glucose administration.[20] Recently Intralipid†, a 10% isotonic soybean emulsion, was approved for pediatric TPN solutions. This oil provides 1.1 kcal per milliliter, is an excellent source of EFAs, and permits an adequate energy intake within the limits of fluid volume that a LBW can tolerate (see Chap. 27 for TPN administration procedures). The recommended level of Intralipid in a TPN solution is approximately 2 g per kilogram per day, but it should be used with caution because plasma clearance time of Intralipid is quite variable in the neonate.[21] There are other concerns related to

---

*USV Pharmaceutical Corp., Tuckahoe, NY 10707
†Cutter Medical, Berkeley, CA

the use of Intralipid in the neonate. Plasma lipid levels must be closely monitored to guard against hyperlipidemia.[21] The consequences of hyperlipidemia during the use of IV feeding when the gastrointestinal tract is bypassed are not known.

Dahms and Halpin[22] recently reported finding liver lipid accumulation in infants who were receiving peripheral Intralipid infusions. The use of Intralipid in the jaundiced newborn is contraindicated because the hydrolyzed free fatty acids displace the unconjugated bilirubin from albumin binding sites and increase the risk of kernicterus. Another concern is that the effect of substituting plant sterols for cholesterol in the developing neurologic system is not known. Intralipid causes a change in pulmonary function in the adult. Whether this also occurs in the neonate is yet to be determined.

The benefits from the use of TPN in the LBW infant are decreased morbidity and an improved survival rate. TPN promotes growth and maintains normal system functions.[23]

However, in addition to the concerns about Intralipid mentioned earlier, there are problems, such as trace mineral deficiencies, and vitamin deficiencies and excesses. The ideal TPN solution has not yet been developed for infants; abnormal plasma aminograms have been noted in some infants receiving TPN. Finally, the long-term effects of bypassing the gastrointestinal tract during periods of rapid growth are not yet known. Much more is yet to be learned about the physiological consequences of our present feeding regimens for LBW infants and how these practices may be improved upon.

### Psychosocial development

Much has been written in the literature about the importance of bonding and its effect on mother–child interaction. The early, and often lengthy, separation of parents from their infant that occurs when an infant is placed in a NICN jeopardizes this bonding process. Separation during this first 12-hour postpartum period has been identified as a contributing factor to child abuse. Prematurely born infants have a three times greater risk of being abused. Many NICNs encourage parental visitation and involve parents in as much of the care of their infant as is feasible.

Parents must be properly prepared for their first visit to the NICN with all of its machines, tubes, and tiny patients. Parental stress is directly related to the illness of their infant, and a visit to the NICN can increase this stress.

Close attention needs to be paid to maternal readiness before her infant is discharged. Fanaroff and coworkers[24] suggest that maternal visitation patterns are a good indicator of maternal readiness. A long-term study is needed to provide a means of identifying high-risk parents early so that appropriate intervention can take place to reduce the potential for abuse of these infants.

### Counseling the mother for discharge

One of the responsibilities of the neonatal dietitian is to counsel the mother or primary caretaker about formula preparation and appropriate feeding techniques prior to the infant's discharge from the hospital. The dietitian must provide well-written and easily understood directions for formula preparation. Many of the special formulas that will be used after discharge are available in powdered form only (although some are in concentrated liquid form), and extreme care must be taken during preparation to reconstitute these formulas correctly and safely. In addition to providing written and verbal directions, it is recommended that the dietitian demonstrate to the parents exactly how to prepare the formula and that the parent repeat the demonstration for the dietitian. This practice should be repeated, if necessary, until the dietitian is certain that the parents are able to prepare the formula exactly as directed. Close follow-up, in the home and in a follow-up clinic, helps to ensure that the formula intake is adjusted as the infant grows.

### Diarrhea

Diarrhea is a word of Greek derivation meaning "to flow through."[25] Clinically, diarrhea is an excessive loss of water or electrolytes or both in the stools. Mild or acute diarrhea may occur in infants and young children for a variety of reasons. The major cause of severe diarrhea throughout the world is intestinal infection.[26] In the United States the human rotovirus (HRV) is the most common cause. Although it is a more common problem in developing countries where lack of sanitation and infection are found more frequently, diarrhea ranks second to respiratory disease as a cause of nonsurgical hospital admissions in the Western hemisphere.[27] There is a close cyclical relationship between malnutrition and diarrhea—malnutrition seems to predispose a child to acute diarrhea, and acute diarrhea is a major cause of malnutrition. Noninfectious diarrhea may be caused by food allergies, emotional problems, excessive ingestion of certain foods and unripe fruits, starvation, or malabsorption syndromes, such as celiac sprue and cystic fibrosis. Celiac sprue is discussed in Chapter 26 and cystic fibrosis later in this chapter. Chronic diarrhea is a less threatening problem to the older child. The pattern of growth and development is usually normal, and there is no evidence of infection. Chronic intractable diarrhea in the newborn is a serious problem, however, and may be treated by hyperalimentation[28] to support growth and development in the first weeks or months of life.

### Acute diarrhea

Severe dehydration resulting from the abnormal loss of water and electrolytes can threaten the infant's life. The risk is greater for infants because approximately 70% of their total body weight is water compared to 60% in the adult. Also, the infant has more exposed surface area relative to his weight. Severe dehydration and febrile seizures may damage the infant's central nervous system. The essential elements of therapy for acute diarrhea are rapid replacement of sodium, chloride, base (bicarbonate or lactate), and potassium; replacement of the volume losses; and maintenance of nutrition. If no vomiting is occurring, fluid and electrolyte balance may be reestablished using an oral electrolyte-glucose solution.* If the infant is vomiting, an intravenous glucose and electrolyte solution may be used. Glucose is recommended for the oral solution to avoid aggravating the diarrhea.[29] Some concern has been expressed about the composition of the two most commonly used oral electrolyte solutions for the treatment of acute diarrhea because they do not contain bicarbonate and are low in sodium.[29]

After reestablishing fluid and electrolyte balances, the nutritional needs to support normal growth must be met. These needs can be met orally, if tolerated, or by hyperalimentation (discussed earlier in this chapter).

When the infant is ready for oral feeding a dilute formula is offered, usually 10 kcal to 13 kcal per oz (30 ml). After the infant has demonstrated a tolerance for oral feedings, gradual progression to a standard dilution formula, 20 kcal per oz, may be made. Depending upon the infant's age, cereal and vegetables may also be offered. Records should be kept of the amount of food taken and retained. Calculations of energy, protein, and fluid intake per kilogram of body weight should be made and recorded daily in the medical record. An infant can be expected to consume more than the normal 110 kcal to 115 kcal per kilogram in order to achieve catch-up growth.

Following acute diarrhea some infants may be lactose-intolerant. These infants require a soy-based, lactose-free formula, such as Isomil, Prosobee or Soyalac (see Table 35-4 for a listing of special formulas). After 3 to 4 months a regular milk-based formula is usually well tolerated again. Another factor in selecting a postdiarrheal formula may be the electrolyte composition, especially the sodium and potassium content of the formula.

In the past, boiled skim milk was offered to infants with diarrhea. This is no longer recommended because the boiling reduces the total water content of the milk, resulting in an increase in the total amount of protein, sodium, and potassium per ounce. This concentration of protein and electrolytes may be hazardous in the very young infant because of his immature kidney function and may further contribute to the problem of hypernatremia.

Acute diarrhea with dehydration is critical in the young child, ages 1 to 4; however, it is not as devastating as it is in the infant unless it is accompanied by meningitis or encephalitis. Children 1 to 2 years of age who have previously been weaned may prefer to take fluids from a nursing bottle, and older children may more readily accept fluids other than milk. In addition to water and milk, fruit juices, fruit drinks fortified with vitamin C, ice pops, and carbonated beverages are commonly used to meet fluid needs. Some clinicians use cola syrups to supply glucose and potassium.

Carbonated beverages are usually more acceptable to the toddler if offered at room temperature and poured far enough ahead of serving time to reduce the fizziness. Before carbonated beverages are offered to a child, it is a good idea to check with the parents. They may not serve these beverages to the child at home and may not want them used in the hospital. Because there are various other fluids with which the child is familiar and which he usually accepts, there is no reason why the parent's wishes cannot be met.

As these children recover, they usually tolerate a soft or simple regular diet adequate to support the nutritional needs of their age group (see Chap. 18). Fluid and food intake, both in kind and amount, should be recorded after each meal.

### Chronic nonspecific diarrhea

This type of diarrhea is characterized by a normal pattern of growth and development, and there is no evidence of malabsorption. Chronic nonspecific diarrhea (CNSD) may last as long as 2 years and is a very common outpatient problem in children under 5 years of age. Cohen and co-workers[30] found that children affected by CNSD consumed a lower percentage of total calories as fat than did non-CNSD children. Their recommendation for treatment was to increase the fat intake to 4 g per kilogram per day. (Fat is a potent inhibitor of gastric emptying, although the exact role it plays in decreasing stool frequency is not well understood.) This high-fat regimen has proven successful in reestablishing a normal stooling pattern. The fat intake is then gradually reduced to a normal level for the age of the child.

### Mild diarrhea

Infants and children with mild diarrhea of 1 to 3 or 4 days' duration are usually treated in the home, especially if the problem is not complicated by continued vomiting. Food may be withheld for up to 24 hours, but fluid and electrolyte intake must be maintained. If required, electrolyte solutions with minimal amounts of glucose (Lytren* or Pedialyte†) are available for home use with infants. The use of electrolyte solutions in the home must be closely monitored. Mothers need precise directions for their use. They should keep accurate records of the

---

*Lytren—Mead Johnson Laboratories, Evansville, IN 47721, or Pedialyte—Ross Laboratories, Columbus, OH 43216

---

*Mead Johnson Laboratories, Evansville, IN 47721
†Ross Laboratories, Columbus, OH 43216

amount taken and retained and report this information to the pediatrician as requested; also they should discontinue use when advised to do so.

In the past, mothers were advised to offer their infants a homemade glucose and electrolyte solution containing water, Karo syrup, and a specified amount of salt (NaCl). This practice has been discontinued because it is potentially dangerous. Not only does the processing of Karo syrup add sodium to the mixture, but inaccuracy in measuring the NaCl could result in an excess of Na leading to hypernatremia and dehydration.

When an infant's diarrhea subsides, the mother may be advised to offer a dilute (10 to 13 calories per 30 ml) lactose-free formula. Some physicians, however, prefer to keep infants on a cow-milk based formula. Close follow-up needs to be maintained with the mother and precise directions given about increasing the strength of the formula to a standard dilution. Growth retardation has been noted in infants who were still on the dilute formula 2 weeks or more after recovery from diarrhea. The mother did not understand that she should resume the normal feeding program.

Water and electrolyte intake can be maintained in the 1 to 4 year old child with mild diarrhea by use of such fluids as fruit juice or plain tomato juice, carbonated beverages, dilute tea made from instant tea with sugar added, dilute broth from meat, vegetable soups, or milk, if tolerated. Broths made from bouillon cubes are to be avoided because they contain excessive amounts of sodium and no carbohydrate. Other than the dilute broths, soups, tomato juice, and milk, all other fluids contain potassium and carbohydrate but no sodium. Therefore, a varied selection of fluids, with the addition of saltines or potato chips if tolerated, should be used to ensure an intake of sodium as well as potassium and carbohydrate.

Within 24 hours most young children with mild diarrhea will accept a diet suitable for their age containing their usual food choices. If the diarrhea continues for more than 4 days, it may be indicative of a malabsorption syndrome requiring dietary treatment and a physician should be consulted.

## Surgery or trauma

The most common reasons for surgery in the fullterm infant are pyloric stenosis and cleft palate or lip.

### Pyloric stenosis

The normal function of the pylorus (the distal opening from the stomach) is to control the volume and rate of gastric contents entering the small intestine, thereby allowing optimal mixing of food in the stomach and maximum intraluminal digestion of various foodstuffs in the duodenum. Pyloric stenosis, with ensuing dehydration and malnutrition, occurs when the pylorus fails to empty properly. The incidence of pyloric stenosis, the etiology of

which in unknown, is about 1 in every 150 live births.[31] It occurs more frequently in boys, usually the first born, than in girls.

The symptoms of pyloric stenosis are usually noticed after the second or third week of life when the infant begins to vomit with increased frequency after feeding. The vomiting changes from regurgitation to projectile vomiting, and weight loss, undernutrition, and dehydration can occur rapidly. If these symptoms are noticed, the infant should be seen by a physician as the ensuing problems can be devastating to the young infant due to the rapid central nervous system development occurring at this time.

Before the pylorus valve can be surgically repaired, the infant's fluid and electrolyte balance must be restored. The infant must be in metabolic balance for surgery.

Postsurgical management involves small, frequent oral feedings of glucose water at 4 to 6 hours postoperatively if bowel sounds have returned.[31] The feedings are increased gradually, as tolerated, to a level appropriate to support normal growth and development as well as allow catch-up growth to occur. It is recommended that intravenous supplements be used during the period when oral feeding is first begun. Recovery is usually complete in a relatively short period of time.

### Cleft palate and lip

The incidence of cleft palate or lip is approximately 1 in every 600 to 1250 live births.[32] These infants may require multiple surgical procedures performed over an extended period of time depending upon the degree of clefting. Before and after initial surgical procedures, modifications need to be made in feeding techniques to guard against aspiration and infection and to ensure that the infant receives an adequate intake.

### Feeding techniques

The infant should be held in a fairly upright position, and the nipple shank should be long enough to allow the formula to enter the back of the mouth near the soft palate or against his cheek to help prevent formula from entering the nasal passages. There are several nipples on the market to assist the mother in feeding her infant. Some have longer shanks, and some are flanged to promote suction in the oral cavity. The holes are usually larger to permit the infant to feed rapidly enough that he does not tire, yet slowly enough that aspiration is prevented. One manufacturer* produces a special nurser that allows the mother to squeeze formula gently into her infant's mouth if he has difficulty sucking. Some physicians recommend using a plastic medicine dropper for early feeding after surgery of the lip and restraining the infant's arms with elbow cuffs to prevent possible contamination of the operative site. It will probably be necessary to experiment with the various

---

*Mead Johnson Laboratories, Evansville, IN 47721

devices to find the one most appropriate for each mother and infant. Feeding periods are longer, the infant may become frustrated by the lack of nursing success and more patience is required on the mother's part. The parents need the support and encouragement of the health-care team in caring for their infant and in dealing with their feelings (guilt or anger) of having produced a defective child.

### Tonsillectomy

There are a variety of regimens for feeding the child after a tonsillectomy. These regimens, in general, avoid very hot or cold fluids and any acid juices, such as orange, grapefruit, or tomato juice. Milk is usually avoided immediately after surgery because it coats the incision and causes discomfort.

### Burns

Burns rank third after automobile deaths and drownings as a cause of accidental deaths in children.[33] A burned infant or child presents an even greater challenge to the health care team than the burned adult. Pediatric patients have a greater need for fluid per unit of body mass and are at a greater risk for wound infection than adults.[34] Even a 10% burn is reason to admit a young child to the hospital.

The first goal of treatment for the pediatric burn patient is the replacement of fluid and electrolytes lost during the injury. If possible this should be done during the first 12 hours postburn. Within 4 to 8 hours postburn the child should be able to tolerate small quantities of milk (1 oz–2 oz). By 4 to 8 hours postburn, oral feedings should be well tolerated.[33]

The goal of nutritional management of the postburn pediatric patient is to provide sufficient exogenous energy and nitrogen to prevent prolonged catabolism and to support normal growth and development. Frequently it is difficult to provide all of the necessary nutrients orally, making it necessary to combine enteral and parenteral feedings.[35] Forced feeding, which is possible with some adults, is not a recommended procedure for children.

When a nutritional care plan is developed, for the burned pediatric patient the pre-burn nutritional status must also be considered. Frequently this information is available from a parent or from previous medical records.

Several methods have become available to the dietitian to assist in developing a suitable nutritional care plan for the burned child. These methods for calculating estimated energy needs have been available for use with adult burn patients for several years. The calculations consider not only the normal needs of the growing child but also the additional needs related to the percentage of total body surface that was burned.

Curreri[36] suggests the following method for developing a nutritional care plan for children less than 8 years of age. He recommends using the gastrointestinal tract for feeding if at all possible.

> 60 kcal per kilogram of total body weight (TBW) plus
> 35 kcal per percentage total body surface burned (TBSB)

Example: The patient is a 2 year old girl who weighs 12.5 kg and has a 30% TBSB.

$$\begin{array}{lll} 60 \times 12.5 \text{ TBW} & = & 750 \\ \text{plus} & & \\ 35 \times 30 \text{ TBSB} & = & \underline{1050} \\ \text{Total kcal per day} & = & 1800 \text{ kcal} \end{array}$$

Total protein needs are approximately 4.0 g of protein per kilogram of total body weight per day.

Other methods have also been developed by Larson[37] and Dergnac.[38] The latter formula is for use when total parenteral nutrition is necessary, as in severe burns in the facial area or when the upper gastrointestinal tract is affected.

For many children regular meals as well as high-calorie, high-protein supplements between meals meet the increased needs. Some very young and older children, however, in the early postburn stage may need partial parenteral nutrition to provide the additional nutrients. Close monitoring of the BUN and serum electrolytes is a necessity.

Since burned children may be hospitalized for a few weeks to several months, it is especially important to provide a varied menu and to take into consideration the patient's likes and dislikes. Parents may wish to contribute to their child's care by bringing in a favorite dish from home or from a fast food restaurant.

### Tube feedings

The infant who requires a tube feeding can be fed a formula of standard dilution (20 kcal per 30 ml) by nasogastric or gastrostomy tube. When the volume of formula cannot provide an adequate energy intake as the infant grows, the caloric density may be increased by adding cereal and bananas or by changing the concentration of the formula. Since a nasogastric tube has a smaller bore than a gastrostomy tube due to the size of an infant's nasal passage, the amount of cereal that can be added to a nasogastric feeding will be limited. With too much cereal the mixture will be too thick to pass through the tube into the stomach. A more concentrated formula, which provides 30 kcal per ounce, may be made by mixing 3 parts concentrated infant formula with one part water. Additional water to meet the infant's fluid needs can be used to test the patency of the feeding tube. It is important that the protein provide no more than 10% to 12% of total calories; fat about 35% and carbohydrate the rest, about

50%. This helps to promote normal growth and development of the infant and young child.

For the older infant and the young child, it is necessary to design a tube feeding that meets a patient's specific energy and nutrient needs. Most standard tube feedings, whether commercial products or prepared in the hospital, are designed for adults and cannot be used for the child under 3 years of age. The protein and electrolyte content of most of these formulas may be too high for children under 3 years.

Tube feedings can be formulated for individual children from powdered or concentrated infant formulas that contain the necessary vitamins and minerals and permit adjustment of the total fluid provided. Casec,* dried soluble calcium caseinate made from skim milk curd or strained meat, can also be used as a source of protein. Karo syrup† or Polycose,‡ together with infant fruits and cereals, can be used as additional sources of energy from carbohydrate. Polycose is derived from the acid hydrolysis of cornstarch, while Karo syrup contains hydrolyzed cornstarch with sucrose and salt added.

The tube feeding should contain approximately 100 kcal per 100 ml. For example, a 2 year old child weighing 12 kg requires about 1200 kcal and 1500 ml fluid per day:

100 kcal per kilogram × 12 kg = 1200 kcal
125 ml per kilogram × 12 kg = 1500 ml

(see Tables 35-2 and 35-3). Therefore, 1200 ml of formula containing 1200 kcal plus 420 ml of water for giving medication and for testing the patency of the feeding tube supplies both the fluid and energy needs of this child every 24 hours. Infant formula is about 90% water. The amount taken and retained by means of the tube along with a record of calories, protein, and milliliters per kilogram should be recorded daily in the medical record. The composition per 100 ml of kilocalories of protein, fat, carbohydrate, sodium, potassium, chloride, and phosphorus should be recorded in the patient's record, and the recipe of ingredients should be readily available to the healthcare team.

## Nutritional problems in otherwise normal infants and children

### Growth charts

Growth charts for children have been discussed in Chapter 19. Growth charts for infants (Fig. 35-3) are also available. Longitudinal data derived from the experiences of healthy infants and children and collected by the Fels Institute, Yellow Springs, Ohio, were used to develop the

infant (birth–36 mo) growth charts. An infant's length is measured in the recumbent (supine) position. The accurate measurement of length, especially in the first months of life, requires the appropriate equipment and two people—one to hold the infant's head against the vertical plane of the measuring device and another to extend the normal flexure of an infant's lower extremities and to place the heels against the movable footboard of the measuring device. Beam balance scales, preferably calibrated in grams and kilograms, should be used to weigh the nude infant. These scales should be carefully maintained and accurately read. A head circumference measurement is a valuable anthropometric tool during the first year of life, as brain growth is directly related to an increase in head circumference during this time period. Head circumference is measured using an unstretchable tape, preferably steel, and measuring the distance over the supraorbital ridge anteriorly and that part of the occiput posteriorly that gives the maximum circumference.

It is important to know the exact birth date of an infant to plot data accurately on a growth chart. Inaccurate data can indicate a problem where none exists or cause a problem to be missed. Frequent plottings are more valuable than just one set of plots. Frequent plottings can also help to pinpoint the time when a problem occurred.

As with adults, the measurement of length and weight of infants does not identify body composition and build, but discrepancies between length, weight, and head circumference can be observed. The weight-for-length graph, which disregards age, is a valuable tool in assessing potential under- or overweight problems.

### Underweight

Children vary greatly in their rate of growth. If a child gains weight and grows in height at a regular rate, even though he is somewhat thinner than other children of his height and age, there is no cause for concern. Mothers should be reminded that a child's growth rate declines in velocity at the end of the first year of life and that the child's appetite compensates for this decrease. The child who fails to grow and gain regularly should have his food habits and home environment investigated. Poor housing, inadequate sleeping space, a mother who cannot remain at home, and poverty may contribute to the child's failure to gain.

The school breakfast and lunch programs available in most urban areas can help the child improve his food habits and provide him with as much as half or more of the needed nutrients each day. Under the guidance of the teacher and the school health counselor, underweight children and their parents may be helped to achieve better nutrition as well as better patterns of rest and sleep.

Occasionally, one sees a child who is anorexic as a result of the mother's anxiety about his food intake. If the child is otherwise well, the mother needs to be reassured

---

*Mead Johnson Laboratories, Evansville, IN 47721
†Best Foods, Englewood Cliffs, NJ 07632
‡Ross Laboratories, Columbus, OH 43216

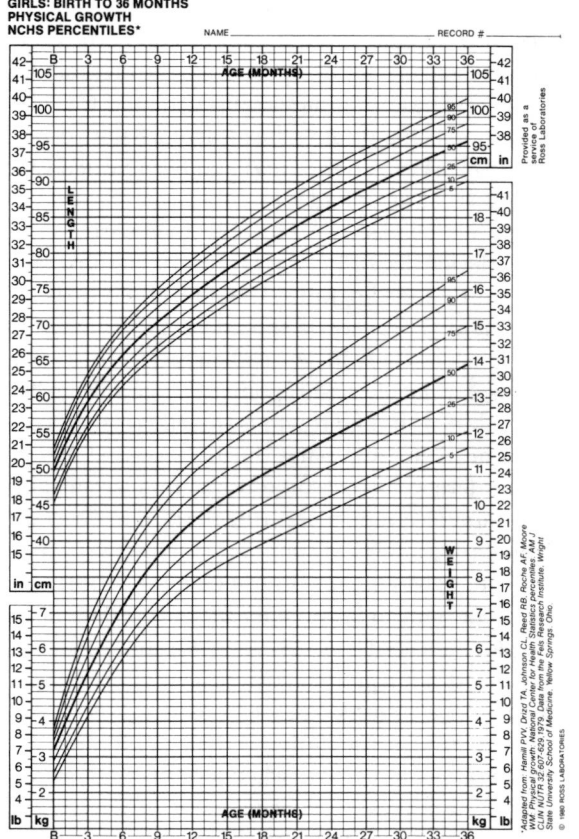

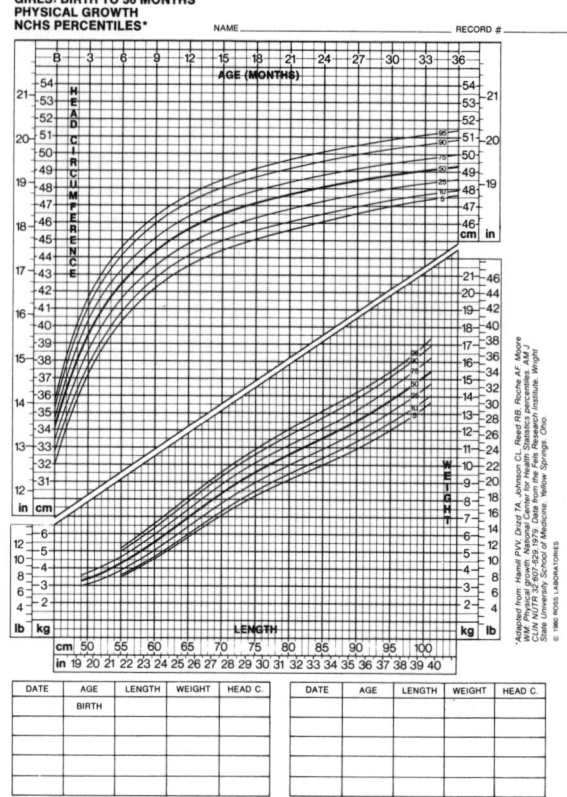

**Fig. 35-3.** Girls: birth to 36 months physical growth. NCHS Percentiles. (Adapted from Hamill PVV, Drizd TA, Johnson CL, Reed RB, Roche AF, Moore WM: Physical growth: National Center for Health Statistics percentiles. Am J Clin Nutr 32:607–629, 1979. Data from the Fels Research Institute. Wright State University School of Medicine, Yellow Springs, Ohio)

that he will eat eventually if tensions are relieved, and he is allowed some choice in deciding how much and what he can eat. For the child who has limited himself to a very few foods this may mean an inadequate diet for a while, but variety in preparation may help to introduce other foods. When the child's appetite has returned to some extent and he begins to look forward to his meals, small quantities of new foods may be tried one at a time. It is always best to serve very small portions and to let the child ask for a second helping. Eventually such a child will eat a varied and adequate diet.

### Growth failure due to psychosocial deprivation

A diagnosis of Failure to Thrive (FTT) may be made for several reasons. The growth failure could be due to an inborn error of amino acid metabolism (see Chap. 36) or a congenital heart anomaly (discussed later in this chapter). Occasionally the FTT is due to no known physical disorder. Some terms that are used to describe these growth-retarded infants include *nonorganic failure to thrive*, *psychosocial growth failure*, and *growth failure due to maternal deprivation*. These infants are not growing because they are not being fed or being provided with the tactile stimulation necessary for normal development to occur. The work of Bowlby,[39] Spitz[40] and others has shown that babies need intimate involvement with other people not merely for their immediate survival, but for their emotional health and normal development. Whitten,[41] however, found that infants grew physically if appropriate intake was provided, even if no change occurred in the mother–child interaction.

### Team approach

The interdisciplinary health-care team approach is most successful in the treatment of these infants and their families. In many hospitals these teams are composed of a

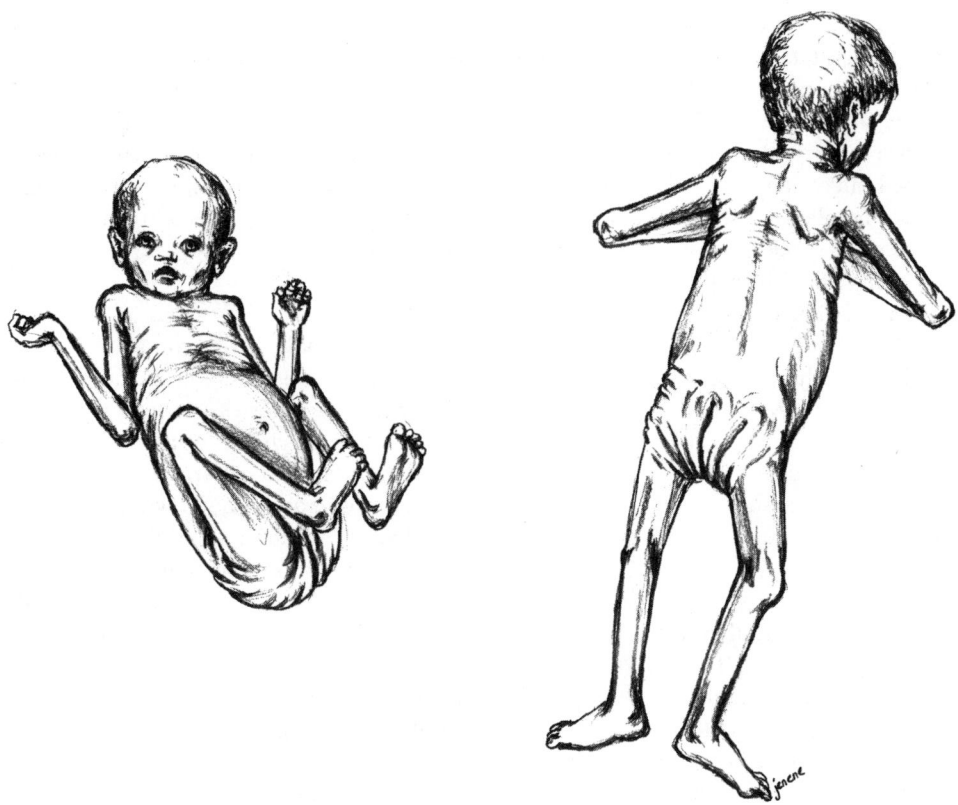

**Fig. 35-4.** "Failure to thrive" child. Copyright © Jenene Warmbier, Medigraphics, Gahanna, OH.

physician, a nurse or nurse practitioner, a psychologist, and social workers. The pediatric dietitian can also play a major role as a member of this interdisciplinary team.

### Parenting problems

The lack of food, as well as stimulation, from which the infant suffers is likely the result of a disturbed mother–child interaction or a parenting disorder. These parenting disorders may have several causes. A mother may lack "mothering skills" because she was never "mothered" and did not have a role model in her own childhood; she may be so burdened with financial or social problems that she simply cannot cope with her new baby; or a young mother may have so many unmet needs of her own that she is incapable of meeting the needs of another person. Many mothers of FTT infants are unaware of the needs of an infant, either nutritional or social. Our society has tended toward the smaller, nuclear family rather than the larger, extended family more common a generation ago. Today's young mothers often have not been exposed to babies, fed them, or watched them grow and reach developmental milestones. Infants who must be admitted to NICNs immediately after birth because of poor weight status, congenital anomalies, or a shortened period of intrauterine life and who consequently are separated from their parents are at increased risk for FTT and abuse. Some researchers[42] believe that FTT without disease and child abuse are part of the same continuum. If FTT infants are

hospitalized, nutritionally rehabilitated, and returned to the untreated environment from which they came, there is a high probability that they will return to the hospital severely or fatally injured.

### Characteristics

Infants diagnosed as FTT due to maternal deprivation are usually less than 1 year old, and nearly always under 2 years of age. The 2 year old can usually fend for himself if food is available. These infants are nearly all delayed in their gross motor and language development when evaluated by the Denver Developmental Screening Test.

Physical characteristics observed in these infants include a protruding abdomen; pipestem limbs; wasted buttocks; and a dull, unresponsive expression (see Fig. 35-4). It is likely that hygiene is poor; frequently a severe diaper rash, as well as general uncleanliness, is noted. There may be a flat, bald spot on the back or on one side of the infant's head indicating the he has spent much time unattended in a crib or playpen and that he has been propped rather then held at feeding time. Often there is a sunken look to the infant's cheeks, evidence of lack of development, or disappearance of, the buccal pads produced from sucking the breast or bottle. If asked to comment, the mother often responds by stating that her baby never cried and he liked just lying in his bed alone, so she decided he wasn't hungry and didn't feed him. Some FTT infants are very fussy, colicky, and resistant to cuddling—babies whom the mothers find it difficult to relate to. These babies may be fed often to keep them quiet, but the feedings may be sweetened water or juices and not formula, which would supply necessary nutrients. These infants probably have well-developed buccal pads.

Weight is affected more than length unless the undernutrition has been of long duration. If previous anthropometric data are available, a falling off of the rate of weight gain is evident. Weight-for-length plots may often be below the 5th percentile.

The FTT infant may be admitted to the hospital with vomiting, diarrhea, and in a state of severe dehydration, so that restoration of fluid and electrolyte balance is of utmost importance. The care needed is similar to that provided any infant admitted with severe diarrhea (see section on diarrhea in this chapter).

### Hospital course

A diet history should be obtained from the mother, if she is available, as soon after admission as possible. If this reported intake appears adequate, it may be used in planning the infant's hospital diet. If weight is gained on this intake, it may be concluded that the infant did not consume the reported amount at home and this information may be used to confirm the diagnosis.

If severe dehydration due to diarrhea, vomiting, or malnutrition is evident, the initial oral feeding should be a dilute formula, 10 kcal to 13 kcal per oz (30 ml). If well tolerated, the concentration may be gradually increased to a standard dilution (20 kcal per oz). The infant may eat voraciously and consume more than the expected 115 kcal per kilogram and, as a result, show a very rapid rate of weight gain. One 5 month old infant gained at the rate of 80 g per day for nearly 2 weeks (the normal expected gain is 20 g to 25 g per day) and consumed nearly 170 kcal per kilogram per day. This intake tapers off as the infant approaches appropriate weight for height. This rapid rate of weight gain also helps to confirm the diagnosis of FTT due to psychosocial deprivation and can save the expense of complicated medical workup.

As part of the family intervention the mother may be encouraged to spend a great deal of time at the hospital helping to care for her infant. During these visits the nursing staff should be aware of the interaction between mother and infant; for example, how and how frequently does mother hold her infant; does she talk to him; does she establish good eye contact? This time can be used to instruct the mother in appropriate techniques of infant care and feeding. It is important that the atmosphere be nonthreatening to avoid further damaging the mother's already low self-esteem. If it is impossible for a mother to spend extensive time at the hospital because of family commitments or work she must not be made to feel guilty because of her time limitations.

In this case it is helpful if a primary caretaker can be provided for the infant. This can be a hospital volunteer or student who is willing to make a commitment of 8 or 9 days to care for the infant. The hospital occupational or physical therapist can assist the mother or primary caretaker with instruction in exercises and appropriate stimulation techniques to guide the infant toward his appropriate developmental level.

### Role of the dietitian

The dietitian should make daily contact with the infant and mother, if the latter is available. Daily intake in milliliters per kilogram, kilocalories per kilogram, and grams of protein per kilogram should be recorded on the patient's chart. The dietitian can assist the mother with such tasks as formula preparation; how, when, and how much to feed her baby; and in planning a daily schedule at home to allow mother time for her baby, for other family members, and for herself. Concrete tasks are more easily managed by these mothers than abstract tasks.[43] The dietitian is nonthreatening to the mother because she is not perceived as someone who will take her baby away, as is the social worker, nurse, or physician. Before the infant's discharge, the dietitian must be certain that the mother can correctly prepare her infant's formula. This is most easily accomplished by a demonstration by the dietitian and return demonstration by the mother until the dietitian is certain that the correct procedure is followed.

Continuity of care is vital for FTT infants. The dietitian can provide this by making home visits and seeing the family during follow-up visits to the physician. During these visits weight and developmental progress can be monitored and necessary changes made to facilitate continued growth and development. Close contact should be established with the public health nurse and social worker involved with the family if such services are provided.

The future of these children depends on three main factors: the age at which the undernutrition occurred; the duration of the undernutrition; and the intervention provided the family and the progress made toward correcting the parenting disorder. Researchers in this area indicate that if nutritional deprivation occurs early in life and is of long duration, the child may never attain his genetic potential. The child's environment and nutritional status are so closely intertwined in their effect on achievement of genetic potential that separation of the two is difficult, if not impossible.

Occasionally, in the best interest of all concerned, the court system must remove the infant from his home and place him in foster care.

## Obesity

At present there is no medically accepted definition of infantile obesity. Part of the problem is conceptual—different cultures and societies have varying concepts about desirable body proportions for infants; the idea that a fat baby is a healthy baby is a very common misconception. Contrary to popular belief, maximum growth is not equal to optimal growth.[44] Frequent plottings on a standard growth chart will give invaluable clues to whether or not an infant is gaining weight too rapidly. A significant discrepancy between height and weight plots on a growth chart is an indication of probable obesity. For example, an infant who plots at the 10th percentile for height and at the 90th percentile for weight is probably obese. One other definition often used is a subscapular or triceps skinfold measurement that is greater than the 90th percentile value for age.[45]

Earlier it was believed that there was a strong correlation between infantile obesity and obesity in adulthood. Hirsch and Knittle[46] expressed the theory that if overfeeding occurred during the hyperplastic phase of growth, more adipose cells would be produced than if appropriate feedings were offered. Because of the excess of adipose cells the infant would be predisposed to obesity. Weight reduction may reduce the size of an adipose cell but will not reduce the number of cells. Fomon and co-workers reported in 1979 that a follow-up study of their infants showed no correlation between overfeeding in infancy and overweight at 8 years of age. There does appear, however, to be a strong correlation between overweight in childhood and overweight in adulthood.[46] Obesity that begins early in life is extremely resistant to treatment.

The problem of infantile obesity can sometimes be attributed to disturbed mother–infant interaction in which the mother uses food to placate her infant rather than offering love and affection. She may be unable to interpret her infant's cries appropriately and, therefore, always offers food in response instead of searching for another reason, such as a wet diaper or a desire to be held. The mother of a very placid, nondemanding infant may not be providing adequate stimulation to her infant, so the obesity is more the result of a low activity level and lack of stimulation rather than overfeeding. It is recommended that the nutrition counselor obtain a typical daily living pattern, including sleep and activity as well as the diet history. The weight status of the infant may reflect lack of activity combined with overfeeding.

Whether or not some children are genetically predisposed to obesity is debatable. Reports show that if a child has one obese parent, the likelihood of his becoming obese is 33%; if both parents are obese, the likelihood rises to 73%. If both parents are of normal weight for height, the possibility of his being obese is only 9%.[47] The basis of the genetic implication may be that overweight persons tend to marry overweight persons, thereby increasing the chances of having an obese child. In a study of 101 twin pairs in 1976 Borjeson[48] found that genetic factors do play a role in the development of some kinds of human obesity.

Problems encountered by obese infants include delay in meeting and surmounting the developmental milestones of infancy, poor response to upper respiratory infections, frequent infections in deep skin folds, and respiratory insufficiency.

## Nutritional intervention

Each case of infantile obesity must be treated individually. It is very helpful for the nutrition counselor to have height and weight data on the parents as well as an understanding of the social and cultural milieu within which the family functions.

The goal of nutritional intervention is to slow the rate at which the infant is gaining weight so that his length can catch up with his weight. Weight control is desired—not weight reduction. A weight reduction diet is not advisable before or during the adolescent growth spurt. A severe dietary restriction could deplete fat-free body tissue, inhibit growth, and deplete energy stores needed to handle stress. Because it is difficult to increase the activity level of an infant, the mother may be counseled on ways to increase stimulation of her infant, including visual, vocal, and tactile stimuli. The mother may need to be educated in differentiating her infant's cries. Demonstrating the differences between the vigorous sucking of a hungry infant and the playful, disinterested mouthing of the nipple by an infant who is not hungry may help the mother distinguish between the two. The mother may also need to distinguish thirst from hunger.

## Exercise

The obese older child probably needs to increase his level of activity. He appears to be less active than his nonobese peers. Although no cause-effect relationship has been established, it may be that the obese child uses less energy to perform a specific task than his nonobese peers.

## Prevention

Wise perinatal and neonatal counseling may help prevent infantile obesity. This counseling should include encouraging breast-feeding and delaying the addition of solid foods to the infant's diet; education about the adverse effects of overfeeding; and encouraging physical activity. Also, it appears that small, frequent meals are more effective in preventing obesity than the same number of calories ingested in one or two larger meals.[60]

## Emotional support

There are psychological and emotional factors that play a role in childhood obesity. Bruch[49] warns that we must not look on obesity as "all of one piece," and suggests that there is great need for a differential diagnosis of the underlying causes of obesity in each person.

One of the problems that the obese child or adolescent faces is the derogatory and rejecting attitudes often exhibited by playmates, parents, and other adults. All who deal with these children should have a supportive approach. The nutrition counselor working with such a child should give him understanding and encouragement, even when the diet has not been strictly followed, so that he may find his own ways of developing mature and independent behavior in his choices of food. The counselor must also be supportive of the mother and elicit her help with the child's problems.

## Nutritional anemias of infancy

Nutritional anemia has been defined as follows:

> . . . a condition in which the hemoglobin concentration is below the level that is normal, for a given individual, due to deficiency of one or more of the nutrients required for hemopoiesis and, conversely, as a condition in which the hemoglobin concentration can be raised by increasing the amount of nutrient(s) absorbed.[50]

The three true nutritional anemias are iron, folate, and vitamin $B_{12}$.[51]

### Iron

Iron deficiency anemia is the most commonly recognized form of a specific nutritional deficiency. Iron deficiency anemia is found in affluent areas of North America as well as in developing countries, although in the United States it is more prevalent in low income families with poor health care. In 1978 Oski[52] reported that 15% to 20% of the population under 18 years of age was iron deficient. However, it is most frequently seen in infants and young children between 6 months and 2 to 3 years of age. Growth velocity is highest in this age group, and the diet is likely to be marginal in iron.

A hemoglobin concentration of less than 11 g per deciliter is the criterion most often used to define iron deficiency anemia in infants and children. However, studies conducted by Dallman and others[53] suggest that there are racial differences in normal hemoglobin concentration. Blacks appear to have a normal hemoglobin concentration that is 0.5 g per deciliter lower than the normal level for whites. Perhaps a more relevant criterion for anemia is an increase in hemoglobin levels in response to a therapeutic dose of iron.

It is not yet known to what extent the iron status of the pregnant woman influences the iron endowment of her fetus, but recent research has demonstrated little, if any, difference between the iron status of infants born to iron-deficient and iron-sufficient mothers.[54] LBW infants and twins are at increased risk for iron deficiency anemia because of lower iron stores at birth.

### Sources of iron

Human milk is relatively low in iron, but approximately 49% of the available iron is absorbed. Therefore, human milk is considered an adequate source of iron until infants have doubled their birth weights. At that time supplemental iron is recommended. However, some physicians recommend iron supplementation from birth if an infant is being breast-fed.

Currently the major manufacturers of proprietary formulas market both an iron-fortified formula and one without iron. The iron-fortified formula contains 10 mg to 12 mg of iron sulfate per liter of formula standard dilution (20 kcal per ounce). About 10% to 12% of this iron is absorbed, probably because ascorbic acid is also added to the formula.[55] Many infantile gastrointestinal problems, from diarrhea to constipation, have been attributed to iron-fortified formula. In a double-blind study conducted with 93 infants from birth to 42 days of age, Oski[56] found no statistically significant difference in the number or consistency of stools or the incidence of colic, or abdominal cramping between infants receiving iron-fortified formula and those receiving formula without iron.

Many researchers suggest that there is little need for exogenous iron before the infant has doubled his birth weight. In fact, Bullen and co-workers[57] have suggested that early iron supplementation may be harmful to the infant because the iron will saturate the lactoferrin (as it does *in vitro*), thereby decreasing the infant's resistance to infection. Others suggest that iron provided from birth augments iron stores and that prevention of iron deficiency anemia offsets any possible increased risk of infection. Because of a lack of information on the role of lactoferrin in the human intestinal tract, the Committee on Nutrition of the American Academy of Pediatrics recommends the use of an iron-fortified formula for the first year of life,[58] if the infant is not breast-fed. All physicians are not in agreement on this policy, and the AAP statement may be revised as new information becomes available.

In infants under 6 months of age, the use of whole cow's milk appears to decrease the absorption of iron from other foods and may even be associated with occult intestinal blood loss.[59] After 6 months of age whole cow's milk is acceptable provided intake is limited to three-fourths of a liter per day.[55] Other factors affecting iron absorption are discussed in Chapters 6 and 18.

Infant cereals, which are usually the first solid food added to an infant's diet, contain an electrolytic iron particle that is believed to be readily absorbed. (No studies have been conducted on the absorption of electrolytic iron in infants.)[55] Frequently, when an infant reaches 6 to 8 months of age, regular adult cereal replaces infant cereal in the diet. This increases the infant's susceptibility to iron deficiency at a time when the needs for iron are increasing. Adult cereals, even if iron-fortified, do not contain a form of iron that is readily available to the infant. This practice has prompted Fomon[60] to recommend continuing the use of iron-fortified infant cereals until the age of 18 months.

### Effects of iron deficiency anemia on the infant

Studies have shown that treatment of iron deficiency in children produces a measurable improvement in developmental and behavioral performance. Oski and Honig's study[52] in which 24 iron-deficient infants were treated suggests that abnormalities are reversible if treated during the first 2 years of life. It is not known if the consequences of long-term iron deficiency anemia have a permanent effect on normal growth and development. Iron deficiency in infancy could produce long-term consequences. The irritable or unresponsive infant could affect the primary caretaker–infant interaction, thereby placing the infant at increased risk for failure to thrive, developmental delay, and abuse.

### Folate

There are few data available concerning the folate requirements of infants and children. The incidence of folate deficiency is greatest in infants 4 to 7 months of age.

### Sources

It appears that for the first 6 months of life human milk provides an adequate supply of folate. Proprietary formulas are fortified with 50 $\mu$g–100 $\mu$g of folate per quart of formula, standard dilution (20 kcal per oz). Folate is heat labile in milk and milk products that are low in ascorbic acid. For this reason, evaporated milk formula is not a good source of folate. Because goat's milk is also an inadequate source, infants receiving either an evaporated milk or a goat's milk formula should receive a folate supplement. The need for folate is based on caloric intake, and the Committee on Nutrition of the American Academy of Pediatrics recommends 4 $\mu$g of folate per 100 kcal per day.

### At risk for deficiency

LBW-infants are at increased risk for folate deficiency due to decreased stores at birth. Because of the role of folate in DNA synthesis, deficiencies can lead to structural abnormalities (see *High Risk Neonate*, in this chapter).

Children who are receiving antiseizure medication also have an increased need for folate due to a drug-nutrient interaction, which interferes with the metabolism of folate. A folate supplement is contraindicated, however, because such supplementation has been found to increase seizure activity in some children. Nevertheless, the child's diet should provide the recommended level of folate intake.

### Vitamin B$_{12}$

As is true for folate, relatively little information is available on vitamin B$_{12}$ requirements for infants and children. Because B$_{12}$ stores at birth are usually sufficient for the first year, a B$_{12}$-deficient infant is rarely seen.

Human milk from a B$_{12}$-sufficient mother provides adequate B$_{12}$ for her infant. Women who are vegans, however, and not receiving a B$_{12}$ supplement are at risk for B$_{12}$ deficiency and for producing B$_{12}$-deficient offspring. At birth such infants are potentially susceptible to irreversible neurologic damage. If these infants are breast-fed with milk low in B$_{12}$ the problem is aggravated.

## Other nutritional deficiency diseases

Frank scurvy and rickets, which were prevalent nutritional deficiency diseases in infants and children in the United States prior to World War II, are seen infrequently today. It appears from recent literature that the number of cases of rickets being reported in the United States is increasing. Rudolf and associates[61] suggest that certain population groups are at increased risk for developing rickets. These include vegetarians, children who are breast-fed for extended periods of time, and black children. Four cases of nutritional rickets were discovered accidentally in Connecticut health centers. Edidin and co-workers[62] also reported two cases of nutritional rickets. Both children were black, offspring of vegetarians, and were breast-fed for prolonged periods of time without supplementation. It appears that nutritional rickets is still a problem, and continued surveillance by health personnel is necessary.

Recent evidence has shown that phenytoin (Dilantin) and phenobarbital, two antiseizure medications, interfere with the synthesis of 1,25-(OH)$_2$ vitamin D.[63] Children being treated with these drugs should be followed closely.

A rare form of rickets, known as vitamin D-resistant, hypophosphatic rickets, is a familial disease. It is not due to deficiency in any of the nutrients needed for bone formation, but to the inability of the kidney tubule to reabsorb phosphate. Since bone consists largely of calcium phosphate, the mineralization of bone is decreased in infants with this disease, with the resultant lesions of rickets and osteomalacia. The problem is medical rather than nutritional, and treatment is accomplished by administering large doses of oral phosphate and 1,25-(OH)$_2$-D$_3$ at a dose of 1 $\mu$g per day[64] (see Chap. 7, *Fat-Soluble Vitamins*).

## Malabsorption syndromes

In this section the malabsorption syndromes with onset in infancy, such as cystic fibrosis, sucrase-isomaltase deficiency, and glucose-galactose malabsorption, are discussed. Lactose intolerance and celiac sprue (gluten-induced enteropathy) are discussed in Chapter 26.

## Cystic fibrosis

Cystic fibrosis (CF), the most common inherited disease in the Western population occurs approximately once in every 2000 live white births. CF has its primary effect on the exocrine glands.[65] The principal manifestations of CF are intestinal malabsorption, frequent and severe respiratory infections, and impaired growth and utilization of calories. Some CF patients develop pulmonary involvement later in life, and some escape pancreatic involvement, but always there is a defect in the reabsorption of the sweat electrolytes, sodium and chloride.[66] Overt diabetes is observed in approximately 5% of CF patients, but one is more apt to observe a carbohydrate intolerance characterized by insulinopenia.[67]

Currently there is little evidence that cystic fibrosis is an inborn error of glycoprotein metabolism as was once thought.[66] There is an increase in the calcium concentration of the glycoprotein, which increases as the disease progresses, but no disturbance in calcium metabolism has been noted. The basic defect that is responsible for CF has not yet been determined, although many hypotheses are being tested. The role of low plasma levels of EFAs found in CF patients and the resulting effect on prostaglandin synthesis is one area of research that appears to be receiving a lot of attention in the literature.[68,69]

Approximately 50% of CF patients die before the age of 21, but others live into adulthood. The increased longevity is attributed to physiotherapeutic techniques to clear the lungs of mucus; to antibiotics, which control secondary infection; and to use of oral pancreatic enzymes and an adequate diet moderately restricted in fat, which reduces malabsorption.

Even with effective treatment mild to moderate growth retardation occurs in most children with cystic fibrosis; and Lapey and co-workers[70] have shown that adolescents and young adults excrete significant quantities of fat and nitrogen in their stools. At this time the two problems—malabsorption of nutrients and poor utilization of nutrients in intermediary metabolism—are also being carefully studied in various research centers.

### Dietary treatment

In cystic fibrosis the digestion of fats presents more problems than the digestion of protein and carbohydrates. For the infant, either a formula high in protein and containing long-chain triglycerides, or one containing medium-chain triglycerides (MCT) may be used. Probana* is one example of the former (24% of total calories from protein and 29% from fat), and Portagen* and Pregestimil* are examples of the latter (14%–15% of total calories from protein and 35%–40% from fat). In the older child, protein and carbohydrate are increased in the diet

and fat is restricted. Excessively fatty foods, such as peanut butter, cream, ice cream, fatty meats, mayonnaise, fried foods, and pastry rich in shortening, are avoided. Moderate amounts of butter or margarine and homogenized whole milk, if tolerated, may be used.

Berry and co-workers[71] recommend the use of MCTs in the diets of all children with cystic fibrosis to provide an adequate energy intake. However, the work of Partin and co-workers[72] suggests that MCTs should not be used by children with liver damage. Durie and associates[73] report that MCT oil was malabsorbed in their nine study infants, and they suggest that if a formula containing MCT oil is used for cystic fibrosis patients, pancreatic enzyme should be added to ensure adequate absorption. Since the older child with cystic fibrosis may also develop cirrhosis, the long-term use of MCT may be contraindicated in cystic fibrosis.

Preparations of water-miscible forms of fat-soluble vitamins and the water-soluble vitamins, together with supplementary iron, are prescribed. Whenever there is excessive loss of sodium chloride in the sweat due to activity or climate, extra salt must be added to the food to compensate for the loss.

Pancreatic enzymes must be given with each infant feeding or each meal or snack for the older child. Powdered forms of the enzymes can be added to fruits, such as applesauce for the infant and young child, while the older child can take the enzymes in capsule form. The powdered forms should not be added to protein foods since they change the consistency of the food if the infant or child is a slow eater.

The child with cystic fibrosis hospitalized for the treatment of an acute infection presents numerous problems. A major one is the scheduling of meals and physiotherapy treatments, especially postural drainage. To prevent regurgitation when the child is clearing mucus from his lungs, postural drainage should not be done too soon after a meal. Also, food and beverages should be available whenever these children request them because they are often anorexic. The diet may need to be modified in the older patient if he also has diabetes or cirrhosis (see Chap. 29, *Diabetes Mellitus*, and Chap. 33, *Liver Disease*).

The team responsible for helping the patient with cystic fibrosis and his family should include the physician, the nurse, the physiotherapist, the dietitian, and the social worker. The team must communicate not only with the family but also with the school teacher or nurse, and any community agencies working with the child and his family. In many instances a psychologist or psychiatrist is needed to help the family and the patient cope with what may be a fatal illness.

## Sucrase-Isomaltase deficiency

This rare inherited disorder of infancy in which there is a lack both of sucrase and isomaltase is the most common congenital disaccharidase deficiency. Sucrase is required to hydrolyze sucrose and isomaltase, to hydrolyze the 1-6

*Mead Johnson Laboratories, Evansville, IN 47721

linkage in the amylopectin of starches. The infant develops a watery diarrhea when sucrose, dextrin, or starch is introduced into the diet. Abdominal distention and cramping are also frequently noted.

Breast milk or formulas free of sucrose or starch such as Enfamil* or Similac[†] are used to feed these infants. All fruits, vegetables, and cereals naturally contain some sucrose or starch. Ament and co-workers[74] report that fruits and vegetables with less than 2% sucrose are usually tolerated by these infants. Donaldson and Gryboski[75] have observed that with age, the tolerance for amylopectin improves, and small quantities of starch can be added to the diet. Strained meats, without sugar or starch added, and eggs can be used.

## Glucose-galactose malabsorption

In this very rare genetic disorder of carbohydrate absorption the mechanism for the active transport of glucose and galactose through the intestinal mucosa is impaired. The hydrolysis of starch yields *glucose.* Lactose is hydrolyzed to *glucose* and *galactose,* and sucrose is hydrolyzed to *glucose* and *fructose.* Therefore, all sources of carbohydrate with the exception of pure fructose must be excluded from the diets of these infants.

RCF[†] with fructose added is used to feed the infant. As the infant grows older, meat, fish, and eggs are added to the diet, and limited amounts of carbohydrates containing glucose and galactose can be added without producing symptoms.[75]

# Chronic illnesses

## Diabetes mellitus

The dietary treatment of diabetes mellitus in children is discussed in Chapter 29.

## Congenital heart disease

Failure to thrive is characteristic of the infant with a congenital cardiac anomaly. Frequently this results from inadequate intake caused by rapid fatigue during feeding or by labored respiration, which interferes with deglutition. Children in congestive heart failure may also have an increased metabolic requirement and inadequate gastrointestinal absorption. Children with a ventral septal defect or patent ductus arteriosus are also likely to exhibit growth failure and have a greater susceptibility to infection.

### Nutritional therapy

The challenge to the dietitian is to provide a diet sufficient in energy, protein, sodium, and other nutrients to support growth, yet not to disturb the fluid balance in these infants.

Because many of these infants are able to take only a small volume of fluid, the caloric density of their formula

must be increased. This can be accomplished by giving a formula containing 100 kcal per 100 ml (30 kcal per oz). Three parts of a commercial liquid formula (133 kcal per 100 ml) and one part of water yield a formula containing 100 kcal per 100 ml. To avoid compromising optimal growth, it is important to keep the protein intake at 8% to 10% of the total energy intake. Therefore, it may be advisable to use a more concentrated formula, such as Similac 24,[†] and to dilute it to 100 kcal per 100 ml. The renal solute load presented must not tax the infant's renal concentrating ability. It is frequently advisable to provide a multivitamin supplement. Iron, folic acid, and, frequently, calcium supplements are also necessary.

Many cardiac anomalies can be corrected by surgery after infancy. Before surgery the child may also require a moderately sodium-restricted diet. The sodium-restricted diet is discussed in Chapter 31.

Mothers need guidance in feeding infants with this condition because they become tired easily and need to rest frequently during a feeding. Therefore, the mother must devote more time to feeding her infant than is usual and may need help in planning a daily schedule so that she can give adequate care to the other members of her family.

A child with a chronic illness often becomes manipulative of his environment. Therefore close follow-up is necessary to provide parents with needed support so they can care for their child.

## Myelomeningocele

Myelomeningocele (spina bifida) is a congenital anomaly occurring approximately once in every 2000 births. It is characterized by defective closure of the vertebral column surrounding the spinal cord in which portions of the spinal cord and meninges protrude. This anomaly affects the child's ability to walk. Some patients are able to manipulate swing-through crutches as they get older, but most are confined to wheelchairs.

The most important dietary consideration in these infants and children is the prevention of obesity. It is possible that these infants are predisposed to obesity from birth because they are unable to increase their activity level. These children have a higher than normal proportion of fat in their total body mass. They are highly susceptible to fractures, probably due to disuse atrophy, and neurologic sensory deprivation of the legs, rather than to other causes, such as scurvy.

A high fluid intake is recommended to reduce the likelihood of kidney infections and constipation. A reduction diet is not recommended until after the prepubertal growth spurt (as is true for the normal child). The goal is to achieve a slower rate of weight gain than would be considered appropriate for a normal child of the same age. Because these patients tend to use food as a means of self-assertion, a positive relationship among dietitian, parents, and patient, along with close follow-up, is essential to ensure dietary compliance.

---

*Mead Johnson, Evansville, IN 47721

[†]Ross Laboratories, Columbus, OH 43216

## Renal disease

Renal disease is discussed in Chapter 32.

The objective in treating children with chronic renal disease is the achievement of normal growth during the first 2 years and greater than normal growth in the older child.[76] The actual protein requirement of children in renal failure is not known and may differ from the requirement of normal children. Because protein intake must be restricted in the affected child's diet, the protein that is provided should be of high biologic value to permit tissue synthesis for growth. Energy levels need to be sufficiently high to prevent catabolism of protein as an energy source. De Luca and associates[77] report that growth retardation in these children can be corrected to a great degree by supplementing the diet with $1-\alpha-OH-D_3$, the analogue of the active form of vitamin D, if normal phosphorus levels are restored before supplementation and if calcium intake is adequate.

## Allergy

Allergy in infants and children is discussed in Chapter 34.

## Hyperactivity

*Hyperactivity, hyperkinesis, learning disabilities,* and *minimal brain dysfunction* are all terms frequently used to describe children who have difficulty behaving, have short attention spans, or are disruptive in the classroom. The most recent term to be added to the list is *attention deficit disorder* (ADD). It is not always the case that the activity level is elevated; it may be the choice of activity that is inappropriate.[78]

Hyperactivity is not a disease state but a deviation from normal behavioral patterns in children. Hyperactive children may be characterized as being inattentive and impulsive; they demonstrate social ineptness; they make hasty, ill-advised decisions; and they are emotionally bland and defensive.

These children do not respond to usual modes of treatment for behavior disorders, such as psychotherapy. The most common treatment for hyperactive children is the administration of stimulant drugs, such as dextroamphetamine (Dexedrine) or methylphenidate (Ritalin). Frequently, an observed improvement in the child's behavior while he is receiving stimulant drug therapy is used as a tool in diagnosing hyperactivity. However, not all children respond favorably to this therapy. Multimodal treatment is frequently recommended, including behavior therapy, psychotherapy, parent-involved intervention, and drug therapy.

The possible connection between diet and hyperactivity was noted in 1973 when Dr. Ben Feingold,[79] then a pediatric allergist with the Kaiser-Permanente Foundation in California, reported that hyperactive behavior in children could be related to the ingestion of certain chemicals in food, namely salicylates and chemically related artificial flavors and colors. The validity of his reports was immediately questioned as were the nutritional implications of long-term use of his diet.

The original Feingold diet excluded all foods that contain artificial flavors and artificial colors as well as all foods that contain high levels of naturally occurring salicylates. Foods that are artificially flavored and colored include prepared and manufactured convenience foods, vitamin preparations, toothpaste, and cough drops. Two vegetables, tomatoes and cucumbers, and many fruits, including oranges, apples and peaches, contain naturally occurring salicylates. The diet does not exclude chocolate and sugar. Adherence to the diet necessitates major changes in eating habits.

Many studies to test the validity of the Feingold hypothesis have depended on subjective observation of behavioral changes by parents and teachers, and the evidence is inconclusive.

As no relationship has been found between naturally occurring salicylates and hyperactivity, research is now focusing on the relationship between artificial colors and flavorings and hyperactivity.

Swanson[80] found that the performance of hyperactive children was adversely affected by the ingestion of 100-mg and 150-mg doses of a blend of FDA-approved food dyes, whereas normal children were not affected by these dosage levels. Not all children exhibit symptoms as a result of ingesting food additives, and improvement on an additive-free diet is not universal. The intermediary metabolism of many drug reactions is controlled by genetic factors, and in some children metabolism may have been altered by mutation.[78] It is postulated that this may be the basis of childhood hyperactivity.

Weiss[81] performed a double-blind study of 22 hyperactive children already on an additive-free diet; he administered a blend of artificial colors. He found no convincing evidence of a reaction to the challenge diet.

In 1978 Harper and associates[82] carried out a study to determine the nutritional adequacy of a diet free of artificial food colors and flavors. They found no significant difference in intake of energy and nutrients between their base-line diet and the hyperactivity diet.

The dietitian's role in treating a child who is being successfully managed on an additive-free diet is to make sure that he is receiving adequate nutrients. This is possible on a diet free of artificial flavors and colors, as Harper reported.

No valid cause and effect relationship between diet and hyperactivity has yet been established, and there is great need for research in this area. Stare[83] raised a real concern when he questioned whether the potential benefits from such diet therapy are worth the cost of having the affected children believe, incorrectly, that their behavior is controlled by what they eat. He and his associates are of the opinion that this psychological damage outweighs any possible benefits from the dietary treatment.

## Epilepsy

Epilepsy is a disease of the central nervous system. It occurs in both children and adults, although it is more frequent in children. The chief symptom is momentary loss of consciousness, so short it may hardly be noticed, in petit mal seizures; or the loss of consciousness may be of longer duration, accompanied by convulsions, as in grand mal seizures.

### Drug therapy

The majority of patients with epilepsy respond to therapy with phenobarbital and other anticonvulsant drugs. Low serum folate levels with or without megaloblastic anemia have been observed in patients with epilepsy taking phenytoin (Dilantin), an anticonvulsant drug, over long periods of time. It is suspected that the drug interferes with metabolism of folic acid. Large doses of folic acid are contraindicated in the patient controlled by phenytoin therapy, however, because they have been observed to induce seizures. Patients taking this drug should be advised to follow a diet that supplies the recommended daily amount of folic acid.

### The ketogenic diet

Before anticonvulsant drugs were available, it was observed that starvation with ketosis had a favorable effect on epileptic seizures. From this observation a diet high in fat, which promotes mild ketosis, was used in the treatment of epilepsy before the development of drug therapy. The exact mechanism for the effectiveness of the ketogenic diet is not known. It is known that the brain of a younger child is better able to use ketone bodies as an energy source than the brain of an adult. Accordingly, the ketogenic diet is more effective in treating children with seizure disorders than in treating adults. It is most effective in controlling petit mal seizures in the preschool and early school-aged child. If epileptic seizures cannot be controlled by drug therapy alone, or if there is evidence of drug toxicity, the ketogenic diet may be prescribed. Rarely are patients treated by the ketogenic diet alone; in most cases the diet is prescribed in conjunction with drug therapy.

There are many drawbacks to the use of the diet, however, and these should be considered before the regimen is attempted. The high fat content of the diet makes it unacceptable to many patients.

The diet should be initiated in the hospital where ketosis can be established under close supervision. The patient is given nothing by mouth except 500 ml to 1000 ml of water daily for approximately 24 to 72 hours. Dodson[84] states that he rarely fasts a child more than 24 hours. Hunger disappears as ketosis develops.

When ketosis has been established the diet is begun. Nausea and vomiting may be present at first but will

## Table 35-6. Method for Calculating a Ketogenic Diet

*Calorie Requirements, Rounded to the Nearest 100*

| Age (years) | Cal/kg body weight |
|---|---|
| 2-3 | 100-80 |
| 3-5 | 80-60 |
| 5-10 | 75-55 |

*Protein Requirement*
1 g/kg body weight for young children
1.5 g/kg body weight for older children

| *To Calculate for a 3:1 Ratio* | *To Calculate for a 4:1 Ratio* |
|---|---|
| 1 g fat = 9 cal × 3 = 27 cal | 1 g fat = 9 cal × 4 = 36 cal |
| 1 g P + C = 4 cal × 1 = <u>4 cal</u> | 1 g P + C = 4 cal × 1 = <u>4 cal</u> |
| 31 cal | 40 cal |
| per unit | per unit |

Example: 4 year old child, weighing 18 kg × 70 cal = 1260 or 1300 cal

For a 3:1 K-AK ratio (31 cal/unit)
  1300 cal: 31 cal = 42 units
  Fat 42 × 3 = 126 g
  P + C 42 × 1 = 42 g
  P (1 g/kg) 18 g
  C (by difference) 24 g

For a 4:1 K-AK ratio (40 cal/unit)
  1300 cal: 40 cal = 32.5 units
  Fat 32.5 × 4 = 130 g
  P + C 32.5 × 1 = 32.5 g
  P (1 g/kg) = 18 g
  C (by difference) = 14.5 g

The diet prescription with a 3:1 K-AK ratio will therefore contain 18 g protein, 126 g fat, and 24 g carbohydrate.

The diet prescription for a 4:1 K-AK ratio will contain 18 g protein, 130 g fat, and 14.5 g carbohydrate. See menu in Table 35-7.

(From Mike EM: Practical Guide and Dietary Management of Children with Seizures Using the Ketogenic Diet. Am J Clin Nutr 17:399, 1965)

**Table 35-7. Menu for a Ketogenic Diet with a 4:1 K-AK Ratio, Containing 18 g Protein, 130 g Fat, and 14.5 g Carbohydrate**

| Food | Weight (g) | Protein | Fat | Carbohydrate |
|---|---|---|---|---|
| *Breakfast* | | | | |
| Orange | 30 | 0.3 | 0.1 | 3.0 |
| Heavy cream (diluted with water for drinking) | 75 | 1.6 | 28.1 | 2.3 |
| Egg, cooked in | 25 | 3.2 | 2.9 | |
| Butter | 15 | | 12.0 | |
| | | 5.1 | 43.1 | 5.3 |
| *Dinner* | | | | |
| Meat, medium fat, cooked in | 20 | 5.6 | 3.2 | |
| Butter | 15 | | 12.0 | |
| Asparagus | 30 | 0.6 | | 1.5 |
| Lettuce | 20 | 0.4 | | 1.0 |
| Mayonnaise | 20 | 0.2 | 16.0 | |
| Oil (added to mayonnaise) | 10 | | 10.0 | |
| Cantaloupe | 20 | 0.2 | | 2.0 |
| | | 7.0 | 41.2 | 4.5 |
| *Supper* | | | | |
| Egg, hard cooked | 25 | 3.2 | 2.9 | |
| Spinach, cooked in | 30 | 0.6 | | 1.5 |
| Butter | 10 | | 8.1 | |
| Lettuce | 20 | 0.4 | | 1.0 |
| Mayonnaise | 20 | 0.2 | 16.0 | |
| Heavy cream, whipped with | 50 | 1.1 | 18.8 | 1.5 |
| Applesauce | 10 | 0.1 | | 0.5 |
| | | 5.6 | 45.8 | 4.5 |
| Totals for the day | | 17.7 | 130.1 | 14.3 |

(All data obtained from Mike EM: Practical Guide and Dietary Management of Children with Seizures Using the Ketogenic Diet. Am J Clin Nutr 17:399, 1965)

disappear. If dehydration occurs and IV rehydration is used, caution must be taken with electrolyte solutions containing glucose as these could cause the recurrence of seizures. Rigid control is necessary as sustained ketosis is important to the success of the ketogenic diet.

**Table 35-8. Comparison of Approximate Composition of 1600 Kcal MCT Ketogenic Diet with 1600 Kcal Traditional Ketogenic Diet (3:1 ratio)**

| Factor | MCT Diet | | | Traditional Ketogenic Diet | | |
|---|---|---|---|---|---|---|
| | g | Kcal | % Kcal | g | Kcal | % Kcal |
| Protein | 41 | 160 | 10 | 29 | 116 | 7 |
| Carbohydrate | 74 | 296 | 19 | 23 | 92 | 6 |
| Fat | 20 | 180 | 11 | 156 | 1404 | 87 |
| MCT | 116 | 963 | 60 | 0 | 0 | 0 |
| Total | | 1609 | 100 | | 1612 | 100 |

Signore JM: J Am Diet Assoc 62:285, 1973

This hospitalization time may be used to afford the parents the opportunity to observe the care that must be taken in weighing food, in menu planning, and in urinalysis. The dietitian may use this time to give carefully planned diet instruction. It is vital that the parents have full knowledge of all the details of the diet before the patient is discharged.

To produce ketosis, the usual ratio of protein and carbohydrate to fat in the normal diet must be sharply reversed. Fifty percent of protein is glucogenic, and all of the carbohydrate becomes glucose, as does 10% of the fat by way of the glycerol molecule. The remainder of the fat and approximately 50% of the protein are ketogenic. Normally fatty acids are metabolized to carbon dioxide and water. When the ratio of fatty acids to available glucose exceeds 2:1, ketosis occurs. Dodson[84] recommends that a 3:1 (fat to nonfat calories) ratio be used in children under the age of 5 years and a 4:1 ratio in those over 5 years.

The method for calculating such a diet to meet the individual child's needs is given by Mike.[85] Table 35-6, from Mike's article, shows that the first step in calculating the ketogenic diet is to identify the energy and protein needs of the child. The table also demonstrates a method for calculating the protein, fat, and carbohydrate in a 3:1 or 4:1 ketogenic diet.

Mike's article[85] also includes a Table of Food Values, a table of allowed foods, and many suggestions for using the fats to make the diet as palatable as possible. She warns that the Exchange Lists for diabetic diets are not suitable and should not be used. However, more recently Lasser and Brush[86] have published a system of equivalents comparable to an exchange system, which can be used to plan menus for ketogenic diets. Table 35-7 shows a menu using Mike's food tables for an 18-g protein, 130-g fat, and 14.5-g carbohydrate diet, with a ketogenic to anti-ketogenic ratio of 4:1. It illustrates some of the difficulties presented by a ketogenic diet.

It can readily be seen from the menu in Table 35-6 that milk, due to its carbohydrate content, cannot be used. All protein foods have to be sharply limited. Carbohydrate foods other than fruits and vegetables must be omitted. Butter, heavy cream, mayonnaise, and oil form the main part of the diet. The protein, fat, and carbohydrate should be equally divided among the three meals and are calculated to the first decimal point. All foods should be eaten at each meal to maintain ketonuria.

The diet is supplemented with an aqueous solution of multiple vitamins; with calcium gluconate or calcium lactate (not as a syrup which contains carbohydrate); and with an iron medication to provide a daily intake of iron. Even though the diet is high in fat it is deficient in vitamin D so this also must be added. Calcium and vitamin D supplements are especially important in light of recent evidence that some anticonvulsant drugs interfere with calcium and vitamin D metabolism.

A ketogenic diet using MCT oil has been developed.[87] It appears that MCT induces ketosis more readily than regular fats containing primarily long-chain triglycerides. Therefore, the total quantity of fat can be reduced and the total quantity of protein and carbohydrate can be increased in the diet compared with the calculations in Table 35-6. A comparison of the approximate composition of a 1600-kcal MCT ketogenic diet with a 1600-kcal traditional ketogenic diet is given in Table 35-8. Signore's article also gives detailed instructions for calculating a ketogenic diet using MCT oil. She reports that the MCT ketogenic diet is more palatable and requires less rigid control than the traditional ketogenic diet. Also, because of the quantity of protein and carbohydrate that can be used in calculating the diet pattern, milk and larger servings of meat can be used.

The diet is continued for 1 to 3 years, then a gradual return to a normal diet is made by slowly reducing the fat and increasing protein and carbohydrate.

There is no evidence at this time to suggest an increased incidence of atherosclerosis in adults who were treated with a ketogenic diet as children.

## Study questions and activities

1. Using the information in Table 35-1 plan a day's menu for a 2½ year old hospitalized child. Do your food selections meet this child's Recommended Dietary Allowance of protein (see Chap. 11 for NRC-RDA)?
2. Using the recordings in the nursing notes of formula and food intake, estimate the 24-hour fluid, energy and protein intake of an infant. Record the infant's length, daily weight, and head circumference on a growth chart. Is the infant progressing normally?
3. List some causes of a disturbed mother–child interaction. What effects can this disturbed interaction have on her infant?
4. What may one expect of a child's food habits when he is ill?
5. How can a child be helped to adjust to eating his food in the hospital?
6. What are the most common causes of nutritional anemia in young children? How may it be prevented?
7. What should be the relationship between the obese child and the person treating him?
8. What considerations need to be made in planning a feeding regimen for a LBW infant?
9. Why should calories and protein be increased in the diet of a child with cystic fibrosis?
10. When may a ketogenic diet be ordered for epilepsy? How is a condition of ketosis established and maintained?
11. What are some of the difficulties inherent in this diet?
12. What advice would you give a mother whose hyperkinetic child is on the Feingold diet?

## References

1. Snyderman SE et al: J Nutr 78:75, 1962
2. Fomon SJ: Infant Nutrition, 2nd ed. Philadelphia, WB Saunders, 1974
3. Fomon SJ: Infant Nutrition, p 310
4. Battaglia FC, Lubchenco LC: J. Pediatr 71:159, 1967
5. Lubchenco LC et al: Pediatrics 37:403, 1966
6. Committee on Nutrition, American Academy of Pediatrics: Pediatrics 60:519, 1967
7. Zeigler EE et al: Growth 40:329, 1976
8. Zeigler EE et al: In Suskind RM (ed): Textbook of Pediatric Nutrition, pp 29–40. New York, Raven Press, 1981
9. Brady MS et al: Perinatal Press 2, No. 9:125, 1978
10. Fomon SJ et al: Am J Dis Child 131:463, 1977
11. Gross SJ et al: J. Pediatr 96:641, 1980
12. Atkinson SA et al: Am J Clin Nutr 33:811, 1980
13. Goldman HI et al: J Pediatr 85:764, 1974
14. Strelling MK et al: Arch Dis Child 54:271, 1979
15. Roy RN et al: Pediatr Res 10:526, 1976
16. Kozloski AM: Surg Gynecol Obstet 148:259, 1979
17. Schreiner RL et al: Am J Dis Child 133:936, 1979
18. Vaughan VC III, McKay RJ Jr, Behrman RE (eds): Nelson Textbook of Pediatrics, 11th ed, p 409. Philadelphia, WB Saunders, 1979

19. Heird WC, Driscoll JM: Clin Perinatol 2:309, 1975
20. Friedman Z, Rosenberg A: Pediatrics 63:855, 1979
21. Bryan H et al: Pediatrics 58:787, 1976
22. Dahms BB, Halpin TC Jr: J Pediatr 97:800, 1980
23. Dudrick SJ et al: Surgery 64:134, 1968
24. Fanaroff AA et al: Pediatrics 49:287, 1972
25. Levine MM, Edelman R: Hosp Pract 14:89, 1979
26. Hamilton R: In Vaughan, McKay, and Behrman, Nelson Textbook, p 1037
27. Vaughan VC III: In Vaughan, McKay, and Behrman, Nelson Textbook, p 4
28. Heird WC, Winters RW: J Pediatr 86:2, 1975
29. Hirschhorn N: Am J Clin Nutr 33:637, 1980
30. Cohen SA et al: Pediatrics 64:402, 1979
31. Hamilton R: In Vaughan, McKay, and Behrman, Nelson Textbook, p 1050
32. Parkins FM: In Vaughan, McKay, and Behrman, Nelson Textbook, p 1027
33. Clarke AM: World J Surg 2:175, 1978
34. Pruitt BA Jr: World J Surg 2:137, 1978
35. Wilmore DW, Pruitt BA Jr: In Fisher JE (ed): Total Parenteral Nutrition, p 231–252. Boston, Little, Brown, 1976
36. Curreri PW: World J Surg 2:215, 1978
37. Larson DL: World J Surg 2:181, 1978
38. Dergnac M: Scand J Plast Reconstr Surg 13:195, 1979
39. Bowlby J: Attachment and Loss, Vol I. New York, Basic Books, 1969
40. Spitz R: Psychoanal Study Child 1:53, 1945
41. Whitten F et al: JAMA 209:1675, 1969
42. Koel BS: Am J Dis Child 118:565, 1969
43. Fischoff J et al: J Pediatr 79:209, 1971
44. Hammar SL: In Collipp P (ed): Childhood Obesity, pp 281–294. Littleton, MA, PSG, 1980
45. Fomon SJ: Nutritional Disorders of Children. DHEW Publ. No. (HSA) 77-5104. Rockville, MD, 1977
46. Hirsch J, Knittle JL: Fed Proc 29:1516, 1970
47. Greenwood MRC et al: In Winick M (ed): Nutritional Management of Genetic Disorders, p 143. New York, John Wiley & Sons, 1979
48. Borjeson M: Acta Paediatr Scand 65:279, 1976
49. Bruch H: Am J Public Health 48:1349, 1958
50. Baker SJ, DeMaeyer EM: Am J Clin Nutr 32:368, 1979
51. Herbert V: Hosp Pract 15:65, 1980
52. Oski FA, Honig AS: J Pediatr 92:21, 1978
53. Dallman PR et al: Am J Clin Nutr 31:377, 1978
54. Singla PN et al: Acta Paediatr Scand 67:645, 1978
55. Dallman PR et al: Am J Clin Nutr 33:86, 1980
56. Oski FA: Pediatrics 66:168, 1980
57. Bullen JJ et al: Curr Top Microbiol Immunol 80:1, 1978
58. Committee on Nutrition, American Academy of Pediatrics: Pediatrics 58:765, 1976
59. Woodruff CW: JAMA 240:657, 1978
60. Fomon SJ et al: Pediatrics 63:52, 1979
61. Rudolf M et al: Pediatrics 66:70, 1980
62. Edidin DV et al: Pediatrics 65:232, 1980
63. Harrison HE, Harrison HC: J Pediatr 87:1144, 1975
64. De Luca HF: In Winick, Nutritional Management of Genetic Disorders, p 3
65. Holslaw DS: Pediatr Ann 7:9, 1978
66. di Sant Agnese PA, Davis PB: N Eng J Med 295:481, 1976
67. Lippe BM et al: Pediatrics 65:1018, 1980
68. Rosenlund ML et al: Pediatrics 59:428, 1977
69. Chase HP, Dupont J: Lancet 2:236, 1978
70. Lapey A et al: J Pediatr 84:328, 1974
71. Berry HK et al: Am J Dis Child 129:165, 1975
72. Partin JC et al: Pediatr Res 8:384, 1974
73. Durie PR et al: J Pediatr 96:862, 1980
74. Ament ME et al: J Pediatr 83:721, 1973
75. Donaldson RM Jr, Gryboski JD: In Sleisenger MH, Fordtran JS (eds): Gastrointestinal Disease — Pathophysiology — Diagnosis—Management, pp 1015–1031. Philadelphia, WB Saunders, 1973
76. Chantler C et al: Am J Clin Nutr 33:1682, 1980
77. Chan JCM et al: JAMA 234:47, 1975
78. Conners CK: Food Additives and Hyperactive Children. New York, Plenum Press, 1980
79. Feingold BF: Paper presented at the annual meeting of the American Medical Association (section on allergy), Chicago, June 24, 1974
80. Swanson JM, Kinsbourne M: Science 207:1485, 1980
81. Weiss B et al: Science 207:1487, 1980
82. Harper PH et al: J Am Diet Assoc 73:515, 1978
83. Stare FJ et al: Pediatrics 66:521, 1980
84. Dodson WE et al: J Pediatr 89:695, 1976
85. Mike EM: Am J Clin Nutr 17:399, 1965
86. Lasser JL, Brush MK: J Am Diet Assoc 62:281, 1973
87. Signore JM: J Am Diet Assoc 62:285, 1973

## Supplementary readings
### General

Authausen TR, Lesh D: Parents need TLC too. Hospitals 47:88, Apr, 1973
Farrel E Sr, Kierhan BS: A positive approach to nutrition for hospitalized children. Am J Matern Child Nurs 2:113, 1977
Glany K: Strategies for nutritional counseling. J Am Diet Assoc 74:431, 1979
Mead J: The lemonade party. Nurs Outlook 21:104, 1973

### The acutely ill child

Babson SG, Benda GI: Growth graphs for the clinical assessment of infants of varying gestational age. J Pediatr 89:814, 1976
Bell EF et al: High volume fluid intake predisposes premature infants to necrotizing enterocolitis. Lancet 2:90, 1979
Candy DCA: Parenteral nutrition in pediatric practice: A review. J Hum Nutr 34:287, 1980
Grant JP: Handbook of Total Parenteral Nutrition. Philadelphia, WB Saunders, 1980
Hack M et al: The low birth weight infant. Evaluation of a changing outlook. N Engl J Med 301:1152, 1979
Heird WC: Total parenteral nutrition. In Lebenthal E (ed): Textbook of Gastroenterology and Nutrition in Infancy. New York, Raven Press, 1981
Klaus MH, Fanaroff AA: Care of the High-Risk Neonate, 2nd ed. Philadelphia, WB Saunders, 1979
Lemons JA et al: Differences in the composition of preterm and term human milk during early lactation. Pediatr Res (in press)
Levy JS et al: Total parenteral nutrition in pediatric patients. Pediatr in Review 2(4):99, 1980
Pearce JL et al: Breast milk and breast feeding in very low birth-weight infants. Arch Dis Child 54:897, 1979

Rickard K et al: Care of children with conditions characterized by high nutritional risks. J Am Diet Assoc 68:546, 1976

Schreiner RL et al: An evaluation of methods to monitor infants receiving intravenous lipids. J Pediatr 94:197, 1979

Schreiner RL et al: Lack of occurrence of lactobezoars with predominately whey protein formulas. Am J Clin Nutr (in press)

Shenai JP et al: Nutritional balance studies on very low birthweight infants: Enhanced nutrient retention rates by an experimental formula. Pediatrics 66:233, 1980

Shils ME et al: Guidelines for essential trace element preparations for parenteral use: A statement by an expert panel. AMA Department of Foods and Nutrition. JAMA 241:2051, 1979

Yu VYH et al: Total parenteral nutrition in very low birth weight infants: A controlled study. Arch Dis Child 54:653, 1979

## The Pediatric Burn Patient

Magrath HL: Nursing pediatric burns from a growth and development perspective. In Wagner MM (ed): Care of the Burned-Injured Patient. Littleton, MA, PSG, 1981

## Cystic fibrosis

Roy CC et al: Abnormal biliary lipid composition in cystic fibrosis: Effect of pancreatic enzymes. N Eng J Med 297:1301, 1977

Shwachman H et al: Cystic fibrosis: A new outlook. Medicine 56:129, 1977

## Diarrhea

Fisher SE et al: Chronic protracted diarrhea: Intolerance to dietary glucose polymers. Pediatrics 67:271, 1981

McGrath BJ: Fluid, electrolyte and replacement therapy in pediatric nursing. Am J Matern Child Nurs 5:58, 1980

Nichols BL, Soriano HA: A critique of oral therapy of dehydration due to diarrheal syndromes. Am J Clin Nutr 30:1457, 1977

Portney BL et al: Antidiarrheal agents in the treatment of acute diarrhea in children. JAMA 236:844, 1976

## Weight status

Coates TJ, Thoresen CE: Treating obesity in children and adolescents: A review. Am J Public Health 68, No. 2:143, 1978

Davies DP: Is inadequate breast-feeding an important cause of failure to thrive? Lancet 1:541, 1979

Heald FP: Juvenile obesity. In Winick M (ed): Childhood Obesity, pp 81–100. New York, John Wiley & Sons, 1975

Holm VA, Pipes PL: Food and children with Prader-Willi syndrome. Am J Dis Child 130:1063, 1976

Knittle JL et al: Adipose tissue development in man. Am J Clin Nutr 30:762, 1977

Miller WL et al: Child abuse as a cause of post traumatic hypopituitarism. N Engl J Med 302:724, 1980

## Nutritional anemias

Garn SM et al: Lifelong differences in hemoglobin levels between blacks and whites. Natl Med Assoc 67:91, 1975

Stevens D et al: Folic acid supplementation in low birth weight infants. Pediatrics 64:333, 1979

## Rickets

De Luca HF: Vitamin D-resistant rickets. A prototype of nutritional management of a genetic disorder. In Winick M (ed): Nutritional Management of Genetic Disorders, pp 3–32. New York, John Wiley & Sons, 1979

Lovinger RD: Rickets. Pediatrics 66:359, 1980

## Renal disease

Burton BT: Nutritional implications of renal disease. J Am Diet Assoc 70:479, 1977

Chantler C et al: 10 years experience with regular haemodialysis and renal transplantation. Arch Dis Child 55:435, 1980

Fennell RS et al: Renal transplantation in children and adolescents. Clin Pediatr 18:518, 1979

Potter DE et al: Measurement of growth in children with renal insufficiency. Kidney Int 14:378, 1978

## Hyperkinesis

Harley JP et al: Synthetic food colors and hyperactivity in children: A double-blind challenge experiment. Pediatrics 62:975, 1978

Lucas B, Sells CJ: Nutrient intake and stimulant drugs in hyperactive children. J Am Diet Assoc 70:373, 1977

Wender EH: Food additives and hyperkinesis. Am J Dis Child 131:1204, 1977

Wender EH: New evidence on food additives and hyperkinesis. Am J Dis Child 134:1122, 1980

*For further references see Bibliography in Part 4.*

## Epilepsy

The Presbyterian Hospital: Part II: The Babies Hospital Diet Manual. In The Diet Manual, 2nd ed. New York, Columbia Presbyterian Medical Center, 1981

# Inborn Errors of Metabolism in Infancy and Childhood

# 36

Galactosemia
Phenylketonuria (PKU)
Maple Syrup Urine Disease (MSUD)
Other Inborn Errors of Metabolism

Linda J. Boyne

In the past 40 years, as more has been learned about the genetic control of metabolism, disorders of carbohydrate, amino acids, lipid, and mineral and vitamin metabolism have been identified. The more common diseases, such as diabetes mellitus, familial hyperlipoproteinemia and cystic fibrosis, are discussed in other chapters in this book. Those relatively rare metabolic disorders with onset in early infancy that respond to dietary management are presented in this chapter.

A specific metabolic defect is caused by one, or possibly more than one, mutant gene, and there is considerable variation in the effects of the mutations on the affected person. Some conditions, such as Tay-Sachs disease, an abnormality of glycosphingolipid metabolism, are incompatible with life, and death occurs by 3 to 4 years. In other conditions, such as phenylketonuria, discussed later in this chapter, the abnormality in intermediary metabolism can be modified by manipulating the exogenous (dietary) source of the metabolite(s) throughout infancy and childhood. Some dietary restrictions may be advisable throughout life. In a few conditions, such as alcaptonuria, due to the lack of homogentisic acid oxidase, the effects of the mutant gene are minimal in infancy, although some effects may be observed in later life. A common problem of infants and children with inborn errors of metabolism is damage to the developing central nervous system, resulting in mental retardation and accompanied in some conditions by growth retardation. It is suspected that central nervous system damage is caused by the biochemical abnormality.

The prevention of mental retardation and growth failure is the goal of therapy in inborn errors of metabolism. In the conditions that respond to diet therapy, the best results have been reported in those infants who were diagnosed during the first week of life with treatment instituted at the time of, or shortly after, diagnosis. Newborn screening programs and positive family histories for

**BCAA:** Branched-chain Amino Acid
**MSUD:** Maple Syrup Urine Disease
**PKU:** Phenylketonuria
**UDP:** Uridine Diphosphate

mental retardation or early infant deaths are used to identify the newborn infant at risk for a metabolic defect. Genetic screening is possible in many areas of the United States, and genetic counseling is advised for those persons found to be carriers of inherited metabolic disorders. Many abnormalities can be detected by amniocentesis if conception has already occurred.

The treatment of these infants and their families is carried out in major medical centers. These centers have a team of specialists with resources for diagnosing genetic diseases and for monitoring the infant's response to therapy. The team consists of a physician and a biochemist who are experts in genetics, a nutrition counselor, a pediatric nurse practitioner, a social worker, and a psychologist. Such teams also need access to a psychiatrist and genetic counselor. The team works not only with the family but also with the family physician and other health resources in the local community.

In those conditions in which diet therapy has proven to be effective, the intake of a specific nutrient is manipulated but, at the same time, the diet must be adequate in energy and all essential nutrients to support normal growth and development. Infants with inborn errors of metabolism present a special challenge to the nutrition counselor and an even greater challenge to their families. The results of the treatment of an infant depend, in many instances, on the relationship that the nutrition counselor establishes and maintains with the mother.

Galactosemia, phenylketonuria, maple syrup urine disease, homocystinuria, and leucine-sensitive hypoglycemia are discussed in the following sections. For more detailed information on these and other inborn errors, the reader is referred to the supplementary readings at the end of this chapter and the bibliography in Part 4.

## Galactosemia

*Galactosemia* is a term used to describe a rare syndrome of inherited disorders involving the utilization of galactose. Galactose is required for the synthesis of cerebrosides, certain mucopolysaccharides, and lactose by the mammary glands of lactating women. However, a dietary source of galactose is not required because uridine diphosphate (UDP) glucose can be converted to UDP galactose in the body (Fig. 36-1, Reaction 3), and the UDP galactose can supply the body's needs for galactose.

### Types of galactosemia

There are two known types of galactosemia—transferase deficiency galactosemia and galactokinase deficiency galactosemia[1] (Fig. 36-1, Reactions 1 and 2). Historically the term has referred to the transferase deficiency that is more prevalent. Both types are transmitted by autosomal recessive genes, and prenatal diagnosis of the transferase deficiency is possible through examination of amniotic fluid cells. The feasibility of prenatal diag-

nosis of the kinase deficiency has not yet been established. The major alternate pathway of galactose metabolism in both types of galactosemia is the conversion of galactose by aldose reductase to the polyol, galactitol.

### Transferase deficiency galactosemia

Vomiting and diarrhea with growth failure start a few days after birth with the ingestion of human or cow milk. This is followed in approximately 1 week by disordered liver function, which can progress to hepatomegaly and ascites. The infants have high blood galactose levels and intermittent galactosuria. Infantile cataracts have been observed within a few days of birth and, if the infant is not treated, mental retardation can develop. Cataracts develop due to the collection of galactitol in the lens. Accumulation of galactose-1-phosphate is believed to be responsible for the mental retardation.[2] The prognosis is generally favorable for those infants who are diagnosed early and who follow a galactose-restricted diet. The galactose-restricted diet is discussed later in this section.

### Kinase deficiency galactosemia

Infants with kinase deficiency do not present all the same symptoms as those observed in transferase deficiency. They do not have vomiting and diarrhea with growth retardation or liver disease and are not mentally retarded. They have high blood galactose levels and galactosuria; and cataracts appear later in childhood. Early diagnosis and treatment with a galactose-restricted diet may prevent cataracts; however the diagnosis is frequently not made until the cataracts are identified later in childhood. Dietary restriction of galactose will not reverse cataract formation but is a recommended treatment for children with a kinase deficiency.

### Galactose-restricted diets

#### Food sources of galactose

The major dietary source of galactose is the disaccharide, lactose, in mammalian milk; human, cow, goat, and the milk of any other mammal used by humans any place in the world. Therefore, all forms of milk—whole milk, nonfat milk, buttermilk, cream, cheese, yogurt, ice cream, and milk sherbets—must be excluded from the diet. Also excluded are foods made with milk—breads, some breakfast cereals, rolls, muffins, biscuits, doughnuts, pastries, cookies, pies, puddings, pancakes, waffles, pizza with cheese, cheese sauces, breaded and creamed items, salad dressings, milk sauces and gravies, margarine, and lunch meats and frankfurters with milk solids added. Liver, pancreas, and brain, animal organs which contain galactose, are excluded. The labels on convenience foods, infant foods, and any other packaged foods must be inspected carefully for the words, *milk*, *milk solids*, or *lactose*. Medications containing lactose as a filler must also be avoided.

Foods other than milk also contain galactose. Peaches, pears, and apples contain 0.2 g galactose per 100-g edible portion.[3] Cow peas, chick peas, lentils, lima beans, defatted wheat germ, and dry mung beans contain raffinose and stachyose, two sugars containing galactose, while rutabagas, navy beans, and soybeans contain galactan, a polysaccharide-containing galactose.[3] Pectin used in jelly-making also contains galactose. Some clinicians responsible for the treatment of galactosemic children exclude the fruits, vegetables, and legumes listed above, while other clinicians do not. Gitzelman and Auricchio[4] have demonstrated that the raffinose and stachyose in soybeans are not hydrolyzed in the gastrointestinal tract and, therefore, the galactose in these two sugars is not available for absorption.

### The infant's diet

Formulas made with soy-isolate or casein hydrolysate without lactose added are essentially galactose-free. These are Isomil, Prosobee and Nutramigen (see Table 35-4). The labels on all infant foods must be inspected carefully because some of these products are unexpected sources of galactose. For example, Gerber High Protein Cereal with Apple and Orange contains nonfat dry milk, while Gerber High Protein (dry) Cereal does not.* The producers of infant foods make available information about the ingredients in their products* and update this information whenever they change their recipes. Rusks, or teething biscuits, for the older infant can be made by drying slices of bread made without milk in a 200° oven until done. Some crackers and simple cookies are also made without milk.

### The older child and adult

As the child grows older he will eat foods from the family table. All foods considered sources of galactose must be avoided. In addition to meat, fish, poultry and eggs, nuts, and fruits and vegetables, bread made without milk and cereal products, such as rice, macaroni, noodles, and spaghetti, can be used to provide an adequate energy and protein intake. Italian and French breads are usually, but not always, made with water rather than milk or nonfat milk solids. Most saltine and graham crackers are acceptable. Some brands of butter as well as many margarines contain nonfat dry milk. Angel food cake and sponge cake and sugar cookies made without milk, as well as gelatin, can be used for desserts. Label reading is a very important part of grocery shopping for the family of a galactosemic child.

### Nutritional adequacy of the diet

Through the use of a galactose-free infant formula with minerals and vitamins added and infant foods free of galactose, the energy and nutrient needs of the infant can

---

*Ingredients, Gerber Baby Foods, June, 1980. Gerber Products Co., Fremont, Michigan 49412

1. Galactose + ATP $\xrightarrow{\blacksquare A}$ Galactose-1-Phosphate + ADP

2. Galactose-1-Phosphate + UDP Glucose $\xrightarrow{\blacksquare B}$ UDP Galactose + Glucose-1-Phosphate

3. UDP Galactose $\xrightarrow{C}$ UDP Glucose

4. UDP Glucose + PP $\xrightarrow{D}$ UTP + Glucose-1-Phosphate

    A = Galactokinase
    B = Galactose-1-Phosphate Uridyltransferase
    C = UPD Galactose-4-Epimerase
    D = UDP Glucose Pyrophosphorylase

**Fig. 36-1.** Metabolic reactions for the interconversion of galactose and glucose. A = galactokinase deficiency galactosemia. B = transferase deficiency galactosemia.

be met. Unless the formula is continued as a beverage or in food preparation as the child grows older, the diet can be inadequate in calcium, vitamin D, and riboflavin because it is difficult to achieve an adequate intake of these three nutrients without some milk in the diet. Supplements of these nutrients may be needed to ensure an adequate intake.

### Liberalization of the diet

Because no acceptable alternate pathway for the metabolism of galactose develops with age, many physicians restrict galactose throughout life. Some physicians, however, feel that by the time the child reaches school age some liberalization of the diet is acceptable provided that careful monitoring for galactosuria and the accumulation of erythrocyte galactose-1-phosphate is carried out. Liberalization means that some baked goods and processed foods containing small amounts of milk products may be allowed in the child's diet.[1]

## Phenylketonuria (PKU)

Phenylketonuria (PKU) is an inborn error in the metabolism of the essential amino acid phenylalanine (Phe) and is transmitted through an autosomal recessive gene. The incidence of PKU is estimated to be about 1 in 14,000 live births. Approximately 400 cases of PKU are diagnosed each year.[5] Those who are affected lack the hepatic enzyme, phenylalanine hydroxylase, which converts Phe, in excess of the quantity required for structural proteins, to tyrosine. The alternate pathway of Phe metabolism is the keto acid of Phe, phenylpyruvic acid, accounting for the name *phenylketonuria* (Fig. 36-2).

The defect is present at birth, and the metabolic abnormalities occur when the infant begins to ingest protein (milk). The abnormalities are elevated blood levels of Phe in excess of 20 mg per 100 ml (normal, 1 mg–3 mg per 100 ml) and of phenylpyruvic acid (normal, 0-trace). Subsequently, phenylalanine, phenylpyruvic acid, phenyllactic acid, and other metabolites are excreted in the urine.[6] These metabolites give a musty odor to the urine.

The infant appears normal at birth but, if the disease goes undetected and untreated, neurologic symptoms such as irritability, hyperactivity, and convulsive seizures usually develop between 6 to 18 months of age, and more than 90% will be moderately to severely mentally retarded. The continued high blood levels of Phe and its metabolites are believed to be responsible for the damage to the neurological system during its development in infancy and early childhood. Because melanin, the pigment of hair and skin, is derived from tyrosine (see Fig. 36-2), the untreated infant with PKU has a lighter coloration of skin and hair than the unaffected members of his family.

The disease was first described by Følling in 1934, but its treatment was delayed for many years because there was no method for limiting the dietary intake of Phe to an infant's requirements and providing an otherwise nutritionally adequate intake. At the same time, it was not possible to identify these infants at birth. During the late 1950s, with the development of a special formula, Lofenalac (see Table 35-4), it became possible to limit an infant's intake of Phe. The phenylalanine-restricted diet is discussed later in this section. It was observed that if the dietary treatment was started in the first months of life it was possible for the child to achieve his growth potential both mentally and physically. When the disease is discovered later, dietary treatment is not effective in preventing mental retardation, although the behavior of the child appears to improve with delayed treatment.

In the early 1960s Guthrie developed an inhibition assay test that detected elevated blood levels of phenylalanine in the newborn. This test gives qualitative, not quantitative, results. Since it has been proven that early treatment of PKU prevents mental retardation, today most of the United States has compulsory PKU screening programs using the Guthrie test. Blood is drawn from the infant after feeding has been offered for a period of 24 to 48 hours and before discharge from the newborn nursery, if possible. Tests taken before feeding has begun must be repeated 2 to 4 weeks after discharge from the nursery. The result of the test is reported to the infant's physician. Prior to the development of methods to detect and treat the disease, it was estimated that $\frac{1}{2}$ to 1% of all patients in institutions for the mentally retarded were phenylketonurics. One survey[7] indicates there has been a significant reduction since the mid 1960s in the admission of patients with PKU to institutions for the mentally retarded.

### Types of PKU

The Guthrie Screening Test is confirmed by the quantitative analysis of blood Phe before diet therapy is initiated. From experience it has been discovered that not all infants with a positive Guthrie test have classical phe-

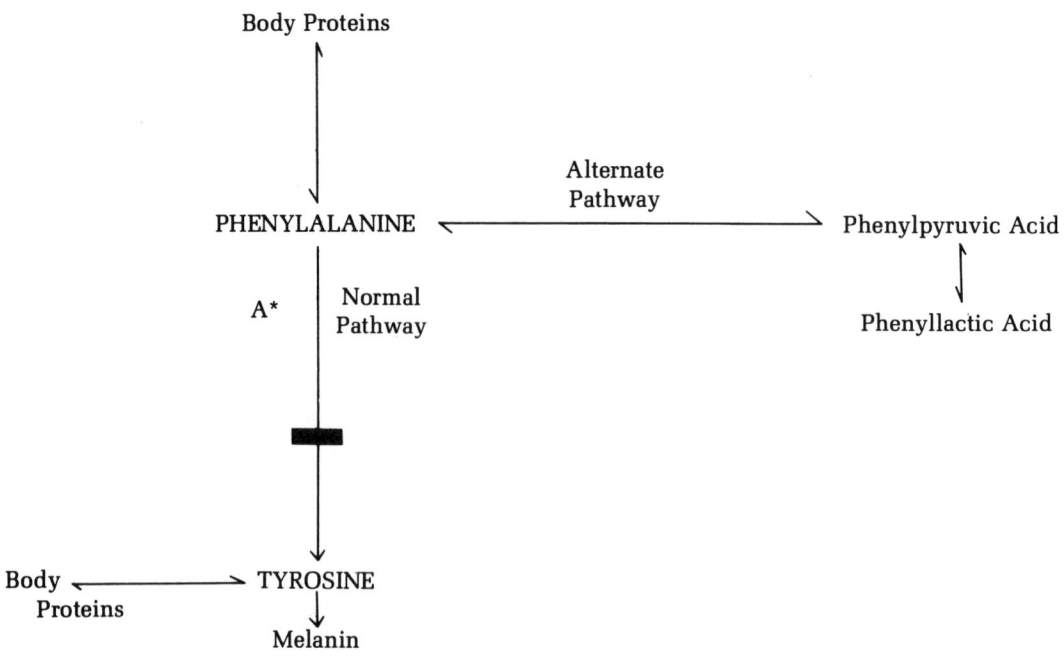

* A = Phenylalanine hydroxylase

**Fig. 36-2.** Normal pathway of phenylalanine metabolism showing block in PKU due to lack of phenylalanine hydroxylase.

nylketonuria. Three types of hyperphenylalaninemia (elevated Phe levels) have been identified. Type I, classical PKU, is characterized by a Phe blood level persistently greater than 20 mg per 100 ml, with the excretion of Phe and its metabolites in the urine. Type II hyperphenylalaninemia is characterized by an elevated blood level (less than 15 mg–20 mg per 100 ml) of Phe accompanied by excretion of phenylpyruvic acid. These infants also have abnormal phenylalanine hydroxylase enzyme activity but have retained between 1% and 35% of normal activity. These infants usually develop normally without dietary treatment. Type III, transient mild hyperphenylalaninemia, is characterized by an elevated Phe level above 20 mg per 100 ml, which eventually approaches normal. It is suspected that Type III may be due to a possible delay in the development of hepatic Phe hydroxylase. It is estimated that approximately 1% to 3% of infants with blood Phe levels greater than 20 mg per 100 ml have a deficiency in tetrahydrobiopterin (BH$_4$), the cofactor of Phe hydroxylase.[8] These infants do not respond to dietary treatment. This variant is referred to as malignant hyperphenylalaninemia. Although current research is being conducted on screening techniques and treatment of malignant hyperphenylalaninemia, BH$_4$, the missing enzyme, is not yet available for use in humans.[9]

About 25% of premature and LBW infants on a high protein diet have transient elevations of blood Phe and tyrosine levels with transient excretion of tyrosine in the urine. It is suspected that the defect is the inhibition of p-hydroxyphenylpyruvic oxidase activity. These infants respond to vitamin C therapy.

All infants with a persistent elevation of blood Phe levels above 20 mg per 100 ml have PKU and are treated with a phenylalanine-restricted diet. Generally, with Phe blood levels between 10 mg to 20 mg per 100 ml, the patient may be treated by diet. Before the types of hyperphenylalaninemia were identified, Type III patients treated with a Phe-restricted diet failed to gain weight and were developmentally delayed. They gained weight with a normal infant diet.[10]

## The phenylalanine-restricted diet
### Principles of diet therapy

Phenylalanine is an essential amino acid required for the synthesis of structural proteins. As one example, the B-chain of insulin contains 3 molecules of Phe; accordingly, Phe must be available for the continuous synthesis of insulin. The diet for a PKU infant is planned to provide his daily requirement of Phe without an excess to be metabolized through the phenylpyruvic acid pathway. At the same time, an adequate intake of energy, protein, and all other nutrients must be provided by the diet to support growth and development.

The diet is planned, and continuously revised as the infant grows, to maintain a blood level of 5 mg to 9 mg of Phe per 100 ml. The quantity of Phe required to maintain this level varies with each infant, depending on his size and rate of growth. The Phe requirement of infants 2 to 4 months of age, as defined by Holt and Snyderman (see Table 36-1), is used as a guide for determining the amount of Phe to be included in the first feedings. In general, the newly diagnosed PKU infant under 2 months of age is offered 70 mg of Phe per kilogram of body weight per day. Seventy mg of Phe is the midpoint in the range of values given by Holt and Snyderman and comparable with Fomon's preliminary estimates of the amino acid requirements of infants.[11] Weekly monitoring of the blood levels of Phe indicate whether or not this quantity is appropriate for a particular infant; if not, the diet is adjusted accordingly.

As the infant progresses through the first year of life, the quantity of Phe per kilogram of body weight decreases because the rate of growth decreases. By 2 years of age the Phe requirement decreases to 25 mg to 35 mg per kilogram of body weight, and children 2 to 10 years of age require on the average 30 mg of Phe per kilogram.[12] Experience with the treatment of adolescents has been limited. However, the work of Nakagawa and co-workers suggests that the Phe requirement of children 10 to 12 years old is approximately 27 mg per kilogram.[13]

### The diet prescription

The diet prescription defines the calories, grams of protein, milliliters of fluid, and the milligrams of phenylalanine required by the infant. For example, the diet order for a two month old infant weighing 4.5 kg requiring 70 mg Phe per kg would be:

> 518 kcal (115 kcal $\times$ 4.5 kg = 518 kcal), 13.5 g to 15 g protein (3.0 or 3.5 $\times$ 4.5 kg = 13.5 g to 15 g protein),* 315 mg Phe (70 mg Phe $\times$ 4.5 kg = 315 mg Phe) and 675 to 900 ml fluid (150 to 200 $\times$ 4.5 kg = 675 to 900 ml).

*Because much of the protein in the PKU diet is provided by amino acids rather than intact protein, it is generally agreed that PKU infants should receive a higher protein intake than is normally recommended for a non-PKU infant.

## Table 36-1. Essential Amino Acid Daily Requirements of Infants 2 to 4 Months of Age

| Amino Acid | Requirement (mg/kg/day) |
| --- | --- |
| Histidine | 16 < 34 |
| Isoleucine | 80 < 100 |
| Leucine | 76 < 229 |
| Lysine | 88 < 103 |
| Methionine (in presence of cystine) | 33 < 45 |
| Phenylalanine (in presence of tyrosine) | 47 < 90 |
| Threonine | 45 < 87 |
| Tryptophan | 15 < 22 |
| Valine | 85 < 105 |

(Adapted from Snyderman S: In Nyhan WL (ed): Heritable Disorders of Amino Acid Metabolism, p 642. New York, John Wiley & Sons, 1974)

As the child grows, the diet prescription will be modified according to his blood Phe level and his changing requirements for energy, protein, and Phe. Early in infancy the diet prescription may be changed as frequently as every 2 weeks and during later infancy, every month.

### Food for the phenylalanine-restricted diet

All foods, with the exception of fats and sugars, contain protein, and 3% to 5% of the protein is phenylalanine. Five percent of the protein is phenylalanine in foods of animal origin and in cereals, dry legumes, nuts, potatoes, sweet potatoes, and fresh vegetables that are immature seeds, such as lima beans, sweet corn, peas, cow peas, and other fresh shelled beans. The protein in dark green leaves contains 4% Phe and, in other fruits and vegetables, 3% phenylalanine.[14]

Since Phe is present to some extent in all food proteins, whether animal or vegetable, it is not possible to design a diet using only normal foods that is restricted in Phe yet adequate in total protein, energy, and all other nutrients. A specially formulated food, Lofenalac* (low-

---

*Mead Johnson, Evansville, Ind. 47721

phenylalanine-milk), is available in the United States for feeding infants and children with PKU. A similar product, Albumaid, is available in England and, to a limited extent, for research purposes in the United States. The protein equivalents in Lofenalac are supplied by an enzymatically digested casein hydrolysate from which most of the Phe has been removed by charcoal filtration. This process also removes the aromatic amino acid, tyrosine. Tyrosine together with tryptophan, histidine, and methionine is added to give an adequate mixture of amino acids. Some amino acids are present in small peptides. Carbohydrate is supplied by corn syrup solids and tapioca starch, and fat is supplied by corn oil. Minerals and vitamins are also added to meet an infant's needs for these nutrients (see Table 36-3).

Lofenalac is marketed as a powder to which water is added to prepare a formula. When reconstituted, it has almost the same appearance and consistency as milk, but a markedly different flavor, which is typical of any amino acid mixture. Most infants and children accept it without difficulty. It is the main source of energy and protein throughout the first 2 years of life and is nutritionally complete, with the possible exception of fluoride.

For the older child (2 yr and above) Phenyl Free*

### Table 36-2. Phenylalanine, Leucine, Isoleucine, and Valine Content of 100 g Portions of Selected Foods

| Food | Energy (Kcal) | Protein (g) | Phenylalanine (mg) | Isoleucine (mg) | Leucine (mg) | Valine (mg) |
|---|---|---|---|---|---|---|
| Milk, whole, 3.3% butterfat | 61 | 3.29 | 159 | 199 | 322 | 220 |
| Milk, whole, 3.7% butterfat | 64 | 3.28 | 158 | 198 | 321 | 220 |
| Milk, 2% low fat | 50 | 3.33 | 161 | 201 | 326 | 223 |
| Milk, 1% low fat | 42 | 3.29 | 159 | 199 | 322 | 220 |
| Milk, skim | 35 | 3.41 | 165 | 206 | 334 | 228 |
| Milk, skim, non-fat milk solids added | 37 | 3.57 | 172 | 216 | 350 | 239 |
| Milk, evaporated whole, unsweetened | 134 | 6.81 | 329 | 412 | 667 | 456 |
| Egg, whole, raw | 158 | 12.14 | 686 | 759 | 1066 | 874 |
| Butter | 717 | 0.85 | 41 | 51 | 83 | 57 |
| Meat | | | | | | |
| Beef | 185 | 29.4 | 711 | 905 | 1417 | 960 |
| Pork, medium fat | 596 | 9.99 | 555 | 724 | 1038 | 733 |
| Chicken | 173 | 30.9 | 1226 | 1632 | 2319 | 1533 |
| Fruits | | | | | | |
| Apple, raw | 58 | 0.4 | 6 | 13 | 23 | 15 |
| Banana, raw | 86 | 1.2 | 34 | 32 | 52 | 44 |
| Orange, raw | 49 | 0.8 | 12 | 23 | 22 | 31 |
| Peach, raw | 38 | 0.6 | 12 | 13 | 29 | 30 |
| Peaches, canned in syrup | 78 | 0.4 | 8 | 7.5 | 15 | 15 |
| Pear, raw | 61 | 0.7 | 12 | 20 | 30 | 26 |
| Pears, canned in syrup | 76 | 0.2 | 6 | 5.7 | 8.7 | 7 |
| Pineapple | 52 | 0.4 | 8 | 11.5 | 17.5 | 15 |
| Strawberries, raw | 37 | 0.7 | 17 | 17.5 | 40 | 21 |
| Tangerine | 46 | 0.8 | 12 | 23 | 22 | 31 |
| Vegetables | | | | | | |
| Beans, green, cooked | 18 | 1.0 | 24 | 45 | 58 | 48 |
| Beets, cooked | 35 | 1.0 | 12 | 32 | 34 | 31 |
| Cabbage, raw | 24 | 1.3 | 27 | 51 | 52 | 39 |
| Carrots, raw | 42 | 1.1 | 38 | 42 | 59 | 51 |
| Corn, canned | 66 | 1.9 | 112 | 74 | 220 | 125 |
| Carrots, cooked, drained | 31 | 0.9 | 31 | 34 | 48 | 41 |
| Celery, raw | 16 | 0.8 | 14 | 34 | 58 | 44 |

## Table 36-2. Phenylalanine, Leucine, Isoleucine, and Valine Content of 100 g Portions of Selected Foods (Continued)

| Food | Energy (Kcal) | Protein (g) | Phenylalanine (mg) | Isoleucine (mg) | Leucine (mg) | Valine (mg) |
|---|---|---|---|---|---|---|
| **Vegetables (Continued)** | | | | | | |
| Lettuce | 15 | 1.3 | 35 | 48 | 80 | 68 |
| Pickles, dill | 11 | 0.7 | 16 | 22 | 30 | 24 |
| Spinach, cooked, frozen | 24 | 2.9 | 125 | 136 | 223 | 160 |
| Tomato, raw | 22 | 1.1 | 31 | 32 | 45 | 31 |
| Tomato juice | 20 | 0.9 | 22 | 26 | 38 | 25 |
| Turnip greens, cooked | 20 | 2.2 | 110 | 81 | 156 | 112 |
| Peas | 71 | 5.4 | 211 | 248 | 340 | 221 |
| Potato, baked | 95 | 2.6 | 114 | 114 | 130 | 138 |
| **Cereals** | | | | | | |
| Cream of Wheat | 60 | 1.7 | 93 | 77 | 110 | 70 |
| Oatmeal | 57 | 2.2 | 110 | 104 | 152 | 118 |
| Cheerios | 500 | 16.7 | 900 | 567 | 1100 | 767 |
| Cornflakes | 563 | 10.9 | 509 | 333 | 1020 | 400 |
| Raisin Bran | 360 | 7.0 | 440 | 300 | 600 | 440 |
| Rice Krispies | 428 | 7.1 | 400 | 257 | 500 | 343 |
| Wheaties | 380 | 10 | 124 | 460 | 700 | 580 |
| **Crackers** | | | | | | |
| Graham | 385 | 8 | 271 | 371 | 621 | 343 |
| Saltines | 467 | 10 | 483 | 417 | 617 | 383 |
| **Bread** | | | | | | |
| White, enriched (3%–4% milk solids) | 270 | 8.7 | 470 | 418 | 692 | 400 |
| Whole wheat | 270 | 10.4 | 509 | 461 | 722 | 492 |
| Rye, American | 280 | 10.5 | 505 | 450 | 705 | 545 |
| **Infant Foods—Strained and Junior** | | | | | | |
| Cereal, dry | | | | | | |
| Barley | 365 | 11.1 | 657 | 419 | 810 | 592 |
| High Protein | 362 | 36 | 1893 | 1755 | 2940 | 1856 |
| Mixed | 379 | 12.2 | 672 | 477 | 1041 | 653 |
| Oatmeal | 398 | 13.6 | 545 | 550 | 1072 | 771 |
| Rice | 391 | 7.1 | 364 | 290 | 559 | 446 |
| Fruits, strained and junior | | | | | | |
| Applesauce | 43 | 0.2 | 9.8 | 6.5 | 11.5 | 7.5 |
| Apricots | 72 | 0.4 | 8.1 | 7.5 | 11.8 | 10.2 |
| Bananas and Tapioca | 67 | 0.4 | 7.2 | 14 | 23 | 20 |
| Peaches | 70 | 0.6 | 9.5 | 7.9 | 17.9 | 25 |
| Pears | 46 | 0.4 | 6.8 | 8.2 | 11.8 | 11.8 |
| Pears and Pineapple | 47 | 0.4 | 9.5 | 11.4 | 17.1 | 15 |
| Vegetables, strained and junior | | | | | | |
| Beans, green | 25 | 1.3 | 53 | 58 | 85 | 71 |
| Beets | 34 | 1.3 | 18 | 38 | 46 | 45 |
| Carrots | 27 | 0.8 | 24 | 24 | 32 | 30 |
| Corn | 57 | 1.4 | 49 | 65 | 140 | 77 |
| Mixed vegetables | 41 | 1.2 | 47 | 47 | 77 | 58 |
| Peas | 40 | 3.5 | 143 | 151 | 235 | 169 |
| Spinach, creamed | 37 | 2.5 | 96 | 112 | 221 | 151 |
| Squash | 24 | 0.8 | 29 | 33 | 47 | 36 |
| Sweet potatoes | 57 | 1.1 | 62 | 51 | 78 | 73 |
| Juices | | | | | | |
| Orange-pineapple | 59 | 0.5 | 13 | 14 | 22 | 19 |
| Orange | 54 | 0.5 | 13 | 14.3 | 14.3 | 19.4 |
| Meats, strained | | | | | | |
| Beef | 91 | 13.5 | 563 | 619 | 1091 | 453 |
| Beef liver | 98 | 14.2 | 586 | 701 | 1320 | 907 |
| Chicken | 134 | 13.6 | 562 | 645 | 1058 | 689 |
| Lamb | 97 | 14.6 | 503 | 662 | 1112 | 714 |
| Pork | 115 | 13.4 | 538 | 680 | 1127 | 702 |
| Egg yolks | 196 | 9.7 | 434 | 566 | 846 | 641 |

(Information compiled from USDA Handbook No. 8 series; Gerber Products Co., Fremont, MI 49412; and Acosta PB, Elsas LJ: Dietary Management of Inherited Metabolic Disease, ACELMU Publishers, Atlanta, GA 30307) (formerly Product 3229) may be used as a primary source of energy and protein. The use of Phenyl Free permits a greater variety of foods to be included in the diet to supply energy as well as to meet the Phe restrictions. Like Lofenalac, Phenyl Free supplies all of the essential amino acids (except Phe), vitamins and minerals needed by the child. (Refer to Table 36-3.)

The quantity of 9.4 g of Lofenalac powder (or one packed scoop supplied by the manufacturer) contains 43 kcal, nitrogen equivalent to 1.4 g protein, and approximately 7.5 mg Phe. Due to the processing method, the amount of Phe in Lofenalac can vary from 0.06% to 0.1%, or from 5.7 mg to 9.5 mg Phe per 9.4 g powder. A formula of normal dilution (20 kcal per 30 ml) can be prepared by

adding 9.4 g of Lofenalac to 60 ml of water. However, it may not be reconstituted routinely to this dilution, but, rather, mixed according to the amount of Phe required and the volume of formula needed to meet the infant's fluid requirement.

Although Lofenalac can supply an infant's energy and protein needs, it cannot supply the Phe requirement. This is discussed in the following section, *Calculating the diet pattern.* Cow's milk, which contains 47 mg Phe per 30 ml, and other foods of known Phe content but of low protein content are used with Lofenalac to provide the Phe requirement.

Table 36-2 lists the quantity of Phe in 100-g portions of selected foods. This list has been compiled from a

### Table 36-3. Composition of Special Formulas for Inborn Errors of Amino Acid Metabolism

| | Lofenalac | | Phenyl-Free | | MSUD Diet Powder | | Product 3200 K | |
| | Per 100 g Powder | Per Quart of Formula * | Per 100 g Powder | Per 16 fl oz ‖ of Formula † | Per 100 g Powder | Per Quart of Formula ‡ | Per 100 g Powder | Per Quart of Formula § |
|---|---|---|---|---|---|---|---|---|
| Kilocalories | 460 | 640 | 406 | 400 | 473 | 640 | 518 | 640 |
| Protein, equivalent, g | 15.0 | 20.8 | 20.3 | 20.0 | 8.2 | 11.1 | 15.8 | 19.5 |
| Carbohydrate, g | 59.6 | 82.8 | 66.0 | 65.0 | 63.3 | 85.6 | 51.1 | 63.1 |
| Fat, g | 18.0 | 25.0 | 6.8 | 6.7 | 20.0 | 27.1 | 28.0 | 34.6 |
| Ash, g | 3.6 | 5.0 | 3.8 | 3.7 | 3.5 | 4.7 | 3.0 | 3.7 |
| Caloric distribution | | | | | | | | |
| Protein, % of calories | 13 | 13 | 20 | 20 | 8 | 8 | 12 | 12 |
| Fat, % of calories | 35 | 35 | 15 | 15 | 38 | 38 | 49 | 49 |
| Carbohydrate, % of calories | 52 | 52 | 65 | 65 | 54 | 54 | 39 | 39 |
| Vitamin A, IU | 1151 | 1600 | 2030 | 2000 | 1183 | 1600 | 1296 | 1600 |
| Vitamin D, IU | 288 | 400 | 406 | 400 | 296 | 400 | 324 | 400 |
| Vitamin E, IU | 7 | 10 | 10 | 10 | 7 | 10 | 8 | 10 |
| Vitamin C (ascorbic acid), mg | 37 | 52 | 53 | 52 | 38 | 52 | 42 | 52 |
| Folic acid (folacin), mcg | 72 | 100 | 102 | 100 | 74 | 100 | 81 | 100 |
| Thiamine (vitamin B$_1$), mg | 0.36 | 0.5 | 0.6 | 0.6 | 0.37 | 0.5 | 0.40 | 0.5 |
| Riboflavin (vitamin B$_2$), mg | 0.43 | 0.6 | 1 | 1 | 0.44 | 0.6 | 0.49 | 0.6 |
| Niacin, mg | 5.8 | 8 | 8 | 8 | 5.9 | 8 | 6.5 | 8 |
| Vitamin B$_6$, mg | 0.3 | 0.4 | 0.5 | 0.5 | 0.3 | 0.4 | 0.3 | 0.4 |
| Vitamin B$_{12}$, mcg | 1.4 | 2.0 | 2.5 | 2.5 | 1.5 | 2.0 | 1.6 | 2.0 |
| Biotin, mg | 0.04 | 0.05 | 0.03 | 0.03 | 0.04 | 0.05 | 0.04 | 0.05 |
| Pantothenic acid, mg | 2.2 | 3.0 | 3.0 | 3.0 | 2.2 | 3.0 | 2.4 | 3.0 |
| Vitamin K, mcg | 72 | 100 | 102 | 100 | 74 | 100 | 81 | 100 |
| Choline, mg | 61 | 85 | 86 | 85 | 63 | 85 | 69 | 85 |
| Inositol, mg | 22 | 30 | 30 | 30 | 22 | 30 | 24 | 30 |
| Calcium, mg | 432 | 600 | 609 | 600 | 488 | 660 | 446 | 550 |
| Phosphorus, mg | 324 | 450 | 457 | 450 | 266 | 360 | 324 | 400 |
| Iodine, mcg | 32 | 45 | 46 | 45 | 33 | 45 | 36 | 45 |
| Iron, mg | 9 | 12 | 12 | 12 | 9 | 12 | 10 | 12 |
| Magnesium, mg | 50 | 70 | 71 | 70 | 52 | 70 | 41 | 60 |
| Copper, mg | 0.4 | 0.6 | 0.6 | 0.6 | 0.4 | 0.6 | 0.5 | 0.6 |
| Zinc, mg | 3 | 4 | 4 | 4 | 3 | 4 | 4 | 5 |
| Manganese, mg | 0.7 | 1 | 1 | 1 | 0.7 | 1 | 0.8 | 1 |
| Chloride, mg | 324 | 450 | 508 | 500 | 370 | 500 | 324 | 400 |
| Potassium, mg | 468 | 650 | 711 | 700 | 448 | 660 | 445 | 550 |
| Sodium, mg | 216 | 300 | 254 | 250 | 185 | 250 | 202 | 250 |

*Lofenalac formula (20 Kcal/fl oz)—139 g powder + 29 fl oz (858 ml) water.

†Phenyl-Free formula (25 Kcal/fl oz)—98.5 g powder + approximately 13.5 fl oz water.

‡MSUD formula (20 Kcal/fl oz)—134.5 g powder + 29 fl oz (858 ml) water.

§Product 3200 K (20 Kcal/fl oz)—123.5 g powder + 850 ml water.

‖Sixteen fluid ounces is equivalent to a normal day's intake of Phenyl-Free formula for the older PKU patient.

(From Nutritional Science Resources, Mead-Johnson Laboratories, Evansville, IN 47721)

variety of sources. It is recommended that as the USDA Handbook 8 series is completed, this reference be used as the source of current amino acid analysis data. Table 36-3 lists Phe-free foods that may be used as desired.

In addition to Table 36-2 and Table 3, Part 4, there are other sources that may be used as guides to the Phe content of foods. Information about the Phe content of some foods is available from the producers. Several state health departments and PKU treatment centers make available guides for the management of PKU, including tables of the Phe content of many foods (see list of sources at the end of chapter).

### Calculating the diet pattern

When formula is the only source of energy and nutrients for an infant, Lofenalac, cow's milk, and Karo syrup or other sources of carbohydrate are used. For example, a newborn infant weighing 3.5 kg needs 405 kcal, 10.5 g protein, 245 mg Phe, and approximately 525 ml fluid per day (Table 36-4).

As the child grows and solids are added to his diet, cereals, fruits, and vegetables will supply some Phe and energy, while Lofenalac and milk continue to be his major source of energy, protein, and Phe. For example, a 6 month old infant weighing 7 kg needs 735 kcal, 18 g to 20 g protein, 280 mg Phe (40 mg per kg) and 875 ml of fluid (Table 36-5).

As the infant becomes older his intake of cereal, fruits, and vegetables increases. At this time, Lofenalac is his major source of protein, and the amount of cow's milk in the formula decreases as the intake of Phe from other foods increases. With each revision in the calculation of the diet pattern, the mineral and vitamin content must be checked for adequacy because an infant's need for these nutrients increases as he grows larger. As dietary changes are made, it is extremely important to monitor closely blood levels of Phe to be certain that Phe levels remain within the acceptable range of 5 mg to 9 mg Phe per 100 ml.

As the very young child progresses to table foods, Lofenalac continues to be the major source of dietary protein and supplies part of the energy needs. Cereals, fruits, vegetables, sugars and fats, with small amounts of animal protein if the diet prescription permits, are used to provide Phe and energy. At this stage, part of the Lofenalac is usually reconstituted for drinking, and part may be used in making puddings, cookies, and white sauce.[15,16] If the Phe prescription requires it, cornstarch or low-protein wheat starch (see Chap. 32) is used in place of wheat flour in these dishes.

After the child reaches his second birthday Phenyl Free* may be offered as a beverage replacing Lofenalac. To provide the recommended intake of 16 oz per day, 98.5 g of the Phenyl Free powder is mixed with 13 oz of water.

No cow's milk is added to Phenyl Free. However, some dietitians recommend mixing some Lofenalac powder with Phenyl Free to increase the energy content of the diet. As was mentioned previously, the use of Phenyl Free allows a greater variety of foods to be included in the child's diet.

### Special problems in dietary treatment
First feedings

When the first feedings are initiated, the quantity of Phe in the diet may be less than the estimated requirement for an infant. The Phe blood levels are monitored daily, and as the level approaches 20 mg per 100 ml or less, the Phe in the feedings is increased to meet the infant's requirement. This can be achieved most readily by adjusting the quantity of cow's milk in the formula.

Excursions in the Phe blood levels
in the treated PKU patient

An elevated Phe blood level in a treated PKU infant or child may reflect an excessive intake of Phe or an inadequate energy intake. Without an adequate energy intake from fats and carbohydrates, body proteins are catabolized to provide energy. Also, an elevated Phe level may be due to a hypermetabolic state caused by infection. Therefore, not only dietary management but, also the infant's or child's physical condition must be assessed when blood Phe levels are elevated in a previously well controlled patient.

### Table 36-4. Quantities of Formula Ingredients Necessary for Newborn Infant

|  | Energy (kcal) | Pro. (gm) | Phe. (mg) | Fluid (ml) |
|---|---|---|---|---|
| 55 g Lofenalac | 253 | 8.3 | 44 |  |
| 4 oz (120 ml) whole cow's milk | 80 | 4.4 | 200 | 120 |
| 4 tsp Karo Syrup | 80 |  |  |  |
| Water |  |  |  | 405 |
| Totals | 413 | 12.7 | 244 | 525 |

### Table 36-5. Quantity of Formula and Solid Foods Necessary for 6-Month-Old Infant

|  | Energy (kcal) | Pro. (gm) | Phe (mg) | Fluid (ml) |
|---|---|---|---|---|
| 80 g Lofenalac | 368 | 12.0 | 64.0 | 0 |
| 3 oz (90 ml) whole cow's milk | 60 | 3.3 | 150.0 | 90 |
| 4 tsp Karo syrup | 80 | 0 | 0 | 0 |
| Water | 0 | 0 | 0 | 785 |
| 10 g rice cereal | 39 | 0.7 | 36.4 | 0 |
| 100 g strained peaches | 70 | 0.6 | 9.5 | 0 |
| 100 g strained green beans | 25 | 1.3 | 5.3 | 0 |
| 100 g strained plums with tapioca | 84 | 0.3 | 9.7 | 0 |
| Totals | 726 | 18.2 | 274.9 | 875 |

*Mead Johnson, Evansville, IN 47721

Very low blood Phe levels, less than 2 mg per 100 ml, are avoided because a blood level this low can result in a condition similar to kwashiorkor or energy-protein malnutrition (see Chap. 21).

## Expense of the diet

In some treatment centers funding is available to provide Lofenalac free of cost to the family. In other situations funding is not available, and the family must purchase the product. In 1980 a $2\frac{1}{2}$-lb can cost approximately $20.80 or $1.44 each day for a 3 month old infant. The cost of Phenyl Free in 1980 was approximately $25.00 for a $2\frac{1}{2}$-lb can. The cost per day for 16 fluid oz of ready-to-drink Phenyl Free was $2.10. Phenyl Free is also provided free of charge at some treatment centers. If any of the wheat starch products are used, these also increase the cost of feeding the infant or child with PKU.

## Liberalization of the diet

Smith and co-workers[17] report on studies conducted in London, England, and Heidelberg, West Germany, which demonstrated that normalization of the diet of PKU children between the ages of 5 and 15 years resulted in a decrease in intellectual progress for many patients. This decrease occurred even if initial dietary treatment had begun before the age of 4 months. However, a relaxed low-Phe diet showed smaller and insignificant changes in intellectual performance in a similar population. Based on these findings, it appears that complete liberalization of the diet of a PKU child, even after myelinization of the central nervous system is essentially complete would be inadvisable.

PKU treatment centers are especially concerned about the liberalization of the diet of PKU girls. It has been observed that mothers with untreated PKU produce nonphenylketonuric children, who are mentally retarded.[18] There is general agreement that dietary restrictions of female children with PKU should be continued through-out the childbearing years if there is to be any possibility of bearing a normal child. Pueschel[19] suggests that special emphasis needs to be placed on ensuring nutritional adequacy of the Phe-restricted diet during pregnancy.

## Counseling the mother

The mother and, whenever possible, the father of the infant with PKU needs to be seen by the same nutrition counselor at each visit to the treatment center and have access to the counselor between visits by either telephone or correspondence. If the blood Phe analysis is not available during the time the mother is at the center, the counselor may need to adjust the diet after the visit. If someone other than the mother is responsible for the child's care, that person should also be instructed by telephone and correspondence.

When the dietary treatment is initiated, the mother needs careful instruction in formula preparation. Errors in the proportions of Lofenalac powder, water, and cow's milk can be hazardous to the infant. It is strongly recommended that the complete preparation of the formula be demonstrated to the mother and that, under supervision, she return the demonstration. If the mother does not have a standard measuring cup and a set of standard measuring spoons, these should be provided, and their correct use in measuring infant foods should be demonstrated.

A copy of the calculated diet pattern with the date noted should be typed so that no error can be made in interpreting the counselor's handwriting. If diet adjustments are made by telephone, a written copy should be mailed immediately to avoid any error in interpreting the oral instructions.

The mother should be helped to understand that the infant must consume the prescribed formula each day and that the quantity of each feeding should be as consistent as possible. For example, if at all possible, she should avoid feeding the infant 90 ml of formula at one feeding and 200 ml at the next, especially when the formula is the

## Table 36-6. Phenylalanine-Free Foods

*(Contain little or no phenylalanine. May be used as desired.)*

| | | |
|---|---|---|
| Apple juice | Cherries, maraschino | Popsicles, with artificial fruit |
| Beverages, carbonated | Fruit ices (if no more than $\frac{1}{2}$ | flavor |
| Gingerbread* | cup used daily) | Rich's Topping |
| Guava butter | Cornstarch | Salt |
| Candy | Jell-quik | Shortening, vegetable |
|   Butterscotch | Jellies | Soy sauce |
|   Cream mints | Kool-aid | Sugar, brown, white, or |
|   Fondant | Lemonade | confectioner's |
|   Gum drops | Molasses | Syrups, corn or maple |
|   Hard | Oil | Tang |
|   Jelly beans | Pepper, black, ground | Tapioca, granulated |
|   Lollipops | | |

*Special recipe must be used (in Phenylalanine-Restricted Diet Recipe Book).

most significant dietary source of energy, protein, and Phe.

Between visits to the treatment center the mother records the quantity and kind of formula and foods consumed by the infant each day. A form that simplifies this task for the mother should be supplied by the center. At each visit the nutrition counselor reviews the record with the mother and correlates the estimation of the infant's daily energy, protein, and Phe intakes with the Phe blood levels. This information is shared with the physician so that, if necessary, adjustments can be made in the diet prescription.

Some mothers prefer an exchange system to plan daily menus. Others prefer to have the values per average serving of food* for older infants and toddlers, in order to calculate the energy, protein, and Phe of the daily menus. With this method a mother can adjust her plans more readily to the child's appetite. For example, on the day a child seems to have a small appetite the mother can offer foods that have more energy and Phe per serving and thus achieve the recommended intake. Also, some mothers are more comfortable using a scale to weigh foods as the child progresses to table foods.

The mother also needs help to prevent other children in the family, or relatives, friends, and neighbors, from offering the child with PKU any kinds of food or beverages without her knowledge. As the child enters kindergarten or elementary school, the mother needs to communicate with teachers about the child's dietary restrictions.

The instructional methods and materials vary with each mother, depending on her ability to learn and to manage her infant's diet. Many mothers need practical suggestions for organizing their daily schedules so that other members of the family as well as the infant with PKU receive her attention and care.

## Maple syrup urine disease (MSUD)

Maple syrup urine disease (MSUD) is a rare inborn error in the metabolism of the keto acids of the three branched-chain essential amino acids, leucine, isoleucine, and valine. The name is derived from the maple syrup-like odor of the urine. MSUD is transmitted through an autosomal recessive gene of unknown frequency. Approximately 50 cases have been reported in the literature. However, it is suspected that the diagnosis is often missed because of early infant deaths. The affected infant appears to lack the three decarboxylases required by the three keto acids derived from the transamination of branched-chain amino acids (Fig. 36-3).

The defect is present at birth, and the biochemical abnormalities occur as soon as the infant begins to take

food protein (milk). The abnormalities are elevated blood levels of the branched-chain amino acids and the three keto acids. The fact that keto acids are also excreted in the urine gives another term for the disease, *branched-chain ketoaciduria.*

The infant is normal at birth but at the end of the first week of life the first symptoms of poor feeding, hypoglycemia, and apathy occur. As early as the fifth day of life the maple syrup-like odor of the urine is detectable. Neurologic symptoms with convulsions appear early and, if the disease is untreated, death occurs during the first few months of life, sometimes as early as the first week. To avoid neurologic damage, diet therapy must be initiated in the first week of life and, from present experience, it appears that the dietary restrictions must be maintained throughout life.

### Types of MSUD

In addition to the classical form of MSUD described above there are two variant forms; one is episodic in nature, and the other is a milder form of the classical type. In the episodic form the biochemical abnormalities are only present during major stress, such as infection. These children do well on a normal diet without excessive protein. In the mild form, the infant responds to a protein intake limited to requirement. One case of a third variant has been reported.[20] The biochemical abnormality in this child responded to massive doses of thiamin.

### Dietary treatment
#### Principles of diet therapy

Leucine, isoleucine, and valine are essential amino acids. Therefore, in the treatment of MSUD the diet must supply the infant's requirement of these three amino acids without an excess to be catabolized through the branched-chain keto acid pathway. At the same time, the diet, as in PKU, must supply adequate energy, total protein, and all other nutrients required for normal growth.

The normal blood levels are leucine, 1.5 mg to 3.0 mg per 100 ml; isoleucine, 0.8 mg to 1.5 mg per 100 ml; and valine, 2.0 mg to 3.0 mg per 100 ml. Smith and Waisman[21] report good control in one patient by the criterion of normal growth when blood levels of leucine were maintained between 3 mg to 9 mg per 100 ml. With this range in leucine levels the blood level of isoleucine is between 1.5 mg to 3.0 mg per 100 ml and of valine, between 3 mg to 6 mg per 100 ml. The amino acid requirements of infants as defined by Holt and Snyderman (see Table 36-1) are used as guides in establishing therapy. Smith and Waisman[21] report that in infancy their patient required 130 mg of leucine per kilogram of body weight during the first months of life and that this decreased to 80 mg per kilogram by the first year.

It has been observed that, to support normal growth, the MSUD infant has a higher energy requirement than

---

*Calculated by the nutrition counselor using Table 3, Part 4 or other resources

normal infants. For example, some patients require 155 kcal to 175 kcal per kilogram of body weight to keep plasma levels normal and to prevent the breakdown of endogenous protein.

## Food for the MSUD diet

All food proteins contain the branched-chain amino acid (BCAA) with a greater percentage in animal than vegetable protein. As in the treatment of PKU, a special formula and low-protein foods are used to feed these infants and children.

One formula, MSUD Diet Powder,* is a mixture of synthetic amino acids free of the branched-chain amino acid (BCAA), with carbohydrate, fat, vitamins, and minerals added. MSUD Diet Powder is similar to Lofenalac and can be used as the sole source of nutrients until plasma levels of the BCAAs approach normal. Whole cow's milk is then added to the MSUD Diet Powder to provide the daily requirements of BCAAs needed for normal growth and development. To prepare 1 qt of formula 134.5 g of powder is added to 29 oz of water. This produces a formula with a caloric density of 20 kcal per ounce

*Mead Johnson Laboratories, Evansville, IN 47721

(30 ml). One hundred ml of homogenized milk contains 322 mg of leucine, 199 mg of isoleucine, and 220 mg of valine (see Table 3, Part 4). Snyderman[22] reports that without a source of natural protein added to the synthetic amino acid mixture, the infant does not gain weight.

Many clinicians prescribe and calculate only leucine intake levels for MSUD infants and children because the relationship between the levels of the BCAAs is approximately the same in foods with leucine levels, usually slightly higher than isoleucine or valine. However, this practice can lead to inadequate or excessive intakes of isoleucine or valine and, for this reason, is not recommended.

Various investigators[21,23] have developed leucine-equivalent tables comparable to an Exchange System. These systems have equated a serving of food with either 15 mg or 30 mg of leucine. Table 36-2 lists the isoleucine, leucine, and valine content in 100-g portions of selected food items, including infant foods. Rice cereal, low-protein fruits, and vegetables are the foods used to supplement the infant's formula. Low-protein wheat starch products (see Chap. 32) may be used as the child grows older as a source of energy.

The MSUD diet is also expensive. In 1980 MSUD Diet

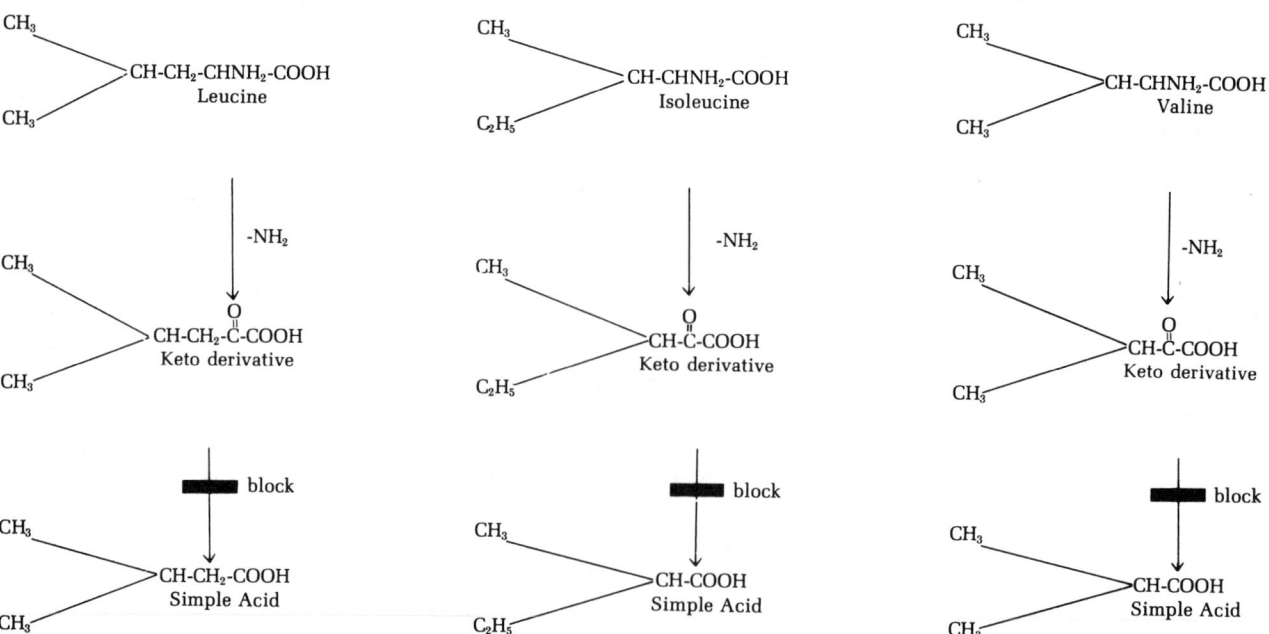

**Fig. 36-3.**   Metabolism of branched-chain amino acids, showing the site of block in maple syrup urine disease.

Powder for a 5 month old infant with MSUD cost approximately $43.75 per month compared with the cost of approximately $26.00 a month for a standard formula. If low-protein wheat starch products are used, this also increases the cost of the diet. As in PKU, some states provide the special foods, while others do not.

## Calculating the diet

The first feedings for the infant with MSUD are made using MSUD Diet Powder with no addition of cow's milk. When the elevated BCAA blood levels return to normal, cow's milk is added to the formula to supply the infant's requirement for these essential amino acids. For example, an infant weighing 3.5 kg requires approximately 532 mg of leucine (3.5 × 152 mg); 315 mg of isoleucine (3.5 × 90 mg); and 333 mg valine (3.5 × 95 mg). These requirements can be met by adding 165 ml (5½ oz) of homogenized milk to the MSUD Diet Powder formula. Calculations are made using the same system as with Lofenalac, being certain that the infant's fluid needs are met to prevent dehydration.

When the child is ready for infant foods, low-protein cereals, fruits, and vegetables can be used, in addition to homogenized milk, to supply the daily requirements of BCAA. Refer to Table 36-2. The MSUD Diet Powder provides the infant's needs for protein, energy, and other nutrients.

### Counseling the mother

The mother of the infant with MSUD needs the same assistance as the mother of an infant with PKU (see preceding discussion on phenylketonuria).

The mother needs a demonstration on formula preparation and a written recipe at the beginning and with every change in formula. She may need to be reminded how important it is to shake the bottle with each feeding, especially the first formula without milk added, because the ingredients may settle to the bottom of the bottle on standing.

## Other inborn errors of metabolism

### Homocystinuria

Homocystinuria is an inborn error in the metabolism of the essential sulfur-containing amino acid, methionine, due to a marked deficiency in the activity of the hepatic enzyme cystathionine synthase. In the untreated patient the disease is characterized by skeletal and ocular abnormalities and mental retardation. There is an elevated blood level of both methionine and homocystine, with the urinary excretion of significant amounts of homocystine and lesser amounts of methionine.

There are two types of homocystinuric patients. One group responds to massive doses of pyridoxine (vitamin $B_6$), possibly due to the stimulation of hepatic cystathio-

nine synthase by pyridoxine. These patients can tolerate a diet with a moderate reduction in methionine.[24]

Another group of patients responds to a diet low in methionine with supplemental L-cystine added. Perry recommends[25] Metinaid,* a product low in methionine, as the major source of dietary protein for the homocystinuric patient. The Metinaid is dissolved in orange juice or lemonade. Fruits, vegetables, bread, cereals, and fats are used to supply energy (see Table 3, Part 4).

Product 3200K† (see Table 36-3) is a soy protein isolate formula that contains no added methionine and is therefore recommended for the dietary treatment of homocystinuria. Product 3200K contains 34 mg of methionine per 100 kcal of formula. Similar to Lofenalac and MSUD Diet Powder, Product 3200K provides all other nutrients, except methionine, to meet the needs of the growing infant. One infant with homocystinuria, reported by Perry,[25] required 40 mg of methionine per kilogram of body weight. This value is in agreement with the figure of Holt and Snyderman of 45 mg per kilogram in the presence of cystine in the diet (see Table 36-1). As the child grows, the requirement per kilogram of body weight decreases.

### Leucine-sensitive hypoglycemia

Hypoglycemic reactions in infancy induced by the essential amino acid leucine may be another inborn error of metabolism. The inheritance pattern is uncertain at present but may be autosomal recessive. In normal children the administration of leucine stimulates a small rise in circulating blood insulin and a small decrease in blood glucose. In leucine-sensitive infants with hypoglycemia there is some evidence that the infant has an increased number of pancreatic beta cells, which may respond by an increase in insulin release when stimulated by leucine, for example, a high-protein diet.

The condition may be manifested from birth, usually appearing within the first 6 months of life. The symptoms are precipitated by a high-protein meal or a state of fast. In the early stages there are irritability and twitching movements of the extremities, and, if the disease is not treated, hypoglycemic convulsions, with blood sugar levels as low as 20 mg per deciliter. Eventually, failure to thrive and mental and psychomotor retardation occur.

The infant with leucine-sensitive hypoglycemia responds to a diet restricted in leucine, although not as restricted as in the treatment of maple syrup urine disease. Snyderman suggests 150 mg of leucine per kilogram of body weight per day (see Table 36-1).

Hsia[26] suggests a more liberal allowance of 150 mg to 230 mg of leucine per kilogram of body weight. A special

---

*Milner Scientific and Medical Research Co., Ltd., 37 Ganung Dr., Ossining, N.Y.

†Mead Johnson Laboratories, Evansville, IN 47721

formula, SMA S-14* (see Table 35-4), is restricted in leucine and is used to feed these infants. As the child grows older, foods of low leucine content are added to the diet (see Table 36-2 for leucine levels in selected foods).

Roth and Segal have devised a dietary regimen for older children consisting of a leucine-restricted diet with extra carbohydrate (between 10 g–30 g carbohydrate) after each meal to prevent hypoglycemic reactions. This regimen has controlled the symptoms, and the children have developed normally.[27,28] The importance of good dental hygiene, such as brushing the teeth after each meal, must be stressed with these patients.

Some clinicians recommend using the drug, diazoxide, in conjunction with a more liberalized intake of leucine in the diet.[29] Diazoxide suppresses insulin secretion, resulting in an increase in plasma glucose levels. Hirsutism is a side effect of this drug.

### Histidinemia

Histidinemia is an inborn error of the metabolism of the amino acid histidine due to a deficiency of the enzyme, histidase. High levels of histidine are found in the blood and urine. Clinical symptoms are manifested in speech disorders, both in articulation and language, though not in all of the patients known to have this disease. There is mental retardation in some patients, although again, not in all. A diet restricted in protein was not effective in lowering histidine in the blood or urine. However, a high-protein diet should be avoided in infancy.[30]

## Study questions and activities

1. What is the metabolic defect in phenylketonuria? Why is it important that it be treated early?
2. List some of the problems that a family may encounter daily in maintaining a 3 year old child with PKU on a phenylalanine-restricted diet.
3. Plan a diet for a 3 year old with PKU.
4. Plan the formula demonstration for a mother with a PKU infant.
5. Why must medications be closely scrutinized when an infant or child is on a galactose-free diet?

## References

1. Segal S: In Stanbury JB, Wyngaarden JB, Fredrickson DS (eds): The Metabolic Basis of Inherited Disease, 4th ed, pp 160–181. New York, McGraw-Hill, 1978
2. Hug G: In Vaughan VC III, McKay RJ Jr, Behrman RE (eds): Nelson Textbook of Pediatrics, 11th ed, pp 520–547. Philadelphia, WB Saunders, 1979
3. Hardinge MG et al: J Am Diet Assoc 46:197, 1965
4. Gitzelman R, Auricchio S: Pediatrics 36:231, 1965
5. Committee on Nutrition, American Academy of Pediatrics:

New developments in hyperphenylalaninemia. Pediatrics 65:844, 1980
6. Knox WE: In Stanbury JB, Wyngaarden JB, Fredrickson DS (eds): Metabolic Basis of Inherited Diseases, 3rd ed, pp 266–295. New York, McGraw-Hill, 1972
7. MacCready RA: Pediatrics 85:383, 1974
8. Morrow G III, Auerbach VH: In Vaughan, McKay, and Behrman (eds): Nelson Textbook, pp 497–520
9. Danks DM: J Pediatr 96:854, 1980
10. Rouse BM: J Pediatr 69:246, 1966
11. Fomon SJ: Infant Nutrition, 2nd ed, p 143. Philadelphia, WB Saunders, 1974
12. Hunt MH et al: Am J Dis Child 122:1, 1971
13. Nakagawa I et al: J Nutr 77:61, 1962
14. McCarthy MA et al: J Am Diet Assoc 52:130, 1968
15. Diet Guide for Parents of Children with Phenylketonuria. Berkeley, CA, California Department of Health, 1966
16. Rinic MM, Rogers PJ: J Am Diet Assoc 55:353, 1969
17. Smith I et al: Br Med J 2:723, 1978
18. Mabry CC et al: N Engl J Med 275:1331, 1966
19. Pueschel SM et al: Am J Clin Nutr 30:1153, 1977
20. Scriver CR et al: Lancet 1:310, 1971
21. Smith BA, Waisman HA: J Am Diet Assoc 59:342, 1971
22. Snyderman SE: In Nyhan WL (ed): Heritable Disorders of Amino Acid Metabolism, New York, John Wiley & Sons, 1974
23. Levy HL, Erickson AM: In Nyhan: Heritable Disorders of Amino Acid Metabolism
24. Mudd SH et al: J Clin Invest 49:1762, 1970
25. Perry TL: In Nyhan: Heritable Disorders of Amino Acid Metabolism
26. Hsia DY-Y: Inborn Errors of Metabolism, Part I, Clinical Aspects, 2nd ed. Chicago, Yearbook. 1966
27. Roth H et al: Pediatrics 34:831, 1964
28. Snyder RD, Robinson A: Am J Dis Child 113:566, 1967
29. Hack S: In Palmer S, Ekvall S (eds): Pediatric Nutrition in Developmental Disorders. Springfield, IL, Charles C Thomas, 1978
30. Ghadmi H: In Nyhan, Heritable Disorders of Amino Acid Metabolism

## Supplementary readings
### General

Committee on Nutrition, American Academy of Pediatrics: Special diets for infants born with inborn errors of amino acid metabolism. Pediatrics 57:783, 1976

Editorial: Heterozygote advantage—and disadvantage? Lancet 1:786, 1977

Kindt E, Halvorsen S: The need of essential amino acids in children. Am J Clin Nutr 33:279, 1980

Nayman R et al: Observations on the composition of milk-substitute products for treatment of inborn errors of amino acid metabolism. Comparisons with human milk. Am J Clin Nutr 32:1279, 1979

O'Brien D: Inborn errors of metabolism. Am J Clin Nutr 32:482, 1979

Scriver CR: Diet and genes: Euphenic nutrition. N Engl J Med 297:202, 1977

Segal S: Disorders of renal amino acid transport. N Engl J Med 294:1044, 1976

---

*Wyeth Laboratories, Philadelphia, PA 19101

## Phenylketonuria

Marino MA: Developing and testing a programmed instruction unit on PKU. J Am Diet Assoc 76:29, 1980

Scriver CR, Clow CL: Phenylketonuria: Epitome of human biochemical genetics. N Engl J Med 303:1336, 1980

Smith I et al: Effect of stopping low-phenylalanine diet on intellectual progress of children with phenylketonuria. Br Med J 2:723, 1978

Wyatt R: Phenylketonuria: The problems vary during different developmental stages. Am J Matern Child Nurs 3:296, 1978

## Maple syrup urine disease

Bell L et al: Dietary management of maple-sirup-urine disease: Extension of equivalency systems. J Am Diet Assoc 74:357, 1979

Cox RP et al: Antenatal diagnosis of maple syrup urine disease. Lancet 2:212, 1978

## Other inborn errors of metabolism

Fischler K et al: Developmental aspects of galactosemia from infancy to childhood. Clin Pediatr 19:38, 1980

Froesch ER: Disorders of fructose metabolism. Clin Endocrinol Metab 5, No. 3:599, 1976

Michals K et al: Dietary treatment of tyrosinemia type I. J Am Diet Assoc 73:507, 1978

Yudkoff M et al: Errors of carbohydrate metabolism in infants and children. Clin Pediatr 17:820, 1978

## Resources for parents of children with PKU

Acosta PB et al: A Parent's Guide to the Child with Maple Syrup Urine Disease. 1980. Department of Pediatrics and Graduate Programs in Dietetics, School of Medicine, Emory University, Atlanta, GA 30322 ($5.00 per copy)

Acosta PB et al: Parents' Guide to the Child with PKU, 1979. Programs in Dietetics, Division of Allied Health Professions, 2040 Ridgewood Dr., N.E., Emory University, Atlanta GA 30322 ($5.00 per copy)

Acosta PB, Elsas LJ: Dietary Management of Inherited Metabolic Disease, 1975. ACELMU Publishers, 1939 Westminster Way, Atlanta, GA 30307 ($10.00)

Hunt MM: The Phenylalanine, Protein and Calorie Content of Selected Foods. 1977. Children's Hospital Research Foundation, Cincinnati, OH 45229

Parents' Guide to the Galactose Restricted Diet. 1976. Maternal and Child Health Bureau, California Department of Health, 2151 Berkeley Way, Berkeley, CA 94704

Read E et al: The PKU Cookbook. P.K.U. Collaborative Study, University of New Mexico, Surge Bldg., Room 236, Albuquerque, NM 87131

Schuett VE: Low Protein Cookery for Phenylketonuria. Madison, University of Wisconsin Press, 1977

Taylor M, Schuett VE: You and PKU. 1978. Waisman Center on Mental Retardation and Human Development, 1500 Highland Ave., Madison WI 53706

*For further references see Bibliography in Part 4.*

# Tabular Material and Bibliography

## Part 4

# *Tables*

## Explanation of Tables

### Table 1. Nutritive values of the edible part of foods

This table of food values gives proximate composition and mineral and vitamin content in 730 foods in common use in the United States. It includes processed and prepared foods where such foods would not be consumed in the natural state. The foods are arranged under the following main headings: Dairy Products; Eggs, Fats, and Oils; Fish; Shellfish; Meat and Poultry; Fruits and Fruit Products; Grain Products; Legumes, Nuts, and Seeds; Sugars and Sweets; Vegetables and Vegetable Products; and Miscellaneous Items. The weight in grams for an approximate measure of each food is shown. The approximate measure shown for each food is in cups, ounces, pounds, some other well-known unit, or a piece of certain size. These values are taken from USDA Home and Garden Bulletin No. 72, 1981.[1]

### Table 2. Cholesterol in common foods

This table gives the total fat and the cholesterol content of common foods. Values are taken from USDA Handbook No. 8 and USDA Handbooks No. 8-1, 8-4, 8-5, 8-6, and 8-7.[2,3-7]

### Table 3. Amino acid content of foods per 100 grams—edible portion

The essential amino acid content of selected foods is listed in an order convenient for nutrition counselors dealing with inborn errors of metabolism. The values are given in micrograms rather than milligrams to avoid the use of decimals.

### Table 4. Sodium and magnesium content of foods

Copper values are omitted in this table because the values given in the literature are conflicting and incomplete. References to pertinent articles are given at the end of Table 4.

### Table 5. Zinc content of foods per 100 grams—edible portion

This table lists the total zinc content in milligrams of 100 g edible portions of raw and cooked foods. It includes the foods that are consumed in greatest quantities by U.S. households and certain other foods that are important sources of zinc. Many values in this table were derived from a limited number of analyses and hence are called provisional.[8]

## Table 6. Vitamin E content of (a) animal products, (b) plant products, and (c) processed, mixed, and miscellaneous foods

This table lists the vitamin E content of most foods. These values will be used in the revised USDA Handbook No. 8 series when it is complete.

## Table 7. Alcoholic and carbonated beverages

The calorie, carbohydrate, and alcohol content of common alcoholic and carbonated beverages are listed in this table to assist the nutrition counselor in planning and assessing dietary intake.

## Table 8. Equivalent weights and measures

This table, which lists weight, volume, and linear equivalents; comparative temperatures for centigrade and Fahrenheit scales; and approximate weights for common measures, should serve as a ready reference.

## Table 9. Percentiles for weight and height of males and females 0–18 years of age

The weights and heights of males and females from 1 month to 18 years in this table are the reference points that were used by the Food and Nutrition Board to establish the 1980 Recommended Dietary Allowances. This table permits the nutrition counselor to compare and evaluate height and weight in terms of percentile when assessing growth.

## Table 10. Desirable weights for men and women aged 25 and over

This table gives the desirable adult weight for height according to the size of the individual's frame—small, medium, or large. It is based on the concept that there is no need for an increase in weight once adult height is achieved.

## Table 11. Current guidelines for criteria of nutritional status for laboratory evaluation

Laboratory methods for evaluating nutritional status include biochemical tests that measure levels of nutrients in blood or urine or biochemical functions that are dependent on an adequate supply of essential nutrients. These tests vary in their reproducibility, and nutrient levels may vary from time to time reflecting immediate rather than usual intake. The "cut-off points" used in the table "as representing some degree of deficiency are, and will pre-

sumably always be, a matter of some argument and arbitrary decision."[9] However, evaluating nutritional status by biochemical tests is recognized as a more precise approach than dietary intake studies or clinical examinations.

## Table 12. Dietary standard for Canada, recommended daily nutrient intake (revised 1975)

This table will assist the Canadian reader in making appropriate interpretations of dietary assessments of Canadian population groups.

## Table 13. Canada's food guide

Canada's Food Guide is based on Table 12. Although the groups are similar to the U.S. Four Food Groups, the recommendations listed under serving size and number differ slightly.

## Table 14. Exchange lists—1950

The original exchange lists are included for the convenience of the nutrition counselor who will encounter numerous patients who had been previously instructed with these lists and who may prefer to continue to use them. (See Chapter 24.)

## Table 15. Calculating bioavailable dietary iron

This table was developed by E. R. Monsen and J. L. Balinfy to assist the nutrition counselor in estimating the bioavailable iron in an individual meal or snack. This work was sponsored by the USDA.

## References

1. Nutritive Value of Foods. USDA Home and Garden Bulletin No. 72. Washington, DC, 1981
2. Watt BK, Merrill AL: Composition of Foods—Raw, Processed and Prepared. USDA Agriculture Handbook No. 8, 2nd ed. Washington, DC, 1963
3. Posati LP, Orr ML: Composition of Foods—Dairy and Egg Products—Raw, Processed and Prepared. USDA Agriculture Handbook No. 8-1. Washington, DC, 1976
4. Reeves JB, Weihrauch JL: Composition of Foods—Fats and Oils—Raw, Processed and Prepared. USDA Agriculture Handbook No. 8-4. Washington, DC, 1979
5. Posati LP: Composition of Foods—Poultry Products—Raw, Processed and Prepared. USDA Agriculture Handbook No. 8-5. Washington, DC, 1979
6. Marsh AC: Composition of Foods—Soups, Sauces and Gravies—Raw, Processed and Prepared. USDA Agriculture Handbook No. 8-6. Washington, DC, 1980
7. Richardson M, Posati LP, Anderson BA: Composition of Foods—Sausages and Luncheon Meats—Raw, Processed and Prepared. USDA Agriculture Handbook No. 8-7. Washington, DC, 1980
8. Murphy EW, Willis BW, Watt BK: J Am Diet Assoc 66:345, 1975
9. Christakis G: Nutritional assessment in health programs. Am J Public Health (Suppl) 63:1–62, Nov, 1973

# Table 1. Nutritive Values of the Edible Part of Foods*

(Dashes (—) denote lack of reliable data for a constituent believed to be present in measurable amount)

*Dairy Products (Cheese, Cream, Imitation Cream, Milk; Related Products)*

Butter (See Fats, Oils, and Related Products, items 103–108)

| Item No. (A) | Foods, Approximate Measures, Units, and Weight (edible part unless footnotes indicate otherwise) (B) | Water Per-cent (C) g | Food Energy Cal-ories (D) | Pro-tein (E) g | Fat (F) g | Fatty Acids Satu-rated (Total) (G) g | Unsaturated Oleic (H) g | Unsaturated Lino-leic (I) g | Carbo-hydrate (J) g | Calcium (K) mg | Phos-phorus (L) mg | Iron (M) mg | Potas-sium (N) mg | Vitamin A Value (O) IU | Thiamin (P) mg | Ribo-flavin (Q) mg | Niacin (R) mg | Ascorbic Acid (S) mg |
|---|---|---|---|---|---|---|---|---|---|---|---|---|---|---|---|---|---|---|
| | Cheese | | | | | | | | | | | | | | | | | |
| | Natural | | | | | | | | | | | | | | | | | |
| 1 | Blue .......... 1 oz .......... | 28 | 100 | 6 | 8 | 5.3 | 1.9 | 0.2 | 1 | 150 | 110 | 0.1 | 73 | 200 | 0.01 | 0.11 | 0.3 | 0 |
| 2 | Camembert (3 wedges per 4-oz container) 1 wedge .......... | 38 52 | 115 | 8 | 9 | 5.8 | 2.2 | 0.2 | tr | 147 | 132 | 0.1 | 71 | 350 | 0.01 | 0.19 | 0.2 | 0 |
| | Cheddar | | | | | | | | | | | | | | | | | |
| 3 | Cut pieces .......... 1 oz .......... | 28 37 | 115 | 7 | 9 | 6.1 | 2.1 | 0.2 | tr | 204 | 145 | 0.2 | 28 | 300 | 0.01 | 0.11 | tr | 0 |
| 4 | 1 cu in .......... | 17.2 37 | 70 | 4 | 6 | 3.7 | 1.3 | 0.1 | tr | 124 | 88 | 0.1 | 17 | 180 | tr | 0.06 | tr | 0 |
| 5 | Shredded .......... 1 c .......... | 113 37 | 455 | 28 | 37 | 24.2 | 8.5 | 0.7 | 1 | 815 | 579 | 0.8 | 111 | 1200 | 0.03 | 0.42 | 0.1 | 0 |
| | Cottage (curd not pressed down) | | | | | | | | | | | | | | | | | |
| | Creamed (cottage cheese, 4% fat) | | | | | | | | | | | | | | | | | |
| 6 | Large curd .......... 1 c .......... | 225 79 | 235 | 28 | 10 | 6.4 | 2.4 | 0.2 | 6 | 135 | 297 | 0.3 | 190 | 370 | 0.05 | 0.37 | 0.3 | tr |
| 7 | Small curd .......... 1 c .......... | 210 79 | 220 | 26 | 9 | 6.0 | 2.2 | 0.2 | 6 | 126 | 277 | 0.3 | 177 | 340 | 0.04 | 0.34 | 0.3 | tr |
| 8 | Low fat (2%) .......... 1 c .......... | 226 79 | 205 | 31 | 4 | 2.8 | 1.0 | 0.1 | 8 | 155 | 340 | 0.4 | 217 | 160 | 0.05 | 0.42 | 0.3 | tr |
| 9 | Low fat (1%) .......... 1 c .......... | 226 82 | 165 | 28 | 2 | 1.5 | 0.5 | 0.1 | 6 | 138 | 302 | 0.3 | 193 | 80 | 0.05 | 0.37 | 0.3 | tr |
| 10 | Uncreamed (cottage cheese dry curd, less than ½% fat) 1 c .......... | 145 80 | 125 | 25 | 1 | 0.4 | 0.1 | tr | 3 | 46 | 151 | 0.3 | 47 | 40 | 0.04 | 0.21 | 0.2 | 0 |
| 11 | Cream .......... 1 oz .......... | 28 54 | 100 | 2 | 10 | 6.2 | 2.4 | 0.2 | 1 | 23 | 30 | 0.3 | 34 | 400 | tr | 0.06 | tr | 0 |
| | Mozzarella, made with— | | | | | | | | | | | | | | | | | |
| 12 | Whole milk .......... 1 oz .......... | 28 48 | 90 | 6 | 7 | 4.4 | 1.7 | 0.2 | 1 | 163 | 117 | 0.1 | 21 | 260 | tr | 0.08 | tr | 0 |
| 13 | Part skim milk .......... 1 oz .......... | 28 49 | 80 | 8 | 5 | 3.1 | 1.2 | 0.1 | 1 | 207 | 149 | 0.1 | 27 | 180 | 0.01 | 0.10 | tr | 0 |
| | Parmesan, grated | | | | | | | | | | | | | | | | | |
| 14 | Cup, not pressed down 1 c .......... | 100 18 | 455 | 42 | 30 | 19.1 | 7.7 | 0.3 | 4 | 1376 | 807 | 1.0 | 107 | 700 | 0.05 | 0.39 | 0.3 | 0 |
| 15 | Tablespoon .......... 1 tbsp .......... | 5 18 | 25 | 2 | 2 | 1.0 | 0.4 | tr | tr | 69 | 40 | tr | 5 | 40 | tr | 0.02 | tr | 0 |
| 16 | Ounce .......... 1 oz .......... | 28 18 | 130 | 12 | 9 | 5.4 | 2.2 | 0.1 | 1 | 390 | 229 | 0.3 | 30 | 200 | 0.01 | 0.11 | 0.1 | 0 |
| 17 | Provolone .......... 1 oz .......... | 28 41 | 100 | 7 | 8 | 4.8 | 1.7 | 0.1 | 1 | 214 | 141 | 0.1 | 39 | 230 | 0.01 | 0.09 | tr | 0 |
| | Ricotta, made with— | | | | | | | | | | | | | | | | | |
| 18 | Whole milk .......... 1 c .......... | 246 72 | 430 | 28 | 32 | 20.4 | 7.1 | 0.7 | 7 | 509 | 389 | 0.9 | 257 | 1210 | 0.03 | 0.48 | 0.3 | 0 |
| 19 | Part skim milk .......... 1 c .......... | 246 74 | 340 | 28 | 19 | 12.1 | 4.7 | 0.5 | 13 | 669 | 449 | 1.1 | 308 | 1060 | 0.05 | 0.46 | 0.2 | 0 |
| 20 | Romano .......... 1 oz .......... | 28 31 | 110 | 9 | 8 | — | — | — | 1 | 302 | 215 | — | — | 160 | — | 0.11 | tr | 0 |

(Continued)

*Footnotes to table 1 appear on pages 682–683.

## Table 1. Nutritive Values of the Edible Part of Foods (Continued)

(Dashes (—) denote lack of reliable data for a constituent believed to be present in measurable amount)

| Item No. (A) | Foods, Approximate Measures, Units, and Weight (edible part unless footnotes indicate otherwise) (B) | | Water (C) | Food Energy (D) | Protein (E) | Fat (F) | Fatty Acids | | | Carbohydrate (J) | Calcium (K) | Phosphorus (L) | Iron (M) | Potassium (N) | Vitamin A Value (O) | Thiamin (P) | Riboflavin (Q) | Niacin (R) | Ascorbic Acid (S) |
| | | | | | | | Saturated (Total) (G) | Unsaturated Oleic (H) | Linoleic (I) | | | | | | | | | | |
| | | g | Percent | Calories | g | g | g | g | g | g | mg | mg | mg | mg | IU | mg | mg | mg | mg |
| | *Dairy Products (Cheese, Cream, Imitation Cream, Milk; Related Products) (Continued)* | | | | | | | | | | | | | | | | | | |
| | Cheese (Continued) | | | | | | | | | | | | | | | | | | |
| 21 | Swiss ... 1 oz | 28 | 37 | 105 | 8 | 8 | 5.0 | 1.7 | 0.2 | 1 | 272 | 171 | tr | 31 | 240 | 0.01 | 0.10 | tr | 0 |
| | Pasteurized process cheese | | | | | | | | | | | | | | | | | | |
| 22 | American ... 1 oz | 28 | 39 | 105 | 6 | 9 | 5.6 | 2.1 | 0.2 | tr | 174 | 211 | 0.1 | 46 | 340 | 0.01 | 0.10 | tr | 0 |
| 23 | Swiss ... 1 oz | 28 | 42 | 95 | 7 | 7 | 4.5 | 1.7 | 0.1 | 1 | 219 | 216 | 0.2 | 61 | 230 | tr | 0.08 | tr | 0 |
| 24 | Pasteurized process cheese food, American ... 1 oz | 28 | 43 | 95 | 6 | 7 | 4.4 | 1.7 | 0.1 | 2 | 163 | 130 | 0.2 | 79 | 260 | 0.01 | 0.13 | tr | 0 |
| 25 | Pasteurized process cheese spread, American ... 1 oz | 28 | 48 | 80 | 5 | 6 | 3.8 | 1.5 | 0.1 | 2 | 159 | 202 | 0.1 | 69 | 220 | 0.01 | 0.12 | tr | 0 |
| | Cream, sweet | | | | | | | | | | | | | | | | | | |
| 26 | Half-and-half (cream and milk) ... 1 c | 242 | 81 | 315 | 7 | 28 | 17.3 | 7.0 | 0.6 | 10 | 254 | 230 | 0.2 | 314 | 260 | 0.08 | 0.36 | 0.2 | 2 |
| 27 | 1 tbsp | 15 | 81 | 20 | tr | 2 | 1.1 | 0.4 | tr | 1 | 16 | 14 | tr | 19 | 20 | 0.01 | 0.02 | tr | tr |
| 28 | Light, coffee, or table ... 1 c | 240 | 74 | 470 | 6 | 46 | 28.8 | 11.7 | 1.0 | 9 | 231 | 192 | 0.1 | 292 | 1730 | 0.08 | 0.36 | 0.1 | 2 |
| 29 | 1 tbsp | 15 | 74 | 30 | tr | 3 | 1.8 | 0.7 | 0.1 | 1 | 14 | 12 | tr | 18 | 110 | tr | 0.02 | tr | tr |
| | Whipping, unwhipped (volume about double when whipped) | | | | | | | | | | | | | | | | | | |
| 30 | Light ... 1 c | 239 | 64 | 700 | 5 | 74 | 46.2 | 18.3 | 1.5 | 7 | 166 | 146 | 0.1 | 231 | 2690 | 0.06 | 0.30 | 0.1 | 1 |
| 31 | 1 tbsp | 15 | 64 | 45 | tr | 5 | 2.9 | 1.1 | 0.1 | tr | 10 | 9 | tr | 15 | 170 | tr | 0.02 | tr | tr |
| 32 | Heavy ... 1 c | 238 | 58 | 820 | 5 | 88 | 54.8 | 22.2 | 2.0 | 7 | 154 | 149 | 0.1 | 179 | 3500 | 0.05 | 0.26 | 0.1 | 1 |
| 33 | 1 tbsp | 15 | 58 | 80 | tr | 6 | 3.5 | 1.4 | 0.1 | tr | 10 | 9 | tr | 11 | 220 | tr | 0.02 | tr | tr |
| 34 | Whipped topping, (pressurized) ... 1 c | 60 | 61 | 155 | 2 | 13 | 8.3 | 3.4 | 0.3 | 7 | 61 | 54 | tr | 88 | 550 | 0.02 | 0.04 | tr | 0 |
| 35 | 1 tbsp | 3 | 61 | 10 | tr | 1 | 0.4 | 0.2 | tr | tr | 3 | 3 | tr | 4 | 30 | tr | tr | tr | 0 |
| 36 | Cream, sour ... 1 c | 230 | 71 | 495 | 7 | 48 | 30.0 | 12.1 | 1.1 | 10 | 268 | 195 | 0.1 | 331 | 1820 | 0.08 | 0.34 | 0.2 | 2 |
| 37 | 1 tbsp | 12 | 71 | 25 | tr | 3 | 1.6 | 0.6 | 0.1 | 1 | 14 | 10 | tr | 17 | 90 | tr | 0.02 | tr | tr |
| | Cream products, imitation (made with vegetable fat) | | | | | | | | | | | | | | | | | | |
| | Sweet | | | | | | | | | | | | | | | | | | |
| | Creamers | | | | | | | | | | | | | | | | | | |
| 38 | Liquid (frozen) ... 1 c | 245 | 77 | 335 | 2 | 24 | 22.8 | 0.3 | tr | 28 | 23 | 157 | 0.1 | 467 | 220[1] | 0 | 0 | 0 | 0 |
| 39 | 1 tbsp | 15 | 77 | 20 | tr | 1 | 1.4 | tr | 0 | 2 | 1 | 10 | tr | 29 | 10[1] | 0 | 0 | 0 | 0 |
| 40 | Powdered ... 1 c | 94 | 2 | 515 | 5 | 33 | 30.6 | 0.9 | tr | 52 | 21 | 397 | 0.1 | 763 | 190[1] | 0 | 0.16[1] | tr | 0 |
| 41 | 1 tsp | 2 | 2 | 10 | tr | 1 | 0.7 | tr | 0 | 1 | tr | 8 | tr | 16 | tr | 0 | tr | 0 | 0 |

| (A) | (B) | | (C) | (D) | (E) | (F) | (G) | (H) | (I) | (J) | (K) | (L) | (M) | (N) | (O) | (P) | (Q) | (R) | (S) |
|---|---|---|---|---|---|---|---|---|---|---|---|---|---|---|---|---|---|---|---|
| | **Whipped topping** | | | | | | | | | | | | | | | | | | |
| 42 | Frozen | 1 c ......... | 75 | 240 | 1 | 19 | 16.3 | 1.0 | 0.2 | 17 | 5 | 6 | 0.1 | 14 | 650[1] | 0 | 0 | 0 | 0 |
| 43 | | 1 tbsp ......... | 4 | 50 | 15 | tr | 1 | 0.9 | 0.1 | tr | 1 | tr | tr | tr | 1 | 30[1] | 0 | 0 | 0 | 0 |
| 44 | Powdered, made with whole milk | 1 c ......... | 80 | 67 | 150 | 3 | 10 | 8.5 | 0.6 | 0.1 | 13 | 72 | 69 | tr | 121 | 290[1] | 0.02 | 0.09 | tr | 1 |
| 45 | | 1 tbsp ......... | 4 | 67 | 10 | tr | tr | 0.4 | tr | tr | 1 | 4 | 3 | tr | 6 | 10[1] | tr | tr | tr | tr |
| 46 | Pressurized | 1 c ......... | 70 | 60 | 185 | 1 | 16 | 13.2 | 1.4 | 0.2 | 11 | 4 | 13 | tr | 13 | 330[1] | 0 | 0 | 0 | 0 |
| 47 | | 1 tbsp ......... | 4 | 60 | 10 | tr | 1 | 0.8 | 0.1 | tr | 1 | tr | 1 | tr | 1 | 20[1] | 0 | 0 | 0 | 0 |
| 48 | Sour dressing (imitation sour cream) made with nonfat dry milk | 1 c ......... | 235 | 75 | 415 | 8 | 39 | 31.2 | 4.4 | 1.1 | 11 | 266 | 205 | 0.1 | 380 | 20[1] | 0.09 | 0.38 | 0.2 | 2 |
| 49 | | 1 tbsp ......... | 12 | 75 | 20 | tr | 2 | 1.6 | 0.2 | 0.1 | 1 | 14 | 10 | tr | 19 | tr | 0.01 | 0.02 | tr | tr |
| | **Ice cream** (see Milk desserts, frozen, items 75–80). | | | | | | | | | | | | | | | | | | |
| | **Ice milk** (see Milk desserts, frozen, items 81–83). | | | | | | | | | | | | | | | | | | |
| | **Milk** | | | | | | | | | | | | | | | | | | |
| | Fluid | | | | | | | | | | | | | | | | | | |
| 50 | Whole (3.3% fat) | 1 c ......... | 244 | 88 | 150 | 8 | 8 | 5.1 | 2.1 | 0.2 | 11 | 291 | 228 | 0.1 | 370 | 310[2] | 0.09 | 0.40 | 0.2 | 2 |
| | Low fat (2%) | | | | | | | | | | | | | | | | | | |
| 51 | No milk solids added | 1 c ......... | 244 | 89 | 120 | 8 | 5 | 2.9 | 1.2 | 0.1 | 12 | 297 | 232 | 0.1 | 377 | 500 | 0.10 | 0.40 | 0.2 | 2 |
| | Milk solids added | | | | | | | | | | | | | | | | | | |
| 52 | Label claims less than 10 g protein per cup | 1 c ......... | 245 | 89 | 125 | 9 | 5 | 2.9 | 1.2 | 0.1 | 12 | 313 | 245 | 0.1 | 397 | 500 | 0.10 | 0.42 | 0.2 | 2 |
| 53 | Label claims 10 or more g protein per cup (protein fortified) | 1 c ......... | 246 | 88 | 135 | 10 | 5 | 3.0 | 1.2 | 0.1 | 14 | 352 | 276 | 0.1 | 447 | 500 | 0.11 | 0.48 | 0.2 | 3 |
| | Low fat (1%) | | | | | | | | | | | | | | | | | | |
| 54 | No milk solids added | 1 c ......... | 244 | 90 | 100 | 8 | 3 | 1.6 | 0.7 | 0.1 | 12 | 300 | 235 | 0.1 | 381 | 500 | 0.10 | 0.41 | 0.2 | 2 |
| | Milk solids added | | | | | | | | | | | | | | | | | | |
| 55 | Label claims less than 10 g protein per cup | 1 c ......... | 245 | 90 | 105 | 9 | 2 | 1.5 | 0.6 | 0.1 | 12 | 313 | 245 | 0.1 | 397 | 500 | 0.10 | 0.42 | 0.2 | 2 |
| 56 | Label claims 10 or more g protein per cup (protein fortified) | 1 c ......... | 246 | 89 | 120 | 10 | 3 | 1.8 | 0.7 | 0.1 | 14 | 349 | 273 | 0.1 | 444 | 500 | 0.11 | 0.47 | 0.2 | 3 |
| | Nonfat (skim) | | | | | | | | | | | | | | | | | | |
| 57 | No milk solids added | 1 c ......... | 245 | 91 | 85 | 8 | tr | 0.3 | 0.1 | tr | 12 | 302 | 247 | 0.1 | 406 | 500 | 0.09 | 0.34 | 0.2 | 2 |
| | Milk solids added | | | | | | | | | | | | | | | | | | |
| 58 | Label claims less than 10 g protein per cup | 1 c ......... | 245 | 90 | 90 | 9 | 1 | 0.4 | 0.1 | tr | 12 | 316 | 255 | 0.1 | 418 | 500 | 0.10 | 0.43 | 0.2 | 2 |
| 59 | Label claims 10 or more g protein per cup (protein fortified) | 1 c ......... | 246 | 89 | 100 | 10 | 1 | 0.4 | 0.1 | tr | 14 | 352 | 275 | 0.1 | 446 | 500 | 0.11 | 0.48 | 0.2 | 3 |

(Continued)

**Table 1. Nutritive Values of the Edible Part of Foods (Continued)**

(Dashes (—) denote lack of reliable data for a constituent believed to be present in measurable amount)

| Item No. (A) | Foods, Approximate Measures, Units, and Weight (edible part unless footnotes indicate otherwise) (B) | Water Percent (C) | Food Energy Calories (D) | Protein g (E) | Fat g (F) | Saturated (Total) g (G) | Unsaturated Oleic g (H) | Unsaturated Linoleic g (I) | Carbohydrate g (J) | Calcium mg (K) | Phosphorus mg (L) | Iron mg (M) | Potassium mg (N) | Vitamin A Value IU (O) | Thiamin mg (P) | Riboflavin mg (Q) | Niacin mg (R) | Ascorbic Acid mg (S) |
|---|---|---|---|---|---|---|---|---|---|---|---|---|---|---|---|---|---|---|
| | *Dairy Products (Cheese, Cream, Imitation Cream, Milk; Related Products) (Continued)* | | | | | | | | | | | | | | | | | |
| | Milk (Continued) | | | | | | | | | | | | | | | | | |
| 60 | Buttermilk 1 c | 90 | 100 | 8 | 2 | 1.3 | 0.5 | tr | 12 | 285 | 219 | 0.1 | 371 | 80[3] | 0.08 | 0.38 | 0.1 | 2 |
| | Canned | | | | | | | | | | | | | | | | | |
| | Evaporated, unsweetened | | | | | | | | | | | | | | | | | |
| 61 | Whole milk 1 c | 74 | 340 | 17 | 19 | 11.6 | 5.3 | 0.4 | 25 | 657 | 510 | 0.5 | 764 | 610[3] | 0.12 | 0.80 | 0.5 | 5 |
| 62 | Skim milk 1 c | 79 | 200 | 19 | 1 | .3 | 0.1 | tr | 29 | 738 | 497 | 0.7 | 845 | 1000[4] | 0.11 | 0.79 | 0.4 | 3 |
| 63 | Sweetened, condensed 1 c | 27 | 980 | 24 | 27 | 16.8 | 6.7 | 0.7 | 166 | 868 | 775 | 0.6 | 1136 | 1000[3] | 0.28 | 1.27 | 0.6 | 8 |
| | Dried | | | | | | | | | | | | | | | | | |
| 64 | Buttermilk 1 c | 3 | 465 | 41 | 7 | 4.3 | 1.7 | 0.2 | 59 | 1421 | 1119 | 0.4 | 1910 | 260[3] | 0.47 | 1.90 | 1.1 | 7 |
| | Nonfat instant | | | | | | | | | | | | | | | | | |
| 65 | Envelope, net wt 3.2 oz[5] 1 envelope | 4 | 325 | 32 | 1 | 0.4 | 0.1 | tr | 47 | 1120 | 896 | 0.3 | 1552 | 2160[6] | 0.38 | 1.59 | 0.8 | 5 |
| 66 | Cup[7] 1 c | 4 | 245 | 24 | tr | 0.3 | 0.1 | tr | 35 | 837 | 670 | 0.2 | 1160 | 1610[6] | 0.28 | 1.19 | 0.6 | 4 |
| | Milk beverages | | | | | | | | | | | | | | | | | |
| | Chocolate milk (commercial) | | | | | | | | | | | | | | | | | |
| 67 | Regular 1 c | 82 | 210 | 8 | 8 | 5.3 | 2.2 | 0.2 | 26 | 280 | 251 | 0.6 | 417 | 300[3] | 0.09 | 0.41 | 0.3 | 2 |
| 68 | Low fat (2%) 1 c | 84 | 180 | 8 | 5 | 3.1 | 1.3 | 0.1 | 26 | 284 | 254 | 0.6 | 422 | 500 | 0.10 | 0.42 | 0.3 | 2 |
| 69 | Low fat (1%) 1 c | 85 | 160 | 8 | 3 | 1.5 | 0.7 | 0.1 | 26 | 287 | 257 | 0.6 | 426 | 500 | 0.10 | 0.40 | 0.2 | 2 |
| 70 | Eggnog (commercial) 1 c | 74 | 340 | 10 | 19 | 11.3 | 5.0 | 0.6 | 34 | 330 | 278 | 0.5 | 420 | 890 | 0.09 | 0.48 | 0.3 | 4 |
| | Malted milk, home-prepared with 1 c whole milk and 2 to 3 heaping tsp malted milk powder (about 3/4 oz) | | | | | | | | | | | | | | | | | |
| 71 | Chocolate 1 c milk plus 3/4 oz powder | 81 | 235 | 9 | 9 | 5.5 | — | — | 29 | 304 | 265 | 0.5 | 500 | 330 | 0.14 | 0.43 | 0.7 | 2 |
| 72 | Natural 1 c milk plus 3/4 oz powder | 81 | 235 | 11 | 10 | 6.0 | — | — | 27 | 347 | 307 | 0.3 | 529 | 380 | 0.20 | 0.54 | 1.3 | 2 |
| | Shakes, thick[8] | | | | | | | | | | | | | | | | | |
| 73 | Chocolate, container, net wt 10.6 oz 1 container | 72 | 355 | 9 | 8 | 5.0 | 2.0 | 0.2 | 63 | 396 | 378 | 0.9 | 672 | 260 | 0.14 | 0.67 | 0.4 | 0 |
| 74 | Vanilla, container, net wt 11 oz 1 container | 74 | 350 | 12 | 9 | 5.9 | 2.4 | 0.2 | 56 | 457 | 361 | 0.3 | 572 | 360 | 0.09 | 0.61 | 0.5 | 0 |
| | Milk desserts, frozen | | | | | | | | | | | | | | | | | |
| | Ice cream | | | | | | | | | | | | | | | | | |
| | Regular (about 11% fat) | | | | | | | | | | | | | | | | | |

Weight column (g): 60: 245; 61: 252; 62: 255; 63: 306; 64: 120; 65: 91; 66: 68; 67: 250; 68: 250; 69: 250; 70: 254; 71: 265; 72: 265; 73: 300; 74: 313.

| (A) | (B) | (C) | (D) | (E) | (F) | (G) | (H) | (I) | (J) | (K) | (L) | (M) | (N) | (O) | (P) | (Q) | (R) | (S) |
|---|---|---|---|---|---|---|---|---|---|---|---|---|---|---|---|---|---|---|
| 75 | Hardened .......... ½ gal ........... 1064 | 61 | 2155 | 38 | 115 | 71.3 | 28.8 | 2.6 | 254 | 1406 | 1075 | 1.0 | 2052 | 4340 | 0.42 | 2.63 | 1.1 | 6 |
| 76 | 1 c ......... 133 | 61 | 270 | 5 | 14 | 8.9 | 3.6 | 0.3 | 32 | 176 | 134 | 0.1 | 257 | 540 | 0.05 | 0.33 | 0.1 | 1 |
| 77 | 3 fl oz container .. 50 | 61 | 100 | 2 | 5 | 3.4 | 1.4 | 0.1 | 12 | 66 | 51 | tr | 96 | 200 | 0.02 | 0.12 | 0.1 | tr |
| 78 | Soft serve (frozen custard) 1 c ......... 173 | 60 | 375 | 7 | 23 | 13.5 | 5.9 | 0.6 | 38 | 236 | 199 | 0.4 | 338 | 790 | 0.08 | 0.45 | 0.2 | 1 |
| 79 | Rich (about 16% fat), hardened ½ gal ......... 1188 | 59 | 2805 | 33 | 190 | 118.3 | 47.8 | 4.3 | 256 | 1213 | 927 | 0.8 | 1771 | 7200 | 0.36 | 2.27 | 0.9 | 5 |
| 80 | 1 c ......... 148 | 59 | 350 | 4 | 24 | 14.7 | 6.0 | 0.5 | 32 | 151 | 115 | 0.1 | 221 | 900 | 0.04 | 0.28 | 0.1 | 1 |
| | **Ice milk** | | | | | | | | | | | | | | | | | |
| 81 | Hardened (about 4.3% fat) ½ gal ......... 1048 | 69 | 1470 | 41 | 45 | 28.1 | 11.3 | 1.0 | 232 | 1409 | 1035 | 1.5 | 2117 | 1710 | 0.61 | 2.78 | 0.9 | 6 |
| 82 | 1 c ......... 131 | 69 | 185 | 5 | 6 | 3.5 | 1.4 | 0.1 | 29 | 176 | 129 | 0.1 | 265 | 210 | 0.08 | 0.35 | 0.1 | 1 |
| 83 | Soft serve (about 2.6% fat) 1 c ......... 175 | 70 | 225 | 8 | 5 | 2.9 | 1.2 | 0.1 | 38 | 274 | 202 | 0.3 | 412 | 180 | 0.12 | 0.54 | 0.2 | 1 |
| 84 | Sherbet (about 2% fat) ½ gal ......... 1542 | 66 | 2160 | 17 | 31 | 19.0 | 7.7 | 0.7 | 469 | 827 | 594 | 2.5 | 1585 | 1480 | 0.26 | 0.71 | 1.0 | 31 |
| 85 | 1 c ......... 193 | 66 | 270 | 2 | 4 | 2.4 | 1.0 | 0.1 | 59 | 103 | 74 | 0.3 | 198 | 190 | 0.03 | 0.09 | 0.1 | 4 |
| | **Milk desserts, other** | | | | | | | | | | | | | | | | | |
| 86 | Custard, baked ........ 1 c ......... 265 | 77 | 305 | 14 | 15 | 6.8 | 5.4 | 0.7 | 29 | 297 | 310 | 1.1 | 387 | 930 | 0.11 | 0.50 | 0.3 | 1 |
| | **Puddings** | | | | | | | | | | | | | | | | | |
| | From home recipe | | | | | | | | | | | | | | | | | |
| | Starch base | | | | | | | | | | | | | | | | | |
| 87 | Chocolate ........ 1 c ......... 260 | 66 | 385 | 8 | 12 | 7.6 | 3.3 | 0.3 | 67 | 250 | 255 | 1.3 | 445 | 390 | 0.05 | 0.36 | 0.3 | 1 |
| 88 | Vanilla (blancmange) 1 c ......... 255 | 76 | 285 | 9 | 10 | 6.2 | 2.5 | 0.2 | 41 | 298 | 232 | tr | 352 | 410 | 0.08 | 0.41 | 0.3 | 2 |
| 89 | Tapioca cream ....... 1 c ......... 165 | 72 | 220 | 8 | 8 | 4.1 | 2.5 | 0.5 | 28 | 173 | 180 | 0.7 | 223 | 480 | 0.07 | 0.30 | 0.2 | 2 |
| | From mix (chocolate) and milk | | | | | | | | | | | | | | | | | |
| 90 | Regular (cooked) .... 1 c ......... 260 | 70 | 320 | 9 | 8 | 4.3 | 2.6 | 0.2 | 59 | 265 | 247 | 0.8 | 354 | 340 | 0.05 | 0.39 | 0.3 | 2 |
| 91 | Instant ......... 1 c ......... 260 | 69 | 325 | 8 | 7 | 3.6 | 2.2 | 0.3 | 63 | 374 | 237 | 1.3 | 335 | 340 | 0.08 | 0.39 | 0.3 | 2 |
| | **Yogurt** | | | | | | | | | | | | | | | | | |
| | With added milk solids | | | | | | | | | | | | | | | | | |
| | Made with low fat milk | | | | | | | | | | | | | | | | | |
| 92 | Fruit-flavored[9] ....... 1 container, net wt 8 oz 227 | 75 | 230 | 10 | 3 | 1.8 | 0.6 | 0.1 | 42 | 343 | 269 | 0.2 | 439 | 120[10] | 0.08 | 0.40 | 0.2 | 1 |
| 93 | Plain ........... 1 container, net wt 8 oz 227 | 85 | 145 | 12 | 4 | 2.3 | 0.8 | 0.1 | 16 | 415 | 326 | 0.2 | 531 | 150[10] | 0.10 | 0.49 | 0.3 | 2 |
| 94 | Made with non-fat milk 1 container, net wt 8 oz 227 | 85 | 125 | 13 | tr | 0.3 | 0.1 | tr | 17 | 452 | 355 | 0.2 | 579 | 20[10] | 0.11 | 0.53 | 0.3 | 2 |
| | Without added milk solids | | | | | | | | | | | | | | | | | |
| 95 | Made with whole milk 1 container, net wt 8 oz 227 | 88 | 140 | 8 | 7 | 4.8 | 1.7 | 0.1 | 11 | 274 | 215 | 0.1 | 351 | 280 | 0.07 | 0.32 | 0.2 | 1 |
| | **Eggs** | | | | | | | | | | | | | | | | | |
| 96 | Eggs, large (24 oz per dozen) / Raw / Whole, without shell .. 1 egg ........... 50 | 75 | 80 | 6 | 6 | 1.7 | 2.0 | 0.6 | 1 | 28 | 90 | 1.0 | 65 | 260 | 0.04 | 0.15 | tr | 0 |

(Continued)

## Table 1. Nutritive Values of the Edible Part of Foods (Continued)

(Dashes (—) denote lack of reliable data for a constituent believed to be present in measurable amount)

| Item No. (A) | Foods, Approximate Measures, Units, and Weight (edible part unless footnotes indicate otherwise) (B) | Water (C) Percent | Food Energy (D) Calories | Protein (E) g | Fat (F) g | Fatty Acids Saturated (Total) (G) g | Unsaturated Oleic (H) g | Linoleic (I) g | Carbohydrate (J) g | Calcium (K) mg | Phosphorus (L) mg | Iron (M) mg | Potassium (N) mg | Vitamin A Value (O) IU | Thiamin (P) mg | Riboflavin (Q) mg | Niacin (R) mg | Ascorbic Acid (S) mg |
|---|---|---|---|---|---|---|---|---|---|---|---|---|---|---|---|---|---|---|
| | **Eggs (Continued)** | | | | | | | | | | | | | | | | | |
| 97 | White ......... 1 white ........ 33 g | 88 | 15 | 3 | tr | tr | 0 | 0 | tr | 4 | 4 | tr | 45 | 0 | tr | 0.09 | tr | 0 |
| 98 | Yolk ......... 1 yolk ......... 17 g | 49 | 65 | 3 | 6 | 1.7 | 2.1 | 0.6 | tr | 26 | 86 | 0.9 | 15 | 310 | 0.04 | 0.07 | tr | 0 |
| | Cooked | | | | | | | | | | | | | | | | | |
| 99 | Fried in butter ...... 1 egg ......... 46 g | 72 | 85 | 5 | 6 | 2.4 | 2.2 | 0.6 | 1 | 26 | 80 | 0.9 | 58 | 290 | 0.03 | 0.13 | tr | 0 |
| 100 | Hard-cooked, shell removed ... 1 egg ........ 50 g | 75 | 80 | 6 | 6 | 1.7 | 2.0 | 0.6 | 1 | 28 | 90 | 1.0 | 65 | 260 | 0.04 | 0.14 | tr | 0 |
| 101 | Poached ......... 1 egg ........ 50 g | 74 | 80 | 6 | 6 | 1.7 | 2.0 | 0.6 | 1 | 28 | 90 | 1.0 | 65 | 260 | 0.04 | 0.13 | tr | 0 |
| 102 | Scrambled (milk added) 1 egg ........ 64 g in butter. Also omelet | 76 | 95 | 6 | 7 | 2.8 | 2.3 | 0.6 | 1 | 47 | 97 | 0.9 | 85 | 310 | 0.04 | 0.16 | tr | 0 |
| | **Fats, Oils, and Related Products** | | | | | | | | | | | | | | | | | |
| | Butter | | | | | | | | | | | | | | | | | |
| | Regular (1 brick or 4 sticks per lb) | | | | | | | | | | | | | | | | | |
| 103 | Stick (1/2 cup) ......... 1 stick .......... 113 g | 16 | 815 | 1 | 92 | 57.3 | 23.1 | 2.1 | tr | 27 | 26 | 0.2 | 29 | 3470[11] | 0.01 | 0.04 | tr | 0 |
| 104 | Tablespoon (about 1/8 stick) ... 1 tbsp .......... 14 g | 16 | 100 | tr | 12 | 7.2 | 2.9 | 0.3 | tr | 3 | 3 | tr | 4 | 430[11] | tr | tr | tr | 0 |
| 105 | Pat (1" square, 1/3 high; 90 per lb) ... 1 pat ........... 5 g | 16 | 35 | tr | 4 | 2.5 | 1.0 | 0.1 | tr | 1 | 1 | tr | 1 | 150[11] | tr | tr | tr | 0 |
| | Whipped (6 sticks or two 8-oz containers per lb) | | | | | | | | | | | | | | | | | |
| 106 | Stick (1/2 cup) ......... 1 stick .......... 76 g | 16 | 540 | 1 | 61 | 38.2 | 15.4 | 1.4 | tr | 18 | 17 | 0.1 | 20 | 2310[11] | tr | 0.03 | tr | 0 |
| 107 | Tablespoon (about 1/8 stick) ... 1 tbsp .......... 9 g | 16 | 65 | tr | 8 | 4.7 | 1.9 | 0.2 | tr | 2 | 2 | tr | 2 | 290[11] | tr | tr | tr | 0 |
| 108 | Pat (1 1/4" square, 1/3 high; 120 per lb) ... 1 pat ........... 4 g | 16 | 25 | tr | 3 | 1.9 | 0.8 | 0.1 | tr | 1 | 1 | tr | 1 | 120[11] | 0 | tr | tr | 0 |
| 109 | Fats, cooking (vegetable shortenings) ... 1 c ........... 200 g | 0 | 1770 | 0 | 200 | 48.8 | 88.2 | 48.4 | 0 | 0 | 0 | 0 | 0 | — | 0 | 0 | 0 | 0 |
| 110 | ............ 1 tbsp .......... 13 g | 0 | 110 | 0 | 13 | 3.2 | 5.7 | 3.1 | 0 | 0 | 0 | 0 | 0 | — | 0 | 0 | 0 | 0 |
| 111 | Lard .......... 1 c ........... 205 g | 0 | 1850 | 0 | 205 | 81.0 | 83.8 | 20.5 | 0 | 0 | 0 | 0 | 0 | 0 | 0 | 0 | 0 | 0 |
| 112 | ............ 1 tbsp .......... 13 g | 0 | 115 | 0 | 13 | 5.1 | 5.3 | 1.3 | 0 | 0 | 0 | 0 | 0 | 0 | 0 | 0 | 0 | 0 |
| | Margarine | | | | | | | | | | | | | | | | | |
| | Regular (1 brick or 4 sticks per lb) | | | | | | | | | | | | | | | | | |
| 113 | Stick (1/2 cup) ......... 1 stick .......... 113 g | 16 | 815 | 1 | 92 | 16.7 | 42.9 | 24.9 | tr | 27 | 26 | 0.2 | 29 | 3750[12] | 0.01 | 0.04 | tr | 0 |
| 114 | Tablespoon (about 1/8 stick) ... 1 tbsp .......... 14 g | 16 | 100 | tr | 12 | 2.1 | 5.3 | 3.1 | tr | 3 | 3 | tr | 4 | 470[12] | tr | tr | tr | 0 |
| 115 | Pat (1" square, 1/3 high; 90 per lb) ... 1 pat ........... 5 g | 16 | 35 | tr | 4 | 0.7 | 1.9 | 1.1 | tr | 1 | 1 | tr | 1 | 170[12] | tr | tr | tr | 0 |
| 116 | Soft, two 8-oz containers per lb ... 1 container ...... 227 g | 16 | 1635 | 1 | 184 | 32.5 | 71.5 | 65.4 | tr | 53 | 52 | 0.4 | 59 | 7500[12] | 0.01 | 0.08 | 0.1 | 0 |

| (A) | (B) | | (C) | (D) | (E) | (F) | (G) | (H) | (I) | (J) | (K) | (L) | (M) | (N) | (O) | (P) | (Q) | (R) | (S) |
|---|---|---|---|---|---|---|---|---|---|---|---|---|---|---|---|---|---|---|---|
| 117 | ......... 1 tbsp | 14 | 16 | 100 | tr | 12 | 2.0 | 4.5 | 4.1 | tr | 3 | 3 | tr | 4 | 470[12] | tr | tr | tr | 0 |
| | Whipped (6 sticks per lb) | | | | | | | | | | | | | | | | | | |
| 118 | Stick (½ cup) ......... 1 stick | 76 | 16 | 545 | tr | 61 | 11.2 | 28.7 | 16.7 | tr | 18 | 17 | 0.1 | 20 | 2500[12] | tr | 0.03 | tr | 0 |
| 119 | Tablespoon (about ⅛ stick) ......... 1 tbsp | 9 | 16 | 70 | tr | 8 | 1.4 | 3.6 | 2.1 | tr | 2 | 2 | tr | 2 | 310[12] | tr | tr | tr | 0 |
| | Oils, salad or cooking | | | | | | | | | | | | | | | | | | |
| 120 | Corn ......... 1 c | 218 | 0 | 1925 | 0 | 218 | 27.7 | 53.6 | 125.1 | 0 | 0 | 0 | 0 | 0 | — | 0 | 0 | 0 | 0 |
| 121 | ......... 1 tbsp | 14 | 0 | 120 | 0 | 14 | 1.7 | 3.3 | 7.8 | 0 | 0 | 0 | 0 | 0 | — | 0 | 0 | 0 | 0 |
| 122 | Olive ......... 1 c | 216 | 0 | 1910 | 0 | 216 | 30.7 | 154.4 | 17.7 | 0 | 0 | 0 | 0 | 0 | — | 0 | 0 | 0 | 0 |
| 123 | ......... 1 tbsp | 14 | 0 | 120 | 0 | 14 | 1.9 | 9.7 | 1.1 | 0 | 0 | 0 | 0 | 0 | — | 0 | 0 | 0 | 0 |
| 124 | Peanut ......... 1 c | 216 | 0 | 1910 | 0 | 216 | 37.4 | 98.5 | 67.0 | 0 | 0 | 0 | 0 | 0 | — | 0 | 0 | 0 | 0 |
| 125 | ......... 1 tbsp | 14 | 0 | 120 | 0 | 14 | 2.3 | 6.2 | 4.2 | 0 | 0 | 0 | 0 | 0 | — | 0 | 0 | 0 | 0 |
| 126 | Safflower ......... 1 c | 218 | 0 | 1925 | 0 | 218 | 20.5 | 25.9 | 159.8 | 0 | 0 | 0 | 0 | 0 | — | 0 | 0 | 0 | 0 |
| 127 | ......... 1 tbsp | 14 | 0 | 120 | 0 | 14 | 1.3 | 1.6 | 10.0 | 0 | 0 | 0 | 0 | 0 | — | 0 | 0 | 0 | 0 |
| 128 | Soybean oil, hydrogenated (partially hardened) ......... 1 c | 218 | 0 | 1925 | 0 | 218 | 31.8 | 93.1 | 75.6 | 0 | 0 | 0 | 0 | 0 | — | 0 | 0 | 0 | 0 |
| 129 | ......... 1 tbsp | 14 | 0 | 120 | 0 | 14 | 2.0 | 5.8 | 4.7 | 0 | 0 | 0 | 0 | 0 | — | 0 | 0 | 0 | 0 |
| 130 | Soybean-cottonseed oil blend, hydrogenated ......... 1 c | 218 | 0 | 1925 | 0 | 218 | 38.2 | 63.0 | 99.6 | 0 | 0 | 0 | 0 | 0 | — | 0 | 0 | 0 | 0 |
| 131 | ......... 1 tbsp | 14 | 0 | 120 | 0 | 14 | 2.4 | 3.9 | 6.2 | 0 | 0 | 0 | 0 | 0 | — | 0 | 0 | 0 | 0 |
| | Salad dressings | | | | | | | | | | | | | | | | | | |
| | Commercial | | | | | | | | | | | | | | | | | | |
| | Blue cheese | | | | | | | | | | | | | | | | | | |
| 132 | Regular ......... 1 tbsp | 15 | 32 | 75 | 1 | 8 | 1.6 | 1.7 | 3.8 | 1 | 12 | 11 | tr | 6 | 30 | tr | 0.02 | tr | tr |
| 133 | Low calorie (5 cal per tsp) ......... 1 tbsp | 16 | 84 | 10 | tr | 1 | 0.5 | 0.3 | tr | 1 | 10 | 8 | tr | 5 | 30 | tr | 0.01 | tr | tr |
| | French | | | | | | | | | | | | | | | | | | |
| 134 | Regular ......... 1 tbsp | 16 | 39 | 65 | tr | 6 | 1.1 | 1.3 | 3.2 | 3 | 2 | 2 | 0.1 | 13 | — | — | — | — | — |
| 135 | Low calorie (5 cal per tsp) ......... 1 tbsp | 16 | 77 | 15 | tr | 1 | 0.1 | 0.1 | 0.4 | 2 | 2 | 2 | 0.1 | 13 | — | — | — | — | — |
| | Italian | | | | | | | | | | | | | | | | | | |
| 136 | Regular ......... 1 tbsp | 15 | 28 | 85 | tr | 9 | 1.6 | 1.9 | 4.7 | 1 | 2 | 1 | tr | 2 | tr | tr | tr | tr | — |
| 137 | Low calorie (2 cal per tsp) ......... 1 tbsp | 15 | 90 | 10 | tr | 1 | 0.1 | 0.1 | 0.4 | tr | tr | 1 | tr | 2 | tr | tr | tr | tr | — |
| 138 | Mayonnaise ......... 1 tbsp | 14 | 15 | 100 | tr | 11 | 2.0 | 2.4 | 5.6 | tr | 3 | 4 | 0.1 | 5 | 40 | tr | 0.01 | tr | — |
| | Mayonnaise type | | | | | | | | | | | | | | | | | | |
| 139 | Regular ......... 1 tbsp | 15 | 41 | 65 | tr | 6 | 1.1 | 1.4 | 3.2 | 2 | 2 | 4 | tr | 1 | 30 | tr | tr | tr | — |
| 140 | Low calorie (8 cal per tsp) ......... 1 tbsp | 16 | 81 | 20 | tr | 2 | 0.4 | 0.4 | 1.0 | 2 | 3 | 4 | tr | 1 | 40 | tr | tr | tr | — |
| 141 | Tartar sauce, regular ......... 1 tbsp | 14 | 34 | 75 | tr | 8 | 1.5 | 1.8 | 4.1 | 1 | 3 | 4 | 0.1 | 11 | 30 | tr | tr | tr | tr |
| | Thousand Island | | | | | | | | | | | | | | | | | | |
| 142 | Regular ......... 1 tbsp | 16 | 32 | 80 | tr | 8 | 1.4 | 1.7 | 4.0 | 2 | 2 | 3 | 0.1 | 18 | 50 | tr | tr | tr | tr |
| 143 | Low calorie (10 cal per tsp) ......... 1 tbsp | 15 | 68 | 25 | tr | 2 | 0.4 | 0.4 | 1.0 | 2 | 2 | 3 | 0.1 | 17 | 50 | tr | tr | tr | tr |
| | From home recipe | | | | | | | | | | | | | | | | | | |
| 144 | Cooked type[13] ......... 1 tbsp | 16 | 68 | 25 | 1 | 2 | 0.5 | 0.6 | 0.3 | 2 | 14 | 15 | 0.1 | 19 | 80 | 0.01 | 0.03 | tr | tr |

(Continued)

# Table 1. Nutritive Values of the Edible Part of Foods (Continued)

(Dashes (—) denote lack of reliable data for a constituent believed to be present in measurable amount)

| Item No. (A) | Foods, Approximate Measures, Units, and Weight (edible part unless footnotes indicate otherwise) (B) | (g) | Water (C) Per cent | Food Energy (D) Calories | Pro-tein (E) g | Fat (F) g | Fatty Acids Satu-rated (Total) (G) g | Unsaturated Oleic (H) g | Unsaturated Lino-leic (I) g | Carbo-hydrate (J) g | Calcium (K) mg | Phos-phorus (L) mg | Iron (M) mg | Potas-sium (N) mg | Vitamin A Value (O) IU | Thiamin (P) mg | Ribo-flavin (Q) mg | Niacin (R) mg | Ascorbic Acid (S) mg |
|---|---|---|---|---|---|---|---|---|---|---|---|---|---|---|---|---|---|---|---|
| | **Fish, Shellfish, Meat, Poultry, and Related Products** | | | | | | | | | | | | | | | | | | |
| | Fish and shellfish | | | | | | | | | | | | | | | | | | |
| 145 | Bluefish, baked with butter or margarine ....... 3 oz | 85 | 68 | 135 | 22 | 4 | — | — | — | 0 | 25 | 244 | 0.6 | — | 40 | 0.09 | 0.08 | 1.6 | — |
| | Clams | | | | | | | | | | | | | | | | | | |
| 146 | Raw, meat only ...... 3 oz | 85 | 82 | 65 | 11 | 1 | — | — | — | 2 | 59 | 138 | 5.2 | 154 | 90 | 0.08 | 0.15 | 1.1 | 8 |
| 147 | Canned, solids and liquid ......... 3 oz | 85 | 86 | 45 | 7 | 1 | 0.2 | tr | tr | 2 | 47 | 116 | 3.5 | 119 | — | 0.01 | 0.09 | 0.9 | — |
| 148 | Crabmeat (white or king), canned, not pressed down ........ 1 c | 135 | 77 | 135 | 24 | 3 | 0.6 | 0.4 | 0.1 | 1 | 61 | 246 | 1.1 | 149 | — | 0.11 | 0.11 | 2.6 | — |
| 149 | Fish sticks, breaded, cooked, frozen (stick, 4" × 1" × ½") ..... 1 fish stick or 1 oz | 28 | 66 | 50 | 5 | 3 | — | — | — | 2 | 3 | 47 | 0.1 | — | 0 | 0.01 | 0.02 | 0.5 | — |
| 150 | Haddock, breaded, fried[14] ....... 3 oz | 85 | 66 | 140 | 17 | 5 | 1.4 | 2.2 | 1.2 | 5 | 34 | 210 | 1.0 | 296 | — | 0.03 | 0.06 | 2.7 | 2 |
| 151 | Ocean perch, breaded, fried[14] ......... 1 fillet | 85 | 59 | 195 | 16 | 11 | 2.7 | 4.4 | 2.3 | 6 | 28 | 192 | 1.1 | 242 | — | 0.10 | 0.10 | 1.6 | — |
| 152 | Oysters, raw, meat only (13–19 medium Selects) ........ 1 c | 240 | 85 | 160 | 20 | 4 | 1.3 | 0.2 | 0.1 | 8 | 226 | 343 | 13.2 | 290 | 740 | 0.34 | 0.43 | 6.0 | — |
| 153 | Salmon, pink, canned, solids and liquid ....... 3 oz | 85 | 71 | 120 | 17 | 5 | 0.9 | 0.8 | 0.1 | 0 | 167[15] | 243 | 0.7 | 307 | 60 | 0.03 | 0.16 | 6.8 | — |
| 154 | Sardines, Atlantic, canned in oil, drained solids ....... 3 oz | 85 | 62 | 175 | 20 | 9 | 3.0 | 2.5 | 0.5 | 0 | 372 | 424 | 2.5 | 502 | 190 | 0.02 | 0.17 | 4.6 | — |
| 155 | Scallops, frozen, breaded, fried, reheated, 6 scallops ...... | 90 | 60 | 175 | 16 | 8 | — | — | — | 9 | — | — | — | — | — | — | — | — | — |
| 156 | Shad, baked with butter or margarine, bacon ....... 3 oz | 85 | 64 | 170 | 20 | 10 | — | — | — | 0 | 20 | 266 | 0.5 | 320 | 30 | 0.11 | 0.22 | 7.3 | — |
| | Shrimp | | | | | | | | | | | | | | | | | | |
| 157 | Canned meat ........ 3 oz | 85 | 70 | 100 | 21 | 1 | 0.1 | 0.1 | tr | 1 | 98 | 224 | 2.6 | 104 | 50 | 0.01 | 0.03 | 1.5 | — |
| 158 | French fried[16] ........ 3 oz | 85 | 57 | 190 | 17 | 9 | 2.3 | 3.7 | 2.0 | 9 | 61 | 162 | 1.7 | 195 | — | 0.03 | 0.07 | 2.3 | — |
| 159 | Tuna, canned in oil, drained solids ....... 3 oz | 85 | 61 | 170 | 24 | 7 | 1.7 | 1.7 | 0.7 | 0 | 7 | 199 | 1.6 | — | 70 | 0.04 | 0.10 | 10.1 | — |
| 160 | Tuna salad[17] ......... 1 c | 205 | 70 | 350 | 30 | 22 | 4.3 | 6.3 | 6.7 | 7 | 41 | 291 | 2.7 | — | 590 | 0.08 | 0.23 | 10.3 | 2 |
| | Meat and meat products | | | | | | | | | | | | | | | | | | |
| 161 | Bacon (20 slices per lb, raw), broiled or fried, crisp) ......... 2 slices | 15 | 8 | 85 | 4 | 8 | 2.5 | 3.7 | 0.7 | tr | 2 | 34 | 0.5 | 35 | 0 | 0.08 | 0.05 | 0.8 | — |

| (A) | (B) | (C) | (D) | (E) | (F) | (G) | (H) | (I) | (J) | (K) | (L) | (M) | (N) | (O) | (P) | (Q) | (R) | (S) |  |
|---|---|---|---|---|---|---|---|---|---|---|---|---|---|---|---|---|---|---|---|
|  | Beef,[18] cooked |  |  |  |  |  |  |  |  |  |  |  |  |  |  |  |  |  |  |
|  | Cuts braised, simmered, or pot roasted |  |  |  |  |  |  |  |  |  |  |  |  |  |  |  |  |  |  |
| 162 | Lean and fat (piece, 2½″ × 2½″ × ¾″) 3 oz | 85 | 53 | 245 | 23 | 16 | 6.8 | 6.5 | 0.4 | 0 | 10 | 114 | 2.9 | 184 | 30 | 0.04 | 0.18 | 3.6 | — |
| 163 | Lean only from item 162  2.5 oz | 72 | 62 | 140 | 22 | 5 | 2.1 | 1.8 | 0.2 | 0 | 10 | 108 | 2.7 | 176 | 10 | 0.04 | 0.17 | 3.3 | — |
|  | Ground beef, broiled |  |  |  |  |  |  |  |  |  |  |  |  |  |  |  |  |  |  |
| 164 | Lean with 10% fat  3 oz or patty 3″ × 5/8″ | 85 | 60 | 185 | 23 | 10 | 4.0 | 3.9 | 0.3 | 0 | 10 | 196 | 3.0 | 261 | 20 | 0.08 | 0.20 | 5.1 | — |
| 165 | Lean with 21% fat  2.9 oz or patty 3″ × 5/8″ | 82 | 54 | 235 | 20 | 17 | 7.0 | 6.7 | 0.4 | 0 | 9 | 159 | 2.6 | 221 | 30 | 0.07 | 0.17 | 4.4 | — |
|  | Roast, oven-cooked, no liquid added |  |  |  |  |  |  |  |  |  |  |  |  |  |  |  |  |  |  |
|  | Relatively fat, such as rib |  |  |  |  |  |  |  |  |  |  |  |  |  |  |  |  |  |  |
| 166 | Lean and fat (2 pieces, 4⅛″ × 2¼″ × ¼″) 3 oz | 85 | 40 | 375 | 17 | 33 | 14.0 | 13.6 | 0.8 | 0 | 8 | 158 | 2.2 | 189 | 70 | 0.05 | 0.13 | 3.1 | — |
| 167 | Lean only from item 166  1.8 oz | 51 | 57 | 125 | 14 | 7 | 3.0 | 2.5 | 0.3 | 0 | 6 | 131 | 1.8 | 161 | 10 | 0.04 | 0.11 | 2.6 | — |
|  | Relatively lean, such as heel of round |  |  |  |  |  |  |  |  |  |  |  |  |  |  |  |  |  |  |
| 168 | Lean and fat (2 pieces, 4⅛″ × 2¼″ × ¼″) 3 oz | 85 | 62 | 165 | 25 | 7 | 2.8 | 2.7 | 0.2 | 0 | 11 | 208 | 3.2 | 279 | 10 | 0.06 | 0.19 | 4.5 | — |
| 169 | Lean only from item 168  2.8 oz | 78 | 65 | 125 | 24 | 3 | 1.2 | 1.0 | 0.1 | 0 | 10 | 199 | 3.0 | 268 | tr | 0.06 | 0.18 | 4.3 | — |
|  | Steak |  |  |  |  |  |  |  |  |  |  |  |  |  |  |  |  |  |  |
|  | Relatively fat-sirloin, broiled |  |  |  |  |  |  |  |  |  |  |  |  |  |  |  |  |  |  |
| 170 | Lean and fat (piece, 2½″ × 2½″ × ¾″) 3 oz | 85 | 44 | 330 | 20 | 27 | 11.3 | 11.1 | 0.6 | 0 | 9 | 162 | 2.5 | 220 | 50 | 0.05 | 0.15 | 4.0 | — |
| 171 | Lean only from item 170  2.0 oz | 56 | 59 | 115 | 18 | 4 | 1.8 | 1.6 | 0.2 | 0 | 7 | 146 | 2.2 | 202 | 10 | 0.05 | 0.14 | 3.6 | — |
|  | Relatively lean-round, braised |  |  |  |  |  |  |  |  |  |  |  |  |  |  |  |  |  |  |
| 172 | Lean and fat (piece, 4⅛″ × 2¼″ × ½″) 3 oz | 85 | 55 | 220 | 24 | 13 | 5.5 | 5.2 | 0.4 | 0 | 10 | 213 | 3.0 | 272 | 20 | 0.07 | 0.19 | 4.8 | — |
| 173 | Lean only from item 172  2.4 oz | 68 | 61 | 130 | 21 | 4 | 1.7 | 1.5 | 0.2 | 0 | 9 | 182 | 2.5 | 238 | 10 | 0.05 | 0.16 | 4.1 | — |
|  | Beef, canned |  |  |  |  |  |  |  |  |  |  |  |  |  |  |  |  |  |  |
| 174 | Corned beef  3 oz | 85 | 59 | 185 | 22 | 10 | 4.9 | 4.5 | 0.2 | 0 | 17 | 90 | 3.7 | — | — | 0.01 | 0.20 | 2.9 | — |
| 175 | Corned beef hash  1 c | 220 | 67 | 400 | 19 | 25 | 11.9 | 10.9 | 0.5 | 24 | 29 | 147 | 4.4 | 440 | — | 0.02 | 0.20 | 4.6 | — |
| 176 | Beef, dried, chipped  2½ oz jar | 71 | 48 | 145 | 24 | 4 | 2.1 | 2.0 | 0.1 | 0 | 14 | 287 | 3.6 | 142 | — | 0.05 | 0.23 | 2.7 | 0 |
| 177 | Beef and vegetable stew  1 c | 245 | 82 | 220 | 16 | 11 | 4.9 | 4.5 | 0.2 | 15 | 29 | 184 | 2.9 | 613 | 2400 | 0.15 | 0.17 | 4.7 | 17 |
| 178 | Beef potpie (home recipe), baked[19] (piece, ⅓ of 9″ diam pie) 1 piece | 210 | 55 | 515 | 21 | 30 | 7.9 | 12.8 | 6.7 | 39 | 29 | 149 | 3.8 | 334 | 1720 | 0.30 | 0.30 | 5.5 | 6 |

(Continued)

**Table 1. Nutritive Values of the Edible Part of Foods (Continued)**

(Dashes (—) denote lack of reliable data for a constituent believed to be present in measurable amount)

| Item No. (A) | Foods, Approximate Measures, Units, and Weight (edible part unless footnotes indicate otherwise) (B) | Water (C) Per cent | Food Energy (D) Calories | Protein (E) g | Fat (F) g | Fatty Acids Saturated (Total) (G) g | Unsaturated Oleic (H) g | Linoleic (I) g | Carbohydrate (J) g | Calcium (K) mg | Phosphorus (L) mg | Iron (M) mg | Potassium (N) mg | Vitamin A Value (O) IU | Thiamin (P) mg | Riboflavin (Q) mg | Niacin (R) mg | Ascorbic Acid (S) mg |
|---|---|---|---|---|---|---|---|---|---|---|---|---|---|---|---|---|---|---|
| | *Fish, Shellfish, Meat, Poultry, and Related Products (Cont.)* | | | | | | | | | | | | | | | | | |
| | Meat and meat products (Continued) | | | | | | | | | | | | | | | | | |
| 179 | Chili con carne with beans, canned 1 c | 72 | 340 | 19 | 16 | 7.5 | 6.8 | 0.3 | 31 | 82 | 321 | 4.3 | 594 | 150 | 0.08 | 0.18 | 3.3 | — |
| 180 | Chop suey with beef and pork (home recipe) 1 c | 75 | 300 | 26 | 17 | 8.5 | 6.2 | 0.7 | 13 | 60 | 248 | 4.8 | 425 | 600 | 0.28 | 0.38 | 5.0 | 33 |
| 181 | Heart, beef, lean, braised 3 oz | 61 | 160 | 27 | 5 | 1.5 | 1.1 | 0.6 | 1 | 5 | 154 | 5.0 | 197 | 20 | 0.21 | 1.04 | 6.5 | 1 |
| | Lamb, cooked | | | | | | | | | | | | | | | | | |
| | Chop, rib (cut 3 per lb with bone), broiled | | | | | | | | | | | | | | | | | |
| 182 | Lean and fat 3.1 oz | 43 | 360 | 18 | 32 | 14.8 | 12.1 | 1.2 | 0 | 8 | 139 | 1.0 | 200 | — | 0.11 | 0.19 | 4.1 | — |
| 183 | Lean only from item 182 2 oz | 60 | 120 | 16 | 6 | 2.5 | 2.1 | 0.2 | 0 | 6 | 121 | 1.1 | 174 | — | 0.09 | 0.15 | 3.4 | — |
| | Leg, roasted | | | | | | | | | | | | | | | | | |
| 184 | Lean and fat (2 pieces, 4⅛" × 2¼" × ¼") 3 oz | 54 | 235 | 22 | 16 | 7.3 | 6.0 | 0.6 | 0 | 9 | 177 | 1.4 | 241 | — | 0.13 | 0.23 | 4.7 | — |
| 185 | Lean only from item 184 2.5 oz | 62 | 130 | 20 | 5 | 2.1 | 1.8 | 0.2 | 0 | 9 | 169 | 1.4 | 227 | — | 0.12 | 0.21 | 4.4 | — |
| | Shoulder, roasted | | | | | | | | | | | | | | | | | |
| 186 | Lean and fat (3 pieces, 2½" × 2½" × ¼") 3 oz | 50 | 285 | 18 | 23 | 10.8 | 8.8 | 0.9 | 0 | 9 | 146 | 1.0 | 206 | — | 0.11 | 0.20 | 4.0 | — |
| 187 | Lean only from item 186 2.3 oz | 61 | 130 | 17 | 6 | 3.6 | 2.3 | 0.2 | 0 | 8 | 140 | 1.0 | 193 | — | 0.10 | 0.18 | 3.7 | — |
| 188 | Liver, beef, fried[20] (slice, 6½" × 2⅜" × ⅜") 3 oz | 56 | 195 | 22 | 9 | 2.5 | 3.5 | 0.9 | 5 | 9 | 405 | 7.5 | 323 | 45390[21] | 0.22 | 3.56 | 14.0 | 23 |
| | Pork, cured, cooked | | | | | | | | | | | | | | | | | |
| 189 | Ham, light cure, lean and fat, roasted (2 pieces, 4⅛" × 2¼" × ¼")[22] 3 oz | 54 | 245 | 18 | 19 | 6.8 | 7.9 | 1.7 | 0 | 8 | 146 | 2.2 | 199 | 0 | 0.40 | 0.15 | 3.1 | — |
| | Luncheon meat | | | | | | | | | | | | | | | | | |
| 190 | Boiled ham, slice (8 per 1 oz 8-oz pkg) | 59 | 65 | 5 | 5 | 1.7 | 2.0 | 0.4 | 0 | 3 | 47 | 0.8 | — | 0 | 0.12 | 0.04 | 0.7 | — |
| | Canned, spiced or unspiced | | | | | | | | | | | | | | | | | |
| 191 | Slice, approximately 3" × 2" × ½" 1 slice | 55 | 175 | 9 | 15 | 5.4 | 6.7 | 1.0 | 1 | 5 | 65 | 1.3 | 133 | 0 | 0.19 | 0.13 | 1.8 | — |
| | Pork, fresh,[18] | | | | | | | | | | | | | | | | | |
| | Chop, loin (cut 3 per lb with bone), broiled | | | | | | | | | | | | | | | | | |

| (A) | (B) | Grams | (C) | (D) | (E) | (F) | (G) | (H) | (I) | (J) | (K) | (L) | (M) | (N) | (O) | (P) | (Q) | (R) | (S) |
|---|---|---|---|---|---|---|---|---|---|---|---|---|---|---|---|---|---|---|---|
| 192 | Lean and fat ...... 2.7 oz | 78 | 42 | 305 | 19 | 25 | 8.9 | 10.4 | 2.2 | 0 | 9 | 209 | 2.7 | 216 | 0 | 0.75 | 0.22 | 4.5 | — |
| 193 | Lean only from item 192 ...... 2 oz | 56 | 53 | 150 | 17 | 9 | 3.1 | 3.6 | 0.8 | 0 | 7 | 181 | 2.2 | 192 | 0 | 0.63 | 0.18 | 3.8 | — |
|  | Roast, oven-cooked, no liquid added |  |  |  |  |  |  |  |  |  |  |  |  |  |  |  |  |  |  |
| 194 | Lean and fat (piece, 2½″ × 2½″ × ¾″) ...... 3 oz | 85 | 46 | 310 | 21 | 24 | 8.7 | 10.2 | 2.2 | 0 | 9 | 218 | 2.7 | 233 | 0 | 0.78 | 0.22 | 4.8 | — |
| 195 | Lean only from item 194 ...... 2.4 oz | 68 | 55 | 175 | 20 | 10 | 3.5 | 4.1 | 0.8 | 0 | 9 | 211 | 2.6 | 224 | 0 | 0.73 | 0.21 | 4.4 | — |
|  | Shoulder cut, simmered |  |  |  |  |  |  |  |  |  |  |  |  |  |  |  |  |  |  |  |
| 196 | Lean and fat (3 pieces, 2½″ × 2½″ × ¼″) ...... 3 oz | 85 | 46 | 320 | 20 | 26 | 9.3 | 10.9 | 2.3 | 0 | 9 | 118 | 2.6 | 158 | 0 | 0.46 | 0.21 | 4.1 | — |
| 197 | Lean only from item 196 ...... 2.2 oz | 63 | 60 | 135 | 18 | 6 | 2.2 | 2.6 | 0.6 | 0 | 8 | 111 | 2.3 | 146 | 0 | 0.42 | 0.19 | 3.7 | — |
|  | Sausages (see also Luncheon meat, items 190–191) |  |  |  |  |  |  |  |  |  |  |  |  |  |  |  |  |  |  |  |
| 198 | Bologna, slice (8 per 8-oz pkg) ...... 1 slice | 28 | 56 | 85 | 3 | 8 | 3.0 | 3.4 | 0.5 | tr | 2 | 36 | 0.5 | 65 | — | 0.05 | 0.06 | 0.7 | — |
| 199 | Braunschweiger, slice (6 per 6-oz pkg) ...... 1 slice | 28 | 53 | 90 | 4 | 8 | 2.6 | 3.4 | 0.8 | 1 | 3 | 69 | 1.7 | — | 1850 | 0.05 | 0.41 | 2.3 | — |
| 200 | Brown and serve (10–11 per 8-oz pkg), browned ...... 1 link | 17 | 40 | 70 | 3 | 6 | 2.3 | 2.8 | 0.7 | tr | — | — | — | — | — | — | — | — | — |
| 201 | Deviled ham, canned ...... 1 tbsp | 13 | 51 | 45 | 2 | 4 | 1.5 | 1.8 | 0.4 | 0 | 1 | 12 | 0.3 | — | 0 | 0.02 | 0.01 | 0.2 | — |
| 202 | Frankfurter (8 per 1-lb pkg), cooked (reheated) ...... 1 frankfurter | 56 | 57 | 170 | 7 | 15 | 5.6 | 6.5 | 1.2 | 1 | 3 | 57 | 0.8 | — | 0 | 0.08 | 0.11 | 1.4 | — |
| 203 | Meat, potted (beef, chicken, turkey), canned ...... 1 tbsp | 13 | 61 | 30 | 2 | 2 | — | — | — | 0 | — | — | — | — | — | tr | 0.03 | 0.2 | — |
| 204 | Pork link (16 per 1-lb pkg), cooked ...... 1 link | 13 | 35 | 60 | 2 | 6 | 2.1 | 2.4 | 0.5 | tr | 1 | 21 | 0.3 | 35 | 0 | 0.10 | 0.04 | 0.5 | — |
|  | Salami |  |  |  |  |  |  |  |  |  |  |  |  |  |  |  |  |  |  |  |
| 205 | Dry type, slice (12 per 4-oz pkg) ...... 1 slice | 10 | 30 | 45 | 2 | 4 | 1.6 | 1.6 | 0.1 | tr | 1 | 28 | 0.4 | — | — | 0.04 | 0.03 | 0.5 | — |
| 206 | Cooked type, slice (8 per 8-oz pkg) ...... 1 slice | 28 | 51 | 90 | 5 | 7 | 3.1 | 3.0 | 0.2 | tr | 3 | 57 | 0.7 | — | — | 0.07 | 0.07 | 1.2 | — |
| 207 | Vienna sausage (7 per 4-oz can) ...... 1 sausage | 16 | 63 | 40 | 2 | 3 | 1.2 | 1.4 | 0.2 | tr | 1 | 24 | 0.3 | — | — | 0.01 | 0.02 | 0.4 | — |
|  | Veal, medium fat, cooked, bone removed |  |  |  |  |  |  |  |  |  |  |  |  |  |  |  |  |  |  |  |
| 208 | Cutlet (4⅛″ × 2¼″ × ½″), braised or broiled ...... 3 oz | 85 | 60 | 185 | 23 | 9 | 4.0 | 3.4 | 0.4 | 0 | 9 | 196 | 2.7 | 258 | — | 0.06 | 0.21 | 4.6 | — |

(Continued)

## Table 1. Nutritive Values of the Edible Part of Foods (Continued)

(Dashes (—) denote lack of reliable data for a constituent believed to be present in measurable amount)

| Item No. (A) | Foods, Approximate Measures, Units, and Weight (edible part unless footnotes indicate otherwise) (B) | Water (C) Per cent | Food Energy (D) Calories | Protein (E) g | Fat (F) g | Fatty Acids Saturated (Total) (G) g | Unsaturated Oleic (H) g | Linoleic (I) g | Carbohydrate (J) g | Calcium (K) mg | Phosphorus (L) mg | Iron (M) mg | Potassium (N) mg | Vitamin A Value (O) IU | Thiamin (P) mg | Riboflavin (Q) mg | Niacin (R) mg | Ascorbic Acid (S) mg |
|---|---|---|---|---|---|---|---|---|---|---|---|---|---|---|---|---|---|---|
| | *Fish, Shellfish, Meat, Poultry, and Related Products (Cont.)* | | | | | | | | | | | | | | | | | |
| | Veal (Continued) | | | | | | | | | | | | | | | | | |
| 209 | Rib (2 pieces, 4⅛" × 2¼" × ¼"), roasted ......... 3 oz | 85 | 55 | 230 | 23 | 14 | 6.1 | 5.1 | 0.6 | 0 | 10 | 211 | 2.9 | 259 | — | 0.11 | 0.26 | 6.6 | — |
| | Poultry and poultry products | | | | | | | | | | | | | | | | | |
| | Chicken, cooked | | | | | | | | | | | | | | | | | |
| 210 | Breast, fried,[23] bones removed, ½ breast (3.3 oz with bones) 2.8 oz ......... | 79 | 58 | 160 | 26 | 5 | 1.4 | 1.8 | 1.1 | 1 | 9 | 218 | 1.3 | — | 70 | 0.04 | 0.17 | 11.6 | — |
| 211 | Drumstick, fried,[23] bones removed (2 oz with bones) 1.3 oz ......... | 38 | 55 | 90 | 12 | 4 | 1.1 | 1.3 | 0.9 | tr | 6 | 89 | 0.9 | — | 50 | 0.03 | 0.15 | 2.7 | — |
| 212 | Half broiler, broiled, bones removed (10.4 oz with bones) 6.2 oz ......... | 176 | 71 | 240 | 42 | 7 | 2.2 | 2.5 | 1.3 | 0 | 16 | 355 | 3.0 | 483 | 160 | 0.09 | 0.34 | 15.5 | — |
| 213 | Chicken, canned, boneless ......... 3 oz | 85 | 65 | 170 | 18 | 10 | 3.2 | 3.8 | 2.0 | 0 | 18 | 210 | 1.3 | 117 | 200 | 0.03 | 0.11 | 3.7 | 3 |
| 214 | Chicken a la king, cooked (home recipe) ......... 1 c | 245 | 68 | 470 | 27 | 34 | 2.7 | 14.3 | 3.3 | 12 | 127 | 358 | 2.5 | 404 | 1130 | 0.10 | 0.42 | 5.4 | 12 |
| 215 | Chicken and noodles, cooked (home recipe) ......... 1 c | 240 | 71 | 365 | 22 | 18 | 5.9 | 7.1 | 3.5 | 26 | 26 | 247 | 2.2 | 149 | 430 | 0.05 | 0.17 | 4.3 | tr |
| | Chicken chow mein | | | | | | | | | | | | | | | | | |
| 216 | Canned ......... 1 c | 250 | 89 | 95 | 7 | tr | — | — | — | 18 | 45 | 85 | 1.3 | 418 | 150 | 0.05 | 0.10 | 1.0 | 13 |
| 217 | From home recipe ......... 1 c | 250 | 78 | 255 | 31 | 10 | 2.4 | 3.4 | 3.1 | 10 | 58 | 293 | 2.5 | 473 | 280 | 0.08 | 0.23 | 4.3 | 10 |
| 218 | Chicken potpie (home recipe), baked,[19] piece (⅓ of 9" diam pie) ......... 1 piece | 232 | 57 | 545 | 23 | 31 | 11.3 | 10.9 | 5.6 | 42 | 70 | 232 | 3.0 | 343 | 3090 | 0.34 | 0.31 | 5.5 | 5 |
| | Turkey, roasted, flesh without skin | | | | | | | | | | | | | | | | | |
| 219 | Dark meat, piece, 2½" × 1⅝" × ¼" ......... 4 pieces | 85 | 61 | 175 | 26 | 7 | 2.1 | 1.5 | 1.5 | 0 | — | — | 2.0 | 338 | — | 0.03 | 0.20 | 3.6 | — |
| 220 | Light meat, piece, 4" × 2" × ¼" ......... 2 pieces | 85 | 62 | 150 | 28 | 3 | 0.9 | 0.6 | 0.7 | 0 | — | — | 1.0 | 349 | — | 0.04 | 0.12 | 9.4 | — |
| | Light and dark meat | | | | | | | | | | | | | | | | | |
| 221 | Chopped or diced ......... 1 c | 140 | 61 | 265 | 44 | 9 | 2.5 | 1.7 | 1.8 | 0 | 11 | 351 | 2.5 | 514 | — | 0.07 | 0.25 | 10.8 | — |
| 222 | Pieces (1 slice white meat, 4" × 2" × ¼" with 2 slices dark meat, 2½" × 1⅝" × ¼") ......... 3 pieces | 85 | 61 | 160 | 27 | 5 | 1.5 | 1.0 | 1.1 | 0 | 7 | 213 | 1.5 | 312 | — | 0.04 | 0.15 | 6.5 | — |

*Fruits and Fruit Products*

| (A) | (B) | g | (C) | (D) | (E) | (F) | (G) | (H) | (I) | (J) | (K) | (L) | (M) | (N) | (O) | (P) | (Q) | (R) | (S) |
|---|---|---|---|---|---|---|---|---|---|---|---|---|---|---|---|---|---|---|---|
|  | Apples, raw, unpeeled, without cores |  |  |  |  |  |  |  |  |  |  |  |  |  |  |  |  |  |  |
| 223 | 2³/₄″ diam (about 3 per lb with cores), 1 apple | 138 | 84 | 80 | tr | 1 | — | — | — | 20 | 10 | 14 | 0.4 | 152 | 120 | 0.04 | 0.03 | 0.1 | 6 |
| 224 | 3¹/₄″ diam (about 2 per lb with cores), 1 apple | 212 | 84 | 125 | tr | 1 | — | — | — | 31 | 15 | 21 | 0.6 | 233 | 190 | 0.06 | 0.04 | 0.2 | 8 |
| 225 | Apple juice, bottled or canned[24], 1 c | 248 | 88 | 120 | tr | tr | — | — | — | 30 | 15 | 22 | 1.5 | 250 | — | 0.02 | 0.05 | 0.2 | 2[25] |
|  | Applesauce, canned |  |  |  |  |  |  |  |  |  |  |  |  |  |  |  |  |  |  |
| 226 | Sweetened, 1 c | 255 | 76 | 230 | 1 | tr | — | — | — | 61 | 10 | 13 | 1.3 | 166 | 100 | 0.03 | 0.03 | 0.1 | 3[25] |
| 227 | Unsweetened, 1 c | 244 | 89 | 100 | tr | tr | — | — | — | 26 | 10 | 12 | 1.2 | 190 | 100 | 0.05 | 0.02 | 0.1 | 2[25] |
|  | Apricots |  |  |  |  |  |  |  |  |  |  |  |  |  |  |  |  |  |  |
| 228 | Raw, without pits (about 12 per lb with pits), 3 apricots | 107 | 85 | 55 | 1 | tr | — | — | — | 14 | 18 | 25 | 0.5 | 301 | 2890 | 0.03 | 0.04 | 0.6 | 11 |
| 229 | Canned in heavy syrup (halves and syrup), 1 c | 258 | 77 | 220 | 2 | tr | — | — | — | 57 | 28 | 39 | 0.8 | 604 | 4490 | 0.05 | 0.05 | 1.0 | 10 |
|  | Dried |  |  |  |  |  |  |  |  |  |  |  |  |  |  |  |  |  |  |
| 230 | Uncooked (28 large or 37 medium halves per cup), 1 c | 130 | 25 | 340 | 7 | 1 | — | — | — | 86 | 87 | 140 | 7.2 | 1273 | 14,170 | 0.01 | 0.21 | 4.3 | 16 |
| 231 | Cooked, unsweetened, fruit and liquid, 1 c | 250 | 76 | 215 | 4 | 1 | — | — | — | 54 | 55 | 88 | 4.5 | 795 | 7500 | 0.01 | 0.13 | 2.5 | 8 |
| 232 | Apricot nectar, canned, 1 c | 251 | 85 | 145 | 1 | tr | — | — | — | 37 | 23 | 30 | 0.5 | 379 | 2380 | 0.03 | 0.03 | 0.5 | 36[26] |
|  | Avocados, raw, whole, without skins and seeds |  |  |  |  |  |  |  |  |  |  |  |  |  |  |  |  |  |  |
| 233 | California, mid- and late-winter (with skin and seed, 3¹/₈″ diam; wt, 10 oz), 1 avocado | 216 | 74 | 370 | 5 | 37 | 5.5 | 22.0 | 3.7 | 13 | 22 | 91 | 1.3 | 1303 | 630 | 0.24 | 0.43 | 3.5 | 30 |
| 234 | Florida, late summer and fall (with skin and seed, 3⁵/₈″ diam; wt, 1 lb), 1 avocado | 304 | 78 | 390 | 4 | 33 | 6.7 | 15.7 | 5.3 | 27 | 30 | 128 | 1.8 | 1836 | 880 | 0.33 | 0.61 | 4.9 | 43 |
| 235 | Banana without peel (about 2.6 per lb with peel), 1 banana | 119 | 76 | 100 | 1 | tr | — | — | — | 26 | 10 | 31 | 0.8 | 440 | 230 | 0.06 | 0.07 | 0.8 | 12 |
| 236 | Banana flakes, 1 tbsp | 6 | 3 | 20 | tr | tr | — | — | — | 5 | 2 | 6 | 0.2 | 92 | 50 | 0.01 | 0.01 | 0.2 | tr |
| 237 | Blackberries, raw, 1 c | 144 | 85 | 85 | 2 | 1 | — | — | — | 19 | 46 | 27 | 1.3 | 245 | 290 | 0.04 | 0.06 | 0.6 | 30 |
| 238 | Blueberries, raw, 1 c | 145 | 83 | 90 | 1 | 1 | — | — | — | 22 | 22 | 19 | 1.5 | 117 | 150 | 0.04 | 0.09 | 0.7 | 20 |
|  | Cantaloupe. See Muskmelons (item 271) |  |  |  |  |  |  |  |  |  |  |  |  |  |  |  |  |  |  |
|  | Cherries |  |  |  |  |  |  |  |  |  |  |  |  |  |  |  |  |  |  |
| 239 | Sour (tart), red, pitted, canned, water pack, 1 c | 244 | 88 | 105 | 2 | tr | — | — | — | 26 | 37 | 32 | 0.7 | 317 | 1660 | 0.07 | 0.05 | 0.5 | 12 |
| 240 | Sweet, raw, without pits and stems, 10 cherries | 68 | 80 | 45 | 1 | tr | — | — | — | 12 | 15 | 13 | 0.3 | 129 | 70 | 0.03 | 0.04 | 0.3 | 7 |

(Continued)

## Table 1. Nutritive Values of the Edible Part of Foods (Continued)

(Dashes (—) denote lack of reliable data for a constituent believed to be present in measurable amount)

| Item No. (A) | Foods, Approximate Measures, Units, and Weight (edible part unless footnotes indicate otherwise) (B) | Weight g | Water Per-cent (C) | Food Energy Cal-ories (D) | Pro-tein g (E) | Fat g (F) | Fatty Acids Satu-rated (Total) g (G) | Unsaturated Oleic g (H) | Unsaturated Lino-leic g (I) | Carbo-hydrate g (J) | Calcium mg (K) | Phos-phorus mg (L) | Iron mg (M) | Potas-sium mg (N) | Vitamin A Value IU (O) | Thiamin mg (P) | Ribo-flavin mg (Q) | Niacin mg (R) | Ascorbic Acid mg (S) |
|---|---|---|---|---|---|---|---|---|---|---|---|---|---|---|---|---|---|---|---|
| | *Fruits and Fruit Products (Continued)* | | | | | | | | | | | | | | | | | | |
| 241 | Cranberry juice cocktail, bottled, sweetened  1 c | 253 | 83 | 165 | tr | tr | — | — | — | 42 | 13 | 8 | 0.8 | 25 | tr | 0.03 | 0.03 | 0.1 | 81[27] |
| 242 | Cranberry sauce, sweetened, canned, strained  1 c | 277 | 62 | 405 | tr | 1 | — | — | — | 104 | 17 | 11 | 0.6 | 83 | 60 | 0.03 | 0.03 | 0.1 | 6 |
| | Dates | | | | | | | | | | | | | | | | | | |
| 243 | Whole, without pits  10 dates | 80 | 23 | 220 | 2 | tr | — | — | — | 58 | 47 | 50 | 2.4 | 518 | 40 | 0.07 | 0.08 | 1.8 | 0 |
| 244 | Chopped  1 c | 178 | 23 | 490 | 4 | 1 | — | — | — | 130 | 105 | 112 | 5.3 | 1153 | 90 | 0.16 | 0.18 | 3.9 | 0 |
| 245 | Fruit cocktail, canned, in heavy syrup  1 c | 255 | 80 | 195 | 1 | tr | — | — | — | 50 | 23 | 31 | 1.0 | 411 | 360 | 0.05 | 0.03 | 1.0 | 5 |
| | Grapefruit | | | | | | | | | | | | | | | | | | |
| | Raw, medium, 3¾" diam (about 1 lb 1 oz) | | | | | | | | | | | | | | | | | | |
| 246 | Pink or red  ½ grapefruit with peel[28] | 241 | 89 | 50 | 1 | tr | — | — | — | 13 | 20 | 20 | 0.5 | 166 | 540 | 0.05 | 0.02 | 0.2 | 44 |
| 247 | White  ½ grapefruit with peel[28] | 241 | 89 | 45 | 1 | tr | — | — | — | 12 | 19 | 19 | 0.5 | 159 | 10 | 0.05 | 0.02 | 0.2 | 44 |
| 248 | Canned, sections with syrup  1 c | 254 | 81 | 180 | 2 | tr | — | — | — | 45 | 33 | 36 | 0.8 | 343 | 30 | 0.08 | 0.05 | 0.5 | 76 |
| | Grapefruit juice | | | | | | | | | | | | | | | | | | |
| 249 | Raw, pink, red or white  1 c | 246 | 90 | 95 | 1 | tr | — | — | — | 23 | 22 | 37 | 0.5 | 399 | (29) | 0.10 | 0.05 | 0.5 | 93 |
| | Canned, white | | | | | | | | | | | | | | | | | | |
| 250 | Unsweetened  1 c | 247 | 89 | 100 | 1 | tr | — | — | — | 24 | 20 | 35 | 1.0 | 400 | 20 | 0.07 | 0.05 | 0.5 | 84 |
| 251 | Sweetened  1 c | 250 | 86 | 135 | 1 | tr | — | — | — | 32 | 20 | 35 | 1.0 | 405 | 30 | 0.08 | 0.05 | 0.5 | 78 |
| | Frozen, concentrate, unsweetened | | | | | | | | | | | | | | | | | | |
| 252 | Undiluted, 6-fl oz can  1 c | 207 | 62 | 300 | 4 | 1 | — | — | — | 72 | 70 | 124 | 0.8 | 1250 | 60 | 0.29 | 0.12 | 1.4 | 286 |
| 253 | Diluted with 3 parts water by volume  1 c | 247 | 89 | 100 | 1 | tr | — | — | — | 24 | 25 | 42 | 0.2 | 420 | 20 | 0.10 | 0.04 | 0.5 | 96 |
| 254 | Dehydrated crystals, prepared with water (1 lb yields about 1 gal)  1 c | 247 | 90 | 100 | 1 | tr | — | — | — | 24 | 22 | 40 | 0.2 | 412 | 20 | 0.10 | 0.05 | 0.5 | 91 |
| | Grapes, European type (adherent skin), raw | | | | | | | | | | | | | | | | | | |
| 255 | Thompson Seedless  10 grapes | 50 | 81 | 35 | tr | tr | — | — | — | 9 | 6 | 10 | 0.2 | 87 | 50 | 0.03 | 0.02 | 0.2 | 2 |
| 256 | Tokay and Emperor, seeded types  10 grapes[30] | 60 | 81 | 40 | tr | tr | — | — | — | 10 | 7 | 11 | 0.2 | 99 | 60 | 0.03 | 0.02 | 0.2 | 2 |

| (A) | (B) | (C) | (D) | (E) | (F) | (G) | (H) | (I) | (J) | (K) | (L) | (M) | (N) | (O) | (P) | (Q) | (R) | (S) |
|---|---|---|---|---|---|---|---|---|---|---|---|---|---|---|---|---|---|---|
|  | Grape juice |  |  |  |  |  |  |  |  |  |  |  |  |  |  |  |  |  |
| 257 | Canned or bottled ..... 1 c | 253 | 83 | 165 | 1 | tr | — | — | 42 | 28 | 30 | 0.8 | 293 | — | 0.10 | 0.05 | 0.5 | tr[25] |
|  | Frozen concentrate, sweetened |  |  |  |  |  |  |  |  |  |  |  |  |  |  |  |  |  |
| 258 | Undiluted, 6-fl oz can .. 1 can | 216 | 53 | 395 | 1 | tr | — | — | 100 | 22 | 32 | 0.9 | 255 | 40 | 0.13 | 0.22 | 1.5 | 32[31] |
| 259 | Diluted with 3 parts water by volume ..... 1 c | 250 | 86 | 135 | 1 | tr | — | — | 33 | 8 | 10 | 0.3 | 85 | 10 | 0.05 | 0.08 | 0.5 | 10[31] |
| 260 | Grape drink, canned ..... 1 c | 250 | 86 | 135 | tr | tr | — | — | 35 | 8 | 10 | 0.3 | 88 | — | 0.03[32] | 0.03[32] | 0.3 | ([32]) |
| 261 | Lemon, raw, size 165, without peel and seeds (about 4 per lb with peels and seeds) ..... 1 lemon | 74 | 90 | 20 | 1 | tr | — | — | 6 | 19 | 12 | 0.4 | 102 | 10 | 0.03 | 0.01 | 0.1 | 39 |
|  | Lemon juice |  |  |  |  |  |  |  |  |  |  |  |  |  |  |  |  |  |
| 262 | Raw ..... 1 c | 244 | 91 | 60 | 1 | tr | — | — | 20 | 17 | 24 | 0.5 | 344 | 50 | 0.07 | 0.02 | 0.2 | 112 |
| 263 | Canned, or bottled, unsweetened ..... 1 c | 244 | 92 | 55 | 1 | tr | — | — | 19 | 17 | 24 | 0.5 | 344 | 50 | 0.07 | 0.02 | 0.2 | 102 |
| 264 | Frozen, single-strength, unsweetened, 6-fl oz can ..... 1 c | 183 | 92 | 40 | 1 | tr | — | — | 13 | 13 | 16 | 0.5 | 258 | 40 | 0.05 | 0.02 | 0.2 | 81 |
|  | Lemonade concentrate, frozen |  |  |  |  |  |  |  |  |  |  |  |  |  |  |  |  |  |
| 265 | Undiluted, 6-fl oz can ..... 1 can | 219 | 49 | 425 | tr | tr | — | — | 112 | 9 | 13 | 0.4 | 153 | 40 | 0.05 | 0.06 | 0.7 | 66 |
| 266 | Diluted with 4⅓ parts water by volume ..... 1 c | 248 | 89 | 105 | tr | tr | — | — | 28 | 2 | 3 | 0.1 | 40 | 10 | 0.01 | 0.02 | 0.2 | 17 |
|  | Limeade concentrate, frozen |  |  |  |  |  |  |  |  |  |  |  |  |  |  |  |  |  |
| 267 | Undiluted, 6-fl oz can ..... 1 can | 218 | 50 | 410 | tr | tr | — | — | 108 | 11 | 13 | 0.2 | 129 | tr | 0.02 | 0.02 | 0.2 | 26 |
| 268 | Diluted with 4⅓ parts water by volume ..... 1 c | 247 | 89 | 100 | tr | tr | — | — | 27 | 3 | 3 | tr | 32 | tr | tr | tr | tr | 6 |
|  | Lime juice |  |  |  |  |  |  |  |  |  |  |  |  |  |  |  |  |  |
| 269 | Raw ..... 1 c | 246 | 90 | 65 | 1 | tr | — | — | 22 | 22 | 27 | 0.5 | 256 | 20 | 0.05 | 0.02 | 0.2 | 79 |
| 270 | Canned, unsweetened ..... 1 c | 246 | 90 | 65 | 1 | tr | — | — | 22 | 22 | 27 | 0.5 | 256 | 20 | 0.05 | 0.02 | 0.2 | 52 |
|  | Muskmelons, raw, with rind, without seed cavity |  |  |  |  |  |  |  |  |  |  |  |  |  |  |  |  |  |
| 271 | Cantaloupe, orange-fleshed (with rind and seed cavity, 5″ diam, 2⅓ lb) ..... ½ melon with rind[33] | 477 | 91 | 80 | 2 | tr | — | — | 20 | 38 | 44 | 1.1 | 682 | 9240 | 0.11 | 0.08 | 1.6 | 90 |
| 272 | Honeydew (with rind and seed cavity, 6½″ diam, 5¼ lb) ..... 1/10 melon with rind[33] | 226 | 91 | 50 | 1 | tr | — | — | 11 | 21 | 24 | 0.6 | 374 | 60 | 0.06 | 0.04 | 0.9 | 34 |
|  | Oranges, all commercial varieties, raw |  |  |  |  |  |  |  |  |  |  |  |  |  |  |  |  |  |
| 273 | Whole, 2⅝″ diam, without peel and seeds (about 2½ per lb with peel and seeds) ..... 1 orange | 131 | 86 | 65 | 1 | tr | — | — | 16 | 54 | 26 | 0.5 | 263 | 260 | 0.13 | 0.05 | 0.5 | 66 |

(Continued)

## Table 1. Nutritive Values of the Edible Part of Foods (Continued)

(Dashes (—) denote lack of reliable data for a constituent believed to be present in measurable amount)

| Item No. (A) | Foods, Approximate Measures, Units, and Weight (edible part unless footnotes indicate otherwise) (B) | | Water (C) Per-cent | Food Energy (D) Cal-ories | Pro-tein (E) g | Fat (F) g | Fatty Acids Satu-rated (Total) (G) g | Unsaturated Oleic (H) g | Lino-leic (I) g | Carbo-hydrate (J) g | Calcium (K) mg | Phos-phorus (L) mg | Iron (M) mg | Potas-sium (N) mg | Vitamin A Value (O) IU | Thiamin (P) mg | Ribo-flavin (Q) mg | Niacin (R) mg | Ascorbic Acid (S) mg |
|---|---|---|---|---|---|---|---|---|---|---|---|---|---|---|---|---|---|---|---|
| | | g | | | | | | | | | | | | | | | | | |
| *Fruits and Fruit Products (Continued)* | | | | | | | | | | | | | | | | | | | |
| | Oranges (Continued) | | | | | | | | | | | | | | | | | | | |
| 274 | Sections without membranes | 1 c | 180 | 86 | 90 | 2 | tr | — | — | — | 22 | 74 | 36 | 0.7 | 360 | 360 | 0.18 | 0.07 | 0.7 | 90 |
| | Orange juice | | | | | | | | | | | | | | | | | | | |
| 275 | Raw, all varieties | 1 c | 248 | 88 | 110 | 2 | tr | — | — | — | 26 | 27 | 42 | 0.5 | 496 | 500 | 0.22 | 0.07 | 1.0 | 124 |
| 276 | Canned, unsweetened | 1 c | 249 | 87 | 120 | 2 | tr | — | — | — | 28 | 25 | 45 | 1.0 | 496 | 500 | 0.17 | 0.05 | 0.7 | 100 |
| | Frozen concentrate | | | | | | | | | | | | | | | | | | | |
| 277 | Undiluted, 6-fl oz can | 1 can | 213 | 55 | 360 | 5 | tr | — | — | — | 87 | 75 | 126 | 0.9 | 1500 | 1620 | 0.68 | 0.11 | 2.8 | 360 |
| 278 | Diluted with 3 parts water by volume | 1 c | 249 | 87 | 120 | 2 | tr | — | — | — | 29 | 25 | 42 | 0.2 | 503 | 540 | 0.23 | 0.03 | 0.9 | 120 |
| 279 | Dehydrated crystals, prepared with water (1 lb yields about 1 gal) | 1 c | 248 | 88 | 115 | 1 | tr | — | — | — | 27 | 25 | 40 | 0.5 | 518 | 500 | 0.20 | 0.07 | 1.0 | 109 |
| | Orange and grapefruit juice | | | | | | | | | | | | | | | | | | | |
| | Frozen concentrate | | | | | | | | | | | | | | | | | | | |
| 280 | Undiluted, 6-fl oz can | 1 can | 210 | 59 | 330 | 4 | 1 | — | — | — | 78 | 61 | 99 | 0.8 | 1308 | 800 | 0.48 | 0.06 | 2.3 | 302 |
| 281 | Diluted with 3 parts water by volume | 1 c | 248 | 88 | 110 | 1 | tr | — | — | — | 26 | 20 | 32 | 0.2 | 439 | 270 | 0.15 | 0.02 | 0.7 | 102 |
| 282 | Papayas, raw, 1/2″ cubes | 1 c | 140 | 89 | 55 | 1 | tr | — | — | — | 14 | 28 | 22 | 0.4 | 328 | 2450 | 0.06 | 0.06 | 0.4 | 78 |
| | Peaches | | | | | | | | | | | | | | | | | | | |
| | Raw | | | | | | | | | | | | | | | | | | | |
| 283 | Whole, 2½″ diam, peeled, pitted (about 4 per lb with peels and pits) | 1 peach | 100 | 89 | 40 | 1 | tr | — | — | — | 10 | 9 | 19 | 0.5 | 202 | 1330[34] | 0.02 | 0.05 | 1.0 | 7 |
| 284 | Sliced | 1 c | 170 | 89 | 65 | 1 | tr | — | — | — | 16 | 15 | 32 | 0.9 | 343 | 2260[34] | 0.03 | 0.09 | 1.7 | 12 |
| | Canned, yellow-fleshed, solids and liquid (halves or slices) | | | | | | | | | | | | | | | | | | | |
| 285 | Syrup pack | 1 c | 256 | 79 | 200 | 1 | tr | — | — | — | 51 | 10 | 31 | 0.8 | 333 | 1100 | 0.03 | 0.05 | 1.5 | 8 |
| 286 | Water pack | 1 c | 244 | 91 | 75 | 1 | tr | — | — | — | 20 | 10 | 32 | 0.7 | 334 | 1100 | 0.02 | 0.07 | 1.5 | 7 |
| | Dried | | | | | | | | | | | | | | | | | | | |
| 287 | Uncooked | 1 c | 160 | 25 | 420 | 5 | 1 | — | — | — | 109 | 77 | 187 | 9.6 | 1520 | 6240 | 0.02 | 0.30 | 8.5 | 29 |
| 288 | Cooked, unsweetened, halves and juice | 1 c | 250 | 77 | 205 | 3 | 1 | — | — | — | 54 | 38 | 93 | 4.8 | 743 | 3050 | 0.01 | 0.15 | 3.8 | 5 |
| | Frozen, sliced, sweetened | | | | | | | | | | | | | | | | | | | |
| 289 | 10-oz container | 1 container | 284 | 77 | 250 | 1 | tr | — | — | — | 64 | 11 | 37 | 1.4 | 352 | 1850 | 0.03 | 0.11 | 2.0 | 116[35] |
| 290 | Cup | 1 c | 250 | 77 | 220 | 1 | tr | — | — | — | 57 | 10 | 33 | 1.3 | 310 | 1630 | 0.03 | 0.10 | 1.8 | 103[35] |

| (A) | (B) | (C) | (D) | (E) | (F) | (G) | (H) | (I) | (J) | (K) | (L) | (M) | (N) | (O) | (P) | (Q) | (R) | (S) |
|---|---|---|---|---|---|---|---|---|---|---|---|---|---|---|---|---|---|---|
| | Pears | | | | | | | | | | | | | | | | | |
| | Raw, with skin, cored | | | | | | | | | | | | | | | | | |
| 291 | Bartlett, 2½″ diam (about 2½ per lb with cores and stems) 1 pear ......... 164 | 83 | 100 | 1 | 1 | — | — | — | 25 | 13 | 18 | 0.5 | 213 | 30 | 0.03 | 0.07 | 0.2 | 7 |
| 292 | Bosc, 2½″ diam (about 3 per lb with cores and stems) 1 pear ......... 141 | 83 | 85 | 1 | 1 | — | — | — | 22 | 11 | 16 | 0.4 | 83 | 30 | 0.03 | 0.06 | 0.1 | 6 |
| 293 | D'Anjou, 3″ diam (about 2 per lb with cores and stems) 1 pear ......... 200 | 83 | 120 | 1 | 1 | — | — | — | 31 | 16 | 22 | 0.6 | 260 | 40 | 0.04 | 0.08 | 0.2 | 8 |
| 294 | Canned, solids and liquid, syrup pack, heavy (halves or slices) 1 c ......... 255 | 80 | 195 | 1 | 1 | — | — | — | 50 | 13 | 18 | 0.5 | 214 | 10 | 0.03 | 0.05 | 0.3 | 3 |
| | Pineapple | | | | | | | | | | | | | | | | | |
| 295 | Raw, diced 1 c ......... 155 | 85 | 80 | 1 | tr | — | — | — | 21 | 26 | 12 | 0.8 | 226 | 110 | 0.14 | 0.05 | 0.3 | 26 |
| | Canned, heavy syrup pack, solids and liquid | | | | | | | | | | | | | | | | | |
| 296 | Crushed, chunks, tidbits 1 c ......... 255 | 80 | 190 | 1 | tr | — | — | — | 49 | 28 | 13 | 0.8 | 245 | 130 | 0.20 | 0.05 | 0.5 | 18 |
| | Slices and liquid | | | | | | | | | | | | | | | | | |
| 297 | Large 1 slice; 2¼ tbsp liquid ......... 105 | 80 | 80 | tr | tr | — | — | — | 20 | 12 | 5 | 0.3 | 101 | 50 | 0.08 | 0.02 | 0.2 | 7 |
| 298 | Medium 1 slice; 1¼ tbsp liquid ......... 58 | 80 | 45 | tr | tr | — | — | — | 11 | 6 | 3 | 0.2 | 56 | 30 | 0.05 | 0.01 | 0.1 | 4 |
| 299 | Pineapple juice, unsweetened, canned 1 c ......... 250 | 86 | 140 | 1 | tr | — | — | — | 34 | 38 | 23 | 0.8 | 373 | 130 | 0.13 | 0.05 | 0.5 | 80[27] |
| | Plums | | | | | | | | | | | | | | | | | |
| | Raw, without pits | | | | | | | | | | | | | | | | | |
| 300 | Japanese and hybrid (2⅛″ diam, about 6½ per lb with pits) 1 plum ......... 66 | 87 | 30 | tr | tr | — | — | — | 8 | 8 | 12 | 0.3 | 112 | 160 | 0.02 | 0.02 | 0.3 | 4 |
| 301 | Prune-type (1½″ diam, about 15 per lb with pits) 1 plum ......... 28 | 79 | 20 | tr | tr | — | — | — | 6 | 3 | 5 | 0.1 | 48 | 80 | 0.01 | 0.01 | 0.1 | 1 |
| | Canned, heavy syrup pack (Italian prunes), with pits and liquid | | | | | | | | | | | | | | | | | |
| 302 | Cup 1 c[36] ......... 272 | 77 | 215 | 1 | tr | — | — | — | 56 | 23 | 26 | 2.3 | 367 | 3130 | 0.05 | 0.05 | 1.0 | 5 |
| 303 | Portion 3 plums; 2¾ tbsp liquid[36] ......... 140 | 77 | 110 | 1 | tr | — | — | — | 29 | 12 | 13 | 1.2 | 189 | 1610 | 0.03 | 0.03 | 0.5 | 3 |
| | Prunes, dried, "softenized," with pits | | | | | | | | | | | | | | | | | |
| 304 | Uncooked 4 extra large or 5 large prunes[36] ......... 49 | 28 | 110 | 1 | tr | — | — | — | 29 | 22 | 34 | 1.7 | 298 | 690 | 0.04 | 0.07 | 0.7 | 1 |
| 305 | Cooked, unsweetened, all sizes, fruit and liquid 1 c[36] ......... 250 | 66 | 255 | 2 | 1 | — | — | — | 67 | 51 | 79 | 3.8 | 695 | 1590 | 0.07 | 0.15 | 1.5 | 2 |

(Continued)

**Table 1.  Nutritive Values of the Edible Part of Foods (Continued)**
(Dashes (—) denote lack of reliable data for a constituent believed to be present in measurable amount)

| Item No. (A) | Foods, Approximate Measures, Units, and Weight (edible part unless footnotes indicate otherwise) (B) | (g) | Water (C) Per-cent | Food Energy (D) Cal-ories | Pro-tein (E) g | Fat (F) g | Fatty Acids Satu-rated (Total) (G) g | Unsaturated Oleic (H) g | Lino-leic (I) g | Carbo-hydrate (J) g | Calcium (K) mg | Phos-phorus (L) mg | Iron (M) mg | Potas-sium (N) mg | Vitamin A Value (O) IU | Thiamin (P) mg | Ribo-flavin (Q) mg | Niacin (R) mg | Ascorbic Acid (S) mg |
|---|---|---|---|---|---|---|---|---|---|---|---|---|---|---|---|---|---|---|---|
| | *Fruits and Fruit Products (Continued)* | | | | | | | | | | | | | | | | | | |
| 306 | Prune juice, canned or bottled ............ 1 c | 256 | 80 | 195 | 1 | tr | — | — | — | 49 | 36 | 51 | 1.8 | 602 | — | 0.03 | 0.03 | 1.0 | 5 |
| | Raisins, seedless | | | | | | | | | | | | | | | | | | |
| 307 | Cup, not pressed down ..... 1 c | 145 | 18 | 420 | 4 | tr | — | — | — | 112 | 90 | 146 | 5.1 | 1106 | 30 | 0.16 | 0.12 | 0.7 | 1 |
| 308 | Packet, 1/2 oz (1 1/2 tbsp) ........ 1 packet | 14 | 18 | 40 | tr | tr | — | — | — | 11 | 9 | 14 | 0.5 | 107 | tr | 0.02 | 0.01 | 0.1 | tr |
| | Raspberries, red | | | | | | | | | | | | | | | | | | |
| 309 | Raw, capped, whole .... 1 c | 123 | 84 | 70 | 1 | 1 | — | — | — | 17 | 27 | 27 | 1.1 | 207 | 160 | 0.04 | 0.11 | 1.1 | 31 |
| 310 | Frozen, sweetened, 10-oz container ...... 1 container | 284 | 74 | 280 | 2 | 1 | — | — | — | 70 | 37 | 48 | 1.7 | 284 | 200 | 0.06 | 0.17 | 1.7 | 60 |
| | Rhubarb, cooked, added sugar | | | | | | | | | | | | | | | | | | |
| 311 | From raw ........... 1 c | 270 | 63 | 380 | 1 | tr | — | — | — | 97 | 211 | 41 | 1.6 | 548 | 220 | 0.05 | 0.14 | 0.8 | 16 |
| 312 | From frozen, sweetened ...... 1 c | 270 | 63 | 385 | 1 | 1 | — | — | — | 98 | 211 | 32 | 1.9 | 475 | 190 | 0.05 | 0.11 | 0.5 | 16 |
| | Strawberries | | | | | | | | | | | | | | | | | | |
| 313 | Raw, whole berries, capped ...... 1 c | 149 | 90 | 55 | 1 | 1 | — | — | — | 13 | 31 | 31 | 1.5 | 244 | 90 | 0.04 | 0.10 | 0.9 | 88 |
| | Frozen, sweetened | | | | | | | | | | | | | | | | | | |
| 314 | Sliced, 10-oz container ..... 1 container | 284 | 71 | 310 | 1 | 1 | — | — | — | 79 | 40 | 48 | 2.0 | 318 | 90 | 0.06 | 0.17 | 1.4 | 151 |
| 315 | Whole, 1-lb container (about 1 3/4 cups) ...... 1 container | 454 | 76 | 415 | 2 | 1 | — | — | — | 107 | 59 | 73 | 2.7 | 472 | 140 | 0.09 | 0.27 | 2.3 | 249 |
| 316 | Tangerine, raw, 2 3/8" diam, size 176, without peel (about 4 per lb with peels and seeds) ...... 1 tangerine | 86 | 87 | 40 | 1 | tr | — | — | — | 10 | 34 | 15 | 0.3 | 108 | 360 | 0.05 | 0.02 | 0.1 | 27 |
| 317 | Tangerine juice, canned, sweetened ...... 1 c | 249 | 87 | 125 | 1 | tr | — | — | — | 30 | 44 | 35 | 0.5 | 440 | 1040 | 0.15 | 0.05 | 0.2 | 54 |
| 318 | Watermelon, raw, 4" × 8" wedge with rind and seeds (1/16 of 32 2/3-lb melon, 10" × 16") ...... 1 wedge with rind and seeds[37] | 926 | 93 | 110 | 2 | 1 | — | — | — | 27 | 30 | 43 | 2.1 | 426 | 2510 | 0.13 | 0.13 | 0.9 | 30 |
| | *Grain Products* | | | | | | | | | | | | | | | | | | |
| | Bagel, 3" diam | | | | | | | | | | | | | | | | | | |
| 319 | Egg ............. 1 bagel | 55 | 32 | 165 | 6 | 2 | 0.5 | 0.9 | 0.8 | 28 | 9 | 43 | 1.2 | 41 | 30 | 0.14 | 0.10 | 1.2 | 0 |
| 320 | Water ........... 1 bagel | 55 | 29 | 165 | 6 | 1 | 0.2 | 0.4 | 0.6 | 30 | 8 | 41 | 1.2 | 42 | 0 | 0.15 | 0.11 | 1.4 | 0 |
| 321 | Barley, pearled, light, uncooked ....... 1 c | 200 | 11 | 700 | 16 | 2 | 0.3 | 0.2 | 0.8 | 158 | 32 | 378 | 4.0 | 320 | 0 | 0.24 | 0.10 | 6.2 | 0 |

| (A) | (B) | (C) | (D) | (E) | (F) | (G) | (H) | (I) | (J) | (K) | (L) | (M) | (N) | (O) | (P) | (Q) | (R) | (S) | |
|---|---|---|---|---|---|---|---|---|---|---|---|---|---|---|---|---|---|---|---|
| | **Biscuits, baking powder, 2" diam (enriched flour, vegetable shortening)** | | | | | | | | | | | | | | | | | | |
| 322 | From home recipe ..... 1 biscuit ....... | 28 | 27 | 105 | 2 | 5 | 1.2 | 2.0 | 1.2 | 13 | 34 | 49 | 0.4 | 33 | tr | 0.08 | 0.08 | 0.7 | tr |
| 323 | From mix ..... 1 biscuit ....... | 28 | 29 | 90 | 2 | 3 | 0.6 | 1.1 | 0.7 | 15 | 19 | 65 | 0.6 | 32 | tr | 0.09 | 0.08 | 0.8 | tr |
| | **Breadcrumbs (enriched)[38]** | | | | | | | | | | | | | | | | | | |
| 324 | Dry, grated ..... 1 c ..... | 100 | 7 | 390 | 13 | 5 | 1.0 | 1.6 | 1.4 | 73 | 122 | 141 | 3.6 | 152 | tr | 0.35 | 0.35 | 4.8 | tr |
| | Soft (see White bread, items 349–350) | | | | | | | | | | | | | | | | | | |
| | **Breads** | | | | | | | | | | | | | | | | | | |
| 325 | Boston brown bread, canned, slice (3 1/4" × 1/2")[38]  1 slice ..... | 45 | 45 | 95 | 2 | 1 | 0.1 | 0.2 | 0.2 | 21 | 41 | 72 | 0.9 | 131 | 0[39] | 0.06 | 0.04 | 0.7 | 0 |
| | **Cracked-wheat bread (3/4 enriched wheat flour, 1/4 cracked wheat)[38]** | | | | | | | | | | | | | | | | | | |
| 326 | Loaf, 1 lb ..... 1 loaf ..... | 454 | 35 | 1195 | 39 | 10 | 2.2 | 3.0 | 3.9 | 236 | 399 | 581 | 9.5 | 608 | tr | 1.52 | 1.13 | 14.4 | tr |
| 327 | Slice (18 per loaf) ..... 1 slice ..... | 25 | 35 | 65 | 2 | 1 | 0.1 | 0.2 | 0.2 | 13 | 22 | 32 | 0.5 | 34 | tr | 0.08 | 0.06 | 0.8 | tr |
| | **French or vienna bread, enriched[38]** | | | | | | | | | | | | | | | | | | |
| 328 | Loaf, 1 lb ..... 1 loaf ..... | 454 | 31 | 1315 | 41 | 14 | 3.2 | 4.7 | 4.6 | 251 | 195 | 386 | 10.0 | 408 | tr | 1.80 | 1.10 | 15.0 | tr |
| | Slice | | | | | | | | | | | | | | | | | | |
| 329 | French (5" × 2 1/2" × 1") 1 slice ..... | 35 | 31 | 100 | 3 | 1 | 0.2 | 0.4 | 0.4 | 19 | 15 | 30 | 0.8 | 32 | tr | 0.14 | 0.08 | 1.2 | tr |
| 330 | Vienna (4 3/4" × 4" × 1/2") 1 slice ..... | 25 | 31 | 75 | 2 | 1 | 0.2 | 0.3 | 0.3 | 14 | 11 | 21 | 0.6 | 23 | tr | 0.10 | 0.06 | 0.8 | tr |
| | **Italian bread, enriched** | | | | | | | | | | | | | | | | | | |
| 331 | Loaf, 1 lb ..... 1 loaf ..... | 454 | 32 | 1250 | 41 | 4 | 0.6 | 0.3 | 1.5 | 256 | 77 | 349 | 10.0 | 336 | 0 | 1.80 | 1.10 | 15.0 | 0 |
| 332 | Slice (4 1/2" × 3 1/4" × 3/4") 1 slice ..... | 30 | 32 | 85 | 3 | tr | tr | tr | 0.1 | 17 | 5 | 23 | 0.7 | 22 | 0 | 0.12 | 0.07 | 1.0 | 0 |
| | **Raisin bread, enriched[38]** | | | | | | | | | | | | | | | | | | |
| 333 | Loaf, 1 lb ..... 1 loaf ..... | 454 | 35 | 1190 | 30 | 13 | 3.0 | 4.7 | 3.9 | 243 | 322 | 395 | 10.0 | 1057 | tr | 1.70 | 1.07 | 10.7 | tr |
| 334 | Slice (18 per loaf) ..... 1 slice ..... | 25 | 35 | 65 | 2 | 1 | 0.2 | 0.3 | 0.2 | 13 | 18 | 22 | 0.6 | 58 | tr | 0.09 | 0.06 | 0.6 | tr |
| | **Rye bread** | | | | | | | | | | | | | | | | | | |
| | American, light (2/3 enriched wheat flour, 1/3 rye flour) | | | | | | | | | | | | | | | | | | |
| 335 | Loaf, 1 lb ..... 1 loaf ..... | 454 | 36 | 1100 | 41 | 5 | 0.7 | 05 | 2.2 | 236 | 340 | 667 | 9.1 | 658 | 0 | 1.35 | 0.98 | 12.9 | 0 |
| 336 | Slice (4 3/4" × 3 3/4" × 7/16") 1 slice ..... | 25 | 36 | 60 | 2 | tr | tr | tr | 0.1 | 13 | 19 | 37 | 0.5 | 36 | 0 | 0.07 | 0.05 | 0.7 | 0 |
| | Pumpernickel (2/3 rye flour, 1/3 enriched wheat flour) | | | | | | | | | | | | | | | | | | |
| 337 | Loaf, 1 lb ..... 1 loaf ..... | 454 | 34 | 1115 | 41 | 5 | 0.7 | 0.5 | 2.4 | 241 | 381 | 1039 | 11.8 | 2059 | 0 | 1.30 | 0.93 | 8.5 | 0 |
| 338 | Slice (5" × 4" × 3/8") 1 slice ..... | 32 | 34 | 80 | 3 | tr | 0.1 | tr | 0.2 | 17 | 27 | 73 | 0.8 | 145 | 0 | 0.09 | 0.07 | 0.6 | 0 |
| | **White bread, enriched[38]** | | | | | | | | | | | | | | | | | | |
| | Soft-crumb type | | | | | | | | | | | | | | | | | | |
| 339 | Loaf, 1 lb ..... 1 loaf ..... | 454 | 36 | 1225 | 39 | 15 | 3.4 | 5.3 | 4.6 | 229 | 381 | 440 | 11.3 | 476 | tr | 1.80 | 1.10 | 15.0 | tr |

(Continued)

## Table 1. Nutritive Values of the Edible Part of Foods (Continued)

(Dashes (—) denote lack of reliable data for a constituent believed to be present in measurable amount)

| (A) Item No. | (B) Foods, Approximate Measures, Units, and Weight (edible part unless footnotes indicate otherwise) | | Water (C) | Food Energy (D) | Protein (E) | Fat (F) | Fatty Acids Saturated (Total) (G) | Unsaturated Oleic (H) | Unsaturated Linoleic (I) | Carbohydrate (J) | Calcium (K) | Phosphorus (L) | Iron (M) | Potassium (N) | Vitamin A Value (O) | Thiamin (P) | Riboflavin (Q) | Niacin (R) | Ascorbic Acid (S) |
|---|---|---|---|---|---|---|---|---|---|---|---|---|---|---|---|---|---|---|---|
| | | g | Per-cent | Calories | g | g | g | g | g | g | mg | mg | mg | mg | IU | mg | mg | mg | mg |
| *Grain Products (Continued)* | | | | | | | | | | | | | | | | | | | |
| | Breads (Continued) | | | | | | | | | | | | | | | | | | |
| 340 | Slice (18 per loaf) ... 1 slice | 25 | 36 | 70 | 2 | 1 | 0.2 | 0.3 | 0.3 | 13 | 21 | 24 | 0.6 | 26 | tr | 0.10 | 0.06 | 0.8 | tr |
| 341 | Slice, toasted ....... 1 slice | 22 | 25 | 70 | 2 | 1 | 0.2 | 0.3 | 0.3 | 13 | 21 | 24 | 0.6 | 26 | tr | 0.08 | 0.06 | 0.8 | tr |
| 342 | Slice (22 per loaf) ... 1 slice | 20 | 36 | 55 | 2 | 1 | 0.2 | 0.2 | 0.2 | 10 | 17 | 19 | 0.5 | 21 | tr | 0.08 | 0.05 | 0.7 | tr |
| 343 | Slice, toasted ....... 1 slice | 17 | 25 | 55 | 2 | 1 | 0.2 | 0.2 | 0.2 | 10 | 17 | 19 | 0.5 | 21 | tr | 0.06 | 0.05 | 0.7 | tr |
| 344 | Loaf, 1½ lb ......... 1 loaf | 680 | 36 | 1835 | 59 | 22 | 5.2 | 7.9 | 6.9 | 343 | 571 | 660 | 17.0 | 714 | tr | 2.70 | 1.65 | 22.5 | tr |
| 345 | Slice (24 per loaf) ... 1 slice | 28 | 36 | 75 | 2 | 1 | 0.2 | 0.3 | 0.3 | 14 | 24 | 27 | 0.7 | 29 | tr | 0.11 | 0.07 | 0.9 | tr |
| 346 | Slice, toasted ....... 1 slice | 24 | 25 | 75 | 2 | 1 | 0.2 | 0.3 | 0.3 | 14 | 24 | 27 | 0.7 | 29 | tr | 0.09 | 0.07 | 0.9 | tr |
| 347 | Slice (28 per loaf) ... 1 slice | 24 | 36 | 65 | 2 | 1 | 0.2 | 0.3 | 0.2 | 12 | 20 | 23 | 0.6 | 25 | tr | 0.10 | 0.06 | 0.8 | tr |
| 348 | Slice, toasted ....... 1 slice | 21 | 25 | 65 | 2 | 1 | 0.2 | 0.3 | 0.2 | 12 | 20 | 23 | 0.6 | 25 | tr | 0.08 | 0.06 | 0.8 | tr |
| 349 | Cubes .............. 1 c | 30 | 36 | 80 | 3 | 1 | 0.2 | 0.3 | 0.3 | 15 | 25 | 29 | 0.8 | 32 | tr | 0.12 | 0.07 | 1.0 | tr |
| 350 | Crumbs ............. 1 c | 45 | 36 | 120 | 4 | 1 | 0.3 | 0.5 | 0.5 | 23 | 38 | 44 | 1.1 | 47 | tr | 0.18 | 0.11 | 1.5 | tr |
| | Firm-crumb type | | | | | | | | | | | | | | | | | | |
| 351 | Loaf, 1 lb .......... 1 loaf | 454 | 35 | 1245 | 41 | 17 | 3.9 | 5.9 | 5.2 | 228 | 435 | 463 | 11.3 | 549 | tr | 1.80 | 1.10 | 15.0 | tr |
| 352 | Slice (20 per loaf) ... 1 slice | 23 | 35 | 65 | 2 | 1 | 0.2 | 0.3 | 0.3 | 12 | 22 | 23 | 0.6 | 28 | tr | 0.09 | 0.06 | 0.8 | tr |
| 353 | Slice, toasted ....... 1 slice | 20 | 24 | 65 | 2 | 1 | 0.2 | 0.3 | 0.3 | 12 | 22 | 23 | 0.6 | 28 | tr | 0.07 | 0.06 | 0.8 | tr |
| 354 | Loaf, 2 lb .......... 1 loaf | 907 | 35 | 2495 | 82 | 34 | 7.7 | 11.8 | 10.4 | 455 | 871 | 925 | 22.7 | 1097 | tr | 3.60 | 2.20 | 30.0 | tr |
| 355 | Slice (34 per loaf) ... 1 slice | 27 | 35 | 75 | 2 | 1 | 0.2 | 0.3 | 0.3 | 14 | 26 | 28 | 0.7 | 33 | tr | 0.11 | 0.06 | 0.9 | tr |
| 356 | Slice, toasted ....... 1 slice | 23 | 24 | 75 | 2 | 1 | 0.2 | 0.3 | 0.3 | 14 | 26 | 28 | 0.7 | 33 | tr | 0.09 | 0.06 | 0.9 | tr |
| | Whole-wheat bread | | | | | | | | | | | | | | | | | | |
| | Soft-crumb type[38] | | | | | | | | | | | | | | | | | | |
| 357 | Loaf, 1 lb .......... 1 loaf | 454 | 36 | 1095 | 41 | 12 | 2.2 | 2.9 | 4.2 | 224 | 381 | 1152 | 13.6 | 1161 | tr | 1.37 | 0.45 | 12.7 | tr |
| 358 | Slice (16 per loaf) ... 1 slice | 28 | 36 | 65 | 3 | 1 | 0.1 | 0.2 | 0.2 | 14 | 24 | 71 | 0.8 | 72 | tr | 0.09 | 0.03 | 0.8 | tr |
| 359 | Slice, toasted ....... 1 slice | 24 | 24 | 65 | 3 | 1 | 0.1 | 0.2 | 0.2 | 14 | 24 | 71 | 0.8 | 72 | tr | 0.07 | 0.03 | 0.8 | tr |
| | Firm-crumb type[38] | | | | | | | | | | | | | | | | | | |
| 360 | Loaf, 1 lb .......... 1 loaf | 454 | 36 | 1100 | 48 | 14 | 2.5 | 3.3 | 4.9 | 216 | 449 | 1034 | 13.6 | 1238 | tr | 1.17 | 0.54 | 12.7 | tr |
| 361 | Slice (18 per loaf) ... 1 slice | 25 | 36 | 60 | 3 | 1 | 0.1 | 0.2 | 0.3 | 12 | 25 | 57 | 0.8 | 68 | tr | 0.06 | 0.03 | 0.7 | tr |
| 362 | Slice, toasted ....... 1 slice | 21 | 24 | 60 | 3 | 1 | 0.1 | 0.2 | 0.3 | 12 | 25 | 57 | 0.8 | 68 | tr | 0.05 | 0.03 | 0.7 | tr |
| | Breakfast cereals | | | | | | | | | | | | | | | | | | |
| | Hot type, cooked | | | | | | | | | | | | | | | | | | |
| | Corn (hominy) grits, degermed | | | | | | | | | | | | | | | | | | |
| 363 | Enriched ........... 1 c | 245 | 87 | 125 | 3 | tr | tr | tr | 0.1 | 27 | 2 | 25 | 0.7 | 27 | tr[40] | 0.10 | 0.07 | 1.0 | 0 |
| 364 | Unenriched ......... 1 c | 245 | 87 | 125 | 3 | tr | tr | tr | 0.1 | 27 | 2 | 25 | 0.2 | 27 | tr[40] | 0.05 | 0.02 | 0.5 | 0 |
| 365 | Farina, quick-cooking, enriched 1 c | 245 | 89 | 105 | 3 | tr | tr | tr | 0.1 | 22 | 147 | 113[41] | (42) | 25 | 0 | 0.12 | 0.07 | 1.0 | 0 |
| 366 | Oatmeal or rolled oats 1 c | 240 | 87 | 130 | 5 | 2 | 0.4 | 0.8 | 0.9 | 23 | 22 | 137 | 1.4 | 146 | 0 | 0.19 | 0.05 | 0.2 | 0 |
| 367 | Wheat, rolled ....... 1 c | 240 | 80 | 180 | 5 | 1 | — | — | — | 41 | 19 | 182 | 1.7 | 202 | 0 | 0.17 | 0.07 | 2.2 | 0 |
| 368 | Wheat, whole-meal ... 1 c | 245 | 88 | 110 | 4 | 1 | — | — | — | 23 | 17 | 127 | 1.2 | 118 | 0 | 0.15 | 0.05 | 1.5 | 0 |

| (A) | (B) | (C) | (D) | (E) | (F) | (G) | (H) | (I) | (J) | (K) | (L) | (M) | (N) | (O) | (P) | (Q) | (R) | (S) |
|---|---|---|---|---|---|---|---|---|---|---|---|---|---|---|---|---|---|---|
|  | Ready-to-eat |  |  |  |  |  |  |  |  |  |  |  |  |  |  |  |  |  |
| 369 | Bran flakes (40% bran), added sugar, salt, iron, vitamins  1 c | 35 | 105 | 4 | 1 | 1 | — | — | 28 | 19 | 125 | 5.6 | 137 | 1540 | 0.46 | 0.52 | 6.2 | 0 |
| 370 | Bran flakes with raisins, added sugar, salt, iron, vitamins  1 c | 50 | 145 | 4 | 1 | 1 | — | — | 40 | 28 | 146 | 7.9 | 154 | 2200[43] | (44) | (44) | (44) | 0 |
|  | Corn flakes |  |  |  |  |  |  |  |  |  |  |  |  |  |  |  |  |  |
| 371 | Plain, added sugar, salt, iron, vitamins  1 c | 25 | 95 | 2 | tr | tr | — | — | 21 | (44) | 9 | (44) | 30 | (44) | (44) | (44) | (44) | 13[45] |
| 372 | Sugar-coated, added salt, iron, vitamins  1 c | 40 | 155 | 2 | tr | tr | — | — | 37 | 1 | 10 | (44) | 27 | 1760 | 0.53 | 0.60 | 7.1 | 21[45] |
| 373 | Corn, oat flour, puffed, added sugar, salt, iron, vitamins  1 c | 20 | 80 | 2 | 1 | 1 | — | — | 16 | 4 | 18 | 5.7 | — | 880 | 0.26 | 0.30 | 3.5 | 11 |
| 374 | Corn, shredded, added sugar, salt, iron, thiamin, niacin  1 c | 25 | 95 | 2 | tr | tr | — | — | 22 | 1 | 10 | 0.6 | — | 0 | 0.33 | 0.05 | 4.4 | 13 |
| 375 | Oats, puffed, added sugar, salt, minerals, vitamins  1 c | 25 | 100 | 3 | 1 | 1 | — | — | 19 | 44 | 102 | 4.0 | — | 1100 | 0.33 | 0.38 | 4.4 | 13 |
|  | Rice, puffed |  |  |  |  |  |  |  |  |  |  |  |  |  |  |  |  |  |
| 376 | Plain, added iron, thiamin, niacin  1 c | 15 | 60 | 1 | tr | tr | — | — | 13 | 3 | 14 | 0.3 | 15 | 0 | 0.07 | 0.01 | 0.7 | 0 |
| 377 | Presweetened, added salt, iron, vitamins  1 c | 28 | 115 | 1 | 0 | 0 | — | — | 26 | 3 | 14 | (44) | 43 | 1240[45] | (44) | (44) | (44) | 15[45] |
| 378 | Wheat flakes, added sugar, salt, iron, vitamins  1 c | 30 | 105 | 3 | tr | tr | — | — | 24 | 12 | 83 | 4.8 | 81 | 1320 | 0.40 | 0.45 | 5.3 | 16 |
|  | Wheat, puffed |  |  |  |  |  |  |  |  |  |  |  |  |  |  |  |  |  |
| 379 | Plain, added iron, thiamin, niacin  1 c | 15 | 55 | 2 | tr | tr | — | — | 12 | 4 | 48 | 0.6 | 51 | 0 | 0.08 | 0.03 | 1.2 | 0 |
| 380 | Presweetened, added salt, iron, vitamins  1 c | 38 | 140 | 3 | tr | tr | — | — | 33 | 7 | 52 | (44) | 63 | 1680 | 0.50 | 0.57 | 6.7 | 20[45] |
| 381 | Wheat, shredded, plain  1 oblong biscuit or 1/2 cup spoon-size biscuits | 25 | 90 | 2 | 1 | 1 | — | — | 20 | 11 | 97 | 0.9 | 87 | 0 | 0.06 | 0.03 | 1.1 | 0 |
| 382 | Wheat germ, without salt and sugar, toasted  1 tbsp | 6 | 25 | 2 | 1 | 1 | — | — | 3 | 3 | 70 | 0.5 | 57 | 10 | 0.11 | 0.05 | 0.3 | 1 |
| 383 | Buckwheat flour, light, sifted  1 c | 98 | 340 | 6 | 1 | 1 | 0.2 | 0.4 | 78 | 11 | 86 | 1.0 | 314 | 0 | 0.08 | 0.04 | 0.4 | 0 |
| 384 | Bulgur, canned, seasoned  1 c | 135 | 245 | 8 | 4 | 4 | — | — | 44 | 27 | 263 | 1.9 | 151 | 0 | 0.08 | 0.05 | 4.1 | 0 |
|  | Cake icings (see Sugars and Sweets, items 532–536) |  |  |  |  |  |  |  |  |  |  |  |  |  |  |  |  |  |  |
|  | Cakes made from cake mixes with enriched flour[46] |  |  |  |  |  |  |  |  |  |  |  |  |  |  |  |  |  |  |

(Continued)

# Table 1. Nutritive Values of the Edible Part of Foods (Continued)

(Dashes (—) denote lack of reliable data for a constituent believed to be present in measurable amount)

| Item No. (A) | Foods, Approximate Measures, Units, and Weight (edible part unless footnotes indicate otherwise) (B) | | g | Water (C) Per-cent | Food Energy (D) Cal-ories | Pro-tein (E) g | Fat (F) g | Fatty Acids Satu-rated (Total) (G) g | Unsaturated Oleic (H) g | Lino-leic (I) g | Carbo-hydrate (J) g | Calcium (K) mg | Phos-phorus (L) mg | Iron (M) mg | Potas-sium (N) mg | Vitamin A Value (O) IU | Thiamin (P) mg | Ribo-flavin (Q) mg | Niacin (R) mg | Ascorbic Acid (S) mg |
|---|---|---|---|---|---|---|---|---|---|---|---|---|---|---|---|---|---|---|---|---|
| | *Grain Products (Continued)* | | | | | | | | | | | | | | | | | | | |
| | Cakes made from cake mixes with enriched flour (Continued) | | | | | | | | | | | | | | | | | | | |
| | Angelfood | | | | | | | | | | | | | | | | | | | |
| 385 | Whole cake (9¾" diam tube cake) | 1 cake | 635 | 34 | 1645 | 36 | 1 | — | — | — | 377 | 603 | 756 | 2.5 | 381 | 0 | 0.37 | 0.95 | 3.6 | 0 |
| 386 | Piece, 1/12 of cake | 1 piece | 53 | 34 | 135 | 3 | tr | — | — | — | 32 | 50 | 63 | 0.2 | 32 | 0 | 0.03 | 0.08 | 0.3 | 0 |
| | Coffeecake | | | | | | | | | | | | | | | | | | | |
| 387 | Whole cake (7¾" × 5⅝" × 1¼"in) | 1 cake | 430 | 30 | 1385 | 27 | 41 | 11.7 | 16.3 | 8.8 | 225 | 262 | 748 | 6.9 | 469 | 690 | 0.82 | 0.91 | 7.7 | 1 |
| 388 | Piece, 1/6 of cake | 1 piece | 72 | 30 | 230 | 5 | 7 | 2.0 | 2.7 | 1.5 | 38 | 44 | 125 | 1.2 | 78 | 120 | 0.14 | 0.15 | 1.3 | tr |
| | Cupcakes, made with egg, milk, 2½" diam | | | | | | | | | | | | | | | | | | | |
| 389 | Without icing | 1 cupcake | 25 | 26 | 90 | 1 | 3 | 0.8 | 1.2 | 0.7 | 14 | 40 | 59 | 0.3 | 21 | 40 | 0.05 | 0.05 | 0.4 | tr |
| 390 | With chocolate icing | 1 cupcake | 36 | 22 | 130 | 2 | 5 | 2.0 | 1.6 | 0.6 | 21 | 47 | 71 | 0.4 | 42 | 60 | 0.05 | 0.06 | 0.4 | tr |
| | Devil's food with chocolate icing | | | | | | | | | | | | | | | | | | | |
| 391 | Whole, 2-layer cake (8" or 9"diam) | 1 cake | 1107 | 24 | 3755 | 49 | 136 | 50.0 | 44.9 | 17.0 | 645 | 653 | 1162 | 16.6 | 1439 | 1660 | 1.06 | 1.65 | 10.1 | 1 |
| 392 | Piece, 1/16 of cake | 1 piece | 69 | 24 | 235 | 3 | 8 | 3.1 | 2.8 | 1.1 | 40 | 41 | 72 | 1.0 | 90 | 100 | 0.07 | 0.10 | 0.6 | tr |
| 393 | Cupcake (2½" diam) | 1 cupcake | 35 | 24 | 120 | 2 | 4 | 1.6 | 1.4 | 0.5 | 20 | 21 | 37 | 0.5 | 46 | 50 | 0.03 | 0.05 | 0.3 | tr |
| | White, 2-layer with chocolate icing | | | | | | | | | | | | | | | | | | | |
| 394 | Whole cake (8" square) | 1 cake | 570 | 37 | 1575 | 18 | 39 | 9.7 | 16.6 | 10.0 | 291 | 513 | 570 | 8.6 | 1562 | tr | 0.84 | 1.00 | 7.4 | tr |
| 395 | Piece, 1/9 of cake | 1 piece | 63 | 37 | 175 | 2 | 4 | 1.1 | 1.8 | 1.1 | 32 | 57 | 63 | 0.9 | 173 | tr | 0.09 | 0.11 | 0.8 | tr |
| | Yellow, 2-layer with chocolate icing | | | | | | | | | | | | | | | | | | | |
| 396 | Whole cake (8" or 9" diam) | 1 cake | 1140 | 21 | 4000 | 44 | 122 | 48.2 | 46.4 | 20.0 | 716 | 1129 | 2041 | 11.4 | 1322 | 680 | 1.50 | 1.77 | 12.5 | 2 |
| 397 | Piece, 1/16 of cake | 1 piece | 71 | 21 | 250 | 3 | 8 | 3.0 | 2.9 | 1.2 | 45 | 70 | 127 | 0.7 | 82 | 40 | 0.09 | 0.11 | 0.8 | tr |
| | Cakes made from home recipes using enriched flour[47] | | | | | | | | | | | | | | | | | | | |
| 398 | Whole cake (8" or 9" diam) | 1 cake | 1108 | 26 | 3735 | 45 | 125 | 47.8 | 47.8 | 20.3 | 638 | 1008 | 2017 | 12.2 | 1208 | 1550 | 1.24 | 1.67 | 10.6 | 2 |
| 399 | Piece, 1/16 of cake | 1 piece | 69 | 26 | 235 | 3 | 8 | 3.0 | 3.0 | 1.3 | 40 | 63 | 126 | 0.8 | 75 | 100 | 0.08 | 0.10 | 0.7 | tr |
| | Boston cream pie with custard filling | | | | | | | | | | | | | | | | | | | |
| 400 | Whole cake (8" diam) | 1 cake | 825 | 35 | 2490 | 41 | 78 | 23.0 | 30.1 | 15.2 | 412 | 553 | 833 | 8.2 | 734[48] | 1730 | 1.04 | 1.27 | 9.6 | 2 |
| 401 | Piece, 1/12 of cake | 1 piece | 69 | 35 | 210 | 3 | 6 | 1.9 | 2.5 | 1.3 | 34 | 46 | 70 | 0.7 | 61[48] | 140 | 0.09 | 0.11 | 0.8 | tr |

| (A) | (B) | | (C) | (D) | (E) | (F) | (G) | (H) | (I) | (J) | (K) | (L) | (M) | (N) | (O) | (P) | (Q) | (R) | (S) |
|---|---|---|---|---|---|---|---|---|---|---|---|---|---|---|---|---|---|---|---|
|  | **Fruitcake, dark** | | | | | | | | | | | | | | | | | | |
| 402 | Loaf, 1-lb (7½" × 2" × 1½"), 1 loaf | 454 | 18 | 1720 | 22 | 69 | 14.4 | 33.5 | 14.8 | 271 | 327 | 513 | 11.8 | 2250 | 540 | 0.72 | 0.73 | 4.9 | 2 |
| 403 | Slice, 1/30 of loaf, 1 slice | 15 | 18 | 55 | 1 | 2 | 0.5 | 1.1 | 0.5 | 9 | 11 | 17 | 0.4 | 74 | 20 | 0.02 | 0.02 | 0.2 | tr |
|  | **Plain, sheet cake** | | | | | | | | | | | | | | | | | | |
|  | *Without icing* | | | | | | | | | | | | | | | | | | |
| 404 | Whole cake (9" square), 1 cake | 777 | 25 | 2830 | 35 | 108 | 29.5 | 44.4 | 23.9 | 434 | 497 | 793 | 8.5 | 614[48] | 1320 | 1.21 | 1.40 | 10.2 | 2 |
| 405 | Piece, 1/9 of cake, 1 piece | 86 | 25 | 315 | 4 | 12 | 3.3 | 4.9 | 2.6 | 48 | 55 | 88 | 0.9 | 68[48] | 150 | 0.13 | 0.15 | 1.1 | tr |
|  | *With uncooked white icing* | | | | | | | | | | | | | | | | | | |
| 406 | Whole cake (9" square), 1 cake | 1096 | 21 | 4020 | 37 | 129 | 42.2 | 49.5 | 24.4 | 694 | 548 | 822 | 8.2 | 669[48] | 2190 | 1.22 | 1.47 | 10.2 | 2 |
| 407 | Piece, 1/9 of cake, 1 piece | 121 | 21 | 445 | 4 | 14 | 4.7 | 5.5 | 2.7 | 77 | 61 | 91 | 0.8 | 74[48] | 240 | 0.14 | 0.16 | 1.1 | tr |
|  | **Pound[49]** | | | | | | | | | | | | | | | | | | |
| 408 | Loaf, 8½" × 3½" × 3¼", 1 loaf | 565 | 16 | 2725 | 31 | 170 | 42.9 | 73.1 | 39.6 | 273 | 107 | 418 | 7.9 | 345 | 1410 | 0.90 | 0.99 | 7.3 | 0 |
| 409 | Slice, 1/17 of loaf, 1 slice | 33 | 16 | 160 | 2 | 10 | 2.5 | 4.3 | 2.3 | 16 | 6 | 24 | 0.5 | 20 | 80 | 0.05 | 0.06 | 0.4 | 0 |
|  | **Spongecake** | | | | | | | | | | | | | | | | | | |
| 410 | Whole cake (9¾" diam tube cake), 1 cake | 790 | 32 | 2345 | 60 | 45 | 13.1 | 15.8 | 5.7 | 427 | 237 | 885 | 13.4 | 687 | 3560 | 1.10 | 1.64 | 7.4 | tr |
| 411 | Piece, 1/12 of cake, 1 piece | 66 | 32 | 195 | 5 | 4 | 1.1 | 1.3 | 0.5 | 36 | 20 | 74 | 1.1 | 57 | 300 | 0.09 | 0.14 | 0.6 | tr |
|  | **Cookies made with enriched flour[50,51]** | | | | | | | | | | | | | | | | | | |
|  | **Brownies with nuts** | | | | | | | | | | | | | | | | | | |
|  | *Home-prepared, 1¾" × 1¾" × 7/8"* | | | | | | | | | | | | | | | | | | |
| 412 | From home recipe, 1 brownie | 20 | 10 | 95 | 1 | 6 | 1.5 | 3.0 | 1.2 | 10 | 8 | 30 | 0.4 | 38 | 40 | 0.04 | 0.03 | 0.2 | tr |
| 413 | From commercial recipe, 1 brownie | 20 | 11 | 85 | 1 | 4 | 0.9 | 1.4 | 1.3 | 13 | 9 | 27 | 0.4 | 34 | 20 | 0.03 | 0.02 | 0.2 | tr |
| 414 | Frozen, with chocolate icing[52] (1½" × 1¾" × 7/8"), 1 brownie | 25 | 13 | 105 | 1 | 5 | 2.0 | 2.2 | 0.7 | 15 | 10 | 31 | 0.4 | 44 | 50 | 0.03 | 0.03 | 0.2 | tr |
|  | **Chocolate chip** | | | | | | | | | | | | | | | | | | |
| 415 | Commercial (2¼" diam, 3/8" thick), 4 cookies | 42 | 3 | 200 | 2 | 9 | 2.8 | 2.9 | 2.2 | 29 | 16 | 48 | 1.0 | 56 | 50 | 0.10 | 0.17 | 0.9 | tr |
| 416 | From home recipe, 2⅓" diam, 4 cookies | 40 | 3 | 205 | 2 | 12 | 3.5 | 4.5 | 2.9 | 24 | 14 | 40 | 0.8 | 47 | 40 | 0.06 | 0.06 | 0.5 | tr |
| 417 | Fig bars, square (1⅝" × 1⅝" × 3/8") or rectangular (1½" × 1¾" × ½"), 4 cookies | 56 | 14 | 200 | 2 | 3 | 0.8 | 1.2 | 0.7 | 42 | 44 | 34 | 1.0 | 111 | 60 | 0.04 | 0.14 | 0.9 | tr |
| 418 | Gingersnaps (2" diam, ¼" thick), 4 cookies | 28 | 3 | 90 | 2 | 2 | 0.7 | 1.0 | 0.6 | 22 | 20 | 13 | 0.7 | 129 | 20 | 0.08 | 0.06 | 0.7 | 0 |
| 419 | Macaroons (2¾" diam, ¼" thick), 2 cookies | 38 | 4 | 180 | 2 | 9 | — | — | — | 25 | 10 | 32 | 0.3 | 176 | 0 | 0.02 | 0.06 | 0.2 | 0 |
| 420 | Oatmeal with raisins (2⅝" diam, ¼" thick), 4 cookies | 52 | 3 | 235 | 3 | 8 | 2.0 | 3.3 | 2.0 | 38 | 11 | 53 | 1.4 | 192 | 30 | 0.15 | 0.10 | 1.0 | tr |
| 421 | Plain, prepared from commercial chilled dough (2½" diam, ¼" thick), 4 cookies | 48 | 5 | 240 | 2 | 12 | 3.0 | 5.2 | 2.9 | 31 | 17 | 35 | 0.6 | 23 | 30 | 0.10 | 0.08 | 0.9 | 0 |

(Continued)

**Table 1. Nutritive Values of the Edible Part of Foods (Continued)**

(Dashes (—) denote lack of reliable data for a constituent believed to be present in measurable amount)

| Item No. (A) | Foods, Approximate Measures, Units, and Weight (edible part unless footnotes indicate otherwise) (B) | Water (C) Per-cent | Food Energy (D) Cal-ories | Pro-tein (E) g | Fat (F) g | Fatty Acids Satu-rated (Total) (G) g | Oleic (H) g | Lino-leic (I) g | Carbo-hydrate (J) g | Calcium (K) mg | Phos-phorus (L) mg | Iron (M) mg | Potas-sium (N) mg | Vitamin A Value (O) IU | Thiamin (P) mg | Ribo-flavin (Q) mg | Niacin (R) mg | Ascorbic Acid (S) mg |
|---|---|---|---|---|---|---|---|---|---|---|---|---|---|---|---|---|---|---|
| *Grain Products (Continued)* | | | | | | | | | | | | | | | | | | |
| | Cookies made with enriched flour (Continued) | | | | | | | | | | | | | | | | | |
| 422 | Sandwich type chocolate or vanilla (1¾" diam, ⅜" thick) 4 cookies | 2 | 200 | 2 | 9 | 2.2 | 3.9 | 2.2 | 28 | 10 | 96 | 0.7 | 15 | 0 | 0.06 | 0.10 | 0.7 | 0 |
| 423 | Vanilla wafers, 1¾" diam, ¼" thick 10 cookies | 3 | 185 | 2 | 6 | — | — | — | 30 | 16 | 25 | 0.6 | 29 | 50 | 0.10 | 0.09 | 0.8 | 0 |
| | Cornmeal | | | | | | | | | | | | | | | | | |
| 424 | Whole-ground, unbolted, dry form 1 c | 12 | 435 | 11 | 5 | 0.5 | 1.0 | 2.5 | 90 | 24 | 312 | 2.9 | 346 | 620[53] | 0.46 | 0.13 | 2.4 | 0 |
| 425 | Bolted (nearly whole-grain), dry form 1 c | 12 | 440 | 11 | 4 | 0.5 | 0.9 | 2.1 | 91 | 21 | 272 | 2.2 | 303 | 590[53] | 0.37 | 0.10 | 2.3 | 0 |
| | Degermed, enriched | | | | | | | | | | | | | | | | | |
| 426 | Dry form 1 c | 12 | 500 | 11 | 2 | 0.2 | 0.4 | 0.9 | 108 | 8 | 137 | 4.0 | 166 | 610[53] | 0.61 | 0.36 | 4.8 | 0 |
| 427 | Cooked 1 c | 88 | 120 | 3 | tr | tr | 0.1 | 0.2 | 26 | 2 | 34 | 1.0 | 38 | 140[53] | 0.14 | 0.10 | 1.2 | 0 |
| | Degermed, unenriched | | | | | | | | | | | | | | | | | |
| 428 | Dry form 1 c | 12 | 500 | 11 | 2 | 0.2 | 0.4 | 0.9 | 108 | 8 | 137 | 1.5 | 166 | 610[53] | 0.19 | 0.07 | 1.4 | 0 |
| 429 | Cooked 1 c | 88 | 120 | 3 | tr | tr | 0.1 | 0.2 | 26 | 2 | 34 | 0.5 | 38 | 140[53] | 0.05 | 0.02 | 0.2 | 0 |
| | Crackers[38] | | | | | | | | | | | | | | | | | |
| 430 | Graham, plain (2½" square) 2 crackers | 6 | 55 | 1 | 1 | 0.3 | 0.5 | 0.3 | 10 | 6 | 21 | 0.5 | 55 | 0 | 0.02 | 0.08 | 0.5 | 0 |
| 431 | Rye wafers, whole-grain (1⅞" × 3½") 2 wafers | 6 | 45 | 2 | tr | — | — | — | 10 | 7 | 50 | 0.5 | 78 | 0 | 0.04 | 0.03 | 0.2 | 0 |
| 432 | Saltines, made with enriched flour 4 crackers or 1 packet | 4 | 50 | 1 | 1 | 0.3 | 0.5 | 0.4 | 8 | 2 | 10 | 0.5 | 13 | 0 | 0.05 | 0.05 | 0.4 | 0 |
| | Danish pastry (enriched flour, plain without fruit or nuts[54] | | | | | | | | | | | | | | | | | |
| 433 | Packaged ring, 12 oz 1 ring | 22 | 1435 | 25 | 80 | 24.3 | 31.7 | 16.5 | 155 | 170 | 371 | 6.1 | 381 | 1050 | 0.97 | 1.01 | 8.6 | tr |
| 434 | Round piece (about 4¼" diam × 1") 1 pastry | 22 | 275 | 5 | 15 | 4.7 | 6.1 | 3.2 | 30 | 33 | 71 | 1.2 | 73 | 200 | 0.18 | 0.19 | 1.7 | tr |
| 435 | Ounce 1 oz | 22 | 120 | 2 | 7 | 2.0 | 2.7 | 1.4 | 13 | 14 | 31 | 0.5 | 32 | 90 | 0.08 | 0.08 | 0.7 | tr |
| | Doughnuts, made with enriched flour[38] | | | | | | | | | | | | | | | | | |
| 436 | Cake type, plain (2½" diam, 1" high) 1 doughnut | 24 | 100 | 1 | 5 | 1.2 | 2.0 | 1.1 | 13 | 10 | 48 | 0.4 | 23 | 20 | 0.05 | 0.05 | 0.4 | tr |
| 437 | Yeast-leavened, glazed (3¾" diam, 1¼" high) 1 doughnut | 26 | 205 | 3 | 11 | 3.3 | 5.8 | 3.3 | 22 | 16 | 33 | 0.6 | 34 | 25 | 0.10 | 0.10 | 0.8 | 0 |
| | Macaroni, enriched, cooked (cut lengths, elbows, shells) | | | | | | | | | | | | | | | | | |

| (A) | (B) | | (C) | (D) | (E) | (F) | (G) | (H) | (I) | (J) | (K) | (L) | (M) | (N) | (O) | (P) | (Q) | (R) | (S) |
|---|---|---|---|---|---|---|---|---|---|---|---|---|---|---|---|---|---|---|---|
| 438 | Firm stage (hot) ... 1 c | 130 | 64 | 190 | 7 | 1 | — | — | — | 39 | 14 | 85 | 1.4 | 103 | 0 | 0.23 | 0.13 | 1.8 | 0 |
|  | Tender stage |  |  |  |  |  |  |  |  |  |  |  |  |  |  |  |  |  |  |
| 439 | Cold macaroni ... 1 c | 105 | 73 | 115 | 4 | tr | — | — | — | 24 | 8 | 53 | 0.9 | 64 | 0 | 0.15 | 0.08 | 1.2 | 0 |
| 440 | Hot macaroni ... 1 c | 140 | 73 | 155 | 5 | 1 | — | — | — | 32 | 11 | 70 | 1.3 | 85 | 0 | 0.20 | 0.11 | 1.5 | 0 |
|  | Macaroni (enriched) and cheese |  |  |  |  |  |  |  |  |  |  |  |  |  |  |  |  |  |  |  |
| 441 | Canned[35] ... 1 c | 240 | 80 | 230 | 9 | 10 | 4.2 | 3.1 | 1.4 | 26 | 199 | 182 | 1.0 | 139 | 260 | 0.12 | 0.24 | 1.0 | tr |
| 442 | From home recipe (served hot)[56] ... 1 c | 200 | 58 | 430 | 17 | 22 | 8.9 | 8.8 | 2.9 | 40 | 362 | 322 | 1.8 | 240 | 860 | 0.20 | 0.40 | 1.8 | tr |
|  | Muffins made with enriched flour[38] |  |  |  |  |  |  |  |  |  |  |  |  |  |  |  |  |  |  |  |
|  | From home recipe |  |  |  |  |  |  |  |  |  |  |  |  |  |  |  |  |  |  |  |  |
| 443 | Blueberry (2 3/8″ diam, 1 1/2″ high) ... 1 muffin | 40 | 39 | 110 | 3 | 4 | 1.1 | 1.4 | 0.7 | 17 | 34 | 53 | 0.6 | 46 | 90 | 0.09 | 0.10 | 0.7 | tr |
| 444 | Bran ... 1 muffin | 40 | 35 | 105 | 3 | 4 | 1.2 | 1.4 | 0.8 | 17 | 57 | 162 | 1.5 | 172 | 90 | 0.07 | 0.10 | 1.7 | tr |
| 445 | Corn, enriched degermed cornmeal and flour (2 3/8″ diam, 1 1/2″ high) ... 1 muffin | 40 | 33 | 125 | 3 | 4 | 1.2 | 1.6 | 0.9 | 19 | 42 | 68 | 0.7 | 54 | 120[57] | 0.10 | 0.10 | 0.7 | tr |
| 446 | Plain (3″ diam, 1 1/2″ high) ... 1 muffin | 40 | 38 | 120 | 3 | 4 | 1.0 | 1.7 | 1.0 | 17 | 42 | 60 | 0.6 | 50 | 40 | 0.09 | 0.12 | 0.9 | tr |
|  | From mix, egg, milk |  |  |  |  |  |  |  |  |  |  |  |  |  |  |  |  |  |  |  |  |
| 447 | Corn (2 3/8″ diam, 1 1/2″ high)[58] ... 1 muffin | 40 | 30 | 130 | 3 | 4 | 1.2 | 1.7 | 0.9 | 20 | 96 | 152 | 0.6 | 44 | 100[57] | 0.08 | 0.09 | 0.7 | tr |
| 448 | Noodles (egg noodles), enriched, cooked[58] ... 1 c | 160 | 71 | 200 | 7 | 2 | — | — | — | 37 | 16 | 94 | 1.4 | 70 | 110 | 0.22 | 0.13 | 1.9 | 0 |
| 449 | Noodles, chow mein, canned ... 1 c | 45 | 1 | 220 | 6 | 11 | — | — | — | 26 | — | — | — | — | — | — | — | — | — |
| 450 | Pancakes (4″ diam)[38] — Buckwheat, made from mix (with buckwheat and enriched flours), egg and milk added ... 1 cake | 27 | 58 | 55 | 2 | 2 | 0.8 | 0.9 | 0.4 | 6 | 59 | 91 | 0.4 | 66 | 60 | 0.04 | 0.05 | 0.2 | tr |
|  | Plain |  |  |  |  |  |  |  |  |  |  |  |  |  |  |  |  |  |  |  |  |
| 451 | Made from home recipe using enriched flour ... 1 cake | 27 | 50 | 60 | 2 | 2 | 0.5 | 0.8 | 0.5 | 9 | 27 | 38 | 0.4 | 33 | 30 | 0.06 | 0.07 | 0.5 | tr |
| 452 | Made from mix with enriched flour, egg and milk added ... 1 cake | 27 | 51 | 60 | 2 | 2 | 0.7 | 0.7 | 0.3 | 9 | 58 | 70 | 0.3 | 42 | 70 | 0.04 | 0.06 | 0.2 | tr |
|  | Pies, piecrust made with enriched flour, vegetable shortening (9″ diam) |  |  |  |  |  |  |  |  |  |  |  |  |  |  |  |  |  |  |  |  |
|  | Apple |  |  |  |  |  |  |  |  |  |  |  |  |  |  |  |  |  |  |  |  |
| 453 | Whole ... 1 pie | 945 | 48 | 2420 | 21 | 105 | 27.0 | 44.5 | 25.2 | 360 | 76 | 208 | 6.6 | 756 | 280 | 1.06 | 0.79 | 9.3 | 9 |
| 454 | Sector, 1/7 of pie ... 1 sector | 135 | 48 | 345 | 3 | 15 | 3.9 | 6.4 | 3.6 | 51 | 11 | 30 | 0.9 | 108 | 40 | 0.15 | 0.11 | 1.3 | 2 |

(Continued)

# Table 1. Nutritive Values of the Edible Part of Foods (Continued)

(Dashes (—) denote lack of reliable data for a constituent believed to be present in measurable amount)

| Item No. (A) | Foods, Approximate Measures, Units, and Weight (edible part unless footnotes indicate otherwise) (B) | g | Water (C) Per cent | Food Energy (D) Calories | Protein (E) g | Fat (F) g | Saturated (Total) (G) g | Oleic (H) g | Linoleic (I) g | Carbohydrate (J) g | Calcium (K) mg | Phosphorus (L) mg | Iron (M) mg | Potassium (N) mg | Vitamin A Value (O) IU | Thiamin (P) mg | Riboflavin (Q) mg | Niacin (R) mg | Ascorbic Acid (S) mg |
|---|---|---|---|---|---|---|---|---|---|---|---|---|---|---|---|---|---|---|---|
| | *Grain Products (Continued)* | | | | | | | | | | | | | | | | | | |
| | *Pies (Continued)* | | | | | | | | | | | | | | | | | | |
| | Banana cream | | | | | | | | | | | | | | | | | | |
| 455 | Whole ... 1 pie | 910 | 54 | 2010 | 41 | 85 | 26.7 | 33.2 | 16.2 | 279 | 601 | 746 | 7.3 | 1847 | 2280 | 0.77 | 1.51 | 7.0 | 9 |
| 456 | Sector, 1/7 of pie ... 1 sector | 130 | 54 | 285 | 6 | 12 | 3.8 | 4.7 | 2.3 | 40 | 86 | 107 | 1.0 | 264 | 330 | 0.11 | 0.22 | 1.0 | 1 |
| | Blueberry | | | | | | | | | | | | | | | | | | |
| 457 | Whole ... 1 pie | 945 | 51 | 2285 | 23 | 102 | 24.8 | 43.7 | 25.1 | 330 | 104 | 217 | 9.5 | 614 | 280 | 1.03 | 0.80 | 10.0 | 28 |
| 458 | Sector, 1/7 of pie ... 1 sector | 135 | 51 | 325 | 3 | 15 | 3.5 | 6.2 | 3.6 | 47 | 15 | 31 | 1.4 | 88 | 40 | 0.15 | 0.11 | 1.4 | 4 |
| | Cherry | | | | | | | | | | | | | | | | | | |
| 459 | Whole ... 1 pie | 945 | 47 | 2465 | 25 | 107 | 28.2 | 45.0 | 25.3 | 363 | 132 | 236 | 6.6 | 992 | 4160 | 1.09 | 0.84 | 9.8 | tr |
| 460 | Sector, 1/7 of pie ... 1 sector | 135 | 47 | 350 | 4 | 15 | 4.0 | 6.4 | 3.6 | 52 | 19 | 34 | 0.9 | 142 | 590 | 0.16 | 0.12 | 1.4 | tr |
| | Custard | | | | | | | | | | | | | | | | | | |
| 461 | Whole ... 1 pie | 910 | 58 | 1985 | 56 | 101 | 33.9 | 38.5 | 17.5 | 213 | 874 | 1028 | 8.2 | 1247 | 2090 | 0.79 | 1.92 | 5.6 | 0 |
| 462 | Sector, 1/7 of pie ... 1 sector | 130 | 58 | 285 | 8 | 14 | 4.8 | 5.5 | 2.5 | 30 | 125 | 147 | 1.2 | 178 | 300 | 0.11 | 0.27 | 0.8 | 0 |
| | Lemon meringue | | | | | | | | | | | | | | | | | | |
| 463 | Whole ... 1 pie | 840 | 47 | 2140 | 31 | 86 | 26.1 | 33.8 | 16.4 | 317 | 118 | 412 | 6.7 | 420 | 1430 | 0.61 | 0.84 | 5.2 | 25 |
| 464 | Sector, 1/7 of pie ... 1 sector | 120 | 47 | 305 | 4 | 12 | 3.7 | 4.8 | 2.3 | 45 | 17 | 59 | 1.0 | 60 | 200 | 0.09 | 0.12 | 0.7 | 4 |
| | Mince | | | | | | | | | | | | | | | | | | |
| 465 | Whole ... 1 pie | 945 | 43 | 2560 | 24 | 109 | 28.0 | 45.9 | 25.2 | 389 | 265 | 359 | 13.3 | 1682 | 20 | 0.96 | 0.86 | 9.8 | 9 |
| 466 | Sector, 1/7 of pie ... 1 sector | 135 | 43 | 365 | 3 | 16 | 4.0 | 6.6 | 3.6 | 56 | 38 | 51 | 1.9 | 240 | tr | 0.14 | 0.12 | 1.4 | 1 |
| | Peach | | | | | | | | | | | | | | | | | | |
| 467 | Whole ... 1 pie | 945 | 48 | 2410 | 24 | 101 | 24.8 | 43.7 | 25.1 | 361 | 95 | 274 | 8.5 | 1408 | 6900 | 1.04 | 0.97 | 14.0 | 28 |
| 468 | Sector, 1/7 of pie ... 1 sector | 135 | 48 | 345 | 3 | 14 | 3.5 | 6.2 | 3.6 | 52 | 14 | 39 | 1.2 | 201 | 990 | 0.15 | 0.14 | 2.0 | 4 |
| | Pecan | | | | | | | | | | | | | | | | | | |
| 469 | Whole ... 1 pie | 825 | 20 | 3450 | 42 | 189 | 27.8 | 101.0 | 44.2 | 423 | 388 | 850 | 25.6 | 1015 | 1320 | 1.80 | 0.95 | 6.9 | tr |
| 470 | Sector, 1/7 of pie ... 1 sector | 118 | 20 | 495 | 6 | 27 | 4.0 | 14.4 | 6.3 | 61 | 55 | 122 | 3.7 | 145 | 190 | 0.26 | 0.14 | 1.0 | tr |
| | Pumpkin | | | | | | | | | | | | | | | | | | |
| 471 | Whole ... 1 pie | 910 | 59 | 1920 | 36 | 102 | 37.4 | 37.5 | 16.6 | 223 | 464 | 628 | 7.3 | 1456 | 22,480 | 0.78 | 1.27 | 7.0 | tr |
| 472 | Sector, 1/7 of pie ... 1 sector | 130 | 59 | 275 | 5 | 15 | 5.4 | 5.4 | 2.4 | 32 | 66 | 90 | 1.0 | 208 | 3210 | 0.11 | 0.18 | 1.0 | tr |
| 473 | Piecrust (home recipe) made with enriched flour and vegetable shortening, baked ... 1 pie shell, 9"diam | 180 | 15 | 900 | 11 | 60 | 14.8 | 26.1 | 14.9 | 79 | 25 | 90 | 3.1 | 89 | 0 | 0.47 | 0.40 | 5.0 | 0 |
| 474 | Piecrust mix with enriched flour and vegetable shortening, 10-oz pkg prepared and baked ... Piecrust for 2-crust pie, 9"diam | 320 | 19 | 1485 | 20 | 93 | 22.7 | 39.7 | 23.4 | 141 | 131 | 272 | 6.1 | 179 | 0 | 1.07 | 0.79 | 9.9 | 0 |
| 475 | Pizza (cheese) baked (4³/₄" sector; 1/8 of 12" diam pie)[19] ... 1 sector | 60 | 45 | 145 | 6 | 4 | 1.7 | 1.5 | 0.6 | 22 | 86 | 89 | 1.1 | 67 | 230 | 0.16 | 0.18 | 1.6 | 4 |

| (A) | (B) | (g) | (C) | (D) | (E) | (F) | (G) | (H) | (I) | (J) | (K) | (L) | (M) | (N) | (O) | (P) | (Q) | (R) | (S) |
|---|---|---|---|---|---|---|---|---|---|---|---|---|---|---|---|---|---|---|---|
| | Popcorn, popped | | | | | | | | | | | | | | | | | | |
| 476 | Plain, large kernel ...... 1 c | 6 | 4 | 25 | 1 | tr | tr | 0.1 | 0.1 | 5 | 1 | 17 | 0.2 | — | — | — | 0.01 | 0.1 | 0 |
| 477 | With oil (coconut) and salt added, large kernel ...... 1 c | 9 | 3 | 40 | 1 | 2 | 1.5 | 0.2 | 0.2 | 5 | 1 | 19 | 0.2 | — | — | — | 0.01 | 0.2 | 0 |
| 478 | Sugar coated ......... 1 c | 35 | 4 | 135 | 2 | 1 | 0.5 | 0.2 | 0.2 | 30 | 2 | 47 | 0.5 | — | — | — | 0.02 | 0.4 | 0 |
| | Pretzels, made with enriched flour | | | | | | | | | | | | | | | | | | |
| 479 | Dutch, twisted (2¾" × 2⅝") ......... 1 pretzel | 16 | 5 | 60 | 2 | 1 | — | — | — | 12 | 4 | 21 | 0.2 | 21 | 0 | 0.05 | 0.04 | 0.7 | 0 |
| 480 | Thin, twisted (3¼" × 2¼" × ¼") ...... 10 pretzels | 60 | 5 | 235 | 6 | 3 | — | — | — | 46 | 13 | 79 | 0.9 | 78 | 0 | 0.20 | 0.15 | 2.5 | 0 |
| 481 | Stick (2¼" long) ...... 10 pretzels | 3 | 5 | 10 | tr | tr | — | — | — | 2 | 1 | 4 | tr | 4 | 0 | 0.01 | 0.01 | 0.1 | 0 |
| | Rice, white, enriched | | | | | | | | | | | | | | | | | | |
| 482 | Instant, ready-to-serve, hot ...... 1 c | 165 | 73 | 180 | 4 | tr | tr | tr | tr | 40 | 5 | 31 | 1.3 | — | 0 | 0.21 | (59) | 1.7 | 0 |
| | Long grain | | | | | | | | | | | | | | | | | | |
| 483 | Raw ...... 1 c | 185 | 12 | 670 | 12 | 1 | 0.2 | 0.2 | 0.2 | 149 | 44 | 174 | 5.4 | 170 | 0 | 0.81 | 0.06 | 6.5 | 0 |
| 484 | Cooked, served hot ...... 1 c | 205 | 73 | 225 | 4 | tr | 0.1 | 0.1 | 0.1 | 50 | 21 | 57 | 1.8 | 57 | 0 | 0.23 | 0.02 | 2.1 | 0 |
| | Parboiled | | | | | | | | | | | | | | | | | | |
| 485 | Raw ...... 1 c | 185 | 10 | 685 | 14 | 1 | 0.2 | 0.1 | 0.1 | 150 | 111 | 370 | 5.4 | 278 | 0 | 0.81 | 0.07 | 6.5 | 0 |
| 486 | Cooked, served hot ...... 1 c | 175 | 73 | 185 | 4 | tr | 0.1 | 0.1 | 0.1 | 41 | 33 | 100 | 1.4 | 75 | 0 | 0.19 | 0.02 | 2.1 | 0 |
| | Rolls, enriched[38] | | | | | | | | | | | | | | | | | | |
| | Commercial | | | | | | | | | | | | | | | | | | |
| 487 | Brown-and-serve (12 per 12-oz pkg), browned ......... 1 roll | 26 | 27 | 85 | 2 | 2 | 0.4 | 0.7 | 0.5 | 14 | 20 | 23 | 0.5 | 25 | tr | 0.10 | 0.06 | 0.9 | tr |
| 488 | Cloverleaf or pan (2½" diam, 2" high) ......... 1 roll | 28 | 31 | 85 | 2 | 2 | 0.4 | 0.6 | 0.4 | 15 | 21 | 24 | 0.5 | 27 | tr | 0.11 | 0.07 | 0.9 | tr |
| 489 | Frankfurter and hamburger (8 per 11½-oz pkg) ......... 1 roll | 40 | 31 | 120 | 3 | 2 | 0.5 | 0.8 | 0.6 | 21 | 30 | 34 | 0.8 | 38 | tr | 0.16 | 0.10 | 1.3 | tr |
| 490 | Hard (3¾" diam, 2" high) ......... 1 roll | 50 | 25 | 155 | 5 | 2 | 0.4 | 0.6 | 0.5 | 30 | 24 | 46 | 1.2 | 49 | tr | 0.20 | 0.12 | 1.7 | tr |
| 491 | Hoagie or submarine (11½" × 3" × 2½") ......... 1 roll | 135 | 31 | 390 | 12 | 4 | 0.9 | 1.4 | 1.4 | 75 | 58 | 115 | 3.0 | 122 | tr | 0.54 | 0.32 | 4.5 | tr |
| | From home recipe | | | | | | | | | | | | | | | | | | |
| 492 | Cloverleaf (2½" diam, 2" high) ......... 1 roll | 35 | 26 | 120 | 3 | 3 | 0.8 | 1.1 | 0.7 | 20 | 16 | 36 | 0.7 | 41 | 30 | 0.12 | 0.12 | 1.2 | tr |
| | Spaghetti, enriched, cooked | | | | | | | | | | | | | | | | | | |
| 493 | Firm stage, "al dente," served hot ...... 1 c | 130 | 64 | 190 | 7 | 1 | — | — | — | 39 | 14 | 85 | 1.4 | 103 | 0 | 0.23 | 0.13 | 1.8 | 0 |
| 494 | Tender stage, served hot ...... 1 c | 140 | 73 | 155 | 5 | 1 | — | — | — | 32 | 11 | 70 | 1.3 | 85 | 0 | 0.20 | 0.11 | 1.5 | 0 |
| | Spaghetti (enriched) in tomato sauce with cheese | | | | | | | | | | | | | | | | | | |
| 495 | From home recipe ...... 1 c | 250 | 77 | 260 | 9 | 9 | 2.0 | 5.4 | 0.7 | 37 | 80 | 135 | 2.3 | 408 | 1080 | 0.25 | 0.18 | 2.3 | 13 |
| 496 | Canned ...... 1 c | 250 | 80 | 190 | 6 | 2 | 0.5 | 0.3 | 0.4 | 39 | 40 | 88 | 2.8 | 303 | 930 | 0.35 | 0.28 | 4.5 | 10 |

(Continued)

**Table 1. Nutritive Values of the Edible Part of Foods (Continued)**
(Dashes (—) denote lack of reliable data for a constituent believed to be present in measurable amount)

| (A) | (B) | (C) | (D) | (E) | (F) | Fatty Acids (G) | (H) | (I) | (J) | (K) | (L) | (M) | (N) | (O) | (P) | (Q) | (R) | (S) |
|---|---|---|---|---|---|---|---|---|---|---|---|---|---|---|---|---|---|---|
| Item No. | Foods, Approximate Measures, Units, and Weight (edible part unless footnotes indicate otherwise) | Water | Food Energy | Protein | Fat | Saturated (Total) | Unsaturated Oleic | Unsaturated Linoleic | Carbohydrate | Calcium | Phosphorus | Iron | Potassium | Vitamin A Value | Thiamin | Riboflavin | Niacin | Ascorbic Acid |
|  |  | Percent | Calories | g | g | g | g | g | g | mg | mg | mg | mg | IU | mg | mg | mg | mg |
|  |  | g |  |  |  |  |  |  |  |  |  |  |  |  |  |  |  |  |
| *Grain Products (Continued)* | | | | | | | | | | | | | | | | | | |
|  | Spaghetti (enriched) with meat balls and tomato sauce | | | | | | | | | | | | | | | | | |
| 497 | From home recipe ..... 1 c | 248 | 70 | 330 | 19 | 12 | 3.3 | 6.3 | 0.9 | 39 | 124 | 236 | 3.7 | 665 | 1590 | 0.25 | 0.30 | 4.0 | 22 |
| 498 | Canned ............ 1 c | 250 | 78 | 260 | 12 | 10 | 2.2 | 3.3 | 3.9 | 29 | 53 | 113 | 3.3 | 245 | 1000 | 0.15 | 0.18 | 2.3 | 5 |
| 499 | Toaster pastries ...... 1 pastry | 50 | 12 | 200 | 3 | 6 | — | — | — | 36 | 54[60] | 67[60] | 1.9 | 74[60] | 500 | 0.16 | 0.17 | 2.1 | (66) |
|  | Waffles, made with enriched flour, 7"diam[38] | | | | | | | | | | | | | | | | | |
| 500 | From home recipe ..... 1 waffle | 75 | 41 | 210 | 7 | 7 | 2.3 | 2.8 | 1.4 | 28 | 85 | 130 | 1.3 | 109 | 250 | 0.17 | 0.23 | 1.4 | tr |
| 501 | From mix, egg and milk added 1 waffle | 75 | 42 | 205 | 7 | 8 | 2.8 | 2.9 | 1.2 | 27 | 179 | 257 | 1.0 | 146 | 170 | 0.14 | 0.22 | 0.9 | tr |
|  | Wheat flours | | | | | | | | | | | | | | | | | |
|  | All-purpose or family flour, enriched | | | | | | | | | | | | | | | | | |
| 502 | Sifted, spooned ...... 1 c | 115 | 12 | 420 | 12 | 1 | 0.2 | 0.1 | 0.5 | 88 | 18 | 100 | 3.3 | 109 | 0 | 0.74 | 0.46 | 6.1 | 0 |
| 503 | Unsifted, spooned .... 1 c | 125 | 12 | 455 | 13 | 1 | 0.2 | 0.1 | 0.5 | 95 | 20 | 109 | 3.6 | 119 | 0 | 0.80 | 0.50 | 6.6 | 0 |
| 504 | Cake or pastry flour, enriched, sifted, spooned 1 c | 96 | 12 | 350 | 7 | 1 | 0.1 | 0.1 | 0.3 | 76 | 16 | 70 | 2.8 | 191 | 0 | 0.61 | 0.38 | 5.1 | 0 |
| 505 | Self-rising, enriched, unsifted, spooned 1 c | 125 | 12 | 440 | 12 | 1 | 0.2 | 0.1 | 0.5 | 93 | 331 | 583 | 3.6 | — | 0 | 0.80 | 0.50 | 6.6 | 0 |
| 506 | Whole-wheat, from hard wheats, stirred 1 c | 120 | 12 | 400 | 16 | 2 | 0.4 | 0.2 | 1.0 | 85 | 49 | 446 | 4.0 | 444 | 0 | 0.66 | 0.14 | 5.2 | 0 |
| *Legumes (Dry), Nuts, Seeds, and Related Products* | | | | | | | | | | | | | | | | | | |
|  | Almonds, shelled | | | | | | | | | | | | | | | | | |
| 507 | Chopped (about 130 almonds) 1 c | 130 | 5 | 775 | 24 | 70 | 5.6 | 47.7 | 12.8 | 25 | 304 | 655 | 6.1 | 1005 | 0 | 0.31 | 1.20 | 4.6 | tr |
| 508 | Slivered, not pressed down (about 115 almonds) 1 c | 115 | 5 | 690 | 21 | 62 | 5.0 | 42.2 | 11.3 | 22 | 269 | 580 | 5.4 | 889 | 0 | 0.28 | 1.06 | 4.0 | tr |
|  | Beans, dry | | | | | | | | | | | | | | | | | |
|  | Common varieties as Great Northern, navy, and others | | | | | | | | | | | | | | | | | |

| (A) | (B) | (C) | (D) | (E) | (F) | (G) | (H) | (I) | (J) | (K) | (L) | (M) | (N) | (O) | (P) | (Q) | (R) | (S) |
|---|---|---|---|---|---|---|---|---|---|---|---|---|---|---|---|---|---|---|
| | **Cooked, drained** | | | | | | | | | | | | | | | | | |
| 509 | Great Northern, 1 c, 180 | 69 | 210 | 14 | 1 | — | — | — | 38 | 90 | 266 | 4.9 | 749 | 0 | 0.25 | 0.13 | 1.3 | 0 |
| 510 | Pea (navy), 1 c, 190 | 69 | 225 | 15 | 1 | — | — | — | 40 | 95 | 281 | 5.1 | 790 | 0 | 0.27 | 0.13 | 1.3 | 0 |
| | **Canned, solids and liquid** | | | | | | | | | | | | | | | | | |
| | **White with—** | | | | | | | | | | | | | | | | | |
| 511 | Frankfurters (sliced), 1 c, 255 | 71 | 365 | 19 | 18 | — | — | — | 32 | 94 | 303 | 4.8 | 668 | 330 | 0.18 | 0.15 | 3.3 | tr |
| 512 | Pork and tomato sauce, 1 c, 255 | 71 | 310 | 16 | 7 | 2.4 | 2.8 | 0.6 | 48 | 138 | 235 | 4.6 | 536 | 330 | 0.20 | 0.08 | 1.5 | 5 |
| 513 | Pork and sweet sauce, 1 c, 255 | 66 | 385 | 16 | 12 | 4.3 | 5.0 | 1.1 | 54 | 161 | 291 | 5.9 | — | — | 0.15 | 0.10 | 1.3 | — |
| 514 | Red kidney, 1 c, 255 | 76 | 230 | 15 | 1 | — | — | — | 42 | 74 | 278 | 4.6 | 673 | 10 | 0.13 | 0.10 | 1.5 | — |
| 515 | Lima, cooked, drained, 1 c, 190 | 64 | 260 | 16 | 1 | — | — | — | 49 | 55 | 293 | 5.9 | 1163 | — | 0.25 | 0.11 | 1.3 | — |
| 516 | Blackeye peas, dry, cooked (with residual cooking liquid), 1 c, 250 | 80 | 190 | 13 | 1 | — | — | — | 35 | 43 | 238 | 3.3 | 573 | 30 | 0.40 | 0.10 | 1.0 | — |
| 517 | Brazil nuts, shelled (6–8 large kernels), 1 oz, 28 | 5 | 185 | 4 | 19 | 4.8 | 6.2 | 7.1 | 3 | 53 | 196 | 1.0 | 203 | tr | 0.27 | 0.03 | 0.5 | — |
| 518 | Cashew nuts, roasted in oil, 1 c, 140 | 5 | 785 | 24 | 64 | 12.9 | 36.8 | 10.2 | 41 | 53 | 522 | 5.3 | 650 | 140 | 0.60 | 0.35 | 2.5 | — |
| 519 | Coconut meat, fresh, Piece (about 2″ × 2″ × 1/2″), 1 piece, 45 | 51 | 155 | 2 | 16 | 14.0 | 0.9 | 0.3 | 4 | 6 | 43 | 0.8 | 115 | 0 | 0.02 | 0.01 | 0.2 | 1 |
| 520 | Shredded or grated, not pressed down, 1 c, 80 | 51 | 275 | 3 | 28 | 24.8 | 1.6 | 0.5 | 8 | 10 | 76 | 1.4 | 205 | 0 | 0.04 | 0.02 | 0.4 | 2 |
| 521 | Filberts (hazelnuts), chopped (about 80 kernels), 1 c, 115 | 6 | 730 | 14 | 72 | 5.1 | 55.2 | 7.3 | 19 | 240 | 388 | 3.9 | 810 | — | 0.53 | — | 1.0 | tr |
| 522 | Lentils, whole, cooked, 1 c, 200 | 72 | 210 | 16 | tr | — | — | — | 39 | 50 | 238 | 4.2 | 498 | 40 | 0.14 | 0.12 | 1.2 | 0 |
| 523 | Peanuts, roasted in oil, salted (whole, halves, chopped), 1 c, 144 | 2 | 840 | 37 | 72 | 13.7 | 33.0 | 20.7 | 27 | 107 | 577 | 3.0 | 971 | — | 0.46 | 0.19 | 24.8 | 0 |
| 524 | Peanut butter, 1 tbsp, 16 | 2 | 95 | 4 | 8 | 1.5 | 3.7 | 2.3 | 3 | 9 | 61 | 0.3 | 100 | — | 0.02 | 0.02 | 2.4 | 0 |
| 525 | Peas, split, dry, cooked, 1 c, 200 | 70 | 230 | 16 | 1 | — | — | — | 42 | 22 | 178 | 3.4 | 592 | 80 | 0.30 | 0.18 | 1.8 | — |
| 526 | Pecans, chopped or pieces (about 120 large halves), 1 c, 118 | 3 | 810 | 11 | 84 | 7.2 | 50.5 | 20.0 | 17 | 86 | 341 | 2.8 | 712 | 150 | 1.01 | 0.15 | 1.1 | 2 |
| 527 | Pumpkin and squash kernels, dry, hulled, 1 c, 140 | 4 | 775 | 41 | 65 | 11.8 | 23.5 | 27.5 | 21 | 71 | 1602 | 15.7 | 1386 | 100 | 0.34 | 0.27 | 3.4 | — |
| 528 | Sunflower seeds, dry, hulled, 1 c, 145 | 5 | 810 | 35 | 69 | 8.2 | 13.7 | 43.2 | 29 | 174 | 1214 | 10.3 | 1334 | 70 | 2.84 | 0.33 | 7.8 | — |
| | **Walnuts** | | | | | | | | | | | | | | | | | |
| | **Black** | | | | | | | | | | | | | | | | | |
| 529 | Chopped or broken kernels, 1 c, 125 | 3 | 785 | 26 | 74 | 6.3 | 13.3 | 45.7 | 19 | tr | 713 | 7.5 | 575 | 380 | 0.28 | 0.14 | 0.9 | — |
| 530 | Ground (finely), 1 c, 80 | 3 | 500 | 16 | 47 | 4.0 | 8.5 | 29.2 | 12 | tr | 456 | 4.8 | 368 | 240 | 0.18 | 0.09 | 0.6 | — |
| 531 | Persian or English, chopped (about 60 halves), 1 c, 120 | 4 | 780 | 18 | 77 | 8.4 | 11.8 | 42.2 | 19 | 119 | 456 | 3.7 | 540 | 40 | 0.40 | 0.16 | 1.1 | 2 |

(Continued)

## Table 1. Nutritive Values of the Edible Part of Foods (Continued)

(Dashes (—) denote lack of reliable data for a constituent believed to be present in measurable amount)

| Item No. (A) | Foods, Approximate Measures, Units, and Weight (edible part unless footnotes indicate otherwise) (B) | | Water (C) | Food Energy (D) | Pro-tein (E) | Fat (F) | Fatty Acids Satu-rated (Total) (G) | Unsaturated Oleic (H) | Lino-leic (I) | Carbo-hydrate (J) | Calcium (K) | Phos-phorus (L) | Iron (M) | Potas-sium (N) | Vitamin A Value (O) | Thiamin (P) | Ribo-flavin (Q) | Niacin (R) | Ascorbic Acid (S) |
|---|---|---|---|---|---|---|---|---|---|---|---|---|---|---|---|---|---|---|---|
| | | g | Per-cent | Cal-ories | g | g | g | g | g | g | mg | mg | mg | mg | IU | mg | mg | mg | mg |
| *Sugars and Sweets* | | | | | | | | | | | | | | | | | | | |
| | Cake icings | | | | | | | | | | | | | | | | | | |
| | Boiled, white | | | | | | | | | | | | | | | | | | |
| 532 | Plain ............ 1 c ............ | 94 | 18 | 295 | 1 | 0 | 0 | 0 | 0 | 75 | 2 | 2 | tr | 17 | 0 | tr | 0.03 | tr | 0 |
| 533 | With coconut ....... 1 c ....... | 166 | 15 | 605 | 3 | 13 | 11.0 | 0.9 | tr | 124 | 10 | 50 | 0.8 | 277 | 0 | 0.02 | 0.07 | 0.3 | 0 |
| | Uncooked | | | | | | | | | | | | | | | | | | |
| 534 | Chocolate made with milk and butter 1 c ....... | 275 | 14 | 1035 | 9 | 38 | 23.4 | 11.7 | 1.0 | 185 | 165 | 305 | 3.3 | 536 | 580 | 0.06 | 0.28 | 0.6 | 1 |
| 535 | Creamy fudge from mix 1 c ... and water | 245 | 15 | 830 | 7 | 16 | 5.1 | 6.7 | 3.1 | 183 | 96 | 218 | 2.7 | 238 | tr | 0.05 | 0.20 | 0.7 | tr |
| 536 | White ............ 1 c ....... | 319 | 11 | 1200 | 2 | 21 | 12.7 | 5.1 | 0.5 | 260 | 48 | 38 | tr | 57 | 860 | tr | 0.06 | tr | tr |
| | Candy | | | | | | | | | | | | | | | | | | |
| 537 | Caramels, plain or 1 oz ... chocolate | 28 | 8 | 115 | 1 | 3 | 1.6 | 1.1 | 0.1 | 22 | 42 | 35 | 0.4 | 54 | tr | 0.01 | 0.05 | 0.1 | tr |
| | Chocolate | | | | | | | | | | | | | | | | | | |
| 538 | Milk, plain ......... 1 oz ... | 28 | 1 | 145 | 2 | 9 | 5.5 | 3.0 | 0.3 | 16 | 65 | 65 | 0.3 | 109 | 80 | 0.02 | 0.10 | 0.1 | tr |
| 539 | Semisweet, small pieces 1 c or 6-oz pkg (60 per oz) | 170 | 1 | 860 | 7 | 61 | 36.2 | 19.8 | 1.7 | 97 | 51 | 255 | 4.4 | 553 | 30 | 0.02 | 0.14 | 0.9 | 0 |
| 540 | Chocolate-coated peanuts 1 oz | 28 | 1 | 160 | 5 | 12 | 4.0 | 4.7 | 2.1 | 11 | 33 | 84 | 0.4 | 143 | tr | 0.10 | 0.05 | 2.1 | tr |
| 541 | Fondant, uncoated 1 oz (mints, candy corn, other) | 28 | 8 | 105 | tr | 1 | 0.1 | 0.3 | 0.1 | 25 | 4 | 2 | 0.3 | 1 | 0 | tr | tr | tr | 0 |
| 542 | Fudge, chocolate, plain 1 oz | 28 | 8 | 115 | 1 | 3 | 1.3 | 1.4 | 0.6 | 21 | 22 | 24 | 0.3 | 42 | tr | 0.01 | 0.03 | 0.1 | tr |
| 543 | Gum drops ......... 1 oz ... | 28 | 12 | 100 | tr | tr | — | — | — | 25 | 2 | tr | 0.1 | 1 | 0 | 0 | tr | tr | 0 |
| 544 | Hard ............ 1 oz ... | 28 | 1 | 110 | 0 | tr | — | — | — | 28 | 6 | 2 | 0.5 | 1 | 0 | 0 | 0 | 0 | 0 |
| 545 | Marshmallows ...... 1 oz ... | 28 | 17 | 90 | 1 | tr | — | — | — | 23 | 5 | 2 | 0.5 | 2 | 0 | 0 | tr | tr | 0 |
| | Chocolate-flavored beverage powders (about 4 heaping tsp per oz) | | | | | | | | | | | | | | | | | | |
| 546 | With non-fat dry milk .. 1 oz .. | 28 | 2 | 100 | 5 | 1 | 0.5 | 0.3 | tr | 20 | 167 | 155 | 0.5 | 227 | 10 | 0.04 | 0.21 | 0.2 | 1 |
| 547 | Without milk ....... 1 oz .... | 28 | 1 | 100 | 1 | 1 | 0.4 | 0.2 | tr | 25 | 9 | 48 | 0.6 | 142 | — | 0.01 | 0.03 | 0.1 | 0 |
| 548 | Honey, strained or 1 tbsp ... extracted | 21 | 17 | 65 | tr | 0 | 0 | 0 | 0 | 17 | 1 | 1 | 0.1 | 11 | 0 | tr | 0.01 | 0.1 | tr |
| 549 | Jams and preserves ..... 1 tbsp .. | 20 | 29 | 55 | tr | tr | — | — | — | 14 | 4 | 2 | 0.2 | 18 | tr | tr | 0.01 | tr | tr |
| 550 | 1 packet ....... | 14 | 29 | 40 | tr | tr | — | — | — | 10 | 3 | 1 | 0.1 | 12 | tr | tr | tr | tr | tr |
| 551 | Jellies ............ 1 tbsp ... | 18 | 29 | 50 | tr | tr | — | — | — | 13 | 4 | 1 | 0.3 | 14 | tr | tr | 0.01 | tr | 1 |
| 552 | 1 packet ....... | 14 | 29 | 40 | tr | tr | — | — | — | 10 | 3 | 1 | 0.2 | 11 | tr | tr | tr | tr | 1 |

| (A) | (B) | (C) | (D) | (E) | (F) | (G) | (H) | (I) | (J) | (K) | (L) | (M) | (N) | (O) | (P) | (Q) | (R) | (S) | (T) |
|---|---|---|---|---|---|---|---|---|---|---|---|---|---|---|---|---|---|---|---|
| | **Syrups** | | | | | | | | | | | | | | | | | | |
| | Chocolate-flavored syrup or topping | | | | | | | | | | | | | | | | | | |
| 553 | Thin type ............ 1 fl oz or 2 tbsp | 38 | 32 | 90 | 1 | 1 | 0.5 | 0.3 | tr | 24 | 6 | 35 | 0.6 | 106 | tr | 0.01 | 0.03 | 0.2 | 0 |
| 554 | Fudge type ......... 1 fl oz or 2 tbsp | 38 | 25 | 125 | 2 | 5 | 3.1 | 1.6 | 0.1 | 20 | 48 | 60 | 0.5 | 107 | 60 | 0.02 | 0.08 | 0.2 | tr |
| | Molasses, cane | | | | | | | | | | | | | | | | | | |
| 555 | Light (first extraction) ... 1 tbsp | 20 | 24 | 50 | — | — | — | — | — | 13 | 33 | 9 | 0.9 | 183 | — | 0.01 | 0.01 | tr | — |
| 556 | Blackstrap (third extraction) ... 1 tbsp | 20 | 24 | 45 | — | — | — | — | — | 11 | 137 | 17 | 3.2 | 585 | — | 0.02 | 0.04 | 0.4 | — |
| 557 | Sorghum ......... 1 tbsp | 21 | 23 | 55 | — | — | — | — | — | 14 | 35 | 5 | 2.6 | — | — | 0.02 | 0.02 | tr | — |
| 558 | Table blends, chiefly corn, light and dark ... 1 tbsp | 21 | 24 | 60 | 0 | 0 | 0 | 0 | 0 | 15 | 9 | 3 | 0.8 | 1 | 0 | 0 | 0 | 0 | 0 |
| | **Sugars** | | | | | | | | | | | | | | | | | | |
| 559 | Brown, pressed down .. 1 c | 220 | 2 | 820 | 0 | 0 | 0 | 0 | 0 | 212 | 187 | 42 | 7.5 | 757 | 0 | 0.02 | 0.07 | 0.4 | 0 |
| | White | | | | | | | | | | | | | | | | | | |
| 560 | Granulated ......... 1 c | 200 | 1 | 770 | 0 | 0 | 0 | 0 | 0 | 199 | 0 | 0 | 0.2 | 6 | 0 | 0 | 0 | 0 | 0 |
| 561 | Granulated ......... 1 tbsp | 12 | 1 | 45 | 0 | 0 | 0 | 0 | 0 | 12 | 0 | 0 | tr | tr | 0 | 0 | 0 | 0 | 0 |
| 562 | ......... 1 packet | 6 | 1 | 23 | 0 | 0 | 0 | 0 | 0 | 6 | 0 | 0 | tr | tr | 0 | 0 | 0 | 0 | 0 |
| 563 | Powdered, sifted, spooned into cup ... 1 c | 100 | 1 | 385 | 0 | 0 | 0 | 0 | 0 | 100 | 0 | 0 | 0.1 | 3 | 0 | 0 | 0 | 0 | 0 |
| | *Vegetable and Vegetable Products* | | | | | | | | | | | | | | | | | | |
| | Asparagus, green | | | | | | | | | | | | | | | | | | |
| | Cooked, drained | | | | | | | | | | | | | | | | | | |
| | Cuts and tips (1½″–2″ lengths) | | | | | | | | | | | | | | | | | | |
| 564 | From raw ......... 1 c | 145 | 94 | 30 | 3 | tr | — | — | — | 5 | 30 | 73 | 0.9 | 265 | 1310 | 0.23 | 0.26 | 2.0 | 38 |
| 565 | From frozen ......... 1 c | 180 | 93 | 40 | 6 | tr | — | — | — | 6 | 40 | 115 | 2.2 | 396 | 1530 | 0.25 | 0.23 | 1.8 | 41 |
| | Spears (½″ diam at base) | | | | | | | | | | | | | | | | | | |
| 566 | From raw ......... 4 spears | 60 | 94 | 10 | 1 | tr | — | — | — | 2 | 13 | 30 | 0.4 | 110 | 540 | 0.10 | 0.11 | 0.8 | 16 |
| 567 | From frozen ......... 4 spears | 60 | 92 | 15 | 2 | tr | — | — | — | 2 | 13 | 40 | 0.7 | 143 | 470 | 0.10 | 0.08 | 0.7 | 16 |
| 568 | Canned, spears (½″ diam at base) ... 4 spears | 80 | 93 | 15 | 2 | tr | — | — | — | 3 | 15 | 42 | 1.5 | 133 | 640 | 0.05 | 0.08 | 0.6 | 12 |
| | Beans | | | | | | | | | | | | | | | | | | |
| | Lima, immature seeds, frozen, cooked, drained | | | | | | | | | | | | | | | | | | |
| 569 | Thick-seeded types (Fordhooks) ... 1 c | 170 | 74 | 170 | 10 | tr | — | — | — | 32 | 34 | 153 | 2.9 | 724 | 390 | 0.12 | 0.09 | 1.7 | 29 |
| 570 | Thin-seeded types (baby limas) ... 1 c | 180 | 69 | 210 | 13 | tr | — | — | — | 40 | 63 | 227 | 4.7 | 709 | 400 | 0.16 | 0.09 | 2.2 | 22 |
| | Snap | | | | | | | | | | | | | | | | | | |
| | Green | | | | | | | | | | | | | | | | | | |
| | Cooked, drained | | | | | | | | | | | | | | | | | | |
| 571 | From raw (cuts and French style) ... 1 c | 125 | 92 | 30 | 2 | tr | — | — | — | 7 | 63 | 46 | 0.8 | 189 | 680 | 0.09 | 0.11 | 0.6 | 15 |

(Continued)

## Table 1. Nutritive Values of the Edible Part of Foods (Continued)

(Dashes (—) denote lack of reliable data for a constituent believed to be present in measurable amount)

| Item No. (A) | Foods, Approximate Measures, Units, and Weight (edible part unless footnotes indicate otherwise) (B) | Weight g | Water (C) Per-cent | Food Energy (D) Cal-ories | Pro-tein (E) g | Fat (F) g | Fatty Acids Satu-rated (Total) (G) g | Unsaturated Oleic (H) g | Lino-leic (I) g | Carbo-hydrate (J) g | Calcium (K) mg | Phos-phorus (L) mg | Iron (M) mg | Potas-sium (N) mg | Vitamin A Value (O) IU | Thiamin (P) mg | Ribo-flavin (Q) mg | Niacin (R) mg | Ascorbic Acid (S) mg |
|---|---|---|---|---|---|---|---|---|---|---|---|---|---|---|---|---|---|---|---|
| | *Vegetable and Vegetable Products (Continued)* | | | | | | | | | | | | | | | | | | |
| | Beans, snap, green, cooked, drained (Continued) | | | | | | | | | | | | | | | | | | |
| | From frozen | | | | | | | | | | | | | | | | | | |
| 572 | Cuts ... 1 c | 135 | 92 | 35 | 2 | tr | — | — | — | 8 | 54 | 43 | 0.9 | 205 | 780 | 0.09 | 0.12 | 0.5 | 7 |
| 573 | French style ... 1 c | 130 | 92 | 35 | 2 | tr | — | — | — | 8 | 49 | 39 | 1.2 | 177 | 690 | 0.08 | 0.10 | 0.4 | 9 |
| 574 | Canned, drained solids 1 c (cuts) | 135 | 92 | 30 | 2 | tr | — | — | — | 7 | 61 | 34 | 2.0 | 128 | 630 | 0.04 | 0.07 | 0.4 | 5 |
| | Yellow or wax | | | | | | | | | | | | | | | | | | |
| | Cooked, drained | | | | | | | | | | | | | | | | | | |
| 575 | From raw (cuts and French style) 1 c | 125 | 93 | 30 | 2 | tr | — | — | — | 6 | 63 | 46 | 0.8 | 189 | 290 | 0.09 | 0.11 | 0.6 | 16 |
| 576 | From frozen (cuts) .. 1 c | 135 | 92 | 35 | 2 | tr | — | — | — | 8 | 47 | 42 | 0.9 | 221 | 140 | 0.09 | 0.11 | 0.5 | 8 |
| 577 | Canned, drained solids 1 c (cuts) | 135 | 92 | 30 | 2 | tr | — | — | — | 7 | 61 | 34 | 2.0 | 128 | 140 | 0.04 | 0.07 | 0.4 | 7 |
| | Beans, mature (see Beans, dry, items 509–515, and Blackeye peas, dry, item 516) | | | | | | | | | | | | | | | | | | |
| | Bean sprouts (mung) | | | | | | | | | | | | | | | | | | |
| 578 | Raw ... 1 c | 105 | 89 | 35 | 4 | tr | — | — | — | 7 | 20 | 67 | 1.4 | 234 | 20 | 0.14 | 0.14 | 0.8 | 20 |
| 579 | Cooked, drained ... 1 c | 125 | 91 | 35 | 4 | tr | — | — | — | 7 | 21 | 60 | 1.1 | 195 | 30 | 0.11 | 0.13 | 0.9 | 8 |
| | Beets | | | | | | | | | | | | | | | | | | |
| | Cooked, drained, peeled | | | | | | | | | | | | | | | | | | |
| 580 | Whole beets (2" diam) 2 beets | 100 | 91 | 30 | 1 | tr | — | — | — | 7 | 14 | 23 | 0.5 | 208 | 20 | 0.03 | 0.04 | 0.3 | 6 |
| 581 | Diced or sliced ... 1 c | 170 | 91 | 55 | 2 | tr | — | — | — | 12 | 24 | 39 | 0.9 | 354 | 30 | 0.05 | 0.07 | 0.5 | 10 |
| | Canned, drained solids | | | | | | | | | | | | | | | | | | |
| 582 | Whole beets, small ... 1 c | 160 | 89 | 60 | 2 | tr | — | — | — | 14 | 30 | 29 | 1.1 | 267 | 30 | 0.02 | 0.05 | 0.2 | 5 |
| 583 | Diced or sliced ... 1 c | 170 | 89 | 65 | 2 | tr | — | — | — | 15 | 32 | 31 | 1.2 | 284 | 30 | 0.02 | 0.05 | 0.2 | 5 |
| 584 | Beet greens, leaves and stems, cooked, drained 1 c | 145 | 94 | 25 | 2 | tr | — | — | — | 5 | 144 | 36 | 2.8 | 481 | 7400 | 0.10 | 0.22 | 0.4 | 22 |
| | Blackeye peas, immature seeds, cooked and drained | | | | | | | | | | | | | | | | | | |
| 585 | From raw ... 1 c | 165 | 72 | 180 | 13 | 1 | — | — | — | 30 | 40 | 241 | 3.5 | 625 | 580 | 0.50 | 0.18 | 2.3 | 28 |
| 586 | From frozen ... 1 c | 170 | 66 | 220 | 15 | 1 | — | — | — | 40 | 43 | 286 | 4.8 | 573 | 290 | 0.68 | 0.19 | 2.4 | 15 |
| | Broccoli, cooked, drained | | | | | | | | | | | | | | | | | | |
| | From raw | | | | | | | | | | | | | | | | | | |
| 587 | Stalk, medium size ... 1 stalk | 180 | 91 | 45 | 6 | 1 | — | — | — | 8 | 158 | 112 | 1.4 | 481 | 4500 | 0.16 | 0.36 | 1.4 | 162 |
| 588 | Stalks cut into 1/2" pieces 1 c | 155 | 91 | 40 | 5 | tr | — | — | — | 7 | 136 | 96 | 1.2 | 414 | 3880 | 0.14 | 0.31 | 1.2 | 140 |
| | From frozen | | | | | | | | | | | | | | | | | | |
| 589 | Stalk (4 1/2"–5"long) ... 1 stalk | 30 | 91 | 10 | 1 | tr | — | — | — | 1 | 12 | 17 | 0.2 | 66 | 570 | 0.02 | 0.03 | 0.2 | 22 |

| (A) | (B) | | (C) | (D) | (E) | (F) | (G) | (H) | (I) | (J) | (K) | (L) | (M) | (N) | (O) | (P) | (Q) | (R) | (S) |
|---|---|---|---|---|---|---|---|---|---|---|---|---|---|---|---|---|---|---|---|
| 590 | Chopped | 1 c | 185 | 92 | 50 | 5 | 1 | — | — | 9 | 100 | 104 | 1.3 | 392 | 4810 | 0.11 | 0.22 | 0.9 | 105 |
| | Brussels sprouts, cooked, drained | | | | | | | | | | | | | | | | | | |
| 591 | From raw, 7–8 sprouts (1¼"–1½" diam) | 1 c | 155 | 88 | 55 | 7 | 1 | — | — | 10 | 50 | 112 | 1.7 | 423 | 810 | 0.12 | 0.22 | 1.2 | 135 |
| 592 | From frozen | 1 c | 155 | 89 | 50 | 5 | tr | — | — | 10 | 33 | 95 | 1.2 | 457 | 880 | 0.12 | 0.16 | 0.9 | 126 |
| | Cabbage | | | | | | | | | | | | | | | | | | |
| | Common varieties | | | | | | | | | | | | | | | | | | |
| | Raw | | | | | | | | | | | | | | | | | | |
| 593 | Coarsely shredded or sliced | 1 c | 70 | 92 | 15 | 1 | tr | — | — | 4 | 34 | 20 | 0.3 | 163 | 90 | 0.04 | 0.04 | 0.2 | 33 |
| 594 | Finely shredded or chopped | 1 c | 90 | 92 | 20 | 1 | tr | — | — | 5 | 44 | 26 | 0.4 | 210 | 120 | 0.05 | 0.05 | 0.3 | 42 |
| 595 | Cooked, drained | 1 c | 145 | 94 | 30 | 2 | tr | — | — | 6 | 64 | 29 | 0.4 | 236 | 190 | 0.06 | 0.06 | 0.4 | 48 |
| 596 | Red, raw, coarsely shredded or sliced | 1 c | 70 | 90 | 20 | 1 | tr | — | — | 5 | 29 | 25 | 0.6 | 188 | 30 | 0.06 | 0.04 | 0.3 | 43 |
| 597 | Savoy, raw, coarsely shredded or sliced | 1 c | 70 | 92 | 15 | 2 | tr | — | — | 3 | 47 | 38 | 0.6 | 188 | 140 | 0.04 | 0.06 | 0.2 | 39 |
| 598 | Cabbage, celery (also called pe-tsai or wongbok), raw, 1" pieces | 1 c | 75 | 95 | 10 | 1 | tr | — | — | 2 | 32 | 30 | 0.5 | 190 | 110 | 0.04 | 0.03 | 0.5 | 19 |
| 599 | Cabbage, white mustard (also called bokchoy or pakchoy), cooked, drained | 1 c | 170 | 95 | 25 | 2 | tr | — | — | 4 | 252 | 56 | 1.0 | 364 | 5270 | 0.07 | 0.14 | 1.2 | 26 |
| | Carrots | | | | | | | | | | | | | | | | | | |
| | Raw, without crowns and tips, scraped | | | | | | | | | | | | | | | | | | |
| 600 | Whole (7½" × 1⅛", or strips, 2½"–3"long) | 1 carrot or 18 strips | 72 | 88 | 30 | 1 | tr | — | — | 7 | 27 | 26 | 0.5 | 246 | 7930 | 0.04 | 0.04 | 0.4 | 6 |
| 601 | Grated | 1 c | 110 | 88 | 45 | 1 | tr | — | — | 11 | 41 | 40 | 0.8 | 375 | 12,100 | 0.07 | 0.06 | 0.7 | 9 |
| 602 | Cooked (crosswise cuts), drained | 1 c | 155 | 91 | 50 | 1 | tr | — | — | 11 | 51 | 48 | 0.9 | 344 | 16,280 | 0.08 | 0.08 | 0.8 | 9 |
| | Canned | | | | | | | | | | | | | | | | | | |
| 603 | Sliced, drained solids | 1 c | 155 | 91 | 45 | 1 | tr | — | — | 10 | 47 | 34 | 1.1 | 186 | 23,250 | 0.03 | 0.05 | 0.6 | 3 |
| 604 | Strained or junior (baby food) | 1 oz (1¾–2 tbsp) | 28 | 92 | 10 | tr | tr | — | — | 2 | 7 | 6 | 0.1 | 51 | 3690 | 0.01 | 0.01 | 0.1 | 1 |
| | Cauliflower | | | | | | | | | | | | | | | | | | |
| 605 | Raw, chopped | 1 c | 115 | 91 | 31 | 3 | tr | — | — | 6 | 29 | 64 | 1.3 | 339 | 70 | 0.13 | 0.12 | 0.8 | 90 |
| | Cooked, drained | | | | | | | | | | | | | | | | | | |
| 606 | From raw (flower buds) | 1 c | 125 | 93 | 30 | 3 | tr | — | — | 5 | 26 | 53 | 0.9 | 258 | 80 | 0.11 | 0.10 | 0.8 | 69 |
| 607 | From frozen (flowerets) | 1 c | 180 | 94 | 30 | 3 | tr | — | — | 6 | 31 | 68 | 0.9 | 373 | 50 | 0.07 | 0.09 | 0.7 | 74 |
| | Celery, Pascal type, raw | | | | | | | | | | | | | | | | | | |
| 608 | Stalk, large outer (8" × 1½" at root end) | 1 stalk | 40 | 94 | 5 | tr | tr | — | — | 2 | 16 | 11 | 0.1 | 136 | 110 | 0.01 | 0.01 | 0.1 | 4 |

(Continued)

## Table 1. Nutritive Values of the Edible Part of Foods (Continued)

(Dashes (—) denote lack of reliable data for a constituent believed to be present in measurable amount)

| Item No. (A) | Foods, Approximate Measures, Units, and Weight (edible part unless footnotes indicate otherwise) (B) | (g) | Water (C) Per-cent | Food Energy (D) Cal-ories | Pro-tein (E) g | Fat (F) g | Fatty Acids Satu-rated (Total) (G) g | Unsaturated Oleic (H) g | Linoleic (I) g | Carbo-hydrate (J) g | Calcium (K) mg | Phos-phorus (L) mg | Iron (M) mg | Potas-sium (N) mg | Vitamin A Value (O) IU | Thiamin (P) mg | Ribo-flavin (Q) mg | Niacin (R) mg | Ascorbic Acid (S) mg |
|---|---|---|---|---|---|---|---|---|---|---|---|---|---|---|---|---|---|---|---|
| | *Vegetable and Vegetable Products (Continued)* | | | | | | | | | | | | | | | | | | |
| | Celery, Pascal type, raw (Continued) | | | | | | | | | | | | | | | | | | |
| 609 | Pieces, diced ........ 1 c | 120 | 94 | 20 | 1 | tr | — | — | — | 5 | 47 | 34 | 0.4 | 409 | 320 | 0.04 | 0.04 | 0.4 | 11 |
| | Collards, cooked, drained | | | | | | | | | | | | | | | | | | |
| 610 | From raw (leaves without stems) 1 c | 190 | 90 | 65 | 7 | 1 | — | — | — | 10 | 357 | 99 | 1.5 | 498 | 14,820 | 0.21 | 0.38 | 2.3 | 144 |
| 611 | From frozen (chopped) 1 c | 170 | 90 | 50 | 5 | 1 | — | — | — | 10 | 299 | 87 | 1.7 | 401 | 11,560 | 0.10 | 0.24 | 1.0 | 56 |
| | Corn, sweet, Cooked, drained | | | | | | | | | | | | | | | | | | |
| 612 | From raw, ear (5" × 1¾") 1 ear[61] | 140 | 74 | 70 | 2 | 1 | — | — | — | 16 | 2 | 69 | 0.5 | 151 | 310[62] | 0.09 | 0.08 | 1.1 | 7 |
| | From frozen | | | | | | | | | | | | | | | | | | |
| 613 | Ear (5" long) 1 ear[61] | 229 | 73 | 120 | 4 | 1 | — | — | — | 27 | 4 | 121 | 1.0 | 291 | 440[62] | 0.18 | 0.10 | 2.1 | 9 |
| 614 | Kernels 1 c | 165 | 77 | 130 | 5 | 1 | — | — | — | 31 | 5 | 120 | 1.3 | 304 | 580[62] | 0.15 | 0.10 | 2.5 | 8 |
| | Canned | | | | | | | | | | | | | | | | | | |
| 615 | Cream style 1 c | 256 | 76 | 210 | 5 | 2 | — | — | — | 51 | 8 | 143 | 1.5 | 248 | 840[62] | 0.08 | 0.13 | 2.6 | 13 |
| | Whole kernel | | | | | | | | | | | | | | | | | | |
| 616 | Vacuum pack 1 c | 210 | 76 | 175 | 5 | 1 | — | — | — | 43 | 6 | 153 | 1.1 | 204 | 740[62] | 0.06 | 0.13 | 2.3 | 11 |
| 617 | Wet pack, drained solids 1 c | 165 | 76 | 140 | 4 | 1 | — | — | — | 33 | 8 | 81 | 0.8 | 160 | 580[62] | 0.05 | 0.08 | 1.5 | 7 |
| | Cowpeas (see Blackeye peas, Items 585–586) | | | | | | | | | | | | | | | | | | |
| | Cucumber slices, ⅛" thick (large, 2⅛" diam; small, 1¾" diam) | | | | | | | | | | | | | | | | | | |
| 618 | With peel .......... 6 large or 8 small slices | 28 | 95 | 5 | tr | tr | — | — | — | 1 | 7 | 8 | 0.3 | 45 | 70 | 0.01 | 0.01 | 0.1 | 3 |
| 619 | Without peel ......... 6½ large or 9 small pieces | 28 | 96 | 5 | tr | tr | — | — | — | 1 | 5 | 5 | 0.1 | 45 | tr | 0.01 | 0.01 | 0.1 | 3 |
| 620 | Dandelion greens, cooked, 1 c | 105 | 90 | 35 | 2 | 1 | — | — | — | 7 | 147 | 44 | 1.9 | 244 | 12,290 | 0.14 | 0.17 | — | 19 |
| 621 | Endive, curly (including escarole), raw, small pieces 1 c | 50 | 93 | 10 | 1 | tr | — | — | — | 2 | 41 | 27 | 0.9 | 147 | 1650 | 0.04 | 0.07 | 0.3 | 5 |
| | Kale, cooked, drained | | | | | | | | | | | | | | | | | | |
| 622 | From raw (leaves without stems and midribs) 1 c | 110 | 88 | 45 | 5 | 1 | — | — | — | 7 | 206 | 64 | 1.8 | 243 | 9130 | 0.11 | 0.20 | 1.8 | 102 |
| 623 | From frozen (leaf style) 1 c | 130 | 91 | 40 | 4 | 1 | — | — | — | 7 | 157 | 62 | 1.3 | 251 | 10,660 | 0.08 | 0.20 | 0.9 | 49 |

| (A) | (B) | | (C) | (D) | (E) | (F) | (G) | (H) | (I) | (J) | (K) | (L) | (M) | (N) | (O) | (P) | (Q) | (R) | (S) |
|---|---|---|---|---|---|---|---|---|---|---|---|---|---|---|---|---|---|---|---|
| | Lettuce, raw | | | | | | | | | | | | | | | | | | |
| | Butterhead, as Boston types | | | | | | | | | | | | | | | | | | |
| 624 | Head, 5" diam | 1 head[63] | 220 | 95 | 25 | 2 | tr | — | — | — | 4 | 57 | 42 | 3.3 | 430 | 1580 | 0.10 | 0.10 | 0.5 | 13 |
| 625 | Leaves | 1 outer, 2 inner, or 3 heart leaves | 15 | 95 | tr | tr | tr | — | — | — | tr | 5 | 4 | 0.3 | 40 | 150 | 0.01 | 0.01 | tr | 1 |
| | Crisphead, as Iceberg | | | | | | | | | | | | | | | | | | | |
| 626 | Head, 6" diam | 1 head[64] | 567 | 96 | 70 | 5 | 1 | — | — | — | 16 | 108 | 118 | 2.7 | 943 | 1780 | 0.32 | 0.32 | 1.6 | 32 |
| 627 | Wedge, ¼ of head | 1 wedge | 135 | 96 | 20 | 1 | tr | — | — | — | 4 | 27 | 30 | 0.7 | 236 | 450 | 0.08 | 0.08 | 0.4 | 8 |
| 628 | Pieces, chopped or shredded | 1 c | 55 | 96 | 5 | tr | tr | — | — | — | 2 | 11 | 12 | 0.3 | 96 | 180 | 0.03 | 0.03 | 0.2 | 3 |
| 629 | Looseleaf (bunching varieties including romaine or cos), chopped or shredded pieces | 1 c | 55 | 94 | 10 | 1 | tr | — | — | — | 2 | 37 | 14 | 0.8 | 145 | 1050 | 0.03 | 0.04 | 0.2 | 10 |
| 630 | Mushrooms, raw, sliced or chopped | 1 c | 70 | 90 | 20 | 2 | tr | — | — | — | 3 | 4 | 81 | 0.6 | 290 | tr | 0.07 | 0.32 | 2.9 | 2 |
| 631 | Mustard greens, without stems and midribs, cooked, drained | 1 c | 140 | 93 | 30 | 3 | 1 | — | — | — | 6 | 193 | 45 | 2.5 | 308 | 8120 | 0.11 | 0.20 | 0.8 | 67 |
| 632 | Okra pods (3" × ⅝"), cooked | 10 pods | 106 | 91 | 30 | 2 | tr | — | — | — | 6 | 98 | 43 | 0.5 | 184 | 520 | 0.14 | 0.19 | 1.0 | 21 |
| | Onions | | | | | | | | | | | | | | | | | | | |
| | Mature | | | | | | | | | | | | | | | | | | | |
| | Raw | | | | | | | | | | | | | | | | | | | |
| 633 | Chopped | 1 c | 170 | 89 | 65 | 3 | tr | — | — | — | 15 | 46 | 61 | 0.9 | 267 | tr[65] | 0.05 | 0.07 | 0.3 | 17 |
| 634 | Sliced | 1 c | 115 | 89 | 45 | 2 | tr | — | — | — | 10 | 31 | 41 | 0.6 | 181 | tr[65] | 0.03 | 0.05 | 0.2 | 12 |
| 635 | Cooked (whole or sliced), drained | 1 c | 210 | 92 | 60 | 3 | tr | — | — | — | 14 | 50 | 61 | 0.8 | 231 | tr[65] | 0.06 | 0.06 | 0.4 | 15 |
| 636 | Young green, bulb (⅜" diam) and white portion of top | 6 onions | 30 | 88 | 15 | tr | tr | — | — | — | 3 | 12 | 12 | 0.2 | 69 | tr | 0.02 | 0.01 | 0.1 | 8 |
| 637 | Parsley, raw, chopped | 1 tbsp | 4 | 85 | tr | tr | tr | — | — | — | tr | 7 | 2 | 0.2 | 25 | 300 | tr | 0.01 | tr | 6 |
| 638 | Parsnips, cooked (diced or 2" lengths) | 1 c | 155 | 82 | 100 | 2 | 1 | — | — | — | 23 | 70 | 96 | 0.9 | 587 | 50 | 0.11 | 0.12 | 0.2 | 16 |
| | Peas, green | | | | | | | | | | | | | | | | | | | |
| | Canned | | | | | | | | | | | | | | | | | | | |
| 639 | Whole, drained solids | 1 c | 170 | 77 | 150 | 8 | 1 | — | — | — | 29 | 44 | 129 | 3.2 | 163 | 1170 | 0.15 | 0.10 | 1.4 | 14 |
| 640 | Strained (baby food) | 1 oz (1¾ to 2 tbsp) | 28 | 86 | 15 | 1 | tr | — | — | — | 3 | 3 | 18 | 0.3 | 28 | 140 | 0.02 | 0.03 | 0.3 | 3 |
| 641 | Frozen, cooked, drained | 1 c | 160 | 82 | 110 | 8 | tr | — | — | — | 19 | 30 | 138 | 3.0 | 216 | 960 | 0.43 | 0.14 | 2.7 | 21 |
| 642 | Peppers, hot, red, without seeds, dried (ground chili powder, added seasonings) | 1 tsp | 2 | 9 | 5 | tr | tr | — | — | — | 1 | 5 | 4 | 0.3 | 20 | 1300 | tr | 0.02 | 0.2 | tr |
| | Peppers, sweet (about 5 per lb, whole), stem and seeds removed | | | | | | | | | | | | | | | | | | | |

(Continued)

# Table 1. Nutritive Values of the Edible Part of Foods (Continued)

(Dashes (—) denote lack of reliable data for a constituent believed to be present in measurable amount)

| Item No. (A) | Foods, Approximate Measures, Units, and Weight (edible part unless footnotes indicate otherwise) (B) | Weight g | Water Per-cent (C) | Food Energy Cal-ories (D) | Pro-tein g (E) | Fat g (F) | Fatty Acids Satu-rated (Total) g (G) | Unsaturated Oleic g (H) | Lino-leic g (I) | Carbo-hydrate g (J) | Calcium mg (K) | Phos-phorus mg (L) | Iron mg (M) | Potas-sium mg (N) | Vitamin A Value IU (O) | Thiamin mg (P) | Ribo-flavin mg (Q) | Niacin mg (R) | Ascorbic Acid mg (S) |
|---|---|---|---|---|---|---|---|---|---|---|---|---|---|---|---|---|---|---|---|
| | *Vegetable and Vegetable Products (Continued)* | | | | | | | | | | | | | | | | | | |
| | Peppers, sweet (Continued) | | | | | | | | | | | | | | | | | | |
| 643 | Raw ... 1 pod | 74 | 93 | 15 | 1 | tr | — | — | — | 4 | 7 | 16 | 0.5 | 157 | 310 | 0.06 | 0.06 | 0.4 | 94 |
| 644 | Cooked, boiled, drained ... 1 pod | 73 | 95 | 15 | 1 | tr | — | — | — | 3 | 7 | 12 | 0.4 | 109 | 310 | 0.05 | 0.05 | 0.4 | 70 |
| | Potatoes, cooked | | | | | | | | | | | | | | | | | | |
| 645 | Baked, peeled after baking (about 2 per lb, raw) ... 1 potato | 156 | 75 | 145 | 4 | tr | — | — | — | 33 | 14 | 101 | 1.1 | 782 | tr | 0.15 | 0.07 | 2.7 | 31 |
| | Boiled (about 3 per lb, raw) | | | | | | | | | | | | | | | | | | |
| 646 | Peeled after boiling ... 1 potato | 137 | 80 | 105 | 3 | tr | — | — | — | 23 | 10 | 72 | 0.8 | 556 | tr | 0.12 | 0.05 | 2.0 | 22 |
| 647 | Peeled before boiling ... 1 potato | 135 | 83 | 90 | 3 | tr | — | — | — | 20 | 8 | 57 | 0.7 | 385 | tr | 0.12 | 0.05 | 1.6 | 22 |
| | French-fried, strip (2 to 3½″ long) | | | | | | | | | | | | | | | | | | |
| 648 | Prepared from raw ... 10 strips | 50 | 45 | 135 | 2 | 7 | 1.7 | 1.2 | 3.3 | 18 | 8 | 56 | 0.7 | 427 | tr | 0.07 | 0.04 | 1.6 | 11 |
| 649 | Frozen, oven-heated ... 10 strips | 50 | 53 | 110 | 2 | 4 | 1.1 | 0.8 | 2.1 | 17 | 5 | 43 | 0.9 | 326 | tr | 0.07 | 0.01 | 1.3 | 11 |
| 650 | Hashed brown, prepared from frozen ... 1 c | 155 | 56 | 345 | 3 | 18 | 4.6 | 3.2 | 9.0 | 45 | 28 | 78 | 1.9 | 439 | tr | 0.11 | 0.03 | 1.6 | 12 |
| | Mashed, prepared from— | | | | | | | | | | | | | | | | | | |
| | Raw | | | | | | | | | | | | | | | | | | |
| 651 | Milk added ... 1 c | 210 | 83 | 135 | 4 | 2 | 0.7 | 0.4 | tr | 27 | 50 | 103 | 0.8 | 548 | 40 | 0.17 | 0.11 | 2.1 | 21 |
| 652 | Milk and butter added ... 1 c | 210 | 80 | 195 | 4 | 9 | 5.6 | 2.3 | 0.2 | 26 | 50 | 101 | 0.8 | 525 | 360 | 0.17 | 0.11 | 2.1 | 19 |
| 653 | Dehydrated flakes (without milk), water, milk, butter, and salt added ... 1 c | 210 | 79 | 195 | 4 | 7 | 3.6 | 2.1 | 0.2 | 30 | 65 | 99 | 0.6 | 601 | 270 | 0.08 | 0.08 | 1.9 | 11 |
| 654 | Potato chips (1¾″ × 2½″ oval cross section) ... 10 chips | 20 | 2 | 115 | 1 | 8 | 2.1 | 1.4 | 4.0 | 10 | 8 | 28 | 0.4 | 226 | tr | 0.04 | 0.01 | 1.0 | 3 |
| 655 | Potato salad, made with cooked salad dressing ... 1 c | 250 | 76 | 250 | 7 | 7 | 2.0 | 2.7 | 1.3 | 41 | 80 | 160 | 1.5 | 798 | 350 | 0.20 | 0.18 | 2.8 | 28 |
| 656 | Pumpkin, canned ... 1 c | 245 | 90 | 80 | 2 | 1 | — | — | — | 19 | 61 | 64 | 1.0 | 588 | 15,680 | 0.07 | 0.12 | 1.5 | 12 |
| 657 | Radishes, raw (prepackaged) stem ends, rootlets cut off ... 4 radishes | 18 | 95 | 5 | tr | tr | — | — | — | 1 | 5 | 6 | 0.2 | 58 | tr | 0.01 | 0.01 | 0.1 | 5 |
| 658 | Sauerkraut, canned, solids and liquid ... 1 c | 235 | 93 | 40 | 2 | tr | — | — | — | 9 | 85 | 42 | 1.2 | 329 | 120 | 0.07 | 0.09 | 0.5 | 33 |
| | Southern peas (see Blackeye peas, items 585–586) | | | | | | | | | | | | | | | | | | |

| (A) | (B) | (C) | (D) | (E) | (F) | (G) | (H) | (I) | (J) | (K) | (L) | (M) | (N) | (O) | (P) | (Q) | (R) | (S) |
|---|---|---|---|---|---|---|---|---|---|---|---|---|---|---|---|---|---|---|
| | **Spinach** | | | | | | | | | | | | | | | | | |
| 659 | Raw, chopped ........ 1 c | 55 | 15 | 2 | tr | — | — | — | 2 | 51 | 28 | 1.7 | 259 | 4460 | 0.06 | 0.11 | 0.3 | 28 |
| | Cooked, drained | | | | | | | | | | | | | | | | | |
| 660 | From raw ......... 1 c | 180 | 40 | 5 | 1 | — | — | — | 6 | 167 | 68 | 4.0 | 583 | 14,580 | 0.13 | 0.25 | 0.9 | 50 |
| | From frozen | | | | | | | | | | | | | | | | | |
| 661 | Chopped ........ 1 c | 205 | 45 | 6 | 1 | — | — | — | 8 | 232 | 90 | 4.3 | 683 | 16,200 | 0.14 | 0.31 | 0.8 | 39 |
| 662 | Leaf .......... 1 c | 190 | 45 | 6 | 1 | — | — | — | 7 | 200 | 84 | 4.8 | 688 | 15,390 | 0.15 | 0.27 | 1.0 | 53 |
| 663 | Canned, drained solids 1 c | 205 | 50 | 6 | 1 | — | — | — | 7 | 242 | 53 | 5.3 | 513 | 16,400 | 0.04 | 0.25 | 0.6 | 29 |
| | Squash, cooked | | | | | | | | | | | | | | | | | |
| 664 | Summer (all varieties), diced, drained ........ 1 c | 210 | 30 | 2 | tr | — | — | — | 7 | 53 | 53 | 0.8 | 296 | 820 | 0.11 | 0.17 | 1.7 | 21 |
| 665 | Winter (all varieties), baked, mashed ....... 1 c | 205 | 130 | 4 | 1 | — | — | — | 32 | 57 | 98 | 1.6 | 945 | 8610 | 0.10 | 0.27 | 1.4 | 27 |
| | Sweet potatoes | | | | | | | | | | | | | | | | | |
| | Cooked (raw, 5" × 2"; about 2½ per lb) | | | | | | | | | | | | | | | | | |
| 666 | Baked in skin, peeled .. 1 potato | 114 | 160 | 2 | 1 | — | — | — | 37 | 46 | 66 | 1.0 | 342 | 9230 | 0.10 | 0.08 | 0.8 | 25 |
| 667 | Boiled in skin, peeled .. 1 potato | 151 | 170 | 3 | 1 | — | — | — | 40 | 48 | 71 | 1.1 | 367 | 11,940 | 0.14 | 0.09 | 0.9 | 26 |
| 668 | Candied, 2½" × 2" piece .. 1 piece | 105 | 175 | 1 | 3 | 2.0 | 0.8 | 0.1 | 36 | 39 | 45 | 0.9 | 200 | 6620 | 0.06 | 0.04 | 0.4 | 11 |
| | Canned | | | | | | | | | | | | | | | | | |
| 669 | Solid pack (mashed) .. 1 c | 255 | 275 | 5 | 1 | — | — | — | 63 | 64 | 105 | 2.0 | 510 | 19,890 | 0.13 | 0.10 | 1.5 | 36 |
| 670 | Vacuum pack, piece (2¾" × 1") ...... 1 piece | 40 | 45 | 1 | tr | — | — | — | 10 | 10 | 16 | 0.3 | 80 | 3120 | 0.02 | 0.02 | 0.2 | 6 |
| | Tomatoes | | | | | | | | | | | | | | | | | |
| 671 | Raw (2⅗" diam, 3 per 12 oz pkg) ..... 1 tomato[66] | 135 | 25 | 1 | tr | — | — | — | 6 | 16 | 33 | 0.6 | 300 | 1110 | 0.07 | 0.05 | 0.9 | 28[67] |
| 672 | Canned, solids and liquid 1 c | 241 | 50 | 2 | tr | — | — | — | 10 | 14[68] | 46 | 1.2 | 523 | 2170 | 0.12 | 0.07 | 1.7 | 41 |
| 673 | Tomato catsup ...... 1 c | 273 | 290 | 5 | 1 | — | — | — | 69 | 60 | 137 | 2.2 | 991 | 3820 | 0.25 | 0.19 | 4.4 | 41 |
| 674 | ............... 1 tbsp | 15 | 15 | tr | tr | — | — | — | 4 | 3 | 8 | 0.1 | 54 | 210 | 0.01 | 0.01 | 0.2 | 2 |
| | Tomato juice, canned | | | | | | | | | | | | | | | | | |
| 675 | Cup .......... 1 c | 243 | 45 | 2 | tr | — | — | — | 10 | 17 | 44 | 2.2 | 552 | 1940 | 0.12 | 0.07 | 1.9 | 39 |
| 676 | Glass (6 fl oz) ...... 1 glass | 182 | 35 | 2 | tr | — | — | — | 8 | 13 | 33 | 1.6 | 413 | 1460 | 0.09 | 0.05 | 1.5 | 29 |
| 677 | Turnips, cooked, diced .. 1 c | 155 | 35 | 1 | tr | — | — | — | 8 | 54 | 37 | 0.6 | 291 | tr | 0.06 | 0.08 | 0.5 | 34 |
| | Turnip greens, cooked, drained | | | | | | | | | | | | | | | | | |
| 678 | From raw (leaves and stems) ......... 1 c | 145 | 30 | 3 | tr | — | — | — | 5 | 252 | 49 | 1.5 | — | 8270 | 0.15 | 0.33 | 0.7 | 68 |
| 679 | From frozen (chopped) .. 1 c | 165 | 40 | 4 | tr | — | — | — | 6 | 195 | 64 | 2.6 | 246 | 11,390 | 0.08 | 0.15 | 0.7 | 31 |
| 680 | Vegetables, mixed, frozen, cooked ....... 1 c | 182 | 115 | 6 | 1 | — | — | — | 24 | 46 | 115 | 2.4 | 348 | 9010 | 0.22 | 0.13 | 2.0 | 15 |

*Miscellaneous Items*

Baking powders for home
  use
Sodium aluminum
  sulfate

(Continued)

## Table 1. Nutritive Values of the Edible Part of Foods (Continued)

(Dashes (—) denote lack of reliable data for a constituent believed to be present in measurable amount)

| Item No. (A) | Foods, Approximate Measures, Units, and Weight (edible part unless footnotes indicate otherwise) (B) | Weight g | Water (C) Per-cent | Food Energy (D) Cal-ories | Pro-tein (E) g | Fat (F) g | Fatty Acids Satu-rated (Total) (G) g | Unsaturated Oleic (H) g | Lino-leic (I) g | Carbo-hydrate (J) g | Calcium (K) mg | Phos-phorus (L) mg | Iron (M) mg | Potas-sium (N) mg | Vitamin A Value (O) IU | Thiamin (P) mg | Ribo-flavin (Q) mg | Niacin (R) mg | Ascorbic Acid (S) mg |
|---|---|---|---|---|---|---|---|---|---|---|---|---|---|---|---|---|---|---|---|
| | *Miscellaneous Items (Continued)* | | | | | | | | | | | | | | | | | | |
| | Baking powders for home use (Continued) | | | | | | | | | | | | | | | | | | |
| 681 | With monocalcium phosphate monohydrate      1 tsp | 3.0 | 2 | 5 | tr | tr | 0 | 0 | 0 | 1 | 58 | 87 | — | 5 | 0 | 0 | 0 | 0 | 0 |
| 682 | With monocalcium phosphate monohydrate, calcium sulfate      1 tsp | 2.9 | 1 | 5 | tr | tr | 0 | 0 | 0 | 1 | 183 | 45 | — | — | 0 | 0 | 0 | 0 | 0 |
| 683 | Straight phosphate      1 tsp | 3.8 | 2 | 5 | tr | tr | 0 | 0 | 0 | 1 | 239 | 359 | — | 6 | 0 | 0 | 0 | 0 | 0 |
| 684 | Low-sodium      1 tsp | 4.3 | 2 | 5 | tr | tr | 0 | 0 | 0 | 2 | 207 | 314 | — | 471 | 0 | 0 | 0 | 0 | 0 |
| 685 | Barbecue sauce      1 c | 250 | 81 | 230 | 4 | 17 | 2.2 | 4.3 | 10.0 | 20 | 53 | 50 | 2.0 | 435 | 900 | 0.03 | 0.03 | 0.8 | 13 |
| 686 | Beverages, alcoholic Beer      12 fl oz | 360 | 92 | 150 | 1 | 0 | 0 | 0 | 0 | 14 | 18 | 108 | tr | 90 | — | 0.01 | 0.11 | 2.2 | — |
| | Gin, rum, vodka, whisky | | | | | | | | | | | | | | | | | | |
| 687 | 80-proof      1½-fl oz jigger | 42 | 67 | 95 | — | — | — | 0 | 0 | tr | — | — | — | 1 | — | — | — | — | — |
| 688 | 86-proof      1½-fl oz jigger | 42 | 64 | 105 | — | — | — | 0 | 0 | tr | — | — | — | 1 | — | — | — | — | — |
| 689 | 90-proof      1½-fl oz jigger | 42 | 62 | 110 | — | — | — | 0 | 0 | tr | — | — | — | 1 | — | — | — | — | — |
| | Wines | | | | | | | | | | | | | | | | | | |
| 690 | Dessert      3½-fl oz glass | 103 | 77 | 140 | tr | 0 | 0 | 0 | 0 | 8 | 8 | — | — | 77 | — | 0.01 | 0.02 | 0.2 | — |
| 691 | Table      3½-fl oz glass | 102 | 86 | 85 | tr | 0 | 0 | 0 | 0 | 4 | 9 | 10 | 0.4 | 94 | — | tr | 0.01 | 0.1 | — |
| | Beverages, carbonated, sweetened, nonalcoholic | | | | | | | | | | | | | | | | | | |
| 692 | Carbonated water      12 fl oz | 366 | 92 | 115 | 0 | 0 | 0 | 0 | 0 | 29 | — | — | — | — | 0 | 0 | 0 | 0 | 0 |
| 693 | Cola-type      12 fl oz | 369 | 90 | 145 | 0 | 0 | 0 | 0 | 0 | 37 | — | — | — | — | 0 | 0 | 0 | 0 | 0 |
| 694 | Fruit-flavored sodas and Tom Collins mixer      12 fl oz | 372 | 88 | 170 | 0 | 0 | 0 | 0 | 0 | 45 | — | — | — | — | 0 | 0 | 0 | 0 | 0 |
| 695 | Ginger ale      12 fl oz | 366 | 92 | 115 | 0 | 0 | 0 | 0 | 0 | 29 | — | — | — | 0 | 0 | 0 | 0 | 0 | 0 |
| 696 | Root beer      12 fl oz | 370 | 90 | 150 | 0 | 0 | 0 | 0 | 0 | 39 | — | — | — | 0 | 0 | 0 | 0 | 0 | 0 |
| | Chili powder (see Peppers, hot, red, item 642) | | | | | | | | | | | | | | | | | | |
| | Chocolate | | | | | | | | | | | | | | | | | | |
| 697 | Bitter or baking      1 oz | 28 | 2 | 145 | 3 | 15 | 8.9 | 4.9 | 0.4 | 8 | 22 | 109 | 1.9 | 235 | 20 | 0.01 | 0.07 | 0.4 | 0 |
| | Semisweet (see Candy, chocolate, item 539) | | | | | | | | | | | | | | | | | | |
| 698 | Gelatin, dry      1 7-g envelope | 7 | 13 | 25 | 6 | tr | 0 | 0 | 0 | 0 | — | — | — | — | — | — | — | — | — |
| 699 | Gelatin dessert prepared with gelatin dessert powder and water      1 c | 240 | 84 | 140 | 4 | 0 | 0 | 0 | 0 | 34 | — | — | — | — | — | — | — | — | — |
| 700 | Mustard, prepared, yellow      1 tsp or individual serving pouch or cup | 5 | 80 | 5 | tr | tr | — | — | — | tr | 4 | 4 | 0.1 | 7 | — | — | — | — | — |

| (A) | (B) | (weight, g) | (C) | (D) | (E) | (F) | (G) | (H) | (I) | (J) | (K) | (L) | (M) | (N) | (O) | (P) | (Q) | (R) | (S) |
|---|---|---|---|---|---|---|---|---|---|---|---|---|---|---|---|---|---|---|---|
| | Olives, pickled, canned | | | | | | | | | | | | | | | | | | |
| 701 | Green ........ 4 medium, 3 extra large, or 2 giant[69] | 16 | 78 | 15 | tr | 2 | 0.2 | 1.2 | 0.1 | tr | 8 | 2 | 0.2 | 7 | 40 | — | — | — | — |
| 702 | Ripe, Mission ......... 3 small or 2 large[69] | 10 | 73 | 15 | tr | 2 | 0.2 | 1.2 | 0.1 | tr | 9 | 1 | 0.1 | 2 | 10 | tr | tr | — | — |
| | Pickles, cucumber | | | | | | | | | | | | | | | | | | |
| 703 | Dill, medium, whole (3¾" long, 1¼" diam) ........ 1 pickle | 65 | 93 | 5 | tr | tr | — | — | — | 1 | 17 | 14 | 0.7 | 130 | 70 | 0.01 | tr | tr | 4 |
| 704 | Fresh-pack, slices (1½" diam, ¼" thick) ........ 2 slices | 15 | 79 | 10 | tr | tr | — | — | — | 3 | 5 | 4 | 0.3 | — | 20 | tr | tr | tr | 1 |
| 705 | Sweet, gherkin, small, whole (about 2½" long, ¾" diam) ........ 1 pickle | 15 | 61 | 20 | tr | tr | — | — | — | 5 | 2 | 2 | 0.2 | — | 10 | tr | tr | tr | 1 |
| 706 | Relish, finely chopped, sweet ........ 1 tbsp | 15 | 63 | 20 | tr | tr | — | — | — | 5 | 3 | 2 | 0.1 | — | — | — | — | — | — |
| | Popcorn (see items 476–478) | | | | | | | | | | | | | | | | | | |
| 707 | Popsicle, 3-fl oz size ..... 1 popsicle | 95 | 80 | 70 | 0 | 0 | 0 | 0 | 0 | 18 | 0 | — | — | — | 0 | 0 | 0 | 0 | 0 |
| | Soups | | | | | | | | | | | | | | | | | | |
| | Canned, condensed | | | | | | | | | | | | | | | | | | |
| | Prepared with equal volume of milk | | | | | | | | | | | | | | | | | | |
| 708 | Cream of chicken ..... 1 c | 245 | 85 | 180 | 7 | 10 | 4.2 | 3.6 | 1.3 | 15 | 172 | 152 | 0.5 | 260 | 610 | 0.05 | 0.27 | 0.7 | 2 |
| 709 | Cream of mushroom ..... 1 c | 245 | 83 | 215 | 7 | 14 | 5.4 | 2.9 | 4.6 | 16 | 191 | 169 | 0.5 | 279 | 250 | 0.05 | 0.34 | 0.7 | 1 |
| 710 | Tomato ..... 1 c | 250 | 84 | 175 | 7 | 7 | 3.4 | 1.7 | 1.0 | 23 | 168 | 155 | 0.8 | 418 | 1200 | 0.10 | 0.25 | 1.3 | 15 |
| | Prepared with equal volume of water | | | | | | | | | | | | | | | | | | |
| 711 | Bean with pork ..... 1 c | 250 | 84 | 170 | 8 | 6 | 1.2 | 1.8 | 2.4 | 22 | 63 | 128 | 2.3 | 395 | 650 | 0.13 | 0.08 | 1.0 | 3 |
| 712 | Beef broth, bouillon, consommé ..... 1 c | 240 | 96 | 30 | 5 | 0 | 0 | 0 | 0 | 3 | tr | 31 | 0.5 | 130 | tr | tr | 0.02 | 1.2 | — |
| 713 | Beef noodle ..... 1 c | 240 | 93 | 65 | 4 | 3 | 0.6 | 0.7 | 0.8 | 7 | 7 | 48 | 1.0 | 77 | 50 | 0.05 | 0.07 | 1.0 | tr |
| 714 | Clam chowder, Manhattan-type (with tomatoes, without milk) ..... 1 c | 245 | 92 | 80 | 2 | 3 | 0.5 | 0.4 | 1.3 | 12 | 34 | 47 | 1.0 | 184 | 880 | 0.02 | 0.02 | 1.0 | — |
| 715 | Cream of chicken ..... 1 c | 240 | 92 | 95 | 3 | 6 | 1.6 | 2.3 | 1.1 | 8 | 24 | 34 | 0.5 | 79 | 410 | 0.02 | 0.05 | 0.5 | tr |
| 716 | Cream of mushroom ..... 1 c | 240 | 90 | 135 | 2 | 10 | 2.6 | 1.7 | 4.5 | 10 | 41 | 50 | 0.5 | 98 | 70 | 0.02 | 0.12 | 0.7 | tr |
| 717 | Minestrone ..... 1 c | 245 | 90 | 105 | 5 | 3 | 0.7 | 0.9 | 1.3 | 14 | 37 | 59 | 1.0 | 314 | 2350 | 0.07 | 0.05 | 1.0 | — |
| 718 | Split pea ..... 1 c | 245 | 85 | 145 | 9 | 3 | 1.1 | 1.2 | 0.4 | 21 | 29 | 149 | 1.5 | 270 | 440 | 0.25 | 0.15 | 1.5 | 1 |
| 719 | Tomato ..... 1 c | 245 | 91 | 90 | 2 | 3 | 0.5 | 0.5 | 1.0 | 16 | 15 | 34 | 0.7 | 230 | 1000 | 0.05 | 0.05 | 1.2 | 12 |
| 720 | Vegetable beef ..... 1 c | 245 | 92 | 80 | 5 | 2 | — | — | — | 10 | 12 | 49 | 0.7 | 162 | 2700 | 0.05 | 0.05 | 1.0 | — |
| 721 | Vegetarian ..... 1 c | 245 | 92 | 80 | 2 | 2 | — | — | — | 13 | 20 | 39 | 1.0 | 172 | 2940 | 0.05 | 0.05 | 1.0 | — |
| | Dehydrated | | | | | | | | | | | | | | | | | | |
| 722 | Bouillon cube (½") ..... 1 cube | 4 | 4 | 5 | 1 | tr | — | — | — | tr | — | — | — | 4 | — | — | — | — | — |
| | Mixes | | | | | | | | | | | | | | | | | | |
| | Unprepared | | | | | | | | | | | | | | | | | | |
| 723 | Onion ............ 1½-oz pkg | 43 | 3 | 150 | 6 | 5 | 1.1 | 2.3 | 1.0 | 23 | 42 | 49 | 0.6 | 238 | 30 | 0.05 | 0.03 | 0.3 | 6 |

(Continued)

# Table 1. Nutritive Values of the Edible Part of Foods (Continued)

(Dashes (—) denote lack of reliable data for a constituent believed to be present in measurable amount)

| Item No. (A) | Foods, Approximate Measures, Units, and Weight (edible part unless footnotes indicate otherwise) (B) | Weight (g) | Water Per-cent (C) | Food Energy Cal-ories (D) | Pro-tein g (E) | Fat g (F) | Fatty Acids Satu-rated (Total) g (G) | Unsaturated Oleic g (H) | Lino-leic g (I) | Carbo-hydrate g (J) | Calcium mg (K) | Phos-phorus mg (L) | Iron mg (M) | Potas-sium mg (N) | Vitamin A Value IU (O) | Thiamin mg (P) | Ribo-flavin mg (Q) | Niacin mg (R) | Ascorbic Acid mg (S) |
|---|---|---|---|---|---|---|---|---|---|---|---|---|---|---|---|---|---|---|---|
| *Miscellaneous Items (Continued)* | | | | | | | | | | | | | | | | | | | |
| | Soups, dehydrated, mixes (Continued) | | | | | | | | | | | | | | | | | | |
| | Prepared with water | | | | | | | | | | | | | | | | | | |
| 724 | Chicken noodle ..... 1 c | 240 | 95 | 55 | 2 | 1 | 1 | — | — | 8 | 7 | 19 | 0.2 | 19 | 50 | 0.07 | 0.05 | 0.5 | tr |
| 725 | Onion ..... 1 c | 240 | 96 | 35 | 1 | 1 | 1 | — | — | 6 | 10 | 12 | 0.2 | 58 | tr | tr | tr | tr | 2 |
| 726 | Tomato vegetable with noodles ..... 1 c | 240 | 93 | 65 | 1 | 1 | 1 | — | — | 12 | 7 | 19 | 0.2 | 29 | 480 | 0.05 | 0.02 | 0.5 | 5 |
| 727 | Vinegar, cider ..... 1 tbsp | 15 | 94 | tr | tr | 0 | 0 | 0 | 0 | 1 | 1 | 1 | 0.1 | 15 | — | — | — | — | — |
| 728 | White sauce, medium, with enriched flour ..... 1 c | 250 | 73 | 405 | 10 | 31 | 19.3 | 7.8 | 0.8 | 22 | 288 | 233 | 0.5 | 348 | 1150 | 0.12 | 0.43 | 0.7 | 2 |
| | Yeast | | | | | | | | | | | | | | | | | | |
| 729 | Baker's, dry, active ..... 1 pkg | 7 | 5 | 20 | 3 | tr | — | — | — | 3 | 3 | 90 | 1.1 | 140 | tr | 0.16 | 0.38 | 2.6 | tr |
| 730 | Brewer's, dry ..... 1 tbsp | 8 | 5 | 25 | 3 | tr | — | — | — | 3 | 17[70] | 140 | 1.4 | 152 | tr | 1.25 | 0.34 | 3.0 | tr |

## Footnotes to table 1

[1] Vitamin A value is largely from beta-carotene used for coloring. Riboflavin value for items 40–41 applies to products with added riboflavin.

[2] Applies to product without added vitamin A. With added vitamin A, value is 500 International Units (IU).

[3] Applies to product without vitamin A added.

[4] Applies to product with added vitamin A. Without added vitamin A, value is 20 IU.

[5] Yields 1 qt fluid milk when reconstituted according to package directions.

[6] Applies to product with added vitamin A.

[7] Weight applies to product with label claim of 1⅓ cups equal 3.2 oz.

[8] Applies to products made from thick shake mixes and those that do not contain added ice cream. Products made from milk shake mixes are higher in fat and usually contain added ice cream.

[9] Content of fat, vitamin A, and carbohydrate varies. Consult the label when precise values are needed for special diets.

[10] Applies to product made with milk containing no added vitamin A.

[11] Based on year-round average.

[12] Based on average vitamin A content of fortified margarine. Federal specifications for fortified margarine require a minimum of 15,000 IU vitamin A per pound.

[13] Fatty acid values apply to product made with regular-type margarine.

[14] Dipped in egg, milk or water, and breadcrumbs; fried in vegetable shortening.

[15] If bones are discarded, value for calcium will be greatly reduced.

[16] Dipped in egg, breadcrumbs, and flour or batter.

[17] Prepared with tuna, celery, salad dressing (mayonnaise type), pickle, onion, and egg.

[18] Outer layer of fat on the cut was removed to within approximately ½″ of the lean. Deposits of fat within the cut were not removed.

[19] Crust made with vegetable shortening and enriched flour.

[20] Regular-type margarine used.

[21] Value varies widely.

[22] About one-fourth of the outer layer of fat on the cut was removed. Deposits of fat within the cut were not removed.

[23] Vegetable shortening used.

[24] Also applies to pasteurized apple cider.

[25] Applies to product without added ascorbic acid. For value of product with added ascorbic acid, refer to label.

[26] Based on product with label claim of 45% of U.S. RDA in 6 fl oz.

[27] Based on product with label claim of 100% of U.S. RDA in 6 fl oz.

[28] Weight includes peel and membranes between sections. Without these parts the weight of the edible portion is 123 g for item 246 and 118 g for item 247.

[29] For white-fleshed varieties, value is about 20 IU per cup; for red-fleshed varieties, 1080 IU.

[30] Weight includes seeds. Without seeds, weight of the edible portion is 57 g.

[31] Applies to product without added ascorbic acid. With added ascorbic acid, based on claim that 6 fl oz of reconstituted juice contains 45% or 50% of the U.S. RDA, value is 108 mg or 120 mg for a 6-fl oz can (item 258), 36 or 40 for 1 cup of diluted juice (item 259).

[32] For products with added thiamin and riboflavin but without added ascorbic acid, values would.. be 0.60 mg for thiamin, 0.80 mg for riboflavin, and trace for ascorbic acid. For products with only ascorbic acid added, value varies with the brand. Consult the label.

[33] Weight includes rind. Without rind, the weight of the edible portion is 272 g for item 271 and 149 g for item 272.

[34] Represents yellow-fleshed varieties. For white-fleshed varieties, value is 50 IU for 1 peach, 90 IU for 1 cup of slices.

[35] Value represents products with added ascorbic acid. For products without added ascorbic acid, value is 116 mg for a 10-oz container, 103 mg for 1 cup.

[36] Weight includes pits. After removal of the pits, the weight of the edible portion is 258 g for item 302, 133 g for item 303, 43 g for item 304, and 213 g for item 305.

[37] Weight includes rind and seeds. Without rind and seeds, weight of the edible portion is 426 g.

[38] Made with vegetable shortening.

[39] Applies to product made with white cornmeal. With yellow cornmeal, value is 30 IU.

[40] Applies to white varieties. For yellow varieties, value is 150 IU.

[41] Applies to products that do not contain disodium phosphate. If disodium phosphate is an ingredient, value is 162 mg.

[42] Value may range from less than 1 mg to about 8 mg depending on the brand. Consult the label.

[43] Applies to product with added nutrient. Without added nutrient, value is trace.

[44] Value varies with the brand. Consult the label.

[45] Applies to product with added nutrient. Without added nutrient, value is trace.

[46] Excepting angelfood cake, cakes were made from mixes containing vegetable shortening; icings, with butter.

[47] Excepting spongecake, vegetable shortening was used for cake portion; butter, for icing. If butter or margarine was used for cake portion, vitamin A values would be higher.

[48] Applies to product made with a sodium aluminum-sulfate type baking powder. With a low-sodium-type baking powder containing potassium, value would be about twice the amount shown.

[49] Equal weights of flour, sugar, eggs, and vegetable shortening.

[50] Products are commercial unless otherwise specified.

[51] Made with enriched flour and vegetable shortening except for macaroons, which do not contain flour or shortening.

[52] Icing made with butter.

[53] Applies to yellow varieties; white varieties contain only a trace.

[54] Contains vegetable shortening and butter.

[55] Made with corn oil.

[56] Made with regular margarine.

[57] Applies to product made with yellow cornmeal.

[58] Made with enriched degermed cornmeal and enriched flour.

[59] Product may or may not be enriched with riboflavin. Consult the label.

[60] Value varies with the brand. Consult the label.

[61] Weight includes cob. Without cob, weight is 77 g for item 612, 126 g for item 613.

[62] Based on yellow varieties. For white varieties, value is trace.

[63] Weight includes refuse of outer leaves and core. Without these parts, weight is 163 g.

[64] Weight includes core. Without core, weight is 539 g.

[65] Value based on white-fleshed varieties. For yellow-fleshed varieties, value is 70 IU for item 633, 50 IU for item 634, and 80 IU for item 635.

[66] Weight includes cores and stem ends. Without these parts, weight is 123 g.

[67] Based on year-round average. For tomatoes marketed from November through May, value is about 12 mg, from June through October, 32 mg.

[68] Applies to product without calcium salts added. Value for products with calcium salts added may be as much as 63 mg for whole tomatoes, 241 mg for cut forms.

[69] Weight includes pits. Without pits, weight is 13 g for item 701, 9 g for item 702.

[70] Value may vary from 6 to 60 mg.

(From USDA Home and Garden Bulletin No. 72. Washington, DC, 1981)

## Table 2. Cholesterol in Common Foods (Amount in 100-g Edible Portion)

| Item and Description | Total Fat g | Cholesterol mg | Item and Description | Total Fat g | Cholesterol mg |
|---|---|---|---|---|---|
| Bacon, broiled or fried | 52.0 | 100 | Eggnog | 7.5 | 59 |
| Beef, raw | | | Frankfurter | | |
|   Chuck | 31.4 | 70 |   Beef | 29.4 | 48 |
|   Porterhouse steak | 36.2 | 70 |   Beef and pork | 29.1 | 50 |
|   Round, entire | 11.9 | 70 |   Chicken | 19.5 | 101 |
|   Rump | 25.3 | 70 | Goose, flesh, skin, roasted | 21.9 | 91 |
|   Hamburger, regular | 21.2 | 70 | Ham, sliced | | |
| Bologna | | |   Lean | 5.0 | 47 |
|   Beef | 28.4 | 56 |   Regular | 11.0 | 57 |
|   Pork | 19.9 | 59 | Herring, raw | 11.3 | 85 |
| Butter | 81.1 | 219 | Ice cream, 10% fat | | |
| Cake, yellow, mixed with eggs, | | |   Vanilla | 10.8 | 45 |
|   water, and chocolate icing | 11.3 | 48 |   French vanilla | 13.2 | 89 |
| Cheese | | | Ice milk | 4.3 | 14 |
|   Cheddar | 33.1 | 105 | Kidney, raw, beef | 6.7 | 375 |
|   Cottage | | | Lamb | | |
|     Creamed | 4.5 | 15 |   Leg, raw | 16.2 | 70 |
|     Low fat 2% | 1.9 | 8 |   Shoulder, raw | 23.9 | 70 |
|   Cream | 34.9 | 110 | Lard | 100.0 | 95 |
|   American, processed | 31.2 | 94 | Liverwurst, pork | 28.5 | 158 |
| Chicken | | | Lobster | 8.6 | 200 |
|   Fat | 99.8 | 85 | Luncheon meat, pork and beef | 32.2 | 55 |
|   Fryers or broilers | | | Mayonnaise, commercial | 79.4 | 59 |
|     Flesh, skin, raw | 15.1 | 75 | Milk | | |
|     Roasted | 13.6 | 88 |   Whole, fluid | 3.3 | 14 |
|   Roasting | | |   Low fat, 2% | 1.9 | 8 |
|     Flesh, skin, raw | 15.9 | 73 |   Low fat, 1% | 1.1 | 4 |
|     Roasted | 13.4 | 76 |   Evaporated, whole, canned | 7.6 | 29 |
|   Stewing | | | Oysters, raw or canned | 2.0 | 200 |
|     Flesh, skin, raw | 20.3 | 71 | Oyster stew, prepared with | | |
|     Stewed | 18.9 | 79 |   water | 1.6 | 6 |
|   Liver, cooked | 5.5 | 631 | Pork | | |
|   Roll | 7.4 | 50 |   Fresh, raw, ham | 26.6 | 70 |
| Clam chowder | | |   Liver, raw | 3.7 | 300 |
|   Manhattan, prepared with | | |   Sausage, fresh, cooked | 31.2 | 83 |
|     water | 0.9 | 1 | Salami, cooked, beef and pork | 20.1 | 65 |
|   New England, prepared with | | | Salmon, canned, pink | 5.9 | 35 |
|     water | 1.2 | 2 | Sherbet, orange | 2.0 | 7 |
| Crab meat | 1.9 | 125 | Shrimp, raw | 0.8 | 125 |
| Cream | | | Sweetbreads, thymus, beef, raw | 16.0 | 250 |
|   Half and half | 11.5 | 37 | Turkey | | |
|   Light-coffee | 20.6 | 66 |   Flesh, skin, roasted | 9.7 | 82 |
|   Heavy-whipping | 37.0 | 137 |   Roll, light and dark meat | 7.0 | 55 |
|   Sour, cultured | 21.0 | 44 | Veal, raw | 10.0 | 90 |
| Cream of chicken soup, | | | Vegetable-with-beef soup, | | |
|   prepared with water | 4.6 | 11 |   prepared with water | 0.8 | 2 |
| Cream of mushroom soup, | | | Yogurt | | |
|   prepared with water | 3.7 | 1 |   Plain | 3.3 | 13 |
| Custard, baked, milk and egg | 5.0 | 105 |   Plain, low fat | 1.6 | 6 |
| Duck, flesh, skin, roasted | 28.3 | 84 | | | |
| Eggs | | | | | |
|   Whole | 11.2 | 548 | | | |
|   Yolk | 32.9 | 1602 | | | |

(Data taken from Table 3, Handbook No. 8, 1963; Handbooks No. 8-1, 1976; No. 8-4, 1979; No. 8-5, 1979; No. 8-6, 1980; No. 8-7, 1980. Washington, DC, USDA.)

## Table 3. Amino Acid Content of Foods per 100 Grams—Edible Portion

| Food Item | Nitrogen Conversion Factor | Protein Content Percent | Phenyl-alanine mg | Iso-leucine mg | Leucine mg | Valine mg | Sulfur Containing | | | Trypto-phan mg | Threo-nine mg | Lysine mg | Tyro-sine mg | Argi-nine mg | Histi-dine mg |
| | | | | | | | Methio-nine mg | Cystine mg | Total mg | | | | | | |
|---|---|---|---|---|---|---|---|---|---|---|---|---|---|---|---|
| *Milk, Milk Products* | | | | | | | | | | | | | | | |
| Fluid, whole | 6.38 | 3.5 | 170 | 223 | 344 | 240 | 86 | 31 | 117 | 49 | 161 | 272 | 178 | 128 | 92 |
| Canned, evaporated, unsweetened | 6.38 | 7.0 | 340 | 447 | 688 | 481 | 171 | 63 | 234 | 99 | 323 | 545 | 357 | 256 | 185 |
| Dried, non-fat | 6.38 | 35.6 | 1724 | 2271 | 3493 | 2444 | 870 | 318 | 1188 | 502 | 1641 | 2768 | 1814 | 1300 | 937 |
| Cheese | | | | | | | | | | | | | | | |
| Cheddar, processed | 6.38 | 23.2 | 1244 | 1563 | 2262 | 1665 | 604 | 131 | 735 | 316 | 862 | 1702 | 1109 | 847 | 756 |
| Cottage | 6.38 | 17.0 | 917 | 989 | 1826 | 978 | 469 | 147 | 616 | 179 | 794 | 1428 | 917 | 802 | 549 |
| *Eggs, whole* | | | | | | | | | | | | | | | |
| fresh or stored | 6.25 | 12.8 | 739 | 850 | 1126 | 950 | 401 | 299 | 700 | 211 | 637 | 819 | 551 | 840 | 307 |
| *Meat, Poultry, Fish* | | | | | | | | | | | | | | | |
| Beef, chuck, medium fat | 6.25 | 18.6 | 765 | 973 | 1524 | 1033 | 461 | 235 | 696 | 217 | 821 | 1625 | 631 | 1199 | 646 |
| Hamburger, regular | 6.25 | 16.0 | 658 | 837 | 1311 | 888 | 397 | 202 | 599 | 187 | 707 | 1398 | 543 | 1032 | 556 |
| Rib roast | 6.25 | 17.4 | 715 | 910 | 1425 | 590 | 432 | 220 | 652 | 203 | 768 | 1520 | 590 | 1122 | 604 |
| Round | 6.25 | 19.5 | 802 | 1020 | 1597 | 1083 | 484 | 246 | 730 | 228 | 861 | 1704 | 661 | 1257 | 677 |
| Rump | 6.25 | 16.2 | 666 | 848 | 1327 | 899 | 402 | 205 | 607 | 189 | 715 | 1415 | 550 | 1045 | 562 |
| Lamb, medium fat | | | | | | | | | | | | | | | |
| Leg | 6.25 | 18.0 | 732 | 933 | 1394 | 887 | 432 | 236 | 668 | 233 | 824 | 1457 | 625 | 1172 | 501 |
| Rib | 6.25 | 14.9 | 606 | 772 | 1154 | 734 | 358 | 195 | 553 | 193 | 682 | 1206 | 517 | 970 | 415 |
| Pork, fresh, medium fat | | | | | | | | | | | | | | | |
| Ham | 6.25 | 15.2 | 598 | 781 | 1119 | 790 | 379 | 178 | 557 | 197 | 705 | 1248 | 542 | 931 | 525 |
| Loin | 6.25 | 16.4 | 646 | 842 | 1207 | 853 | 409 | 192 | 601 | 213 | 761 | 1346 | 585 | 1005 | 567 |
| Pork, cured | 6.25 | | | | | | | | | | | | | | |
| Bacon, medium fat | 6.25 | 9.1 | 434 | 399 | 728 | 434 | 141 | 106 | 247 | 95 | 306 | 587 | 234 | 622 | 246 |
| Ham | 6.25 | 16.9 | 646 | 841 | 1306 | 879 | 411 | 273 | 684 | 162 | 692 | 1420 | 652 | 1068 | 544 |
| Luncheon meat, canned, spiced | 6.25 | 14.9 | 570 | 741 | 1151 | 775 | 362 | 241 | 603 | 143 | 610 | 1252 | 879 | 942 | 479 |
| Veal, medium fat | 6.25 | | | | | | | | | | | | | | |
| Round | 6.25 | 19.5 | 792 | 1030 | 1429 | 1008 | 446 | 231 | 677 | 256 | 846 | 1629 | 702 | 1270 | 627 |
| Poultry, flesh only | 6.25 | | | | | | | | | | | | | | |
| Chicken, fryer | 6.25 | 20.6 | 811 | 1088 | 1490 | 1012 | 537 | 277 | 814 | 250 | 877 | 1810 | 725 | 1302 | 593 |
| Turkey | 6.25 | 24.0 | 960 | 1260 | 1836 | 1187 | 664 | 330 | 994 | | 1014 | 2173 | | 1513 | 649 |
| Fish | 6.25 | | | | | | | | | | | | | | |
| Cod, fresh, raw | 6.25 | 16.5 | 612 | 837 | 1246 | 879 | 480 | 222 | 702 | 164 | 715 | 1447 | 446 | 929 | |
| Haddock, raw | 6.25 | 18.2 | 676 | 923 | 1374 | 930 | 530 | 245 | 775 | 181 | 789 | 1596 | 492 | 1025 | |
| Halibut, raw | 6.25 | 18.6 | 690 | 943 | 1405 | 991 | 542 | 250 | 792 | 185 | 806 | 1631 | 503 | 1048 | |
| Salmon, Pacific, raw | 6.25 | 17.4 | 646 | 883 | 1314 | 927 | 507 | 234 | 741 | 173 | 754 | 1526 | 470 | 980 | |
| Canned, sockeye or red | 6.25 | 20.2 | 750 | 1025 | 1526 | 1076 | 588 | 271 | 859 | 200 | 876 | 1771 | 546 | 1138 | |
| Meat products | 6.25 | | | | | | | | | | | | | | |
| Liver, calf | 6.25 | 19.0 | 958 | 994 | 1754 | 1195 | 447 | 234 | 681 | 286 | 903 | 447 | 711 | 1158 | 505 |
| Bologna sausage | 6.25 | 14.8 | 540 | 718 | 1061 | 744 | 313 | 185 | 498 | 126 | 606 | 1191 | 481 | 1028 | 398 |

(Continued)

**Table 3.  Amino Acid Content of Foods per 100 Grams—Edible Portion (Continued)**

| Food Item | Nitrogen Conversion Factor | Protein Content Percent | Phenyl-alanine mg | Iso-leucine mg | Leucine mg | Valine mg | Sulfur Containing Methio-nine mg | Cystine mg | Total mg | Trypto-phan mg | Threo-nine mg | Lysine mg | Tyro-sine mg | Argi-nine mg | Histi-dine mg |
|---|---|---|---|---|---|---|---|---|---|---|---|---|---|---|---|
| *Meat, Poultry, Fish (Continued)* | | | | | | | | | | | | | | | |
| Meat products (Continued) | | | | | | | | | | | | | | | |
| Frankfurters | 6.25 | 14.2 | 518 | 688 | 1018 | 713 | 300 | 177 | 477 | 120 | 582 | 1143 | 461 | 986 | 382 |
| Liverwurst | 6.25 | 16.7 | 759 | 818 | 1400 | 1037 | 347 | 203 | 550 | 187 | 724 | 1301 | 510 | 1034 | 497 |
| *Legumes (dry) and Nuts* | | | | | | | | | | | | | | | |
| Bean, red kidney, canned | 6.25 | 5.7 | 315 | 324 | 490 | 346 | 57 | 57 | 114 | 53 | 247 | 423 | 220 | 343 | 162 |
| Peanuts | 5.46 | 26.9 | 1557 | 1266 | 1872 | 1532 | 271 | 463 | 734 | 340 | 828 | 1099 | 1104 | 3296 | 749 |
| Peanut butter | 5.46 | 26.1 | 1510 | 1228 | 1816 | 1487 | 263 | 449 | 712 | 330 | 803 | 1066 | 1071 | 3198 | 727 |
| Pecans | 5.30 | 9.4 | 564 | 553 | 773 | 525 | 153 | 216 | 369 | 138 | 389 | 435 | 316 | 1185 | 273 |
| Walnuts | 5.30 | 15.0 | 767 | 767 | 1228 | 974 | 306 | 320 | 626 | 175 | 589 | 441 | 583 | 2287 | 405 |
| *Grains and Their Products* | | | | | | | | | | | | | | | |
| Bread, white | | | | | | | | | | | | | | | |
| 4% milk solids | 5.70 | 8.5 | 465 | 429 | 668 | 435 | 142 | 200 | 342 | 91 | 282 | 225 | 243 | 340 | 192 |
| Cereal combinations | | | | | | | | | | | | | | | |
| Infant food, precooked mixed cereal and dry milk | 6.25 | 19.4 | 543 | | | | 310 | 137 | 447 | 118 | | 273 | 447 | 447 | 233 |
| Oat-corn-rye, puffed | 5.83 | 14.5 | 933 | 841 | 1368 | 900 | 388 | 234 | 622 | 172 | 545 | 343 | 622 | 776 | 326 |
| Corn products | 6.25 | | | | | | | | | | | | | | |
| Corn grits | 6.25 | 8.7 | 395 | 402 | 1128 | 444 | 161 | 113 | 274 | 53 | 347 | 251 | 532 | 306 | 180 |
| Corn meal, degermed | 6.25 | 7.9 | 359 | 365 | 1024 | 403 | 147 | 102 | 249 | 48 | 315 | 228 | 483 | 278 | 163 |
| Cornflakes | 6.25 | 8.1 | 354 | 306 | 1047 | 386 | 135 | 152 | 287 | 52 | 275 | 154 | 283 | 231 | 226 |
| Hominy | 6.25 | 8.7 | 333 | 349 | 810 | 398 | 99 | | | 84 | 316 | 358 | 331 | 444 | 203 |
| Oatmeal, rolled oats | 5.83 | 14.2 | 758 | 733 | 1065 | 845 | 209 | 309 | 518 | 183 | 470 | 521 | 524 | 935 | 261 |
| Rice, white or converted | 5.95 | 7.6 | 382 | 356 | 655 | 531 | 137 | 103 | 240 | 82 | 298 | 300 | 347 | 438 | 128 |
| Rice products | | | | | | | | | | | | | | | |
| Flakes or puffed | 5.95 | 5.9 | 286 | | | | | 44 | | 46 | | 56 | 124 | 137 | 137 |
| Wheat products | 5.70 | | | | | | | | | | | | | | |
| Farina | 5.70 | 10.9 | 579 | 496 | 891 | 572 | 143 | 184 | 327 | 124 | | 199 | 447 | 424 | 268 |
| Flakes | 5.70 | 10.8 | 478 | 642 | 849 | 728 | 127 | 191 | 318 | 121 | 356 | 360 | 311 | 559 | 231 |
| Macaroni or spaghetti | 5.70 | 12.8 | 669 | 621 | 834 | 745 | 193 | 243 | 436 | 150 | 499 | 413 | 422 | 582 | 303 |
| Noodles, made with egg | 5.70 | 12.6 | 610 | | | | 212 | 245 | 457 | 133 | 533 | 411 | 312 | 621 | 301 |
| Shredded wheat | 5.83 | 12.8 | 755 | | | | | 246 | | 136 | | 466 | 481 | 742 | 371 |
| *Fruits* | | | | | | | | | | | | | | | |
| Bananas, ripe | 6.25 | 1.2 | | | | | 11 | | | 18 | | 55 | 31 | | |
| Grapefruit | 6.25 | 0.5 | | | | | 10 | | | 1 | | 30 | | | |
| Muskmelon | 6.35 | 0.6 | | | | | 2 | | | 1 | | 15 | | | |
| Oranges or orange juice | 6.25 | 0.9 | | | | | 2 | | | 3 | | 22 | | | |
| Pineapple | 6.25 | 0.4 | | | | | 1 | | | 5 | | 9 | | | |

# Table 3. Amino Acid Content of Foods per 100 Grams—Edible Portion (Continued)

| Food Item | Nitrogen Conversion Factor | Protein Content Percent | Phenyl-alanine mg | Iso-leucine mg | Leucine mg | Valine mg | Sulfur Containing — Methio-nine mg | Sulfur Containing — Cystine mg | Sulfur Containing — Total mg | Trypto-phan mg | Threo-nine mg | Lysine mg | Tyro-sine mg | Argi-nine mg | Histi-dine mg |
|---|---|---|---|---|---|---|---|---|---|---|---|---|---|---|---|
| *Vegetables* | | | | | | | | | | | | | | | |
| Asparagus, canned | 6.25 | 1.9 | 60 | 69 | 83 | 92 | 27 | | | 23 | 57 | 89 | | 106 | 31 |
| Beans, snap, canned | 6.25 | 1.0 | 24 | 45 | 58 | 48 | 14 | 10 | 24 | 14 | 38 | 52 | 21 | 42 | 19 |
| lima, canned | 6.25 | 3.8 | 197 | 233 | 306 | 246 | 41 | 42 | 83 | 49 | 171 | 240 | 131 | 230 | 125 |
| Beets, canned | 6.25 | 0.9 | 15 | 29 | 31 | 28 | 3 | | | 8 | 19 | 48 | | 16 | 12 |
| Beet greens | 6.25 | 2.0 | 116 | 84 | 129 | 101 | 34 | | | 24 | 76 | 108 | | 83 | 26 |
| Broccoli | 6.25 | 3.3 | 119 | 126 | 163 | 170 | 50 | | | 37 | 122 | 147 | | 192 | 63 |
| Cabbage | 6.25 | 1.4 | 30 | 40 | 57 | 43 | 13 | 28 | 41 | 11 | 39 | 66 | 30 | 105 | 25 |
| Carrots, raw | 6.25 | 1.2 | 42 | 46 | 65 | 56 | 10 | 29 | 39 | 10 | 43 | 52 | 20 | 41 | 17 |
| Cauliflower | 6.25 | 2.4 | 75 | 104 | 162 | 144 | 47 | | | 33 | 102 | 134 | 34 | 110 | 48 |
| Celery | 6.25 | 1.3 | | | | | 15 | 6 | 21 | 12 | | | | | |
| Corn, sweet, white or yellow, canned | 6.25 | 2.0 | 112 | 74 | 220 | 125 | 39 | 33 | 72 | 12 | 82 | 74 | 67 | 94 | 52 |
| Cucumber | 6.25 | 0.7 | | | | | 8 | | | 14 | | | | | |
| Eggplant | 6.25 | 1.1 | 48 | 56 | 68 | 65 | 6 | | | 10 | 38 | 30 | | 37 | 19 |
| Lettuce | 6.25 | 1.2 | | | | | 4 | | | | | 70 | | | |
| Onions, mature | 6.25 | 1.4 | 39 | 21 | 37 | 31 | 13 | 37 | 64 | 21 | 22 | 64 | 46 | 180 | 14 |
| Peas, canned | 6.25 | 3.4 | 131 | 156 | 212 | 139 | 27 | | | 28 | 125 | 160 | 83 | 302 | 55 |
| Potatoes, cooked or canned | 6.25 | 1.7 | 75 | 75 | 85 | 91 | 21 | 16 | 37 | 18 | 67 | 91 | 30 | 84 | 24 |
| Pumpkin | 6.25 | 1.2 | 32 | 44 | 63 | 45 | 11 | | | 16 | 28 | 58 | 16 | 43 | 19 |
| Radishes | 6.25 | 1.2 | | | | 30 | 2 | | | 5 | 59 | 34 | | | |
| Spinach | 6.25 | 2.3 | 99 | 107 | 176 | 126 | 39 | 46 | 85 | 37 | 102 | 142 | 73 | 116 | 49 |
| Squash, summer | 6.25 | 0.6 | 16 | 19 | 27 | 22 | 8 | | | 5 | 14 | 23 | 14 | 27 | 9 |
| Tomatoes, all types | 6.25 | 1.0 | 28 | 29 | 41 | 28 | 7 | | | 9 | 33 | 42 | | 29 | 15 |
| Turnips | 6.25 | 1.1 | 20 | 20 | | | 12 | | | | | 57 | 29 | | |

(Data from Orr ML, Watt BK: Amino Acid Content of Foods. Home Economics Research Report No. 4. Washington, DC, USDA, 1957. Amino acid content is given in milligrams, using whole numbers, rather than in grams, using decimals. The order of listing the amino acids has been arranged for the convenience of dietitians dealing with inborn errors of metabolism. For further explanation of the nitrogen conversion factors see reference above.)

## Table 4. Sodium and Magnesium Content of Foods

| Food | Na | Mg | Food | Na | Mg |
|---|---|---|---|---|---|
| | **(mg per 100 g)** | | | **(mg per 100 g)** | |
| Acerola | 8 | | Buttermilk, cultured | 130 | 14 |
| Almonds, shelled | 4 | 270 | Cabbage | | |
| Apples | | | Common | 20 | 13 |
| Raw, pared | 1 | 5 | Chinese | 23 | 14 |
| Frozen slices, sweetened | 14 | 4 | Candy | | |
| Apple juice, canned | 1 | 4 | Butterscotch | 66 | |
| Applesauce, canned, sweetened | 2 | 5 | Caramels | 226 | |
| Apricots | | | Chocolate, milk | 94 | |
| Raw | 1 | 12 | Fudge | 190 | |
| Canned | 1 | 7 | Hard candy | 32 | tr |
| Dried | 26 | 62 | Peanut brittle | 31 | |
| Frozen | 4 | 9 | Cantaloupe or honeydew | 12 | 16 |
| Nectar | tr | | Carrots, raw | 47 | 23 |
| Asparagus | | | Cashew nuts | 15 | 267 |
| Fresh, cooked | 1 | 20 | Cauliflower, raw | 13 | 24 |
| Frozen, cooked | 1 | 14 | Celery, raw | 126 | 22 |
| Avocados | 4 | 45 | Cereals | | |
| Bacon | | | Corn flakes | 1005 | 16 |
| Broiled or fried | 1021 | 25 | Corn grits, cooked | | 3 |
| Canadian, broiled or fried | 2555 | 24 | Cornmeal, yellow or white | 1 | 106 |
| Baking powders* | | | Farina, cooked | 690 | 3 |
| Bananas | 1 | 33 | Oatmeal, cooked | 218 | 21 |
| Barley, pearled | 3 | 37 | Rice, puffed, unsalted | 2 | |
| Beans, baked | | | Wheat, shredded, unsalted | 3 | 133 |
| canned, no pork | 338 | 37 | Wheat, puffed, unsalted | 4 | |
| Beans | | | Chard, raw | 147 | 65 |
| Snap, canned | 236 | 14 | Cheese | | |
| Canned, low sodium | 2 | 14 | Cheddar | 700 | 45 |
| Frozen, cooked | 1 | 21 | Cottage, creamed | 229 | |
| Lima, cooked, frozen | 101 | 48 | Parmesan | 734 | 48 |
| Beef | | | Cherries, sweet or sour | 2 | 8–14 |
| Lean, cooked | 60 | 29 | Chestnuts, fresh | 6 | 41 |
| Heart, raw | 86 | 18 | Chicken, cooked, | | |
| Liver, cooked | 184 | 18 | White meat | 64 | 19 |
| Tongue, raw | 73 | 16 | Dark meat | 86 | |
| Beets | | | Liver | 61 | 16 |
| Canned, solids | 236 | 15 | Chicory greens, raw | | 13 |
| Cooked, unsalted | 46 | 15 | Chives, raw | | 32 |
| Beet greens, raw | 130 | 106 | Chocolate, bitter | 4 | 292 |
| Beverages, carbonated† | | | Chocolate syrup | 52 | 63 |
| Blackberries | 1 | 30 | Clams, meat only | 120 | |
| Blueberries, raw or frozen | 1 | 6 | Coconut, shredded | | 77 |
| Boysenberries, frozen | 1 | 18 | Coffee, instant dry powder | 72 | 456 |
| Brazil nuts | 1 | 225 | Collards, raw | 43 | 57 |
| Breads | | | Corn | | |
| Boston, brown | 251 | | Sweet, cooked | 15 | |
| Cracked, wheat | 529 | 35 | Frozen, cooked | 1 | 22 |
| Rye | | | Canned | 236 | 19 |
| Regular | 557 | 42 | Cornbread, from mix | 744 | 13 |
| Unsalted | 30 | 42 | Crab, cooked meat, canned | 1000 | 34 |
| White | | | Crackers | | |
| Enriched | 507 | 22 | Graham | 670 | 51 |
| Unsalted | 30 | 22 | Soda | 1100 | 29 |
| Whole wheat | | | Cranberries | | |
| Regular | 527 | 78 | Juice | 1 | 2 |
| Unsalted | 30 | 78 | Sauce | 1 | 2 |
| Raisin | 365 | 24 | Cream, light, coffee | 43 | 11 |
| Broccoli, frozen | 13 | 21 | Cress, garden | 14 | |
| Brussels sprouts, raw | 14 | 29 | Cucumbers | 6 | 11 |
| Butter | | | Currants, raw, red | 2 | 15 |
| Salted | 987 | 2 | Dates, natural and dry | 1 | 58 |
| Unsalted | 10 | 2 | Eggplant, cooked | 1 | 16 |

## Table 4. Sodium and Magnesium Content of Foods (Continued)

| Food | Na (mg per 100 g) | Mg (mg per 100 g) | Food | Na (mg per 100 g) | Mg (mg per 100 g) |
|---|---|---|---|---|---|
| Eggs | | | Parsnips, cooked | 8 | 32 |
| Whole | 122 | 11 | Peaches | | |
| Whites | 146 | 9 | Raw | 1 | 10 |
| Yolk | 52 | 16 | Canned | 2 | 6 |
| Endive or escarole | 14 | 10 | Peanuts, roasted, unsalted | 5 | 175 |
| Figs, dried | 34 | 71 | Peanut butter | 606 | 173 |
| Filberts (hazelnuts) | 2 | 184 | Pears | | |
| Fish | | | Raw | 2 | 7 |
| Cod, broiled | 110 | 28 | Canned | 1 | 5 |
| Haddock, fried | 177 | 24 | Peas | | |
| Halibut, broiled | 134 | | Canned, regular | 236 | 20 |
| Salmon, baked, broiled | 116 | 30 | Frozen | 115 | 24 |
| Sardines, canned in oil | 823 | 24 | Low sodium, canned | 3 | 24 |
| Tuna, canned, water | 41 | | Pecans | tr | 142 |
| Gooseberries | 1 | 9 | Peppers, raw | 13 | 18 |
| Grapefruit | | | Persimmons | 6 | 8 |
| Pulp | 1 | 12 | Pickles | | |
| Juice | 1 | 12 | Dill | 1428 | 12 |
| Grapes | | | Sweet | 527 | 1 |
| American type | 3 | 13 | Pineapple | | |
| European type | 3 | 6 | Raw | 1 | 13 |
| Grape juice, canned | 2 | 12 | Canned, heavy syrup | 1 | 8 |
| Guava, common, raw | 4 | 13 | Juice, unsweetened | 1 | 12 |
| Honey, strained | 5 | 3 | Pistachio nuts | | 158 |
| Ice cream, regular | 63 | 14 | Plums | | |
| Ice milk | 68 | | Raw | 1 | 9 |
| Jams, jellies, average | 15 | 12 | Purple, canned, in syrup | 1 | 5 |
| Lamb, any cut, broiled or roasted | 70 | 19 | Pork | | |
| Leeks, raw | 5 | 23 | All cuts, fresh cooked | 65 | 23 |
| Lemon juice, fresh or frozen | 1 | 7 | Ham, cured, cooked | 930 | 17 |
| Lettuce, iceberg | 9 | 11 | Sausage, pork, cooked | 958 | 16 |
| Lime juice | 1 | | Potatoes | | |
| Lobster, cooked | 210 | 22 | Peeled, boiled, unsalted | 2 | 22 |
| Loganberries, raw | 1 | 25 | French fried, unsalted | 6 | 25 |
| Macaroni, plain, cooked | 1 | 18 | Mashed, milk added | 301 | 12 |
| Mangos, raw | 7 | 18 | Potato chips | 1000‡ | |
| Margarine | | | Pretzels | 1680 | |
| Regular | 987 | | Prunes | | |
| Unsalted | 10 or less | | Dried, uncooked | 8 | 40 |
| | | | Cooked | 4 | 20 |
| Marmalade, citrus | 14 | 4 | Pumpkin, canned, unsalted | 2 | 12 |
| Milk | | | Radishes, raw | 18 | 15 |
| Whole or skim | 50 | 13 | Raisins, uncooked | 27 | 35 |
| Evaporated, unsweetened | 118 | 25 | Raspberries | | |
| Molasses, light | 15 | 46 | Raw, red | 1 | 20 |
| Mushrooms | | | Black | 1 | 30 |
| Canned | 400 | 8 | Rhubarb, cooked | 2 | 13 |
| Fresh | 15 | 13 | Rice | | |
| Mussels | 289 | 24 | Cooked, regular, salted | 374 | 8 |
| Mustard greens, cooked | 18 | 25 | Cooked without salt | 2 | 8 |
| Nectarines | 6 | 13 | Rutabagas, cooked, unsalted | 4 | 15 |
| Noodles, cooked | 2 | | Salad dressings | | |
| Okra, fresh or frozen | 2 | 47 | French | 1370 | 10 |
| Olives | | | Italian | 2092 | |
| Green | 2400 | 22 | Mayonnaise | 597 | 2 |
| Ripe | 750 | | Russian | 868 | |
| Onions, mature, raw | 10 | 12 | Scallops, cooked | 265 | |
| Oranges or orange juice | 1 | 11 | Shrimp, cooked | 186 | 51 |
| Oysters, raw | 73 | 32 | Syrup, maple | 10 | 11 |
| Pancakes, from mix | 451 | | Soybean curd (tofu) | 7 | 111 |
| Papaya, raw | 3 | | Spinach, cooked | 50 | 63 |
| Parsley | 45 | 41 | | | (Continued) |

## Table 4. Sodium and Magnesium Content of Foods (Continued)

| Food | Na | Mg | Food | Na | Mg |
|------|----|----|------|----|----|
| | *(mg per 100 g)* | | | *(mg per 100 g)* | |
| Squash | | | Turnips | | |
|   Summer, cooked, unsalted | 1 | 16 |   Raw | 49 | 20 |
|   Winter, cooked, unsalted | 1 | 17 |   Cooked, unsalted | 34 | 20 |
| Strawberries, raw | 1 | 12 | Turnip greens, frozen | 17 | 26 |
| Sweet potato, baked | 12 | 31 | Veal, all cuts, cooked | 80 | 18 |
| Tangerine, raw | 1 | | Walnuts, English | 2 | 131 |
| Tomatoes, raw | 3 | 14 | Watercress | 52 | 20 |
| Tomato juice | | | Watermelon | 1 | 8 |
|   Canned | 200 | 10 | Wheat | | |
|   Canned, low sodium | 3 | 10 |   Flour | 2 | 25 |
| Tomato catsup | | |   Bran | 9 | 490 |
|   Regular | 1338 | 21 |   Germ | 3 | 336 |
|   Low sodium | 5–35 | 21 | Yams | | |
| Turkey, roasted | 130 | 28 | Yogurt | 51 | |
| | | | Zweiback | 250 | |

*Baking powders vary greatly in sodium and potassium content. The label on the package tells the type. One tsp or 5 g of baking power contains:

| | Mg Na | Mg K |
|---|---|---|
| Alum type ............................................... | 500 | 8 |
| Phosphate type ......................................... | 450 | 9 |
| Tartrate type ........................................... | 360 | 250 |
| Low-sodium type ....................................... | 2 | 500 |

†The sodium content of carbonated beverages depends upon the sodium content of the water in the area where they are manufactured. (See JAMA 195:236, 1966.)

‡Potato chips vary in sodium according to amount of salt added.

Values for these minerals in canned and processed foods are subject to variation because of methods of processing. *Additional References on Sodium and Magnesium Content of Foods*

(Sodium and magnesium figures from Composition of Food, Raw Processed and Prepared. Agriculture Handbook No. 8 Washington, D.C., USDA 1963; and Church CE, Church HN: Food Values of Portions Commonly Used, 11th ed. Philadelphia, JB Lippincott, 1970.)

Cancio M: Sodium and potassium in Puerto Rican meats and fish. J Am Diet Assoc 38:341, 1961

Cancio M, Leon JM: Sodium and potassium in Puerto Rican foods and waters. J Am Diet Assoc 35:1165, 1959

Chan SL, Kennedy BM: Sodium in Chinese vegetables. J Am Diet Assoc 37:573, 1960

Clifford PA: Sodium content of food. J Am Diet Assoc 31:21, 1955

Dahl LK: Sodium in foods for a 100 mg diet. J Am Diet Assoc 34:717, 1958

Davidson CS *et al:* Sodium-restricted diets. The rationale, complications, and practical aspects of their use. National Academy of Science–National Research Council Publ. No. 325. Washington, DC, 1954

Holinger BW *et al:* Analyzed sodium values in foods ready to serve. J Am Diet Assoc 48:501, 1966

Hopkins HT: Minerals and proximate composition of organ meats. J Am Diet Assoc 38:344, 1961

Hopkins HT, Eisen J: Mineral elements in fresh vegetables from different geographical areas. J Agric Food Chem 7:633, 1959

Nelson GY, Gram MR: Magnesium content of accessory foods. J Am Diet Assoc 38:437, 1961

Oglesby LM, Bannister AC: Sodium and potassium in salt-water fish. J Am Diet Assoc 35:1163, 1959

Thurston CE: Sodium and potassium content of 34 species of fish. J Am Diet Assoc 34:396, 1958

Thurston CE, Osterhaug KL: Sodium content of fish flesh. J Am Diet Assoc 36:212, 1960

*Copper Content of Foods*

Tables giving the copper content of certain foods are too conflicting and incomplete to be included in the above table. The following references are listed for persons interested in the copper content of foods in dealing with Wilson's disease:

Hook L, Brandt IK: Copper content of some low copper foods. J Am Diet Assoc 49:202, 1966

Pennington JT, Calloway DH: Copper content of foods. Factors affecting reported values. J Am Diet Assoc 63:143, 1973

Review: Dietary copper in Wilson's disease. Nutr Rev 23:301, 1965

Silverberg M, Gellis SS: Wilson's disease. Am J Dis Child 113:178, 1967 (Lists foods to be avoided)

Silverberg M, Gellis SS: Preventing Wilson's disease sequelae. JAMA 200:41, 1967

## Table 5. Zinc Content of Foods Per 100 Grams—Edible Portion

| Item No. | Food and Description | Zinc mg | Item No. | Food and Description | Zinc mg |
|---|---|---|---|---|---|
| 1 | Apples, raw | 0.05 | 14 |   Cooked, moist heat | 6.2 |
| 2 | Applesauce, unsweetened | 0.1 | 15 | Beef, separable fat, raw | 0.5 |
| 3 | Bananas, raw | 0.2 | | Beef, ground (77% lean) | |
| | Beans, common, mature, dry | | 16 |   Raw | 3.4 |
| 4 |   Raw | 2.8 | 17 |   Cooked | 4.4 |
| 5 |   Boiled, drained | 1.0 | | Beverages, carbonated, nonalcoholic | |
| | Beans, lima, mature, dry | | 18 |   Bottled | 0.01 |
| 6 |   Raw | 2.8 | 19 |   Canned | 0.08 |
| 7 |   Boiled, drained | 0.9 | | Bran (see wheat) | |
| | Beans, snap, green | | | Breads | |
| 8 |   Raw | 0.4 | 20 |   Rye | 1.6 |
| 9 |   Boiled, drained | 0.3 | 21 |   White | 0.6 |
| 10 |   Canned, solids and liquid | 0.2 | 22 |   Whole wheat | 1.8 |
| 11 |   Canned, drained solids | 0.3 | 23 | Butter | 0.1 |
| | Beef, separable lean | | | Cabbage, common | |
| 12 |   Raw | 4.2 | 24 |   Raw | 0.4 |
| 13 |   Cooked, dry heat | 5.8 | 25 |   Boiled, drained | 0.4 |

## Table 5.  Zinc Content of Foods Per 100 Grams—Edible Portion (Continued)

| Item No. | Food and Description | Zinc mg | Item No. | Food and Description | Zinc mg |
|---|---|---|---|---|---|
| 26 | Cake, white, without icing | 0.2 | 65 | Bolted (nearly whole grain) | 1.8 |
| | Carrots | | | Degermed | |
| 27 | Raw | 0.4 | 66 | Dry form | 0.8 |
| 28 | Cooked or canned, drained solids | 0.3 | 67 | Cooked | 0.1 |
| 29 | Cheese, cheddar type | 4.0 | 68 | Cornstarch | 0.03 |
| | Chicken, broiler-fryer | | | Cowpeas (blackeyes), mature, dry | |
| | Breast, meat only | | 69 | Raw | 2.9 |
| 30 | Raw | 0.7 | 70 | Boiled, drained | 1.2 |
| 31 | Cooked, dry heat | 0.9 | | Crabs, blue and Dungeness | |
| | Breast | | 71 | Raw | 4.0 |
| 32 | Raw (81% meat, 12% skin, 7% fat) | 0.7 | 72 | Steamed | 4.3 |
| 33 | Cooked, dry heat (89% meat, 11% skin) | 0.9 | | Crackers | |
| | Drumstick, thigh, back, meat only | | 73 | Graham | 1.1 |
| 34 | Raw | 1.8 | 74 | Saltines | 0.5 |
| 35 | Cooked, dry heat | 2.8 | 75 | Doughnuts, cake-type | 0.5 |
| | Drumstick | | | Eggs, fresh | |
| 36 | Raw (85% meat, 13% skin, 2% fat) | 1.7 | 76 | Whites | 0.02 |
| | | | 77 | Yolks | 3.0 |
| 37 | Cooked, dry heat (84% meat, 16% skin) | 2.5 | 78 | Whole | 1.0 |
| | Wing, meat only | | | Farina, regular | |
| 38 | Raw | 1.6 | 79 | Dry form | 0.5 |
| 39 | Cooked, dry heat | 2.4 | 80 | Cooked | 0.06 |
| | Neck, meat only | | | Fish, white varieties, flesh only | |
| 40 | Raw | 2.7 | 81 | Raw | 0.7 |
| 41 | Cooked, moist heat | 3.0 | 82 | Cooked, fillet | 1.0 |
| | Skin | | 83 | Cooked, steak | 0.8 |
| 42 | Raw | 1.0 | | Gizzard | |
| 43 | Cooked, dry heat | 1.2 | | Chicken | |
| | Chickpeas or garbanzos, mature seeds, dry | | 84 | Raw | 2.9 |
| | | | 85 | Cooked, drained | 4.3 |
| 44 | Raw | 2.7 | | Turkey | |
| 45 | Boiled, drained | 1.4 | 86 | Raw | 2.8 |
| 46 | Chocolate syrup | 0.9 | 87 | Cooked, drained | 4.1 |
| | Clams | | 88 | Granola | 2.1 |
| | Soft shell | | | Heart | |
| 47 | Raw | 1.5 | | Chicken | |
| 48 | Cooked | 1.7 | 89 | Raw | 2.9 |
| | Hard shell | | 90 | Cooked, drained | 4.8 |
| 49 | Raw | 1.5 | | Turkey | |
| 50 | Cooked | 1.7 | 91 | Raw | 2.8 |
| 51 | Surf, canned, solids and liquid | 1.2 | 92 | Cooked, drained | 4.8 |
| 52 | Cocoa, dry powder | 5.6 | 93 | Ice cream | 0.5 |
| | Coffee | | | Lamb | |
| 53 | Dry, instant | 0.6 | | Separable lean | |
| 54 | Fluid beverage | 0.03 | 94 | Raw | 3.0 |
| 55 | Cookies, vanilla wafers | 0.3 | 95 | Cooked, dry heat | 4.3 |
| | Cooking oil (see oils) | | 96 | Cooked, moist heat | 5.0 |
| 56 | Corn, field, whole-grain, yellow, or white | 2.1 | 97 | Separable fat, raw | 0.5 |
| | | | 98 | Lard | 0.2 |
| | Corn, sweet, yellow | | | Lentils, mature, dry | |
| 57 | Raw | 0.5 | 99 | Raw | 3.1 |
| 58 | Boiled, drained | 0.4 | 100 | Boiled, drained | 1.0 |
| | Corn, canned, whole kernel, yellow | | 101 | Lettuce, head or leaf | 0.4 |
| 59 | Brine pack, solids and liquid | 0.3 | | Liver | |
| 60 | Brine pack, drained solids | 0.4 | | Beef | |
| 61 | Vacuum pack, solids and liquid | 0.4 | 102 | Raw | 3.8 |
| 62 | Corn chips | 1.5 | 103 | Cooked | 5.1 |
| 63 | Corn grits, white, degermed, dry form | 0.4 | | Calf | |
| 64 | Corn flakes | 0.3 | 104 | Raw | 3.8 |
| | Cornmeal, white or yellow | | 105 | Cooked | 6.1 |

(Continued)

## Table 5.  Zinc Content of Foods Per 100 Grams—Edible Portion (Continued)

| Item No. | Food and Description | Zinc mg | Item No. | Food and Description | Zinc mg |
|---|---|---|---|---|---|
| | Chicken | | 148 | Cooked | 3.1 |
| 106 | Raw | 2.4 | 149 | Separable fat, raw | 0.5 |
| 107 | Cooked | 3.4 | | Potatoes | |
| | Turkey | | 150 | Raw | 0.3 |
| 108 | Raw | 2.7 | 151 | Boiled, drained | 0.3 |
| 109 | Cooked | 3.4 | | Rice | |
| | Lobster, crayfish | | | Brown | |
| 110 | Raw | 1.8 | 152 | Dry form | 1.8 |
| 111 | Cooked or canned | 2.2 | 153 | Cooked | 0.6 |
| | Macaroni | | | White, regular | |
| 112 | Dry form | 1.5 | 154 | Dry form | 1.3 |
| 113 | Cooked, tender stage | 0.5 | 155 | Cooked | 0.4 |
| 114 | Margarine | 0.2 | | White, parboiled | |
| | Milk | | 156 | Dry form | 1.1 |
| 115 | Fluid, whole or skim | 0.4 | 157 | Cooked | 0.3 |
| 116 | Canned, evaporated | 0.8 | | White, precooked, quick | |
| 117 | Dry, non-fat | 4.5 | 158 | Dry form | 0.7 |
| | Oatmeal or rolled oats | | 159 | Cooked | 0.2 |
| 118 | Dry form | 3.4 | 160 | Cereal, ready-to-eat, puffed, | |
| 119 | Cooked | 0.5 | | or flakes | 1.4 |
| 120 | Oat cereal, puffed, ready-to-eat | 3.0 | 161 | Rolls, hamburger | 0.6 |
| 121 | Oil, salad or cooking | 0.2 | 162 | Salad dressing | 0.2 |
| 122 | Onions, mature or green, raw | 0.3 | 163 | Salmon, canned (77% solids, | |
| 123 | Oranges, raw | 0.2 | | 23% liquid) | 0.9 |
| | Orange juice | | | Sausages and cold cuts | |
| 124 | Canned, unsweetened | 0.07 | 164 | Bologna, beef | 1.8 |
| 125 | Fresh or frozen | 0.02 | 165 | Braunschweiger | 2.8 |
| | Oysters, raw or frozen | | | Frankfurters | |
| 126 | Atlantic | 74.7 | 166 | Made with beef | 2.0 |
| 127 | Pacific | 9.0 | 167 | Made with beef and pork | 1.6 |
| | Peaches | | | Shrimp | |
| 128 | Raw | 0.2 | 168 | Raw | 1.5 |
| 129 | Canned, drained slices | 0.1 | 169 | Boiled, peeled, deveined | 2.1 |
| | Peanuts | | 170 | Canned, drained solids | 2.1 |
| 130 | Raw | 2.9 | | Spinach | |
| 131 | Roasted | 3.0 | 171 | Raw | 0.8 |
| 132 | Peanut butter | 2.9 | 172 | Boiled, drained | 0.7 |
| | Peas, green, immature | | | Canned | |
| 133 | Raw | 0.9 | 173 | Solids and liquid | 0.6 |
| 134 | Boiled, drained | 0.7 | 174 | Drained solids | 0.8 |
| 135 | Canned, drained solids | 0.8 | 175 | Sugar, white, granulated | 0.06 |
| | Peas, green, mature seeds, dry | | | Tea | |
| 136 | Raw | 3.2 | 176 | Dry leaves | 3.3 |
| 137 | Boiled, drained | 1.1 | 177 | Fluid beverage | 0.02 |
| | Popcorn | | | Tomatoes, ripe | |
| 138 | Unpopped | 3.9 | 178 | Raw | 0.2 |
| | Popped | | 179 | Boiled, solids and liquid | 0.2 |
| 139 | Plain | 4.1 | 180 | Canned, solids and liquid | 0.2 |
| 140 | Oil and salt added | 3.0 | | Tunafish, canned in oil | |
| | Pork | | 181 | (85% solids, 15% oil) | 1.0 |
| | Trimmed lean cuts, separable lean | | 182 | Drained solids | 1.1 |
| 141 | Raw | 2.7 | | Turkey | |
| 142 | Cooked | 3.8 | | Light meat | |
| | Boston butt, separable lean | | 183 | Raw | 1.6 |
| 143 | Raw | 3.2 | 184 | Cooked, dry heat | 2.1 |
| 144 | Cooked | 4.5 | | Dark meat | |
| | Ham or picnic, separable lean | | 185 | Raw | 3.1 |
| 145 | Raw | 2.8 | 186 | Cooked, dry heat | 4.4 |
| 146 | Cooked | 4.0 | | Neck meat | |
| | Loin, separable lean | | 187 | Raw | 5.0 |
| 147 | Raw | 2.2 | 188 | Cooked | 6.4 |

## Table 5.  Zinc Content of Foods Per 100 Grams—Edible Portion (Continued)

| Item No. | Food and Description | Zinc mg | Item No. | Food and Description | Zinc mg |
|---|---|---|---|---|---|
| | Skin | | 200 | 80% extraction | 1.5 |
| 189 | Raw | 1.3 | 201 | All-purpose | 0.7 |
| 190 | Cooked | 2.1 | 202 | Bread flour | 0.8 |
| | Veal | | 203 | Cake or pastry flour | 0.3 |
| | Separable lean | | 204 | Wheat bran, crude | 9.8 |
| 191 | Raw | 2.8 | 205 | Wheat germ, crude | 14.3 |
| 192 | Cooked, dry heat | 4.1 | | Wheat cereal, whole-meal | |
| 193 | Cooked, moist heat | 4.2 | 206 | Dry form | 3.6 |
| 194 | Separable fat, raw | 0.5 | 207 | Cooked | 0.5 |
| | Wheat, whole grain | | | (Also see Farina) | |
| 195 | Hard | 3.4 | | Wheat cereals, ready-to-eat | |
| 196 | Soft | 2.7 | 208 | Bran flakes, 40% | 3.6 |
| 197 | White | 2.2 | 209 | Flakes | 2.3 |
| 198 | Durum | 2.7 | 210 | Germ, toasted | 15.4 |
| | Wheat flours | | 211 | Puffed | 2.6 |
| 199 | Whole | 2.4 | 212 | Shredded | 2.8 |

(Provisional table prepared by Murphy EW, Willis BW, Watt BK: J Am Diet Assoc 66:345, 1975)

Data are given to two decimal places if food contains less than 0.1 mg zinc.

## Table 6-A. Vitamin E Content of Animal Products

| Food and Description | Number of Samples | Total Vitamin E | Tocopherols | | | |
|---|---|---|---|---|---|---|
| | | | Alpha | Beta | Gamma | Delta |
| | | ←———————————— mg/100 g food ————————————→ | | | | |
| *Meat (mammalian)* | | | | | | |
| Beef | | | | | | |
| Muscle, skeletal, raw | 9 | 0.43 | 0.41 | | 0.02 | |
| Ground | | | | | | |
| Raw | 1 | | 0.79 | | | |
| Fried | 1 | 0.63 | 0.37 | | | |
| Canned | 3 | | 0.60 | | | |
| Roast, cooked | 3 | | 0.14 | | | |
| Steak | | | | | | |
| Raw | 1 | 0.63 | 0.47 | | | <0.16 |
| Broiled | 1 | 0.55 | 0.13 | | | |
| Heart, raw | 5 | | 0.60 | | | |
| Liver | | | | | | |
| Raw | 115 | 0.67 | 0.67 | 0 | 0 | 0 |
| Broiled | 1 | 1.62 | 0.63 | | | |
| Veal | | | | | | |
| Muscle, skeletal | | | | | | |
| Raw | 33 | 0.15 | | | | |
| Very young, raw | 12 | | 0.08 | | | |
| Cutlet | | | | | | |
| Raw | 2 | 0.08 | | | | |
| Pan fried | 1 | 0.24 | 0.05 | | | |
| Heart, raw | 20 | 0.34 | 0.33 | tr | tr | |
| Liver, raw | 16 | 0.35 | 0.33 | tr | tr | |
| Lamb | | | | | | |
| Chop | | | | | | |
| Raw | 1 | 0.77 | 0.62 | | | 0.15 |
| Broiled | 1 | 0.32 | 0.16 | | | |
| Cutlet, broiled | 1 | | 0.22 | | | |
| Roast, leg, precooked, reheated | 1 | | 0.05 | | | |
| Liver, raw | 10 | 0.79 | | | | |
| Mutton | | | | | | |
| Muscle, skeletal, raw | 4 | 0.46 | 0.43 | | 0.03 | |
| Kidney, raw | 4 | 0.41 | | | | |

(Continued)

## Table 6-A. Vitamin E Content of Animal Products (Continued)

| Food and Description | Number of Samples | Total Vitamin E | Tocopherols | | | |
|---|---|---|---|---|---|---|
| | | | Alpha | Beta | Gamma | Delta |
| | | ←————————————— mg/100 g food —————————————→ | | | | |
| **Meat (mammalian) (Continued)** | | | | | | |
| Pork | | | | | | |
| Muscle, skeletal, raw | 7 | 0.10 | 0.08 | | 0.02 | |
| Chop | | | | | | |
| Raw | 3 | 0.48 | | | | |
| Pan fried | 1 | 0.60 | 0.16 | | | |
| Loin | | | | | | |
| Raw | 1 | | 0.40 | | | |
| Canned | 3 | | 0.29 | | | |
| Ham, fried | 1 | 0.52 | 0.28 | | | |
| Bacon | | | | | | |
| Raw | 3 | 0.57 | 0.48 | | | |
| Fried | 1 | 0.59 | 0.53 | | | |
| Heart, raw | 200 | 0.63 (range: 0.3–1.34) | | | | |
| Liver, raw | 263 | 0.47 (range: 0.06–1.76) | | | | |
| Rabbit | | | | | | |
| Muscle, skeletal | | | | | | |
| Mature, raw | 4 | | 0.40 | | | |
| Young, raw | 4 | 0.54 | | | | |
| Liver | | | | | | |
| Mature, raw | 6 | | 1.69 | | | |
| Young, raw | 9 | 1.46 | | | | |
| Caribou, muscle, raw | 2 | | 0.02 | | | |
| Polar bear, meat, raw | 1 | | 0.04 | | | |
| Seal, meat, raw | 3 | | 0.15 | | | |
| Whale | | | | | | |
| Meat, frozen, raw | 13 | | 0.28 | | | |
| Liver, frozen, raw | 10 | | 0.81 | | | |
| Sausage and Luncheon meats | | | | | | |
| Bologna | 1 | 0.49 | 0.06 | | | |
| Knockwurst, knackwurst | 10 | 0.57 | | | | |
| Liver paste, canned | 10 | 0.35 | | | | |
| Liverwurst | 1 | 0.69 | 0.35 | | | |
| Luncheon meat, canned | 10 | 0.52 | | | | |
| Salami | 1 | 0.68 | 0.11 | | | |
| Sausage | | | | | | |
| Pork, fried | 2 | 0.32 | 0.16 | | | |
| Beef, fried | 1 | | 0.15 | | | |
| **Poultry** | | | | | | |
| Chicken | | | | | | |
| Meat | | | | | | |
| Raw | 23 | 0.34 | 0.29 | | | |
| Cooked | 3 | 0.55 | 0.35 | | | |
| Frozen fried, not heated | 2 | 1.12 | 0.25 | | | |
| Frozen fried, oven heated | 3 | 0.94 | 0.19 | | | |
| Frozen raw | 1 | | 0.42 | | | |
| Cooked, canned | 3 | | 0.28 | | | |
| Eviscerated carcass, raw | >2 | 0.98 | | | | |
| Heart, raw | 3 | | 1.19 | | | |
| Liver, raw | 75 | 1.44 | | | | |
| Duck, white Peking, eviscerated | | | | | | |
| Carcass | | | | | | |
| Adult, raw | >2 | 2.80 | | | | |
| Young, raw | >2 | 0.70 | | | | |
| Goose, Toulouse, eviscerated carcass, raw | >2 | 1.74 | | | | |

## Table 6-A. Vitamin E Content of Animal Products (Continued)

| Food and Description | Number of Samples | Total Vitamin E | Tocopherols | | | |
|---|---|---|---|---|---|---|
| | | | Alpha | Beta | Gamma | Delta |
| | | ← | | mg/100 g food | | → |
| **Poultry (Continued)** | | | | | | |
| Pigeon | | | | | | |
| Breast, raw | 4 | | 0.06 | | | |
| Liver, raw | 4 | | 1.54 | | | |
| Quail, Japanese domesticated, | | | | | | |
| eviscerated carcass, raw | >2 | 0.70 | | | | |
| Turkey, raw | | | | | | |
| Eviscerated carcass | >2 | 1.43 | | | | |
| Breast | 33 | | 0.09 | | | |
| Thigh | 1 | | 0.64 | | | |
| Skin | 1 | | 0.40 | | | |
| Heart | 1 | | 0.16 | | | |
| Liver | 5 | 2.90 | | | | |
| **Eggs** | | | | | | |
| Chicken | | | | | | |
| Yolk, raw | 66 | 3.12 | 2.05 | | 1.03 | 0.03 |
| Whole large, raw | 66 | 1.06 | 0.70 | | 0.35 | 0.01 |
| Whole, cooked | 8 | | 0.77 | | | |
| Powder | 3 | 5.46 | | | | |
| Pheasant, yolk, raw | 2 | | 4.86 | | | |
| Turkey, yolk, raw | 290 | 2.90 | | | | |
| **Dairy products** | | | | | | |
| Butter | | | | | | |
| United States (U.S.) | 4 | 1.58 | 1.58 | | | |
| Foreign | 644 | 2.40 (range: 0.5–5.0) | 2.40 | | | |
| Cheese, various | 3 | | 0.64 | | | |
| Cream, sweet, fluid | 7 | 0.63 | | | | |
| Ice cream, chocolate | 2 | 1.06 | 0.37 | | | |
| Ice cream, vanilla | 2 | 0.35 | 0.06 | | | |
| Milk, cow—fluid, whole | | | | | | |
| U.S. commercial | 3 | 0.09 | 0.06 | | 0.01 | 0 |
| U.S. producer | 1644 | 0.11 | | | | |
| U.S. producer calculated at milk fat content of 3.34% | 1636 | 0.09 | | | | |
| Foreign, commercial | 206 | | 0.16 | | 0.03 | |
| Chocolate | 1 | | 0.09 | | | |
| Buttermilk | 2 | 0.07 | | | | |
| Condensed, reconstituted | 8 | 0.11 | | | | |
| Evaporated | 16 | 0.18 | | | | |
| Skim | 4 | tr | tr | | | |
| Dry | | | | | | |
| Whole | 4 | 1.08 | | | | |
| Buttermilk | 3 | 0.40 | | | | |
| Milk, human, fluid | 448 | 0.99 | 0.88 | 0.02 | 0.07 | 0.02* |
| Milk, sheep, fluid, whole | 41 | 0.14 | | | | |
| **Finfish** | | | | | | |
| Fillet | | | | | | |
| Carp (Cyprinus carpio) | | | | | | |
| Raw | 1 | | 0.63 | | | |
| With skin, raw | 1 | 0.31 | | | | |
| Cod, Atlantic (Gadus morhua) | | | | | | |
| Raw | 10 | | 0.23 | | | |
| Dark meat, raw | 3 | | 1.16 | | | |
| White meat, frozen | 1 | | 0.24 | | | |
| Flounder, winter (Pseudopleuronectes americanus), frozen | 20 | | 0.36 | | | (Continued) |

## Table 6-A. Vitamin E Content of Animal Products (Continued)

| Food and Description | Number of Samples | Total Vitamin E | Tocopherols | | | |
|---|---|---|---|---|---|---|
| | | | Alpha | Beta | Gamma | Delta |
| | | ←————————— mg/100 g food —————————→ | | | | |
| **Finfish (Continued)** | | | | | | |
| Haddock (*Melanogrammus aeglefinus*) | | | | | | |
| Raw | 2 | | 0.39 | | | |
| Broiled | 1 | 1.20 | 0.60 | | | |
| Halibut, Atlantic (*Hippoglossus hippoglossus*), raw | 2 | | 0.85 | | | |
| Halibut, bastard (*Paralichthys olivaceus*), raw | 1 | | 0.14 | | | |
| Herring (*Clupea harengus*) | | | | | | |
| Raw | 3 | | 1.07 | | | |
| Light meat, frozen 4–5 months | 10 | 2.00 | 2.00 | | | |
| Dark meat, frozen 4–5 months | 4 | 2.30 | 2.30 | | | |
| Ling (*Molva molva*), raw | 1 | | 0.30 | | | |
| Mackerel, Atlantic (*Scomber scombrus*) | | | | | | |
| Dark meat, raw | 1 | | 1.52 | | | |
| Canned | 6 | 1.2 | | | | |
| Mackerel, jack (*Trachurus japonicus*) | | | | | | |
| Raw | 1 | | 0.36 | | | |
| Ocean perch (*Sebastes marinus*), raw | 1 | | 1.25 | | | |
| Pollock (*Pollachius virens*), raw | 2 | | 0.31 | | | |
| Sablefish (*Anaplopoma fimbria*), frozen | 1 | | 4.35 | | | |
| Salmon, unspecified, steak, broiled | 1 | 1.81 | 1.35 | | | |
| Skipjack, unspecified, with skin, raw | 1 | 1.47 | | | | |
| Trout, rainbow (*Salmo gairdneri*), with skin, raw | 1 | 0.20 | | | | |
| Wolffish, Atlantic (*Anarhichas lupus*), raw | 1 | | 2.1 | | | |
| Wrasse, European (*Labrus bergylta*), raw | 1 | | 0.60 | | | |
| Yellowtail (*Seriola quinqueradiata*) | | | | | | |
| Raw | 2 | | 0.18 | | | |
| Frozen, 60 days | 3 | | 0.11 | | | |
| Liver | | | | | | |
| Carp, raw | 1 | | 0.84 | | | |
| Cod, Atlantic | | | | | | |
| Raw | 4 | | 15.85 | | | |
| Canned | 2 | | 2.45 | | | |
| Haddock | | | | | | |
| Raw | 2 | | 6.25 | | | |
| Canned | 4 | 17.5 | | | | |
| Halibut, bastard, raw | 1 | | 0.34 | | | |
| Herring, raw | 3 | | 5.97 | | | |
| Mackerel, Atlantic, raw | 1 | | 3.10 | | | |
| Mackerel, jack, raw | 1 | | 1.21 | | | |
| Ocean perch, raw | 1 | | 16.5 | | | |
| Pollock, raw | 4 | | 8.40 | | | |
| Skipjack, raw | 1 | 2.61 | | | | |
| Trout, rainbow, raw | 1 | 0.12 | | | | |
| Tuna (*Thunnus thynnus*), raw | 1 | | 5.0 | | | |
| Turbot (*Rhombus lupus*), raw | 1 | | 3.0 | | | |
| Wolffish, Atlantic, raw | 2 | | 29.50 | | | |

## Table 6-A. Vitamin E Content of Animal Products (Continued)

| Food and Description | Number of Samples | Total Vitamin E | Tocopherols | | | |
|---|---|---|---|---|---|---|
| | | | Alpha | Beta | Gamma | Delta |
| | ← | | mg/100 g food | | | → |
| **Finfish (Continued)** | | | | | | |
| Wrasse, European, raw | 2 | | 14.40 | | | |
| Yellowtail | | | | | | |
|   Raw | 2 | | 0.94 | | | |
|   Frozen, 60 days | 3 | | 0.64 | | | |
| **Shellfish** | | | | | | |
| Mollusks | | | | | | |
|   Mussel, common (Mytilus edulis) | | | | | | |
|     Fresh, raw | 7 | | 0.74 | | | |
|     Frozen | 1 | | 2.5 | | | |
|   Mussel, horse (Volsella modiolus), | | | | | | |
|     Fresh, raw | 1 | | 0.58 | | | |
|   Mussel, ribbed (Volsella demissa), | | | | | | |
|     Fresh, raw | 1 | | 0.50 | | | |
|   Oyster (Crassostrea virginica), | | | | | | |
|     Fresh, raw | 3 | | 0.85 | | | |
|   Oyster, Australian, raw | 1 | | 0.26 | | | |
|   Limpet (Patella vulgata), raw | 2 | | 14.00 | | | |
|   Periwinkle, common (Littorina | | | | | | |
|     litorea), fresh, raw | 4 | | 3.90 | | | |
|   Squid (Ommestrephes todarus), raw | 1 | | 1.2 | | | |
|   Whelk (Bucinnum undatum), raw | 1 | | 0.8 | | | |
| Crustaceans | | | | | | |
|   Crab, queen (Chioncectes opilio) | | | | | | |
|     Frozen, raw | 2 | 2.25 | | | | |
|     Frozen, cooked | 1 | 1.22 | | | | |
|   Lobster (Homarus americanus), | | | | | | |
|     Muscle, raw | 3 | | 1.47 | | | |
|   Prawn (Pandalus borealis), raw | 1 | | 2.85 | | | |
| **Fats and oils** | | | | | | |
| Mammalian | | | | | | |
|   Beef tallow | 1 | | 2.65 | | | |
|   Butter oil, cow | | | | | | |
|     U.S. | 1643 | 2.83 | | | | |
|     Japanese | 28 | 2.61 | 2.48 | 0 | 0.13 | 0 |
|     Foreign, summer | 300 | 3.71 | | | | |
|     Foreign, winter | 297 | 2.28 | | | | |
|   Caribou tallow | 3 | | 0.37 | | | |
|   Ghee, cow or buffalo, fresh | 34 | 3.00 | | | | |
|   Pork lard, commercial | 12 | 1.34 | 1.20 | | 0.07* | |
|   Seal oil | 5 | | 8.9 | | | |
|   Whale, commercial oil | 3 | | 4.53 | | | |
| Poultry | | | | | | |
|   Chicken fat, raw | 83 | 2.73 (range: 0.1–30.0) | | | | |
|   Turkey fat, raw | 17 | 2.87 | | | | |
| Finfish, commercial oil | | | | | | |
|   Anchovy (Engraulis ringens) | 3 | | 29.08 | | | |
|   Capelin (Mallotus villosus) | 2 | | 14.0 | | | |
|   Cod, Atlantic, liver | 7 | 21.96 | 21.96 | | | |
|   Herring | 5 | | 9.22 | | | |
|   Menhaden, Atlantic (Brevoortia | | | | | | |
|     tyrannus) | 1 | | 7.5 | | | |
|   Dogfish, spiny, liver | 2 | | 25.0 | | | |
|   Shark, Greenland (Somniosus | | | | | | |
|     microcephalus), liver | 2 | | 50.0 | | | |

(Continued)

## Table 6-A. Vitamin E Content of Animal Products (Continued)

| Food and Description | Number of Samples | Total Vitamin E | Tocopherols | | | |
|---|---|---|---|---|---|---|
| | | | Alpha | Beta | Gamma | Delta |
| | | ←——————— mg/100 g food ———————→ | | | | |
| **Fats and oils (Continued)** | | | | | | |
| Finfish, noncommercial oil | | | | | | |
| Anchovy | 2 | | 74.55 | | | |
| Haddock | 1 | 0.7 | 0.6 | | | |
| Haddock, liver | 1 | | 18.0 | | | |
| Ocean perch | 5 | 18.74 | | | | |
| Salmon, chinook (*Oncorhynchus* | | | | | | |
| *tshawytscha*) | 2 | | 19.15 | | | |
| Skipjack | | | | | | |
| Liver | 1 | 90.0 | | | | |
| Trout, rainbow | | | | | | |
| Meat and skin | 1 | 12.5 | | | | |
| Liver | 1 | 5.2 | | | | |
| Wolffish, Atlantic | | | | | | |
| Liver | 1 | | 185.5 | | | |
| Meat | 2 | | 35.5 | | | |
| Wrasse, European, liver | 3 | 250.67 | 250.67 | | | |
| Shellfish oil | | | | | | |
| Limpet | 1 | | 150.0 | | | |
| Prawn | 1 | | 95.0 | | | |
| Squid, commercial oil | 1 | | 21.0 | | | |

Blanks indicate a lack of information. Zeros indicate that an author tested for that form and stated that none was present. A dash means no detectable amount was reported. Trace (tr) means an amount too small to be measured was present.

*Also present, trace of gamma-tocotrienol.

## Table 6-B. Vitamin E Content of Plant Products

| Food and Description | Number of Samples | Total Vitamin E | Tocopherols | | | | Tocotrienols | | |
|---|---|---|---|---|---|---|---|---|---|
| | | | Alpha | Beta | Gamma | Delta | Alpha | Beta | Gamma |
| | | ←————————————————— mg/100 g food —————————————————→ | | | | | | | |
| **Beans and peas** | | | | | | | | | |
| Beans | | | | | | | | | |
| Broad (*Vicia faba*) | | | | | | | | | |
| Raw | 1 | | 0.05 | 0 | 0.40 | | | | |
| Flour, dry | 1 | | 1.00 | | 2.50 | 0 | | 0 | |
| Chickpea (*Cicer- arietinum*), | | | | | | | | | |
| Dry | 5 | 3.11 | | | | | | | |
| French (*Phaseo- lus vulgaris*), | | | | | | | | | |
| Raw | 3 | <0.10 | | | | | | | |
| Great Northern (*P. vulgaris*) | | | | | | | | | |
| Dry | 1 | 2.30 | | | | | | | |
| Sprouts only | 1 | 0.06 | | | | | | | |
| Green (*P. vul- garis*) | | | | | | | | | |
| Fresh | 1 | 0.11 | 0.02 | — | 0.09 | — | — | — | — |
| Dry | 2 | 0.51 | | | | | | | |
| Sprouts only | 2 | 0.04 | | | | | | | |
| Canned | 1 | 0.05 | 0.03 | | | | | | |
| Freeze dried | 1 | | 6.25 | | | | | | |
| Frozen, not cooked | 1 | 0.24 | 0.09 | | | | | | |
| Frozen, cooked | 6 | 0.25 | 0.13 | | | | | | |

## Table 6-B. Vitamin E Content of Plant Products (Continued)

| Food and Description | Number of Samples | Total Vitamin E | Tocopherols | | | | Tocotrienols | | |
|---|---|---|---|---|---|---|---|---|---|
| | | | Alpha | Beta | Gamma | Delta | Alpha | Beta | Gamma |
| | | | ←————————————————mg/100 g food————————————————→ | | | | | | |
| ***Beans and peas (Continued)*** | | | | | | | | | |
| Kidney *(P. vulgaris)* | | | | | | | | | |
| Dry | 2 | 2.08 | tr | — | 2.08 | tr | — | — | — |
| Sprouts only | 1 | 0.05 | | | | | | | |
| Lima *(P. lunatus)* | | | | | | | | | |
| Large | | | | | | | | | |
| Dry | 1 | 7.68 | tr | — | 7.15 | 0.53 | — | — | — |
| Mung *(P. aureus)* | | | | | | | | | |
| Dry | 1 | 1.97 | | | | | | | |
| Navy *(P. vulgaris)* | | | | | | | | | |
| Dry | 3 | 2.26 | 0.34 | | ⁀1.92 | | | | |
| Sprouts only | 1 | 0.06 | | | | | | | |
| Pinto *(P. vulgaris)* | | | | | | | | | |
| Dry | 1 | 1.40 | | | | | | | |
| Sprouts only | 1 | 0.21 | | | | | | | |
| Snap *(P. vulgaris)* | | | | | | | | | |
| Dry | 3 | 1.55 | | | | | | | |
| Sprouts only | 3 | 0.11 | | | | | | | |
| Wax *(P. vulgaris)*, canned | | | | | | | | | |
| Boiled | 1 | | 0.29 | | | | | | |
| Sprouts only | 1 | 0.20 | | | | | | | |
| Scarlet runner | | | | | | | | | |
| *(P. coccineus)* | | | | | | | | | |
| Raw | 2 | | <0.1 | | | | | | |
| Soy *(Glycine max)* | | | | | | | | | |
| Dry | 4 | 20.43 | 0.85 | — | 10.97 | 8.61 | — | — | — |
| Sprouts only | 1 | 0.09 | | | | | | | |
| Sulphur | | | | | | | | | |
| Dry | 1 | 0.78 | | | | | | | |
| Sprouts only | 1 | 0.07 | | | | | | | |
| Lentils, *(Lens culinaris)*, | | | | | | | | | |
| Dry | 1 | 1.27 | | | | | | | |
| Peas *(Pisum sativum)* | | | | | | | | | |
| Fresh | 13 | 2.71 | 0.13 | | 2.58 | | | | |
| Dry | 8 | 2.27 | 0.09 | 0 | 2.09 | 0.09 | | | |
| Canned | 5 | 2.63 | | | | | | | |
| Frozen | | | | | | | | | |
| Uncooked | 4 | 0.64 | 0.12 | | ⁀0.52 | 0 | | | |
| Cooked | 1 | 0.65 | 0.12 | | | | | | |
| Sprouts only | 6 | 0.14 | | | | | | | |
| ***Cocoa products*** | | | | | | | | | |
| Butter, natural and Dutch | 9 | 19.86 | 1.79 | tr | 17.39 | 0.43 | 0.25 | | — |
| Powder, natural and Dutch | 4 | 2.25 | 0.2 | | | | | | |
| Chocolate | | | | | | | | | |
| Dark, sweet | 2 | 6.0 | 0.7 | | | | | | |
| Milk | | | | | | | | | |
| 12%, milk | 2 | 5.6 | 0.7 | | | | | | |
| 20%, milk | 2 | 6.3 | 0.7 | | | | | | |
| Bar | 1 | 4.2 | 1.1 | | | | | | |
| ***Fruits*** | | | | | | | | | |
| Apple *(Pyrus* sp.) | | | | | | | | | |
| Whole, raw | 9 | 0.66 | 0.59 | | | | | | |
| Fresh only, raw | 9 | | 0.27 | | | | | | |
| Stewed with sugar | 1 | | 0.05 | | | | | | |
| Juice, canned | 1 | | 0.01 | | | | | | |

(Continued)

## Table 6-B. Vitamin E Content of Plant Products (Continued)

| Food and Description | Number of Samples | Total Vitamin E | Tocopherols | | | | Tocotrienols | | |
|---|---|---|---|---|---|---|---|---|---|
| | | | Alpha | Beta | Gamma | Delta | Alpha | Beta | Gamma |
| | | | ←————————————————— mg/100 g food —————————————————→ | | | | | | |
| **Fruits (Continued)** | | | | | | | | | |
| Apricot (*Prunus armeniaca*), Canned, sweetened | 1 | | 0.89 | | | | | | |
| Avocado (*Persea americana*) California Fuerte, raw | 4 | | 1.61 | | | | | | |
| California Hass, raw | 2 | | 1.07 | | | | | | |
| Banana (*Musa sapientum*), raw | 6 | 0.32 | 0.27 | | | | | | |
| Blackberry (*Rubus* sp.) Wild, raw | 2 | | 3.5 | | 4.7 | 4.5 | | | |
| Cultivated, raw | 3 | | 0.6 | | 1.1 | 1.0 | | | |
| Cherry (*Prunus avium*), raw | 1 | | 0.13 | | | | | | |
| Current Black (*Ribes nigrum*), raw | 1 | | 1.0 | | | | | | |
| Red (*R. rubrum*), raw | 1 | | 0.1 | | | | | | |
| Damson (*Prunus instititia*), raw | 1 | | 0.7 | | | | | | |
| Gooseberry (*Ribes grossularia, uva-crispa*), raw | 7 | | 0.37 | | | | | | |
| Grapefruit (*Citrus paradisi*) Raw | 1 | 0.26 | 0.25 | | $\widetilde{<0.01}$ | | | | |
| Juice, canned | 1 | 0.18 | 0.04 | | | | | | |
| Mango, (*Mangifera indica*), raw | 1 | | 1.12 | | | | | | |
| Muskmelon (*Cucumis melo*), raw | 2 | 0.31 | 0.14 | | | | | | |
| Orange (*Citrus sinensis*) Raw | 2 | 0.24 | 0.24 | | $\widetilde{\phantom{x}}$ | — | | | |
| Juice, fresh | 1 | 0.2 | 0.04 | | | | | | |
| Pear (*Pyrus communis*) Flesh and skin, raw | 3 | | 0.5 | | | | | | |
| Flesh, raw | 3 | | <0.1 | | | | | | |
| Pineapple (*Ananas omosus*), flesh | 5 | 0.10 | 0.10 | | | | | | |
| Raspberry (*Rubus idaeus*), raw | 1 | | 0.3 | | 1.5 | 2.7 | | | |
| Strawberry (*Fragaria* sp.) Raw | 3 | 0.26 | 0.12 | | $\widetilde{0.08}$ | — | | | |
| Frozen, sliced | 1 | 0.40 | 0.21 | | | | | | |
| Tomato (*Lycopersicum esculentum*) Raw | 10 | 0.49 | 0.34 | | $\widetilde{0.13}$ | 0.02 | | | |
| Juice, canned | 1 | 0.71 | 0.22 | | | | | | |

## Table 6-B. Vitamin E Content of Plant Products (Continued)

| Food and Description | Number of Samples | Total Vitamin E | Tocopherols | | | | Tocotrienols | | |
|---|---|---|---|---|---|---|---|---|---|
| | | | Alpha | Beta | Gamma | Delta | Alpha | Beta | Gamma |
| | | | ← | | | mg/100 g food | | | → |
| ***Cereal grains and their products*** | | | | | | | | | |
| Barley (*Hordeum vulgare*) | | | | | | | | | |
| Whole grain | 8 | 2.98 | 0.57 | | 0.27 | tr | 1.23 | 0.90 | |
| Pearled | 2 | 0.76 | 0.02 | tr | tr | — | 0.37 | 0.27 | 0.10 |
| Buckwheat (*Fagopyrum* sp.), flour | 1 | 7.91 | 0.32 | — | 7.14 | 0.45 | — | — | — |
| Bulgur | 1 | 1.40 | 0.06 | 0.12 | — | — | 0.14 | 1.08 | — |
| Corn (*Zea mays*) | | | | | | | | | |
| Whole | 127 | 5.81 (range: 0.9–11.16) | 0.49 | 0 | 4.56 | tr | 0.21 | 0.09 | 0.46 |
| Flour | 1 | 1.47 | 0.12 | | 0.33 | | 0.32 | | 0.70 |
| Grits | 1 | 1.38 | 0.12 | | 0.36 | | 0.34 | | 0.56 |
| Meal | 5 | 1.80 | 0.15 | | 0.52 | | 0.41 | | 0.72 |
| Meal, cooked | 1 | 0.42 | 0.08 | | | | | | |
| Starch | 1 | 0 | | | | | | | |
| Processed products | | | | | | | | | |
| Flakes | 4 | | 0.10 | | 0.29 | | | | |
| Puffed | 1 | | 0.09 | | 0.34 | | | | |
| Shredded | 1 | | 0.08 | | 0.26 | | | | |
| Hominy grits, cooked | 1 | 0.15 | 0.04 | | | | | | |
| Millet, unspecified | 1 | 1.75 | 0.05 | tr | 1.3 | 0.4 | — | — | — |
| Oats (*Avena sativa*) | | | | | | | | | |
| Whole grain | 9 | 2.05 | 1.09 | | 0.20 | 0.01 | 0.67 | 0.08 | — |
| Dry cereal | 1 | 1.53 | 0.60 | | | | | | |
| Granular | 2 | | 0.09 | | 0.23 | | 0.11 | | |
| Meal | 6 | 2.31 | 1.51 | | 0.11 | — | 0.63 | 0.05 | |
| Shredded | 1 | | 0.08 | | 0.06 | | 0 | | |
| Rice (*Oryza sativa*) | | | | | | | | | |
| Brown, de-hulled | 6 | 2.04 | 0.68 | — | 0.37 | tr | — | — | 0.98 |
| White, milled | 5 | 0.39 | 0.11 | — | 0.07 | tr | 0.05 | — | 0.15 |
| Bran | 1 | 14.92 | | | | | | | |
| Germ | 1 | 8.73 | | | | | | | |
| Grits | 1 | | 0.04 | | 0.10 | | | | |
| Meal | 1 | | 0.10 | | 0.27 | | | | |
| Processed cereal, dry | 1 | 0.28 | 0.04 | | | | | | |
| Puffed or expanded | 5 | | 0.06 | | 0.35 | | | | |
| Shredded | 1 | | 0.02 | | 0.02 | 0.01 | | | |
| Rye (*Secale cereale*) | | | | | | | | | |
| Whole grain | 5 | 3.80 | 1.28 | 0.53 | — | — | 1.07 | 0.91 | — |
| Flour | | | | | | | | | |
| Dark | 1 | 6.68 | 1.41 | 0.60 | — | — | 2.89 | 1.78 | — |
| Light | 3 | 0.93 | 0.43 | 0.16 | — | — | 0.17 | 0.16 | — |
| Medium | 1 | 3.18 | 0.79 | 0.56 | — | — | 0.85 | 0.98 | — |
| Semolina, boiled | 1 | | 0.06 | | | | | | |
| Triticale (*Triticum aestivum x Secale cereale*) | | | | | | | | | |
| Whole grain | 5 | | 0.90 | | | | | | |
| Flour | 5 | | 0.20 | | | | | | |
| Wheat (*Triticum aestivum*) | | | | | | | | | |

(Continued)

## Table 6-B. Vitamin E Content of Plant Products (Continued)

| Food and Description | Number of Samples | Total Vitamin E | Tocopherols | | | | Tocotrienols | | |
|---|---|---|---|---|---|---|---|---|---|
| | | | Alpha | Beta | Gamma | Delta | Alpha | Beta | Gamma |
| | | | ←——————————————————— mg/100 g food ——————————————————→ | | | | | | |
| **Cereal grains and their products (Continued)** | | | | | | | | | |
| Whole grain | 106 | 4.57 (range: 0.58–5.2) | 1.01 | 0.68 | — | — | 0.31 | 2.56 | — |
| Bran | 65 | 9.12 | 1.49 | 1.11 | | | 0.91 | 5.60 | |
| Flour | | | | | | | | | |
| Unbleached | 71 | 2.31 | 0.25 | 0.17 | 0 | 0 | 0.12 | 1.77 | |
| Bleached | 21 | 0.42 | 0.03 | 0.04 | 0 | 0 | 0 | 0.35 | |
| Cake | 6 | 0.23 | 0.04 | 0.03 | — | — | tr | 0.17 | |
| Cracker | 7 | 2.81 | 0.65 | 0.38 | — | — | 0.15 | 1.63 | |
| Whole wheat | 1 | 3.95 | 0.82 | 0.66 | — | — | 0.27 | 2.20 | — |
| Low grade | 61 | 4.24 | 1.08 | 0.82 | — | — | 0.20 | 2.14 | — |
| Germ | 20 | 27.56 (range: 21.8–33.2) | 14.07 | 8.14 | 0 | 0 | 0 | 1.06 | |
| Breakfast cereals | | | | | | | | | |
| Farina | 2 | 0.94 | | | | | | | |
| Flakes | 13 | 2.11 | 0.42 | 0.24 | 0.23 | tr | 0.03 | 1.18 | — |
| Puffed | 3 | 0.67 | | | | | | | |
| Shredded | 10 | 2.15 | 0.36 | 0.28 | 0.26 | | | 1.25 | |
| Whole wheat | 10 | 4.05 | 1.06 | 0.52 | 0.30 | | | 2.17 | |
| Wheat, durum (T. durum) | | | | | | | | | |
| Whole grain | 2 | 5.20 | 0.89 | 0.43 | — | — | 0.60 | 3.28 | |
| Flour | 2 | 2.12 | 0.26 | 0.13 | — | — | 0.21 | 1.52 | |
| **Nuts, peanuts, and seeds** | | | | | | | | | |
| Almond (Prunus amygdalus) | | | | | | | | | |
| Shelled, raw | 5 | 24.48 | 23.96 | | 0.51 | | | | |
| Blanched | 1 | 20.63 | | | | | | | |
| Roasted | 1 | 5.65 | | | | | | | |
| Meal | 1 | 33.4 | 31.7 | 0.3 | 0.9 | — | 0.5 | — | — |
| Brazil nut (Bertholletia excelsa), raw | 1 | | 6.5 | | 11.0 | | | | |
| Cashew (Anacardium occidentale) | | | | | | | | | |
| Shelled, raw | 1 | 4.20 | 0.19 | — | 3.84 | 0.17 | — | — | — |
| Roasted, dry or oil | 1 | 11 | | | | | | | |
| Chestnut (Castanea sativa), raw | 1 | | 0.5* | | 7.0 | | | | |
| Coconut (Cocos nucifera), raw | 1 | | 0.7 | | 0.25 | | tr | | |
| Filbert (Corylus sp.), raw | 2 | | 23.75 | | 1.7* | | tr | | |
| Mixed | | | | | | | | | |
| Dry roasted | 1 | 12 | | | | | | | |
| Oil roasted | 1 | 12 | | | | | | | |
| Peanut (Arachis hypogaea)† | | | | | | | | | |
| Shelled, raw | 5 | 16.37 | 8.33 | — | 8.04 | — | — | — | — |
| Oil roasted | 2 | 11.60 | 6.94 | | | | | | |
| Dry roasted | 2 | 11.85 | 7.80 | | | | | | |
| Paprika seed (Capsicum annum), raw | 1 | 9.60 | | | | | | | |
| Pecan (Carya illincensis), Shelled, raw | 3 | 19.86 | 1.24 | — | 18.62 | — | — | — | — |

## Table 6-B. Vitamin E Content of Plant Products (Continued)

| Food and Description | Number of Samples | Total Vitamin E | Tocopherols | | | | Tocotrienols | | |
|---|---|---|---|---|---|---|---|---|---|
| | | | Alpha | Beta | Gamma | Delta | Alpha | Beta | Gamma |
| | | | ← | | | mg/100 g food | | | → |
| ***Nuts, peanuts, and seeds (Continued)*** | | | | | | | | | |
| Pistachio (*Pistacia vera*), shelled, raw | 1 | | 5.21 | | | | | | |
| Poppy seed (*Papaver somniferum*), raw | 1 | 11.0 | 1.8 | — | 9.2 | — | — | — | — |
| Sesame seed (*Sesamum indicum*), raw | 1 | 22.7 | — | — | 22.7 | — | — | — | — |
| Sunflower seed (*Helianthus annuus*), hulled, raw | 1 | 52.18 | 49.45 | | 2.73 | — | — | — | — |
| Walnut, English (*Juglans regia*), shelled, raw | 3 | 19.62 | 0.84 | — | 17.84 | 0.94 | — | — | — |
| ***Vegetables*** | | | | | | | | | |
| Artichoke, Jerusalem (*Helianthus tuberosus*), Tuber, raw | 4 | | 0.19 | | | | | | |
| Asparagus (*Asparagus officinalis*) | | | | | | | | | |
| Fresh, raw | 5 | 2.10 | 1.98 | 0.05 | 0.07 | — | | | |
| Canned | 2 | 0.38 | | | | | | | |
| Frozen | 1 | 1.59 | 1.40 | 0.07 | 0.12 | — | — | — | — |
| Beet (*Beta vulgaris*) | | | | | | | | | |
| Root, raw | 1 | | <0.03 | | | | | | |
| Root, canned | 1 | | 0.03 | | | | | | |
| Leaf, raw | 4 | | 1.5 | | | | | | |
| Broccoli (*Brassica oleracea*), fresh | 1 | 0.64 | 0.46 | — | 0.18 | — | — | — | — |
| Brussels sprouts (*B. oleracea*) | | | | | | | | | |
| Fresh, raw | 11 | 0.88 | 0.88 | | | | | | |
| Cooked | 2 | 0.85 | 0.85 | | | | | | |
| Cabbage, common (*B. oleracea*), Raw | 23 | 1.67 | 1.67 | — | tr | tr | — | — | — |
| Cabbage, Chinese (*B. Chinensis*), Raw | 1 | 0.13 | 0.12 | | 0.01 | — | | | |
| Carrot (*Daucus carota*) | | | | | | | | | |
| Raw | 13 | 0.51 | 0.44 | 0.02 | — | 0.01 | 0.04 | tr | |
| Cooked | 1 | 0.46 | 0.42 | | | | | | |
| Cauliflower (*B. oleracea*), fresh | 2 | 0.09 | 0.03 | — | 0.05 | 0.01 | — | — | — |
| Celery (*Apium graveolens*), Stalk and pale Leaf, raw | 10 | 0.73 | 0.36 | | 0.01 | 0.36 | | | |
| Corn, sweet (*Zea mays*) | | | | | | | | | |
| Canned | 1 | 0.62 | 0.04 | — | 0.16 | tr | 0.12 | — | 0.30 |
| Frozen | 1 | 0.64 | 0.03 | — | 0.09 | tr | 0.14 | — | 0.38 |

(Continued)

## Table 6-B. Vitamin E Content of Plant Products (Continued)

| Food and Description | Number of Samples | Total Vitamin E | Tocopherols | | | | Tocotrienols | | |
| --- | --- | --- | --- | --- | --- | --- | --- | --- | --- |
| | | | Alpha | Beta | Gamma | Delta | Alpha | Beta | Gamma |
| | | | ←――――――――――――――――― mg/100 g food ―――――――――――――――――→ | | | | | | |
| ***Vegetables (Continued)*** | | | | | | | | | |
| Cress (*Lepid-ium, sativum*), raw | 5 | | 0.7 | | | | | | |
| Cucumber (*Cucumis sativus*), whole, raw | 4 | 0.31 | 0.15 | | 0.11 | 0.05 | | | |
| Dandelion leaf (*Taraxacum officinalè*), raw | 4 | | 2.5 | | | | | | |
| Eggplant (*So-lanum me-longena*), raw | 1 | | 0.03 | | tr | — | | | |
| Garlic (*Allium sativum*), raw | 1 | | 0.01 | | tr | 0.09 | | | |
| Leek (*A. porrum*), white, raw | 10 | | 0.92 | | | | | | |
| Lettuce (*Lac-tuca sativa*), raw | 17 | 0.75 | 0.40 | | 0.35 | — | | | |
| Mint (*Mentha spicata*), leaf, raw | 3 | | 5.0 | | | | | | |
| Mushroom (*Agaricus bisporus*), raw | 6 | 0.29 | 0.08 | | 0.09 | — | 0.12 | | |
| Boletus, edible yellow (steinpilz), raw | 1 | 0.60 | 0.04 | | 0.11 | 0.06 | 0.39 | | |
| Chanterelle (pfifferling), raw | 1 | 0.08 | 0.03 | | 0.02 | 0 | 0.03 | | |
| Morel, raw | 1 | 0.63 | 0.05 | | 0.12 | 0 | 0.46 | | |
| Lorchel, raw | 1 | 0.14 | 0.03 | | 0 | 0 | 0.11 | | |
| Mustard greens (*Sinapis alba*), raw | 10 | | 2.01 | | | | | | |
| Nasturtium (*Tropaeo-lum majus*), leaf, raw | 6 | | 2.5 | | | | | | |
| Nettle (*Urtica dioica*), leaf, raw | 21 | | 14.5 | | | | | | |
| Onion (*Allium cepa*) | | | | | | | | | |
| Raw | 8 | 0.31 | 0.12 | | 0.01 | 0.18 | | | |
| Frozen | | | | | | | | | |
| French fried rings, not heated | 2 | 5.4 | 0.56 | | | | | | |
| Oven heated | 2 | 6.3 | 0.69 | | | | | | |
| White, pickled in vinegar | 1 | | 0.19 | | | | | | |
| Parsley (*Pe-troselinum hortense*), raw | 15 | 2.53 | 1.74 | | 0.18 | 0.61 | | | |
| Parsnip (*Pastinaca sativa*), raw | 2 | | 1.0 | | | | | | |
| Pepper, sweet (*Coaosicum* sp.), raw | 2 | | 0.68 | | 0.01 | — | | | |

## Table 6-B. Vitamin E Content of Plant Products (Continued)

| Food and Description | Number of Samples | Total Vitamin E | Tocopherols | | | | Tocotrienols | | |
|---|---|---|---|---|---|---|---|---|---|
| | | | Alpha | Beta | Gamma | Delta | Alpha | Beta | Gamma |
| | | | ←——————————————— mg/100 g food ———————————————→ | | | | | | |
| ***Vegetables (Continued)*** | | | | | | | | | |
| Potato, white *(Solanum tuberosum)* | | | | | | | | | |
| Raw | 5 | 0.07 | 0.06 | | ⁓tr⁓ | — | | | |
| Baked | 1 | 0.06 | 0.03 | | | | | | |
| Boiled | 1 | 0.06 | 0.04 | | | | | | |
| Chips | 2 | 7.31 | 4.27 | | | | | | |
| French fried | 2 | | 0.19 | | | | | | |
| Potato, sweet *(Ipomoea batatas)*, raw | 4 | 4.60 | 4.56 | | ⁓0.03⁓ | 0.01 | | | |
| Pumpkin *(Cucurbita pepo)*, raw | 1 | | 1.02 | | ⁓0.14⁓ | — | | | |
| Radish *(Raphanus sativus)* | | | | | | | | | |
| Root, raw | 4 | | — | | ⁓tr⁓ | tr | | | |
| Leaf, raw | 2 | 3.76 | 3.06 | | 0.02 | 0.68 | | | |
| Raisin, Sultana *(Vitis vinifera)*, raw | 1 | | 0.7 | | | | | | |
| Rhubarb *(Rheum hybridum)*, raw | 3 | | 0.2 | | | | | | |
| Rutabaga *(Brassica napus)* | | | | | | | | | |
| Raw | 3 | | <0.03 | | | | | | |
| Steamed | 1 | | 0.15 | | | | | | |
| Shallots *(Allium ascalonicum)*, Green, raw | 1 | | 0.21 | | | | | | |
| Spinach *(Spinacia oleracea)* | | | | | | | | | |
| Fresh, raw | 11 | 3.00 | 1.88 | — | 0.14 | 0.98 | — | — | — |
| Leaf, canned | 1 | 0.06 | 0.02 | | | | | | |
| Squash, mar-row type *(Cucurbito pepo)*, steamed | 1 | | 0.12 | | | | | | |
| Tea leaf *(Camellia)* | 1 | | 25.90 | | ⁓0.07⁓ | 1.02 | | | |
| Turnip *(Brassica rapa)* | | | | | | | | | |
| Root, raw | 2 | | <0.03 | | | | | | |
| Greens, raw | 1 | 2.30 | 2.24 | | ⁓0.06⁓ | | | | |
| Watercress *(Nasturtium officinale)*, Leaf and stalk, raw | 6 | | 1.0 | | | | | | |
| ***Vegetable oils*** | | | | | | | | | |
| Almond | 4 | 40.09 | 39.17 | — | 0.92 | — | | | |
| Apricot kernel | 6 | 50.48 | 3.99 | | 43.03 | 2.72 | | | |
| Avocado | 15 | 17.23 | 12.55 | — | 4.23 | tr | — | | — |
| Barley | 11 | 150.29 | 25.77 | 5.59 | 5.05 | tr | 67.25 | 40.21 | 6.41 |
| Brazil nut | 4 | 24.22 | 7.10 | — | 17.12 | — | | | |
| Castor bean *(Ricinus communis)*, Refined | 6 | 67.40 | 1.91 | | ⁓26.04‡⁓ | 38.64* | | | |
| Cherry seed *(Prunus* sp.) | 2 | 35.14 | 6.5 | | 21.1 | 7.5 | | | (Continued) |

## Table 6-B. Vitamin E Content of Plant Products (Continued)

| Food and Description | Number of Samples | Total Vitamin E | Tocopherols | | | | Tocotrienols | | |
|---|---|---|---|---|---|---|---|---|---|
| | | | Alpha | Beta | Gamma | Delta | Alpha | Beta | Gamma |
| | | | ← | | | mg/100 g food | | | → |
| **Vegetable oils (Continued)** | | | | | | | | | |
| Coconut, refined | 13 | 3.58 | 0.35 | 0 | 0.17 | 0.35 | 1.29 | 0.10 | 1.32 |
| Corn, refined commercial | 46 | 83.17 (range: 40.0–150.88) | 14.26 | 0.38 | 64.90 | 2.75 | 0.58 | — | — |
| Crude commercial | 8 | 116.71 | 13.71 | tr | 98.04 | 4.95 | | | |
| Partially hydrogenated commercial | 2 | 47.45 | 17.30 | | | | | | |
| Cottonseed (*Gossypium* sp.) | | | | | | | | | |
| Refined | 22 | 65.24 (range: 25.9–94.0) | 35.26 | 0 | 29.98 | 0 | 0 | 0 | 0 |
| Crude | 42 | 105.52 (range: 34.4–147.5) | 51.34 | 0 | 54.17 | 0 | | | |
| Filbert | 14 | 47.24 | 47.24 | | | | | | |
| Grapefruit | 1 | | 26.5 | | | | | | |
| Grapeseed (*Vitis vinifera*) | 17 | 61.82 (range: 19.4–115.6) | 28.82 | | 30.79 | 2.01 | | | |
| Oat (*Avena sativa*) | 12 | 40.89 | 9.54 | | 14.69 | 2.47 | 11.20 | 2.50 | 0.49 |
| Olive (*Olea europaea*) | 31 | 12.64 (range: 0–24.0) | 11.92 | 0 | 0.72 | 0 | — | — | — |
| Orange flavedo | 1 | 390 | 390 | | | | | | |
| Palm (*Elaeis guineensis*) | | | | | | | | | |
| Refined | 10 | 35.53 | 18.32 | 0 | 0 | 0 | 11.46 | 0 | 5.75 |
| Nonhydrogenated | 9 | 38.40 | 19.12 | 0 | 0 | 0 | 13.10 | 0 | 6.18 |
| Hydrogenated | 1 | 9.7 | 5.58 | 0 | 0 | 0 | 2.52 | 0 | 1.60 |
| Crude | 15 | 58.74 (range: 9.42–80.45) | 16.72 | tr | 0 | 0 | 11.18 | 2.46 | 22.74§ |
| Palm kernel | | | | | | | | | |
| Refined | 3 | 6.20 | | | | | | | |
| Crude | 3 | 21.06 | | | | | | | |
| Peach kernel (*Amygdalus persica*) | 1 | 15.00 | 13.35 | | 1.65 | — | | | |
| Peanut | | | | | | | | | |
| Refined | 24 | 25.00 (range: 9.4–54.0) | 11.62 | — | 12.98 | 0.33 | 0 | 0 | 0 |
| Crude | 23 | 37.88 (range: 14.8–93.4) | 14.41 | — | 22.52 | 0.94 | | | |
| Hydrogenated | 4 | 22.89 | 10.04 | 0 | 12.85 | 0 | 0 | — | 0 |
| Pecan | 2 | 23.34 | 0.89 | — | 22.45 | — | — | — | — |

## Table 6-B. Vitamin E Content of Plant Products (Continued)

| Food and Description | Number of Samples | Total Vitamin E | Tocopherols | | | | Tocotrienols | | |
|---|---|---|---|---|---|---|---|---|---|
| | | | Alpha | Beta | Gamma | Delta | Alpha | Beta | Gamma |
| | | | ⟵———————————————— mg/100 g food ————————————————⟶ | | | | | | |
| *Vegetable oils (Continued)* | | | | | | | | | |
| Rapeseed (*Brassica* sp.) | | | | | | | | | |
| Refined | 45 | 44.81 (range: 14.6–85.3) | 17.65 | | 27.04 | 0.04 | — | — | — |
| Crude | 38 | 62.75 (range: 36.6–100.0) | 25.79 | — | 36.56 | 0.40 | | | |
| Hydrogen-ated | 2 | 50.10 | 16.24 | | 33.86 | 0 | | | |
| Rice | | | | | | | | | |
| Bran | 4 | 51.0 | 36.39 | tr | present | tr | tr | | |
| Germ | 2 | 171.87 | 103.12 | — | 34.89 | 18.41 | | | |
| Rye | 3 | 192.11 | 71.42 | | 16.74 | 0 | 53.24 | 50.55 | — |
| Safflower seed (*Carthamus tinctorius*) | | | | | | | | | |
| Refined | 22 | 38.10 (range: 24.8–69.77) | 34.05 | | 3.50 | 0.49 | — | — | — |
| Crude | 4 | 51.63 | 38.25 | | 7.45 | 5.93 | | | |
| Hydrogen-ated | 2 | 23.2 | 18.8 | | | | | | |
| Sesame | | | | | | | | | |
| Refined | 5 | 29.07 | 1.38 | 0.37 | 25.24 | 2.08 | — | — | — |
| Crude | 5 | 74.60 | 28.82 | 0 | 45.66 | tr | | | |
| Soybean (*Glycine* sp.) | | | | | | | | | |
| Refined | 84 | 93.74 (range: 25.0–163.9) | 10.99 | | 62.40 | 20.38 | 0 | 0 | 0 |
| Crude | 34 | 110.56 (range: 52.9–166.6) | 10.47 | — | 66.69 | 33.40 | — | — | — |
| Hydrogen-ated | 3 | 103.0 | 9.58 | | 66.27 | 27.15 | | | |
| Sunflower seed | | | | | | | | | |
| Refined | 33 | 63.62 (range: 26.8–90.0) | 59.50 | | 3.54 | tr | — | — | — |
| Crude | 35 | 68.19 (range: 27.1–124.3) | 62.26 | — | 5.85 | tr | | | |
| Tomato seed | 2 | 59.3 | 3.8 | | 20.5 | 35.0 | | | |
| Walnut (*Juglans* sp.) | 4 | 32.07 | 0.44 | — | 27.83 | 3.80 | | | |
| Wheat germ | 22 | 254.58 (range: 165.6–300.0) | 149.44 | 81.19 | — | | | | |
| *Margarine* | | | | | | | | | |
| Coconut, sun-flower, palm oils, stick | 1 | 11.1 | 8.8 | 0.6 | 0.8 | 0.4 | 0.5 | tr | tr |
| Corn oil, stick | 6 | 57.65 | 12.89 | | 42.46 | 2.30 | | | |
| Corn oil, tub | 3 | 46.38 | 10.91 | | 33.86 | 1.61 | | | |
| Corn oil, diet imitation, tub | 2 | 30.0 | | | | | | | |

(Continued)

## Table 6-B. Vitamin E Content of Plant Products (Continued)

| Food and Description | Number of Samples | Total Vitamin E | Tocopherols | | | | Tocotrienols | | |
|---|---|---|---|---|---|---|---|---|---|
| | | | Alpha | Beta | Gamma | Delta | Alpha | Beta | Gamma |
| | | | ←——————————————— mg/100 g food ———————————————→ | | | | | | |
| ***Margarine (Continued)*** | | | | | | | | | |
| Corn, soybean, cottonseed oils, stick | 7 | 68.18 | 11.38 | | 49.09 | 7.71 | | | |
| Safflower, soybean oils | | | | | | | | | |
| Stick | 1 | | 17.75 | | | | | | |
| Tub | 1 | 48.8 | 11.7 | | 29.0 | 8.1 | | | |
| Safflower, soybean, cottonseed oils, stick | 1 | | 16.43 | | | | | | |
| Soybean oil | | | | | | | | | |
| Stick | 1 | | 3.14 | | | | | | |
| Tub | 1 | 32.4 | 2.3 | | 24.2 | 5.9 | | | |
| Diet imita-tion tub | 1 | 9.71 | 0.8 | | 7.11 | 1.8 | | | |
| Soybean, cot-tonseed oils | | | | | | | | | |
| Stick | 18 | 45.49 | 11.15 | | 26.43 | 7.91 | | | |
| Tub | 9 | 74.32 | 8.60 | | 50.11 | 15.61 | | | |
| Liquid | 2 | | 2.53 | | | | | | |
| Diet | 2 | | 5.62 | | | | | | |
| ***Other oil products*** | | | | | | | | | |
| Mayonnaise | 4 | 58.0 | 20.74 | | | | | | |
| Salad dressing, mayonnaise type | 2 | 30.0 | | | | | | | |
| Salad dressing, other (Italian, French, Thousand Island) | 4 | 47.5 | | | | | | | |
| Sandwich spread | 2 | 34.5 | | | | | | | |
| Shortening, vegetable, soybean | 4 | 98.28 | 13.97 | — | 76.07 | 7.67 | | | |
| Tartar sauce | 2 | 51.5 | | | | | | | |

See first footnote, Table 6-A.

*Approximately.

†A legume.

‡Nearly all gamma-tocopherol.

§In addition, 5.64 mg/100 g delta-tocotrienol is present in crude palm oil. None was found in refined palm oil.

## Table 6-C. Vitamin E Content of Processed, Mixed, and Miscellaneous Foods

| Food and Description | Number of Samples | Total Vitamin E | Tocopherols | | | | Tocotrienols | | |
|---|---|---|---|---|---|---|---|---|---|
| | | | Alpha | Beta | Gamma | Delta | Alpha | Beta | Gamma |
| | | | ←——————————————— mg/100 g food ———————————————→ | | | | | | |
| ***Baked products*** | | | | | | | | | |
| Bread | | | | | | | | | |
| White, U.S. | 55 | 1.19 | 0.12 | 0.01 | 0.43 | 0.20 | 0.05 | 0.38 | |
| Whole wheat, U.S. | 10 | 0.90 | 0.10 | 0.09 | 0.23 | 0.13 | | 0.35 | |
| Biscuit mix, dry | 10 | 2.48 | 0.27 | tr | 1.60 | 0.50 | | 0.11 | |

## Table 6-C. Vitamin E Content of Processed, Mixed, and Miscellaneous Foods (Continued)

| Food and Description | Number of Samples | Total Vitamin E | Tocopherols | | | | Tocotrienols | | |
|---|---|---|---|---|---|---|---|---|---|
| | | | Alpha | Beta | Gamma | Delta | Alpha | Beta | Gamma |
| | | | ←———————————————— mg/100 g food ————————————————→ | | | | | | |
| **Baked products (Continued)** | | | | | | | | | |
| Cake—from soft | | | | | | | | | |
|   wheat flour | 6 | 7.27 | 0.85 | | 4.86 | 1.56 | | tr | |
|   various, un- | | | | | | | | | |
|   frosted | 3 | 8.49 | 2.69 | | 5.80 | | | | |
| Cookies, various | 8 | 5.45 | 2.57 | | | | | | |
| Crackers from soft | | | | | | | | | |
|   wheat flour | 7 | 1.82 | 0.37 | 0.24 | 0.09 | 0.03 | 0.09 | 1.00 | |
| Cupcakes, choco- | | | | | | | | | |
|   late | 1 | 2.0 | 0.14 | | | | | | |
| Doughnuts | 10 | 4.05 | 0.72 | tr | 2.23 | 0.74 | | 0.36 | |
| Pies, apple | | | | | | | | | |
|   blueberry, and | | | | | | | | | |
|   lemon cream | 6 | 7.29 | 1.59 | | 0.38 | | | | |
| Pie shell | 1 | 0.87 | 0.49 | | | | | | |
| Pretzel sticks | 1 | 0.77 | 0.15 | | | | | | |
| Rolls | | | | | | | | | |
|   Hamburger | 10 | 0.53 | 0.04 | 0.01 | 0.26 | 0.11 | | 0.11 | |
|   From white | | | | | | | | | |
|   patent flour | 25 | 6.65 | 0.78 | tr | 3.57 | 1.23 | 0.21 | 0.86 | |
|   Dough before | | | | | | | | | |
|   baking | | | | | | | | | |
|   from white | | | | | | | | | |
|   patent flour | 25 | 5.43 | 0.66 | tr | 2.70 | 1.05 | 0.18 | 0.84 | |
| **Infant and baby foods** | | | | | | | | | |
| Infant formulas, | | | | | | | | | |
|   Normal dilution | | | | | | | | | |
|   Milk-fat based, | | | | | | | | | |
|   unfortified | 14 | 0.04 | 0.03 | 0 | tr | | | | |
|   Vitamin E-forti- | | | | | | | | | |
|   fied | 1 | 0.70 | 0.70 | 0 | 0 | | | | |
|   Non-milk fat | | | | | | | | | |
|   based, made | | | | | | | | | |
|   with soybean | | | | | | | | | |
|   oil, unforti- | | | | | | | | | |
|   fied | 11 | 1.94 | 0.46 | 0 | 1.32 | 0.06 | | | |
|   Soybean oil, | | | | | | | | | |
|   vitamin E- | | | | | | | | | |
|   fortified | 4 | 2.20 | 0.55 | 0 | 1.33 | 0.32 | | | |
|   Corn oil, un- | | | | | | | | | |
|   fortified | 1 | 1.87 | 0.28 | | 1.55 | 0.02 | | | |
|   Corn, coconut, | | | | | | | | | |
|   and olive oils, | | | | | | | | | |
|   unfortified | 2 | 1.49 | 0.20 | | 1.27 | 0 | | | |
|   Soybean, | | | | | | | | | |
|   corn, and | | | | | | | | | |
|   coconut oils, | | | | | | | | | |
|   vitamin E- | | | | | | | | | |
|   fortified | 1 | 1.14 | 0.51 | | 0.57 | 0.06 | | | |
|   Coconut, | | | | | | | | | |
|   corn, and | | | | | | | | | |
|   soybean | | | | | | | | | |
|   oils, vita- | | | | | | | | | |
|   min E- | | | | | | | | | |
|   fortified | 1 | 1.38 | 0.44 | | 0.87 | 0.06 | | | |
|   Assorted fat | | | | | | | | | |
|   based | 53 | 0.87 (range: 0.003–1.94) | 0.32 | 0 | 0.51 | 0.03 | tr | tr | |

(Continued)

## Table 6-C. Vitamin E Content of Processed, Mixed, and Miscellaneous Foods (Continued)

| Food and Description | Number of Samples | Total Vitamin E | Tocopherols | | | | Tocotrienols | | |
| --- | --- | --- | --- | --- | --- | --- | --- | --- | --- |
| | | | Alpha | Beta | Gamma | Delta | Alpha | Beta | Gamma |
| | | | ← | | | mg/100 g food | | | → |
| **Infant and baby foods (Continued)** | | | | | | | | | |
| Infant cereals | | | | | | | | | |
| Barley | 2 | 0.64 | 0.10 | | 0.57 | | | | |
| High protein | 2 | 1.36 | 0.27 | | 0.13 | 0.12 | 0.32 | | 0.08 |
| Mixed | 2 | 1.01 | 0.16 | | 0.38 | 0 | 0.40 | | 0.32 |
| Oat flakes | 1 | 2.72 | 0.90 | | | | 1.39 | | 0.05 |
| Oatmeal | 2 | 0.85 | 0.19 | | 0.35 | | | | |
| Rice | 2 | 0.83 | 0.26 | | | | | | |
| Baby foods, strained | | | | | | | | | |
| Breakfast cereal with fruit or egg | 8 | 0.39 | 0.25 | | 0.08 | 0.04 | | | |
| Desserts | 8 | 0.23 | 0.23 | | 0 | 0 | | | |
| Fruits | 14 | 0.68 | 0.58 | | 0.06 | 0.04 | | | |
| Meats | 14 | 0.42 | 0.39 | | 0.02 | 0.01 | | | |
| Dinners, meat and vegetable mixtures | 29 | 0.31 | 0.22 | | 0.05 | 0.02 | | | |
| Egg yolk | 3 | 1.66 | 0.60 | | 0.59 | 0.47 | | | |
| Vegetables | 40 | 0.73 | 0.45 | | 0.22 | 0.06 | | | |
| **Mixed dishes*** | | | | | | | | | |
| Canned convenience foods | | | | | | | | | |
| Beans | | | | | | | | | |
| Lima, with ham | 2 | 0.47 | 0 | | 0.47 | 0 | | | |
| Refried | 2 | 0.50 | 0 | | tr | 0.50 | | | |
| Beef | | | | | | | | | |
| Corned, hash | 4 | 0.04 | 0.03 | | 0.01 | 0 | | | |
| Mexican | 4 | 0.14 | 0.06 | | 0.08 | 0 | | | |
| Sloppy Joe | 2 | 0.27 | 0.13 | | 0.14 | 0 | | | |
| Stew | 4 | 0.38 | 0.15 | | 0.19 | 0.04 | | | |
| Chicken with dumplings | 2 | 0.10 | tr | | 0.10 | tr | | | |
| Ravioli | 2 | 0.48 | 0.16 | | 0.26 | 0.06 | | | |
| Chow Mein and meat | 3 | 0.05 | tr | | tr | 0.05 | | | |
| Frozen convenience foods | | | | | | | | | |
| Beef and vegetables | 19 | | 0.56 | | | | | | |
| Chicken and vegetables | 17 | | 0.38 | | | | | | |
| Pasta and cheese or beef | 5 | | 0.16 | | | | | | |
| Pork or ham and vegetables | 2 | | 0.43 | | | | | | |
| Scallops, deep fried | 1 | 6.4 | 0.6 | | | | | | |
| Shrimp, deep fried | 1 | 6.6 | 0.4 | | | | | | |

## Table 6-C. Vitamin E Content of Processed, Mixed, and Miscellaneous Foods (Continued)

| Food and Description | Number of Samples | Total Vitamin E | Tocopherols | | | | Tocotrienols | | |
|---|---|---|---|---|---|---|---|---|---|
| | | | Alpha | Beta | Gamma | Delta | Alpha | Beta | Gamma |
| | | | ←————————————————— mg/100 g food —————————————————→ | | | | | | |
| *Mixed dishes (Continued)* | | | | | | | | | |
| Home prepared foods | | | | | | | | | |
| Beans | | | | | | | | | |
| Baked | 2 | 1.08 | 0.22 | | 0.86 | 0 | | | |
| Lima with ham | 1 | 1.55 | 0.20 | | 1.13 | 0.22 | | | |
| Beef and vegetable stew | 10 | 0.55 | 0.21 | | 0.17 | 0.17 | | | |
| Chicken and dumplings | 1 | 1.27 | 0.08 | | 0.98 | 0.20 | | | |
| Sandwiches | | | | | | | | | |
| Beef | 2 | 0.50 | 0.07 | | 0.35 | 0.08 | | | |
| Beef and cheese | 2 | 0.18 | 0.05 | | 0.10 | 0.03 | | | |
| Egg salad | 1 | 1.14 | 0.09 | | 0.94 | 0.11 | | | |
| Ham | | | | | | | | | |
| Plain | 1 | 1.86 | 0.88 | | 0.82 | 0.17 | | | |
| Salad | 1 | 0.59 | tr | | 0.47 | 0.12 | | | |
| With cheese | 2 | 0.65 | 0.04 | | 0.50 | 0.11 | | | |
| Pork, hot dog | 1 | 0.14 | 0.14 | | tr | tr | | | |
| Tuna salad | 1 | 1.49 | tr | | 1.27 | 0.22 | | | |
| Turkey | 1 | 1.05 | 0.04 | | 0.84 | 0.17 | | | |
| *Miscellaneous* | | | | | | | | | |
| Candy, toffee | 1 | | 0.17 | | | | | | |
| Coffee, instant | 1 | 0.48 | 0 | | | | | | |
| Jam and jelly | 2 | | 0.09 | | | | | | |
| Molasses, cane | 4 | | 0.41 | | | | | | |
| Mustard, prepared | 1 | 4.15 | 1.75 | | | | | | |
| Pasta | | | | | | | | | |
| Macaroni | 2 | 0.27 | 0.02 | 0.02 | | | 0.02 | 0.21 | |
| Spaghetti | 1 | 1.20 | | | | | | | |
| Peanut butter | 2 | 20.0 | 7.0 | | 11.0 | 0.5 | | | |
| Seaweed (dry) | | | | | | | | | |
| Kelp (*Laminaria* sp.) | 3 | 0.87 | 0.87 | | | | | | |
| Dulse (*Rhodymenia palmata*) | 1 | 3.5 | 3.5 | | | | | | |
| Laver (*porphyra umbilicalis*) | 1 | <1.0 | <1.0 | | | | | | |
| Yeast, baker's (*Saccharomyces* sp.) dried or compressed | 5 | | 0.08 | | | | | | |

*Listed by type and main ingredients.

(Data from Mclaughlin PJ, Weihrauch JL: Vitamin E content of foods. J Am Diet Assoc 75:647, 1979)

## Table 7.  Alcoholic and Carbonated Beverages

| Beverage | Average Portion | Weight g | Energy (Calories) | Carbohydrate g | Alcohol* g |
|---|---|---|---|---|---|
| Alcoholic beverages | | | | | |
| Ale, mild | 8 oz glass | 230 | 100 | 8 | 9 |
| Beer, average | 8 oz glass | 240 | 114 | 11 | 9 |
| Beer, light | 8 oz glass | 240 | 64 | 2 | 8 |
| Benedictine | cordial glass | 20 | 70 | 7 | 7 |
| Brandy, California | brandy glass | 30 | 73 | 0 | 11 |
| Cider, fermented | 6 oz glass | 180 | 71 | 2 | 9 |
| Cordial, anisette | cordial glass | 20 | 75 | 7 | 7 |
| Creme de menthe | cordial glass | 20 | 67 | 6 | 7 |
| Curaçao | cordial glass | 20 | 54 | 6 | 6 |
| Daiquiri | cocktail glass | 100 | 125 | 5 | 15 |
| Eggnog, Christmas | 4 oz punch cup | 123 | 335 | 18 | 15 |
| Gin rickey | 8 oz glass | 120 | 150 | 1 | 21 |
| Gin, dry, 86 proof | 1 jigger, 1–1½ oz | 45 | 112 | 0 | 16 |
| Highball, average | 8 oz glass | 240 | 165 | 0 | 24 |
| Manhattan | cocktail glass, 3½ oz | 100 | 165 | 8 | 19 |
| Old fashioned | 4 oz glass | 100 | 180 | 4 | 24 |
| Planter's punch | 4 oz glass | 100 | 175 | 8 | 22 |
| Rum, 80 proof | 1 jigger, 1–1½ oz | 43 | 104 | 0 | 15 |
| Tom Collins | 10 oz glass | 300 | 180 | 9 | 22 |
| Whiskey | | | | | |
|   Rye, 90 proof | 1 jigger, 1–1½ oz | 45 | 118 | 0 | 17 |
|   Scotch, 100 proof | 1 jigger, 1–1½ oz | 45 | 133 | 0 | 19 |
| Wines | | | | | |
|   Champagne | 4 oz glass | 120 | 85 | 3 | 11 |
|   Muscatel or port | 3½ oz glass | 100 | 158 | 14 | 15 |
|   Sauterne | 3½ oz glass | 100 | 85 | 4 | 11 |
|   Sherry, domestic | 2 oz glass | 60 | 85 | 5 | 9 |
|   Vermouth, dry | 3½ oz glass | 100 | 105 | 1 | 15 |
|   Vermouth, sweet | 3½ oz glass | 100 | 167 | 12 | 18 |
| Carbonated beverages | | | | | |
|   Coca-cola | 6 oz bottle | 180 | 72 | 18 | 0 |
|   Ginger ale | 6 oz bottle | 180 | 68 | 17 | 0 |
|   Pepsi-cola | 8 oz bottle | 240 | 104 | 26 | 0 |
|   Soda, orange | 8 oz bottle | 240 | 111 | 30 | 0 |
|   Root beer | 8 oz bottle | 240 | 102 | 26 | 0 |

*Alcohol yields 7 calories per g.

(Values from Pennington JAT, Church HN: Bowes and Church's Food Values of Portions Commonly Used, 13th ed. Philadelphia, JB Lippincott, 1980)

## Table 8.  Equivalent Weights and Measures

| | *Weight Equivalents* | | | | | |
|---|---|---|---|---|---|---|
| | Milligram | Gram | Kilogram | Grain | Ounce | Pound |
| 1 microgram (mcg) | 0.001 | 0.000001 | | | | |
| 1 milligram (mg) | 1 | 0.001 | | 0.0154 | | |
| 1 gram(g) | 1000 | 1 | 0.001 | 15.4 | 0.035 | 0.0022 |
| 1 kilogram (kg) | 1,000,000 | 1000 | 1 | 15,400 | 35.2 | 2.2 |
| 1 grain (gr) | 64.8 | 0.065 | | 1 | | |
| 1 ounce (oz) | | 28.3 | | 437.5 | 1 | 0.063 |
| 1 pound (lb) | | 453.6 | 0.454 | | 16.0 | 1 |

| | *Volume Equivalents* | | | | | |
|---|---|---|---|---|---|---|
| | Cubic Millimeter | Cubic Centimeter | Liter | Fluid Ounce | Pint | Quart |
| 1 cubic millimeter (cu mm) | 1 | 0.001 | | | | |
| 1 cubic centimeter (cc) | 1000 | | 0.001 | | | |
| 1 liter (L) | 1,000,000 | 1000 | 1 | 33.8 | 2.1 | 1.05 |
| 1 fluid ounce | | 30(29.57) | 0.03 | 1 | | |
| 1 pint (pt) | | 473 | 0.473 | 16 | 1 | |
| 1 quart (qt) | | 946 | 0.946 | 32 | 2 | 1 |

## Table 8.  Equivalent Weights and Measures (Continued)

### Linear Equivalents

|  | Millimeter | Centimeter | Meter | Inch | Foot | Yard |
|---|---|---|---|---|---|---|
| 1 millimeter (mm) | 1 | 0.1 | 0.001 | 0.039 | 0.00325 | 0.0011 |
| 1 centimeter (cm) | 10 | 1 |  | 0.39 | 0.0325 | 0.011 |
| 1 meter (M) | 1,000 | 100 | 1 | 39.37 | 3.25 | 1.08 |
| 1 inch (in) | 25.4 | 2.54 | 0.025 | 1 | 0.083 | 0.028 |
| 1 foot (ft) | 304.8 | 30.48 | 0.305 | 1.12 | 1 | 0.33 |
| 1 yard (yd) | 914.4 | 91.44 | 0.914 | 36.0 | 3 | 1 |

### Comparative Values of Weight and Volume of Water

| 1 liter | = | 1 kilo | = 2.2  lbs |
|---|---|---|---|
| 1 fluid ounce | = | 30 g | = 1.04 ozs |
| 1 pint | = | 473 g | = 1.04 lbs |
| 1 quart | = | 0.946 kilo | = 2.1  lbs |

### Table of Common Measures and Metric Equivalents

| 1 tsp | = | 5 cc |
|---|---|---|
| 1 tbsp | = | 14 cc (approximately 15 g) |
| 1 cup | = | 225 cc (approximately 240 g) |

### Comparative Temperatures

|  | Centigrade | Fahrenheit |
|---|---|---|
| Boiling water, sea level | 100 | 212 |
| Body temperature | 37 | 98.6 |
| Tropical temperature | 30 | 89 |
| Room temperature, average | 20 | 70 |
| Freezing | 0 | 32 |

### Table of Measures and Approximate Weights

| 3 teaspoons | 1 tbsp | 1 tablespoon liquid* | 1/2 oz |
|---|---|---|---|
| 16 tablespoons | 1 cup | 1 tablespoon flour | 1/4 oz |
| 1/2 cup | 1 gill | 1 tablespoon sugar | 3/5 oz |
| 2 cups | 1 pt | 1 cup liquid* | 8 oz |
| 4 cups | 1 qt | 1 cup flour | 4 1/2 oz |
| 2 pints | 1 qt | 1 cup butter | 8 oz |
| 4 quarts | 1 gal | 1 cup sugar | 10 oz |
| 1 tablespoon butter | 1/2 oz | | |

*Water or milk.

## Table 9.  Percentiles for Weight and Height of Males and Females 0–18 Years of Age

| | Males | | | | | | Females | | | | | |
|---|---|---|---|---|---|---|---|---|---|---|---|---|
| | Weight (kg) | | | Height (cm) | | | Weight (kg) | | | Height (cm) | | |
| Age | 5 | 50 | 95 | 5 | 50 | 95 | 5 | 50 | 95 | 5 | 50 | 95 |
| (Months) | | | | | | | | | | | | |
| 1 | 3.16 | 4.29 | 5.38 | 50.4 | 54.6 | 58.6 | 2.97 | 3.98 | 4.92 | 49.2 | 53.5 | 56.9 |
| 3 | 4.43 | 5.98 | 7.37 | 56.7 | 61.1 | 65.4 | 4.18 | 5.40 | 6.74 | 55.4 | 59.5 | 63.4 |
| 6 | 6.20 | 7.85 | 9.46 | 63.4 | 67.8 | 72.3 | 5.79 | 7.21 | 8.73 | 61.8 | 65.9 | 70.2 |
| 9 | 7.52 | 9.18 | 10.93 | 68.0 | 72.3 | 77.1 | 7.00 | 8.56 | 10.17 | 66.1 | 70.4 | 75.0 |
| 12 | 8.43 | 10.15 | 11.99 | 71.7 | 76.1 | 81.2 | 7.84 | 9.53 | 11.24 | 69.8 | 74.3 | 79.1 |
| 18 | 9.59 | 11.47 | 13.44 | 77.5 | 82.4 | 88.1 | 8.92 | 10.82 | 12.76 | 76.0 | 80.9 | 86.1 |
| (Years) | | | | | | | | | | | | |
| 2 | 10.49 | 12.34 | 15.50 | 82.5 | 86.8 | 94.4 | 9.95 | 11.80 | 14.15 | 81.6 | 86.8 | 93.6 |
| 3 | 12.05 | 14.62 | 17.77 | 89.0 | 94.9 | 102.0 | 11.61 | 14.10 | 17.22 | 88.3 | 94.1 | 100.6 |
| 4 | 13.64 | 16.69 | 20.27 | 95.8 | 102.9 | 109.9 | 13.11 | 15.96 | 19.91 | 95.0 | 101.6 | 108.3 |
| 5 | 15.27 | 18.67 | 23.09 | 102.0 | 109.9 | 117.0 | 14.55 | 17.66 | 22.62 | 101.1 | 108.4 | 115.6 |
| 6 | 16.93 | 20.69 | 26.34 | 107.7 | 116.1 | 123.5 | 16.05 | 19.52 | 25.75 | 106.6 | 114.6 | 122.7 |
| 7 | 18.64 | 22.85 | 30.12 | 113.0 | 121.7 | 129.7 | 17.71 | 21.84 | 29.68 | 111.8 | 120.6 | 129.5 |
| 8 | 20.40 | 25.30 | 34.51 | 118.1 | 127.0 | 135.7 | 19.62 | 24.84 | 34.71 | 116.9 | 126.4 | 136.2 |
| 9 | 22.25 | 28.13 | 39.58 | 122.9 | 132.2 | 141.8 | 21.82 | 28.46 | 40.64 | 122.1 | 132.2 | 142.9 |
| 10 | 24.33 | 31.44 | 45.27 | 127.7 | 137.5 | 148.1 | 24.36 | 32.55 | 47.17 | 127.5 | 138.3 | 149.5 |
| 11 | 26.80 | 35.30 | 51.47 | 132.6 | 143.3 | 154.9 | 27.24 | 36.95 | 54.00 | 133.5 | 144.8 | 156.2 |

(Continued)

## Table 9. Percentiles for Weight and Height of Males and Females 0–18 Years of Age (Continued)

| | Males | | | | | | Females | | | | | |
|---|---|---|---|---|---|---|---|---|---|---|---|---|
| | Weight (kg) | | | Height (cm) | | | Weight (kg) | | | Height (cm) | | |
| Age | 5 | 50 | 95 | 5 | 50 | 95 | 5 | 50 | 95 | 5 | 50 | 95 |
| (Years) (Continued) | | | | | | | | | | | | |
| 12 | 29.85 | 39.78 | 58.09 | 137.6 | 149.7 | 162.3 | 30.52 | 41.53 | 60.81 | 139.8 | 151.5 | 162.7 |
| 13 | 33.64 | 44.95 | 65.02 | 142.9 | 156.5 | 169.8 | 34.14 | 46.10 | 67.30 | 145.2 | 157.1 | 168.1 |
| 14 | 38.22 | 50.77 | 72.13 | 148.8 | 163.1 | 176.7 | 37.76 | 50.28 | 73.08 | 148.7 | 160.4 | 171.3 |
| 15 | 43.11 | 56.71 | 79.12 | 155.2 | 169.0 | 181.9 | 40.99 | 53.68 | 77.78 | 150.5 | 161.8 | 172.8 |
| 16 | 47.74 | 62.10 | 85.62 | 161.1 | 173.5 | 185.4 | 43.41 | 55.89 | 80.99 | 151.6 | 162.4 | 173.3 |
| 17 | 51.50 | 66.31 | 91.31 | 164.9 | 176.2 | 187.3 | 44.74 | 56.69 | 82.46 | 152.7 | 163.1 | 173.5 |
| 18 | 53.97 | 68.88 | 95.76 | 165.7 | 176.8 | 187.6 | 45.26 | 56.62 | 82.47 | 153.6 | 163.7 | 173.6 |

Data have been used to derive weight and height reference points in the present report. It is not intended that they necessarily be considered standards of normal growth and development. Data pertaining to infants 2–18 months of age are taken from longitudinal growth studies at Fels Research Institute. Ages are exact, and infants were measured in the recumbent position. The measurements were based on some 867 children followed longitudinally at the institute between 1929 and 1975. Data pertaining to children between 2 and 18 years of age were collected between 1962 and 1974 by the National Center for Health Statistics and involve some 20,000 individuals comprising nationally representative samples in three studies conducted between 1960 and 1974. In these studies, children were measured in the standing position with no upward pressure exerted on the mastoid processes. In the previous edition of this report, data for children up to 6 years of age were taken from longitudinal growth studies in Iowa and Boston, where children were measured in the recumbent position. This explains the systematically smaller heights for 2–5-year-old children in this current table compared with those represented in previous editions. In this table, actual age is represented.

(From Food and Nutrition Board, Recommended Daily Allowances, 9th ed, pp 20–21. Washington, DC, National Academy of Sciences, 1980)

## Table 10. Desirable Weights for Men and Woman Aged 25 and Over (Weight in Pounds According to Frame in Indoor Clothing)

| Height | | Small Frame | Medium Frame | Large Frame | | Height | | Small Frame | Medium Frame | Large Frame |
|---|---|---|---|---|---|---|---|---|---|---|
| | | | Men | | | | | | Women* | |
| Feet | Inches | | | | | Feet | Inches | | | |
| 5 | 2 | 112–120 | 118–129 | 126–141 | | 4 | 10 | 92– 98 | 96–107 | 104–119 |
| 5 | 3 | 115–123 | 121–133 | 129–144 | | 4 | 11 | 94–101 | 98–110 | 106–122 |
| 5 | 4 | 118–126 | 124–136 | 132–148 | | 5 | 0 | 96–104 | 101–113 | 109–125 |
| 5 | 5 | 121–129 | 127–139 | 135–152 | | 5 | 1 | 99–107 | 104–116 | 112–128 |
| 5 | 6 | 124–133 | 130–143 | 138–156 | | 5 | 2 | 102–110 | 107–119 | 115–131 |
| 5 | 7 | 128–137 | 134–147 | 142–161 | | 5 | 3 | 105–113 | 110–122 | 118–134 |
| 5 | 8 | 132–141 | 138–152 | 147–166 | | 5 | 4 | 108–116 | 113–126 | 121–138 |
| 5 | 9 | 136–145 | 142–156 | 151–170 | | 5 | 5 | 111–119 | 116–130 | 125–142 |
| 5 | 10 | 140–150 | 146–160 | 155–174 | | 5 | 6 | 114–123 | 120–135 | 129–146 |
| 5 | 11 | 144–154 | 150–165 | 159–179 | | 5 | 7 | 118–127 | 124–139 | 133–150 |
| 6 | 0 | 148–158 | 154–170 | 164–184 | | 5 | 8 | 122–131 | 128–143 | 137–154 |
| 6 | 1 | 152–162 | 158–175 | 168–189 | | 5 | 9 | 126–135 | 132–147 | 141–158 |
| 6 | 2 | 156–167 | 162–180 | 173–194 | | 5 | 10 | 130–140 | 136–151 | 145–163 |
| 6 | 3 | 160–171 | 167–185 | 178–199 | | 5 | 11 | 134–144 | 140–155 | 149–168 |
| 6 | 4 | 164–175 | 172–190 | 182–204 | | 6 | 0 | 138–148 | 144–159 | 153–173 |

*For girls between 18 and 25, subtract 1 pound for each year under 25.

(From Metropolitan Life Insurance Company)

## Table 11. Current Guidelines for Criteria of Nutritional Status for Laboratory Evaluation

| Nutrient and Units | Age of Subject (Years) | Criteria of Status | | |
|---|---|---|---|---|
| | | Deficient | Marginal | Acceptable |
| Hemoglobin | 6–23 mos | Up to  9.0 | 9.0– 9.9 | 10.0+ |
| (g/100 ml)* | 2–5 | Up to 10.0 | 10.0–10.9 | 11.0+ |
| | 6–12 | Up to 10.0 | 10.0–11.4 | 11.5+ |
| | 13–16M | Up to 12.0 | 12.0–12.9 | 13.0+ |
| | 13–16F | Up to 10.0 | 10.0–11.4 | 11.5+ |
| | 16+M | Up to 12.0 | 12.0–13.9 | 14.0+ |
| | 16+F | Up to 10.0 | 10.0–11.9 | 12.0+ |
| | Pregnant (after 6+ mos) | Up to  9.5 | 9.5–10.9 | 11.0+ |

## Table 11. Current Guidelines for Criteria of Nutritional Status for Laboratory Evaluation (Continued)

| Nutrient and Units | Age of Subject (Years) | Deficient | Marginal | Acceptable |
|---|---|---|---|---|
| Hematocrit | Up to 2 | Up to 28 | 28–30 | 31+ |
| (Packed cell volume | 2–5 | Up to 30 | 30–33 | 34+ |
| in percent)* | 6–12 | Up to 30 | 30–35 | 36+ |
| | 13–16M | Up to 37 | 37–39 | 40+ |
| | 13–16F | Up to 31 | 31–35 | 36+ |
| | 16+M | Up to 37 | 37–43 | 44+ |
| | 16+F | Up to 31 | 31–37 | 33+ |
| | Pregnant | Up to 30 | 30–32 | 33+ |
| Serum albumin | Up to 1 | | Up to 2.5 | 2.5+ |
| (g/100 ml)* | 1–5 | | Up to 3.0 | 3.0+ |
| | 6–16 | | Up to 3.5 | 3.5+ |
| | 16+ | Up to 2.8 | 2.8– 3.4 | 3.5+ |
| | Pregnant | Up to 3.0 | 3.0– 3.4 | 3.5+ |
| Serum protein | Up to 1 | | Up to 5.0 | 5.0+ |
| (g/100 ml)* | 1–5 | | Up to 5.5 | 5.5+ |
| | 6–16 | | Up to 6.0 | 6.0+ |
| | 16+ | Up to 6.0 | 6.0– 6.4 | 6.5+ |
| | Pregnant | Up to 5.5 | 5.5– 5.9 | 6.0+ |
| Serum ascorbic acid (mg/100 ml)* | All ages | Up to 0.1 | 0.1–0.19 | 0.2+ |
| Plasma vitamin A (mcg/100 ml)* | All ages | Up to 10 | 10–19 | 20+ |
| Plasma carotene | All ages | Up to 20 | 20–39 | 40+ |
| (mcg/100 ml)* | Pregnant | | 40–79 | 80+ |
| Serum iron | Up to 2 | Up to 30 | | 30+ |
| (mcg/100 ml)* | 2–5 | Up to 40 | | 40+ |
| | 6–12 | Up to 50 | | 50+ |
| | 12+M | Up to 60 | | 60+ |
| | 12+F | Up to 40 | | 40+ |
| Transferrin saturation | Up to 2 | Up to 15.0 | | 15.0+ |
| (percent)* | 2–12 | Up to 20.0 | | 20.0+ |
| | 12+M | Up to 20.0 | | 20.0+ |
| | 12+F | Up to 15.0 | | 15.0+ |
| Serum folacin (ng/ml)† | All ages | Up to 2.0 | 2.1– 5.9 | 6.0+ |
| Serum vitamin B$_{12}$ (pg/ml)† | All ages | Up to 100 | | 100+ |
| Thiamine in urine | 1–3 | Up to 120 | 120–175 | 175+ |
| (mcg/g creatinine)* | 4–5 | Up to 85 | 85–120 | 120+ |
| | 6–9 | Up to 70 | 70–180 | 180+ |
| | 10–15 | Up to 55 | 55–150 | 150+ |
| | 16+ | Up to 27 | 27– 65 | 65+ |
| | Pregnant | Up to 21 | 21– 49 | 50+ |
| Riboflavin in urine | 1–3 | Up to 150 | 150–499 | 500+ |
| (mcg/g creatinine)* | 4–5 | Up to 100 | 100–299 | 300+ |
| | 6–9 | Up to 85 | 85–269 | 270+ |
| | 10–16 | Up to 70 | 70–199 | 200+ |
| | 16+ | Up to 27 | 27– 79 | 80+ |
| | Pregnant | Up to 30 | 30– 89 | 90+ |
| RBC transketolase-TPP-effect (ratio)† | All ages | 25+ | 15– 25 | Up to 15 |
| RBC glutathione reductase-FAD-effect (ratio)† | All ages | 1.2+ | | Up to 1.2 |
| Tryptophan load | Adults | 25+(6 hr) | | Up to 25 |
| (mg xanthurenic | (Dose: 100 mg/kg | 75+(24 hr) | | Up to 75 |
| acid excreted)† | body weight) | | | (Continued) |

## Table 11. Current Guidelines for Criteria of Nutritional Status for Laboratory Evaluation (Continued)

| Nutrient and Units | Age of Subject (Years) | Criteria of Status | | |
|---|---|---|---|---|
| | | Deficient | Marginal | Acceptable |
| Urinary pyridoxine (mcg/g creatinine)† | 1–3 | Up to 90 | | 90+ |
| | 4–6 | Up to 80 | | 80+ |
| | 7–9 | Up to 60 | | 60+ |
| | 10–12 | Up to 40 | | 40+ |
| | 13–15 | Up to 30 | | .30+ |
| | 16+ | Up to 20 | | 20+ |
| Urinary N'methyl nicotinamide (mg/g creatinine)* | All ages | Up to 0.2 | 0.2–5.59 | 0.6+ |
| | Pregnant | Up to 0.8 | 0.8–2.49 | 2.5+ |
| Urinary pantothenic acid (mcg)† | All ages | Up to 200 | | 200+ |
| Plasma vitamin E (mg/100 ml)† | All ages | Up to 0.2 | 0.2– 0.6 | 0.6+ |
| Transaminase index (ratio)† | | | | |
| EGOT‡ | Adult | 2.0+ | | Up to 2.0 |
| EGPT§ | Adult | 1.25+ | | Up to 1.25 |

*Adapted from the Ten-State Nutrition Survey.

†Criteria may vary with different methodology.

‡Erythrocyte glutamic oxalacetic transaminase.

§Erythrocyte glutamic pyruvic transaminase.

(Am J Public Health [Suppl] 63:34, Nov, 1973)

# Table 12. Dietary Standard for Canada, Recommended Daily Nutrient Intake (Revised 1975)

| Age | Sex | Weight (kg) | Height (cm) | Energy* (kcal) | Energy (MJ)† | Protein (g) | Thiamin (mg) | Niacin (NE)# | Riboflavin (mg) | Vitamin B6 (mg)** | Folate (µg)†† | Vitamin B12 (µg) | Vitamin C (mg) | Vitamin A (RE)§§ | Vitamin D (µg cholecalciferol)|||| | Vitamin E (mg d-α-tocopherol) | Calcium (mg) | Phosphorus (mg) | Magnesium (mg) | Iodine (µg) | Iron (mg) | Zinc (mg) |
|---|---|---|---|---|---|---|---|---|---|---|---|---|---|---|---|---|---|---|---|---|---|---|
| 0–6 mo | Both | 6 | | kg × 117 | kg × 0.49 | kg × 2.2 (2.0)|| | 0.3 | 5 | 0.4 | 0.3 | 40 | 0.3 | 20‡‡ | 400 | 10 | 3 | 500*** | 250*** | 50*** | 35*** | 7*** | 4*** |
| 7–11 mo | Both | 9 | | kg × 108 | kg × 0.45 | kg × 1.4 | 0.5 | 6 | 0.6 | 0.4 | 60 | 0.3 | 20 | 400 | 10 | 3 | 500 | 400 | 50 | 50 | 7 | 5 |
| 1–3 yr | Both | 13 | 90 | 1400 | 5.9 | 22 | 0.7 | 9 | 0.8 | 0.8 | 100 | 0.9 | 20 | 400 | 10 | 4 | 500 | 500 | 75 | 70 | 8 | 5 |
| 4–6 yr | Both | 19 | 110 | 1800 | 7.5 | 27 | 0.9 | 12 | 1.1 | 1.3 | 100 | 1.5 | 20 | 500 | 5 | 5 | 500 | 500 | 100 | 90 | 9 | 6 |
| 7–9 yr | M | 27 | 129 | 2200 | 9.2 | 33 | 1.1 | 14 | 1.3 | 1.6 | 100 | 1.5 | 30 | 700 | 2.5## | 6 | 700 | 700 | 150 | 110 | 10 | 7 |
| 7–9 yr | F | 27 | 128 | 2000 | 8.4 | 33 | 1.0 | 13 | 1.2 | 1.4 | 100 | 1.5 | 30 | 700 | 2.5## | 6 | 700 | 700 | 150 | 100 | 10 | 7 |
| 10–12 yr | M | 36 | 144 | 2500 | 10.5 | 41 | 1.2 | 17 | 1.5 | 1.8 | 100 | 3.0 | 30 | 800 | 2.5## | 7 | 900 | 900 | 175 | 130 | 11 | 8 |
| 10–12 yr | F | 38 | 145 | 2300 | 9.6 | 40 | 1.1 | 15 | 1.4 | 1.5 | 100 | 3.0 | 30 | 800 | 2.5## | 7 | 1000 | 1000 | 200 | 120 | 11 | 9 |
| 13–15 yr | M | 51 | 162 | 2800 | 11.7 | 52 | 1.4 | 19 | 1.7 | 2.0 | 200 | 3.0 | 30 | 1000 | 2.5## | 9 | 1200 | 1200 | 250 | 140 | 13 | 10 |
| 13–15 yr | F | 49 | 159 | 2200 | 9.2 | 43 | 1.1 | 15 | 1.4 | 1.5 | 200 | 3.0 | 30 | 800 | 2.5## | 7 | 800 | 800 | 250 | 110 | 14 | 10 |
| 16–18 yr | M | 64 | 172 | 3200 | 13.4 | 54 | 1.6 | 21 | 2.0 | 2.0 | 200 | 3.0 | 30 | 1000 | 2.5## | 10 | 1000 | 1000 | 300 | 160 | 14 | 12 |
| 16–18 yr | F | 54 | 161 | 2100 | 8.8 | 43 | 1.1 | 14 | 1.3 | 1.5 | 200 | 3.0 | 30 | 800 | 2.5## | 6 | 700 | 700 | 250 | 110 | 14 | 11 |
| 19–35 yr | M | 70 | 176 | 3000 | 12.6 | 56 | 1.5 | 20 | 1.8 | 2.0 | 200 | 3.0 | 30 | 1000 | 2.5## | 9 | 800 | 800 | 300 | 150 | 10 | 10 |
| 19–35 yr | F | 56 | 161 | 2100 | 8.8 | 41 | 1.1 | 14 | 1.3 | 1.5 | 200 | 3.0 | 30 | 800 | 2.5## | 6 | 700 | 700 | 250 | 110 | 14 | 9 |
| 36–50 yr | M | 70 | 176 | 2700 | 11.3 | 56 | 1.4 | 18 | 1.7 | 2.0 | 200 | 3.0 | 30 | 1000 | 2.5## | 8 | 800 | 800 | 300 | 140 | 10 | 10 |
| 36–50 yr | F | 56 | 161 | 1900 | 7.9 | 41 | 1.0 | 13 | 1.2 | 1.5 | 200 | 3.0 | 30 | 800 | 2.5## | 6 | 700 | 700 | 250 | 100 | 14 | 9 |
| 51 + yr | M | 70 | 176 | 2300‡ | 9.6‡ | 56 | 1.4 | 18 | 1.7 | 2.0 | 200 | 3.0 | 30 | 1000 | 2.5## | 8 | 800 | 800 | 300 | 140 | 10 | 10 |
| 51 + yr | F | 56 | 161 | 1800‡ | 7.5‡ | 41 | 1.0 | 13 | 1.2 | 1.5 | 200 | 3.0 | 30 | 800 | 2.5## | 6 | 700 | 700 | 250 | 100 | 9 | 10 |
| Pregnancy | | | | +300§ | +1.3§ | +20 | +0.2 | +2 | +0.3 | +0.5 | +50 | +1.0 | +20 | +100 | +2.5## | 1 | +500 | +500 | +25 | +15 | +1††† | +3 |
| Lactation | | | | +500 | 2.1 | +24 | +0.4 | +7 | +0.6 | +0.6 | +50 | +0.5 | +30 | +400 | +2.5## | +2 | +500 | +500 | +75 | +25 | +1††† | +7 |

*Recommendations assume characteristic activity pattern for each age group.

†Megajoules (106 joules). Calculated from the relation 1 kilocalorie = 4.184 kilojoules and rounded to 1 decimal place.

‡Recommended energy intake for age 66 + years reduced to 2000 kcal (8.4 MJ) for men and 1500 kcal (6.3 MJ) for women.

§Increased energy intake recommended during second and third trimesters. An increase of 100 kcal (418.4 kJ) per day is recommended during the first trimester.

||Recommended protein intake of 2.2 g/kg body wt. for infants age 0.2 mo and 2.0 g/kg body wt. for those age 3–5 mo. Protein recommendation for infants 0–11 mo assumes consumption of breast milk or protein of equivalent quality.

#1 NE (niacin equivalent) is equal to 1 mg of niacin or 60 mg of tryptophan.

**Recommendations are based on estimated average daily protein intake of Canadians.

††Recommendation given in terms of free folate.

‡‡Considerably higher levels may be prudent for infants during the first week of life to guard against neonatal tyrosinemia.

§§1 RE (retinol equivalent) corresponds to a biological activity in humans equal to 1 µg retinol (3.33 IU) or 6 µg β-carotene (40 IU vitamin A activity).

||||One µg cholecalciferol is equivalent to 1 µg ergocalciferol (40 IU ergocalciferol is equivalent to 1 µg ergocalciferol (40 IU vitamin D activity).

##Most older children and adults receive vitamin D from irradiation, but 2.5 µg daily is recommended. This intake should be increased to 5.0 µg daily during pregnancy and lactation and for those confined indoors or otherwise deprived of sunlight for extended periods.

***The intake of breast-fed infants may be less than the recommendation but is considered to be adequate.

†††A recommended total intake of 15 mg daily during pregnancy and lactation assumes the presence of adequate stores of iron. If stores are suspected of being inadequate, additional iron as a supplement is recommended.

(From Committee for the Revision of the Canadian Dietary Standard, Bureau of Nutritional Sciences, Department of National Health and Welfare: Dietary Standard for Canada, rev ed. Hull, Quebec, Canadian Publishing Center, Supply and Services Canada, 1975)

## Table 13.  Canada's Food Guide

| Food Group | Recommended Number of Servings (Adult) | Serving Size | Food Group | Recommended Number of Servings (Adult) | Serving Size |
|---|---|---|---|---|---|
| Meat and alternates | 2 | 60–90 g (2–3 oz) cooked lean meat, poultry, liver, or fish<br>60 ml (4 tbsp) peanut butter<br>250 ml (1 c) cooked dried peas, beans, or lentils<br>80–250 ml (⅓–1 c) nuts or seeds<br>60 g (2 oz) cheddar, processed, or cottage cheese<br>2 eggs | Fruits and vegetables | 4–5† | 125 ml (½ c) vegetables or fruits<br>125 ml (½ c) juice<br>1 medium potato, carrot, tomato, peach, apple, orange, or banana |
|  |  |  | Bread and cereals | 3–5‡ | 1 slice bread<br>125–250 ml (½–1 c) cooked or ready-to-eat cereal<br>1 roll or muffin<br>125–200 ml (½–¾ c) cooked rice, macaroni, or spaghetti |
| Milk and milk products | 2* | 250 ml (1 c) milk, yogurt, or cottage cheese<br>45 g (1½ oz) cheddar or processed cheese |  |  |  |

*Children up to 11 years, 2–3 servings; adolescents, 3–4 servings; pregnant and nursing women, 3–4 servings. Skim, 2%, whole, buttermilk, reconstituted dry, or evaporated milk may be used as a beverage or as the main ingredient in other foods. Cheese may also be chosen. In addition, a supplement of vitamin D is recommended when the milk that is consumed does not contain added vitamin D.

†Include at least two vegetables. Choose a variety of both vegetables and fruits—cooked, raw, or their juices. Include yellow or green or green, leafy vegetables.

‡Whole-grain or enriched. Whole-grain products are recommended.

(From Canadian Ministry of Health and Welfare: Canada's Food Guide: Handbook Catalogue No. H21-74/1977. Ottawa, Canadian Ministry of Health & Welfare, 1977)

## Table 14.  Exchange Lists—1950

**Foods That Need Not Be Measured**
**(Insignificant carbohydrate or calories)**

| | |
|---|---|
| Coffee | Cranberries (unsweetened) |
| Tea | Mustard (dry) |
| Clear broth | Pickle (unsweetened) |
| Bouillon (fat free) | Saccharin |
| Lemon | Pepper and other spices |
| Gelatin (unsweetened) | Vinegar |
| Rennet tablets | Seasonings |

Chopped parsley, mint, garlic, onion, celery salt, nutmeg, mustard, cinnamon, pepper and other spices, lemon, saccharin, and vinegar may be used freely.

### List 1.  Milk Exchanges

One exchange of milk contains 8 g protein, 10 g fat, 12 g carbohydrate, and 170 calories.

This list shows the different types of milk to use for one exchange.

| Type of Milk | Amount to Use |
|---|---|
| Whole milk (plain or homogenized) | 1 c |
| Skim milk* | 1 c |
| Evaporated milk | ½ c |
| Powdered whole milk | ¼ c |

*Skim milk and buttermilk have the same food values as whole milk, except that they contain less fat. Two fat exchanges are added when 1 cup of skim milk or buttermilk made from skim milk is used in place of whole milk calculated in a diet pattern.

### List 1.  Milk Exchanges (Continued)

| Type of Milk | Amount to Use |
|---|---|
| Powdered skim milk (non-fat dried milk)* | ¼ c |
| Buttermilk (made from whole milk) | 1 c |
| Buttermilk (made from skim milk)* | 1 c |

One type of milk may be used instead of another, for example, ½ cup of evaporated milk in place of 1 cup of whole milk.

### List 2.  Vegetable Exchanges: Group A

Group A contains little protein, carbohydrate, or calories; 1 cup at a time may be used without counting it.

| | |
|---|---|
| Asparagus | Kale* |
| Beet greens* | Lettuce |
| Broccoli* | Mushrooms |
| Brussels sprouts | Mustard* |
| Cabbage | Okra |
| Cauliflower | Pepper* |
| Celery | Radishes |
| Chard* | Sauerkraut |
| Chicory* | Spinach* |
| Collard* | String beans, young |
| Cucumbers | Summer squash |
| Dandelion greens* | Tomatoes* |
| Eggplant | Turnip greens* |
| Escarole* | Watercress* |

*Good source of vitamin A.

# Table 14. Exchange Lists—1950 (Continued)

## List 2. Vegetable Exchanges: Group B

Each exchange contains 2 g protein, 7 g carbohydrate, and 35 calories.

$1/2$ cup of vegetable equals 1 exchange

| | |
|---|---|
| Beets | Pumpkin* |
| Carrots* | Rutabagas |
| Onions | Squash, winter* |
| Peas, green | Turnip |

*Good source of vitamin A.

## List 3. Fruit Exchanges

One exchange of fruit contains 10 g carbohydrate and 40 calories.

This list shows the different amounts of fruits to use for one fruit exchange:

| Fruit | Amount to Use |
|---|---|
| Apple (2″ diam) | 1 small |
| Applesauce | $1/2$ c |
| Apricots, fresh | 2 medium |
| Apricots, dried | 4 halves |
| Banana | $1/2$ small |
| Blackberries | 1 c |
| Raspberries | 1 c |
| Strawberries* | 1 c |
| Blueberries | $2/3$ c |
| Cantaloupe (6″ diam)* | $1/4$ |
| Cherries | 10 large |
| Dates | 2 |
| Figs, fresh | 2 large |
| Figs, dried | 1 small |
| Grapefruit* | $1/2$ small |
| Grapefruit juice* | $1/2$ c |
| Grapes | 12 |
| Grape juice | $1/4$ c |
| Honeydew melon | $1/8$ medium |
| Mango | $1/2$ small |
| Orange* | 1 small |
| Orange juice* | $1/2$ c |
| Papaya | $1/3$ medium |
| Peach | 1 medium |
| Pear | 1 small |
| Pineapple | $1/2$ c |
| Pineapple juice | $1/3$ c |
| Plums | 2 medium |
| Prunes, dried | 2 medium |
| Raisins | 2 tbsp |
| Tangerine* | 1 large |
| Watermelon | 1 c |

*Rich source of vitamin C.

## List 4. Bread Exchanges

One exchange contains 2 g protein, 15 g carbohydrate, and 70 calories.

This list shows the different amounts of foods to use for one bread exchange.

| Bread, Cereal, and Others | Amount to Use |
|---|---|
| Bread | 1 slice |
| Biscuit, roll (2″ diam) | 1 |
| Muffin (2″ diam) | 1 |

## List 4. Bread Exchanges (Continued)

| Bread, Cereal, and Others | Amount to Use |
|---|---|
| Bread (Continued) | |
| Cornbread (1$1/2$″ cube) | 1 |
| Cereals, cooked | $1/2$ c |
| Dry, flake, and puff types | $3/4$ c |
| Rice, grits, cooked | $1/2$ c |
| Spaghetti, noodles, cooked | $1/2$ c |
| Macaroni, and so on, cooked | $1/2$ c |
| Crackers, graham (2$1/2$″ sq) | 2 |
| Oyster ($1/2$ c) | 20 |
| Saltines (2″ sq) | 5 |
| Soda (2$1/2$″ sq) | 3 |
| Round, thin (1$1/2$″) | 6 |
| Flour | 2$1/2$ tbsp |
| Vegetables | |
| Beans and peas, dried, cooked (Lima, navy, split pea, cowpeas, and so on) | $1/2$ c |
| Baked beans, no pork | $1/4$ c |
| Corn | $1/3$ c |
| Popcorn | 1 c |
| Parsnips | $2/3$ c |
| Potatoes, white | 1 small |
| Potatoes, white, mashed | $1/2$ c |
| Potatoes, sweet, or yams | $1/4$ c |
| Sponge cake, plain (1$1/2$″ cube) | 1 |
| Ice cream (omit 2 fat exchanges) | $1/2$ c |

These foods are measured carefully because they contain significant amounts of carbohydrate.

## List 5. Meat Exchanges

One meat exchange contains 7 g protein, 5 g fat, and 75 calories.

This list shows the different amounts of foods to use for one meat exchange.

| Meat | Amount to Use |
|---|---|
| Meat and poultry (medium fat) beef, lamb, pork, liver, chicken, and so on | 1 oz cooked |
| Cold cuts (4$1/2$″ × $1/8$″) (Salami, minced ham, bologna, liverwurst, luncheon loaf) | 1 slice |
| Frankfurter (8–9 per lb) | 1 |
| Egg | 1 |
| Fish | |
| Haddock, and so on | 1 oz |
| Salmon, tuna, crab, lobster | $1/4$ c |
| Shrimp, clams, oysters, and so on | 5 small |
| Sardines | 3 medium |
| Cheese | |
| Cheddar type | 1 oz |
| Cottage | $1/4$ c |
| Peanut butter* | 2 tbsp |

*Peanut butter is limited to 1 exchange a day unless the carbohydrate in it is allowed for in the calculated diet pattern.

(Continued)

## Table 14.  Exchange Lists—1950 (Continued)

*List 6.  Fat Exchanges*

One fat exchange contains 5 g fat and 45 calories.

This list shows the different foods to use for one fat exchange.

| Fat | Amount to Use |
|---|---|
| Butter or margarine | 1 tsp |
| Bacon, crisp | 1 slice |
| Cream, light | 2 tbsp |
| Cream, heavy | 1 tbsp |
| Cream cheese | 1 tbsp |
| Avocado (4″ diam) | $\frac{1}{8}$ |
| French dressing | 1 tbsp |
| Mayonnaise | 1 tsp |
| Oil or cooking fat | 1 tsp |
| Nuts | 6 small |
| Olives | 5 small |

(Adapted from Meal Planning with Exchange Lists. American Dietetic Association, 430 N. Michigan Ave., Chicago, IL 60611, in J Am Diet Assoc 62:575, 1950)

## Table 15.  Calculating Bioavailable Dietary Iron

1. For each individual meal or snack, determine

    Total iron

    Heme iron (40% of meat, fish, and poultry iron)

    Nonheme iron (60% of meat, fish, and poultry iron, *and* all other food iron)

    Milligrams ascorbic acid of foods as ingested

    Grams cooked meat/fish/poultry (MFP)

    Note: 1 g raw MFP $\div$ 1.3 = 1 g cooked MFP

2. Milligrams heme iron $\times$ 23% = milligrams heme iron bioavailable.

3. Add the milligrams of ascorbic acid to the grams of cooked MFP. The sum equals the enhancing factors (EF) for nonheme iron bioavailability. Consult *the chart below* for percentage of nonheme iron bioavailability.

4. Add (2) and (3) to determine total bioavailable iron for the individual meal or snack.

5. Add individual meal and snack bioavailable iron for day's bioavailable iron.

### Percent Bioavailable Nonheme Dietary Iron for Individual with 500-mg Body Iron Stores

| $\sum EF$ | % | $\sum EF$ | % | $\sum EF$ | % | $\sum EF$ | % | $\sum EF$ | % |
|---|---|---|---|---|---|---|---|---|---|
| 0 | 3.00 | | | | | | | | |
| 1 | 3.09 | 16 | 4.33 | 31 | 5.41 | 46 | 6.38 | 61 | 7.26 |
| 2 | 3.18 | 17 | 4.40 | 32 | 5.48 | 47 | 6.44 | 62 | 7.31 |
| 3 | 3.26 | 18 | 4.48 | 33 | 5.55 | 48 | 6.50 | 63 | 7.37 |
| 4 | 3.35 | 19 | 4.55 | 34 | 5.61 | 49 | 6.56 | 64 | 7.42 |
| 5 | 3.44 | 20 | 4.63 | 35 | 5.68 | 50 | 6.62 | 65 | 7.47 |
| 6 | 3.52 | 21 | 4.70 | 36 | 5.75 | 51 | 6.68 | 66 | 7.53 |
| 7 | 3.60 | 22 | 4.78 | 37 | 5.81 | 52 | 6.74 | 67 | 7.58 |
| 8 | 3.69 | 23 | 4.85 | 38 | 5.88 | 53 | 6.80 | 68 | 7.64 |
| 9 | 3.77 | 24 | 4.92 | 39 | 5.94 | 54 | 6.86 | 69 | 7.69 |
| 10 | 3.85 | 25 | 5.00 | 40 | 6.01 | 55 | 6.92 | 70 | 7.74 |
| 11 | 3.93 | 26 | 5.06 | 41 | 6.07 | 56 | 6.97 | 71 | 7.79 |
| 12 | 4.01 | 27 | 5.14 | 42 | 6.13 | 57 | 7.03 | 72 | 7.85 |
| 13 | 4.09 | 28 | 5.21 | 43 | 6.20 | 58 | 7.09 | 73 | 7.90 |
| 14 | 4.17 | 29 | 5.28 | 44 | 6.26 | 59 | 7.14 | 74 | 7.95 |
| 15 | 4.25 | 30 | 5.34 | 45 | 6.32 | 60 | 7.20 | 75 | 8.00 |

(Courtesy of Elaine R. Monsen, Ph.D., R.D., University of Washington DL-10, Seattle, WA 98112; and Joseph L. Balintfy, Eng. D., University of Massachusetts, Amherst, MA)

# Bibliography

## Part One
## Principles of Nutrition

### General references
### Books

Alfin-Slater RB, Kritchevsky D: Nutrition and the Adult: Macronutrients. New York, Plenum Press, 1980

Altschule MD: Nutritional Factors in General Medicine: Effects of Stress and Distorted Diets. Springfield, IL, Charles C Thomas, 1978

Arlin M: The Science of Nutrition, 2nd ed. New York, Macmillan, 1977

Ashwell M (ed): Clinical and Scientific Aspects of the Regulation of Metabolism. Boca Raton, FL, CRC Press, 1980

Briggs GM, Calloway DH: Bogert's Nutrition and Physical Fitness, 10th ed. Philadelphia, WB Saunders, 1979

Calloway DH, Carpenter KO: Nutrition and Health. Philadelphia, WB Saunders, 1981

Chaney M et al: Nutrition, 9th ed. Boston, Houghton Mifflin, 1979

Davidson S et al: Human Nutrition and Dietetics, 7th ed. New York, Churchill Livingstone, 1978

Fleck H: Introduction to Nutrition. New York, Macmillan, 1981

Goodhart RS, Shils ME (eds): Modern Nutrition in Health and Disease, 6th ed. Philadelphia, Lea & Febiger, 1980

Gussow JD: Feeding Web: Issues in Nutritional Ecology. Palo Alto, CA, Bull, 1978

Guthrie HA: Introductory Nutrition, 4th ed. St Louis, CV Mosby, 1979

Hamilton EM, Whitney E: Nutrition: Concepts and Controversies. St Paul, West, 1979

Hodges RE: Nutrition in Medical Practice. Philadelphia, WB Saunders, 1980

Howard RB, Herbold NH: Nutrition in Clinical Care. New York, McGraw-Hill, 1978

Hunt SM, Groff JL, Holbrook JM: Nutrition Principles and Clinical Practice. New York, John Wiley & Sons, 1980

Krause MV, Maham LK: Food, Nutrition and Diet Therapy. Philadelphia, WB Saunders, 1979

Kreutler PA: Nutrition in Perspective. Englewood Cliffs, NJ, Prentice-Hall, 1980

Moghissi KS, Evans TN (eds): Nutritional Impacts on Women. Hagerstown, MD, Harper & Row, 1977

Randolph PM, Dennison CI: Diet, Nutrition and Dentistry. St Louis, CV Mosby, 1980

Reed PB: Nutrition: An Applied Science. St Paul, West, 1980

Robinson CH, Lawler MR: Normal and Therapeutic Nutrition. New York, Macmillan, 1977

Roe DA: Drug-Induced Nutritional Deficiencies. Westport, CT, Avi, 1976

Schneider HA, Anderson CE, Coursin DB (eds): Nutritional Support of Medical Practice. Hagerstown, MD, Harper & Row, 1977

Stare FJ, McWilliams M: Living Nutrition, 3rd ed. New York, John Wiley & Sons, 1981

Suitor CW, Hunter MF: Nutrition: Principles and Application in Health Promotion. Philadelphia, JB Lippincott, 1980

Tobias AL, Thompson PJ: Issues in Nutrition for the 1980s. Monterey, CA, Wadsworth Health Sciences Division, 1980

Vitamin–Mineral Safety, Toxicity and Misuse. Chicago, IL, American Dietetic Association, 1978

Wenck DA, Baren M, Dewan SP: Nutrition: The Challenge of Being Well Nourished. Reston, VA, Reston, 1980

Whitney ER, Hamilton EMN: Understanding Nutrition, 2nd ed. St Paul, West, 1981

Williams SR: Nutrition and Diet Therapy, 4th ed. St Louis, CV Mosby, 1981

Wilson ED, Fisher KH, Garcia PA: Principles of Nutrition, 4th ed. Somerset, NJ, John Wiley & Sons, 1979

Worthington-Roberts BS: Contemporary Developments in Nutrition. St Louis, CV Mosby, 1980

### Journals and Annuals

American Journal of Clinical Nutrition
American Journal of Nursing
American Journal of Public Health
Cajanus
Ecology of Food and Nutrition
Family Economics Review
FDA Consumer
Food and Nutrition Notes and Reviews
Food Technology
Indian Journal of Nutrition and Dietetics
Journal of the American Dietetic Association
Journal of the Canadian Dietetic Association
Journal of Food Protection
Journal of Home Economics
Journal of Human Nutrition
Journal of the New Zealand Dietetic Association
Journal of Nutrition
Journal of Nutrition Education
Metabolism
National Food Situation Economic Research Service (quarterly)
Nutrition Abstracts and Reviews
Nutrition Reviews
Nutrition Today
Obesity and Bariatric Medicine
World Review of Nutrition and Dietetics

## Reliable sources for nutrition information

American Dietetic Association, 420 N. Michigan Ave., Chicago, IL 60611

American Home Economics Association, 1600 Twentieth St., Washington, DC 20009

Better Business Bureaus

Cooperative Extension—State and Federal (USDA), State and County Cooperative Extension Service

Council on Foods and Nutrition, or Bureau of Investigation, American Medical Association, 535 N. Dearborn St., Chicago, IL 60610

Federal Trade Commission, Bureau of Investigation, State and Local Health Departments, Washington, DC

Food and Drug Administration, U.S. Department of Health and Human Services, Washington, DC 20204

Food and Nutrition Board, National Academy of Sciences—National Research Council, 2101 Constitution Ave., Washington, DC 20418

Food and Nutrition Departments of State University

Food and Nutrition Section, American Public Health Association, 1740 Broadway, New York, NY 10019

The Nutrition Foundation, Inc., 99 Park Ave., New York, NY 10016

United States Department of Agriculture, Washington, DC

United States Department of Health and Human Services, Washington, DC

## National nutrition policies and nutritional status surveys

### Books and pamphlets

Austin JE, Hitt C: Nutrition Intervention in the United States. Cambridge, MA, Ballinger, 1979

Berg A: The Nutrition Factor. Washington, DC, Brookings Institution, 1973

Dietary Intake Findings—U.S. 1971–74 Health and Nutrition Examination Survey, National Center for Health Statistics, Series II, No. 202. Hyattsville, MD, Public Health Resources Administration, 1978

Food Consumption Profiles of White and Black Persons Aged 1–74 Years: U.S. 1971–74. Vital and Health Statistics Series 11, No. 210. DHEW Publ. No. (PHS) 79-1658. Hyattsville, MD, Science and Technological Information Bureau, National Center for Health Statistics, 1979

Food and Nutrient Intakes of Individuals in 1 Day in the U.S., Spring, 1977. Nationwide Food Consumption Survey, 1977–78. Preliminary Report No. 2. Washington, DC, Consumer Nutrition Center, Human Nutrition, 1980

Hemoglobin and Selected Iron-Related Findings of Persons 1–74 Years of Age: U.S., 1971–74. Washington, DC, National Center for Health Statistics, DHEW, Advancedata, Jan 26, 1979

Mayer J, Dwyer JT (eds): Food and Nutrition Policy in a Changing World. New York, Oxford University Press, 1979

Nutrient Levels in Food Used by Households in the U.S., Spring, 1977. Nationwide Food Consumption Survey 1977–78. Preliminary Report No. 3. Washington, DC, Consumer Nutrition Center, Human Nutrition, 1980

Plan and Operation of the Health and Nutrition Examination Survey: U.S. 1971–73. Vital and Health Statistics Series 1 (10a and 10b). DHEW Publ. No. (HSM) 73-1310, 1973

Rizek RL, Jackson EM: Current Food Consumption Practices and Nutrient Sources in the American Diet. Nationwide Food Consumption Survey, 1977–78. Washington, DC, Consumer Nutrition Center, Human Nutrition, 1980

Schmandt J et al: Nutrition Policy in Transition. Lexington, MA, Lexington Books, 1980

Ten-State Nutrition Survey, 1968–70. Highlights. DHEW Publ. No. (HSM)72-8134, 1972

Weight by Height and Age of Adults 18–74 Years: U.S. 1971–74. Washington, DC, National Center for Health Statistics, DHEW, Advancedata, Nov 30, 1977

Winikoff B (ed): Nutrition and National Policy. Cambridge, MA, MIT Press, 1978

### Journal articles

Dwyer JT, Mayer J: Beyond economics and nutrition: The complex basis of food policy. Science 188:566, 1975

Evans DJ: The role of the state governments in educating the public about health. J Med Educ 50:130, 1975

Habicht JP et al: National nutrition surveillance. Fed Proc 37:1181, 1978

McNutt K: Dietary advice to the public: 1957 to 1980. Nutr Rev 38:353, 1980

Quelch JA: The role of nutrition information in national nutrition policy. Nutr Rev 35:289, 1977

Sims LS, Smiciklas-Wright H: An ecological systems perspective: Its application to nutrition policy, program design and evaluation. Ecol Food Nutr 7:173, 1978

Sabry ZI et al: Nutrition Canada—A national nutrition survey. Nutr Rev 32:105, 1974

## Carbohydrates

### Books

Blanshard JMV, Mitchell JR: Polysaccharides in Foods. Woburn, MA, Butterworth, 1979

Counsell JN: Xylitol. London, Applied Science, 1978

Heaton KW (ed): Dietary Fiber—Current Developments of Importance to Health. Westport, CT, Food and Nutrition Press, 1979

Inglett GE, Falkehag SI (eds): Dietary Fibers: Chemistry and Nutrition. New York, Academic Press, 1979

Lieber CS: Nutrition and alcoholism. In Goodhart RS, Shils ME (eds): Modern Nutrition in Health and Disease, 6th ed, pp 1220–1243. Philadelphia, Lea & Febiger, 1980

Roe DA: Alcohol and the Diet. Westport, CT, Avi, 1979

Spiller GA (ed): Topics in Dietary Fiber Research. New York, Plenum Press, 1978

### Journal articles

Ad Hoc Committee on Hypoglycemia: Statement on hypoglycemia. Arch Intern Med 131:591, 1973

Albrink MJ et al: Effects of high- and low-fiber diets on plasma lipids and insulin. Am J Clin Nutr 32:1486, 1979

Anderson JW, Chen WJH: Plant fiber: Carbohydrate and lipid metabolism. Am J Clin Nutr 32:346, 1979

Ayres JC: Manioc. Food Tech 26:128, 1972

Beyer PH, Flynn MA: Effects of high- and low-fiber diets on human feces. J Am Diet Assoc 72:271, 1978

Brown AT: The role of dietary carbohydrate in plaque formation and oral disease. Nutr Rev 33:353, 1975

Brunzell J: Use of fructose, sorbitol, or xylitol as a sweetener in diabetes mellitus. A review. J Am Diet Assoc 73:499, 1978

Bunce GE: Nutrition and cataracts. Nutr Rev 37:337, 1979

Cardello AV et al: Relative sweetness of fructose and sucrose in model solutions, lemon beverages and white cake. J Food Sci 44:748, 1979

Cohn RM, Segal S: Galactose metabolism and its regulation. Metabolism 22:627, 1973

Crapo PA, Olefsky JM: Fructose—Its characteristics, physiology and metabolism. Nutr Today 15:10, 1980

Dietary fiber. A Scientific Status Summary by the IFT's Expert Panel on Food Safety and Nutrition. Food Tech 33:35, 1979

Eastwood MA, Kay RM: An hypothesis for the action of dietary fiber along the gastrointestinal tract. Am J Clin Nutr 32:364, 1979

Edgar WM et al: Acid production in plaque after eating snacks: Modifying factors in food. J Am Dent Assoc 90:418, 1975

Gallagher CR et al: Lactose intolerance and fermented dairy products. J Am Diet Assoc 65:418, 1974

Gilat T: Lactose deficiency: The world pattern today. Israel J Med Sci 15:369, 1979

Hamed MGE et al: Preparation and chemical composition of sweet potato flour. Cereal Chem 50:133, 1973

Hardy SL: Fructose: Comparison with sucrose as sweetener in four products. J Am Diet Assoc 74:41, 1979

Jensen OM, MacLennan R: Dietary factors and colorectal cancer in Scandinavia. Israel J Med Sci 15:329, 1979

Lieber CS: The metabolism of alcohol. Sci Am 234:25, 1976

Lorenz K: Food uses of triticale. Food Tech 26:66, 1972

Marabou Symposium: Food and fiber. Nutr Rev 35:1, 1977

McDonald JL, Stookey GK: Animal studies concerning the cariogenicity of dry breakfast cereals. J Dent Res 56:1001, 1977

Morris C: Batter-Lite blasts consumer charges. (Fructose) Food Engineering 52:30, 1980

O'Brien PJ: The sweet potato: Its origin and dispersal. Am Anthropologist 74:342, 1972

Review: Alcohol-induced brain damage and its reversibility. Nutr Rev 38:11, 1980

Review: Evaluation of the caries-producing ability of human foods. Nutr Rev 36:249, 1978

Robbins GS, Pomeranz Y: Composition and utilization of milled barley products. Cereal Chem 49:240, 1972

Shaw JH: Influence of cereal incorporation in a caries-producing diet on caries activity in rats. J Dent Res 53:397, 1974

Sugars and nutritive sweeteners in processed foods. A Scientific Status Summary by the Institute of Food Technologists' Expert Panel on Food Safety and Nutrition. Food Tech 33:101, 1979

Symposium on role of dietary fiber in health. Am J Clin Nutr (Suppl) 31:1–255, 1978

Toepfer EW et al: Nutrient composition of selected wheats and wheat products. II. Summary. Cereal Chem 49:173, 1972

# Fats and Other Lipids

## Books

Sabine JR (ed): Cholesterol. New York, Marcel Dekker, 1977

Somogyy JC, Francois A (eds): Nutritional Aspects of Fats. Basel, Switzerland, S Karger AG, 1977

## Journal articles

Babayan VK: Medium-chain triglycerides. Their composition, preparation and application. J Am Oil Chem Soc 45:23, 1968

Clegg AJ: Composition and related nutritional and organoleptic aspects of palm oil. J Am Oil Chem Soc 50:321, 1973

Crawford AG et al: Essential fatty acid requirements in infancy. Am J Clin Nutr 32:2181, 1978

de Groat I et al: Lipids in school children, aged 6–17: Upper normal limits. Pediatrics 60:437, 1977

Hirono H et al: Essential fatty acid deficiency induced by total parenteral nutrition and by medium-chain triglyceride feeding. Am J Clin Nutr 30:1670, 1977

Itoh T, Tamura T, Matsumoto T: Sterol composition of 19 vegetable oils. J Am Oil Chem Soc 50:122, 1973

Jensen RG: Composition of bovine milk lipids. J Am Oil Chem Soc 50:186, 1973

Lundberg WO: The significance of cis, cis, cis, 5, 8, 11 eicosatrienoic acid in essential fatty acid deficiency. Nutr Rev 38:233, 1980

Massiello FJ: Changing trends in consumer margarines. J Am Oil Chem Soc 55:262, 1978

McKenna MC, Campagnoni AT: Effect of pre- and postnatal essential fatty acid deficiency on brain development and myelination. J Nutr 109:1195, 1979

Mishkel MA, Nazir DJ, Baere-Rogers JL: Letter: The linoleic and trans fatty acids of margarines. Am J Clin Nutr 33:2055, 1980

Paulsrud JR et al: Essential fatty acid deficiency in infants induced by fat-free intravenous feeding. Am J Clin Nutr 25:897, 1972

Review: Does eicosapentenoic acid prevent thrombosis and atheroslerosis? Nutr Rev 37:316, 1979

Review: Effects of feeding dihomo-$\gamma$-linolenic acid (20:3 $\omega$6) in man. Nutr Rev 37:286, 1979

Review: Essential fatty acid deficiency in continuous-drip alimentation. Nutr Rev 33:329, 1975

Review: Essential fatty acids and water permeability of the skin. Nutr Rev 35:303, 1977

Review: Is essential fatty acid deficiency part of the syndrome of abetalipoproteinemia? Nutr Rev 38:244, 1980

Review: Linolenic acid, an essential fatty acid? Nutr Rev 37:296, 1979

Review: The multiple pathways of arachidonic acid metabolism. Nutr Rev 36:10, 1978

Review: Prostacyclin and coronary vasodilation. Nutr Rev 36:222, 1978

Vergroesen AJ: Physiological effects of dietary linoleic acid. Nutr Rev 35:1, 1977

# Proteins

## (See also references under digestion, absorption, and metabolism)

### Books and pamphlets

FAO: Amino Acid Content of Foods and Biological Data on Proteins. Nutrition Studies No. 24. Rome, FAO, 1970

FAO/WHO Joint Expert Group: Protein Requirements. Rome, FAO, 1965

## Journal articles

Allen LH et al: Reduction of renal calcium reabsorption in man by consumption of dietary protein. J Nutr 109:1345, 1979

Bessman SP: The justification theory: The essential nature of the non-essential amino acids. Nutr Rev 37:209, 1979

Brewer JD et al: Nitrogen retention of young men who consumed selected patterns of essential amino acids at a constant nitrogen intake. Am J Clin Nutr 31:786, 1978

Chopra JG et al: Protein in the U.S. diet. J Am Diet Asoc 72:253, 1978

Hegsted DM: Assessment of nitrogen requirements. Am J Clin Nutr 31:1669, 1978

Hegsted DM, Irwin MI: A conspectus of research on protein requirements of man. J Nutr 101:385, 1971

Hilton MA: Nutrition need for sulfur amino acids in the "liquid protein" diet—An hypothesis. Obesity Bariatric Med 8:49, 1979

Hoffman-Goetz L, Kluger MJ: Protein deficiency: Its effects on body temperature in health and disease states. Am J Clin Nutr 32:1423, 1979

Holt LE, Snyderman SE: Protein and amino acid requirements of infants and children. Nutr Abstr Rev 35:1, 1965

Jones AOL et al: Elemental content of predigested liquid protein products. Am J Clin Nutr 33:2545, 1980

Lantigua RA et al: Cardiac arrhythmias associated with a liquid protein diet for the treatment of obesity. N Engl J Med 303:735, 1980

Lockmiller NR: What are textured protein products? Food Tech 26:59, 1972

Matthews DM, Adibi SA: Peptide absorption. Gastroenterology 71:151, 1976

Michiel RR et al: Sudden death in a patient on a liquid protein diet. N Engl J Med 298:1005, 1978

Review: High protein diets and bone homeostasis. Nutr Rev 38:11, 1981

Review: Sulfur amino acids and the calciuretic effect of dietary protein. Nutr Rev 39:127, 1981

Review: Urinary calcium and dietary protein. Nutr Rev 38:9, 1980

Rose WC: Amino acid requirements of adult man. Nutr Abstr Rev 27:631, 1957

Scrimgeour M: Unconventional sources of protein. J Hum Nutr 32:439, 1979

Scrimshaw NS et al: Protein requirements of man: Variations in obligatory urinary and fecal nitrogen losses in young men. J Nutr 102:1595, 1972

Spencer H et al: Effect of high protein (meat) intake on calcium metabolism in man. Am J Clin Nutr 32:2167, 1978

Sukhatme PV, Margen S: Models for protein deficiency. Am J Clin Nutr 31:1237, 1978

Uauy R et al: Human protein requirements: Nitrogen balance response to graded levels of egg protein in elderly men and women. Am J Clin Nutr 31:779, 1978

Uauy R et al: Human protein requirements: Obligatory urinary and fecal nitrogen losses and the factorial estimation of protein needs in elderly males. J Nutr 108:97, 1978

Valencia ME et al: Protein quality evaluation of corn tortillas, wheat flour tortillas, pinto beans, soybeans, and their combination. Nutr Rep Int 19:195, 1979

Young VR et al: Plasma tryptophan response curve and its relation to tryptophan requirements in young adult men. J Nutr 101:45, 1971

Young VR et al: Protein requirements of man: Efficiency of egg protein utilization at maintenance levels in young men. J Nutr 103:1164, 1973

Young VR et al: Plasma amino acid response curve and amino acid requirements in young men: Valine and lysine. J Nutr 102:1159, 1972

# Water and Electrolyte Metabolism

## Journal articles

Aladjem M et al: Changes in the electrolyte content of serum and urine during total parenteral nutrition. J Pediatr 97:437, 1980

Almroth SG: Water requirements of breast-fed infants in a hot climate. Am J Clin Nutr 31:1154, 1978

Andersson B: Thirst and brain control of water balance. Am Sci 59:408, 1971

Baldetorp L et al: Urinary excretion of inorganic sulfate, ester sulfate, total sulfur and taurine in cancer patients. Acta Med Scand 208:293, 1980

Briscoe J: The role of water supply in improving health in poor countries (with special reference to Bangladesh). Am J Clin Nutr 31:2100, 1978

Corbett WT et al: Utilization of swine to study risk factor of an elevated salt diet on blood pressure. Am J Clin Nutr 32:2068, 1979

Cumming AM et al: Severe hypokalemia with paralysis induced by small doses of liquorice. Postgrad Med J 56:526, 1980

Food and Nutrition Board: Water deprivation and performance of athletes. Nutr Rev 32:314, 1974

Grigorev AI et al: Effect of duration of bed rest on water and mineral metabolism and kidney function. Hum Physiol 5:483, 1979

Hofman A et al: Increased blood pressure in school children related to high sodium levels in drinking water. J Epidemiol Community Health 34:179, 1980

Jourdan M et al: Sulphate, acid-base, and mineral balances of obese women during weight loss. Am J Clin Nutr 33:236, 1980

Klahr S, Slatopolsky E: Renal regulation of sodium excretion. Arch Intern Med 131:780, 1973

Klahr S, Wessler S, Avioli LV: Acid-base disorders in health and disease. JAMA 222:567, 1972

Korolkov UI et al: Water and mineral metabolism and kidney function in man at high altitudes. Hum Physiol 5:634, 1979

Krehl WA: The potassium depletion syndrome. Nutr Today 1:20, June, 1966

Krehl WA: Sodium: A most extraordinary dietary essential. Nutr Today 1:16, 1966

Letteri JM et al: Serial measurement of total body potassium in chronic renal disease. Am J Clin Nutr 31:1937, 1978

McDonald JT, Margen S: Wine versus ethanol in human nutrition. II. Fluid, sodium and potassium balance. Am J Clin Nutr 32:817, 1979

Mortimer JG: Acute water intoxication as another unusual manifestation of child abuse. Arch Dis Child 55:401, 1980

Nalin DR et al: Comparison of low and high sodium and potassium content in oral rehydration solutions. J Pediatr 97:848, 1980

Nicolis GL et al: Glucose-induced hyperkalemia in diabetic subjects. Arch Intern Med 141:49, 1981

Nolten WE et al: Sodium and mineralocorticoids in normal pregnancy. Kidney Int 18:162, 1980

Oliver WJ et al: Hormonal adaptation to the stresses imposed upon sodium balance by pregnancy and lactation in the Yanomama Indians, a culture without salt. Circulation 63:110, 1981

Patrick J, Golden M: Leukocyte electrolytes and sodium transport in protein-energy malnutrition. Am J Clin Nutr 30:1478, 1977

Rado JP et al: Renal response to graded intravenous hypertonic NaCl infusion in healthy and hypertensive subjects: Close-related impairment in distal NaCl reabsorption. Am Heart J 100:183, 1980

Rolls BJ et al: Thirst following water deprivation in humans. Am J Physiol 239:R476, 1980

Review: Development of gut water transport in rats. Nutr Rev 37:118, 1979

Review: Renal failure, acidosis and glutamine metabolism in man. Nutr Rev 37:224, 1979

Schachter J et al: Comparison of sodium and potassium intake with excretion. Hypertension 2:695, 1980

Schneider RE et al: The potential effect of water on gastrointestinal infections prevalent in developing countries. Am J Clin Nutr 31:2089, 1978

Schoeller DA et al: Total body water measurement in humans with $^{18}O$ and $^2H$ labelled water. Am J Clin Nutr 33:2686, 1980

Symposium on fluid, electrolyte, and acid-base balance. Nurs Clin North Am 15:535–646, Sept, 1980

Tobian L: The relationship of salt to hypertension. Am J Clin Nutr 32:2739, 1979

Torun B et al: Effect of isometric exercises on body potassium and dietary protein requirements of young men. Am J Clin Nutr 30:1983, 1977

Tuomilehto J et al: Sodium and potassium excretion in a sample of normotensive and hypertensive persons in eastern Finland. J Epidemiol Community Health 34:174, 1980

# Mineral Metabolism
## Calcium, phosphorus and magnesium
### Books and pamphlets

Avioli LV, Krane SM (eds): Metabolic Bone Disease. New York, Academic Press, 1977

FAO/WHO Expert Committee on Calcium Requirements: Calcium Requirements. Rome, FAO, 1962

Nordin BEC (ed): Calcium, Phosphate and Magnesium Metabolism. Edinburgh, Churchill Livingstone, 1976

### Journal articles

Ashe JR et al: The retention of calcium, iron, phosphorus, and magnesium during pregnancy: The adequacy of prenatal diets with and without supplements. Am J Clin Nutr 32:286, 1979

Bell RP et al: Long term effects of calcium, phosphorus and forced exercise on bones of mature mice. J Nutr 110:1161, 1980

Dennis VW et al: Renal handling of phosphate and calcium. Annu Rev Physiol 41:257, 1979

Draper HH, Scythes CA: Calcium, phosphorus, and osteoporosis. Fed Proc 40:2434, 1981

Ismail-Bergi F et al: Effects of cellulose added to diets of low and high fiber content upon the metabolism of calcium, magnesium, zinc and phosphorus in man. J Nutr 107:510, 1977

Reinhold JG et al: Decreased absorption of calcium, magnesium, zinc, and phosphorus by humans due to increased fiber and phosphorus consumption as wheat bread. J Nutr 106:493, 1976

Robeson BL et al: Muscle changes in rats fed magnesium and calcium deficient diets. J Nutr 109:1383, 1979

Schaafsma G, Visser R: Nutritional interrelationships between calcium, phosphorus and lactose in rats. J Nutr 110:1101, 1980

## Calcium
### Journal articles

American Academy of Pediatrics: Calcium requirements in infancy and childhood. Pediatrics 62:826, 1978

Block GD et al: A comparison of effects of feeding sulfur amino acids and protein on urine calcium in man. Am J Clin Nutr 33:2128, 1980

Chu J-Y et al: Integumentary loss of calcium. Am J Clin Nutr 32:1699, 1979

Cummings JH et al: The digestion of pectin in the human gut and its effect on calcium absorption and large bowel function. Br J Nutr 41:477, 1979

Fayez KG et al: Maturation of calcium transport in the rat small and large intestine. J Nutr 110:1622, 1980

Heaney RP et al: Calcium balance and calcium requirements in middle-aged women. Am J Clin Nutr 30:1603, 1977

Hegsted M, Linkswiler HM: Long-term effects of low level of protein intake on calcium metabolism of young adult women. J Nutr 111:244, 1981

Kim Y, Linkswiler HM: Effect of level of protein intake on calcium metabolism and on parathyroid and renal function in the adult human male. J Nutr 109:1399, 1979

Linkswiler HM et al: Protein-induced hypercalciuria. Fed Proc 40:2429, 1981

Massry SG, Goldstein DA: Calcium metabolism in patients with nephrotic syndrome. Am J Clin Nutr 31:1572, 1978

Pansu D et al: Effect of lactose on duodenal calcium-binding protein and calcium absorption. J Nutr 109:508, 1979

Petith MM, Schedl HP: Effect of semistarvation on large intestinal calcium transport: In vivo studies in the rat. Am J Clin Nutr 32:1006, 1979

Pingle U, Ramasastri BV: Absorption of calcium from a leafy vegetable rich in oxalates. Br J Nutr 39:119, 1978

Pingle U, Ramasastri BV: Effect of water-soluble oxalates in *Amaranthus* spp. leaves on the absorption of milk calcium. Br J Nutr 40:591, 1978

Raman L et al: Effect of calcium supplementation to undernourished mothers during pregnancy on the bone density of the neonates. Am J Clin Nutr 31:466, 1978

Review: Calcium absorption by way of the vacuolar apparatus. Nutr Rev 37:359, 1979

Review: Diet and urinary calculi. Nutr Rev 38:74, 1980

Review: Metabolic bone disease as a result of lactase deficiency. Nutr Rev 37:72, 1979

Review: Urinary calcium and dietary protein. Nutr Rev 38:9, 1980

Spencer H et al: Effect of a high protein (meat) intake on calcium metabolism in man. Am J Clin Nutr 31:2167, 1978

Toverud SU, Boss A: Hormonal control of calcium metabolism during lactation. Vitam Horm 37:303, 1979

Wrobel J, Nagel G: Diurnal rhythm of active calcium transport in rat intestine. Experientia 35:1581, 1979

Zemel B, Linkswiler HM: Calcium metabolism in the young adult male as affected by the level and form of phosphorus intake and level of calcium intake. J Nutr 111:315, 1981

## Phosphorus
### Journal articles

Bell RR et al: Physiological responses of human adults to foods containing phosphate additives. J Nutr 107:42, 1977

Draper HH et al: Osteoporosis in aging rats induced by high phosphorus diets. J Nutr 102:1133, 1972

Ferraro C et al: Intestinal absorption of phosphate: Action of protein synthesis inhibitors and glucocorticoids in the rat. J Nutr 106:1752, 1976

Freeman RM, Lawton WJ: Phosphorus metabolism in potassium deficient rats. Am J Clin Nutr 30:549, 1977

Henry Y et al: Influence of the level of dietary phosphorus on the voluntary intake of energy and metabolic utilization of nutrients in the growing rat. Br J Nutr 42:127, 1979

Kohaut EC et al: Reduced renal acid excretion in malnutrition: A result of phosphate depletion. Am J Clin Nutr 30:861, 1977

Maschio G et al: Early dietary phosphorus restriction and calcium supplementation in the prevention of renal osteodystrophy. Am J Clin Nutr 33:1546, 1980

Sie T-L et al: Hypocalcemia, hyperparathyroidism and bone resorption in rats induced by dietary phosphate. J Nutr 104:1195, 1974

Spencer H et al: Effect of phosphorus on the absorption of calcium and on the calcium balance in man. J Nutr 108:447, 1978

## Magnesium
### Journal articles

Abdulla M: Letter: Clinical signs of magnesium deficiency. Nutr Rev 38:99, 1980 (Reply: Caddell J, pp 100–102)

Abraham AS et al: Magnesium levels in patients with chronic ischemic heart disease. Am J Clin Nutr 31:1400, 1978

Aikawa JK: Biochemistry and physiology of magnesium. World Rev Nutr Diet 28:112, 1978

Ebel H, Gunther T: Magnesium metabolism—A review. J Clin Chem Clin Biochem 18:257, 1980

Forbes RM, Parker HM: Effect of magnesium deficiency on rat bone and kidney sensitivity to parathyroid hormone. J Nutr 110:1610, 1980

Freude KA et al: Splenic protein synthesis in magnesium deficiency: Mechanism of the inhibition. J Nutr 108:1635, 1978

Johnson CJ et al: Myocardial tissue concentrations of magnesium and potassium in men dying suddenly from ischemic heart disease. Am J Clin Nutr 32:967, 1979

Kraeuter SL, Schwartz R: Blood and mast cell histamine levels in magnesium-deficient rats. J Nutr 110:851, 1980

Krehl WA: Magnesium. Nutr Today 2:16, Sept, 1967

Lo GS et al: Effect of isolated soybean protein on magnesium bioavailability. J Nutr 110:829, 1980

McNair P et al: Hypomagnesemia, a risk factor in diabetic retinopathy. Diabetes 27:1075, 1978

Medalle R et al: Vitamin D resistance in magnesium deficiency. Am J Clin Nutr 29:854, 1976

Mordes JP, Wacker WE: Excess magnesium. Pharmacol Rev 29:273, 1978

Nichols BL et al: Magnesium supplementation in protein calorie malnutrition. Am J Clin Nutr 31:176, 1978

Ophaug RH, Singer L: Effect of fluoride on the mobilization of skeletal magnesium and soft-tissue calcinosis during acute magnesium deficiency in the rat. J Nutr 106:771, 1976

Schwartz R et al: Magnesium absorption from leafy vegetables intrinsically labeled with the stable isotope. J Nutr 110:1365, 1980

Zieve FJ et al: Effects of magnesium deficiency on protein and nucleic acid synthesis in vivo. J Nutr 107:2178, 1977

## Trace minerals—general
### Books and pamphlets

Levander OA, Cheng L (eds): Micronutrient Interactions: Vitamins, Minerals and Hazardous Elements. Ann NY Acad Sci 355:1–371, 1980

Prasad AS (ed): Trace Elements in Human Health and Disease, Vol I, Zinc and Copper, Vol II, Essential and Toxic Elements. New York, Academic Press, 1976

Prasad AS (ed): Trace Elements and Iron in Human Metabolism. New York, Plenum Medical, 1978

Underwood EJ: Trace Elements in Human and Animal Nutrition, 4th ed. New York, Academic Press, 1977

WHO Expert Committee: Trace Elements in Human Nutrition. WHO Tech Rep Ser, no. 532. Geneva, World Health Organization, 1973

### Journal articles

Beisel WR: Trace elements in infectious processes. Med Clin North Am 60:831, 1976

Casey CE, Hambidge KM: Trace element deficiencies in man. In Draper HH (ed): Advances in Nutritional Research, Vol 3, pp 23–63. New York, Plenum Press, 1980

Chesters JK: Trace elements: Adventitious yet essential dietary ingredients. Proc Nutr Soc 35:15, 1976

Hauer EC, Kaminski MV Jr: Trace metal profile of parenteral nutrition solutions. Am J Clin Nutr 31:264, 1978

Jacobson S, Wester PO: Balance study of twenty trace elements during total parenteral nutrition in man. Br J Nutr 37:107, 1977

Moses HA: Trace elements: An association with cardiovascular diseases and hypertension. J Natl Med Assoc 71:227, 1979

Review: Metallothionein in trace metal metabolism. Nutr Rev 38:286, 1980

Ulmer DD: Trace elements. N Engl J Med 297:318, 1977

Williams RB: Trace elements and congenital abnormalities. Proc Nutr Soc 36:25, 1977

## Iron
### Pamphlets

Committee on Nutrition of the Mother and Preschool Child, Food and Nutrition Board, National Research Council, National Academy of Sciences: Iron Nutriture in Adolescence. DHEW Publ. No. (HSA)77-5100. Washington, DC, 1976

International Nutritional Anemia Consultive Group: Guidelines for the Eradication of Iron Deficiency Anemia. New York, Nutrition Foundation, 1977

## Journal articles

Basta SS et al: Iron deficiency anemia and the productivity of adult males in Indonesia. Am J Clin Nutr 32:916, 1979

Bjorn-Rasmussen E, Hallberg L: Effect of animal proteins on the absorption of food iron in man. Nutr Metab 23:192, 1979

Bowering J et al: A conspectus of research on iron requirements of man. J Nutr 106:985, 1976

Czajka-Narins DM et al: Nutrition and social correlates in iron deficiency anemia. Am J Clin Nutr 31:955, 1978

Dallman PR: New approaches to screening for iron deficiency. J Pediatr 90:678, 1977

Derman DP et al: Serum ferritin as an index of iron nutrition in rural and urban South African children. Br J Nutr 39:383, 1978

Gardner GR et al: Physical work capacity and metabolic stress in subjects with iron deficiency anemia. Am J Clin Nutr 30:910, 1977

Gershoff SN et al: Studies of the elderly in Boston. I. The effects of iron fortification on moderately anemic people. Am J Clin Nutr 30:226, 1977

Gross SJ et al: Malabsorption of iron in children with iron deficiency. J Pediatr 88:795, 1976

Hallberg L et al: Dietary heme in iron absorption. A discussion of possible mechanisms for iron absorption-promoting effect of meat and for the regulation of iron absorption. Scand J Gastroenterol 14:769, 1979

Hallberg L et al: Iron absorption from South-East Asian diets and the effect of iron fortification. Am J Clin Nutr 31:1403, 1978

Hazell T et al: Iron availability from meat. Br J Nutr 39:631, 1978

Koerper MA, Dallman PR: Serum iron concentration and transferrin saturation in diagnosis of iron deficiency in children—Normal development changes. J Pediatr 91:870, 1977

Martinez-Torres C et al: Effect of cysteine on iron absorption in man. Am J Clin Nutr 34:322, 1981

Matseshe JW et al: Recovery of dietary iron and zinc from the proximal intestine of healthy man: Studies of different meals and supplements. Am J Clin Nutr 33:1946, 1980

Monnier L et al: Evidence of mechanism for pectin-reduced intestinal inorganic iron absorption in idiopathic hemochromatosis. Am J Clin Nutr 33:1225, 1980

Ohira Y et al: Oxygen consumption and work capacity of iron-deficient anemic rats. J Nutr 111:17, 1981

Olszon E et al: Food iron absorption in iron deficiency. Am J Clin Nutr 31:106, 1978

Oski FA: The nonhematologic manifestations of iron deficiency. Am J Clin Dis Child 133:315, 1979

Oski F, Landaw SA: Inhibition of iron absorption from human milk by baby food. Am J Dis Child 134:459, 1980

Picciano MF, Deering RH: The influence of feeding regimens on iron status during infancy. Am J Clin Nutr 33:746, 1980

Rao BSN, Prabhavathi T: An in vitro method for predicting the bioavailability of iron from foods. Am J Clin Nutr 31:169, 1978

Rao BSN, Vijayasarathy C: An alternate formula for the fortification of common salt with iron. Am J Clin Nutr 31:1112, 1978

Review: A specific skeletal muscle dysfunction in iron deficiency. Nutr Rev 35:76, 1977

Rothenbacher H, Sherman AR: Target organ pathology in iron-deficient suckling rats. J Nutr 110:1648, 1980

Saarinen UM et al: Iron absorption in infants: High bioavailability of breast milk iron as indicated by the extrinsic tag method of iron absorption and by the concentration of serum ferritin. J Pediatr 91:36, 1977

Sacks PV, Houchin DN: Comparative bioavailability of elemental iron powders for repair of iron deficiency anemia in rats. Studies on efficiency and toxicity of carbonyl iron. Am J Clin Nutr 31:566, 1978

Siimes MA et al: Manifestation of iron deficiency at various levels of dietary iron intake. Am J Clin Nutr 33:570, 1980

Strauss RG: Iron deficiency, infections and immune function: A reassessment. Am J Clin Nutr 31:660, 1978

Van Campen DR, Welch RM: Availability to rats of iron from spinach: Effects of oxalic acid. J Nutr 110:1618, 1980

Weinberg ED: Infection and iron metabolism. Am J Clin Nutr 30:1485, 1977

## Zinc

### Books

Brewer GJ, Prasad AS (eds): Zinc Metabolism: Current Aspects in Health and Disease. New York, Alan R Liss, 1977

Subcommittee on Zinc, Committee on Medical and Biologic Effects of Environmental Pollutants, Division of Medical Sciences, Assembly of Life Sciences, National Research Council: Zinc. Baltimore, University Park Press, 1979

### Journal articles

Bettger WJ et al: Interaction of zinc and polyunsaturated fatty acids in the chick. J Nutr 110:50, 1980

Butrimowitz GP, Purdy WC: Zinc nutrition and growth in a childhood population. Am J Clin Nutr 31:1409, 1978

Clinical cases: Correction of impaired immunity in Down's syndrome by zinc. Nutr Rev 38:365, 1980

Davies NT: Studies on the absorption of zinc by rat intestine. Br J Nutr 43:189, 1980

Deeming SB, Weber CW: Evaluation of hair analysis for determination of zinc status using rats. Am J Clin Nutr 30:2047, 1977

Erten J et al: Hair zinc levels in healthy and malnourished children. Am J Clin Nutr 31:1172, 1978

Evans GW, Johnson EC: Effect of iron, vitamin $B_6$ and picolinic acid on zinc absorption in the rat. J Nutr 111:68, 1981

Evans GW, Johnson EC: Zinc absorption in rats fed a low-protein diet and a low-protein diet supplemented with tryptophan and picolinic acid. J Nutr 110:1076, 1980

Freeland-Graves JH: Salivary zinc as index of zinc status in women fed a low-zinc diet. Am J Clin Nutr 34:312, 1981

Golden BA, Golden MHN: Plasma zinc and the clinical features of malnutrition. Am J Clin Nutr 32:2490, 1979

Greger JL et al: Zinc and nitrogen balance in adolescent females fed varying levels of zinc and soy protein. Am J Clin Nutr 31:112, 1978

Greger JL, Geissler AH: Effect of zinc supplementation on taste acuity of the aged. Am J Clin Nutr 31:633, 1978

Greger JL, Sickles VS: Saliva zinc levels: Potential indicators of zinc status. Am J Clin Nutr 32:1859, 1979

Hambidge KM et al: Zinc nutrition in preschool children in Denver Head Start Program. Am J Clin Nutr 29:734, 1976

Hambidge KM et al: Zinc nutritional status of young middle-income children and effects of consuming zinc-fortified breakfast cereals. Am J Clin Nutr 33:2532, 1979

Janghorbani M et al: Measurement of $^{68}$Zn and $^{70}$Zn in human blood in reference to the study of zinc metabolism. Am J Clin Nutr 34:581, 1981

Johnson PE, Evans GW: Relative zinc availability in human breast milk, infant formulas and cow's milk. Am J Clin Nutr 31:416, 1978

Kasarskis EJ, Schuna A: Serum alkaline phosphatase after treatment of zinc deficiency in humans. Am J Clin Nutr 33:2609, 1980

McClain C et al: Zinc deficiency: A complication of Crohn's disease. Gastroenterology 78:272, 1980

Nishi Y et al: Zinc status and its relation to growth retardation in children with chronic inflammatory bowel disease. Am J Clin Nutr 33:2613, 1980

Prasad AS: Nutritional zinc today. Nutr Today 16:4, Mar-Apr, 1981

Review: Clinical application of an oral zinc tolerance test. Nutr Rev 39:129, 1981

Solomons NW et al: Studies on the bioavailability of zinc in man. III. Effects of ascorbic acid on zinc absorption. Am J Clin Nutr 32:2495, 1979

Solomons NW, Jacob RA: Studies on the bioavailability of zinc in humans: Effects of heme and nonheme iron on the absorption of zinc. Am J Clin Nutr 34:475, 1981

## Copper, iron, and zinc
### Journal articles

Crews MG et al: Effects of oral contraceptive agents on copper and zinc balance in young women. Am J Clin Nutr 33:1940, 1980

Danks DM: Diagnosis of trace metal deficiency—With emphasis on copper and zinc. Am J Clin Nutr 34:278, 1981

Fleming CR et al: A prospective study of serum copper and zinc levels in patients receiving total parenteral nutrition. Am J Clin Nutr 29:70, 1976

Greger JL, Snedeker SM: Effect of dietary protein and phosphorous levels on the utilization of zinc, copper, and manganese by adult males. J Nutr 110:2243, 1980

Jacob RA et al: Hair as a biopsy material. V. Hair metal as an index of hepatic metal in rats: Copper and zinc. Am J Clin Nutr 31:477, 1978

Keen CL et al: Effect of dietary iron, copper, and zinc chelates of nitrilotriacetic acid (NTA) on trace metal concentrations in rat milk and maternal and pup tissues. J Nutr 110:897, 1980

King JC et al: Absorption of stable isotopes of iron, copper and zinc during oral contraceptive use. Am J Clin Nutr 31:1198, 1978

Klevay LM: Diets deficient in copper and zinc. Med Hypotheses 5:1323, 1979

McKenzie JM: Alteration of the zinc and copper concentration of hair. Am J Clin Nutr 31:470, 1978

Morris ER, Ellis R: Bioavailability to rats of iron and zinc in wheat bran: Response to low phytate bran and effect of phytate/zinc molar ratio. J Nutr 110:2000, 1980

O'Dell BL: Biochemistry of copper. Med Clin North Am 60:687, 1976

Prasad AS: Trace elements: Biochemical and clinical effects of zinc and copper. Am J Hematol 6:77, 1979

Sherman AR, Tissue NT: Tissue iron, copper and zinc levels in offspring of iron-sufficient and iron-deficient rats. J Nutr 110:266, 1980

Vir SC, Love HG: Zinc and copper status of the elderly. Am J Clin Nutr 32:1472, 1979

Vuori E et al: The effect of the dietary intakes of copper, iron, manganese and zinc on the trace element content of human milk. Am J Clin Nutr 33:227, 1980

## Chromium, manganese, and selenium
### Journal articles

Bunk MJ, Combs GF: Effect of selenium on appetite in the selenium-deficient chick. J Nutr 110:743, 1980

deRosa G et al: Regulation of superoxide dismutase activity by dietary manganese. J Nutr 110:795, 1980

Gurson CT: Metabolic significance of dietary chromium. In Draper HH (ed): Advances in Nutritional Research, Vol 1. New York, Plenum Press, 1977

Kumpulainen J, Vuori E: Longitudinal study of chromium in human milk. Am J Clin Nutr 33:2299, 1980

Leach RM, Lilburn MS: Manganese metabolism and its function. World Rev Nutr Diet 32:123, 1978

Lee YH et al: Glutathione peroxidase activity in iron-deficient rats. J Nutr 111:194, 1981

Lifschitz ML et al: Radiochromium distribution in thyroid and parathyroid gland. Am J Clin Nutr 33:57, 1980

Liu VJK, Morris JS: Relative chromium response as an indicator of chromium status. Am J Clin Nutr 31:972, 1978

McKenzie RL et al: Selenium concentration and glutathione peroxidase activity in blood of New Zealand infants and children. Am J Clin Nutr 31:1413, 1978

Miller JA: Manganese deficit may cause seizure. Science News 112:171, 1977

Paynter DI: Changes in activity of the manganese superoxide dismutase enzyme in tissues of the rat with changes in dietary manganese. J Nutr 110:437, 1980

Rabinowitz MB et al: Comparisons of chromium status in diabetic and normal men. Metabolism 29:355, 1980

Review: Blood selenium in cystic fibrosis patients. Nutr Rev 39:14, 1981

Review: Selenium-containing glutathione peroxidase: Its synthesis and function in arachidonate metabolism. Nutr Rev 39:21, 1981

Robinson MF et al: Blood selenium and glutathione peroxidase activity in normal subjects and in surgical patients with and without cancer in New Zealand. Am J Clin Nutr 32:1477, 1979

Saner G et al: Effect of chromium on insulin secretion and glucose removal rate in the newborn. Am J Clin Nutr 33:232, 1980

Sargent T et al: Reduced chromium retention in patients with hemochromatosis, a possible basis of hemochromatic diabetes. Metabolism 28:70, 1979

Sunde RA et al: Effect of dietary methionine on the biopotency of selenite and selenomethionine in the rat. J Nutr 111:76, 1981

## Other trace minerals
### Journal articles
Bello-Reuss EN et al: Serum vanadium levels in chronic renal disease. Ann Intern Med 91:743, 1979

Carlisle EM: Silicon requirement for normal skull formation in chicks. J Nutr 110:352, 1980

Cymbaluk NF: Influence of dietary molybdenum on copper metabolism in ponies. J Nutr 111:96, 1981

Flanagan PR et al: Comparative effects of iron deficiency induced by bleeding and a low-iron diet on the intestinal absorptive interactions of iron, cobalt, manganese, lead and cadmium. J Nutr 110:1754, 1980

Felgal KM et al: Dietary selenium and cadmium interrelationships in growing swine. J Nutr 110:1255, 1980

Fox MRS: Safe levels of cadmium in intravenous diets. Am J Clin Nutr 32:725, 1979

Gibson RS, DeWolfe MS: Cooper, zinc, manganese, vanadium, and iodine concentrations in the hair of Canadian low birth weight neonates. Am J Clin Nutr 32:1728, 1979

Hsu JM: Lead toxicity as related to glutathione metabolism. J Nutr 111:26, 1981

Hsu JM: Current knowledge of zinc, copper and chromium in aging. World Rev Nutr Diet 33:42, 1979

Myron DR et al: Intake of nickel and vanadium by humans. A survey of selected diets. Am J Clin Nutr 31:527, 1978

Nielsen FH: Evidence of the essentiality of arsenic, nickel, and vanadium and their possible nutritional significance. In Draper HH (ed): Advances in Nutritional Research, Vol 3, pp 157–172. New York, Plenum Press, 1980

Perry HM et al: The biology of cadmium. Med Clin North Am 60:759, 1976

Review: The effect of oral cadmium on the pregnant rat and embryo. Nutr Rev 39:26, 1981

## Fat-soluble Vitamins
### General references
#### Books
DeLuca HF (ed): The Fat-Soluble Vitamins, Handbook of Lipid Research, Vol 2. New York, Plenum Press, 1978

## Vitamin A
### Pamphlets
Agency for International Development: Guidelines for the Eradication of Vitamin A Deficiency and Xerophthalmia. A report of the International Vitamin A Consultative Group. Washington, DC, Nutrition Foundation, 1976

Agency for International Development: The Safe Use of Vitamin A. A report of the International Vitamin A Consultative Group. Washington, DC, Nutrition Foundation, 1980

WHO: Vitamin A deficiency and xerophthalmia. Report of a Joint WHO/USAID Meeting. WHO Tech Rep Ser, no. 590. Geneva, World Health Organization, 1976

### Journal articles
Anzano MA et al: Growth, appetite sequence and pathological signs and survival following the induction of rapid, synchronous vitamin A deficiency in the rat. J Nutr 109:1419, 1979

Arroyave G et al: The effect of vitamin A fortification of sugar on the serum vitamin A levels of preschool Guatemalan children: A longitudinal study. Am J Clin Nutr 34:41, 1981

Broske SP et al: Vitamin A status of children in Sri Lanka. Am J Clin Nutr 32:84, 1979

Brown KH et al: Failure of a large dose of vitamin A to enhance the antibody response to tetanus toxoid in children. Am J Clin Nutr 33:212, 1980

Chase HP et al: Low vitamin A and zinc concentrations in Mexican-American migrant children with growth retardation. Am J Clin Nutr 33:2395, 1980

Goodman DS: Vitamin A metabolism. Fed Proc 39:2716, 1980

Mejia LA et al: Clinical signs of anemia in vitamin A-deficient rats. Am J Clin Nutr 32:1439, 1979

Menon K, Vijayaraghavan K: Sequelae of severe xerophthalmia— A follow-up study. Am J Clin Nutr 33:218, 1980

Mohanram M et al: Hematological studies in vitamin A deficient children. Int J Vitam Nutr Res 47:389, 1977

Olson JA: The distribution of vitamin A in human liver. Am J Clin Nutr 32:2500, 1979

Ott DB, Lachance PA: Retinoic acid—A review. Am J Clin Nutr 32:2522, 1979

Palin D et al: The effect of oral zinc supplementation on plasma levels of vitamin A and retinol-binding protein in cystic fibrosis. Am J Clin Nutr 32:1253, 1979

Pirie A, Anbunathan P: Early serum changes in severely malnourished children with corneal xerophthalmia after injection of water-miscible vitamin A. Am J Clin Nutr 34:34, 1981

Review: A cell-surface receptor for plasma retinol-binding protein on pigment epithelium and intestinal mucosal cells. Nutr Rev 35:220, 1977

Review: Cirrhosis, abnormal dark adaptation and vitamin A. Nutr Rev 37:73, 1979

Review: Depression of serum levels of retinol and retinol binding protein during infection. Nutr Rev 39:165, 1981

Review: Effect of growth hormone on vitamin A storage and release. Nutr Rev 39:139, 1981

Review: Interaction of retinol and retinoic acid with the nucleus. Nutr Rev 38:23, 1980

Review: Mobilization of vitamin A by zinc supplementation in zinc deficiency associated with protein-energy malnutrition. Nutr Rev 38:275, 1980

Review: Plasma vitamin A homeostasis: The relative dose response as a measure of liver vitamin A reserves. Nutr Rev 37:361, 1979

Review: The role of vitamin A deficiency in endemic goiter. Nutr Rev 38:15, 1980

Review: "Turnover" of vitamin A. Nutr Rev 35:310, 1977

Review: Vitamin A and the thyroid. Nutr Rev 37:90, 1979

Rojanapo W et al: The prevalance, metabolism and migration of goblet cells in rat intestine following the induction of rapid, synchronous vitamin A deficiency. J Nutr 110:178, 1980

Russell RM: Vitamin A and zinc metabolism in alcoholism. Am J Clin Nutr 33:2741, 1980

Solomons NW, Russell RM: The interaction of vitamin A and zinc: Implications for human nutrition. Am J Clin Nutr 33:2031, 1980

Solon F et al: An evaluation of strategies to control vitamin A deficiency in the Philippines. Am J Clin Nutr 32:1445, 1979

Sommer A et al: History of night-blindness: A simple tool for xerophthalmia screening. Am J Clin Nutr 33:887, 1980

Sporn MB: Retinoids and carcinogenesis. Nutr Rev 35:65, 1977

Symposium: Vitamin A and retinoids—Recent advances. Fed Proc 38:2501, 1979

Vahlquist A et al: Vitamin A transporting plasma proteins and female sex hormones. Am J Clin Nutr 32:1433, 1979

Vahlquist A, Nilsson S: Mechanism of vitamin A transfer from blood to milk in rhesus monkeys. J Nutr 109:1456, 1979

Wolf G: Retinol-linked sugars in glycoprotein synthesis. Nutr Rev 35:97, 1977

## Vitamin D

### Books

DeLuca HF: Vitamin D: Metabolism and Function. Monog Endocrinol, Vol 13. New York, Springer-Verlag, 1979

Lawson DEM: Vitamin D. New York, Academic Press, 1978

Norman AW et al (eds): Vitamin D: Basic Research and Its Clinical Application. Berlin, Walter de Gruyter, 1979

Norman AW et al (eds): Vitamin D: Biochemical, Chemical and Clinical Aspects Related to Calcium Metabolism. Berlin, Walter de Gruyter, 1977

### Journal articles

Brickman AS et al: Actions of 1-$\alpha$-hydroxyvitamin $D_3$ and 1,25-dihydroxy vitamin $D_3$ on mineral metabolism in man. I. Effects on net absorption of phosphorus. Am J Clin Nutr 30:1064, 1977

Frazer DR: Regulation of metabolism of vitamin D. Physiol Rev 60:551, 1980

Haussler MR, McCain TA: Basic and clinical concepts related to vitamin D metabolism and action, Part I. N Engl J Med 297:974, 1977

Haussler MR, McCain TA: Basic and clinical concepts related to vitamin D metabolism and action, Part II. N Engl J Med 297:1041, 1977

Heckmatt JZ et al: Plasma 25-hydroxy vitamin D in pregnant Asian women and their babies. Lancet II:546, 1979

Hobden AN et al: 1,25-dihydroxycholecalciferol stimulation of a mitochondrial protein in chick intestinal cells. Nature 288:718, 1980

Holick MF, Clark MB: The photobiogenesis and metabolism of vitamin D. Fed Proc 37:2567, 1978

Hollander D: Mechanism and site of small intestinal uptake of vitamin $D_3$ in pharmacological concentrations. Am J Clin Nutr 29:970, 1976

Holmberg I, Larsson A: Seasonal variation of vitamin $D_3$ and 25-hydroxy vitamin $D_3$ in human serum. Clin Chim Acta 100:173, 1980

Konishi F, Harrison SL: Vitamin D for adults. J Nutr Educ 11:120, 1979

Kowarski S, Schachter D: Vitamin D-dependent membrane component of the intestinal calcium transport mechanism. J Biol Chem 255:10834, 1980

Lakdawala DR, Widdowson EM: Vitamin D in human milk. Lancet I:167, 1977

Lapatsanis P et al: Two types of nutritional rickets in infants. Am J Clin Nutr 29:1222, 1976

Massry SG: Requirements of vitamin D metabolites in patients with renal disease. Am J Clin Nutr 33:1530, 1980

Pietrek J et al: Kinetics of serum 25-OH-vitamin D in patients with acute renal failure. Am J Clin Nutr 31:1919, 1978

Review: A vitamin D-dependent, membrane-derived intestinal calcium-binding protein. Nutr Rev 39:175, 1981

Review: Growth hormone and vitamin D. Nutr Rev 37:57, 1979

Review: Presence of 1,25-dihydroxyvitamin $D_3$ receptor in rat pituitary. Nutr Rev 39:140, 1981

Review: Vitamin D deficiency rickets revisited. Nutr Rev 38:116, 1980

Review: Vitamin D intoxication treated with glucocorticoids. Nutr Rev 37:323, 1979

Review: Vitamin D metabolism in patients with small-bowel resection. Nutr Rev 35:297, 1977

Ritz E et al: Effects of vitamin D and parathyroid hormone on muscle: Potential role in uremic myopathy. Am J Clin Nutr 33:1522, 1980

Stamp TC: Factors in human vitamin D nutrition and in the production and cure of classical rickets. Proc Nutr Soc 34:119, 1975

## Vitamin E

### Journal articles

Bell EF, Filer LJ Jr: The role of vitamin E in the nutrition of premature infants. Am J Clin Nutr 34:424, 1981

Bieri JG et al: Factors affecting the exchange of tocopherol between red blood cells and plasma. Am J Clin Nutr 30:686, 1977

Bieri JG, Evarts RP: Vitamin E adequacy of vegetable oils. J Am Diet Assoc 66:134, 1975

Desai ID et al: Vitamin E status of agricultural migrant workers in southern Brazil. Am J Clin Nutr 34:2669, 1980

Drake JR, Fitch CD: Status of vitamin E as an erythropoietic factor. Am J Clin Nutr 33:2386, 1980

Horwitt JK: Relative biological value of d-$\alpha$-tocopherol acetate and all-rac-$\alpha$-tocopherol acetate in man. Am J Clin Nutr 33:1856, 1980

Jansson L et al: Vitamin E and fatty acid composition of human milk. Am J Clin Nutr 34:8, 1981

Jansson L et al: Vitamin E requirements of preterm infants. Acta Pediatr Scand 67:459, 1978

Mason KE: The first two decades of vitamin E. Fed Proc 36:1906, 1977

Natta C, Machlin L: Plasma levels of tocopherol in sickle cell anemia subjects. Am J Clin Nutr 32:1359, 1979

Nockels CF: Protective effects of supplemental vitamin E against infection. Fed Proc 38:2134, 1979

Ogunmekan AO: Relationship between age and vitamin E level in epileptic and normal children. Am J Clin Nutr 32:2269, 1979

Paceasciak CR, Carrara MC: Reduction in vitamin E prevents onset of hypertension in developing spontaneously hypertensive rats. Experientia 35:1561, 1979

Packer L, Smith JR: Extension of the life span of cultured human diploid cells by vitamin E: A reevaluation. Proc Natl Acad Sci 74:1640, 1977

Prasad JS: Effect of vitamin E supplementation on leukocyte function. Am J Clin Nutr 33:606, 1980

Rachmilewilz EA et al: Vitamin E deficiency in β-thalassemia major: Changes in hematological and biochemical parameters after a therapeutic trial with α-tocopherol. Am J Clin Nutr 32:1850, 1979

Review: Effect of dietary α-tocopherol in aging rats. Nutr Rev 35:50, 1977

Review: Possible role of vitamin E in the conversion of cyanocobalamine to its coenzyme form. Nutr Rev 37:332, 1979

Review: Safety of vitamin E therapy in low birth weight infants. Nutr Rev 39:121, 1981

Review: Vitamin E. Nutr Rev 35:57, 1977

Review: Vitamin E. A scientific status summary. Food Tech 31:77, 1977

Review: Vitamin E in the prevention of chronic bronchopulmonary dysplasia in low birth weight infants. Nutr Rev 37:11, 1979

Scott ML: Advances in our understanding of vitamin E. Fed Proc 39:2736, 1980

Sheffy BE, Schults RD: Influence of vitamin E and selenium on immune response mechanisms. Fed Proc 38:2139, 1979

Vatassery GT, Chiang T: Serum α-tocopherol, lipids, potassium, creatine phosphokinase in normal and malabsorption patients. Am J Clin Nutr 32:2061, 1979

Witting LA et al: Dietary levels of vitamin E and polyunsaturated fatty acids and plasma vitamin E. Am J Clin Nutr 28:571, 1975

Witting LA et al: RDA for vitamin E. Am J Clin Nutr 28:577, 1975

# Vitamin K

## Journal articles

Almquist HT: The early history of vitamin K. Am J Clin Nutr 28:656, 1975

American Academy of Pediatrics, Committee on Nutrition: Vitamin K supplementation for infants receiving mild substitute infant formulas and for those with fat malabsorption. Pediatrics 48:483, 1971

Bell RG: Metabolism of vitamin K and prothrombin synthesis: Anticoagulants and the vitamin K-epoxide cycle. Fed Proc 37:2599, 1978

Larsen JF et al: Intrauterine injection of vitamin K before delivery during anticoagulant therapy of the mother. Acta Obstet Gynecol Scand 57:227, 1978

Olson RE, Suttie JW: Vitamin K and carboxyglutamate biosynthesis. Vitam Horm 35:59, 1977

Review: The functional significance of vitamin K action. Nutr Rev 34:182, 1976

Review: Interaction between vitamin K and fat absorption. Nutr Rev 34:314, 1976

Review: Vitamin K and the carboxylation of glutamyl residues. Nutr Rev 33:25, 1975

Review: Vitamin K reduction precedes epoxidation and prothrombin synthesis. Nutr Rev 36:20, 1978

Sadowsky JA et al: Vitamin K epoxidase: Properties and relationship to prothrombin synthesis. Biochemistry 16:3856, 1977

Stenflo J, Suttie JW: Vitamin K-dependent formation of α-carboxyglutamic acid. Annu Rev Biochem 46:157, 1977

Suttie JW: The metabolic role of vitamin K. Fed Proc 39:2730, 1980

Symposium: Vitamin K. Fed Proc 37:2598, 1978

# Water-soluble Vitamins

## Books

Barker BM, Bender DA (eds): Vitamins in Medicine. Vol 1, 4th ed. London, William Heinemann Medical Books, 1980

## Ascorbic acid

### Journal articles

Cameron E et al: Ascorbic acid and cancer: A review. Cancer Res 39:663, 1979

Cook JD, Monsen ER: Vitamin C, the common cold, and iron absorption. Am J Clin Nutr 30:235, 1977

Coulehan JL et al: Vitamin C and acute illness in Navajo schoolchildren. N Engl J Med 295:973, 1976

Cummings M: Can some people synthesize ascorbic acid? Am J Clin Nutr 34:297, 1981

Davis MG et al: Ascorbic acid absorption in rat intestine and kidney. Nutr Metab (Suppl 1) 21:266, 1977

Ginter E et al: Effect of ascorbic acid on plasma cholesterol in humans in a long-term experiment. Int J Vitam Nutr Res 47:123, 1977

Ginter E et al: Tissue levels and optimum dosage of vitamin C in guinea pigs. Nutr Metab 23:217, 1979

Goldman HM et al: The antiscorbutic action of L-ascorbic acid and D-isoascorbic acid (erythroic acid) in the guinea pig. Am J Clin Nutr 34:24, 1981

Hoffer J: Synergistic effect of vitamin C and aspirin. Am J Clin Nutr 32:280, 1979

Irwin MI, Hutchins BK: A conspectus of research on vitamin C requirements of man. J Nutr 106:821, 1976

Kallner A et al: Determination of body pool size and turnover rate of ascorbic acid in man. Nutr Metab (Suppl 1) 21:31, 1977

Keltz FR et al: Urinary ascorbic acid excretion in the human as affected by dietary fiber and zinc. Am J Clin Nutr 31:1167, 1978

King CG, Burns JJ (eds): Second Conference on Vitamin C. Ann NY Acad Sci 258:5–552, 1975

Knodell RG et al: Vitamin C prophylaxis for posttransfusion hepatitis: Lack of effect in a controlled trial. Am J Clin Nutr 34:20, 1981

Lukes TH et al: Vitamin C and growth. JAMA 238:937, 1977

Machlin LJ et al: Lack of antiscorbutic activity of ascorbate 2—sulfate in the rhesus monkey. Am J Clin Nutr 29:825, 1976

Miller JZ et al: Therapeutic effect of vitamin C; A co-twin control study. JAMA 237:248, 1977

Myres AW: Serum vitamin C levels in infants. Am J Clin Nutr 30:133, 1977

Puistola U et al: Studies on the lysyl hydroxylase reaction. I. Initial velocity kinetics and related aspects. Biochim Biophys Acta 611:40, 1980

Puistola U et al: Studies on the lysyl hydroxylase reaction. II. Inhibition kinetics and the reaction mechanism. Biochim Biophys Acta 611:51, 1980

Review: Ascorbic acid and catecholamines. Nutr Rev 34:181, 1976

Review: The function of ascorbic acid in collagen formation. Nutr Rev 36:118, 1978

Review: New information on synthesis and metabolism of ascorbic acid. Nutr Rev 35:22, 1977

Review: Vitamin C and phagocyte function. Nutr Rev 36:183, 1978

Review: Vitamin C toxicity. Nutr Rev 34:236, 1976

Shilotri PG, Bhat KS: Effect of megadoses of vitamin C on bactericidal activity of leucocytes. Am J Clin Nutr 30:1077, 1977

## Thiamin

### Books

Gubler CJ et al (eds): Thiamine. New York, John Wiley & Sons, 1974

### Journal articles

Basu TK, Dickerson JW: The thiamin status of early cancer patients with particular reference to those with breast and bronchial carcinomas. Oncology 33:250, 1976

Centerwall BS: Prevention of the Wernicke-Korsakoff syndrome: A cost–benefit analysis. N Engl J Med 299:285, 1978

Chan AW: Combined metabolic effects of ethanol and thiamine deficiency in the central nervous system. Biochem Pharmacol 27:1259, 1978

Gontzea I et al: Biochemical assessment of thiamin status in patients with neurosis. Nutr Metab 19:153, 1975

Henderson GI et al: Effects of thiamine deficiency on cerebral and visceral protein synthesis. Biochem Pharmacol 27:1677, 1978

Kjosen B, Seim SH: The transketolase assay of thiamin in some diseases. Am J Clin Nutr 30:1591, 1977

Labadarious D et al: Thiamine deficiency in fulminant hepatic failure and effects of supplementation. Int J Vitam Nutr Res 47:17, 1977

Long A: Thiamine in vegetarian diets. Br Med J 2:47, 1976

Lonsdale D, Shamberger RJ: Red cell transketolase as an indicator of nutritional deficiency. Am J Clin Nutr 33:205, 1980

Lumeng LJ et al: Transport and metabolism of thiamin in isolated rat hepatocytes. J Biol Chem 254:7265, 1979

Meinen M et al: Studies on the absorption of thiamine, riboflavin and pyridoxine in vitro. Nutr Metab (Suppl 1) 21:264, 1977

Neumann CG et al: Biochemical evidence of thiamin deficiency in young Ghanaian children. Am J Clin Nutr 32:99, 1979

Niwa T et al: Plasma level and transfer capacity of thiamin in patients undergoing long-term hemodialysis. Am J Clin Nutr 28:1105, 1975

Penttinen HK: Determination of thiamine and its phosphate esters by electrophoresis and fluorometry. Acta Chem Scand B32:609, 1978

Plaitakis A et al: The effect of acute thiamine deficiency on brain tryptophan, serotonin and 5-hydroxyindoleacetic acid. J Neurochem 31:1087, 1978

Read DJ: The aetiology of the sudden infant death syndrome: Current ideas on breathing and sleep and possible links to deranged thiamine neurochemistry. Aust NZ J Med 8:322, 1978

Schenker S et al: Hepatic and Wernicke's encephalopathies: Current concepts of pathogenesis. Am J Clin Nutr 33:2719, 1980

Viana MB et al: Thiamine-responsive megaloblastic anemia, sensorineural deafness and diabetes mellitus: A new syndrome? J Pediatr 93:235, 1978

Vimokesant SL: Effects of betel nut and fermented fish on the thiamin status of northeastern Thais. Am J Clin Nutr 28:1458, 1975

Waldenlind L: Studies on thiamine and neuromuscular transmission. Acta Physiol Scand (Suppl) 459:1, 1978

Waldenlind L: Studies on thiamine and neuromuscular transmission. Acta Physiol Scand 105:1, 1979

Weinstein MC: Editorial: Prevention that pays for itself. N Engl J Med 299:307, 1978

Wood B et al: A study of partial thiamin restriction in human volunteers. Am J Clin Nutr 33:848, 1980

## Riboflavin

### Books

Rivlin RS (ed): Riboflavin. New York, Plenum Press, 1975

Singer TP (ed): Flavins and Flavoproteins. Amsterdam, Elsevier, 1976

### Journal articles

Boni H et al: Assessment of the vitamin $B_2$ status by means of the glutathione reductase test. Nutr Metab (Suppl 1) 21:20, 1977

Brady PS et al: Effects of riboflavin deficiency on growth and glutathione peroxidase system enzymes in the baby pig. J Nutr 109:1615, 1979

Buzina R et al: The effect of riboflavin administration on iron metabolism parameters in a school-age population. Int J Vitam Nutr Res 49:136, 1979

Decker K et al: Riboflavin status and anaemia in pregnant women. Nutr Metab (Suppl 1) 21:17, 1977

Garry PJ, Owen GM: An automated flavin adenine dinucleotide-dependent glutathione reductase assay for assessing riboflavin nutriture. Am J Clin Nutr 29:663, 1976

Gromisch DS et al: Light (phototherapy) induced riboflavin deficiency in the neonate. J Pediatr 90:118, 1977

Guggenheim K, Segal S: Oral contraceptives and riboflavin nutriture. Int J Vitam Nutr Res 47:234, 1977

Hoppel C et al: Riboflavin and rat hepatic cell structure and function. Mitochondrial oxidative metabolism in deficiency status. J Br Chem 254:4164, 1979

Hughes J et al: Riboflavin levels in the diet and breast milk of vegans and omnivores. Proc Nutr Soc 38:95A, 1979

Kramer V et al: Applicability of blood and urine analysis for the determination of nutritional status of riboflavin. Nutr Metab (Suppl 1) 21:22, 1977

Lakshmi AV, Bamji MS: Regulation of blood pyridoxal phosphate in riboflavin deficiency in man. Nutr Metab 20:228, 1976

Lewis JA et al: Urinary riboflavin and creatinine excretion in children treated with anticonvulsant drugs. Am J Dis Child 129:394, 1975

Lopez R: Riboflavin deficiency in a pediatric population of low socio-economic status in New York City. J Pediatr 87:420, 1975

Merrill AH Jr et al: Purification of riboflavin-binding proteins from bovine plasma and discovery of a pregnancy-specific riboflavin-binding protein. J Biol Chem 254:9362, 1979

Newman LJ: Riboflavin deficiency in women taking oral contraceptives. Am J Clin Nutr 31:247, 1978

Pascale JA et al: Riboflavin and bilirubin response during phototherapy. Pediatr Res 10:854, 1976

Powers HJ et al: Physiological effects of marginal riboflavin deficiency in young adults and geriatrics: A reduction in the in vivo survival time of erythrocytes. Proc Nutr Soc 39:17A, Feb, 1980

Prentice AM et al: Biochemical evaluation of the erythrocyte glutathione reductase test for riboflavin deficiency. Proc Nutr Soc 37:49A, 1978

Redd AS et al: The role of riboflavin in carbohydrate metabolism. Adv Exp Med Biol 119:243, 1979

Review: Influence of red cell age on the measurement of riboflavin status. Nutr Metab (Suppl 1) 21:155, 1977

Review: The interrelationship between riboflavin and pyridoxine. Nutr Rev 35:237, 1977

Review: Riboflavin deficiency in rats and fatty acid oxidation. Nutr Rev 38:90, 1980

Review: Riboflavin and thiamine binding proteins: Their physiological significance and hormonal specificity. Nutr Rev 37:261, 1979

Review: Urinary riboflavin metabolites from rats. Nutr Rev 35:281, 1977

Rutishauser IH et al: Long-term vitamin status and dietary intake of healthy elderly subjects. 1. Riboflavin. Br J Nutr 42:33, 1979

Vir SC et al: Riboflavin nutriture of oral contraceptive users. Int J Vitam Nutr Res 49:286, 1979

## Niacin
### Books
Roe DA: A Plague of Corn. The Social History of Pellagra. Ithaca, Cornell University Press, 1973

### Journal articles
Crouinard et al: Tryptophan–nicotinamide combination in the treatment of newly admitted depressed patients. Commun Psychopharmacol 2:311, 1978

Henderson LM et al: Transport of niacin and niacinamide in perfused rat intestine. J Nutr 109:646, 1979

Henderson LM et al: Metabolism of niacin and niacinamide in perfused rat intestine. J Nutr 109:654, 1979

Horwitt MK et al: Niacin–tryptophan relationships for evaluating niacin equivalents. Am J Clin Nutr 34:423, 1981

Labadarias D et al: Metabolic abnormalities of tryptophan and nicotinic acid in patients with rheumatoid arthritis. Rheumatol Rehabil 17:227, 1978

Manson JA et al: The effect of a high level of dietary leucine on the niacin status of chicks and rats. J Nutr 108:1883, 1978

Manson JA et al: The effect of a high level of dietary leucine on the niacin status of dogs. J Nutr 108:1889, 1978

Review: Effect of high intake of leucine on urinary tryptophan and niacin metabolites. Nutr Rev 34:105, 1976

Sadoogh-Abasian F et al: Absorption of nicotinic acid and nicotinamide from rat small intestine in vitro. Biochim Biophys Acta 598:385, 1980

Spector R: Niacin and niacinamide transport in the central nervous system. In vitro studies. J Neurochem 33:895, 1979

Vannucchi H et al: Effect of corn and sorghum diets in $N^1$-methylnicotinamide excretion and hepatic enzymes in rats. Int J Vitam Nutr Res 48:352, 1978

## Vitamin $B_6$
### Booklets
Food and Nutrition Board: Human Vitamin $B_6$ Requirements. Washington, DC, National Academy of Sciences, 1978

### Journal articles
Alton-Mackey MG, Walker BL: The physical and neuromotor development of progeny of female rats fed graded levels of pyridoxine during lactation. Am J Clin Nutr 31:76, 1978

Alton-Mackey MG, Walker BL: Physical and neuromotor development of pyridoxine-restricted rats cross-fostered with control of isonutritional dams. Am J Clin Nutr 31:241, 1978

Bapurao S, Krishnaswany K: Vitamin $B_6$ nutritional status of pellagrins and their leucine tolerance. Am J Clin Nutr 31:819, 1978

Kirksey A et al: Vitamin $B_6$ nutritional status of a group of female adolescents. Am J Clin Nutr 31:946, 1978

Kleiner MJ et al: Vitamin $B_6$ deficiency in maintenance dialysis patients: Metabolic effects of repletion. Am J Clin Nutr 33:1612, 1980

Labadarios D et al: Vitamin $B_6$ deficiency in chronic liver disease—Evidence for increased degradation of pyridoxal-5-phosphate. Gut 18:23, 1977

Lewis JS, Nunn KP: Vitamin $B_6$ intake and 24 hr. 4-pyridoxic acid excretions of children. Am J Clin Nutr 30:2023, 1977

Livingston JE et al: Vitamin $B_6$ status in women with postpartum depression. Am J Clin Nutr 31:886, 1978

Middleton HM: Effect of vitamin $B_6$ deficiency on in vitro uptake and metabolism of pyridoxine HCL by rat jejunum. Am J Clin Nutr 33:2168, 1980

Potera C et al: Vitamin $B_6$ deficiency in cancer patients. Am J Clin Nutr 30:1677, 1977

Reinken L, Zieglauer H: Vitamin $B_6$ absorption in children with acute celiac disease and in control subjects. J Nutr 108:1562, 1978

Review: Does pyridoxal phosphate have a non-coenzymatic role in steroid hormone action? Nutr Rev 38:93, 1980

Review: Nature and activity of vitamin $B_6$ bound in heat-processed foods. Nutr Rev 36:346, 1978

Review: Phosphorylase response to vitamin $B_6$ feeding. Nutr Rev 36:55, 1978

Review: Pyridoxine and its metabolism in chronic liver disease. Nutr Rev 35:136, 1977

Review: Pyridoxine (Pyridoxamine)5'-phosphate oxidase in human red cells. Nutr Rev 38:380, 1980

Review: The role of growth hormone in the action of vitamin $B_6$ on cellular transfer of amino acids. Nutr Rev 37:30, 1979

Review: Vitamin $B_6$ deficiency and immune responses. Nutr Rev 34:188, 1976

Roepke LLB, Kirksey A: Vitamin B$_6$ nutriture during pregnancy and lactation. I. Vitamin B$_6$ intake, levels of the vitamin in biological fluids, and condition of the infant at birth. Am J Clin Nutr 32:2249, 1979

Roepke LLB, Kirksey A: Vitamin B$_6$ nutriture during pregnancy and lactation. II. The effect of long-term use of oral contraceptives. Am J Clin Nutr 32:2257, 1979

Solomon RS, Hillman RS: Regulation of vitamin B$_6$ metabolism in human red cells. Am J Clin Nutr 32:1824, 1979

Spannuth CL Jr et al: Increased plasma clearance of pyridoxal-5-phosphate in vitamin B$_6$ deficient uremic man. J Lab Clin Med 90:632, 1977

Teehan BP et al: Plasma pyridoxal-5'-phosphate levels and clinical correlations in chronic hemodialysis patients. Am J Clin Nutr 31:1932, 1978

Vir SC, Love AHG: Vitamin B$_6$ status of the hospitalized aged. Am J Clin Nutr 31:1383, 1978

Wheatley D: Treatment of pregnancy sickness. Br J Obstet Gynecol 84:444, 1977

## Folacin—folic acid

### Booklets

Food and Nutrition Board: Folic Acid: Biochemistry and Physiology in Relation to the Human Nutrition Requirement. Washington, DC, National Academy of Sciences, 1977

### Journal articles

Bailey LB et al: Folacin and iron status and hematological findings in predominantly black elderly persons from urban low-income households. Am J Clin Nutr 32:2346, 1979

Bailey LB et al: Folacin and iron status in low-income pregnant adolescents and mature women. Am J Clin Nutr 33:1997, 1980

Eichner ER et al: Elevated serum levels of unsaturated folate-binding protein: Clinical correlates in a general hospital population. Am J Clin Nutr 31:1988, 1978

Gerson CD, Cohen N: Folic acid absorption in regional enteritis. Am J Clin Nutr 29:182, 1976

Hoppner K, Lampi B: Folate levels in human liver from autopsies in Canada. Am J Clin Nutr 33:862, 1980

Rasmussen KM et al: Folacin deficiency and requirement in the squirrel monkey (Saimiri Sciureus). Am J Clin Nutr 32:2508, 1979

Review: Accumulation of 5-methyltetra-hydrofolic acid in ethanol-treated hepatocytes. Nutr Rev 38:223, 1980

Review: The deoxyuridine suppression test for the diagnosis of masked or previous folate deficiency. Nutr Rev 37:77, 1979

Review: Folate-losing gastropathy in giant hypertrophic gastritis. Nutr Rev 36:185, 1978

Review: Inhibition of the hemopoietic activity of folic acid. Nutr Rev 37:254, 1979

Review: Intestinal enzymes in folate deficiency and tropical sprue. Nutr Rev 36:135, 1978

Review: Methionine and the "methyl folate trap." Nutr Rev 36:255, 1978

Review: Pterin-6-aldehyde production from folic acid by malignant tissues. Nutr Rev 35:169, 1977

Tamura T et al: Absorption of mono- and polyglutamyl folates in zinc-depleted men. Am J Clin Nutr 31:1984, 1978

## Vitamin B$_{12}$

### Journal articles

Brandt LT et al: The effect of bacterially produced vitamin B$_{12}$ analogues (cobamides) on the in vitro absorption of cyanocobalamin. Am J Clin Nutr 32:1832, 1979

Chen SC, Oace SM: Methylmalonic acid metabolism in germ free and conventional B-12 deprived rats fed precursors of methylmalonte. J Nutr 109:1205, 1979

Jacob E et al: Vitamin B$_{12}$-binding proteins. Physiol Rev 60:918, 1980

Marcoullis G et al: Cobalamin malabsorption due to non-degradation of R proteins in the human intestine: Inhibited cobalamin absorption in exocrine pancreatic dysfunction. J Clin Invest 66:430, 1980

Marcus M et al: Stability of vitamin B$_{12}$ in the presence of ascorbic acid in food and serum: Restoration by cyanide of apparent loss. Am J Clin Nutr 33:137, 1980

Review: Dietary fiber and vitamin B-12 balance. Nutr Rev 37:116, 1979

Review: Hyperpigmentation in pernicious anemia. Nutr Rev 37:137, 1979

Review: Pitfalls in the diagnosis of vitamin B$_{12}$ deficiency by radiodilution assay. Nutr Rev 37:313, 1979

Review: Possible role of vitamin E in the conversion of cyanocobalamin to its coenzyme form. Nutr Rev 37:332, 1979

Review: Vegetarian diet and vitamin B$_{12}$ deficiency. Nutr Rev 36:243, 1978

## Biotin

### Journal articles

Balnave D: Clinical symptoms of biotin deficiency in animals. Am J Clin Nutr 30:1408, 1977

Bayer EA et al: The biotin transport system. Methods Enzymol 46:613, 1977

Bitsch R et al: Effect of different biotin supply in rats. Nutr Metab (Suppl 1) 21:27, 1977

McCormick DB: Biotin. Nutr Rev 33:97, 1975

Meolar HW et al: Biotin-binding protein from egg yolk. A protein distinct from egg white avidin. J Biol Chem 253:6979, 1978

Murphy PN et al: Biotin. Prog Food Nutr Sci 2:405, 1977

Petrelli F et al: Effects of biotin deficiency on serum proteins and plasma amino acids. Experientia 34:1481, 1978

Review: A role of biotin in fatty liver and kidney syndrome in chicks. Nutr Rev 34:217, 1976

Review: Multiple biotin-dependent carboxylase deficiencies associated with defects in immunity. Nutr Rev 37:289, 1979

Schrijver T et al: Some biochemical observations on biotin deficiency in the rat as a model for human pyruvate carboxylase deficiency. Nutr Metab 23:179, 1979

Volpe JJ et al: Mechanism and regulation of biosynthesis of saturated fatty acids. Physiol Rev 56:339, 1976

## Pantothenic acid

### Journal articles

Cohenour SH, Calloway DH: Blood, urine and dietary pantothenic acid levels of pregnant teenagers. Am J Clin Nutr 25:512, 1972

Fry PC et al: Metabolic response to a pantothenic acid deficient diet in humans. J Nutr Sci Vitaminol 22:339, 1976

Ellestad-Soyed JJ et al: Pantothenic acid, coenzyme A, and human chronic ulcerative and granulomatous colitis. Am J Clin Nutr 29:1333, 1976

Smith CM et al: The effect of metabolic state on incorporation of $^{14}$C-pantothenate into CoA in rat liver and heart. J Nutr 108:863, 1978

Mahboob S, Estes LW: Effect of pantothenic acid deficiency on rat hepatocytes. Nutr Metab 22:177, 1978

Pietrzik K, Hotzel D: Studies for the evaluation of pantothenic acid requirement. Nutr Metab (Suppl 1) 21:23, 1977

# Nutrient Utilization: Digestion, Absorption, and Metabolism

## Books and pamphlets

Davenport HW: Physiology of the Digestive Tract. Chicago, Yearbook, 1977

Dietary Sugars in Health and Disease. I. Fructose. FASEB Publ. No. 262-764. Bethesda, MD, Life Sciences Research Office, 1976

McMurray WC: Essentials of Human Metabolism. Hagerstown, MD, Harper & Row, 1977

Vergroesen AJ (ed): The Role of Fats in Human Nutrition. New York, Academic Press, 1975

## Journal articles

Agbedana EO et al: Studies on hepatic and extra hepatic lipoprotein lipases in protein-calorie malnutrition. Am J Clin Nutr 32:292, 1979

Balasse EO: Kinetics of ketone body metabolism in fasting humans. Metabolism 28:41, 1979

Balint JA: Ileal uptake of oleic acid: Evidence for adaptive response to high fat feeding. Am J Clin Nutr 33:2276, 1980

Barr SI et al: Postprandial exchange of apolipoprotein C-III between plasma lipoproteins. Am J Clin Nutr 34:191, 1981

Barrett AJ: The many forms and functions of cellular proteinases. Fed Proc 39:10, 1980

Beck-Nielsen H et al: Impaired cellular insulin binding and insulin sensitivity induced by high-fructose feeding in normal subjects. Am J Clin Nutr 33:273, 1980

Bierman EL: Carbohydrates, sucrose and human disease. Am J Clin Nutr 32:2712, 1979

Bird JWC et al: Proteinases in cardiac and skeletal muscle. Fed Proc 39:20, 1980

Bronsgeest-Schante DC et al: Dependence of the effects of dietary cholesterol and experimental conditions on serum lipids in man. I. Effects of dietary cholesterol in linoleic acid-rich diet. Am J Clin Nutr 32:2183, 1979; II. Effects of dietary cholesterol in a linoleic acid-poor diet. 32:2188, 1979; III. The effect on serum cholesterol of removal of eggs from the diet of free living habitually egg-eating people. Am J Clin Nutr 32:2193, 1979

Brunner D et al: Serum lipid response to a high-caloric, high-fat diet in agricultural workers during 12 months. Am J Clin Nutr 32:1342, 1979

Bursztein S et al: Utilization of protein, carbohydrate and fat in fasting and post absorptive subjects. Am J Clin Nutr 33:998, 1980

Chey WY, Gutierrez JG: The endocrine control of gastro-intestinal function. Adv Intern Med 23:61, 1978

Coulston A et al: Effect of source of dietary carbohydrate on plasma glucose and insulin response to test meals in normal subjects. Am J Clin Nutr 33:1279, 1980

Crapo PA et al: Comparison of serum glucose, insulin, and glucagon responses to different types of complex carbohydrate in noninsulin-dependent diabetic patients. Am J Clin Nutr 34:184, 1981

Crapo PA et al: Postprandial hormonal responses to different types of complex carbohydrates in individuals with impaired glucose tolerance. Am J Clin Nutr 33:1723, 1980

Dockray GJ: Comparative biochemistry and physiology of gut hormones. Annu Rev Physiol 41:83, 1979

Feingold KR et al: Sex difference in human mevalonate metabolism. J Clin Invest 66:361, 1980

Flynn MA et al: Effect of dietary egg on human serum cholesterol and triglycerides. Am J Clin Nutr 32:1051, 1979

Gardner JD: Regulation of pancreatic endocrine function in vitro: Initial steps in the actions of secretagogues. Annu Rev Physiol 41:55, 1979

Gastrointestinal hormones. Clin Gastroenterol 9:483–798, Sept, 1980

Giordano C: Amino acids and keto-acids—Advantages and pitfalls. Am J Clin Nutr 33:1649, 1980

Glueck GJ et al: Effects of alcohol ingestion on lipids and lipoproteins in normal men: Isocaloric metabolic studies. Am J Clin Nutr 33:2287, 1980

Glueck CJ et al: Effect of sucrose polyester on fecal bile acid excretion and composition in normal men. Am J Clin Nutr 33:2177, 1980

Goldberg AL et al: Hormonal regulation of protein degradation and synthesis in skeletal muscle. Fed Proc 39:31, 1980

Harris WS et al: Bile acid metabolism in ascorbic acid-deficient guinea pigs. Am J Clin Nutr 32:1837, 1979

Hatch TF: Effect of postnatal malnutrition on pancreatic zymogen enzymes in the rat. Am J Clin Nutr 32:1224, 1979

Hayford JT et al: Triglyceride integrated concentrations: Effect of variation of source and amount of dietary carbohydrate. Am J Clin Nutr 32:1670, 1979

Hems DA, Whitton PD: Control of hepatic glycogenolysis. Physiol Rev 60:1, 1980

Henning SJ: Biochemistry of intestinal development. Environ Health Perspect 33:9, 1979

Holt PR et al: Effect of sucrose feeding upon intestinal and hepatic lipid synthesis. Am J Clin Nutr 32:1792, 1979

Hutson SM, Harper AE: Blood and tissue branched-chain amino and $\alpha$-keto acid concentrations: Effect of diet, starvation and disease. Am J Clin Nutr 34:173, 1981

Jones RS, Meyers WC: Regulation of hepatic biliary secretion. Annu Rev Physiol 41:67, 1979

Kelly TJ et al: Effect of sucrose on intestinal very low-density lipoprotein production. Am J Clin Nutr 33:1033, 1980

Kissileff HR et al: C-terminal octapeptide of cholecystokinin decreases food intake in man. Am J Clin Nutr 34:154, 1981

Lack L: Properties and biological significance of the ileal bile salt transport system. Environ Health Perspect 33:79, 1979

Lecce JG: Intestinal barriers to water-soluble macromolecules. Environ Health Perspect 33:57, 1979

Lombardo D et al: Studies on substrate specificity of a carboxyl ester hydrolase from human pancreatic juice. I. Action of carboxyl esters, glycerides and phospholipids. Biochim Biophys Acta 611:136, 1980; II. Action on cholesterol esters and lipid solution vitamin esters. Biochim Biophys Acta 611:147, 1980

McGill HC: The relationship of dietary cholesterol to serum cholesterol concentration and to atherosclerosis in man. Am J Clin Nutr 32:2664, 1979

Nestel PJ et al: Changes in cholesterol metabolism in infants in response to dietary cholesterol and fat. Am J Clin Nutr 32:2177, 1979

Oguenshina SO, Hussain MA: Plasma thyroxine binding prealbumin as an index of mild protein-energy malnutrition in children. Am J Clin Nutr 33:794, 1980

Pearse AGE et al: The newer gut hormones: Cellular sources, physiology, pathology, and clinical aspects. Gastroenterology 72:746, 1977

Potter JG et al: Effect of test meals of varying dietary fiber content of plasma insulin and glucose response. Am J Clin Nutr 34:328, 1981

Price SF et al: Food sensitivity in reflux esophagitis. Gastroenterology 75:240, 1978

Reaven GM: Effects of differences in amount and kind of dietary carbohydrate on plasma glucose and insulin responses in man. Am J Clin Nutr 32;2568, 1979

Review: Carnitine metabolism in man. Nutr Rev 38:338, 1980

Review: Gastrin: A G.I. tract growth hormone. Nutr Dev 38:155, 1980

Review: Hormone regulation of hepatic ketogenesis—Pivotal role of malonyl CoA. Nutr Rev 37:236, 1979

Review: Lipases and lipid absorption in the newborn. Nutr Rev 37:104, 1979

Review: The regulation of fatty acid synthesis and oxidation by malonyl CoA and carnitine. Nutr Rev 38:25, 1980

Review: Routes of neutral amino acid transport in intestinal basolateral membrane vesicles. Nutr Rev 38:255, 1980

Review: Tissue levels and synthesis of coenzyme A in different metabolic states. Nutr Rev 37:200, 1979

Richardson DP et al: The effect of dietary sucrose on protein utilization in healthy young men. Am J Clin Nutr 33:264, 1980

Robinson AM, Williamson DH: Physiological roles of ketone bodies as substrates and signals in mammalian tissues. Physiol Rev 60:143, 1980

Rossoura JE et al: The effect of skim milk, yoghurt and full cream milk on human serum lipids. Am J Clin Nutr 34:351, 1981

Schulz I, Stolze HH: The exocrine pancreas: The role of secretagogues, cyclic nucleotides and calcium in enzyme secretion. Annu Rev Physiol 42:127, 1980

Soll HA, Walsh JH: Regulation of gastric acid secretion. Annu Rev Physiol 41:35, 1979

Tan MH et al: The effect of a high cholesterol, and saturated fat diet on serum high-density lipoprotein-cholesterol, apoprotein A-I, and apoprotein E levels in normolipidemic humans. Am J Clin Nutr 33:2559, 1980

Turner JL et al: Effect of dietary fructose on triglyceride transport and glucoregulatory hormones in hypertriglyceridemic men. Am J Clin Nutr 32:1043, 1979

Visek WJ: Ammonia metabolism, urea cycle capacity and their biochemical assessment. Nutr Rev 37:273, 1979

Ward SD et al: Determinants of plasma cholesterol in children— A family study. Am J Clin Nutr 33:63, 1980

Yonoszai MK et al: Intestinal disaccharidases in newborn and mother rats; Effect of dietary protein deficiency during pregnancy. Am J Clin Nutr 31:931, 1978

# Energy Metabolism
## Books and pamphlets

FAO/WHO: *Energy and protein requirements.* WHO Tech Rep Ser, no 522. Geneva, World Health Organization, 1973

Richardson M, McCracken EC: *Energy Expenditures of Women Performing Selected Activities.* Home Economics Research Report No. 11. Washington, DC, Agriculture Research Service, 1960

Sargent DW: *An Evaluation of Basal Metabolic Data for Children and Youth in the United States.* Home Economics Research Report No. 14. Washington, DC, Agriculture Research Service, 1961

Sargent DW: *An Evaluation of Basal Metabolic Data for Infants in the United States.* Home Economics Research Report No. 18. Washington, DC, Agriculture Research Service, 1962

## Journal articles

Ashworth A: Malnutrition and metabolic rates. Nutr Rev 28:279, 1970

Bell FB: Hypothalamic control of food intake. Proc Nutr Soc 30:103, 1971

Bradfield RB: A technique for determination of usual daily energy expenditure in the field. Am J Clin Nutr 24:1148, 1971

Bradford RB, Jourdain MH: Relative importance of specific dynamic action in weight-reduction diets. Lancet 22:640, Sept, 1973

Bray GA: Physiological control of energy balance. Int J Obes 4:287, 1980

Bray GA et al: The acute effects of food intake on energy expenditure during cycle erogometry. Am J Clin Nutr 27:254, 1974

Brooke OG: Energy balance and metabolic rate in preterm infants fed with standard and high-energy formulas. Br J Nutr 44:13, 1980

Buskirk ER et al: Comparison of two assessments of physical activity and a survey method for caloric intake. Am J Clin Nutr 24:1119, 1971

Buskirk ER et al: Human energy expenditure studies in the National Institute of Arthritis and Metabolic Disease. I. Interaction of cold environment and special dynamic effect. II. Sleep. Am J Clin Nutr 8:602, 1960

Calloway DH, Zanni E: Energy expenditure of elderly men. Am J Clin Nutr 33:2088, 1980

Consolazio CF et al: Body weight, heart rate, and ventilatory volume relationships to oxygen uptakes. Am J Clin Nutr 24:1180, 1971

Cunningham JJ: A reanalysis of the factors influencing basal metabolic rate in normal adults. Am J Clin Nutr 33:2372, 1980

Edmundson W: Individual variations in basal metabolic rate and work efficiency in East Java. Ecol Food Nutr 8:189, 1979

Edmundson W: Individual variations in work output per unit energy intake in East Java. Ecol Food Nutr 6:147, 1977

Flodin NW: The energetic joule. Am J Clin Nutr 30:302, 1977

Haisman MF: Energy expenditure of soldiers in a warm humid climate. Br J Nutr 27:375, 1972

Hamilton CL: Physiologic control of food intake. J Am Diet Assoc 62:35, 1973

Hanson JS: Exercise responses following production of experimental obesity. J Appl Physiol 35:587, 1973

Harrison SL: Body weight-gain equivalents of selected foods. J Am Diet Assoc 70:367, 1977

Havel RJ: Caloric homeostasis and disorders of fuel transport. N Engl J Med 287:1186, 1972

Hawkins WW: The calorie, the joule. J Nutr 102:1553, 1972

Hegsted DM: Energy needs and energy utilization. Nutr Rev 32:33, 1974

Hervey GR: Physiological mechanisms for the regulation of energy balance. Proc Nutr Soc 30:109, 1971

Hommes FA: The energy requirement for growth. A reevaluation. Nutr Metab 24:110, 1980

Hunscher HA: Pertinent factors in interpreting metabolic data. J Am Diet Assoc 39:209, 1961

Khan MA, Bender AE: Adaptation to restricted intake of protein and energy. Nutr Metab 23:449, 1979

Kleiber M: Joules vs. calories in nutrition. J Nutr 102:309, 1972

Konishi F: Food energy equivalents of various activities. J Am Diet Assoc 46:186, 1965

Koong LJ: A new method for estimating energetic efficiencies. J Nutr 107:1724, 1977

LeDividich J et al: Effects of environmental temperature on heat production, energy retention, protein and fat gain in early weaned piglets. Br J Nutr 44:313, 1980

Margaria R: The sources of muscular energy. Sci Am 226, No. 3:84, 1972

Mason ED et al: Racial group differences in basal metabolism and body composition of Indian and European women in Bombay. Hum Biol 26:374, 1964

Maxfield ME: The indirect measurement of energy expenditure in industrial situations. Am J Clin Nutr 24:1126, 1971

McCance RA: The composition of the body: Its maintenance and regulation. Nutr Abstr Rev 42:1269, 1972

Montoye HJ: Estimation of habitual physical activity by questionnaire and interview. Am J Clin Nutr 24:1113, 1971

Moore FD: Energy and maintenance of body cell mass. J Parent Ent Nutr 4:228, 1980

Naismith DJ, Holdsworth MD: Utilization of proteins at submaintenance energy intakes. Nutr Metab 24:13, 1980

Pahud P et al: Energy expenditure during oxygen deficit of submaximal concentric and eccentric exercise. J Appl Physiol 49:16, 1980

Passmore R: The regulation of body-weight in man. Proc Nutr Soc 30:122, 1971

Payne PR, Dugdale AE: A model for the prediction of energy balance and body weight. Ann Hum Biol 4:525, 1977

Payne PR, Wheeler EF, Salvosa CB: Prediction of daily energy expenditure from average pulse rate. Am J Clin Nutr 24:1164, 1971

Pittet PH et al: Thermic effect of glucose and amino acids in man studied by direct and indirect calorimetry. Br J Nutr 31:343, 1974

Review: Energy requirements: How much is enough? Nutr Rev 38:337, 1980

Review: Work output in undernourished adolescents: Effect of early malnutrition. Nutr Rev 38:143, 1980

Schutz Y et al: Energy expenditures and food intakes of lactating women in Guatemala. Am J Clin Nutr 33:892, 1980

Southgate DAT: Assessing the energy value of the human diet. Nutr Rev 29:131, 1971

Spurr GB et al: Energy expenditure, productivity, and physical work capacity of sugarcane loaders. Am J Clin Nutr 30:1740, 1977

Symposium: The application of human and animal calorimetry. Proc Nutr Soc 37:1, 1978

Warnold I et al: Energy intake and expenditure in selected groups of hospital patients. Am J Clin Nutr 31:742, 1978

Weaver EI, Elliot DE: Factors affecting energy expended in home-making tasks. J Am Diet Assoc 39:205, 1961

Whipp BJ et al: Exercise energetics in normal man following acute weight gain. Am J Clin Nutr 26:1284, 1973

Wilmore JH, Haskell WL: Use of the heart rate–energy relationship in the individualized prescription of exercise. Am J Clin Nutr 24:1186, 1971

Yoshimura M et al: Climatic adaptation of basal metabolism. Fed Proc 25, No. 2:1169, 1966

# Meeting Nutritional Norms
## Books

Committee on Dietary Allowances, Food and Nutrition Board: Recommended Dietary Allowances, 9th ed. National Research Council-National Academy of Sciences, Washington, DC, 1980

National Nutrition Consortium: Nutrition Labeling: How It Can Work For You. P.O. Box 4110, Kankakee, IL, National Nutrition Consortium, 1978

Osbourne DR, Voogt P: The Analysis of Nutrients in Foods. New York, Academic Press, 1978

## Journal articles

Graham DM, Hertzler AA: Why enrich or fortify foods? J Nutr Educ 9:166, 1977

Guthrie HA, Scheer JC: Validity of a dietary score for assessing nutrient adequacy. J Am Diet Assoc 78:240, 1981

Hansen G, Sorenson AW: Nutritional Quality Index of Foods. Westport, CT, Avi, 1979

Harper AE: Meeting recommended dietary allowances. J FL Med Assoc 66:419, 1979

Harper AE: Recommended dietary allowances—1980. Nutr Rev 38:290, 1980

Hegsted DM: On dietary standards. Nutr Rev 36:33, 1978

Young VR, Scrimshaw NS: Genetic and biological variability in human nutrition requirements. Am J Clin Nutr 32:486, 1979

# Food Composition
## Journal articles

Anderson BA et al: Comprehensive evaluation of fatty acids in foods. II. Beef products. J Am Diet Assoc 67:35, 1975

Anderson BA et al: Comprehensive evaluation of fatty acids in foods. XIII. Sausages and luncheon meats. J Am Diet Assoc 72:48, 1978

Appledorf H, Kelly LS: Proximate and mineral content of fast foods. Pizza, Mexican-American-style foods and submarine sandwiches. J Am Diet Assoc 74:35, 1979

Bang HO, Dyerberg J, Sinclair HM: The composition of the Eskimo food in north-western Greenland. Am J Clin Nutr 33:2657, 1980

Bunker ML, McWilliams M: Caffeine content of common beverages. J Am Diet Assoc 74:28, 1979

Clements RS, Darnell B: Myo-inositol content of common foods. Am J Clin Nutr 33:1954, 1980

Deeming SB, Weber CW: Trace minerals in commercially prepared baby foods. J Am Diet Assoc 75:149, 1979

Dong MH, McGown EL, Schwenneker BW et al: Thiamin, riboflavin, and vitamin B₆ contents of selected foods as served. J Am Diet Assoc 76:156, 1980

Freeland-Graves JH, Ebangit ML, Bodzy PW: Zinc and copper content of foods used in vegetarian diets. J Am Diet Assoc 77:648, 1980

Gormican A: Inorganic elements in food used in hospital menus. J Am Diet Assoc 56:397, 1970

Groisser DS: A study of caffeine in tea. I. A new spectrophotometric micromethod. II. Concentration of caffeine in various strengths, brands, blends and types of teas. Am J Clin Nutr 31:1727, 1978

Hanson JM, Kinsella JE: Fatty acid content and composition of infant formulas and cereals. J Am Diet Assoc 78:250, 1981

Hawley LE et al: Fatty acid composition of prepared infant formulas. J Am Diet Assoc 72:170, 1978

Hoppner K et al: Nutrient levels of some foods of Eskimos from Arctic Bay, N.W.T., Canada. J Am Diet Assoc 73:257, 1978

Kinsella JE et al: Fatty acid content and composition of fresh water finfish. J Am Oil Chem Soc 54:424, 1977

Korsrud GO, Truk KD: Sucrose, fructose and glucose contents of infant cereals. J Can Diet Assoc 40:56, 1979

Kuhnlein HV, Calloway DH, Harland BF: Composition of traditional Hopi foods. J Am Diet Assoc 75:37, 1979

Mathews RH, Workman MY: Nutrient content of selected baby foods. J Am Diet Assoc 72:27, 1978

McLaughin PJ, Weihrauch JL: Vitamin E content of foods. J Am Diet Assoc 75:647, 1979

Murphy EW et al: Nutrient content of spices and herbs. J Am Diet Assoc 72:174, 1978

Pennington JAT, Church HN: Bowes and Church's Food Values of Portions Commonly Used, 13th ed. Philadelphia, JB Lippincott, 1980

Southgate DAT et al: Free sugars in foods. J Hum Nutr 32:335, 1978

Staroscik JA, Gregorio FU, Reeder SE: Nutrients in fresh peeled oranges and grapefruit from California and Arizona. J Am Diet Assoc 77:567, 1980

USDA: Agriculture Handbook No. 8 Composition of Foods—Raw, Processed, Prepared. Washington, DC, United States Government Printing Office; 8-1 Dairy and Egg Products, 1976; 8-2 Spices and Herbs, 1977; 8-3 Baby Foods, 1978; 8-4 Fats and Oils, 1979; 8-5 Poultry Products, 1979; 8-6 Soups, Sauces and Gravies, 1980; 8-7 Sausages and Luncheon Meats, 1980

USDA: Nutritive Value of Foods. Home and Garden Bulletin No. 72. Washington, DC, United States Government Printing Office, 1981

Walsh JH, Wyse BW, Hansen RG: Pantothenic acid content of 75 processed and cooked foods. J Am Diet Assoc 78:140, 1981

Watt BK, Merrill AL: Composition of Foods—Raw, Processed, Prepared. USDA Handbook No. 8. Washington, DC, United States Government Printing Office, 1963

Weihrauch JL, Gardner JM: Sterol content of foods of plant origin. J Am Diet Assoc 73:39, 1978

Wong NA et al: Mineral content of dairy products. I. Milk and milk products. J Am Diet Assoc 72:288, 1978

Wong NA et al: Mineral content of dairy products. II. Cheeses. J Am Diet Assoc 72:608, 1978

# Meal Management
## Books and pamphlets

Fonosch GG, Kvitka EF: Meal Management: Concepts and Applications. San Francisco, Harper & Row, 1978

Kinder F, Green NR: Meal Management, 5th ed. New York, Macmillan, 1978

McWilliams M: Food Fundamentals. 3rd ed. Somerset, NJ, John Wiley & Sons, 1979

Medved E: Food in Theory and Practice. Fullerton, CA, Plycon Press, 1977

Peckham GC, Freeland-Graves JH: Foundations of Food Preparation, 4th ed. New York, Macmillan, 1979

Sexauer BH, Mann JS: Food Expenditure Patterns of Single-Person Households. Agricultural Economics Report No. 428. Washington, DC, USDA, Economics, Statistics, and Cooperatives Service

## Journal articles

Jensen GR et al: Menu evaluation—A nutrient approach for consumers. J Nutr Educ 9:162, 1977

Lane S, Vermeersch V: Evaluation of Thrifty Food Plan. J Nutr Educ 11:96, 1979

Schafer RB: Factors affecting food behavior and the quality of husbands' and wives' diet. J Am Diet Assoc 72:138, 1978

# The Helping Process in Nutrition Services
## Books

Aronson V, Fitzgerald B: Guidebook for Nutrition Counselors. Quincy, MA, Christopher, 1980

Bernstein L, Bernstein RS: Interviewing; A Guide for Health Professionals. New York, Appleton-Century-Crofts, 1980

Bigge ML: Learning Theories for Teachers. New York, Harper & Row, 1976

Brill NI: Working with People. The Helping Process. New York, JB Lippincott, 1973

Collins M: Communication in Health Care. St Louis, CV Mosby, 1977

Danish SJ, D'Augelli AR, Hauer AL: Helping Skills. A Basic Training Program. New York, Human Sciences Press, 1980

D'Augelli AR, Danish SJ, Hauer AL et al: Helping Skills. A Basic Training Program—Leader's Manual. New York, Human Sciences Press, 1980

Mager RF: Preparing Instructional Objectives. Belmont, CA, Lear Siegler, 1962

Mason M, Wenberg BG, Welsch PK: The Dynamics of Clinical Dietetics. New York, John Wiley & Sons, 1977

Skipper JK, Leonard RC: Social Interaction and Patient Care. Philadelphia, JB Lippincott, 1965

Sundel M, Sundel SS: Behavior Modification in the Human Services. A Systematic Introduction to Concepts and Applications. New York, John Wiley & Sons, 1975

### Journal articles

Carruth BR, Mangel M, Anderson HL: Assessing change-proneness and nutrition-related behaviors. J Am Diet Assoc 70:47, 1977

Danish SJ, Ginsberg MR, Terrell AH et al: The anatomy of a dietetic counseling interview. J Am Diet Assoc 75:626, 1979

Detmer DG: The nutrition component of training for the physician's assistant and his education. J Am Diet Assoc 66:269, 1975

Erkel EA: The implications of cultural conflict for health care. Health Values: Achieving High Level Wellness 4:51, 1980

Hauser ST, Pollets D, Turner BL et al: Ego development and self-esteem in diabetic adolescents. Diabetes Care 2:465, 1979

Hill DH, Madison R: A health education program for weight reduction in a hypertension clinic. Public Health Rep 95:271, 1980

Kocher RE: Monitoring nutritional care of the long term patient. I. Policies and systems that support the on-going evaluation of care. J Am Diet Assoc 67:45, 1975

Laquatra I, Danish SJ: Effect of a helping skills transfer program on dietitians' helping behavior. J Am Diet Assoc 78:22, 1981

Ling L, Spragg D, Stein P et al: Guidelines for diet counseling. J Am Diet Assoc 66:571, 1975

Mandriota R, Bunkers B, Wilcox ME: Nutrition intervention strategies in the multiple risk factor intervention trial (MRFIT). J Am Diet Assoc 77:138, 1980

Ronnestad MH: The effects of modeling, feedback and experimental methods on counselor empathy. Counsel Educ Supervis 16:194, 1977

Ruffing MA: Preventive health behavior: A theoretical review. Health Values: Achieving High Level Wellness 3:235, 1979

Spooner SE, Stone SC: Maintenance of specific counseling skills over time. J Counsel Psychol 24:66, 1977

Wylie J, Singer J: Growth process in nutrition counseling. J Am Diet Assoc 69:505, 1976

Zifferblatt SM, Wilbur CS: Dietary counseling: Expectations and guidelines. J Am Diet Assoc 70:591, 1977

# Regional, Cultural, and Religious Food Patterns

## Books and pamphlets

Chang KC (ed): Food in Chinese Culture: Anthropological and Historical Perspectives. New Haven, Yale University Press, 1977

Editors of Consumer Reports Books: Health Quackery: Consumers Union's Report on False Health Claims, Worthless Remedies, and Unproved Therapies. Mount Vernon, NY, Consumers Reports Books, 1980

Go K, Moore I: Food Habits and Practices of Southeast Asians (Primarily Cambodians and Laotians) 2837 Aledi St., Oakland CA, Food Habits Guide, 1979

Herbert V: Nutrition Cultism: Facts and Fictions. Philadelphia, George F Stickley, 1980

Moore ST, Byers MP: A Vegetarian Diet. Santa Barbara, CA. Woodbridge Press, 1978

Nutrition, Growth and Development of North American Indian Children. Publ. No. (NIH) 72-26. Washington, DC, Department of Health, Education and Welfare, 1972

Root W: Food: An Authoritative and Visual History and Directory of the Foods of the World. New York, Simon & Schuster, 1980

Southeast Asian American Nutrition Education Materials. Washington, DC, USDA, Nutrition and Technical Services Division, Food and Nutrition Service, 1980

### Journal articles

Abiaka MH: Japanese-American food equivalents for calculating exchange diets. J Am Diet Assoc 62:173, 1973

Acosta PB et al: Nutritional status of Mexican-American preschool children in a border town. Am J Clin Nutr 27:1359, 1974

American Academy of Pediatrics, Committee on Nutrition: Nutritional aspects of vegetarianism, health foods, and fad diets. Nutr Rev 35:153, 1977

Berkes F, Farkas CS: Eastern James Bay Cree Indians: Changing patterns of wild food use and nutrition. Ecol Food Nutr 7:155, 1978

Council on Foods and Nutrition: Zen macrobiotic diets. JAMA 218:397, Oct 18, 1971

Day M-L et al: Food acceptance patterns of Spanish-speaking New Mexicans. J Nutr Educ 10:121, 1978

Dwyer JT et al: The new vegetarians: Group affiliation and dietary strictures related to attitudes and life style. J Am Diet Assoc 64:376, 1974

Frankle RT, Heussenstamm FK: Food zealotry and youth: New dilemmas for professionals. Am J Public Health 64:11, 1974

Galli N: The influence of cultural heritage on the health status of Puerto Ricans. J Sch Health 45:10, 1975

Grivetti LE, Paquette MD: Nontraditional ethnic food choices among first generation Chinese in California. J Nutr Educ 10:109, 1978

Hunt S: Traditional Asian food customs. J Hum Nutr 31:245, 1977

James SM: When your patient is black West Indian. Am J Nurs 78:1908, 1978

Joseph S et al: Composition of Israeli mixed dishes. J Am Diet Assoc 40:125, 1962

Kuhnlein HV, Calloway DH: Adventitious mineral elements in Hopi Indian diets. J Food Sci 44:282, 1979

Kuhnlein HV, Calloway DH: Contemporary Hopi food intake patterns. Ecol Food Nutr 6:159, 1977

Larson LB et al: Nutritional status of children of Mexican-American migrant families. J Am Diet Assoc 64:29, 1974

Our cooking heritage: African foods. What's New in Home Economics. 35:28, 1971

Ping Yang GI, Lox HM: Food habit changes of Chinese persons living in Lincoln, Nebraska. J Am Diet Assoc 79:420, 1979

Regenstein JM, Regenstein CE: An introduction to the kosher dietary laws for food scientists and food processors. Food Tech 33:89, 1979

Sakr AH: Dietary regulations and food habits of Muslims. J Am Diet Assoc 58:123, 1971

Soulsby T: Russian-American food patterns. J Nutr Educ 4:170, 1972

Van Duzen J, Carter JP, Vander Zwaag R: Protein and calorie malnutrition among preschool Navajo Indian children. Am J Clin Nutr 29:657, 1976

Wheeler M Sr, Haider SQ: Buying and food preparation patterns of ghetto blacks and Hispanics in Brooklyn. J Am Diet Assoc 75:560, 1979

White HS: The organic foods movement. Food Tech 26:29, 1972

## Factors influencing food habits

### Books and pamphlets

Darby WJ et al: Food: The Gift of Osiris. New York, Academic Press, 1977

Fitzgerald TK (ed): Nutrition and Anthropology in Action. Assen, Amsterdam, Van Gorcum, 1977

Kandel RF, Pelto GH: Nutritional Anthropology. Pleasantville, NY, Redgrave, 1980

Larsen E: Food: Past, Present and Future. New York, Crane, Russack, 1978

Lowenberg ME, Todhunter EN, Wilson ED et al: Food and People, 3rd ed. New York, John Wiley & Sons, 1979

Mead M: Food Habits Research: Problems of the 60's. National Academy of Sciences—National Research Council Publ. No. 1225. Washington, DC, NAS-NRC, 1964

Turner M (ed): Nutrition and Lifestyles. Essex, England, Applied Science, 1980

Walcher DN et al (eds): Food, Man and Society. New York, Plenum, 1976

Wilson C: Food-Custom and Nurture: An Annotated Bibliography on Sociocultural and Biocultural Aspects of Nutrition. Berkeley, CA, Society Nutrition Education, 1979

### Journal articles

Barlow DH, Tillotson JT: Behavioral science and nutrition: A new perspective. J Am Diet Assoc 72:368, 1978

Evans RI, Hall Y: Social psychological perspective on motivating changes in eating behavior. J Am Diet Assoc 72:378, 1978

Hertzler AA: Sociologic study of food habits—A review. 1. Diversity in diet and scalogram analysis. J Am Diet Assoc 69:377, 1976

Keen S: Eating our way to enlightenment. Psychology Today 12:62, Oct, 1978

Keen S: The pure, the impure, and the paranoid. Psychology Today 12:67, Oct, 1978

Krondl M, Law D: Food habit modification as a public health measure. Can J Public Health 69:39, 1978

Mahoney MJ, Caggiula AW: Applying behavioral methods to nutrition counseling. J Am Diet Assoc 72:372, 1978

Reaburn JA et al: Social determinants in food selection. J Am Diet Assoc 74:637, 1979

Smiciklas-Wright H, Krondl M: Dietary counseling and the behavioral sciences. J Can Diet Assoc 40:99, 1979

## Ecology of food
## General references

### Books and pamphlets

Baxter K (ed): Food Chains and Human Nutrition. Essex, England, Applied Science, 1979

Bernarde MA: The Chemicals We Eat. New York, American Heritage, 1971

Clydeside F (ed): Food Science and Nutrition: Current Issues and Answers. Englewood Cliffs, NJ, Prentice-Hall, 1979

Evaluation of certain food additives and the contaminants mercury, lead, and cadmium. Sixteenth Report of the Joint FAO/WHO Expert Committee on Food Additives. WHO Tech Rep Ser, no. 505. FAO Nutrition Meeting Report Series No. 51. Geneva, FAO/WHO 1972

International Commission on Microbiological Specifications for Foods: Microbial Ecology of Foods, Vols I and II. New York, Academic Press, 1980

Pimentel D, Pimentel M: Food, Energy and Society. New York, Halsted Press, 1979

Rhodes ME (ed): Food Mycology. Boston, GK Hall, 1979

Riemann H, Bryan FL: Food-Borne Infections and Intoxications. New York, Academic Press, 1979

Taylor RJ: Food Additives. New York, John Wiley & Sons, 1980

We Want You to Know What We Know about Salmonella and Food Poisoning. DHEW Publ. No. (FDA) 73-2004. Washington, DC, Food and Drug Administration, 1973

## Food processing

### Journal articles

Erdman JW: Effect of preparation and service of food on nutrient value. Food Tech 33:38, 1979

Hurt HD: Effect of canning on the nutritive value of vegetables. Food Tech 33:62, 1979

Karel M: Effect of storage on nutrient retention of foods. Food Tech 33:36, 1979

Kramer A: Effects of freezing and frozen storage on the nutrient retention of fruits and vegetables. Food Tech 33:58, 1979

Lund DB: Effect of commercial processing on nutrients. Food Tech 33:28, 1979

Rodricks JV: Food hazards of natural origin. Fed Proc 37:2587, 1978

Taub IA et al: Effect of irradiation on meat proteins. Food Tech 33:184, 1979

## Foodborne diseases

### Journal articles

Beuchat LR, Jones WK: Growth of Vibrio parahaemolyticus in seafoods extended with soy protein concentrate, structured protein fiber and textured vegetable protein. J Food Sci 44:1114, 1979

Blake PA et al: Disease caused by a marine Vibrio: Clinical characteristics and epidemiology. N Engl J Med 300:1, 1979

Bryan FL: Factors that contribute to outbreaks of foodborne disease. J Food Protection 41:816, 1978

Bullerman LB: Significance of mycotoxins to food safety and human health. J Food Protection 41:65, 1979

Cohen ML, Blake PA: Trends in foodborne salmonellosis outbreaks: 1963–1975. J Food Protection 40:798, 1977

Duitschaever CL, Buteau C: Incidence of salmonella in pork and poultry products. J Food Protection 42:662, 1979

Formal SB et al: Mechanisms of shigella pathogenesis. Am J Clin Nutr 25:1427, 1972

Foster EM: Foodborne hazards of microbial origin. Fed Proc 37:2577, 1978

Haddock RL: Vibrio parahaemolyticus food poisoning incidents in the Territory of Guam. J Environ Health 41:329, 1979

Harsanyi YL: Paralytic shellfish poisoning. FDA Consumer 7:22, 1973

IFT Expert Panel on Food Safety and Nutrition: Botulism. A scientific status summary. J Food Sci 37:985, 1972

Kauter DA, Lynt RR: Botulism. Nutr Rev 31:265, 1973

Overview: Update on food spoilage organisms. Food Tech 33:52, 1979

## Food additives, intentional and accidental
### Journal articles

Bauerman JF: Processing of poultry products with and without sodium nitrite. Food Tech 33:42, 1979

Cassens RG et al: Reactions of nitrite in meat. Food Tech 33:46, 1979

Dales LG: The neurotoxicity of alkyl mercury compounds. Am J Med 53:219, 1972

Dickinson L et al: Lead poisoning in family due to cocktail glasses. Am J Nurs 52:391, 1972

IFT Expert Panel on Food Safety and Nutrition: Nitrites, nitrates and nitrosamines in foods—A dilemma. J Food Sci 37:989, 1972

Ingredients report. Food Engineer 51:93, 1979

Johnson PE: Misuse in foods of useful chemicals. Nutr Rev 35:225, 1977

Lin-Fu JS: Vulnerability of children to lead exposure and toxicity. N Engl J Med 289:1289, Dec 13, 1974

Mitchell DG: Increased lead absorption: Paint is not the only problem. Pediatrics 53:142, 1974

Sebranek JG: Advances in the technology of nitrite use and consideration of alternatives. Food Tech 33:58, 1979

Special report: The use of chemicals in food production, processing, storage, and distribution. Nutr Rev 31:191, 1973

Takizawa Y et al: Studies on the causes of the Niigata episode of Minamata disease outbreak. Acta Med Biol 19:193, 1972

Wilson BJ: Naturally occurring toxicants in foods. Nutr Rev 37:305, 1979

## Safeguarding the food supply
### Journal articles

Balsley M: Technologists look ahead to food safety. Hospitals 53:107, 1979

Darby WJ, Hambraeus L: Proposed nutritional guidelines for utilization of industrially produced nutrients. Nutr Rev 36:65, 1978

Doull J: Assessment of food safety. Fed Proc 37:2594, 1978

Irving GW: Safety evaluation of the food ingredients called GRAS. Nutr Rev 36:321, 1978

Jukes TH: Carcinogens in food and the Delaney Clause. JAMA 241:617, 1979

Rucker MH et al: Food safety—What do the experts say? J Nutr Educ 9:158, 1977

Seligsohn M: Cancer and the food industry. A struggle for sane regulation. Food Engineer 51:22, 1979

Seligsohn M: Is GRAS safe? Food Engineer 52:20, 1980

Special report: Perspectives on food safety. Nutr Rev 37:29, 1979

Symposium: Risk versus benefits: The future of food safety. Nutr Rev 38:35, 1980

Ward AG: Safeguarding our food. Nutr Rev 35:116, 1977

# Part Two
# Application of Nutrition to Critical Periods Throughout the Life Span
## General references

American Dietetic Association: Position paper on the scope and thrust of nutrition education. J Am Diet Assoc 72:302, 1978

Bass MA, Wakefield L, Kolasa K: Community Nutrition and Individual Food Behavior. Minneapolis, Burgess, 1979

Caliendo MA: Nutrition and Preventive Health Care. New York, Macmillan, 1980

Frankle RT, Owen AY: Nutrition in the Community: The Art of Delivering Services. St Louis, CV Mosby, 1978

Obert JC: Community Nutrition. New York, John Wiley & Sons, 1978

# Growth and Development
## General references
### Books and pamphlets

Falkner F, Tanner JM (eds): Human Growth. New York, Plenum Press, 1979

Hurley LS: Developmental Nutrition. Englewood Cliffs, NJ, Prentice-Hall, 1979

Jelliffe DB, Jelliffe EFP (eds): Human Nutrition: A Comprehensive Treatise, Vol 2, Nutrition and Growth. New York, Plenum Press, 1979

McWilliams M: Nutrition for the Growing Years, 3rd ed. New York, John Wiley & Sons, 1980

NCHS Growth Curves for Children: Birth–18 Years. U.S. Vital and Health Statistics, Series 11, No. 165. DHEW Publ. No. (PHS) 78:1650. Washington, DC, National Center for Health Statistics, 1978

Oski FA, Pearson HA (eds): Iron Nutrition Revisited—Infancy, Childhood, Adolescence. Report of the Eighty-Second Ross Conference on Pediatric Research. Columbus, OH, Ross Laboratories, 1981

Springer NS: An Annotated Bibliography—Nutrition and Mental Retardation (1964–1970). Ann Arbor, ISMR, University of Michigan, 1970

Winick M (ed): Human Nutrition: A Comprehensive Treatise, Vol I, Nutrition: Pre- and Postnatal Development. New York, Plenum Press, 1979

Winick M (ed): Nutrition and Development, Vol I, Current Concepts in Nutrition. New York, John Wiley & Sons, 1972

Winick M (ed): Nutrition and Fetal Development, Vol II, Current Concepts in Nutrition. New York, John Wiley & Sons, 1974

Winick M (ed): Childhood Obesity, Vol III, Current Concepts in Nutrition. New York, John Wiley & Sons, 1975

Wurtman RJ, Wurtman JJ: Nutrition and the Brain, Vol 1, Determinants of the Availability of Nutrients to the Brain; Vol 2, Control of Feeding Behavior and Biology of the Brain in Protein-Calorie Malnutrition; Vol 3, Disorders of Eating and Nutrients in Treatment of Brain Diseases. New York, Raven Press, 1977, 1979

### Journal articles

Brozek J: Malnutrition and behavior. A decade of conferences. J Am Diet Assoc 72:17, 1978

Deren JS: Development of structure and function in the fetal and newborn stomach. Am J Clin Nutr 24:144, 1971

Fernstrom JD, Faller DV: Neutral amino acids in the brain: Changes in response to food ingestion. J Neurochem 30:1531, 1978

Growdon JH, Wurtman RJ: Dietary influences on the synthesis of neurotransmitters in the brain. Nutr Rev 37:129, 1979

Lien NM et al: Early malnutrition and "late" adoption: A study of their effects on the development of Korean orphans adopted into American families. Am J Clin Nutr 30:1734, 1977

Lytle LD, Alter A: Diet, central nervous system and aging. Fed Proc 38:2017, 1979

Review: Growth hormone and sex steroid stimulated growth at puberty. Nutr Rev 35:268, 1977

Review: Growth rate, body size and onset of puberty. Nutr Rev 35:302, 1977

Review: Nutrition and transmitter amines in rat brain. Nutr Rev 35:283, 1977

Review: Tryptophan entry into the brain: Modifications in response to food ingestion and albumin binding. Nutr Rev 36:343, 1978

Roche AF, Hines JH: Incremental growth charts. Am J Clin Nutr 33:2041, 1980

Ross MH: Dietary behavior and longevity. Nutr Rev 35:257, 1977

Special report: Committee on Nutrition of the Mother and Pre-school Child: Summary of a Workshop: Fetal and infant nutrition and susceptibility to obesity. Nutr Rev 36:122, 1978

Tizard J: Early malnutrition, growth and mental development in man. Br Med Bull 30:169, 1974

## Nutrition in Pregnancy and Lactation
### Books and pamphlets

Annis LF: The Child Before Birth. Ithaca, Cornell University Press, 1978

Burrow GN, Ferris TF: Medical complications during pregnancy. Philadelphia, WB Saunders, 1975

Committee on Maternal Nutrition, Food and Nutrition Board: Maternal Nutrition and the Course of Pregnancy. Washington, DC, National Academy of Sciences-National Research Council, 1970

Committee on Maternal Nutrition, Nutritional supplementation and the outcome of pregnancy. Washington, DC, National Academy of Sciences-National Research Council, 1975

Committee on Nutrition of the Mother and the Preschool Child, Food and Nutrition Board, NRC-NAS: Laboratory Indices of Nutrition Status in Pregnancy. Washington, DC, United States Government Printing Office, 1978

Food, Pregnancy and Family Health. Chicago, American College of Obstetrics and Gynecology Publ. No. R-37, 1976

Giroud A: The Nutrition of the Embryo. Springfield, IL, Charles C Thomas, 1970

Goldfarb J, Tibbets E: Breastfeeding Handbook: A Practical Reference for Physicians, Nurses and Other Health Professionals. Hillside, NJ, Enslow, 1980

Hurley LS: Developmental Nutrition. Englewood Cliffs, NJ, Prentice-Hall, 1980

Worthington-Roberts BS, Vermeersch J, Williams SR: Nutrition in Pregnancy and Lactation. St Louis, CV Mosby, 1981

Zackler J, Brandstadt W (eds): The Teenage Pregnant Girl. Springfield, IL, Charles C Thomas, 1975

### Journal articles

Adams S et al: Effect of nutritional supplementation in pregnancy. II. Effect on diet. J Am Diet Assoc 73:630, 1978

Adams SO, Barr GD, Huenemann RL: Effect of nutritional supplementation in pregnancy. I. Effect on outcome of pregnancy. J Am Diet Assoc 72:144, 1978

Arthur LJH, Gray H: Management of maternal phenylketonuria. Br Med J 2:498, 1979

Aubry RH et al: Assessment of maternal nutrition. Clin Perinatol 2:207, 1975

Beal VA: Assessment of nutritional status in pregnancy. II. Am J Clin Nutr 34:691, 1981

Blumenthal I: Diet and diuretics in pregnancy and subsequent growth of offspring. Br Med J 2:733, 1976

Bowering J et al: Role of EFNEP aides in improving diets of pregnant women. J Nutr Educ 8:111, 1976

Brennan RE, Caldwell M, Richard KA: Assessment of maternal nutrition. J Am Diet Assoc 75:152, 1979

Buist NRM et al: Maternal phenylketonuria. Lancet 2:589, 1979

Clarren SK, Smith DW: The fetal alcohol syndrome. N Engl J Med 298:1063, 1978

Cleary RE, Lumeng L, Li T: Maternal and fetal plasma levels of pyridoxal phosphate at term: Adequacy of vitamin $B_6$ supplementation during pregnancy. Am J Obstet Gynecol 121:25, 1975

Committee on Adolescence, American Academy of Pediatrics: Statement on teenage pregnancy. Pediatrics 63:795, 1979

Duenhoelter JH, Jimenez JM, Baumann G: Pregnancy performance of patients under fifteen years of age. Obstet Gynecol 46:49, 1975

Edwards LE et al: Pregnancy in the underweight woman: Course, outcome, and growth patterns of the infant. Am J Obstet Gynecol 135:297, 1979

Elsborg L, Rosenquist A, Helms P: Iron intake by teenage girls and by pregnant women. Int J Vitam Nutr Res 49:210, 1979

Falkner F: Maternal nutrition and fetal growth. Am J Clin Nutr 34:769, 1981

Farquhar JW: Conception in a phenylketonuric woman. Lancet 1:322, 1979

Fielding JE: Adolescent pregnancy revisited. N Engl J Med 299:893, 1978

Fielding JE, Yankauer A: The pregnant drinker. Am J Public Health 68:836, 1978

Filer LJ: Maternal nutrition in lactation. Clin Perinatol 2:353, 1975

Graham DM: Caffeine—Its identity, dietary sources, intake and biological effects. Nutr Rev 36:97, 1977

Green JW: Diabetes mellitus in pregnancy. Obstet Gynecol 46:6, 1975

Gugliucci CL et al: Intensive care of the pregnant diabetic. Am J Obstet Gynecol 125:435, 1976

Hanson JW, Streissguth KL, Smith DW: The effects of moderate alcohol consumption during pregnancy on fetal growth and morphogenesis. J Pediatr 92:457, 1978

Hook EB: Dietary cravings and aversions during pregnancy. Am J Clin Nutr 31:1355, 1978

Hunt IF et al: Effect of nutrition education on the nutritional status of low income pregnant women of Mexican descent. Am J Clin Nutr 29:675, 1976

Hutchins FL, Kendall N, Rubino J: Experience with teenage pregnancy. Obstet Gynecol 54:1, 1979

Jackson RL: Maternal and infant nutrition and health in later life. Nutr Rev 37:33, 1979

Jacobson HN: Diet in pregnancy: New perspectives. N Engl J Med 297:1051, 1977

Jacobson HN: Weight and weight gain in pregnancy. Clin Perinatol 2:233, 1975

Jelliffe DB, Jelliffe EFP: "Breast is best": Modern meanings. N Engl J Med 297:912, 1977

Johnstone FD et al: Measurement of variables: Data quality control. Am J Clin Nutr 34:804, 1981

Jouganatos DM, Gabbe SG: Diabetes in pregnancy: Metabolic changes and current management. J Am Diet Assoc 73:168, 1978

King JC: Assessment of nutritional status in pregnancy. I. Am J Clin Nutr 34:685, 1981

King JC: Protein metabolism during pregnancy. Clin Perinatol 2:243, 1975

Kitay DZ, Harbort RA: Iron and folic acid deficiency in pregnancy. Clin Perinatol 2:255, 1975

Komrower GM et al: Management of maternal phenylketonuria: An emerging clinical problem. Br Med J 1:1383, 1979

Lechtig A: Research design. Am J Clin Nutr 34:814, 1981

Lechtig A et al: Effect of food supplementation during pregnancy on birth weight. Pediatrics 56:508, 1975

Lind T: Nutrient requirements during pregnancy. I. Am J Clin Nutr 34:669, 1981

Malone JI: Vitamin passage across the placenta. Clin Perinatol 2:295, 1975

Mellies MJ et al: Effects of varying maternal dietary cholesterol and phytosterol in lactating women and their infants. Am J Clin Nutr 31:1347, 1978

Mellies MJ et al: Effects of varying maternal dietary fatty acids in lactating women and their infants. Am J Clin Nutr 32:299, 1979

Metcoff J et al: Maternal nutrition and fetal outcome. Am J Clin Nutr 34:708, 1981

Morriss FH: Placental factors conditioning fetal nutrition and growth. Am J Clin Nutr 34:760, 1981

Munro HN: Nutrient requirements during pregnancy. II. Am J Clin Nutr 34:679, 1981

Munro HN: Placental factors conditioning fetal nutrition and development. Am J Clin Nutr 34:756, 1981

Naeye RL: Nutritional/nonnutritional interactions that affect the outcome of pregnancy. Am J Clin Nutr 34:727, 1981

Naeye RL: Weight gain and the outcome of pregnancy. Am J Obstet Gynecol 135:3, 1979

Newcomb RG: Nonnutritional factors affecting fetal growth. Am J Clin Nutr 34:732, 1981

Nielson KB, Wamburg E, Weber J: Successful outcome of pregnancy in a phenylketonuric woman after low-phenylalanine diet introduced before conception. Lancet 1:1245, 1979

Orr RD, Simmons JJ: Nutritional care in pregnancy. J Am Diet Assoc 75:126, 1979

Pitkin RM: Assessment of nutritional status of mother, fetus and newborn. Am J Clin Nutr 34:658, 1981

Pitkin RM: Calcium metabolism in pregnancy: A review. Am J Obstet Gynecol 121:724, 1975

Pueschel SM, Hum C, Andrews M: Nutritional management of the female with phenylketonuria during pregnancy. Am J Clin Nutr 30:1153, 1977

Raman L: Influence of maternal nutritional factors affecting birthweight. Am J Clin Nutr 34:775, 1981

Review: A controlled trial of prenatal nutritional supplementation. Nutr Rev 38:210, 1980

Review: The importance of carnitine in the perinatal period. Nutr Rev 38:310, 1980

Review: Nutritional composition of breast milk produced by mothers of preterm infants. Nutr Rev 38:312, 1980

Review: Toxemia of pregnancy: The dietary calcium hypothesis. Nutr Rev 39:124, 1981

Robertson E, Monkus E: Methods for determining nutrient requirements in pregnancy. II. Am J Clin Nutr 34:705, 1981

Rosette HL et al: Therapy of heavy drinking during pregnancy. Obstet Gynecol 52:41, 1978

Rosso P: Nutrition and maternal–fetal exchange. Am J Clin Nutr 34:744, 1981

Rush D et al: A randomized control trial of prenatal nutritional supplementation in New York City. Pediatrics 65:683, 1980

Sanstead HH: Methods for determining nutrient requirements in pregnancy. I. Am J Clin Nutr 34:697, 1981

Smith GV et al: Breast feeding and infant nutrition. Am Fam Physician 17:92, 1978

Smith I et al: Fetal damage despite low phenylalanine diet after conception in a phenylketonuric woman. Lancet 1:17, 1979

Snowman MK, Dibble MV: Nutrition component in a comprehensive child development program. J Am Diet Assoc 74:119, 1979

Spearing GJ: Diabetes in pregnancy. J Hum Nutr 31:329, 1977

Special Report: Second International Caffeine Workshop. Nutr Rev 38:196, 1980

Susser M: Prenatal nutrition, birthweight, and psychological development: An overview of experiments, quasi-experiments, and natural experiments in the past decade. Am J Clin Nutr 34:784, 1981

Task Force Report: Nutrition Assessment of Maternal Nutrition. Chicago, American College of Obstetrics and Gynecology, 1978

Theodoropoulas LE et al: Iodide-induced hypothyroidism: A potential hazard during prenatal life. Science 205:502, 1979

Van den Berg BJ: Maternal variables affecting fetal growth. Am J Clin Nutr 34:722, 1981

Waber DP et al: Nutritional supplementation, maternal education, and cognitive development of infants at risk of malnutrition. Am J Clin Nutr 34:807, 1981

Warshaw JB, Curry E: Comparison of serum carnitine and ketone body concentration in breast- and formula-fed newborn infants. J Pediatr 97:122, 1980

Weigley ES: The pregnant adolescent: A review of nutritional resources and programs. J Am Diet Assoc 66:588, 1975

Young M: Placental factors and fetal nutrition. Am J Clin Nutr 34:738, 1981

Youngs DD et al: Experience with an adolescent pregnancy program. Obstet Gynecol 50:212, 1977

Zaleski LA, Casey RE, Zaleski W: Maternal phenylketonuria dietary treatment during pregnancy. Can Med Assoc J 121:1591, 1979

# Nutrition During Infancy and Early Childhood—From Birth to Three Years

## Books and pamphlets

Current Practices in Infant Feeding. Fremont, MI, Gerber Products, 1980

Fomon SJ: Infant Nutrition, 2nd ed. Philadelphia, WB Saunders, 1974

Henderson JO, Collins SM, Muller LL et al: Bibliography of Infant Foods and Nutrition 1938–1977. Forest Grove, OR, International Scholarly Book Services, 1979

Heslin J, Natow AB, Raven BC: No-Nonsense Nutrition for Your Baby's First Year. Boston, CBI, 1978

Jelliffe DB, Jelliffe EFP: Human Milk in the Modern World. Oxford, Oxford University Press, 1978

Larson BL (ed): Lactation. New York, Academic Press, 1978

Lawrence R: Breast-Feeding: A Guide for the Medical Profession. St Louis, CV Mosby, 1980

Ogra PL, Dayton DH (eds): Immunology of Breast Milk. New York, Raven Press, 1979

Pipes PL: Nutrition in Infancy and Childhood, 2nd ed. St Louis, CV Mosby, 1981

## Journal articles

Abbey LM: Is breast feeding a likely cause of dental caries in young children? J Am Dent Assoc 98:21, 1979

Abrams CAL et al: Hazards of overconcentrated milk formula. JAMA 232:1136, 1975

Aitchison JM et al: Influence of diet on trans fatty acids in human milk. Am J Clin Nutr 30:2006, 1977

Alfin-Slater RB, Jelliffe DB: Nutritional requirements with special reference to infancy. Pediatr Clin North Am 24:3, 1977

Almroth SG: Water requirements of breast fed infants in a hot climate. Am J Clin Nutr 31:1154, 1978

American Academy of Pediatrics: Breast-feeding. Pediatrics 62:591, 1978

Anderson TA: Commercial infant foods: Content and composition. Pediatr Clin North Am 24:37, 1977

Arnold RR, Cole MF, McGhee JR: A bactericidal effect for human lactoferrin. Science 197:263, 1977

Aroun SS et al: Honey and other environmental risk factors for infant botulism. Pediatrics 94:331, 1979

Asfour R et al: Folacin requirements of children. III. Normal infants. Am J Clin Nutr 30:1098, 1977

Atkinson SA, Bryan MH, Anderson GH: Human milk: Differences in nitrogen concentration in milk from mothers of term and premature infants. J Pediatr 93:67, 1978

Bachrach S, Fisher J, Parks JS: An outbreak of vitamin D deficiency in a susceptible population. Pediatrics 64:871, 1979

Bode HH, Vanjonack WJ, Crawford JB: Mitigation of cretinism by breast feeding. Pediatrics 62:13, 1978

Bowering J et al: Infant feeding practices in East Harlem. J Am Diet Assoc 72:648, 1978

Bullen JJ: Iron-binding proteins in milk and resistance to Escherichia coli infection in infants. Postgrad Med J 51:67, 1975

Castile RG, Marks LJ, Stickler GB: Vitamin D deficiency, rickets, two cases with faulty infant feeding practices. Am J Dis Child 129:964, 1975

Chandra RK: Immunological aspects of human milk. Nutr Rev 36:265, 1978

Choi MW: Breast milk for infants who can't breastfeed. Am J Nurs 78:852, 1978

Committee on Nutrition, American Academy of Pediatrics: Calcium requirements in infancy and childhood. Pediatrics 62:826, 1978

Committee on Nutrition, American Academy of Pediatrics: Commentary on breast feeding and infant formulas, including proposed standards for formulas. Pediatrics 57:278, 1976

Committee on Nutrition, American Academy of Pediatrics: Fluoride supplementation. Revised dosage schedule. Pediatrics 63:150, 1979

Committee on Nutrition, American Academy of Pediatrics: Iron supplementation for infants. Pediatrics 58:765, 1976

Committee on Nutrition, American Academy of Pediatrics: Relationship between iron status and incidence of infection in infancy. Pediatrics 62:246, 1978

Committee on Nutrition, American Academy of Pediatrics: Zinc. Pediatrics 62:408, 1978

Conner AE: Elevated levels of sodium and chloride in milk from mastitic breast. Pediatrics 63:910, 1979

Crawford MA, Hassam AG, Rivers JPW: Essential fatty acid requirements in infancy. Am J Clin Nutr 31:2181, 1978

DeVizin B et al: Digestibility of starches in infants and children. J Pediatr 86:50, 1975

Easthan E et al: Further decline in breastfeeding. Br Med J 1:305, 1976

Eckhert CD: Zinc binding: A difference between human and bovine milk. Science 195:789, 1977

Edidin DV et al: Resurgence of nutritional rickets associated with breastfeeding and special dietary practices. Pediatrics 65:232, 1980

Edozren JC, Switzer BR, Bryan RV: Medical evaluation of the special supplemental food program for women, infants, and children. Am J Clin Nutr 32:677, 1979

Ferris AG et al: Diets in the first six months of infants in western Massachusetts. I. Energy-yielding nutrients. II. Semi-solid foods. J Am Diet Assoc 72:155; 160, 1978

Fomon SJ: Nutritional deficiency in breastfed infants. N Engl J Med 299:355, 1978

Fomon SJ: What are infants fed in the United States? Pediatrics 56:350, 1975

Fomon SJ et al: Recommendations for feeding normal infants. Pediatrics 63:52, 1979

Fomon SJ, Strauss RG: Nutrient deficiencies in breast-fed infants. N Engl J Med 299:355, 1978

Forsum E, Lonnerdal B: Variation in the contents of nutrients of breast milk during one feeding. Nutr Rep Int 19:815, 1979

Gardner DE, Norwood JR, Eisenson JE: At-will breastfeeding and dental caries. J Dent Child 13:186, 1977

Gerrard JW: Allergy in breast-fed babies to ingredients in breast milk. Ann Allergy 42:69, 1979

Gilmore HE, Rowland TW: Critical malnutrition in breast-fed infants. Am J Dis Child 132:885, 1978

Goldblum RM et al: Antibody-forming cells in human colostrum after oral immunization. Nature 257:797, 1975

Gromish DS: Light (phototherapy)-induced riboflavin deficiency in the neonate. J Pediatr 90:118, 1977

Guthrie HA, Picciano MF, Sheehe D: Fatty acid patterns of human milk. J Pediatr 90:39, 1977

Hall B: Changing composition of human milk and early development of an appetite control. Lancet 1:779, 1975

Hambidge KM: Trace elements in pediatric nutrition. Adv Pediatr 24:191, 1977

Hambidge KM et al: Plasma zinc concentrations of breast fed infants. J Pediatr 94:607, 1979

Hambraeus L: Proprietary milk versus human milk in infant feeding: A critical approach from a nutritional point of view. Pediatr Clin North Am 24:17, 1977

Hamosh M: A review: Fat digestion in the newborn: Role of lingual lipase and preduodenal digestion. Pediatr Res 13:615, 1979

Head JR: Immunobiology of lactation. Semin Perinatol 1:195, 1977

Higginbottom L, Sweetman L, Nyhan WL: A syndrome of methyl-malonic aciduria, homocystinuria, megaloblastic anemia and neurological abnormalities of a vitamin $B_{12}$-deficient breast fed infant of a strict vegetarian. N Engl J Med 299:317, 1978

Jelliffe DB, Jelliffe EFP: The volume and composition of human milk in poorly nourished communities: A review. Am J Clin Nutr 31:492, 1978

Jensen RG, Hagerty MM, McMahon KE: Lipids of human milk and infant formulas: A review. Am J Clin Nutr 31:990, 1978

Johnson PE, Evans GW: Relative zinc availability in human milk, infant formulas and cows milk. Am J Clin Nutr 31:416, 1978

Kabara JJ: Lipids as host-resistance factors of human milk. Nutr Rev 38:65, 1980

Kafatas AG, Zee P: Nutritional benefits from federal food assistance. Am J Dis Child 131:265, 1977

Kemberling SR: Supporting breast-feeding. Pediatrics 63:60, 1979

Kerr CM, Reisinger KC, Plankey FW: Sodium concentration of home-made baby food. Pediatrics 62:331, 1978

Knapp J et al: Growth and nitrogen balance in infants fed cereal proteins. Am J Clin Nutr 26:586, 1973

Kooh SW et al: Rickets due to calcium deficiency. N Engl J Med 297:1264, 1977

Lakdawala DR, Widdowson EM: Vitamin-D in human milk. Lancet 1:167, 1977

Lamm E, Delancy J, Dwyer JT: Economy in the feeding of infants. Pediatr Clin North Am 24:71, 1977

Lapatsanis P et al: Two types of nutritional rickets in infants. Am J Clin Nutr 29:1222, 1976

Larsen SA, Homer DR: Relation of breast versus bottle feeding to hospitalization for gastroenteritis in a middle-class U.S. population. J Pediatr 92:417, 1978

Lebenthal E: Use of modified food starch in infant nutrition. Am J Dis Child 132:850, 1978

Liebhaber M et al: Alterations of lymphocytes and of antibody content of human milk after processing. J Pediatr 91:897, 1977

Lonnerdal B, Forsum E, Gebre-Medhin M et al: Breast milk composition in Ethiopian and Swedish mothers, Part II. Lactase, nitrogen and protein contents. Am J Clin Nutr 29:1134, 1976

Lozy M, Hegsted DM: Calculation of the amino acid requirements of children at different ages by the factorial method. Am J Clin Nutr 28:1052, 1975

Martinez GA, Nalezienski JP: The recent trend in breast-feeding. Pediatrics 64:686, 1979

Mata L: Breast-feeding: Main promoter of infant health. Am J Clin Nutr 31:2058, 1978

Mayer J: A new look at old formulas. Family Health/Today's Health Oct:38, 1976

Nayman R et al: Observation on the composition of milk-substitute products for treatment of inborn errors of amino acid metabolism: Comparison with human milk: A proposal to rationalize nutrient content of treatment products. Am J Clin Nutr 32:1279, 1979

McKenzie RL et al: Seleniun concentration and glutathione peroxidase activity in blood of New Zealand infants and children. Am J Clin Nutr 31:1413, 1978

McMillan JA et al: Iron absorption from human milk, simulated human milk and proprietary formulas. Pediatrics 60:896, 1977

McMillan JA, Landaw SA, Oski FA: Iron sufficiency in breast-fed infants and the availability of iron from human milk. Pediatrics 58:686, 1976

Mellics MJ et al: Cholesterol, phytosterols and polyunsaturated/saturated fatty acid ratios during the first 12 months of lactation. Am J Clin Nutr 32:2383, 1979

O'Connor P: Vitamin D deficiency rickets in two breast-fed infants who were not receiving vitamin D supplements. Clin Pediatr 16:361, 1977

Oski FA, Honig AS: The effects of therapy on the developmental scores of iron-deficient infants. J Pediatr 92:21, 1978

Owen G, Lippman G: Nutritional status of infants and young children: U.S.A. Pediatr Clin North Am 24:211, 1977

Paxson CL, Adcock EW, Morris FH: Osmolalities of infant formulas. Am J Dis Child 131:139, 1977

Picciano MF: Mineral content of human milk during a single nursing. Nutr Rep Int 18:5, 1978

Picciano MF, Guthrie HA: Copper, iron and zinc contents of mature human milk. Am J Clin Nutr 29:242, 1976

Picciano MF, Guthrie HA, Shecke DM: The cholesterol content of human milk. Clin Pediatr 17:359, 1978

Pipes P: When should semisolid foods be fed to infants? J Nutr Educ 9:57, 1977

Pittar WB: Breast milk immunology. Am J Dis Child 133:83, 1979

Review: Acrodermatitis enteropathica, zinc and human milk. Nutr Rev 36:241, 1978

Review: Breast feeding and avoidance of food antigens in the prevention and management of allergic disease. Nutr Rev 36:181, 1978

Review: The development of adipose tissue in infancy. Nutr Rev 37:194, 1979

Review: Diet and iron absorption in the first year of life. Nutr Rev 37:195, 1979

Review: The importance of carnitine in the perinatal period. Nutr Rev 38:310, 1980

Review: Lipases and lipid absorption in the newborn. Nutr Rev 37:104, 1979

Review: Morbidity in breast fed and artificially fed infants. Nutr Rev 38:115, 1980

Review: Nutritional adequacy of breast feeding. Nutr Rev 38:145, 1980

Review: The role of milk leukocytes in protection from necrotizing enterocolitis. Nutr Rev 36:190, 1978

Robertson NRC, Smith MA: Early neonatal hypocalcemia. Arch Dis Child 50:604, 1975

Roy S, Arant BS: Alkalosis from chloride-deficient Neo-Mull Soy. N Engl J Med 301:615, 1979

Saarinen UM: Iron absorption from breast milk, cow's milk, and iron supplemented formula: An opportunistic use of changes in total body iron determined by hemoglobin, ferritin and body weight in 132 infants. Pediatr Res 13:143, 1979

Sauls HS: Potential effect of demographic and other variables in studies comparing morbidity of breast-fed and bottle-fed infants. Pediatrics 64:523, 1979

Schedewh HK et al: Parathormone and perinatal calcium homeostasis. Pediatr Res 13:1, 1979

Shapiro Y, Ben AB, Slater MS: Folic acid deficiency: A reversible cause of infantile hypotonia. J Pediatr 93:984, 1978

Simopoulos AP, Bartter FC: The metabolic consequences of chloride deficiency. Nutr Rev 38:201, 1980

Smith GV, Calvert LJ, Kanto WP Jr: Breast feeding and infant nutrition. Am Fam Physician 17:92, 1978

Stewart D, Gaiser C: Supporting lactation when mothers and infants are separated. Nurs Clin North Am 13:47, 1978

Thomas MD et al: The effects of vitamin C, vitamin $B_6$ and vitamin $B_{12}$ supplementation on the breast milk and maternal status of well-nourished women. Am J Clin Nutr 32:1679, 1979

Thomson CA, Sheremeta IS: Current issues in infant feeding. J Can Diet Assoc 39:189, 1978

Tsang RC et al: Studies in calcium metabolism in infants with intrauterine growth retardation. J Pediatr 86:936, 1975

Tyrala EE, Dodson E: Caffeine secretion into breast milk. Arch Dis Child 54:787, 1979

Vaughan LA, Weber CW, Kemberling SR: Longitudinal changes in the mineral content of human milk. Am J Clin Nutr 32:2301, 1979

Welsh JK, May JT: Anti-infection properties of breast milk. J Pediatr 94:1, 1979

Wolfsdorf JI, Senior B: Failure to thrive and metabolic alkalosis. Adverse effects of a chloride-deficient formula in two infants. JAMA 243:1068, 1980

Woodruff CW: The science of infant nutrition and the art of infant feeding. JAMA 240:657, 1978

Zabel NL et al: Selenium content of commercial formula diets. Am J Clin Nutr 31:850, 1978

Ziegler EE et al: Nitrogen balance studies with normal children. Am J Clin Nutr 30:939, 1977

# Nutrition for Children and Youth
## General references
### Books and pamphlets

Committee on Nutrition of the Mother and Preschool Child, Food and Nutrition Board, National Academy of Sciences: Iron Nutriture in Adolescence. DHEW Publ. No. (HBA) 77-5100. Washington, DC, United States Government Printing Office, 1977

Daniels WA: Adolescents in Health and Disease. St Louis, CV Mosby, 1977

Endres JB, Rockwell RE: Food, Nutrition and the Young Child. St Louis, CV Mosby, 1980

Fomon SJ: Nutritional Disorders of Children. Prevention, Screening and Follow-up. DHEW Publ. No. (HSA) 77-5104. Washington, DC, United States Government Printing Office, 1977

Fomon SJ, Anderson TA, Stephen HYW et al: Nutritional Disorders of Children: Prevention, Screening and Follow-up. DHEW Publ. No. (HSA) 76-5612. Washington, DC, United States Government Printing Office, 1976

Food and Nutrition Board: Oral Contraception and Nutrition. Washington, DC, NRC-NAS, 1975

Gaillard B, Haskell W, Smith NJ et al: Handbook for the Young Athlete. Palo Alto, CA, Bull, 1978

Huenemann RL et al: Teenaged Nutrition and Physique. Springfield, IL, Charles C Thomas, 1974

Martin EA, Beal VA: Roberts' Nutrition Work with Children, 4th ed. Chicago, University of Chicago Press, 1978

McKegney J, Munro HN (eds): Nutrient Requirements in Adolescence. Cambridge, MIT Press, 1976

Preschool Nutrition Education Monograph. 2140 Shattuck Ave., Suite 1110, Berkeley, CA, Society for Nutrition Education, 1979

Smith NJ: Food for Sport. Palo Alto, CA, Bull, 1977

Vonde DAA, Beck J: Food Adventures for Children. Redondo Beach, CA, Plycon Press, 1980

Wanamaker N et al: More than Graham Crackers: Nutrition Education and Food Preparation with Young Children. Washington, DC, National Association for the Education of Young Children, 1979

Winick M (ed): Childhood Obesity. New York, John Wiley & Sons, 1975

Young DR: Physical Performance, Fitness and Diet. Springfield, IL, Charles C Thomas, 1977

### Journal articles

American Dietetic Association: Nutrition and physical fitness. J Am Diet Assoc 76:437, 1980

Blakeway SF, Knickrehm ME: Nutrition education in the Little Rock school lunch program. J Am Diet Assoc 72:389, 1978

Breakfast: A second look. School Foodservice J 31:36, 1977

Butrimovitz BP, Purdy WC: Zinc nutriture and growth in children. Am J Clin Nutr 31:1409, 1978

Crawford L: Junk food in our schools: A look at student spending in school vending machines and concessions. J Can Diet Assoc 38:193, 1977

Galst JP, White MA: The unhealthy persuader: The reinforcing value of television and children's purchase-influencing attempts at the supermarket. Child Dev 47:1089, 1976

Greulich WW: Some secular changes in the growth of American-born and native Japanese children. Am J Phys Anthropol 45:553, 1976

Morrison JA et al: Lipids and lipoproteins in 927 school children ages 6–17 years. Pediatrics 62:990, 1978

Trahms CM et al: Restriction of growth and elevated protoporphyrin in children deprived of animal protein. Clin Res 25:179, 1977

Zavaleta AN, Malina RM: Growth, fatness and leanness in Mexican-American children. Am J Clin Nutr 33:2008, 1980

## Preschoolers
### Journal articles

Birch LL: Dimensions of preschool children's food preferences. J Nutr Educ 11:77, 1979

Burt JV, Hertzler AA: Parental influence on the child's food preference. J Nutr Educ 10:127, 1978

Caliendo MA et al: Nutritional status of preschool children. J Am Diet Assoc 71:20, 1977

Caliendo MA, Sanjur D: The dietary status of preschool children: An ecological approach. J Nutr Educ 10:69, 1978

Crawford PB, Hankin JH, Huenemann RL: Environmental factors associated with preschool obesity. J Am Diet Assoc 72:589, 1978

Dwyer JT et al: Preschoolers on alternate lifestyle diets. J Am Diet Assoc 72:264, 1978

Hambidge KM et al: Zinc nutrition of preschool children in the Denver Headstart Program. Am J Clin Nutr 29:734, 1976

Owen GM et al: A study of nutritional status of preschool children in the U.S. 1968–70. Pediatrics 53:597, 1974

Shull MW et al: Velocities of growth in vegetarian preschool children. Pediatrics 60:410, 1977

Stolley H, Schlage C: Water balance and water requirement of preschool children. Nutr Metab (Suppl 1) 21:15, 1977

Trahms CM, Feeney MC: Evaluation of diet and growth of vegans, vegetarian and non-vegetarian preschool children. Fed Proc 34:675, 1975

Williams S, Henneman A, Fox H: Contributions of food service programs in preschool centers to children's nutritional needs. J Am Diet Assoc 71:610, 1977

## The school-age child
### Journal articles

Barnes L: Preadolescent training: How young is too young? Phys Sports Med 7:114, 1979

Coates TJ, Thoresen CE: Treating obesity in children and adolescents: A review. Am J Public Health 68:143, 1978

Committee on Nutrition, American Academy of Pediatrics: Calcium requirements in infancy and childhood. Pediatrics 62:826, 1978

Fisk D: A successful program for changing children's eating habits. Nutr Today 14:6, May-June, 1979

Frank GC et al: Dietary studies of rural school children in a cardiovascular study. J Am Diet Assoc 71:31, 1977

Jansen GR, Harper JM: Consumption and plate waste of menu items served in the National School Lunch Program. J Am Diet Assoc 73:395, 1978

Karp R et al: Effects of rise in food costs on hemoglobin concentrations of early school-age children. Public Health Rep 93:456, 1978

Kondo S et al: Secular trends in height and weight of Japanese pupils. Tohoku J Exp Med 126:203, 1978

Meiners CR et al: The relationship of zinc to protein utilization in the preadolescent child. Am J Clin Nutr 30:879, 1977

Voichick J: School lunch in Chicago. J Nutr Educ 9:102, 1977

Yperman AM, Vermeersch JA: Factors associated with children's food preferences. J Nutr Educ 11:72, 1979

## Adolescents
### Journal articles

Aftergood L, Alexander AF, Alfin-Slater RB: Effect of oral contraceptives on plasma lipoproteins, cholesterol and $\alpha$-tocopherol levels in young women. Nutr Rep Int 11:295, 1975

Alcohol and athletes. Phys Sports Med 7:39, 1979

Alexson JM, Del Campo DS: Improving teenagers' nutrition knowledge through the mass media. J Nutr Educ 10:30, 1978

Barnes HV (ed): Symposium on adolescent medicine. Med Clin North Am 50:1279, 1975

Basse TR, Donald EA: The vitamin $B_6$ requirement in oral contraceptive users. I. Assessment of pyridoxal level and transferase activity in erythrocytes. Am J Clin Nutr 32:1015, 1979

Burman D: Adolescent nutrition. Practitioner 222:615, 1979

Cho M, Fryer BA: Nutritional knowledge of collegiate physical education majors. J Am Diet Assoc 65:30, 1974

Clancy KL et al: Snack food intakes of adolescents and caries development. J Dent Res 56:568, 1977

Committee on Adolescence, American Academy of Pediatrics: Statement on teenage pregnancy. Pediatrics 63:795, 1979

Consolazio CF et al: Protein metabolism of intensive physical training in the young adult. Am J Clin Nutr 28:29, 1975

Costill DL et al: Effects of elevated plasma free fatty acids and insulin on muscle glycogen usage during exercise. J Appl Physiol 43:695, 1977

Costill DL, Dalsky GP, Fink WJ: Effects of caffeine ingestion on metabolism and exercise performance. Med Sci Sports 10:155, 1978

Crews MG, Taper LJ, Ritchey SJ: Effects of oral contraceptive agents on copper and zinc balance in young women. Am J Clin Nutr 33:1940, 1980

Daniel WA, Gaines EG, Bennett DL: Dietary intakes and plasma concentrations of folate in healthy adolescents. Am J Clin Nutr 28:363, 1975

Daniel WA, Gaines EG, Bennett DL: Iron intake and transferrin saturation in adolescents. J Pediatr 86:288, 1975

Esterly NB, Furey NL: Acne: Current concepts. Pediatrics 62:1044, 1978

Gregor JL et al: Calcium, magnesium, phosphorus, copper and magnesium balance in adolescent females. Am J Clin Nutr 31:117, 1978

Gregor JL, Buckley S: Menstrual loss of zinc, copper, magnesium, and iron by adolescent girls. Nutr Rep Int 16:639, 1977

Gregor JL et al: Nutritional status of adolescent girls in regard to zinc, copper and iron. Am J Clin Nutr 31:269, 1978

Greenwood CT, Richardson DP: Nutrition during adolescence. World Rev Nutr Diet 33:1, 1979

Heald FP: Adolescent nutrition. Med Clin North Am 59:1329, 1975

Hess FM, King JC, Mergen S: Zinc excretion in young women on low zinc intakes and oral contraceptive agents. J Nutr 107:1610, 1977

Hickson RC et al: Effects of increasing plasma free fatty acids on endurance. Fed Proc 36:450, 1977

Hursh LM: Food and water restriction in the wrestler. JAMA 241:915, 1979

Ikeda J: For teenagers only: Change your habits to change your shape. Palo Alto, CA, Bull, 1978

Jette M: Physiological aspects of fitness and physical activity. J Can Diet Assoc 39:116, 1978

Jette M et al: The nutritional and metabolic effects of a carbohydrate-rich diet in a glycogen supercompensation training regimen. Am J Clin Nutr 32:2140, 1978

Kirksey A et al: Vitamin B$_6$ nutritional status of a group of female adolescents. Am J Clin Nutr 31:946, 1978

Lane HW et al: Effect of physical activity on human potassium metabolism in a hot and humid climate. Am J Clin Nutr 31:838, 1978

Lane HW, Cerda JJ: Potassium requirements and exercise. J Am Diet Assoc 73:64, 1978

Lee CJ: Nutritional status of selected teenagers in Kentucky. Am J Clin Nutr 31:1453, 1978

Mapes MC: Gulp: An alternate method for reaching teens. J Nutr Educ 9:12, 1977

Massey LK, Davison MA: Effects of oral contraceptives on nutritional status. Am Fam Physician 19:119, 1979

Morrissey ER: Alcohol-related problems in adolescents and women. Postgrad Med 64:111, 1978

Parizkova J: Growth and growth velocity of lean body mass and fat in adolescent boys. Pediatr Res 10:647, 1976

Review: Nutrition in adolescence. Nutr Rev 39:37, 1981

Richardson BD, Pieters L: Menarche and growth. Am J Clin Nutr 30:2088, 1977

Schwartz NE: Nutritional knowledge, attitudes and practices of high school graduates. J Am Diet Assoc 66:28, 1975

Smith NJ: Gaining and losing weight in athletes. JAMA 236:149, 1976

Tanner JM, Whitehouse RH: Clinical longitudinal standards for height, weight, height velocity and stages of puberty. Arch Dis Child 51:170, 1976

Vaccaro P, Zauner CW, Cade JR: Changes in body weight, hematocrit and plasma protein concentration due to dehydration and rehydration in wrestlers. J Sports Med 16:45, 1976

## Nutrition for Older Persons

Albanese AA: An introduction. Nutrition of the elderly. Postgrad Med 63:117, 1978

Albanese AA: Calcium nutrition in the elderly. Postgrad Med 63:167, Mar, 1978

Albanese AA: Osteoporosis. J Am Pharm Assoc 17:252, 1977

Albanese AA, Edelson AH, Lorenze E et al: Problems of bone health in the elderly—A ten-year study. NY State J Med 75:326, 1975

Anderson EL: Eating patterns before and after dentures. J Am Diet Assoc 58:421, 1971

Baltes PB, Schaie KW: The myth of the twilight years. Psychology Today 8:35, Mar, 1974

Barboriak JJ, Rooney CB, Leitschuh TH et al: Alcohol and nutrient intake of elderly men. J Am Diet Assoc 72:493, 1978

Beauchene RE, Davis TA: The nutritional status of the aged in the U.S.A. Age 2:23, 1979

Bradshaw BR: Community based residential care for the minimally impaired elderly: A survival analysis. J Am Geriatr Soc 24:423, 1976

Brin M, Bauernfeind JC: Vitamin needs of the elderly. Postgrad Med 63:155, 1978

Brown EL: Factors influencing food choices and intake. Geriatrics 31:89, Sept, 1976

Busse EW: Eating in late life: Physiologic and psychologic factors. Contemp Nutr 4:1, Nov, 1979

Busse EW: How mind, body and environment influence nutrition in the elderly. Postgrad Med 63:118, 1978

Butler RN, Engel BT: Psychosomatic medicine and aging research. Psychosom Med 40:365, 1978

Cape RDT, Henschke PJ: Perspective of health in old age. J Am Geriatr Soc 28:295, 1980

Chen AHR, Gomez A, Bergan JG et al: Comparative nitrogen balance study between young and aged adults using three levels of protein intake from a combination wheat-soy-milk mixture. Am J Clin Nutr 31:12, 1978

Combs KL: Preventive care in the elderly. Am J Nurs 78:1339, 1978

Crocco S: Feeding the elderly: Packaging is the problem. Food Engineer 47:31, June, 1975

Dibble MV, Brin M, Thiele VF et al: Evaluation of the nutritional status of elderly subjects with a comparison between fall and spring. J Am Geriatr Soc 15:1031, 1967

Dobihal SV: Enabling a patient to die at home. Am J Nurs 80:1448, 1980

Domencia AD: Implementing a "2 +3" meal plan. Hospitals 42:89, Mar 16, 1968

Exton-Smith AN: Physiological aspects of aging: Relationship to nutrition. Am J Clin Nutr 25:853, 1972

Feldman RS, Kapur KK, Alman JE et al: Aging and mastication: Changes in performance and in the swallowing threshold with natural dentition. J Am Geriatr Soc 28:97, Mar, 1980

Ferrero E, Casale G, DeNicola P: Serum glucagon after arginine infusion in aged and young subjects. J Am Geriatr Soc 28:285, 1980

Finch CE: The brain and aging. In Behnke JA, Finch CE, Moment GB (eds): The Biology of Aging, pp 301–309. New York, Plenum Press, 1978

Fitzgibbons JJ, Garcia PA, Connolly CP: Nutrition education for the elderly: Using television PSAs. J Home Econ 71:43, Fall, 1979

Gershoff SN, Brusis OA, Nino HV et al: Studies of the elderly in Boston. I. The effects of iron fortification on moderately anemic people. Am J Clin Nutr 30:226, 1977

Gillespie NG, Mena I, Cotzias GC et al: Diets affecting treatment of parkinsonism with levodopa. J Am Diet Assoc 62:525, 1973

Gioiella EC: Give the older person space. Am J Nurs 80:898, 1980

Gorrod JW: Absorption, metabolism and excretion of drugs in geriatric subjects. Gerontol Clin 16:30, 1974

Gotz BE, Gotz VP: Drugs and the elderly. Am J Nurs 78:1347, 1978

Grotkowski ML, Sims LS: Nutrition knowledge, attitudes, and dietary practices of the elderly. J Am Diet Assoc 72:499, 1978

Growdon JH, Wurtman RJ: Nutrients and neurotransmitters. Contemp Nutr 4:1, Dec, 1979

Guthrie HA, Black K, Madden JP: Nutritional practices of elderly citizens in rural Pennsylvania. Gerontologist 12:330, 1972

Hackley JA: Full-service hospice offers home, day and inpatient care. Hospitals 51:84, Nov 1, 1977

Hain MJ, Chen SPC: Health needs of the elderly. Nurs Res 25:433, 1976

Hamilton M, Reid HA (eds): A Hospice Handbook. A New Way to Care for the Dying. Grand Rapids, MI, William B Eerdmans, 1980

Hanson RG: Considering "social nutrition" in assessing geriatric nutrition. Geriatrics 3:49, 1978

Harper AE: Recommended dietary allowances for the elderly. Geriatrics 33:13, 1978

Harrill I, Cervone N: Vitamin status of older women. Am J Clin Nutr 30:431, 1977

Harris CS: Fact Book on Aging: A Profile of America's Older Population. Washington, DC, National Council on Aging, 1978

Hayflick L: The cell biology of human aging. N Engl J Med 295:1302, 1976

Hodgson JL, Buskirk ER: Physical fitness and age, with emphasis on cardiovasular function in the elderly. J Am Geriatr Soc 25:385, 1977

Holmes D: Nutrition and health-screening services for the elderly. J Am Diet Assoc 60:301, 1972

Kateri M: Scheduling five-a-day. Hosp Nurs Home Food Mgt 6:32, Jan, 1970

Kohrs MB, O'Neal R, Preston A et al: Nutritional status of elderly residents in Missouri. Am J Clin Nutr 31:2186, 1978

Lamb MJ: Biology of Aging. New York, John Wiley & Sons, 1977

Lane MM: Five meals a day: A reassessment. Nurs Homes 17:25, Feb, 1968

Lee CJ, Johnson GH: Effect of supplementary calcium and calcium-rich foods on bone density of elderly females with osteoporosis. Fed Proc 38:772, 1979

Madden JP, Goodman SJ, Guthrie HA: Validity of the 24-hour recall. Analysis of data obtained from elderly subjects. J Am Diet Assoc 68:143, 1976

Marrs DC: Milk drinking by the elderly of three races. J Am Diet Assoc 72:495, 1978

Mason JB, Bearden WO: Profiling the shopping behavior of elderly consumers. Gerontologist 18:454, 1978

McDermott JR, Smith AI, Iqbal K et al: Brain aluminum in aging and Alzheimer disease. Neurology 29:809, 1979

McGandy RB, Barrows CH, Spanias A et al: Nutrient intakes and energy expenditure in men of different ages. J Gerontol 21:581, 1966

Metress J, Kart C: A system for observing the potential nutritional risks of elderly people living at home. J Geriatr Psychiatry 11:67, 1978

Miller DB: Physician's attitudes toward the ill aged and nursing homes. J Am Geriatr Soc 24:498, 1976

Moss JM: Pitfalls to avoid in diagnosing diabetes in the elderly. Geriatrics 31:52, 1976

Munro HN: Major gaps in nutrient allowances. J Am Diet Assoc 76:137, 1980

Munro HN, Young VR: Protein metabolism in the elderly. Postgrad Med 63:143, 1978

Murray WI: Nutritional problems in the aged: Consumer advocate views. J Natl Med Assoc 70:133, 1978

Myers TW: Nutritional programming for the elderly. J Natl Med Assoc 70:335, 1978

Natow AB, Heslin JA, Natow AJ: Geriatric Nutrition. Boston, CBI, 1980

Nutrition, longevity, and aging. Dairy Council Digest 50:1, July–Aug, 1979

Nutrition of the elderly. Dairy Council Digest 48:1, Jan, 1977

Paige RL, Looney JF: Hospice care for the adult. Am J Nurs 77:1812, 1977

Paradise lost. Nutr Today 13:6, 1978

Polanska N, Wills MR: Factors contributing to osteomalacia in the elderly and in Asian communities in the United Kingdom. J Hum Nutr 30:371, 1976

Posner BM: Nutrition and the Elderly. Policy Development, Program Planning and Evaluation. Lexington, MA, Lexington Books, 1979

Rae J, Burke AL: Counseling the elderly on nutrition in a community health care system. J Am Geriatr Soc 26:130, 1978

Rao DB: Problems of nutrition in the aged. J Am Geriatr Soc 21:362, 1973

Rapp JW: Five-meal plan tried, found wanting. Hospitals 42:108, Oct 11, 1968

Rawson IG, Weinberg EI, Herold JA et al: Nutrition of rural elderly in southwestern Pennsylvania. Gerontologist 18:24, 1978

Reid WR: New hospital uses four-meal plan with success. Hospitals 43:77, Feb 16, 1969

Ross MH: Dietary behavior and longevity. Nutr Rev 35:257, 1977

Ross MH: Nutrition and longevity in experimental animals. In Winick M (ed): Nutrition and Aging, pp 43–57. New York, John Wiley & Sons, 1976

Rossman I: Clinical Geriatrics. Philadelphia, JB Lippincott, 1979

Rossman P: Hospice: Creating New Models of Care for the Terminally Ill. New York, Association Press, 1977

Rountree JL, Tinklin GL: Food beliefs and practices of selected senior citizens. Gerontologist 15:537, 1975

Rowe JW: The aging process: Characteristics and clinical relevance. Professional Nurse 1:3, May 10, 1980

Schaefer AE: Nutrition problems of the elderly. Nutr News 43:9, Oct, 1980

Schieffman S: Food recognition by the elderly. J Gerontol 32:586, 1977

Shanas E: The family as a social support system in old age. Gerontologist 19:169, 1979

Shephard RJ: Exercise and aging. In Behnke JA, Finch CE, Moment GB (eds): The Biology of Aging, pp 131–149. New York, Plenum Press, 1978

Sherwood S: Sociology of food and eating: Implications for action for the elderly. Am J Clin Nutr 26:1108, 1973

Shock NW: Physiologic aspects of aging. J Am Diet Assoc 56:491, 1970

Sidney KH, Shephard RJ, Harrison JE: Endurance training and body composition of the elderly. Am J Clin Nutr 30:326, 1977

Sniadach R: Care of the elderly. N Engl J Med 296:1070, 1977

Spritzler M: Editorial: Three versus five. Hosp Nurs Home Food Mgt 6:27, Aug, 1970

Stare FJ: Three score and ten plus more. J Am Geriatr Soc 25:529, 1977

Stoddard S: The Hospice Movement. A Better Way of Caring for the Dying. Briarcliff Manor, NY, Stein & Day, 1978

Templeton, CL: Nutrition counseling needs in a geriatric population. Geriatrics 4:59, 1978

Tempro WA: Nutritional problems in the aged: Dietary aspects. J Natl Med Assoc 70:281, 1978

Timiras PS: Biological perspectives on aging. Am Sci 66:605, 1978

Todhunter EN, Darby WJ: Guidelines for maintaining adequate nutrition in old age. Geriatrics 33:49, June, 1978

Triche MK: Nutritional care in a geriatric hospital. J Am Diet Assoc 66:377, 1975

Uauy R: Human protein requirements: Obligatory urinary and fecal nitrogen losses and the factorial estimation of protein needs in elderly males. J Nutr 108:90, 1978

Uauy R, Scrimshaw NS, Young VR: Human protein requirements: Nitrogen balance response to graded levels of egg protein in elderly men and women. Am J Clin Nutr 31:799, 1978

Unklesbay N: Students in food systems management contribute to nutrition programs for the elderly. J Am Diet Assoc 70:516, 1977

U.S. Bureau of Census: Current Population Reports, Series P-23, No. 69. Survey of Institutionalized Persons. A Survey of Persons Receiving Long-Term Care. Washington, DC, United States Government Printing Office, 1976

U.S. Bureau of Census: Current Population Reports, Series P-25, No. 704. Projections of the Population of the United States: 1977 to 2050. Washington, DC, United States Government Printing Office, 1977

Velardo CG: Geriatric psycho-social history outline. J Am Geriatr Soc 24:470, 1976

Watson RR: Nutrition, disease resistance, and age. Food Nutr News 51:1, Oct–Nov, 1979

Wurtman R: Brain muffin. Psychology Today 12:140, Oct, 1978

Wurtman RJ, Wurtman JJ: Nutrition and the Brain. New York, Raven Press, 1977

Yearick ES: Nutritional status of the elderly: Anthropometric and clinical findings. J Gerontol 33:657, 1978

Young VR: Diet as a modulator of aging and longevity. Fed Proc 38:1994, 1979

Young VR, Steffee WP, Pencharz PB et al: Total human body protein requirements at various ages. Nature 253:192, 1975

Zanni E, Calloway DH, Zezuka AY: Protein requirements of elderly men. J Nutr 109:513, 1979

## Malnutrition—A World Problem
### Books
### General

Altschul AM, Wilcke HL: New Protein Foods, Vol 3, Animal Protein Supplies. New York, Academic Press, 1978

Brozek J (ed): Behavioral Effects of Energy and Protein Deficits. National Institute of Arthritis. Metabolism and Digestive Diseases, NIH Publ. No. 79-1906, Washington, DC, NIH, 1979

Caliendo MA: Nutrition and the World Food Crisis. New York, Macmillan, 1979

Chandra RK, Newberne PM: Nutrition, Immunity and Infection: Mechanisms of Interactions. New York, Plenum Press, 1977

Child Growth and Nutrition in Jordan: A Study of Factors and Patterns. Amman, Jordan, Royal Scientific Society Press, 1977

De Mayer EM et al: Control of Endemic Goitre. Geneva, World Health Organization, 1979 (available from WHO Publications Center, Albany, NY)

den Hartog AP, van Staveren WA: Field Guide on Food Habits and Food Consumption: A Practical Introduction to Social Surveys on Food and Nutrition in Third World Communities. Wageningen, Netherlands, International Course in Food Science and Nutrition, 1979

de Ville de Goyet C et al: Management of Nutritional Emergencies in Large Populations. Geneva, World Health Organization, 1978 (available from WHO Publications Center, Albany, NY)

FAO/WHO: Handbook on human nutrition requirements. WHO Monogr Ser, no. 61. Rome, FAO/WHO, 1974

Greene LS (ed): Malnutrition, Behavior, and Social Organization. New York, Academic Press, 1977

Hakim P, Solimano G: Development, Reform and Malnutrition in Chile. Cambridge, MIT Press, 1978

Hopkins RF et al (eds): Food, Politics, and Agricultural Development: Case Studies in the Public Policy of Rural Modernization. Boulder, CO, Westview Press, 1979

Mata LJ: The Children of Santa Maria Cauque: A Prospective Field Study of Health and Growth. Cambridge, MIT Press, 1978

May JM, McLellan DL: The Ecology of Malnutrition in the Caribbean. New York, Hafner Press, 1973

May JM, McLellan DL: The Ecology of Malnutrition in Seven Countries in Southern Africa and in Portuguese Guinea—Studies in Medical Geography, Vol 10. New York, Hafner Press, 1971

Miller ME: Host Defenses in the Human Neonate. New York, Grune & Stratton, 1978

Pariser ER, Corkery CJ, Wallenstein MB et al: Fish Protein Concentrate: Panacea for Protein Malnutrition. Cambridge, MIT Press, 1978

Patwardhan VN, Darby WI: The State of Nutrition in the Arab Middle East. Nashville, Vanderbilt University Press, 1972

Pearcy E: World Food Scene. Redondo Beach, CA, Plycon Press, 1980

Rechcigl M (ed): CRC Handbook Series in Nutrition and Food. Section E Nutritional Disorders, Vol III, Effect of Nutrient Deficiencies in Man. West Palm Beach, FL, CRC Press, 1978

Schultz GO: Malnutrition in the Levant 1. Protein Energy Malnutrition (PEM). Beirut, Lebanon, A Oustayan, P.O. Box 6807, 1979

Winikoff B (ed): Nutrition and National Policy. Cambridge, MIT Press, 1978

### Journal articles
### General

An action-oriented research, development, and training programme in nutrition. WHO Chron 33:225, 1979

Arena JM: Nutritional status of China's children: An overview. Nutr Rev 32:289, 1974

Bang FB: The role of disease in the ecology of famine. Ecol Food Nutr 7:1, 1978

Clark WF: The rural to urban nutritional gradient: Application and interpretation in a developing nation and urban situation. Soc Sci Med 14D:31, 1980

Freij L et al: Ascariasis and malnutrition. A study in Ethiopian children. Am J Clin Nutr 32:1545, 1979

Gebre-Medhin M, Vahlquist B: Famine in Ethiopia—The period 1973–75. Nutr Rev 35:194, 1977

Katz M, Stiehm DR: Host defenses in malnutrition. Pediatrics 59:1977

Kielmann AA et al: The Narangwal Nutrition Study: A summary review. Am J Clin Nutr 31:2040, 1978

Latham M: Nutrition and infection in national development. Science 188:561, 1975

Lechtig A et al: Maternal nutrition and fetal growth in developing societies: Socioeconomic factors. Am J Dis Child 129:434, 1975

Lynch L: Nutrition-planning methodologies: A comparative review of types and applications. Food Nutr Bull 1:1, 1979

Mejia LA, Hodges RE, Arroyave G et al: Vitamin A deficiency and anemia in Central American children. Am J Clin Nutr 30:1175, 1977

Parrack DW: Famine symposium: Ecosystems and famine. Ecol Food Nutr 7:17, 1978

Review: Changes in composition of tears of malnourished children. Nutr Rev 36:147, 1978

Review: Evaluation of the impact of mothercraft centers on therapy and prevention of malnutrition. Nutr Rev 36:275, 1978

Review: How useful are supplementary feeding programs? Nutr Rev 36:278, 1978

Review: Impaired cellular immunity associated with fetal growth retardation. Nutr Rev 37:42, 1979

Review: Metabolic and enzyme activities of neutrophils in malnutrition. Nutr Rev 35:230, 1977

Review: Moves to cities: Nutritional causes and consequences. Nutr Rev 38:367, 1980

Review: Nutritional consequences of giardiasis. Nutr Rev 38:369, 1980

Review: Work output in undernourished adolescents: Effect of early malnutrition. Nutr Rev 38:143, 1980

Satyanarayana AN et al: Nutritional deprivation in childhood and the body size, activity, and physical work capacity of young boys. Am J Clin Nutr 32:1769, 1979

Stoch MB, Smythe PM: Fifteen year developmental study on effects of severe undernutrition on subsequent physical growth and intellectual functioning. Arch Dis Child 51:327, 1976

Valverde V et al: Relationship between family land availability and nutritional status. Ecol Food Nutr 6:1, 1977

## Infant feeding

Abrahamsson L et al: The nutritional value of home-prepared and industrially produced weaning foods. J Hum Nutr 32:279, 1978

Brown RE: Weaning foods in developing countries. Am J Clin Nutr 31:2066, 1978

Gueri M et al: Breast feeding practices in Trinidad. Bull Pan Am Health Organ 12:316, 1978

Knodel J: Breast-feeding and population growth. Science 198:1111, 1977

Mata L: Breast feeding: Main promoter of infant health. Am J Clin Nutr 31:2058, 1978

## Protein energy malnutrition

FAO/WHO: Protein and energy requirements. Bull WHO 57:65, 1979

John TJ et al: Kwashiorkor not associated with poverty. Pediatrics 90:730, 1977

Payne RP: Safe protein–calorie ratios in diets. The relative importance of protein and energy intake as a causal factor in malnutrition. Am J Clin Nutr 28:281, 1975

Protein energy requirements under conditions prevailing in developing countries: Current knowledge and research needs. Food Nutr Bull (Suppl 1) July, 1979

Review: Adaptation in protein calorie malnutrition. Nutr Rev 37:250, 1979

Review: A "new" protein food from a traditional process. Nutr Rev 39:9, 1981

Review: Scrimshaw NS: Through a glass darkly: Discerning the practical implications of human dietary protein-energy interrelationships. Nutr Rev 35:321, 1977

Review: Special report: Energy-protein malnutrition and behavior. Nutr Rev 38:164, 1980

Whitehead PG: Protein and energy requirements of young children living in developing countries to allow for catch-up growth after infections. Am J Clin Nutr 30:1545, 1977

## Vitamin deficiencies

Brink EW et al: Vitamin A status of children in Sri Lanka. Am J Clin Nutr 32:84, 1979

Liem ITH et al: Production of vitamin $B_{12}$ in tempeh, a fermented soybean food. Appl Environ Microbiol 34:773, 1977

Neumann CG et al: Biochemical evidence of thiamin deficiency in young Ghanian children. Am J Clin Nutr 32:99, 1979

Review: The biochemical abnormality of transketolase in patients with Wernicke-Korsakoff syndrome. Nutr Rev 37:226, 1979

Solon F et al: An evaluation of strategies to control vitamin A deficiency in the Philippines. Am J Clin Nutr 32:1445, 1979

Sommer A: Field Guide to the Detection and Control of Xerophthalmia. Albany NY, World Health Organization, 1978

Underwood BA: Strategies for the prevention of vitamin A deficiency. Food Nutr Bull 2:11, 1980

## Mineral deficiencies

Baker SJ, De Maeyer EM: Nutritional anemia: Its understanding and control with special reference to the work of the World Health Organization. Am J Clin Nutr 32:368, 1979

Czajka-Narins DM, Haddy TB, Kallen DJ: Nutrition and social correlates of iron deficiency anemia. Am J Clin Nutr 31:955, 1978

Kook SW et al: Rickets due to calcium deficiency. N Engl J Med 297:1264, 1977

Nadiger HA, Krishnamachari KAVR, Naidu AN et al: The use of common salt (sodium chloride) fortified with iron to control anemia. Br J Nutr 43:45, 1980

Review: Iron-fortified salt to combat anemia. Nutr Rev 38:308, 1980

Stanbury JB, Hetzel BS: Endemic Goiter and Endemic Cretinism: Iodine Nutrition in Health and Disease. New York, John Wiley & Sons, 1980

Trowbridge FL et al: Iodine and goiter in children. Pediatrics 56:82, 1975

## Dental caries

Johnson NW: Aetiology of dental disease and theoretical aspects of dietary control. J Hum Nutr 33:98, 1979

Review: Daily fluoride supplements and dental caries. Nutr Rev 36:329, 1978

Special report: Prevention of major dental disorders. Nutr Rev 38:134, 1980

# Part Three
# Diet in Disease

## Nutritional care and diet therapy for the hospitalized patient

### Feeding the hospitalized patient
### Books and pamphlets

Bernstein L, Bernstein RS: Interviewing: A Guide for Health Professionals, 3rd ed. New York, Appleton-Century-Crofts, 1980

Mason M, Wenberg BG, Welsch PK: The Dynamics of Clinical Dietetics, 2nd ed. New York, John Wiley & Sons (in press)

Neelon FA, Ellis GJ: A Syllabus of Problem-Oriented Patient Care. Boston, Little, Brown, 1974

Walters FM, Crumley SJ (eds): Patient Care Audit: A Quality Assurance Procedure Manual for Dietitans. Chicago, American Dietetic Association, 1978

### Journal articles
### Problem-oriented record

Ometer JL: Documentation of nutritional care. J Am Diet Assoc 76:35, 1980

Rodgers TV, Clark ME: Sharing information by means of the patient's medical record. J Am Diet Assoc 63:42, 1973

Voytovich AE: The dietitian/nutritionist and the problem-oriented medical record. I. A physician's viewpoint. J Am Diet Assoc 63:639, 1973

Walters FM, DeMarco M: The dietitian/nutritionist and the problem-oriented medical record. II. The role of the dietitian. J Am Diet Assoc 63:641, 1973

Weed LL: Medical records that guide and teach. N Engl J Med 278:593, 652, 1968

### Quality assurance

Donabedian A: The Definition of Quality and Approaches to its Assessment: Exploring in Quality Assessment and Monitoring. Ann Arbor, Health Administration Press, 1980

Drexler L Sr, Caliendo MA: Developing and implementing a nutritional care audit. J Am Diet Assoc 76:374, 1980

Gormican A: Audit of dietary care shows better documentation needed. Hospitals 55:107, Mar 16, 1981

Kendrick EMJ: Professional standards review for dietitians. Dietetic Currents 6:5, Mar-Apr, 1979

Krejci CB: Quality assurance audit. J Am Diet Assoc 76:378, 1980

Krikorian J: Quality control enhanced by chart review. Hospitals 53:97, Nov 1, 1979

Looney DH, Gibson C: Standard of practice: Nutritional quality assurance in acute-care hospitals. J Am Diet Assoc 79:64, 1981

Ometer JL: An intradepartmental process audit to measure quality of care. J Am Diet Assoc 75:563, 1979

O'Regan DJ: Quality assurance: Consensus reached on assessment but not on assurance. Hospitals 52:150, Apr 1, 1978

Ostrow PC, Jones E: Peer review for nonphysicians. Hospitals 53:66, Dec 1, 1979

Weed JE, Molleson AL: Establishing guidelines for peer review of the clinical dietitian. J Am Diet Assoc 70:157, 1977

## Assessment of Patient Needs
### Journal articles

Barac-Nietro M et al: Body composition during nutritional repletion of severely undernourished men. Am J Clin Nutr 32:981, 1979

Beisel WR: Effects of infection on nutritional status and immunity. Fed Proc 39:3105, 1980

Bistrian BR: Letter: Anthropometric norms used in assessment of hospitalized patients. Am J Clin Nutr 33:2211, 1980

Bistrian BR et al: Cellular immunity in semistarved states in hospitalized adults. Am J Clin Nutr 28:1148, 1975

Bistrian BR et al: Prevalence of malnutrition in general medical patients. JAMA 235:1567, 1976

Bistrian BR et al: Protein status of general surgical patients. JAMA 230:858, 1974

Blackburn GL, Thornton PA: Nutritional assessment of the hospitalized patient. Med Clin North Am 63:1103, 1979

Brozek J, Kinzey W: Age changes in skinfold compressibility. J Gerontol 15:45, 1960

Burget SL, Anderson CF: An evaluation of upper arm measurements used in nutritional assessment. Am J Clin Nutr 32:2136, 1979

Chandra RK: Cell-mediated immunity in nutritional imbalance. Fed Proc 39:3088, 1980

Copeland EM et al: Nutrition as an adjunct to cancer treatment in the adult. Cancer Res 37:2451, 1977

Driver AG, McAlvey MT: Letter: Creatinine height index as a function of age. Am J Clin Nutr 33:2057, 1980

Dugdale AE, Griffiths M: Estimating fat body mass from anthropometric data. Am J Clin Nutr 32:2400, 1979

Gray GE, Gray LK: Validity of anthropometric norms used in the assessment of hospitalized patients. J Parent Ent Nutr 3:366, 1979

Grundfest S: Home parenteral nutrition. JAMA 244:1701, 1980

Hill GL et al: Malnutrition in surgical patients. An unrecognized problem. Lancet 1:689, 1977

Himes JH et al: Compressibility of skinfolds and the measurement of subcutaneous fatness. Am J Clin Nutr 32:1734, 1979

Long CL, Blakemore WS: Energy and protein requirements in the hospitalized patient. J Parent Ent Nutr 3:69, 1979

McMurray DN et al: Development of impaired cell-mediated immunity in mild and moderate malnutrition. Am J Clin Nutr 34:68, 1981

Merritt RJ, Suskind RM: Nutritional survey of hospitalized pediatric patients. Am J Clin Nutr 32:1320, 1979

Murray RL et al: Body composition in the critically ill patient: Emphasis on water balance. J Parent Ent Nutr 3:219, 1979

Newman CG: Interaction of malnutrition and infection—A neglected clinical concept. Arch Intern Med 137:1364, 1977

Parsons HG et al: The nutritional status of hospitalized children. Am J Clin Nutr 33:1140, 1980

Reed ML et al: Height and weight data in the patient's medical record. J Am Diet Assoc 72:409, 1978

Salmond SW: How to assess the nutritional status of acutely ill patients. Am J Nurs 80:922, 1980

Shapiro LR: Streamlining and implementing nutritional assessment: The dietary approach. J Am Diet Assoc 75:230, 1979

Tobias AL, Van Itallie TB: Nutritional problems of hospitalized patients. J Am Diet Assoc 71:253, 1977

Watson FE et al: Total body water volumes for adult males and females estimated from simple anthropometric measurements. Am J Clin Nutr 33:27, 1980

Young GA, Hill GL: Assessment of protein-calorie malnutrition in surgical patients from plasma proteins and anthropometric measurements. Am J Clin Nutr 31:429, 1978

## Food Composition—A Basic Tool of Diet Therapy

### Books and pamphlets

Arbogast KK: Exchange Lists and Diet Patterns. New York, Van Nostrand Reinhold, 1980

Convenience Foods Update for Calculated Diets. Park Ridge, IL, Lutheran General Hospital, 1980

Hansen RG, Wyse BW, Sorenson AW: Nutritional Quality Index of Foods. Westport, CT, Avi, 1979

Harris RS, Karmas E: Nutritional Evaluation of Food Processing, 2nd ed. Westport, CT, Avi, 1975

Nutritional Analyses of Foods Served at McDonald's Restaurants. McDonald Corporation, Oak Brook, IL 60521

Pennington JAT, Church HN: Bowes and Church's Food Values of Portions Commonly Used, 13th ed. Philadelphia, JB Lippincott, 1980

### Journal articles

Appledorf H, Kelly LS: Proximate and mineral content of fast foods. Pizzas, Mexican-American-style of foods and submarine sandwiches. J Am Diet Assoc 74:35, 1979

Lilyblade A et al: Composition of and cholesterol in Araucana and commercial eggs. J Am Diet Assoc 72:45, 1978

Rosenfield D: Nutritional optimization of new foods. J Am Diet Assoc 72:475, 1978

Scott LW et al: A low-cholesterol menu in a steak restaurant. J Am Diet Assoc 74:54, 1979

Shannon BM, Park SC: Fast foods: A prospective on their nutritional impact. J Am Diet Assoc 76:242, 1980

Slover HT et al: Lipids in fast foods. J Food Sci 45:1583, 1980

Underwood EJ: Trace element imbalances of interest to the dietitian. J Am Diet Assoc 72:177, 1978

Wyse BW, Hansen RG: Nutrient analysis of exchange lists for meal planning. II. Nutrient density food profiles. J Am Diet Assoc 75:242, 1979

## Handicapping Problems—Self-Feeding, Chewing, and Swallowing

### Books and pamphlets

Amary IB: Effective Meal Planning and Food Preparation for the Mentally Retarded/Developmentally Disabled. Springfield, IL, Charles C Thomas, 1979

Howard RB et al: The nervous system and handicapping conditions. In Howard RB, Herbold NH (eds): Nutrition in Clinical Care, pp 462–492. New York, McGraw-Hill, 1978

Palmer S, Ekvall S (eds): Pediatric Nutrition in Developmental Disorders. Springfield, IL, Charles C Thomas, 1978

Pipes PL: Nutrition in Infancy and Childhood, 2nd ed, pp 275–293. St Louis, CV Mosby, 1981

### Journal articles

Gasek G: Communicating with the communicatively impaired person. J Can Diet Assoc 40:106, 1979

Hyman LR et al: Immobilization hypercalcemia. Am J Dis Child 124:723, 1972

Katz WA et al: Salivary gland dysfunction in systemic lupus erythematosus and rheumatoid arthritis. Arch Intern Med 140:949, 1980

Overcoming barriers: Serving the handicapped patron. Food Service Marketing 40:82, Nov, 1978

Peskett EJ: Hospitals for the mentally ill and handicapped in Melbourne, Australia. J Hum Nutr 33:70, 1979

Schneider M: Los Angeles schools feed handicapped and teach self-feeding in developmental centers. Institutions/Volume Feeding 82:45, May 1, 1978

Springer NS: Ascorbic acid status of children with developmental disabilities. J Am Diet Assoc 75:425, 1979

Training that works: Patience and enlightened instruction transform handicapped into hires. Institutions 84:42, June 15, 1979

## Diet in Gastrointestinal Disease

### Books and pamphlets

Davenport HW: A Digest of Digestion, 2nd ed. Chicago, Yearbook, 1978

Davenport HW: Physiology of the Digestive Tract, 4th ed. Chicago, Yearbook, 1977

Sleisenger MH, Fordtran JS: Gastrointestinal Disease, 2 vols, 2nd ed. Philadelphia, WB Saunders, 1978

Spiro HM: Clinical Gastroenterology, 2nd ed. New York, Macmillan, 1977

Winick M: Nutrition and Gastroenterology. New York, John Wiley & Sons, 1980

## Physiology

### Journal articles

Dockray GJ: Molecular evolution of gut hormones: Application of comparative studies of the regulation of digestion. Gastroenterology 72:344, 1977

Clain J et al: Inhibitory role of the distal small intestine on the gastric inhibitory response to meals in man. Gastroenterology 74:704, 1978

Eastwood GL: Gastrointestinal epithelial renewal. Gastroenterology 72:962, 1977

Gershon MD, Erde SM: The nervous system of the gut. Gastroenterology 80:1571, 1981

Grotzinger U et al: Effect of fundic distention on gastric acid secretion in man. Gut 18:105, 1977

Johnson LR: The trophic action of gastrointestinal hormones. Gastroenterology 70:278, 1976

Malagelada JR et al: Measurement of gastric functions during digestion of ordinary solid meals in man. Gastroenterology 70:203, 1976

Miller LJ et al: Postprandial duodenal function in man. Gut 19:699, 1978

Moore JG, Motok D: Gastric secretory and humoral responses to anticipated feeding in five men. Gastroenterology 76:71, 1979

Pearse AGE et al: The newer gut hormones: Cellular sources, physiology, pathology, and clinical aspects. Gastroenterology 72:746, 1977

Rayford PL et al: Secretin, cholecystokinin and newer gastrointestinal hormones. N Engl J Med 294:1093, 1976

Richardson CT et al: Studies on the mechanisms of food-stimulated gastric acid secretion in normal human subjects. J Clin Invest 58:623, 1976

Richardson CT et al: Studies on the role of cephalic-vagal stimulation on the acid secretory response to eating in normal human subjects. J Clin Invest 60:435, 1977

Singh M, Webster PD III: Neurohormonal control of pancreatic secretion. Gastroenterology 74:294, 1978

Walker WA, Isselbacher KJ: Intestinal antibodies. N Engl J Med 297:767, 1977

Walsh JH, Grossman I: Gastrin. N Engl J Med 292:1324, 1975

Williamson REM: Intestinal adaptation: Structural, functional and cytokinetic change. N Engl J Med 298:1393, 1444, 1978

Wolf S: The psyche and the stomach: A historical vignette. Gastroenterology 80:605, 1981

## Peptic ulcer disease

Cargill JM et al: Very long-term treatment of peptic ulcer with cimetidine. Lancet 2:1113, 1978

Chang HK, Morrison SL: Bone marrow suppression associated with cimetidine. Ann Intern Med 91:580, 1979

Faber RG, Hobsley M: Basal gastric secretion: Reproducibility and relationship with duodenal ulceration. Gut 18:57, 1977

Fordtran JS: Placebo, antacid and cimetidine for duodenal ulcer. N Engl J Med 298:1080, 1978

Hastings PR et al: Antacid titration in the prevention of acute gastrointestinal bleeding. N Engl J Med 298:1041, 1978

Ippoliti AF et al: Cimetidine versus intensive antacid therapy for duodenal ulcer: A multicenter trial. Gastroenterology 74:393, 1978

Johnson AG: Peptic ulcer and the pylorus. Lancet 1:710, 1979

Korman MG et al: Relapse rate of duodenal ulcer after cessation of long-term cimetidine treatment: A double-blind controlled study. Dig Dis Sci 25:88, 1980

Priebe HJ et al: Antacid versus cimetidine in preventing acute gastrointestinal bleeding. N Engl J Med 302:426, 1980

Rotter JI et al: Duodenal-ulcer disease associated with elevated serum pepsinogen I: An inherited autosomal disorder. N Engl J Med 300:63, 1979

Shields HM: Rapid fall of serum phosphorus secondary to antacid therapy. Gastroenterology 75:1137, 1978

Tormey WR et al: Nocturnal ulcer pain associated with slow-wave sleep. Lancet 1:1340, 1978

Walsh JH: New look at peptic ulcer. Ann Intern Med 84:57, 1976

Woodings EP et al: Rantidine—A new $H_2$-receptor antagonist. Gut 21:187, 1980

## Other upper gastrointestinal problems

Behar J et al: Cimetidine in treatment of symptomatic gastroesophageal reflux. Gastroenterology 74:441, 1978

Hanson RE, Pries JM: Synthesis and enterohepatic circulation of bile salts. Gastroenterology 73:611, 1977

Kaye MD: On the relationship between gastric pH and pressure in the normal human lower oesophageal sphincter. Gut 20:59, 1979

Marshall JB, Settles RH: Zollinger-Ellison syndrome: A clinical update. Postgrad Med 68:38, July, 1980

McCallum RW, Walsh JH: Relationship between lower esophageal sphincter pressure and serum gastrin concentration in Zollinger-Ellison syndrome and other clinical settings. Gastroenterology 76:76, 1979

Regan PT et al: Comparative effects of antacids, cimetidine and enteric coating on the therapeutic response to oral enzymes in severe pancreatic insufficiency. N Engl J Med 297:854, 1977

Sedaghat A, Grundy SM: Cholesterol crystals and the formation of cholesterol gallstones. N Engl J Med 302:1274, 1980

Toskes PP et al: Non-diabetic retinal abnormalities in chronic pancreatitis. N Engl J Med 300:942, 1979

## Lactose malabsorption

Brown KH et al: Lactose malabsorption in Bangladeshi village children: Relation with age, history of recent diarrhea, nutritional status, and breast feeding. Am J Clin Nutr 32:1962, 1979

Brown KH et al: Nutritional consequences of low dose milk supplements consumed by lactose-malabsorbing children. Am J Clin Nutr 33:1054, 1980

Fernandes J et al: Respiratory hydrogen excretion as a parameter for lactose malabsorption in children. Am J Clin Nutr 31:597, 1978

Jones DV et al: Symptom response to lactose-reduced milk in lactose-intolerant adults. Am J Clin Nutr 29:633, 1976

Lacassie Y et al: Poor predictability of lactose-malabsorption from clinical symptoms for Chilian populations. Am J Clin Nutr 31:799, 1978

Paige DM et al: Lactose hydrolyzed milk. Am J Clin Nutr 28:818, 1975

Phillips AD et al: Microvillous surface area in secondary disaccharide deficiency. Gut 21:44, 1980

Solomons NW et al: Hydrogen breath test of lactose absorption in adults: The application of physiological doses and whole cow's milk sources. Am J Clin Nutr 33:545, 1980

Turner SJ et al: Utilization of a low-lactose milk. Am J Clin Nutr 29:739, 1976

## Celiac sprue

Katz AJ, Falchuk ZM: Current concepts in gluten sensitive enteropathy. Pediatr Clin North Am 22:767, 1975

Vuoristo M et al: Serum lipids and fecal steroids in patients with celiac disease: Effects of gluten-free diet and cholestyramine. Gastroenterology 78:1518, 1980

## Dietary fiber

Anderson NE, Clydesdale FM: Effects of processing on the dietary fiber content of wheat bran, pureed green beans, and carrots. J Food Sci 45:1533, 1980

Baker D, Holden JM: Fiber in breakfast cereals. J Food Technology 46:396, 1981

Cummings JH et al: Colonic response to dietary fibre from carrots, cabbage, apple, bran and guar gum. Lancet 1:5, 1978

Devroede G: Dietary fiber, bowel habits, and colonic function. Am J Clin Nutr (Suppl) 31:S157, 1978

Eastwood MA et al: Colonic function in patients with diverticular disease. Lancet 1:1181, 1978

Heaton KW et al: Treatment of Crohn's disease with an unrefined-carbohydrate, fiber-rich diet. Br Med J 2:764, 1979

Holloway WD et al: The humicellulose component of dietary fiber. Am J Clin Nutr 33:260, 1980

Holloway WD et al: Digestion of certain fractions of dietary fiber in humans. Am J Clin Nutr 31:923, 1978

Kelsay JL et al: Effect of fiber from fruits and vegetables on metabolic responses of human subjects. Am J Clin Nutr 31:1149, 1978

Leeds AR: Gastric emptying, fibre and absorption. Lancet 1:872, 1979

Williams GA: A study of the laxative action of wheat bran. Am J Physiol 83:1, 1927

# Nutrition Care—Surgery and Burn Therapy

## Books

Deitel M (ed): Nutrition in Clinical Surgery. Baltimore, Williams & Wilkins, 1980

## Journal articles
### Metabolic response to injury

Askanazi J et al: Muscle and plasma amino acids after injury: The role of inactivity. Ann Surg 188:797, 1978

Askari A et al: Urinary zinc, copper, nitrogen, and potassium losses in response to trauma. J Parent Ent Nutr 3:151, 1979

Blanchard J et al: Effect of protein depletion and repletion on liver structures, nitrogen content and serum proteins. Ann Surg 190:144, 1979

Cuthbertson DP: The metabolic response to injury and its nutritional implications: Retrospect and prospect. J Parent Ent Nutr 3:108, 1979

Daniel PM: The metabolic homeostatic role of muscle and its function as a store of protein. Lancet 2:446, 1977

Holbrook IB et al: Response of plasma amino acids to elective surgical trauma. J Parent Ent Nutr 3:424, 1979

Hoover-Plow JL et al: The effects of surgical trauma on plasma amino acid levels in humans. Surg Gynecol Obstet 150:161, 1980

Imamura M et al: Liver metabolism and gluconeogenesis in trauma and sepsis. Surgery 77:868, 1975

Irvin TT et al: Ascorbic acid requirement in postoperative patients. Surg Gynecol Obstet 147:49, 1978

Kinney JM et al: Tissue fuel and weight loss after injury. J Clin Pathol (Suppl 4) 23:65, 1978

Long CL et al: Contribution of skeletal muscle protein in elevated rates of whole body protein catabolism in trauma patients. Am J Clin Nutr 34:1087, 1981

Powanda MC: Changes in body balances of nitrogen and other key nutrients: Description and underlying mechanisms. Am J Clin Nutr 30:1254, 1977

Tweedle DE: Metabolism of amino acids after trauma. J Parent Ent Nutr 4:165, 1980

Udupa KN: The neurohormonal response to trauma. Am J Surg 135:403, 1978

### Infection and sepsis

Beisel WR: Magnitude of the host nutritional response to infection. Am J Clin Nutr 30:1236, 1977

Beisel WR, Wannemacher RW Jr: Gluconeogenesis, ureagenesis, and ketogenesis during sepsis. J Parent Ent Nutr 4:277, 1980

Bistrian BR: Interaction of nutrition and infection in the hospital setting. Am J Clin Nutr 30:1228, 1977

Christou NV et al: The predictive role of delayed hypersensitivity in preoperative patients. Surg Gynecol Obstet 152:297, 1981

Christou NV, Meakins JL: Delayed hypersensitivity, a mechanism for energy in surgical patients. Surgery 86:78, 1979

Clowes GHA et al: Amino acid and energy metabolism in septic and traumatized patients. J Parent Ent Nutr 4:195, 1980

Clowes GHA et al: Blood insulin responses to blood glucose levels in high output sepsis and septic shock. Am J Surg 135:577, 1978

Daly JM et al: Effect of protein depletion and repletion on cell-mediated immunity in experimental animals. Ann Surg 188:791, 1978

Dionigi R et al: Nutrition and infection. J Parent Ent Nutr 3:62, 1979

Freund HR et al: Amino acid derangements in patients with sepsis: Treatment with branched chain amino acid rich infusions. Ann Surg 188:423, 1978

Long CL: Energy balance and carbohydrate metabolism in infection and sepsis. Am J Clin Nutr 30:1301, 1977

Long CL: Whole body protein synthesis and catabolism in septic man. Am J Clin Nutr 30:1341, 1977

Meakins JL et al: Indicator of acquired failure of host defense in sepsis and trauma. Ann Surg 186:241, 1977

Mullen JL et al: Implications of malnutrition in the surgical patient. Arch Surg 114:121, 1979

Rhoads JE: The impact of nutrition on infection. Surg Clin North Am 60:41, 1980

Wannemacher RW Jr: Key role of various individual amino acids in host response to infection. Am J Clin Nutr 30:1269, 1977

### Total parenteral nutrition

Barr LH et al: Essential fatty acid deficiency during total parenteral nutrition. Ann Surg 193:304, 1981

Borgen L: Total parenteral nutrition in adults. Am J Nurs 78:224, 1978

Collins JP et al: Intravenous amino acids and intravenous hyperalimentation as protein-sparing therapy after major surgery: A controlled clinical trial. Lancet 1:788, 1978

Hauer EC, Kaminski MV Jr: Trace metal profile of parenteral nutrition solutions. Am J Clin Nutr 31:264, 1978

Herlihy P et al: Total parenteral nutrition. J Am Diet Assoc 70:279, 1977

Hickey MM et al: Parenteral nutrition utilization: Evaluation of an educational protocol and consult service. J Parent Ent Nutr 3:433, 1979

Hill GL et al: Changes in body weight and body protein with intravenous nutrition. J Parent Ent Nutr 3:215, 1979

Hoover HC Jr et al: Nutritional benefits of immediate postoperative jejunal feeding of an elemental diet. Am J Surg 139:153, 1980

Howard L et al: A comparison of administering protein alone and protein plus glucose on nitrogen balance. Am J Clin Nutr 31:226, 1978

Irvin TT: Effects of malnutrition and hyperalimentation on wound healing. Surg Gynecol Obstet 146:33, 1978

Isaacs JW et al: Parenteral nutrition of adults with a 900 milliosmolar solution via peripheral veins. Am J Clin Nutr 30:552, 1977

Jurgens P: Parenteral nutrition studies with four L-amino acid solutions in metabolically normal adults. J Parent Ent Nutr 3:374, 1979

Kim CW et al: Urinary excretion of amino acids in patients receiving intravenous hyperalimentation. Clin Chim Acta 83:151, 1978

Koffler DP, Levine GM: Reversible gastric and pancreatic hyposecretion after long-term total parenteral nutrition. N Engl J Med 300:241, 1979

Levine GM et al: Effect of total parenteral nutrition on gastric acid secretion. Dig Dis Sci 25:284, 1980

Long MG III et al: Effect of carbohydrate and fat intake on nitrogen excretion during total intravenous feeding. Ann Surg 185:417, 1977

Lowry SF et al: Parenteral vitamin requirements during intravenous feedings. Am J Clin Nutr 31:2149, 1978

Mascioli EA et al: Effect of total parenteral nutrition with cycling on essential fatty acid deficiency. J Parent Ent Nutr 3:171, 1979

Nube M et al: Simultaneous and consecutive administration of nutrients in parenteral nutrition. Am J Clin Nutr 32:1505, 1979

Paradis C et al: Total parenteral nutrition with lipids. Am J Surg 135:164, 1978

Powell-Tuck J et al: Team approach to long-term intravenous feeding in patients with gastrointestinal disorders. Lancet 2:825, 1978

Silberman J: Hyperalimentation in patients with cancer. Surg Gynecol Obstet 150:755, 1980

Sims AJW et al: Glucose promotes whole-body protein synthesis from infused amino acids in fasting man. Lancet 1:68, 1979

Wells FE, Smits BJ: Plasma amino acid relationships during parenteral nutrition. J Parent Ent Nutr 4:268, 1980

Wolman SL et al: Zinc in total parenteral nutrition: Requirements and metabolic effects. Gastroenterology 76:458, 1979

Young GA et al: Plasma proteins in patients receiving intravenous amino acids or intravenous hyperalimentation after major surgery. Am J Clin Nutr 32:1192, 1979

## Home parenteral nutrition

Bryne WJ et al: Home parenteral nutrition: An alternative approach to the management of complicated gastrointestinal fistulas not responding to conventional medical or surgical therapy. J Parent Ent Nutr 3:355, 1979

Dudrick SJ et al: New concept of ambulatory home hyperalimentation. J Parent Ent Nutr 3:72, 1979

Jonsea AR: Ethical problems in home total parenteral nutrition. J Parent Ent Nutr 3:169, 1979

Perl M et al: Psychological aspects of long-term home hyperalimentation. J Parent Ent Nutr 4:554, 1980

Rault RMJ, Scribner BH: Treatment of Crohn's disease with home parenteral nutrition. Gastroenterology 72:1249, 1977

Scribner BH, Cole JJ: Evaluation of the technique of home parenteral nutrition. J Parent Ent Nutr 3:58, 1979

## Enteral nutrition

Bayless E: Taste tray increases acceptance of nutritional supplements. J Am Diet Assoc 73:543, 1978

Bondy RA et al: Comparison of two commercial low residue diets and a low residue diet of common foods. J Parent Ent Nutr 3:226, 1979

Cha C-JM, Randall HT: Osmolality of liquid and defined formula diets: The effect of hydrolysis by pancreatic enzymes. J Parent Ent Nutr 5:7, 1981

Chernoff R, Bloch AS: Liquid feedings: Considerations and alterations. J Am Diet Assoc 70:389, 1977

Cortot A et al: Gastric emptying of lipids after ingestion of a solid-liquid meal in humans. Gastroenterology 80:922, 1981

Fairclough PD et al: Comparison of the absorption of two protein hydrolysates and their effects on water and electrolyte movements in the human jejunum. Gut 21:829, 1980

Fairclough PD et al: Major differences in intestinal assimilation of two protein hydrolysates: Potential importance for formulation of elemental diets. Gastroenterology 76:1129, 1979

Fairfull-Smith RJ et al: Superiority of nonelemental diets for enteral nutrition in surgical patients. J Parent Ent Nutr 3:297, 1979

Hanson RL: Predictive criteria for length of nasogastric tube insertion for tube feeding. J Parent Ent Nutr 3:160, 1979

Heymsfield SB et al: Enteral hyperalimentation: Alternative to central venous hyperalimentation. Ann Intern Med 90:63, 1979

Huxley EJ et al: Pharyngeal aspiration in normal adults and patients with depressed consciousness. Am J Med 64:564, 1978

Jones BJM et al: Pump assisted enteral feeding system. J Parent Ent Nutr 3:297, 1979

Koretz RL, Meyer JH: Elemental diets—facts and fallacies. Gastroenterology 78:393, 1980

Metz G et al: Simple technique for naso-enteric feeding. Lancet 2:454, 1978

Page CP et al: Safe, cost-effective postoperative nutrition: Defined formula diet via needle-catheter jejunostomy. Am J Surg 138:939, 1979

Silk DBA et al: Use of a peptide rather than free amino acid nitrogen source in chemically defined "elemental" diets. J Parent Ent Nutr 4:548, 1980

Young CK et al: Effect of an elemental diet on body composition: A comparison with intravenous nutrition. Gastroenterology 77:652, 1979

## Gastrointestinal surgery

Block GE: Surgical management of Crohn's colitis. N Engl J Med 302:1068, 1980

Calam J et al: Elemental diets in the management of Crohn's perianal fistulae. J Parent Ent Nutr 4:4, 1980

Cortot A et al: Improved nutrient absorption after cimetidine in short-bowel syndrome with gastric hypersecretion. N Engl J Med 300:79, 1979

Greenberg GR, Jeejeebhoy KN: Intravenous protein-sparing therapy in patients with gastrointestinal disease. J Parent Ent Nutr 3:427, 1979

Hickman DM et al: Serum albumin and body weight as predictors of postoperative course in colorectal cancer. J Parent Ent Nutr 4:314, 1980

MacGregor IM et al: Gastric emptying of solid food in normal man and after subtotal gastrectomy and truncal vagotomy with pyloroplasty. Gastroenterology 72:206, 1977

Murphy JP Jr et al: Treatment of gastric hypersecretion with cimetidine in the short-bowel syndrome. N Engl J Med 300:80, 1979

Schrock TR, Way LW: Total gastrectomy. Am J Surg 135:348, 1978

Schrumpp E et al: Mucosal changes in the gastric stump 20–25 years after partial gastrectomy. Lancet 2:467, 1977

Welch CE, Malt RA: Abdominal surgery. N Engl J Med 300:648, 705, 765, 1979

## Burns

Curreri W, Luterman A: Nutritional support of the burned patient. Surg Clin North Am 58:1151, 1978

Long JC: Energy expenditure of major burns. J Trauma (Suppl) 19:904, 1979

Pennisi VM: Monitoring the nutritional care of burned patients. J Am Diet Assoc 69:531, 1976

Sheldon GF et al: Metabolism, oxygen transport, and erythropoietin synthesis in the anemia of thermal injury. Am J Surg 135:406, 1978

Wilmore DW et al: Catecholamines: Mediator of the hypermetabolic response to thermal injury. Ann Surg 180:653, 1974

Wilmore DW, Aulick LH: Systemic responses to injury and the healing wound. J Parent Ent Nutr 4:147, 1980

Wilmore DW, Aulick LH: Metabolic changes in burned patients. Surg Clin North Am 58:1173, 1978

## Other surgical problems

DeVaul RA, Fallace LA: Persistent pain and illness insistence: A medical profile of proneness to surgery. Am J Surg 135:828, 1978

Rose EA, King TC: Understanding postoperative fatigue. Surg Gynecol Obstet 147:97, 1978

Sherlock S: Halothane hepatitis. Lancet 2:364, 1978

Strauss RJ, Wise L: Operative risks of obesity. Surg Gynecol Obstet 146:286, 1978

Thompson JE, Garrett WV: Peripheral-arterial surgery. N Engl J Med 302:491, 1980

Woods JH et al: Postoperative ileus: A colonic problem? Surgery 84:527, 1978

# Weight Control

## Books

Bray GA (ed): Obesity in America. DHEW NIH Publ. No. 80-359. Washington, DC, U.S. Government Printing Office, 1980

Dally P et al: Anorexia Nervosa. Chicago, Year Book Medical Publishers, 1979

Pariskova J, Rogozkin VA (eds): Nutrition, Physical Fitness, and Health, Vol 7, International Series on Sport Sciences. Baltimore, University Park Press, 1978

Powers PS: Obesity. The Regulation of Weight. Baltimore, Williams & Wilkins, 1980

Stunkard AJ: Obesity. Philadelphia, WB Saunders, 1980

## Journal articles
## Obesity

Bray GA et al: Hepatic sodium-potassium-dependent ATPase in obesity. N Engl J Med 304:1580, 1981

Fuchs RJ et al: A nomogram to predict lean body mass in men. Am J Clin Nutr 31:673, 1978

Harrison LC et al: Correlation between insulin receptor binding of isolated fat cells and insulin sensitivity in obese human subjects. J Clin Invest 58:1435, 1976

Inglett GE: Sweeteners—a review. Food Technol 35:37, 1981

Joffe SN: Surgical management of morbid obesity. Gut 22:242, 1981

Kissileff HR et al: C-terminal octapeptide of cholecystokinin decreases food intake in man. Am J Clin Nutr 34:154, 1981

Knittle JL et al: Adipose tissue development in man. Am J Clin Nutr 30:762, 1977

Nasrallah SM et al: Hepatic morphology in obesity. Dig Dis Sci 26:325, 1981

Newsholme EA: Sounding Board: A possible metabolic basis for the control of body weight. N Engl J Med 302:400, 1980

Pollet RJ, Levey GS: Principles of membrane receptor physiology and their application in clinical medicine. Ann Intern Med 92:663, 1980

Rodin J: Pathogenesis of obesity: Energy intake and expenditure. In Bray GA (ed): Obesity in America. DHEW NIH Publ. No. 80-359. Washington, DC, U.S. Government Printing Office, 1980

Rotter JI, Rimoin DL: The genetics of the glucose intolerance disorders. Am J Med 70:116, 1981

Schumaker JF, Wagner MK: External-cue responsivity as a function of age at onset of obesity. J Am Diet Assoc 70:275, 1977

Swartz RS, Brunzell JD: Increased adipose-tissue lipoprotein-lipase activity in moderately obese men after weight reduction. Lancet 1:1230, 1978

Symposium: Control of endogenous triglyceride metabolism in adipose tissue and muscle. Fed Proc 36:1984, 1977

Van Itallie TB, Hirsch J: Appraisal of excess calories as a factor in the causation of disease. Am J Clin Nutr (Suppl) 32:2648, 1979

Wade J et al: Evidence for a physiological regulation of food selection and nutrient intake in twins. Am J Clin Nutr 34:143, 1981

Warnold I et al: Energy expenditure and body composition during weight reduction in hyperplastic obese women. Am J Clin Nutr 31:750, 1978

Young RL et al: Glucose-insulin response to oral glucose in a healthy obese population. Diabetes 28:208, 1979

## Protein-sparing modified fast

Brown JM et al: Cardiac complications of protein sparing modified fasting. JAMA 240:120, 1978

Michiel RR et al: Sudden death in a patient on a liquid protein diet. N Engl J Med 298:1005, 1978

Singh BN et al: Liquid protein diets and "torsade de pointes." JAMA 240:115, 1978

Young SP et al: Weight reduction utilizing a protein-sparing modified fast. J Am Diet Assoc 76:343, 1980

## Surgery in morbid obesity

Compton JE et al: Osteomalacia after small bowel resection. Lancet 1:9, 1978

Condon SC et al: Role of caloric intake in the weight loss after jejunoileal bypass for obesity. Gastroenterology 74:34, 1978

Drenick EJ et al: Renal damage with intestinal bypass. Ann Intern Med 89:594, 1978

Ellison EC et al: Prevention of early failure of stapled gastric portions in treatment of morbid obesity. Arch Surg 115:528, 1980

Fogel MR et al: Absorptive and digestive function of the jejunum after jejunoileal bypass for treatment of human obesity. Gastroenterology 71:729, 1976

Frances WW, Iannucilli E: Acute fulminating transmural ileocolitis after small bowel bypass for morbid obesity. Am J Surg 135:524, 1978

Hirschman GH, Burton BT (eds): Symposium on surgical treatment of morbid obesity. Am J Clin Nutr (Suppl) 33:353, 1980

Kessler JI et al: Alterations of hepatic triglycerides in patients before and after jejunoileal bypass for morbid obesity. Gastroenterology 76:159, 1979

Kral JG, Bondjers G: Increased arterial-tissue cholesterol after intestinal bypass in severe obesity. Lancet 2:288, 1978

Mason EE et al: Risk reduction in gastric operations for obesity. Ann Surg 190:158, 1979

Parfitt AM et al: Metabolic bone disease after intestinal bypass for treatment of obesity. Ann Intern Med 89:193, 1978

Phillips RB: Small intestinal bypass for the treatment of morbid obesity. Surg Gynecol Obstet 146:455, 1978

Rogers S et al: Jaw wiring in treatment of obesity. Lancet 1:1221, 1977

### Anorexia nervosa

Boyar MR et al: Cortisol secretion and metabolism in anorexia nervosa. N Engl J Med 296:190, 1977

Stordy BJV et al: Weight gain, thermic effect of glucose and resting metabolic rate during recovery from anorexia nervosa. Am J Clin Nutr 30:138, 1977

Vigersky RA et al: Hypothalamic dysfunction in secondary amenorrhea associated with simple weight loss. N Engl J Med 297:1141, 1977

## Diabetes Mellitus

### Books and pamphlets

American Diabetes Association and American Dietetic Association: Exchange Lists for Meal Planning. Chicago, The American Dietetic Association, 1976

American Diabetes Association and American Dietetic Association: A Guide for Professionals: The Effective Application of "Exchange Lists for Meal Planning." Chicago, The American Dietetic Association, 1977

Arbogast KK: Exchange Lists and Diet Patterns. New York, John Wiley & Sons, 1980

Educational Material for and about Young People with Diabetes. DHEW NIH Publ. No. 80-1871. Washington, DC, U.S. Government Printing Office, 1979

Katzen HM, Mahler EJ (eds): Diabetes, Obesity and Vascular Disease: Metabolic and Molecular Interrelationships, Parts 1 and 2. New York, John Wiley & Sons, 1978

Krall LP (ed): Joslin Diabetes Manual, 11th ed. Philadelphia, Lea & Febiger, 1978

West KM: Epidemiology of Diabetes and Its Vascular Lesions. New York, Elsevier, 1978

Williams RH, Porte D Jr: The pancreas. In Textbook of Endocrinology, 5th ed, pp 509–629. Philadelphia, WB Saunders, 1974

### Journal articles
### Diabetes

Bales GS, Entmacher PS: Estimated life expectancy of diabetics. Diabetes 26:434, 1977

Beeken RK: Initiating exercise programs for patients with non-insulin-dependent diabetes. Diabetes Care 5:627, 1980

Bennion LJ, Grundy SM: Effects of diabetes mellitus on cholesterol metabolism in man. N Engl J Med 296:1365, 1977

Bunn HF et al: The glycosylation of hemoglobin: Relevance to diabetes mellitus. Science 200:21, 1978

Cahill GF Jr et al: Blood glucose control in diabetes. Diabetes 25:237, 1976

Cerkoney KAB, Hart LK: The relationship between health care belief model and compliance of persons with diabetes mellitus. Diabetes Care 3:594, 1980

Clarke WL et al: Overnight basal insulin requirements in fasting insulin-dependent diabetes. Diabetes 29:78, 1980

Cudworth AG, Woodrow JD: HL-A system and diabetes mellitus. Diabetes 24:345, 1975

Czech MR: Insulin action and the regulation of hexose transport. Diabetes 29:399, 1980

Ditzel J: Changes in red cell oxygen release capacity in diabetes mellitus. Fed Proc 38:2484, 1979

Flier JS et al: Receptors, antireceptor antibodies and mechanisms of insulin resistance. N Engl J Med 300:413, 1979

Fulop M, Hoberman HD: Phenformin-associated metabolic acidosis. Diabetes 25:292, 1976

Gabbay KH et al: Glycosylated hemoglobins and long-term blood glucose control in diabetes mellitus. J Clin Endocrinol Metab 44:859, 1977

Gale EAM, Tattersall RB: Unrecognized nocturnal hypoglycemia in insulin-treated diabetics. Lancet 1:1049, 1979

Galloway JA, Bressler R: Insulin treatment in diabetes. Med Clin North Am 62:663, 1978

Ganda OP, Soeldner SJ: Genetic, acquired and related factors in the etiology of diabetes mellitus. Arch Intern Med 137:461, 1977

Gelfand RA et al: Dietary carbohydrate and metabolism of ingested protein. Lancet 1:65, 1979

Given BD et al: Diabetes due to secretion of an abnormal insulin. N Engl J Med 302:129, 1980

Hagenfeldt L: Metabolism of free fatty acids and ketone bodies during exercise in normal and diabetic man. Diabetes (Suppl) 28:66, 1979

Henderson JR et al: The pancreas as a single organ: The influence of the endocrine upon the exocrine part of the gland. Gut 22:158, 1981

Ingelfinger FJ: Editorial: Debate on diabetes. N Engl J Med 296:1228, 1977

Livingston JN et al: Insulin induced changes in insulin binding and insulin sensitivity of adipocytes. Metabolism (Suppl 2) 27:2009, 1978

Micossi P et al: Aspirin stimulates insulin and glucagon secretion and increases glucose tolerance in normal and diabetic subjects. Diabetes 27:1196, 1978

Olefsky JM: The insulin receptor: Its role in insulin resistance of obesity and diabetes. Diabetes 25:1154, 1976

Pfeifer MA et al: Insulin secretion in diabetes mellitus. Am J Med 70:579, 1981

Richter EA et al: Diabetes and exercise. Am J Med 70:201, 1981

Rizza RA et al: Control of blood sugar in insulin-dependent diabetes: Comparison of an artificial endocrine pancreas, continuous subcutaneous infusion and intensified conventional insulin therapy. N Engl J Med 303:1313, 1980

Robertson RP, Metz SA: Sounding Board: Prostaglandins, the glucoreceptors, and diabetes. N Engl J Med 301:1446, 1979

Rotter JI, Rimoin DL: The genetics of glucose intolerance disorders. Am J Med 70:116, 1981

Skyler JS et al: Home glucose monitoring as an aid in diabetes management. Diabetes Care 1:150, 1978

Soman VR et al: Increased insulin sensitivity and insulin binding to monocytes after physical training. N Engl J Med 301:1200, 1979

Streja D et al: Nutrition therapy in non-insulin-dependent diabetes mellitus. Diabetic Care 4:81, 1981

Tambourlane WV et al: Insulin-infusion-pump treatment of diabetes: Influence of improved metabolic control on plasma somatomedin levels. N Engl J Med 305:303, 1981

Tambourlane WV et al: Restoration of normal lipid and amino acid metabolism in diabetic patients treated with a portable insulin-infusion pump. Lancet 1:1258, 1979

Vranic M et al (eds): Proceedings of a conference on diabetes and exercise. Diabetes (Suppl 1) 28:1, 1979

Wolfe RR et al: Glucose metabolism in man: Responses to intravenous glucose infusion. Metabolism 28:210, 1979

Yoon J-W et al: Virus-induced diabetes mellitus: Isolation of a virus from the pancreas of a child with diabetic ketoacidosis. N Engl J Med 300:1173, 1979

### Fiber in the diabetic diet

Anderson IH et al: Incomplete absorption of the carbohydrate in all-purpose wheat flour. N Engl J Med 304:891, 1981

Anderson JW: Effect of carbohydrate restriction and high carbohydrate diets on men with chemical diabetes. Am J Clin Nutr 30:402, 1977

Bolton RP et al: The role of dietary fiber in satiety, glucose and insulin: Studies with fruit and fruit juice. Am J Clin Nutr 34:211, 1981

Crapo PA et al: Post-prandial plasma glucose and insulin responses to different complex carbohydrates. Diabetes 26:1178, 1977

Haber GB et al: Depletion and disruption of dietary fibre. Lancet 2:1213, 1975

Miranda PM, Horwitz DL: High-fiber diets in the treatment of diabetes mellitus. Ann Intern Med 88:482, 1978

Munoz JM et al: Effects of some cereal brans on glucose tolerance and plasma lipids in men. Fed Proc 37:755, 1978

Reaven GM et al: Nutritional management of diabetes. Med Clin North Am 63:927, 1979

Simpson HCR et al: A high carbohydrate leguminous fibre diet improves all aspects of diabetic control. Lancet 1:1, 1981

### Diabetes in young patients

Farquhar JW: Juvenile diabetes mellitus. Arch Dis Child 54:569, 1979

Malone JI et al: Good diabetic control—A study in mass delusion. J Pediatr 88:943, 1976

Mann JI et al: Serum lipids in treated diabetic children and their families. Clin Endocrinol 8:27, 1978

White NH et al: Reversal of neuropathic and gastrointestinal complications related to diabetes mellitus in adolescents with improved metabolic control. J Pediatr 99:41, 1981

### Complications of diabetes

Bunn HF: Nonenzymatic glycosylation of protein: Relevance to diabetes. Am J Med 70:325, 1981

Clements RB Jr: Diabetic neuropathy—New concepts of its etiology. Diabetes 28:604, 1979

Cooppan R, Kozak GP: Hyperthyroidism and diabetes mellitus. Arch Intern Med 140:370, 1980

Eschwerge E et al: Delayed progression of diabetic retinopathy by divided insulin administration: A further follow-up. Diabetologia 16:13, 1979

Ewing JD et al: Heart rate changes in diabetes mellitus. Lancet 1:183, 1981

Graf RJ et al: Glycemic control and nerve conduction abnormalities in non-insulin dependent diabetic subjects. Ann Intern Med 94:307, 1981

Job D, Eschwerge E: Effect of multiple daily insulin injections on the course of diabetic retinopathy. Diabetes 25:463, 1976

Jovanovic L, Peterson CM: The clinical utility of glycosylated hemoglobin. Am J Med 70:331, 1981

Knowles WC et al: Increased incidence of retinopathy in diabetics with elevated blood pressure: A six year follow-up study in Pima Indians. N Engl J Med 302:645, 1980

McDonald J: Alcohol and diabetes. Diabetes Care 5:629, 1980

Rosenbloom AL et al: Limited joint mobility in childhood diabetes mellitus indicates increased risk for microvascular disease. N Engl J Med 305:191, 1981

Scarpello JHD, Sladen GE: Diabetes and the gut. Gut 19:1153, 1978

Tchobroutsky G: Relation of diabetic control to development of microvascular complications. Diabetologia 15:143, 1978

Wautier J-L et al: Increased adhesion of erythrocytes to endothelial cells in diabetes mellitus and its relationship to vascular complications. N Engl J Med 305:327, 1981

### Pregnancy in diabetes

Green JW: Diabetes mellitus in pregnancy. Obstet Gynecol 46:6, 1975

Plides RS: Infants of diabetic mothers. N Engl J Med 289:902, 1973

Soler NG, Malins JM: Diabetic pregnancy: Management of diabetes on the day of delivery. Diabetologia 15:411, 1978

## Atherosclerosis
### Books and pamphlets

A Maximal Approach to the Dietary Treatment of the Hyperlipidemias. Physician's Handbook. New York, American Heart Association, 1973

Dawber TR: The Framingham Study: The Epidemiology of Atherosclerotic Disease. Cambridge: Harvard University Press, 1980

Dietary Management of Hyperlipoproteinemia, A Handbook for Physicians and Dietitians, rev ed. Bethesda, MD, NIH, National Heart and Lung Institute, 1973

Feldman EB: Nutrition and Cardiovascular Disease. New York, Appleton-Century-Crofts, 1976

Levy RI, Rifkind BM, Dennis BA, Ernst ND (eds): Nutrition in Health and Disease, Vol 1, Nutrition, Lipids and Coronary Heart Disease. A Global View. New York, Raven Press, 1979

National Center for Health Statistics: Chartboard for the Conference on Decline in Coronary Heart Disease Mortality. Hyattsville, MD, DHEW, Public Health Service, National

Center for Health Statistics, Division of Vital Statistics, Aug, 1978

Rifkind BM, Levy RI (eds): Hyperlipidemia, Diagnosis, and Therapy. New York, Grune & Stratton, 1977

## Journal articles

American Heart Association: Coronary heart disease in seven countries. Circulation (Suppl I) Vols XLI and XLII, Apr, 1970

Barndt R et al: Regression and progression of early femoral atherosclerosis in treated hyperlipoproteinemic patients. Ann Intern Med 86:139, 1977

Bortz WM: The pathogenesis of hypercholesterolemia. Ann Intern Med 80:738, 1974

Cohen L, Morgan J: A rationale for the management of hyperlipoproteinemias in the prevention and treatment of coronary artery disease. J.C.E. Cardiol. 14, No. 6:11, 1979

Dawber TR et al: Coffee and cardiovascular disease: Observations from the Framingham Study. N Engl J Med 291:871, 1974

Dustan HP: Atherosclerosis complicating chronic hypertension. Circulation 50:871, 1974

Farmer RG et al: Hyperlipoproteinemia and pancreatitis. Am J Med 54:161, 1973

Glueck CJ: Dietary fat and atherosclerosis. Am J Clin Nutr 32:2703, 1979

Grundy SM: Effect of polyunsaturated fats on lipid metabolism in patients with hypertriglyceridemia. J Clin Invest 55:269, 1975

Hjermann I et al: The effect of dietary changes on high density lipoprotein cholesterol: The Oslo Study. Am J Med 66:105, 1979

Hjermann I: Smoking and diet intervention in healthy coronary high risk men. Methods and 5-year follow up of risk factors in a randomized trial: The Oslo Study. J Oslo City Hosp 30:3, 1980

Hulley SB et al: Epidemiology as a guide to clinical decisions. The association between triglyceride and coronary heart disease. N Engl J Med 302:1383, 1980

Inter-Society Commission for Heart Disease Resources, Atherosclerosis Study Group and Epidemiology Study Group: Primary prevention of the atherosclerotic diseases. Circulation 42:A55, 1970

Jenkins DJA et al: Effect of pectin, guar gum, and wheat fibre on serum-cholesterol. Lancet 1:1116, 1975

Kannel WB et al: Cholesterol in the prediction of atherosclerotic disease. Ann Intern Med 90:85, 1979

Lauer RM et al: Coronary heart disease risk factors in school children: The Muscatine Study. J Pediatr 86:697, 1975

Levy RI et al: Drug therapy: Treatment of hyperlipidemia. N Engl J Med 290:1295, 1974

Livingston GE: The prudent diet: What? Why? How? Food Tech 28:16, 1974

McGill HC: The relationship of dietary cholesterol to serum cholesterol concentration and to atherosclerosis in man. Am J Clin Nutr 32:2664, 1979

National Diet–Heart Research Group: National Diet–Heart Study final report. Circulation (Suppl 1) 37:1–419, 1968

Olefsky J et al: Effects of weight reduction on obesity: Studies of lipid and carbohydrate metabolism in normal and hyperlipoproteinemic subjects. J Clin Invest 53:64, 1974

Olendzki MC et al: Evaluating nutrition intervention in atherosclerosis: Some theoretical and practical considerations. J Am Diet Assoc 79:9, 1981

Perry HM Jr: Minerals in cardiovascular disease. J Am Diet Assoc 62:631, 1973

Phillips RL et al: Coronary heart disease mortality among Seventh Day Adventists with differing dietary habits: A preliminary report. Am J Clin Nutr 31:191, 1978

Stone NJ et al: Coronary artery disease in 116 kindred with familial type II hyperlipoproteinemia. Circulation 49:476, 1974

Sturdevant RAL et al: Increased prevalence of cholelithiasis in men ingesting a serum-cholesterol-lowering diet. N Engl J Med 288:24, 1973

Wilmore JH, McNamara JJ: Prevalence of coronary heart disease risk factors in boys 8 to 12 years of age. J Pediatr 84:527, 1974

Wynder EL, Hill P: Blood lipids: How normal is normal? Prev Med 1:161, 1972

# Cardiovascular Disease
## Books and pamphlets

Braunwald E (ed): Heart Disease: A Textbook of Cardiovascular Medicine. Philadelphia, WB Saunders, 1980

Braunwald E: Edema. In Isselbacher KJ et al (eds): Harrison's Principles of Internal Medicine, 9th ed., pp 171–175. New York, McGraw-Hill, 1980

Braunwald E: Heart failure. In Isselbacher KJ et al (eds): Harrison's Principles of Internal Medicine, 9th ed., pp 1035–1044. New York, McGraw-Hill, 1980

Williams GH: Hypertensive vascular disease. In Isselbacher KJ et al (eds): Harrison's Principles of Medicine, 9th ed., pp 1167–1178. New York, McGraw-Hill, 1980

## Journal articles

Amery A et al: Glucose intolerance during diuretic therapy: Results of trial by the European working party on hypertension in the elderly. Lancet 1:681, 1978

Calabrese EJ, Tuthill RW: A review of literature to support a sodium drinking water standard. J Environ Health 40:80, 1977

Canessa M et al: Increased sodium–lithium countertransport in red cells of patients with essential hypertension. N Engl J Med 302:772, 1980

DeFronzo RA, Thier SO: Pathophysiologic approach to hyponatremia. Arch Intern Med 140:879, 1980

Feig PU, McCurdy DK: The hypertonic state. N Engl J Med 297:1444, 1977

Freis ED: Salt, volume and the prevention of hypertension. Circulation 53:589, 1976

Garay RP et al: Laboratory distinction between essential and secondary hypertension by measurement of erythrocyte cation fluxes. N Engl J Med 302:769, 1980

Grimm RH et al: Effects of thiazide diuretics on plasma lipids and lipoproteins in mildly hypertensive patients. Ann Intern Med 94:7, 1981

Heller RF et al: Value of blood-pressure measurements in relatives of hypertensive patients. Lancet 1:1206, 1980

Morgan T et al: Hypertension treated by salt restriction. Lancet 1:227, 1978

Mueller HS, Ayres SM: Metabolic responses of the heart in acute myocardial infarction in man. Am J Cardiol 42:363, 1978

Mundth ED, Austin WC: Surgical measures for coronary heart disease. N Engl J Med 293:13, 1975

Newborg B: Sodium-restricted diets: Sodium content of wines and other alcoholic beverages. Arch Intern Med 123:692, 1969

Olesen KH, Faergeman O: Metabolic response to acute myocardial infarction. J Parent Ent Nutr 4:157, 1980

Parfrey PS et al: Blood pressure and hormonal changes following alteration in dietary sodium and potassium in mild hypertension. Lancet 1:59, 1981

Parfrey PS et al: Blood pressure and hormonal changes following alteration in dietary sodium and potassium in young men with and without a familial predisposition to hypertension. Lancet 1:113, 1981

Peart WS: Renin-angiotensin system. N Engl J Med 292:302, 1975

Pietinen PI et al: Electrolyte output, blood pressure, and family history of hypertension. Am J Clin Nutr 32:997, 1979

Reisin E et al: Effect of weight loss without salt restriction on the reduction of blood pressure in overweight hypertensive patients. N Engl J Med 298:1, 1978

Relman AS: Editorial: Mild hypertension: No more benign neglect. N Engl J Med 302:293, 1980

Shorecki KL, Brenner BM: Body fluid homeostasis in man: An overview. Am J Med 70:77, 1981

Sweadner KJ, Goldwin SM: Active transport of sodium and potassium ions. N Engl J Med 302:777, 1980

Tuck ML et al: The effect of weight reduction on blood pressure, plasma renin activity, and plasma aldosterone levels in obese patients. N Engl J Med 304:930, 1981

Warren SE et al: Diet in the coronary care unit. Am Heart J 95:130, 1978

Williams RS et al: Physical conditioning augments the fibrinolytic response to venous occlusion in healthy adults. N Engl J Med 302:987, 1980

# Renal Disease—Nephrolithiasis

## Books and pamphlets

Coe FL (ed): Nephrolithiasis. New York, Churchill Livingstone, 1980

Kopple JD: Nutrition and the kidney. In Hodges RE (ed): Human Nutrition: A Comprehensive Treatise, Vol 4, Metabolic and Clinical Applications, pp 409–457. New York, Plenum Press, 1979

## Journal articles

Bonomini V et al: Atherosclerosis in uremia: A longitudinal study. Am J Clin Nutr 33:1493, 1980

Burton BT, Wineman RJ: Design of clinical studies for evaluation of nutritional therapy in renal failure. Am J Clin Nutr 31:1688, 1978

DeLuca HF: Vitamin D metabolism and function. Arch Intern Med 138:836, 1978

Harvey KB et al: Nutritional assessment and treatment of chronic renal failure. Am J Clin Nutr 33:1586, 1980

Kluthe R et al: Protein requirements in maintenance hemodialysis. Am J Clin Nutr 31:1812, 1978

Kopple JD et al: Amino acid and protein metabolism in renal failure. Am J Clin Nutr 31:1532, 1978

Maschio G et al: Early dietary phosphorus restriction and calcium supplementation in the prevention of renal osteodystrophy. Am J Clin Nutr 33:1546, 1980

Massry SG: Requirements of vitamin D metabolites in patients with renal disease. Am J Clin Nutr 33:1530, 1980

Moncrief JW: Continuous ambulatory peritoneal dialysis. The Kidney 12, No. 3:9, 1979

Reaven GM et al: An inquiry into the mechanism of hypertriglyceridemia in patients with chronic renal failure. Am J Clin Nutr 33:1476, 1980

Ritz E et al: Protein restriction in the conservative management of uremia. Am J Clin Nutr 31:1703, 1978

Sanfelippo M et al: Reduction of plasma triglycerides by diet in subjects with chronic renal failure. Kidney Int 11:54, 1977

Sargent J et al: Mass balance: A quantitative guide to clinical nutritional therapy. I. The predialysis patient with renal disease. II. The dialyzed patient. J Am Diet Assoc 75:547, 1979

Slatopolsky E et al: How important is phosphate in the pathogenesis of renal osteodystrophy? Arch Intern Med 138:848, 1978

Walser M: Principles of keto acid therapy in uremia. Am J Clin Nutr 31:1756, 1978

# Liver Disease

## Books and pamphlets

Davidson CS (ed): Problems in Liver Disease. New York, Stratton Intercontinental, 1979

Galambos JT: Cirrhosis. Philadelphia, WB Saunders, 1979

Roe DA: Alcohol and Diet. Westport, CT, Avi, 1979

## Journal articles

Arch RD et al: Serum alanine aminotransferase of donors in relation to risk of non-A, non-B hepatitis in recipients. The Transfusion-Transmitted Viruses Study. N Engl J Med 304:989, 1981

Fernstrom JD et al: Diurnal variations in plasma neutral amino acid concentrations among patients with cirrhosis: Effect of dietary protein. Am J Clin Nutr 32:1923, 1979

Fischer JE et al: The effect of normalization of plasma amino acids on hepatic encephalopathy in man. Surgery 80:77, 1976

Glover SC et al: Cholestasis in acute alcoholic liver disease. Lancet 2:1305, 1977

Greenberger NJ et al: Effect of vegetable and animal protein diets in chronic hepatic encephalopathy. Am J Dig Dis 22:845, 1977

Korsten MA, Lieber CS: Nutrition in the alcoholic. Med Clin North Am 63:963, 1979

Krawitt EL et al: Absorption, hydroxylation, and excretion of vitamin D in primary biliary cirrhosis. Lancet 2:1246, 1977

James JH et al: Hyperammonaemia, plasma amino acid imbalance, and blood-brain amino acid transport: A unified theory of portal-systemic encephalopathy. Lancet 2:772, 1979

Jones AL, Schmucker DL: Current concepts of liver structure as related to function. Gastroenterology 73:833, 1977

LeVeen HH et al: Peritoneo-venous shunting for ascites. Ann Surg 180:580, 1974

Lieber CS: Alcohol, protein metabolism, and liver injury. Gastroenterology 79:373, 1980

Lifton L, Scheig R: Ethanol-induced hypertriglyceridemia. Prevalence and contributing factors. Am J Clin Nutr 31:614, 1978

Long RG et al: Clinical, biochemical, and histological studies of osteomalacia, osteoporosis, and parathyroid function in chronic liver disease. Gut 19:85, 1978

Malt RA: Portasystemic venous shunts. N Engl J Med 295:24; 80, 1976

Mezey E: Intestinal function in chronic alcoholism. Ann NY Acad Sci 252:215, 1975

Mezey E: Liver disease and nutrition. Gastroenterology 74:770, 1978

Millan MS et al: Villous damage induced by suction biopsy and by acute ethanol intake in normal human small intestine. Dig Dis Sci 25:513, 1980

Morrison SA et al: Zinc deficiency: A cause of abnormal dark adaptation in cirrhotics. Am J Clin Nutr 31:276, 1978

Patek AJ Jr, Hermos JA: Recovery from alcoholism in cirrhotic patients: A study of 45 cases. Am J Med 70:782, 1981

Pitchumoni CS et al: Nutrition in the pathogenesis of alcoholic pancreatitis. Am J Clin Nutr 33:631, 1980

Reynolds JB et al: Results of a 12-year randomized trial of portacaval shunt in patients with alcoholic liver disease and bleeding varices. Gastroenterology 80:1005, 1981

Rosen HM et al: Plasma amino acid patterns in hepatic encephalopathy. Gastroenterology 72:489, 1977

Russell RM: Vitamin A and zinc metabolism in alcoholism. Am J Clin Nutr 33:2741, 1980

Schenker S et al: Hepatic and Wernicke's encephalopathies: Current concepts of pathogenesis. Am J Clin Nutr 33:2719, 1980

Smith AR et al: Alterations in plasma and CSF amino acids, amines and metabolism in hepatic coma. Ann Surg 187:343, 1978

Sternlieb I: Copper and the liver. Gastroenterology 78:1615, 1980

Stone HH, Fabian TC: Peritoneal dialysis in the treatment of acute alcohol pancreatitis. Surg Gynecol Obstet 150:878, 1980

Witte CL et al: The portal triad in hepatic cirrhosis. Surg Gynecol Obstet 146:965, 1978

# Cancer and Special Problems

## Cancer

### Journal articles

Aker SN: Oral feeding in the cancer patient. Cancer 43:2103, 1979

Bartoshuk LM: The psychophysics of taste. Am J Clin Nutr 31:1068, 1978

Bernstein IL, Sigmundi RA: Tumor anorexia: A learned food aversion? Science 209:416, 1980

Brennan MF: Uncomplicated starvation versus cancer cachexia. Cancer Res 37:2359, 1977

Caswell M, Phillips I: Food as a source of Klebsiella species for colonization and infection of intensive care patients. J Clin Pathol 31:845, 1978

Copeland EM III et al: Nutrition as an adjunct to cancer treatment in the adult. Cancer Res 37:2451, 1977

Copeland EM III et al: Nutrition, cancer and intravenous hyperalimentation. Cancer 43:2108, 1979

Costa G: Determination of nutritional needs. Cancer Res 37:2419, 1977

DeWys WD: Changes in taste sensation and feeding behavior in cancer patients: A review. J Hum Nutr 32:447, 1978

DeWys WD, Herbst SH: Oral feeding in the nutritional management of the cancer patient. Cancer Res 37:2429, 1977

DeWys WD, Walters K: Abnormalities of taste sensation in cancer patients. Cancer 36:1888, 1975

Donaldson SS, Lenon RA: Alterations of nutritional status: Impact of chemotherapy and radiation therapy. Cancer 43:2036, 1979

Eriksson B, Douglass HO Jr: Intravenous hyperalimentation. An adjunct to treatment of malignant disease of upper gastrointestinal tract. JAMA 243:2049, 1980

Gale RP: Advances in the treatment of acute myelogenous leukemia. N Engl J Med 300:1189, 1979

Hankin JH, Rawlings V: Diet and breast cancer: A review. Am J Clin Nutr 31:2005, 1978

Lyman NW et al: Cisplatin-induced hypocalcemia and hypomagnesemia. Arch Intern Med 140:1513, 1980

Nauseef WM, Maki DG: A study of the value of simple protective isolation in patients with granulocytopenia. N Engl J Med 304:448, 1981

Ohnuma T, Holland JF: Nutritional consequences of cancer chemotherapy and immunotherapy. Cancer Res 37:2395, 1977

Ota DM et al: The effects of nutrition and treatment of cancer on host immunocompetence. Surg Gynecol Obstet 148:104, 1979

Rosenbaum EH, Rosenbaum IR: Principles of home care for the patient with advanced cancer. JAMA 244:1484, 1980

Russ JE et al: Correction of taste abnormality of malignancy with intravenous hyperalimentation. Arch Intern Med 138:799, 1978

Segaloff A: Managing endocrine and metabolic problems in the patient with advanced cancer. JAMA 245:177, 1981

Sloan GM et al: Nutritional effects of surgery, radiation therapy, and adjuvant chemotherapy for soft tissue sarcomas. Am J Clin Nutr 34:1094, 1981

Swain JF, Hargleroad MJ: Minimal-bacteria diets: An assessment for implementation. J Am Diet Assoc 69:258, 1976

Theologides A: Cancer cachexia. Cancer 43:2004, 1979

Williams LR, Cohen MH: Altered taste thresholds in lung cancer. Am J Clin Nutr 31:122, 1978

## Allergy

### Books

Gerrard JW (ed): Food Allergy: New Perspectives. Springfield, Charles C Thomas, 1980

### Journal articles

Atherton DJ et al: A double-blind controlled crossover trial of an antigen-avoidance diet in atopic eczema. Lancet 1:401, 1978

Belut D et al: IgE levels in intestinal juice. Dig Dis Sci 25:323, 1980

Brostoff J: Complexed IgE in atopy. Lancet 2:741, 1977

Finn R, Cohen HN: "Food allergy": Fact or fiction. Lancet 1:426, 1978

Gallant SP et al: A potential diagnostic method for food allergy: Clinical and immunogenicity evaluation in an elemental diet. Am J Clin Nutr 30:512, 1977

Hosen H: Provocative testing for food allergy diagnosis. J Asthma Res 14:45, 1976

Hughes EC: Use of a chemically defined diet in the diagnosis of food sensitivities and the determination of offending foods. Ann Allergy 40:393, 1978

Zlotlow MJ, Setfipane GA: Allergic potential of food additives: A report of a case of tartrazine sensitivity without aspirin intolerance. Am J Clin Nutr 30:1023, 1977

## Anemia
### Books
Bunn HF: Anemia associated with chronic systemic disorders. In Isselbacher KJ et al (eds): Harrison's Principles of Internal Medicine, 9th ed, pp 1530–1533. New York, McGraw-Hill, 1980

De Vita VT Jr: Principles of cancer therapy. In Isselbacher KJ et al (eds): Harrison's Principles of Internal Medicine, 9th ed, pp 1597–1620. New York, McGraw-Hill, 1980

Erslev AJ: In Williams WJ et al: Hematology, 2nd ed, pp 288–297; 434–442. New York, McGraw-Hill, 1977

### Journal article
Bateman CJ: Editorial: Sideroblastic anemia. Arch Intern Med 140:1278, 1980

## Diseases of the musculoskeletal system
### Journal articles
Glynn LE: Hypothesis: Primary lesion in osteoarthritis. Lancet 1:574, 1977

Lipiello L et al: Collagen synthesis in normal and osteoarthritic human collagen. J Clin Invest 59:593, 1977

Procop DJ et al: The biosynthesis of collagen and its disorders. N Engl J Med 301:13, 77, 1979

## Diet–medication interrelationship
### Books
Hathcock JN, Coon J (eds): Nutrition and Drug Interactions. New York, Academic Press, 1978

Physicians' Desk Reference, 35th ed. Oradell, NJ, Medical Economics, 1981

Roe DA: Drug-Induced Nutritional Deficiencies. Westport, CT, Avi, 1976

### Journal articles
Ioannides C, Parke DV: Effect of diet on the metabolism and toxicity of drugs. J Hum Nutr 33:357, 1979

Kenny AD: Drugs and nutrition. Fed Proc 38:2655, 1979

Kent Smith C, Durack DT: Isoniazid and reaction to cheese. Ann Intern Med 88:520, 1978

Roe DA: Interactions between drugs and nutrients. Med Clin North Am 63:985, 1979

Seixas FA: Alcohol and its drug interactions. Ann Intern Med 83:86, 1975

## Miscellaneous metabolic problems
Boss GR, Seegmiller JE: Hyperuricemia and gout: Classification, complications and management. N Engl J Med 300:1459, 1979

Foa PP et al: Reactive hypoglycemia and A-cell ('pancreatic') glucagon deficiency in the adult. JAMA 244:2281, 1980

Fox IH: Metabolic basis for disorders of purine nucleotide degradation. Metabolism 30:616, 1981

Leichter SB: Alimentary hypoglycemia: A new approach. Am J Clin Nutr 32:2104, 1979

Permutt MA et al: Alimentary hypoglycemia in the absence of gastrointestinal surgery. N Engl J Med 288:1206, 1973

## Nutrition in Diseases of Infancy and Childhood
### Books and pamphlets
Ames LB et al: The Gesell Institute's Child from One to Six. New York, Harper & Row, 1979

Beal VA: Nutrition in the Life Span. New York, John Wiley & Sons, 1980

Klaus ML, Kennell JH: Maternal-Infant Bonding. St Louis, CV Mosby, 1976

Lebenthal E (ed): Textbook of Gastroenterology and Nutrition in Infancy. New York, Raven Press, 1981

Pipes PL: Nutrition in Infancy and Childhood. St Louis, CV Mosby, 1981

Sinclair D: Human Growth After Birth, 2nd ed. London, Oxford University Press, 1973

Suskind RM: Textbook of Pediatric Nutrition. New York, Raven Press, 1981

Tanner JM: Fetus Into Man. Cambridge, Harvard University Press, 1978

Vaughan VC III, McKay RJ, Behrman RE (eds): Nelson Textbook of Pediatrics, 11th ed. Philadelphia, WB Saunders, 1979

### Committee on Nutrition statements
Committee on Nutrition, American Academy of Pediatrics: Iron supplementation for infants. Pediatrics 58:765, 1976

Committee on Nutrition, American Academy of Pediatrics: Nutritional needs of low-birth-weight infants. Pediatrics 60:519, 1977

Committee on Nutrition, American Academy of Pediatrics: On the feeding of supplemental foods to infants. Pediatrics 65:1178, 1980

Committee on Nutrition, American Academy of Pediatrics: Plant fiber intake in the pediatric diet. Pediatrics 67:572, 1981

Committee on Nutrition, American Academy of Pediatrics: Relationship between iron status and incidence of infection in infancy. Pediatrics 62:246, 1978

### Growth
Forbes GB: Nutrition and growth. J Pediatr 91:40, 1977

Harvey MAS et al: Infant growth standards in relation to parental stature. Clin Pediatr 18:602, 1979

Tanner JM, Whitehouse RH: Clinical longitudinal standards for height, weight, height velocity, weight velocity, and stages of puberty. Arch Dis Child 51:170, 1976

### The high-risk neonate

Atkinson SA et al: Human milk: Comparison of the nitrogen composition in milk from mothers of premature and full-term infants. Am J Clin Nutr 33:811, 1980

Brown EG, Sweet AY: Prevention of necrotizing enterocolitis. JAMA 240:2452, 1978

Ehrenkranz RA: Vitamin E and the neonate. Am J Dis Child 134:1157, 1980

Erenberg A et al: Lactobezoar in the low-birth-weight infant. Pediatrics 63:642, 1979

Fomon S et al: Human milk and the small premature infant. Am J Dis Child 131:463, 1977

Friedman Z et al: Rapid onset of essential fatty acid deficiency in the newborn. Pediatrics 58:640, 1976

Heird WC: Feeding the premature infant human milk or artificial formula. Am J Dis Child 131:468, 1977

Kumar SP et al: Follow-up studies of very-low-birth-weight infants (1250 grams or less) born and treated in a perinatal center. Pediatrics 66:438, 1980

Perura GR, Lemons JA: Controlled study of transpyloric and intermittent gavage feeding in the small preterm infant. Pediatrics 67:68, 1981

Shenai JP et al: Nutritional balance studies in very low birth weight infants: Role of soy formula. Pediatrics 67:631, 1981

Zlotkin SH et al: Intravenous nitrogen and energy intakes required to duplicate in utero nitrogen accretion in prematurely born human infants. J Pediatr 99:115, 1981

### Total parenteral nutrition in infants

Benner JW et al: The importance of different calorie sources in the intravenous nutrition of infants and children. Surgery 86:429, 1979

James BE: Total parenteral nutrition of premature infants. 1. Requirement for macro-nutritional element. Aust Paediatr J 15:62, 1979

James BE: Total parenteral nutrition of premature infants. 2. Requirements for micro-nutritional elements. Aust Paediatr J 15:67, 1979

Knight PJ et al: Calcium and phosphate requirements of preterm infants who require prolonged hyperalimentation. JAMA 243:1244, 1980

Law DH: Current concepts in nutrition: Total parenteral nutrition. N Engl J Med 297:1104, 1977

Meng HC et al: The use of a crystalline amino acid mixture for parenteral nutrition in low-birth-weight infants. Pediatrics 59:699, 1977

Periera GR et al: Decreased oxygenation and hyperlipemia during intravenous fat infusions in premature infants. Pediatrics 66:26, 1980

Postuma R, Trevenen CL: Liver disease in infants receiving total parenteral nutrition. Pediatrics 63:110, 1979

Smith L: The use of intravenous fat emulsions in the critically ill neonate. Nutr Sup Serv 1, No. 3:17, 1981

### Renal disease

Betts PR, White RHR: Growth potential and skeletal maturity in children with chronic renal insufficiency. Nephron 16:325, 1976

Broyer M et al: Plasma and muscle free amino acids in children at the early stages of renal failure. Am J Clin Nutr 33:1396, 1980

Cheek DB, Graystone JE: Insulin and growth hormone: Regulators of growth with particular reference to muscle. Kidney Int 14:317, 1978

Fine RN: Treatment of endstage renal disease in children. Pediatr Ann 10:15, 1981

Hetrick A et al: Nutrition in renal disease when the patient is a child. Am J Nurs 79:2152, 1979

Holliday MA, Chantler C: Metabolic and nutritional factors in children with renal insufficiency. Kidney Int 14:306, 1978

Jones WA et al: Oral essential amino acid supplements in children with advanced chronic renal failure. Am J Clin Nutr 33:1096, 1980

Munro HN: Nutritional requirements for health: Their relevance to tissue function in renal failure. Am J Clin Nutr 33:1555, 1980

Nash MA et al: Hyperphosphatemia with insufficient parathyroid response in renal failure. J Pediatr 98:247, 1981

Spinozzi NS, Grupe WE: Nutritional implications of renal disease. J Am Diet Assoc 70:493, 1977

### Growth failure due to psychosocial deprivation

Editorial: Nutrition in critical periods of development. Lancet 2:229, 1977

Gardner LI: The endocrinology of abuse dwarfism. Am J Dis Child 131:505, 1977

Holmes GL: Evaluation and progress in non-organic failure to thrive. South Med J 72:693, 1979

Hunter RS et al: Antecedents of child abuse and neglect in premature infants: A prospective study in a newborn intensive care unit. Pediatrics 61:629, 1978

Lazoff B et al: The mother–newborn relationship: Limits of adaptability. J Pediatr 91:1, 1977

Lynch MA, Roberts J: Predicting child abuse: Signs of bonding failure in the maternity hospital. Br Med J 1:624, 1977

Morse AE et al: Environmental correlates of pediatric social illness: Preventive implications of an advocacy approach. Am J Public Health 67:612, 1977

Neligan GA, Prudham D: Family factors affecting child development. Arch Dis Child 51:853, 1976

Rosenn DW et al: Differentiation of organic from nonorganic failure to thrive syndrome in infancy. Pediatrics 66:698, 1980

ten Bensel RW, Paxson AL: Child abuse following early postpartum separation. J Pediatr 90:490, 1977

Wolfe PH: Mother–infant interaction in the first year. N Engl J Med 295:999, 1976

### The chronically ill child

Rickard K et al: Nutritional management of the chronically ill child. Pediatr Clin North Am 24:157, 1977

### Nutritional anemias

Dallman PR et al: Hemoglobin concentration in white, black and oriental children: Is there a need for separate criteria for screening for anemia? Am J Clin Nutr 31:377, 1978

Driggers DA et al: Iron deficiency in one year old infants: Comparison of results of a therapeutic trial in infants with anemia or low-normal hemoglobin levels. J Pediatr 98:753, 1981

Fomon SJ et al: Cow milk feeding in infancy: Gastrointestinal blood loss and iron nutritional status. J Pediatr 98:540, 1981

Koerper MA, Dallman PR: Serum iron concentration and transferrin saturation in the diagnosis of iron deficiency in children: Normal developmental changes. J Pediatr 91:870, 1977

Saarinen LM et al: Iron absorption in infants: High bioavailability of breast milk iron as indicated by the extrinsic tag method of iron absorption and by the concentration of serum ferritin. J Pediatr 91:36, 1977

Stockman JA III et al: The anemia of prematurity: Factors governing the erythropoietin response. N Engl J Med 296:647, 1977

Wolfe LC, Lux SE: Nutritional anemias of childhood. Pediatr Ann 8:38, 1979

Woodruff CW et al: Iron nutrition in the breast-fed infant. J Pediatr 90:36, 1977

### Cystic fibrosis

Antonowicz I et al: Disaccharidase activities in small intestinal mucosa in patients with cystic fibrosis. J Pediatr 92:214, 1978

Dann LG, Blau K: Exocrine-gland function and the basic biochemical defect in cystic fibrosis. Lancet 2:405, 1978

Hubbaro VS et al: Abnormal fatty-acid composition of plasma lipids in cystic fibrosis. Lancet 2:1302, 1977

Lloyd-Still JD, Ganther HE: Selenium and glutathione peroxidase levels in cystic fibrosis. Pediatrics 65:1010, 1980

### Diarrhea

Chernoff R, Dean JA: Medical and nutritional aspects of intractable diarrhea. J Am Diet Assoc 76:161, 1980

Dagan R et al: Letter: Lactose-free formula for infantile diarrhea. Lancet 1:207, 1980

Eastham EJ, Walker WA: Adverse effect of milk formula ingestion on the gastrointestinal tract: An update. Gastroenterology 76:365, 1979

Ghishan FR et al: Chronic diarrhea of infancy: Nonbeta cell hyperplasia. Pediatrics 64:46, 1979

Liebman WM: Recurrent abdominal pain in children: Lactose and sucrose intolerance, a prospective study. Pediatrics 64:43, 1979

Lloyd-Still JB: Chronic diarrhea of childhood and the misuse of elimination diets. J Pediatr 95:10, 1979

MacLean WC et al: Nutritional management of chronic diarrhea and malnutrition: Primary reliance of oral feeding. J Pediatr 97:316, 1980

Sperotto G et al: Treatment of diarrheal dehydration. Am J Clin Nutr 30:1447, 1979

Waterson T: Fluids for diarrhea in young children. Lancet 1:545, 1977

### Rickets

Brooks H et al: Vitamin D resistant rickets type II: Resistance of target organs to 1,25 Di-hydroxy vitamin D. N Engl J Med 298:996, 1978

Kouh SW et al: Rickets due to calcium deficiency. N Engl J Med 297:1264, 1977

Rowe JC et al: Nutritional hypophosphatemic rickets in a premature infant fed breast milk. N Engl J Med 300:293, 1979

### Burns

Aulick LH et al: The relative significance of thermal and metabolic demands on burn hypermetabolism. J Trauma 19, No. 8:559, 1979

Kien CL et al: Whole body protein synthesis in relation to basal energy expenditure in healthy children and in children recovering from burn injury. Pediatr Res 12, No. 3:211, 1978

Long JC: Energy expenditures of major burns. J Trauma 19:904, 1979

### Epilepsy

Nelson KB, Ellenberg JH: Predictors of epilepsy in children who have experienced febrile seizures. N Engl J Med 295:1029, 1976

### Hyperactivity

Harley JP et al: Hyperkinesis and food additives: Testing the Feingold hypothesis. Pediatrics 62:818, 1978

# Inborn Errors of Metabolism in Infancy and Childhood

## Books and pamphlets

Stanbury JB, Wyngaarden JB, Fredrickson DS (eds): The Metabolic Basis of Inherited Disease, 4th ed. New York, McGraw-Hill, 1978

Winick M (ed): Nutritional Management of Genetic Disorders. New York, John Wiley & Sons, 1979

## Committee on Nutrition statements

Committee on Nutrition, American Academy of Pediatrics: New developments in hyperphenylalaninemia. Pediatrics 65:844, 1980

Committee on Nutrition, American Academy of Pediatrics: Special diets for infants with inborn errors of amino acid metabolism. Pediatrics 57:783, 1976

## Phenylketonuria

Acosta PB et al: Methods of dietary inception in infants with PKU. J Am Diet Assoc 72:164, 1978

Acosta PB et al: Nutrient intake of treated infants with phenylketonuria. Am J Clin Nutr 30:198, 1977

Ford RC, Berman JL: Phenylalanine metabolism and intellectual functioning among carriers of phenylketonuria and hyperphenylalaninemia. Lancet 1:767, 1977

Holm VA, Knox WE: Physical growth in phenylketonuria. I. A retrospective study. Pediatrics 63:694, 1979

Holm VA et al: Physical growth in phenyletonuria. II. Growth of treated children in the PKU collaborative study from birth to 4 years of age. Pediatrics 63:700, 1979

Lenke RR, Levy HL: Maternal phenylketonuria and hyperphenylalaninemia. N Engl J Med 303:1202, 1980

Milstein S et al: Hyperphenylalaninemia due to dihydropteridine reductase deficiency. J Pediatr 89:763, 1976

Milstein S et al: Hyperphenylalaninemia due to dihydropteridine reductase deficiency: Diagnosis by measurement of oxidized and reduced pterins in urine. Pediatrics 65:806, 1980

Smith I et al: Birthweight of infants with phenylketonuria and their unaffected siblings. J Inherited Metab Dis 1:99, 1978

## Maple syrup urine disease

Committee for Improvement of Hereditary Disease Management: Management of maple syrup urine disease in Canada. Can Med Assoc J 115:1005, 1976

Gibson GE: Inhibition of acetylcholine synthesis and of carbohydrate utilization by maple syrup urine disease metabolites. J Neurochem 26:1073, 1976

Naylor EW, Guthrie R: Newborn screening for maple syrup urine disease. Pediatrics 61:262, 1978

Nayman R et al: Observations on the composition of milk substitute products for treatment of inborn errors of amino acid metabolism, comparisons with human milk. Am J Clin Nutr 32:1279, 1979

Noel MB et al: Dietary treatment of MSUD (branched chain ketoaciduria). J Am Diet Assoc 69:62, 1976

Snyderman SE: Branched chain ketoaciduria (MSUD). Clin Perinatol 34:41, 1976

### Other inborn errors of metabolism

Burton BK, Nadler HL: Clinical diagnosis of the inborn errors of metabolism in the neonatal period. Pediatrics 61:398, 1978

Lee CWG et al: Trimethylaminuria: Fishy odor in children. N Engl J Med 295:937, 1976

O'Brien D: Inborn errors of metabolism. Am J Clin Nutr 32:482, 1979

Orkin SH, Nathan DG: Current concepts: The thalassemias. N Engl J Med 295:710, 1976

Thoene J et al: Neonatal citrullinemia: Treatment with keto-analogues of essential amino acids. J Pediatr 90:218, 1977

Van Acker KJ et al: Complete deficiency of adenine phosphoribosyl transferase: Report of a family. N Engl J Med 297:127, 1977

### General references

### Books

Bray GA (ed): Obesity: Comparative Methods of Weight Control. Westport, Technomic Publishing, 1980

Bondy PK, Rosenberg LE: Metabolic Control of Metabolism, 8th ed. Philadelphia, WB Saunders, 1980

Brobeck JR (ed): Best and Taylor's Physiological Basis of Medical Practice, 10th ed. Baltimore, Williams & Wilkins, 1979

Davidson S, Passmore R, Brock JF et al: Human Nutrition and Dietetics, 7th ed. New York, Churchill Livingstone, 1979

DeGroot LJ et al (eds): Endocrinology. New York, Grune & Stratton, 1979

Deitel M (ed): Nutrition in Clinical Surgery. Baltimore, Williams & Wilkins, 1980

Felig P et al: Endocrinology and Metabolism. New York, McGraw-Hill, 1981

Fomon SJ: Infant Nutrition, 2nd ed. Philadelphia, WB Saunders, 1974

Gilman AG, Goodman L, Gilman A: Goodman and Gilman's The Pharmacological Basis of Therapeutics, 6th ed. New York, Macmillan, 1980

Goodhart RS, Shils ME: Modern Nutrition in Health and Disease, 6th ed. Philadelphia, Lea & Febiger, 1980

Guyton AC: Textbook of Medical Physiology, 6th ed. Philadelphia, WB Saunders, 1981

Harper HA, Rodwell VW, Mayes PA: Review of Physiological Chemistry, 18th ed. Los Angeles, Lange, 1981

Harvey A McG et al: Principles and Practice of Medicine, 20th ed. New York, Appleton-Century-Crofts, 1980

Isselbacher KJ et al (eds): Harrison's Principles of Internal Medicine, 9th ed. New York, McGraw-Hill, 1980

Isselbacher KJ et al (eds): Harrison's Principles of Internal Medicine, 9th ed. Update 1. New York, McGraw-Hill, 1981

Pennington JAT, Church HN: Bowes and Church's Food Values of Portions Commonly Used, 13th ed. Philadelphia, JB Lippincott, 1980

Pike RL, Brown ML: Nutrition: An Integrated Approach, 2nd ed. New York, John Wiley & Sons, 1975

Ross G (ed): Essentials of Human Physiology. Chicago, Yearbook, 1978

Sabiston DC Jr (ed): Textbook of Surgery: The Biological Basis of Modern Surgical Practice, 12th ed. Philadelphia, WB Saunders, 1981

Sleisenger MH, Fordtran JS: Gastrointestinal Disease: Pathophysiology, Diagnosis, Management, 2nd ed. Philadelphia, WB Saunders, 1978

Stanbury JB, Wyngaarden JB, Frederickson DS (eds): The Metabolic Basis of Inherited Disease, 4th ed. New York, McGraw-Hill, 1978

Vaughan VC III, McKay RI, Behrman R (eds): Nelson Textbook of Pediatrics, 11th ed. Philadelphia, WB Saunders, 1979

### Journals

American Journal of Clinical Nutrition
American Journal of Diseases of Children
American Journal of Gastroenterology
American Journal of Medicine
American Journal of Nursing
American Journal of Surgery
Archives of Internal Medicine
Diabetes
Diabetes Care
Digestive Diseases and Science
Federation Proceedings
Gastroenterology
Gut
Journal of the American Dietetic Association
Journal of the American Medical Association
Journal of Clinical Investigation
Journal of Food Science
Journal of Human Nutrition
Journal of Parenteral and Enteral Nutrition
Journal of Pediatrics
Lancet
Metabolism
New England Journal of Medicine
Nutrition Reviews
Pediatrics
Postgraduate Medicine
Surgery Gynecology and Obstetrics

# Glossary

**acetylcholine** (as-e-til-ko'len). A chemical transmitter of nerve impulses released upon stimulation of the nerve cell and in the presence of calcium ions.

**acetylcholinesterase** (as-e-til-ko'len-es'ter-as). An enzyme that catalyzes the hydrolysis of acetylcholine into choline and acetic acid.

**acidosis** (as'i-do'sis). A pathological condition resulting from an accumulation of acid or loss of base in the body and characterized by increase in hydrogen ion concentration.

**ACP.** Acyl carrier protein, which contains pantothenic acid, and is involved in the synthesis of fatty acids.

**acrodermatitis enteropathica** (ak'ro-der'mah-ti'tis en'ter-o-path'e-ka). A rare recessive gene disease caused by an inherited defect in zinc metabolism.

**ADH.** An antidiuretic hormone released from the posterior pituitary and also known as *vasopressin*. The primary effect of ADH is on the kidney, where it increases the reabsorption of water by the renal tubules, thereby decreasing water loss by excretion.

**adrenergic** (ad'ren-er'jik). Refers to nerve fibers that release epinephrine (adrenalin) or to drugs that produce effects similar to those of epinephrine or to a stimulation of the sympathetic nervous system.

**aflatoxins** (a'flah-tok'sin). Group of toxic substances produced by the common mold aspergillus flavus, which grows on peanuts and cereals. They have toxic and carcinogenic effects in many species.

**aldosterone** (al'do-ster'ōn). A steroid hormone produced by the adrenal cortex. It regulates electrolyte balance by increasing the renal tubular reabsorption of sodium and increasing the excretion of potassium.

**alkalosis** (al'kah-lo'sis). A pathological condition resulting from accumulation of base or loss of acid in the body and characterized by a decrease in hydrogen ion concentration.

**alginate** (al'ji-nāt). A salt of alginic acid that is extracted from marine kelp and forms a viscous solution or a gel.

**alpha-tocopherol equivalents** (al'fah-to-kof'er-ol i-kwiv'e-lent) αTE. A measure used to express the vitamin E activity of the diet.

**Alzheimer's disease** (altz'hi-merz). Presenile dementia.

**AMC.** Arm muscle circumference.

**amenorrhea** (ah-men-o-re'ah). Absence or abnormal stoppage of the menses.

**aminotransferase** (am'i-no-trans'fer-āz). An enzyme that transfers an amino-group from an amino acid to a keto acid. Also known as *transaminase* (trans-am'i-nās). Common examples include alanine aminotransferase, also known as *glutamate - pyruvate transaminase (GPT)* and *aspartate aminotransferase* or *glutamate - oxaloacetate transaminase (GOT)*.

**amylase** (am'i-lās). A pancreatic or salivary enzyme that catalyzes the hydrolysis of starch into smaller molecules.

**amylopectin** (am'i-lo-pek'tin). The branched chain insoluble form of starch that stains violet red with iodine and forms a paste with hot water.

**amylose** (am'i-lōs). The straight chain soluble form of starch that stains blue with iodine and does not form a paste with hot water.

**anabolism** (ah-nab'o-lizm). Phase of metabolism that synthesizes new molecules.

**angiotensin** (an'je-o-ten'sin). Angiotensin I and II are deca- and octapeptides, respectively, produced by sequential proteolylis from a plasma protein precursor, *angiotensinogen*. Angiotensin II is an active vasoconstrictor that increases blood pressure and also acts as a stimulator of the secretion of *aldosterone* from adrenal cortex.

**anion** (an'i-on). A negatively charged ion.

**anisakiasis** (ah-nis'a-ki'a-ciz). Disease caused by the consumption of raw or pickled fish containing the anisakis larvae.

**antagonist** (an-tag'o-nist). See *antimetabolite.*

**anticholinergic** (an'ti-ko'lin-er'jik). Blocking transmission of nerve impulses through the parasympathetic (cholinergic) nerves.

**anticoagulant** (an'ti-ko-ag'u-lant). A substance that inhibits or prevents blood coagulation by interfering with the clotting mechanism.

**antihemorrhagic** (an'ti-hem'o-raj'ik). An agent that prevents or stops hemorrhage.

**antihistamine** (an'ti-his'tah-min). Refers to drugs that block or counteract the actions of histamine.

**antimetabolite** (an'ti-me-tab'o-lit). A substance bearing a close structural resemblance to one required for normal physiological functioning and perhaps exerting its desired effect by replacing or interfering with the utilization of the essential metabolite.

**antioxidant** (an'ti-ok'se-dant). A substance that prevents or delays oxidation.

**apoenzyme** (ap'o-en'zim). The protein portion of an enzyme to which the prosthetic group or coenzyme is attached.

**aquaculture** (ah'kwah-kul'cher). Growing crops in water.

**arabinose** (ah-rab'i-nōs). A pentose (five carbon sugar) obtained from vegetable gums by acid hydrolysis.

**ash.** Inorganic mineral residue remaining after the burning or oxidation of all organic matter.

**aspergillus flavus** (as'per-jil'us fla-vus). A group of molds found on corn, peanuts, and certain grains when improperly dried and stored; a source of aflatoxin.

**assessment** (ah-ses'ment). The process of collecting and analyzing data for the purpose of identifying client problems and needs as well as the resources available to the client for meeting the needs and solving or ameliorating the problem.

**ataxia** (ah-tak'se-ah). Failure of muscular coordination; irregularity of muscular action.

**audit** (ô'dit). A component of a quality assurance program in which actual performance as recorded in the medical record is compared with established standards.

**autosomal** (au'to-so'mal). Pertaining to an autosome, a paired chromosome, not a sex chromosome.

**avidin** (av'i-din). A protein-like antivitamin isolated from egg white; antagonist of biotin.

**bacillus cereus** (bah-sil'lus sêr'i-us). A large gram-positive, rod-shaped, aerobic, spore-bearing organism.

**bactericidal** (bak'ter-i-si'dal). Ability to destroy bacteria.

**BAO.** Basal (gastric) acid output.

**BE.** Barium enema.

**BEE.** Basal energy expenditure.

**benign** (be-nīn'). Not malignant.

**biocytin** (bi'o-si'tin). A naturally occurring complex of biotin and lysine.

**Bitot's spot** (bi-toz'). A small, triangular, silvery patch of epithelial degeneration, sometimes with a foamy surface, on the conjunctiva.

**botulism** (bot'u-lizm). Poisoning from the toxin produced by the organism *Clostridium botulinum*. The toxin has a selective action on the nervous system.

**bran** (bran). The skin or husk of grains of cereals that are separated from the endosperm.

**CAC.** Citric acid cycle. Also known as *tricarboxylic acid cycle* or *Krebs' cycle*.

**calcitonin** (kal'si-to'nin). A hormone secreted by the thyroid gland that inhibits the release of calcium from bone.

**carrageenan** (kar'ah-gēn'in). From carrageen (Irish moss); the commercial colloid extract from the moss, which forms a gel.

**casein** (ka'se-in). The principal protein of cow's milk, the basis of cheese.

**catabolism** (kah-tab'o-lizm). That aspect of metabolism that converts nutrients or complex substances in living cells into simpler compounds with the release of energy.

**cataract** (kat'ah-rakt). The opacity of the crystalline eye lens or its capsule.

**catecholamine** (kat'e-kol-am'in). Any one of a group of structurally and functionally related compounds, including norepinephrine, epinephrine, and dopamine.

**cation** (kat'i-on). An ion carrying a positive charge that is attracted to the negative pole or cathode (see *anions*, above). Cations include all metals and hydrogen.

**ceruloplasmin** (se-roo"lo-plaz'min). An alpha-globulin of the plasma, being a glycoprotein in which approximately 96% of the plasma copper is transported.

**cheilosis** (ki-lo'sis). A condition marked by lesions on the lips and cracks at the angles of the mouth.

**child abuse** (child ah-buz'). Nonaccidental injury inflicted on a child (under 18 yr of age) by a parent or parent substitute.

**choline** (ko'lēn). A component of lecithin. Necessary for fat transport in the body. Prevents the accumulation of fat in the liver.

**cholinergic** (ko'lin-er'jik). Refers to nerve fibers that release acetylcholine as a neurotransmitter; parasympathetic nerves.

**chromatin** (kro'mah-tin). The more stainable portion of the cell nucleus; contains the chromosomes.

**chylomicrons** (ki'lo-mi'kronz). Particles of emulsified lipoproteins containing primarily triglycerides from dietary fat and very little protein.

**client-managed care** (klī'ent man'ijd kâr). The type of care provided for health maintenance and prevention. In this type of care practitioners offer counseling services to the clients so that they can develop their own objectives as well as implement and evaluate their own care at home.

**clinical dietitian** (klin'e-k'l di-e-tish'an). A registered dietitian who is a member of the health-care team. She assesses nutritional needs, develops and implements nutritional care plans of individuals or groups, and evaluates and reports the results appropriately.

**CMC.** Critical micellar concentration, referring to bile salts. The minimum concentration required for complete solubilization of the digestion products of fats by micelle formation and, therefore, for effective absorption.

**collagen** (kol′a-jen). The main protein constituent of connective tissue and of the organic substance of bones; changed into gelatin by boiling.

**colloidal** (ko-loi′dal). Pertaining to a colloid, which is a substance containing tiny, solid, evenly dispersed particles not dissolved in the medium but which will not settle out.

**colostrum** (ko-los′trum). The thin milky fluid secreted by the mammary glands a few days before or after parturition.

**congenital** (kon-jen′i-tal). Existing at or before birth.

**congregate living** (kon′gre-get liv′ing). Groups of people living together and sharing certain facilities in common.

**corticoid**—See *corticosteroid*.

**corticosteroid** (kor′ti-ko-ste′roid). A term referring to the steroid hormones of the adrenal cortex or other compounds with similar activity.

**CRABP.** Cellular retinoic acid-binding protein.

**CRBP.** Cellular retinol-binding protein.

**creatine** (kre′a-tin). A nitrogenous end product of muscle metabolism.

**creatinine** (kre-at′i-nin). A basic substance, creatine anhydride, derived from creatine.

**cretinism** (kre′tin-izm). A chronic condition due to congenital lack of thyroid secretion.

**crude fiber** (krōōd fi′ber). The ash-free insoluble residue left after boiling a food sample first with dilute acid and then with dilute alkali. Although this term is used to express fiber values in food composition tables, it has little meaning in defining the actual amount of dietary fiber present in foods.

**cyanosis** (si-an-o′sis). Blueness of the skin due to insufficient oxygenation of the blood.

**cyclamate** (si′kla-māt). Sodium or calcium cyclamate, used as an artificial sweetener. Use prohibited by FDA.

**cystine** (sis′tin). A nonessential amino acid containing sulfur.

**cystinuria** (sis′ti-nu′re-ah). The occurrence of excessive cystine in the urine.

**deamination** (de-am′in-a′shun). The process of metabolism during which the nitrogen portion (amine group) is removed from amino acids.

**deciduous** (de-sid′u-us). Not permanent; used in connection of teeth.

**decubitus ulcer** (de-ku′bī′tus ul′ser). An ulceration caused by prolonged pressure in a patient confined to bed for a long period of time.

**DHHS.** United States Department of Health and Human Services, Washington, D.C. (Formerly DHEW—Department of Health Education and Welfare).

**dehydration** (de′hi-dra′shun). Removal of water from food or tissue; or the condition that results from undue loss of water.

**dietary fiber** (di′ĕ-ta′re fi′ber). The plant materials that are resistant to the action of the digestive enzymes of the human small intestines.

**diet pattern** (di′et pat′ern). A daily meal plan stated in terms of food groups (milk, meat, etc.) that interprets a therapeutic diet order.

**DNA, deoxyribonucleic acid** (de-ok′se-ri′bo-nu-kle′ik). Found in the nucleus of living cells, functions in the transfer of genetic characteristics.

**disaccharidase** (di-sak′ah-ri-das). An enzyme that hydrolyzes disaccharides.

**disaccharide** (di-sak′a-rid). Any one of the sugars that yield two monosaccharides on hydrolysis.

**ecchymosis** (ek-im-o′sis). A discoloration of the skin due to extravasation of blood.

**eclampsia** (ek-lamp′se-ah). Convulsions and coma occurring in a pregnant woman and associated with hypertension, edema, or proteinuria.

**ecology** (e-kol′o-je). Study of the environment and life history.

**edema** (e-de′mah). Presence of excess fluid in the intercellular spaces of body tissues.

**EDTA.** Ethylenediamine tetraacetic acid, which has a capacity to form chelates with cations.

**EFA.** Essential fatty acid, linoleic.

**electrolyte** (e-lek′tro-lit). The ionized form of an element. Common electrolytes in the body are sodium, potassium, and chloride.

**electron transport chain** (e-lek′tron trans-port′ chān). Process that occurs in the mitochondria of the cell where hydrogen and then electrons from a substrate are passed from nicotinamide adenine dinucleotide (NAD) to flavin adenine dinucleotide (FAD) to coenzyme $Q_{10}$ to cytochromes and then to oxygen to form water. The series of electron carriers are reduced and oxidized, thereby providing for the regeneration of NAD and FAD. As this occurs, the energy released is trapped by adenosine diphosphate (ADP) to form adenosine triphosphate (ATP). This is called *oxidative phosphorylation.*

**encephalopathy** (en-sef′ah-lop′ah-the). Any degenerative disease of the brain.

**endemic** (en-dem′ik). A disease of low morbidity that is constantly present in a human community.

**endogenous** (en-doj′e-nus). Originating within the organism, for example, nutrients synthesized in intermediary metabolism.

**endosperm** (en′do-sperm). The nutritive substance within the embryo sac of plants.

**enterohepatic cycle** (en′ter-o-hep-ah-tic). Refers to recycling of substances that are secreted by the liver to the intestine in bile, reabsorbed from the intestine, and returned to the liver through the portal vein, that is, enterohepatic circulation (cycling) of bile salts.

**enteropathy** (en′ter-op′ah-the). Any disease of the intestine.

**enterotoxin** (en′ter-o-tok′sin). A toxin specific for the cells of the intestinal mucosa.

**enzyme** (en′zīm). A substance, usually protein in nature and formed in living cells, that brings about chemical changes.

**EPA.** Environmental Protection Agency.

**epinephrine** (ep′i-nef′rin). A hormone secreted by the adrenal medulla and released predominantly in response to hypoglycemia.

**epiphysis** (e-pif′i-sis). A piece of bone separated from a long bone in early life by cartilage, but later becoming a part of the larger bone.

**ERCP.** Endoscopic retrograde cholangio pancreatography.

**erythropoiesis** (e-rith′ro-poi-e′sis). Synthesis of red blood cells.

**evaluation** (e-val′u-a′shun). The process of comparing expected outcomes to actual outcomes to determine whether or not the criteria of care are met and to identify those factors that either facilitate or prevent the meeting of objectives.

**exchange system** (eks-chanj′ sis′tem). A simplified system of grouping foods of comparable energy and nutrient composition to facilitate the calculation of a therapeutic diet pattern.

**exogenous** (eks-oj′e-nus). Originating outside the organism, for example, nutrients in food.

**FAD.** Flavin adenine dinucleotide, a coenzyme form of riboflavin.

**FAO.** Food and Agriculture Organization of the United Nations. Headquarters in Rome, Italy.

**favism** (fa′vism). An acute hemolytic anemia due to contact with the fava or broad bean.

**FDA.** Food and Drug Administration of the Public Health Service, U.S. Department of Health and Human Services, Washington, D.C. 20250.

**ferritin** (fer′i-tin). An iron-containing protein and the form in which iron is stored in the liver, spleen, intestinal mucosa, and reticuloendothelial cells.

**flavoproteins** (fla′vo-pro′te-ins). Compounds containing riboflavin, certain nucleotides, and proteins. They are important as enzymes in the citric acid cycle.

**FMN.** Flavin adenine mononucleotide, a coenzyme form of riboflavin.

**formiminoglutamic acid (FIGLU)** (form-im′i-no′gluta′mik). Intermediary product of histidine metabolism. Since folic acid is necessary for its breakdown, the urinary excretion of FIGLU may be measured to determine folic acid status.

**GABA.** Gamma aminobutyric acid produced by decarboxylation of glutamic acid, especially in the tissues of the central nervous system. Pyridoxal phosphate is required as a coenzyme for its formation.

**galactose** (gah-lak′tos). A monosaccharide derived from lactose by hydrolysis.

**galactosemia** (găh-lak′to-se′me-ah). A hereditary condition characterized by excess galactose in the blood.

**genes** (jēns). Units of hereditary DNA, carried by chromosomes.

**genetic screening** (je-net′ik skrēn′ing). Biochemical testing for inherited metabolic diseases. Screening can identify heterozygous carriers of inherited diseases.

**geriatric** (jer′ĕ-at′rik). Pertaining to the treatment of the aged.

**gliadin** (glī′a-din). One of the proteins found in the gluten of cereal grains.

**glucocorticoid** (gloo′ko-kor′ti-koid). Hormones of the adrenal cortex that stimulate gluconeogenesis.

**gluten** (gloo′ten;-t′n). A protein found in many cereal grains.

**glycogen** (glī′ko-jen). A carbohydrate, similar in composition to the amylopectin form of starch. In this form, carbohydrate is stored in the liver and the muscles.

**glycogen-loading** (glī′ko-jen lod′ing). Process of increasing glycogen stores in the muscles by first depleting muscle glycogen stores and then loading with a high carbohydrate diet.

**goitrin** (goi′trin). A goitrogen present in rutabagas and turnips.

**goitrogen** (goi′tro-jen). A substance that interferes with the production of thyroid hormones and thus is capable of producing goiter.

**GSH.** Reduced glutathione, which is a tripeptide consisting of glutamic acid, cysteine, and glycine.

**GTF.** Glucose tolerance factor. Refers to the biologically active organic form of chromium that facilitates the action of insulin.

**HANES** (hanz). Health and Nutrition Examination Survey conducted by the National Center for Health Statistics, U.S. Department of Health and Human Services.

**Harris-Benedict Formula** (har′is ben′e-dikt). A formula developed to estimate the basal energy expenditure (BEE) of adult men and women using height (cm), weight (kg) and age (yr).

**hematocrit** (he-mat′o-krit). The volume percentage of erythrocytes in whole blood when centrifuged under standardized conditions.

**hemicellulose** (hem′e-sel′u-los). A complex carbohydrate found in the cell wall of plants; it is indigestible but absorbs water, thereby stimulating laxation.

**hemochromatosis** (he′mo-kro-mah-to′sis). A genetic condition characterized by excessive iron deposition in the tissue.

**hemosiderin** (he′mo-sid′er-in). An insoluble storage form of iron in the tissues, found mainly in the liver, spleen, and bone marrow.

**heterozygote** (het′er-o-zi′gōt). An individual possessing different alleles in regard to a given characteristic.

**hexose** (hek′sos). A single sugar containing six carbon atoms.

**HMS.** The hexose monophosphate shunt, a pathway for glucose oxidation. Also known as the phosphogluconate pathway or pentose phosphate pathway.

**high risk infant** (hi risk in′fant). An infant born before 37 or after 40 weeks of gestation; who weighs less than 2500 g or more than 4000 g; whose weight is not appropriate for gestational age; and who is in poor condition at the time of delivery or whose mother has a poor obstetrical history.

**histidine** (his′ti-din). An amino acid required by growing animals.

**homeostasis** (ho′me-o-sta′sis). A tendency to maintain stability and constancy of the various body systems, such as the concentration of specific substances in the body fluids, total body fluid volume, and body temperature.

**homozygote** (ho′mo-zi′gōt). A person possessing an identical pair of alleles in regard to a given characteristic or to all characteristics.

**hormone sensitive lipase** (hor′mōn sen′si-tiv lip′ ās). Refers to an enzyme that releases fatty acids from triglycerides in the adipose tissue. Some hormones stimulate the activity of this enzyme (epinephrine), while others suppress it (insulin).

**hospice** (hos′pis). A home for the sick.

**humectant** (hu-mek′tant). A food additive that prevents foods from drying out, for example, glycerine, mannitol.

**hydrogenation** (hi′dro-jen-a′shun). The process of introducing hydrogen into a compound, as when oils are hydrogenated to produce solid fats.

**hydrolysate** (hi-drol′i-sāt). A product of hydrolysis. Often applied to protein hydrolysate.

**hydrolysis** (hi-drol′i-sis). A chemical reaction in which decomposition is due to the incorporation and splitting of water, resulting in the formation of two new compounds.

**hydroxyproline** (hi-drok′se-pro′lin). An amino acid that occurs in structural proteins, primarily collagen.

**hydrophobic** (hi′dro-fo′bik). Poor affinity for water; does not absorb water.

**hydrophilic** (hi′dro-fil′ik). High affinity for water; absorbs water readily.

**hyperactivity** (hi′per-ak-tiv′i-te). One of the terms used to identify a combination of behavioral symptoms that occur in children of normal intelligence who fail to learn at a normal rate.

**hypercalcemia** (hi′per-kal-se′me-ah). An excess of calcium in the blood.

**hypercholesteremia** (hi′per-ko-les′ter-e′me-a). Excess of cholesterol in the blood.

**hyperglycemia** (hi′per-gli-se′me-a). An increase in the blood sugar level to levels above normal.

**hyperplasia** (hi′per-pla′zhe-a). Increase in number of normal cells in normal arrangement in a tissue.

**hypertrophy** (hi-per′tro-fe). The enlargement or overgrowth of an organ or part of an organ due to an increase in size of its constituent cells.

**hyperuricemia** (hi′per-u-ri-se′me-ah). Excess of uric acid in the blood.

**hypervitaminosis** (hi′per-vi′ta-min-o′sis). A condition due to an excess of one or more vitamins.

**hypoalbuminemia** (hi′po-al-bu′min-e′me-a). Abnormally low albumin content of the blood.

**hypocalcemia** (hi′po-kal-se′me-a). Abnormally low blood calcium.

**hypochloremia metabolic alkalosis** (hi′po-klo-re′me-a met′ah-bol′ik al′kah-lo′sis). Increase in the bicarbonate of the body fluids due to loss of chloride from the body, or inadequate chloride intake.

**hypoglycemia** (hi′po-gli-se′me-a). A decrease in the blood sugar level below normal.

**hypoproteinemia** (hi′po-pro′te-in-e′me-a). A decrease in the normal quantity of serum protein in the blood.

**iatrogenic** (i′at-ro′jen′ik). Resulting from the activity of physicians.

**IDDM.** Insulin-dependent diabetes mellitus. Formerly juvenile onset diabetes mellitus (JODM).

**idiopathic** (id′i-o-path′ik). Self-originated; occurring without known cause.

**IDL.** The intermediate-density lipoprotein fraction of the blood.

**IGT.** Impaired glucose tolerance.

**implementation** (im′ple-men-ta′shun). The process of putting plans into effect. This includes managing resources essential to client care and counseling clients in the management of their own care.

**incontinence** (in-kon′ti-nens). Inability to refrain from yielding to normal impulses, such as the urge to defecate or urinate.

**inositol** (in-o′si-tol). A hexahydroxycyclohexane once considered to be a member of the vitamin B complex.

**INQ.** Index of Nutrition Quality or nutrient density in relation to caloric value.

**interdialytic** (in′ter-di-al-i′tic). Between dialysis treatments.

**intrinsic factor, IF** (in-trin′sik). A glycoprotein present in the normal gastric juice and required for the absorption of vitamin $B_{12}$ (extrinsic factor).

**isoleucine** (i′so-lu′sin). An essential amino acid.

**isomer** (i′so-mer). One of two or more compounds having the same kind and number of atoms but differing in the atomic arrangements in the molecule.

**isotopes** (i′so-topes). Two or more chemical elements which have the same atomic number and identical chemical properties but which differ in atomic weight or in the structure of the nucleus.

**keratin** (ker′ah-tin). A scleroprotein which is the principal constituent of epidermis, hair, nails, and the organic matrix of the enamel of teeth.

**ketogenic** (ke′to-jen′ik). Capable of being converted to ketone bodies. Ketogenic substances in metabolism are the fatty acids and certain amino acids.

**ketone bodies** (ke′tōn). Acetoacetic acid. β-hydroxybutyric acid and acetone.

**ketosis** (ke-to′sis). A condition in which there is an accumulation in the body of the ketone bodies as a result of incomplete oxidation of the fatty acids.

**kwashiorkor** (kwa-shi-or′ker). A severe protein-calorie deficiency disease occurring in small children. Endemic in many parts of the world.

**L-BHT.** Lactose breath hydrogen test.

**LBW.** Low-birth-weight infant. Weighs less than 2500 g.

**LCAT.** Lecithin. Cholesterol acyltransferase, an enzyme found in the blood and tissues. It uses a fatty acid from lecithin to form cholesterol esters.

**lecithin** (les′i-thin). A phospholipid containing glycerol, fatty acids, phosphoric acid, choline.

**LES.** The lower esophageal sphincter, which prevents regurgitation of the contents of the stomach to the esophagus.

**leucine** (lu′sin). An essential amino acid.

**leukocyte** (lu′ko-sīt). Any colorless, amoeboid cell mass. Applied especially to one of the formed elements of the blood, consisting of a colorless granular mass of protoplasm and varying in size between 0.005 and 0.015 mm. in diameter.

**life-style.** That constellation of religious, cultural and aesthetic traditions that finds expression in either a reliance on members of one's own family and close social group or a reliance on broader social groups and institutions.

**ligand** (lig′and). A substance that forms a complex with a metal ion.

**lignin** (lig′nin). Component of dietary fiber from the woody parts of plants that is a phenylpropane branched chain polymer.

**linoleic acid** (lin′o-le′ik as′id). A polyunsaturated fatty acid essential for nutrition.

**linolenic acid** (lin′o-le′nik as′id). A polyunsaturated fatty acid.

**lipase** (li′pās; lip′ās). An enzyme that digests fat.

**lipid** (lip′id). **lipoid** (lip′oid). Fat or fat-like substances.

**lipoprotein** (lip′o-pro′te-in). Combination of a protein with fat, found in both animal and plant tissues.

**lipoprotein lipase** (lip′o-pro′te-in li′pas). An enzyme that catalyzes the hydrolysis of triglycerides present in the lipoproteins of the blood, especially those of chylomicrons and the very low-density lipoproteins. Also known as *clearing factor.*

**lipotrophic** (lip′o-trof′ik). Having an affinity for fats or oils, and thereby acting on fat metabolism by hastening the removal of or decrease in the deposit of fat in the liver.

**LTT.** Lactose tolerance test.

**lupus erythematosus** (lu′pus er′i-them-ah-to-sus). An inflammatory dermatitis.

**lysosomes** (li′so-sōms). Membranous structures in cytoplasm that contain hydrolytic enzymes.

**lysozyme** (li′so-zim). Enzyme that digests certain high molecular weight carbohydrates and some gram-positive bacteria.

**malabsorption syndrome** (mal′ab-sorp′shun). A group of symptoms that result from the inability to digest or absorb food in the intestinal tract.

**MAO.** Maximal (gastric) acid output.

**marasmus** (ma-raz′mus). Wasting and emaciation, especially in infants due to underfeeding or disease.

**medulla** (me-dul′lah). The middle, inmost part, used as a general term in anatomical nomenclature to designate the innermost portion of an organ or structure.

**megaloblast** (meg′ah-lo-blast′). A primitive nucleated red blood cell that is much larger than a mature erythrocyte and is present in increased concentration in the bone marrow and blood of patients with pernicious anemia or anemia due to deficiency of folacin.

**melanin** (mel′ah-nin). The dark amorphous pigment of the skin, hair, and certain other tissues that derives from tyrosine metabolism.

**menadione** (me-an-di′on). Synthetic vitamin K. 2 - methyl - 1, 4 - naphthoquinone.

**metabolism** (me-tab′o-lizm). General term to designate all chemical changes that occur in food nutrients after they have been absorbed from the gastrointestinal tract and to designate the cellular activity involved in using these nutrients.

**metallothionein(s)** (me-tal′o-thi′o-ne′in). Protein(s) that bind trace metals and may be involved in their absorption, storage, and detoxification in the body tissue.

**methionine** (meth-i′o-nin). An essential amino acid containing sulfur.

**mitochondria** (mit′o-kon′dre-ah). Small granules or rod-shaped structures in the cell; the principal site of oxidative reactions by which the energy in foodstuff is made available to the cell.

**moiety** (moi′e-te). Any equal part; a half; also any part or portion.

**monosaccharide** (mon′o-sak′a-rīd). A single sugar that cannot be decomposed by hydrolysis.

**monounsaturated** (mon′o-un-sat′u-rat-ed). An organic compound, such as a fatty acid, in which two carbon atoms are united by a double bond.

**MSUD.** Maple syrup urine disease. An inherited metabolic disorder of the branched chain amino acids, leucine, isoleucine, and valine.

**mucopolysaccharide** (mu′ko-pol′e-sak′ah-rid). A group of polysaccharides that contains hexosamine, which may or may not be combined with protein and which, dispersed in water, form many of the mucins.

**mucoprotein** (mu′ko-pro′te-in). Substance containing a polypeptide chain and disaccharides, found in mucous secretions of the digestive glands.

**mycotoxin** (mi′ko-tox′sin). A fungal or bacterial toxin.

**myelin** (mi′ĕ-lin). The fat-like substance forming a sheath around certain nerve fibers.

**myelination** (mi′ĕ-li-na′shun) or myelinization. The act of furnishing with or taking on myelin.

**myofibrils** (mi-o-fī'brilz). Fine fibers embedded in the sarcoplasm of the muscle cell.

**naphthoquinone** (naf'tho-kwin'on). A derivative of quinone; some of these derivatives have vitamin K activity.

**NAS-NRC.** National Academy of Science-National Research Council, Washington, D.C. 20418.

**neglect** (ni-glekt'). Chronic failure of the primary caretaker to provide the physical necessities of life, that is, food, shelter, clothing, education, medical care, dental care, financial support, and proper supervision.

**neurotransmitters** (nu'ro-trans'mit-erz). Chemical compounds that relay impulses among neurons enabling nerve cells to communicate with each other, such as serotonin, norepinephrine, dopamine.

**neutropenia** (nu'tro-pe'ne-ah). A decrease in the number of neutrophilic leucocytes in the blood.

**NFCS.** National Food Consumption Survey. Conducted by the United States Department of Agriculture.

**NIDDM.** Noninsulin-dependent diabetes mellitus. Formerly called *maturity-onset diabetes mellitus* (MODM) or *adult-onset diabetes mellitus* (AODM).

**nitrosamine** (ni-tros'am'in). Chemicals known to produce cancer in test animals.

**noncellulosic polysaccharides** (non-cel'u-los'ik pol'e-sak'ah-rids). Components of dietary fiber including hemicelluloses, pectin substances, algal polysaccharides, gums, and mucilages.

**NRC-RDA.** National Research Council-Recommended Dietary Allowances.

**nucleoprotein** (nu'kle-o-pro'tein). The conjugated protein found in the nuclei of cells.

**nucleotide** (nu'kle-o-tīd). Compound containing a sugar-phosphate component and a purine or pyrimidine base.

**nutrient** (nu'tre-ent). An organic or inorganic substance in food that is digested and absorbed in the gastrointestinal tract and used in intermediary metabolism.

**nutritional care.** The process of assessing, planning, implementing, and evaluating services for clients. It is concerned with helping persons and populations achieve a level of well-being consistent with their potential.

**nutrition support team.** A multidisciplinary healthcare team responsible for the nutritional care of clients with malnutrition.

**OGTT.** Oral glucose tolerance test.

**oleic acid** (o-le'ik). A monounsaturated fatty acid.

**oligosaccharide** (ol'i-go-sak'ah-rid). A complex carbohydrate that contains two to ten molecules of monosaccharides combined with each other.

**opsin** (op'sin). A protein compound that combines with retinal, vitamin A aldehyde, to form rhodopsin, visual purple.

**oral contraceptive** (o'ral kon'trah-sep-tiv). An agent taken by mouth to prevent conception.

**osteoblast** (os'te-o-blast). Any one of the cells that are developed into bone.

**osteoclast** (os'te-o-clast). A cell that assists in the resorption of bone.

**osteomalacia** (os'te-o-ma-la'she-a). Softening of the bone due to loss of calcium. Occurs chiefly in adults.

**osteoporosis** (os'te-o-po-ro'sis). Abnormal porousness or rarefaction of bone due to failure of the osteoblasts to lay down bone matrix, occurring when resorption dominates over mineral deposition.

**outcome criteria.** The effect of health care on the patient.

**oxaluria** (ok'sah-lu're-ah). The presence of an excess of oxalic acid or of oxalates in the urine.

**oxidation** (ok'si-da'shun). A chemical process during which a substance combines with oxygen. Chemically it is an increase of positive charges on an atom through the loss of electrons.

**parenchymal** (par-eng'ki-mal). Used in reference to the functional tissue of an organ in contrast to its structural framework, connective tissue, or stroma.

**Parkinson's disease** (par'kin-sunz di-sez). Paralysis agitans.

**PBI.** Protein bound iodine.

**PEM.** Protein-energy malnutrition.

**pentose** (pen'tos). A single sugar containing five carbon atoms. Ribose is a pentose.

**peptide** (pep'tid). A compound of two or more amino acids containing one or more peptide bonds. Peptides are formed as intermediary products of protein digestion.

**PER.** Protein Efficiency Ratio. A measure of protein quality determined by measuring the weight gain of a growing rat per amount of protein consumed.

**periodontal disease** (per'e-o-don'tal di-sez'). A disorder or disease of the tissues surrounding the root of a tooth.

**pernicious anemia** (per-nish'us ah-ne'meah). A chronic severe macrocytic anemia caused by the deficiency of vitamin $B_{12}$ due to lack of the intrinsic factor required for absorption of vitamin $B_{12}$.

**pesticide** (pes'ti-sīd). A poison used to destroy pests of any sort. The term includes fungicides, insecticides, and rodenticides.

**petechia** (pe-te'ke-ah). A small spot formed by the effusion of blood.

**phenylalanine** (fen'il-al'a-nen; nin). An essential amino acid.

**phenylketonuria (PKU)** (fen'il-ke'ton-nu're-ah). An inborn error of the metabolism of phenylalanine; phenylpyruvic acid appears in the urine.

**phenylpyruvic acid** (fen'il-pi-ru'vik). An intermediate product in phenylalanine metabolism.

**phospholipid** (fos'fo-lip'id). A fat in which one fatty acid is replaced by phosphorus and a nitrogenous compound.

**phosphorylation** (fos'for-i-la'shun). The process of introducing the trivalent phosphate group into an organic molecule. The phosphate donor is usually ATP.

**photosynthesis** (fo'to-sin'the-sis). Formation of carbohydrate from carbon dioxide and water in the chlorophyll tissue of plants under the influence of light.

**pica** (pi'kah). A craving for unnatural food items, such as clay or laundry starch.

**picolinic acid** (pik'o-lin-ik). A tryptophan metabolite that binds zinc and enhances its absorption from the intestine.

**PKU.** Phenylketonuria. An inherited metabolic disorder of phenylalanine metabolism.

**planning.** The process of establishing objectives and selecting resources and strategies for meeting client needs and establishing criteria for client evaluation.

**polysaccharide** (pol'e-sak'ah-rid). A complex carbohydrate that contains more than ten molecules of monosaccharides combined with each other.

**polyunsaturated** (pol'e-un-sat'u-rat'ed). An organic compound, such as a fatty acid, in which there is more than one double bond.

**POMR.** Problem-oriented medical record. A system of organizing and recording patient data bases.

**postmenopausal** (pōst'men-o'paw'zal). Occurring after the cessation of menstruation in the human female.

**practitioner-managed care.** The type of care provided by practitioners during a health crisis and usually in an institutional setting. It is planned and implemented by the practitioner and is restorative or palliative in nature.

**prealbumin, PA** (pre'al-bu'min). A plasma protein fraction that functions in the transport of the thyroid hormones and vitamin A. It forms a complex with the retinol-binding protein.

**preeclampsia** (pre'e-klamp'se-ah). A toxemia of late pregnancy, characterized by hypertension, albuminuria, and edema.

**precursor** (pre-kur'ser). A substance that is converted into another; for example, $\beta$ carotene to vitamin A.

**pre-term.** Born before 37 weeks of gestation. Used synonymously with the term *premature*.

**process criteria.** A list of what the professional performance should be in the delivery of health care.

**prostaglandins** (pros'tah-glan'dins). A group of hormone-like compounds derived from linoleic and linolenic acids that cause strong contraction of smooth muscle and dilatation of certain vascular beds.

**protein hydrolysate** (pro'te-in hi-drol'i-zat). A solution containing the constituent amino acids of an artificially digested protein, usually milk or beef protein.

**protease** (pro'te-as). An enzyme that digests protein.

**proteinuria** (pro'te-i-nu're-a). Presence of protein in the urine.

**proteolytic** (pro'te-o-lit'ik). Effecting the digestion of proteins.

**provitamin** (pro-vi'ta-min). The forerunner of a vitamin. Provitamin A, for example, is carotene.

**ptyalin** (ti'a-lin). The starch splitting enzyme amylase of saliva.

**PUFA.** Polyunsaturated fatty acid.

**purine(s)** (pu'rēn). A nonprotein heterocyclic nitrogenous base. End products of nucleoprotein metabolism.

**quality assurance.** A method for assessing the quality of care delivered by health professionals.

**RAD.** A unit of measurement of absorbed doses of ionizing radiation.

**registered dietitian.** A dietitian who has successfully completed the examination for registration and maintains continuing education requirements.

**reticuloendothelial system** (re-tik'u-lo-en'do-the'le'al). The cells of the body having both endothelial and reticular attributes and showing a common phagocytic behavior, including cells of the liver and bone marrow. This system is involved in blood cell formation and destruction, storage of fatty materials, the metabolism of iron and pigment; and plays a defensive role in inflammation and immunity.

**retinal** (ret'i-nal). The aldehyde form of vitamin A that is necessary for the synthesis of rhodopsin, visual purple.

**retinoic acid** (ret'i-no-ic). The acid form of vitamin A.

**retinol** (ret'i-nol). The chemical term for vitamin A alcohol.

**retinyl** (ret'i-nel). Refers to the vitamin A portion of the ester form of the vitamin. Retinyl palmitate is hydrolyzed to vitamin A alcohol (retinol) and palmitic acid in the gastrointestinal tract.

**rhodopsin** (ro-dop'sin). Visual purple, formed in the rods of the retina by combining the protein opsin and vitamin A aldehyde. It is necessary for scotopic vision.

**ribonucleic acid (RNA)** (ri-bo-nu-kle'ik). A nucleic acid replicated from DNA and found in cytoplasm.

**saccharine** (sak'ah-rin). An intensely sweet, white crystalline compound used as a substitute for ordinary sugar. It has no food value.

**safflower oil** (saf'flou'er). An edible oil from the seeds of the safflower plant, Carthamus tinctorius; high in linoleic acid.

**saponification** (sah-pon'i-fi-ka'shun). Alkaline hydrolysis of fat to form soap.

**sarcolemma** (sar-ko-lem'ah). Delicate elastic sheath that invests striated muscle fibers.

**sarcomere** (sar'ko-mer). Smallest contractile unit in a myofibril.

**sarcoplasm** (sar'ko-plazm). The interfibrillary substance of the striated muscle in which myofibrils are embedded.

**sequestrants** (se-kwes′trants). Food additives that combine with a substance in a food to prevent physical or chemical changes influencing color, flavor, texture, and appearance of foods.

**senile dementia** (se′nil de-men′she-ah). Mental deterioration seen in the elderly.

**serotonin** (ser′o-to′nin). A derivative of tryptophan that is a neurotransmitter.

**SGA.** Infants who are small for gestational age. They may be fullterm but are shorter, lighter in weight, and appear to have disproportionately large heads relative to body size.

**SGPT.** Serum glutamate-pyruvate transaminase (alanine aminotransferase). Increased level associated with tissue injury, especially with acute damage to liver cells.

**SGOT.** Serum glutamate-oxaloacetate transaminase (aspartate aminotransferase). Increased level associated with tissue damage, such as myocardial infarction or acute liver damage.

**SOAP.** A method for recording progress notes in the problem-oriented medical record. S (subjective), O (objective), A (appraisal), P (plan).

**sphingomyelin** (sfing′go-mi′e-lin). A phospholipid found primarily in brain and lung tissue as a constituent of the myelin sheaths.

**stachyose** (stak′e-os). An indigestible tetrasaccharide containing galactose.

**standards of practice.** Statements that delineate or define norms or expectations of nutritional care, education, research, or management.

**stearic acid** (ste′a-rik). A saturated fatty acid.

**steatorrhea** (ste′a-to-re′a). Presence of an excess of fat in the stools.

**sterol** (ster′ol). Fat-soluble substance with a complex molecular structure.

**substrate** (sub′strāt). A substance upon which an enzyme acts.

**succinic acid** (suk-sin′ik). Intermediary product in metabolism.

**suet** (su′et). Hard fat of beef or mutton.

**synapse** (sin′aps). Anatomical relation of one nerve cell to another, the region of contact between two adjacent neurons forming the place where a nervous impulse is transmitted from one neuron to another.

**synergism** (sin′er-jizm). The joint action of agents so that their combined effect is greater than the algebraic sum of their individual effects.

**T$_3$.** Triiodothyronine, a thyroid hormone.

**T$_4$.** Thyroxine, the tetraiodo form of thyroid hormones.

**thermogenesis** (ther′mo-jen′e-sis). Production of heat in an animal body.

**THFA.** Tetrahydrofolic acid.

**thyroglobulin** (thi-ro-glob′u-lin). The storage form of thyroid hormones in the colloid of the follicles of the thyroid gland.

**thyrotoxicosis** (thi′ro-tok′si-ko′sis). A morbid condition resulting from overactivity of the thyroid gland.

**TIBC.** Total iron-binding capacity, which is a mixture of the concentration of transferrin in the blood.

**toxemia** (toks-e′me-ah). Complication of pregnancy characterized by an elevation in blood pressure, proteinuria, and rapid weight gain due to edema; preeclampsia, eclampsia.

**TPN.** Total parenteral nutrition, refers to total intravenous feeding.

**TPP.** Thiamin pyrophosphate, the coenzyme form of thiamin.

**transamination** (trans′am-i-na′shun). The transferring of an amino group from an amino acid to another compound. By this process the body is able to synthesize the nonessential amino acids as well as to form urea. A vitamin B$_6$-containing enzyme is necessary for this reaction.

**transferrin** (trans′fer-in). A protein compound that is found in the bloodstream and transports iron to the bone marrow for hemoglobin synthesis, to the liver or spleen for storage, or to the other tissues for their use.

**transferrin saturation.** (trans′fer-in sat′u-ra′ shun). The percentage of total iron-binding capacity that is saturated with iron.

**TRF.** The thyrotropin-releasing factor produced by the hypothalamus.

**triacylglycerol** (tri-as′il-glis′er-ol). Term for triglyceride describing its chemical structure.

**trichinosis** (trik′i-no′sis). A disease due to infection with trichinae parasites found in raw pork.

**TSF.** Triceps skinfold.

**TSH.** Thyroid-stimulating hormone secreted by the anterior pituitary. Also known as thyrotropic hormone or thyrotropin.

**tyrosine** (ti-ro′sin). A nonessential amino acid.

**UGI.** Upper gastrointestinal x-ray study.

**UGI-SBFT.** Upper gastrointestinal x-ray test with small bowel follow-through.

**UNESCO.** United Nations Educational, Scientific and Cultural Organization. Headquarters, Paris, France.

**USDA.** United States Department of Agriculture. Washington, D.C. 20250.

**urea** (u-re′a). The chief nitrogenous end product of protein metabolism in the body.

**valine** (val′in). An essential amino acid.

**vibrio cholerae** (vib′re-o- kol′er-a′). Gram-negative, straight or slightly curved rod, facultatively anaerobic bacterium.

**vibrio parahaemolyticus** (vib′re-o par′ah-he′mo-lit-i-kus). A gram-negative generally straight or slightly curved rod, facultatively anaerobic bacterium.

**VLBW.** Very-low-birth-weight infants, weighing at birth less than 1500 g.

**Wernicke-Korsakoff syndrome** (ver′ni-ke-kor′sak′of). A psychosis that is usually based on chronic alcoholism, probably due to prolonged thiamin deficiency.

**WHO.** World Health Organization of the United Nations. Headquarters, Geneva, Switzerland.

**xerophthalmia** (ze′rof-thal′mi-a). A dry and lusterless condition of the conjunctiva of the eyes resulting from a vitamin A deficiency.

**xylose** (zi′lōs). A pentose obtained from wood.

**zein** (ze′in). A protein obtained from corn.

**zygote** (zi′gōt). The cell resulting from the fusion of two gametes.

# Abbreviations

| | |
|---|---|
| **ACP** | Acyl carrier protein |
| **ADD** | Attention deficit disorder |
| **ADI** | Acceptable daily intake |
| **AMC** | Arm muscle circumference |
| | |
| **BAI** | Bureau of Animal Industry |
| **BAO** | Basal acid output |
| **BCAA** | Branched-chain amino acid |
| **BE** | Barium enema |
| **BEE** | Basal energy expenditure |
| **BHA** | Butylated hydroxyanisole |
| **BHT** | Butylated hydroxytoluene |
| **BMR** | Basal metabolic rate |
| **BUN** | Blood urea nitrogen |
| **BV** | Biologic value |
| | |
| **CaBP** | Calcium-binding protein |
| **CAC** | Citric acid cycle |
| **CF** | Cystic fibrosis |
| **CHI** | Creatinine height index |
| **CMC** | Critical micellar concentration |
| **CNSD** | Chronic nonspecific diarrhea |
| **CRABP** | Calcium retinoic acid-binding protein |
| **CRBP** | Cellular retinol-binding protein |
| **CSFP** | Commodity Surplus Food Program |
| **CSM** | Corn soy milk |
| **CVA** | Cerebrovascular accident |
| **CVD** | Cardiovascular disease |
| | |
| **DSM** | Dry skim milk |
| **dU** | Deoxyuridine |
| **dUMP** | Deoxyuridine monophosphate |
| | |
| **ECW** | Extracellular water |
| **EDTA** | Ethylenediamine tetraacetic acid |
| **EFA** | Essential fatty acids |
| **EPA** | Environmental Protection Agency |
| **EPM** | Energy-protein malnutrition |
| **ERCP** | Endoscopic retrograde cholangiopancreatography |

| | |
|---|---|
| **FAD** | Flavin adenine dinucleotide |
| **FDA** | Food and Drug Administration |
| **FFA** | Free fatty acids |
| **FIGLU** | Formiminoglutamic acid |
| **FMN** | Riboflavin mononucleotide |
| **FNIC** | Food and Nutrition Information Center |
| **FTC** | Federal Trade Commission |
| **FTT** | Failure to thrive |
| | |
| **GABA** | Gamma aminobutyric acid |
| **GDP** | Guanosinediphosphate |
| **GFR** | Glomerular filtration rate |
| **GMP** | Good manufacturing practices |
| **GRAS** | Generally Recognized as Safe |
| **GRR** | Glucose removal rate |
| **GSH** | Reduced glutathione |
| **GSH-Px** | Glutathione peroxidase |
| **GTF** | Glucose tolerance factor |
| **GTP** | Guanosinetriphosphate |
| **GTT** | Glucose tolerance test |
| | |
| **HANES** | Health and Nutrition Examination Survey |
| **HDL** | High-density lipoprotein |
| **HFCS** | High-fructose corn syrup |
| **HLP** | Hyperlipoproteinemia |
| **HMS** | Hexose monophosphate shunt |
| **HNIS** | Human Nutrition Information Service |
| **HRV** | Human rotovirus |
| | |
| **ICEA** | International Childhood Education Association |
| **ICW** | Intracellular water |
| **IDDM** | Insulin-dependent diabetes mellitus |
| **IDL** | Intermediate density lipoproteins |
| **IF** | Intrinsic factor |
| **IGT** | Impaired glucose tolerance |
| **ILDL** | Intermediate low-density lipoprotein |
| **INCAP** | Institute of Nutrition in Central America and Panama |
| **ISW** | Interstitial water |
| **IU** | International Units |

| | |
|---|---|
| **JCAH** | Joint Commission on Accreditation of Hospitals |
| **L-BHT** | Lactose breath hydrogen test |
| **LBW** | Low birth weight |
| **LCAT** | Lecithin-cholesterol acyltransferase |
| **LCT** | Long-chain triglycerides |
| **LDL** | Low-density lipoprotein |
| **LES** | Lower esophageal sphincter |
| **LTT** | Lactose tolerance test |
| **MAO** | Monoamine oxidase |
| **MCT** | Medium-chain triglycerides |
| **MDR** | Minimum Daily Requirement |
| **MFP** | Meat, fish, or poultry |
| **MRFIT** | Multiple Risk Factor Intervention Trial |
| **MSUD** | Maple syrup urine disease |
| **NAD** | Nicotinamide adenine dinucleotide |
| **NADH** | Reduced niacin coenzyme |
| **NAS-NRC** | National Academy of Sciences-National Research Council |
| **NDDG** | National Diabetes Data Group |
| **NE** | Niacin equivalent |
| **NEC** | Necrotizing enterocolitis |
| **NEFA** | Nonesterified fatty acids |
| **NFCS** | National Food Consumption Survey |
| **NICN** | Neonatal intensive care nursery |
| **NIDDM** | Noninsulin-dependent diabetes mellitus |
| **NPH** | Neutral protamine Hagedorn |
| **NPU** | Net protein utilization |
| **NSLP** | National School Lunch Program |
| **OAA** | Oxaloacetate |
| **OCA** | Oral contraceptive agents |
| **OGTT** | Oral glucose tolerance test |
| **PA** | Prealbumin |
| **PALP** | Pyridoxal-5-phosphate |
| **PBI** | Protein-bound iodine |
| **PCB's** | Polychlorinated biphenyls |
| **PEM** | Protein-energy malnutrition |
| **PER** | Protein efficiency ratio |
| **PG** | Plasma glucose |
| **PGA** | Pteroylglutaminic acid |
| **PHLA** | Postheparin lipolytic activity |
| **PIR** | Poverty income ratio |
| **PKU** | Phenylketonuria |
| **PL** | Pyridoxal |
| **PM** | Pyridoxamine |
| **PMP** | Pyridoxamine phosphate |
| **PN** | Pyridoxine |

| | |
|---|---|
| **PNP** | Pyridoxine phosphate |
| **PNS** | Preschool Nutrition Survey |
| **PPS** | Pteroylpolyglutamate synthetase |
| **PSRO** | Professional Standards Review Organization |
| **PTH** | Parathyroid hormone |
| **PUFA** | Polyunsaturated fatty acids |
| **RBP** | Retinol-binding protein |
| **RCR** | Relative chromium response |
| **RD** | Registered Dietitian |
| **RDA** | Recommended Dietary Allowances |
| **RE** | Retinol equivalents |
| **RMR** | Resting metabolic rate |
| **SCT** | Short-chain triglycerides |
| **SDA** | Specific dynamic action |
| **SGA** | Small-for-gestational-age |
| **SGOT** | Serum glutamate oxaloacetate transaminase |
| **SK-SD** | Streptokinase-streptodornase |
| **TAG** | Total available glucose |
| **TBSB** | Total body surface burned |
| **TBW** | Total body weight |
| **TC** | Transcobalamin |
| **TCA** | Tricarboxylic acid |
| **TG** | Triglycerides |
| **THFA** | Tetrahydrofolic acid |
| **TIBC** | Total iron-binding capacity |
| **TMP** | Thiamin monophosphate |
| **TPN** | Total parenteral nutrition |
| **TPP** | Thiamin pyrophosphate |
| **TRF** | Thyrotropin-releasing factor |
| **TSF** | Triceps skinfold thickness |
| **TSH** | Thyroid-stimulating factor |
| **TSNS** | Ten-State Nutrition Survey |
| **TXA$_2$** | Thromboxane |
| **UDP** | Uridine diphosphate |
| **UGDP** | University Group Diabetes Program |
| **UGI** | Upper gastrointestinal series |
| **UGI-SBFT** | Upper gastrointestinal series with small bowel follow-through |
| **US-RDA** | United States Recommended Daily Allowances |
| **VLBW** | Very low birth weight |
| **VLDL** | Very low density lipoprotein |
| **WIC** | Special Supplementary Program for Women, Infants and Children |
| **WSB** | Wheat-soy blend |

# *Index*

Numerals in italics indicate a figure; *t* following a page number indicates tabular material.